Feline Orthopedic Surgery and Musculoskeletal Disease

For Elsevier:

Commissioning Editors: *Robert Edwards/Rita Demetriou-Swanwick*
Development Editors: *Louisa Welch/Susan Young*
Project Manager: *Andrew Palfreyman*
Designer: *Charles Gray*
Illustration Manager: *Merlyn Harvey*

Feline Orthopedic Surgery and Musculoskeletal Disease

P.M. Montavon
Vetsuisse Faculty, University of Zurich, Switzerland

K. Voss
Vetsuisse Faculty, University of Zurich, Switzerland

S.J. Langley-Hobbs
Department of Veterinary Medicine, University of Cambridge, UK

Design and layout: Marianne Mathys, Audio-Visual Services, Vetsuisse Faculty, University of Zurich
Project consultant and initial design: Rainer M. Egle and Daniel Erni, Focused Publishing GmbH, Russikon, Switzerland
Drawings ©: Matthias Haab, Scientific Illustrator, Animal Surgery Clinic, Vetsuisse Faculty, University of Zurich
Pictures: Clinic for Small Animal Surgery, Vetsuisse Faculty, University of Zurich; Department of Clinical Veterinary Medicine, University of Cambridge

MOSBY

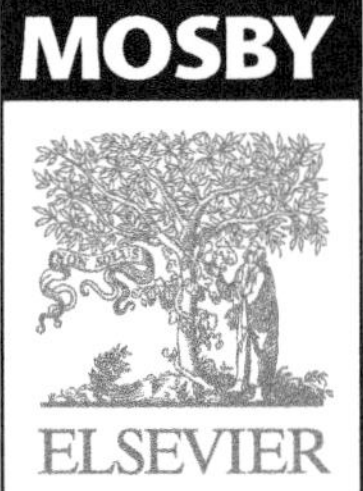

Edinburgh London New York Oxford Philadelphia St Louis Sydney Toronto 2009

SAUNDERS
ELSEVIER

First published 2009

ISBN: 978-0-7020-2986-8

British Library Cataloguing in Publication Data
A catalogue record for this book is available from the British Library

Library of Congress Cataloging in Publication Data
A catalog record for this book is available from the Library of Congress

'I am the cat that walked by himself. ...'
Just So Stories, Rudyard Kipling

Contents

Part 3: Polytrauma

Part 4: Introduction to musculoskeletal injuries

Part 5: The surgical patient

Part 6: Orthopedic materials, instruments, implants, and techniques

Part 7: Treatment of selected surgical diseases and injuries

Preface

The practice of feline surgery has developed markedly over the last 10 years. One cat lives in approximately every fourth household in industrial countries, and the caseload of cats reaches or exceeds 50% of the species seen in many urban practices and clinics in the USA, Europe, and Japan. Development of modern implants and improvement of diagnostic modalities have resulted in an increased knowledge of feline orthopedic conditions, and offer a wider range of treatment options.

The majority of feline orthopedic cases seen in practice have sustained trauma, resulting in many different types of orthopedic injuries. The old saying, that "if two pieces of cat bone are put together in the same room they will heal," is of course not true. Although fixation stability may be of less concern in cats compared to dogs, the small size of the cat bones and the severity of some injuries can make feline orthopedic surgery particularly challenging. Also the choice of implants is different, as many implants used in dogs are too large for cat bones.

Cats are less commonly presented with lameness than dogs. It can be a real diagnostic challenge to determine the cause of lameness if the cat does not suffer from a cat bite abscess or a fracture. Knowledge of feline orthopedic diseases is much lower when compared to dogs. Many feline othopedic diseases are only described in single case reports or small case series, and cats often show non-specific clinical signs with diseases of the musculoskeletal system, which reduces owners and veterinarians' awareness of such conditions.

The goal of this book was to produce a comprehensive and up-to-date textbook on feline orthopedics. There are parts on diagnostics, musculoskeletal diseases and neurological conditions, diagnosis and treatment of polytraumatized cats, basic principles of orthopedic surgery, anesthesia and analgesia, surgical instruments and implants, rehabilitation, and arthroscopy. The main emphasis is on orthopedic surgical techniques. These are described in detail for diseases and injuries of each bone and joint. Common classic surgical techniques are reported, as well as many novel topics specific to feline musculoskeletal disease and orthopedics. This textbook should form a good grounding in orthopedics for veterinary students. It should improve the diagnosis of feline orthopedic conditions, provide detailed explanations of their treatment for small animal practitioners, and it will offer further novel treatment options to specialist surgeons.

P.M. Montavon
K. Voss
S.J. Langley-Hobbs

Acknowledgments

We would like to thank our dear colleagues for their generous contributions in the form of cases, radiographs, inspiration or ideas:

Kenneth Bruecker, DVM, DACVS, Ventura, United States
Stuart Carmichael BVMS, MVM, DSAO, MRCVS, Glasgow, United Kingdom
Jean-Romain Carroz, Dr med. vet., Sion, Switzerland
James L. Cook, DVM, PhD, DACVS, Columbia, USA
Jan Declercq, Dr med. vet., Gent, Belgium
Renate Dennler, Dr med. vet., DECVS, Affoltern, Switzerland
Jean-Christophe Dubuis, Dr med. vet., Lausanne, Switzerland
Erick L. Egger, DVM, DACVS, Loveland, USA
Barbara Haas, Dr med. vet., DECVS, Munich, Germany
Alex Heller, Dr med. vet., Reinach, Switzerland
Gaëlle Mandon, Dr med. vet., Sion, Switzerland
Ulrike Matis, Prof. Dr med. vet., DECVS, Munich, Germany
Alison J. Patricelli, DVM, DACVS, Albuquerque, USA
Matthew Pead, BVetMed, PhD, MRCVS, RVC, London, United Kingdom
Bruno Peirone, Prof. Dr med. vet., Turin, Italy
Rico Vannini, Dr med. vet., DECVS, Watt, Switzerland
Stergios Vlachopoulos, Dr med. vet., Athens, Greece
Urs Weber, Dr med. vet., DECVS, Tenniken Switzerland

Many thanks also to the following friends for their valuable help with the production of figures:

Corina Blecher, Zurich, Switzerland
Anita Hug, Zurich, Switzerland

Sources of illustrations:

Department of Veterinary Medicine, University of Cambridge
Figs 3.07, 3.08, 4.06, 5.05, 5.10, 8.07, 15.06, 22.02, 27.04, 28.01, 28.04, 28.05, 29.03, 29.12, 30.04, 30.16, 31.03, 32.14, 33.04, 33.10, 35.02, 35.08, 35.19, 35.20, 36.08, 37.09, 38.06, 38.07, 38.16A–C

Vetsuisse Faculty, University of Zurich
Figs 1.01, 1.16, 2.01, 2.02, 2.03, 2.04, 2.05, 2.06, 2.07, 2.08, 2.09, 2.10, 2.11, 2.12, 2.13, 2.14, 2.15, 2.16, 3.04, 3.09, 3.10, 3.11, 4.01, 4.04, 4.07, 5.01, 5.02, 5.03, 5.04, 5.06, 5.07, 5.08, 5.09, 5.11, 5.12, 6.01, 6.02, 6.03, 6.05, 6.07, 6.08, 7.01, 7.02, 7.06, 7.07, 7.08, 7.10, 8.01, 8.02, 8.03, 8.04, 8.05, 8.06, 9.01, 9.02, 10.01, 12.02, 12.04, 12.05, 12.06, 12.07, 12.08, 12.09, 12.10, 13.11, 13.12, 13.13, 13.15, 13.24, 13.25, 13.31, 14.02, 14.03, 14.06, 14.07, 15.01, 15.03, 15.04, 15.05, 15.07, 16.03, 16.04, 16.05, 20.02, 20.13, 22.10, 26.01, 26.02, 26.03, 26.09, 26.10, 26.11, 26.15, 26.17, 26.18, 26.20, 27.02, 27.06, 28.02, 29.05, 29.10, 29.16, 30.03, 30.05, 30.06, 30.07, 30.08, 30.11, 30.13, 30.14, 30.15, 31.05, 31.06, 31.07, 31.08, 31.12, 31.15, 32.02, 32.03, 32.05, 32.06, 32.07, 32.08, 32.09, 32.10, 32.12, 32.15, 33.05, 33.06, 33.07, 33.11, 33.13, 34.06, 34.08, 34.10, 34.11, 34.12, 34.13, 34.14, 35.03, 35.07, 35.10, 35.11, 35.13, 35.16, 35.18, 36.02, 36.03, 36.04, 36.05, 36.06, 36.10, 36.12, 36.13, 37.03, 37.04, 37.07, 37.11, 37.13, 37.15, 37.18, 38.01, 38.02, 38.03, 38.04, 38.08, 38.10, 38.12, 38.14, 38.16D–E, 39.03, 39.05, 39.08, 39.10, 39.11, 39.13, 39.15, 40.02, 40.03, 40.04, 40.05, 40.07, 40.09, 40.11, 40.12, 40.14, 40.16, 40.17, 40.19, 40.20, 42.01, 42.02, 42.03, 42.04, 42.05, 42.06, 42.07, 42.08, 42.09, 42.10, 42.11, 42.12, 42.13, 42.14, 42.15, 42.16, 42.17, 42.18, 42.19, 42.20, 42.21, 42.22, 42.23, 42.24, 42.25, 42.26, 42.27, 42.28, 42.29, 42.30, 42.31, 42.32, 42.33, 42.34, 42.35, 42.36, 42.37, 42.38, 42.39, 42.40, 42.41, 42.42, 42.43, 42.44, 42.45, 42.46, 42.47, 42.48, 42.49, 42.50, 42.51

Contributors

Authors

Susi Arnold Prof., Dr med. vet., DECAR
Center for Small Animal Reproduction
Hünenberg, Switzerland

Brian Beale DVM, DACVS
Gulf Coast Veterinary Specialists
Houston, USA

Luc Borer Dr med. vet., DECVS
Cabinet Vétérinaire de Riantbosson
Genève, Switzerland

Claude Favrot DVM, MsSc, DECVD
Clinic for Small Animal Internal Medicine
Vetsuisse Faculty University of Zurich
Zurich, Switzerland

Francesco Gallorini Dr med. vet.
Clinica Veterinaria S. Silvestro
Arezzo, Italy

Stefan Grundmann Dr med. vet., DECVS
Kleintierpraxis Reinle & Grundmann GmbH
Weil am Rhein, Germany

Fredrik Gruenenfelder Dr med. vet., DECVN
Faculty of Veterinary Medicine
University of Glasgow
Glasgow, United Kingdom

Madeleine Hubler Dr med. vet., DECAR
Center for Small Animal Reproduction
Hünenberg, Switzerland

Sandra L. Hudson BS, MBA, CCRP
Canine Rehabilitation & Conditioning Center
Round Rock, USA

Sabine Kaestner Prof., Dr med. vet., DECVA
Small Animal Clinic
University of Veterinary Medicine
Hannover, Germany

Marcel Keller Dr med. vet., DECVS
Kleintierklinik Rigiplatz
Hünenberg, Switzerland

Sorrel Langley-Hobbs MA BVet Med, DSAS(O), DECVS, MRCVS
Department of Veterinary Medicine
University of Cambridge
Cambridge, United Kingdom

Pierre Montavon Prof., Dr med. vet.
Clinic for Small Animal Surgery
Vetsuisse Faculty University of Zurich
Zurich, Switzerland

Stefanie Ohlerth Dr. med. vet. DECVDI
Division of Diagnostic Imaging
Vetsuisse Faculty University of Zurich
Zurich, Switzerland

John Lapish BSc, BVetMed, MRCVS
Veterinary Instrumentation
Sheffield, United Kingdom

Valérie J. Poirier DMV, DACVIM, DECVIM-CA, DACVR
Brisbane Veterinary Specialist Center
Albany Creek, Australia

Frank Steffen PD, Dr med. vet. DECVN
Clinic for Small Animal Surgery
Vetsuisse Faculty University of Zurich
Zurich, Switzerland

Katja Voss Dr med. vet., DECVS
Clinic for Small Animal Surgery
Vetsuisse Faculty University of Zurich
Zurich, Switzerland

Drawings and design

Rainer Egle
Egle Consulting
Russikon, Switzerland

Daniel Erni
Focused Publishing
Russikon, Switzerland

Matthias Haab
Equine Clinic
Vetsuisse Faculty University of Zurich
Zurich, Switzerland

Marianne Mathys
Graphik/AVD
Vetsuisse Faculty University of Zurich
Zurich, Switzerland

Foreword

Over the years many books have been published regarding the surgical and medical care of the dog and cat – some of the dog alone, few of the cat alone. One of the earliest of the latter was *Feline Medicine and Surgery*, edited by Dr. EJ Catcott in 1964. A second edition of that text was published in 1975, in which I had a small contribution. Since that date fortunately the paucity of scientific texts regarding the treatment of many conditions of cats has gradually been reduced. There are now a number of texts solely dedicated to the care of specific systems of the domesticated feline species.

The new text before you is confined to feline orthopedics and traumatology. Using the word "confined" in the context of this text is really an enigma: the term in itself is correct but is contrary to fact, an antithesis of what is to be found in the book, which very competently covers the subjects that come under its title. More so, one ventures to suggest that there are many more "pearls of wisdom" than one might anticipate. Within, the reader will find new information regarding the diagnosis of conditions, including digital radiography and magnetic resonance imaging, and the essential supportive subjects of anesthesia and analgesia – the foreword to the latter two subjects has been written by Dr. William Muir, an eminent colleague in those areas. The reader will also find current information regarding arthroscopy, postoperative care, and rehabilitation. These subjects are described in detail, along with those covering the core subjects of traumatology and orthopedics. The whole is a veritable cornucopia of new and exciting instructive chapters to salve the enquiring mind of practitioners in the art of feline care.

Dr. Pierre Montavon and his co-editors have elected to divide the text into different parts, each with a varying number of conjunctional chapters. The apparent contradiction is solved when one observes that each part has been allocated a separate color for the title page; the same colors have been used as "thumb marks" in the edges of the relevant pages, the marks moving down the page to a new position for the chapters following. The system thus readily aids the reader who, after consulting the list of contents at the beginning of the book, is then readily able to follow the "thumb marks" and rapidly arrives at the material desired. The more one uses the text the more readily one is able to go straight to the material sought.

At this point I should like to pay tribute to the staff at the publishers who were responsible for the layout and printing of the text. The fonts employed are very readable due to their size and spacing, according to what is required by the relevant text. I am also pleased to see the excellent quality of the figures. The reproduction of the radiographs is excellent, as are the colored photographs. The diagrams are simple – clear and colored with two, or sometimes three, pastel tints. The artist has been asked for clarity – not for works of art, as is required in major anatomical texts – and has succeeded handsomely. The diagrams add considerably to the interpretation of the neighboring text. One could comment upon each individual chapter, but I am not going to do so, believing it not within the remit of an individual asked to write the foreword, but being in the realm of a reviewer.

The reader may be either a "tearer" or a "saver" when it comes to professional journals. If one color-codes articles and gives them a page number, relevent to a condition described within this book, then one can – dare one say – write the reference number in the margin of the relevant material in the text. In this way, a cross-reference system will grow on its own, with or without a computer.

Herein, the triumvirate of editors has assembled much that is new in the literature, as well as some material that has originally been published in journals. Nevertheless, it is all brought together – *for the cat.* New procedures and techniques are described, as well as old techniques that have been melded to fit the necessity of the feline traumatized patient. Neophytes to veterinary orthopedics, to trauma in general and the cat in particular, would do well to engage themselves deeply in all that has been written by the cadre of accomplished authors, garnered by the editors, to produce a text that may be used by newcomers to the field who would do well to absorb the material between these covers. To the veterinarian experienced in trauma and orthopedics, I respectfully suggest that you too will find useful ideas and information within. I did!

Learning is but an adjunct to ourself (Shakespeare, *Love's Labour's Lost*).

Finally, looking back over the nearly 60 years of my professional life, I believe that it is mandatory for me to presume to pass on some of that experience by making what one considers some cogent and, one hopes, sagacious advice. I believe that it is mandatory that before attempting to employ a new technique it should be practiced on a cadaver or the clinician should receive instruction alongside someone already vested with experienced in its use. Know your own limitations and do not be afraid to refer the patient to a specialist. In so doing the neophyte to the endeavor will become better advised as to the progress that has been made in the treatment of particular problems. That having been said, in a genuine and dire emergency any method to resolve a critical situation is eminently defendable.

Sometimes the limitations of the owners' ability to fund a procedure may negate its use. In this text, in some instances, you will see different methods for the treatment of the same problem – some more expensive than others. After reading the results of the different techniques available for your choice, some more expensive than others, only one's conscience remains to decide what is to be done.

This new addition to the veterinary literature should be exceedingly helpful to all clinicians finding themselves with a traumatized cat on their examination table.

Geoff. Sumner-Smith DVSc(Liv) MSc FRCVS
University Professor Emeritus of the University of Guelph
Ontario, Canada

Foreword

This, the first edition of the text *Feline Orthopedic Surgery and Musculoskeletal Disease* is a work long overdue. The nuances of feline anatomy, physiology, and behavior in conjunction with the cat's unique responses to disease, surgery, and medications deserve special attention. The aforementioned distinctive characteristics create special challenges when designing and implementing adequate and effective anesthesia and analgesia protocols for cats. Compared to dogs, for example, cats are more easily stressed, oftentimes difficult to restrain, even for minor medical procedures (intravenous catheter placement), harder to intubate orotracheally, easily overdosed or overanesthetized, and more frequently found to be hypotensive and hypothermic. Their size and temperament alone predispose them to accidental drug-related side-effects.

The importance of vigilance, dosing accuracy, and familiarity with species differences in relationship to the anesthetic and analgesic drugs and techniques used in cats cannot be overemphasized. Recent data assessing anesthetic-related mortality suggest that approximately 1:400 (0.24%) anesthetized cats die and that age, weight, procedural urgency, endotracheal intubation, and fluid therapy increase risk. The mortality rate associated with anesthesia in cats is much greater than in dogs and argues for greater vigilance and improved methods for detection of deleterious changes in the cat's physical status during anesthesia. Importantly, the routine use of monitoring devices including, but not limited to, an electrocardiogram, pulse oximeter, and indirect arterial blood pressure decrease anesthetic risk.

Most cats that have suffered an orthopedic injury are stressed, in pain, and dehydrated. Those that have incurred significant injuries secondary to trauma often sustain extensive soft-tissue damage, blood loss, and infection. Those that have experienced severe head or chest wall trauma in addition to appendicular injuries may exhibit signs of central nervous system (stupor, depression), respiratory (labored breathing), or cardiovascular (arrhythmias) problems.

The feline orthopedic surgical candidate presents special anesthetic risks, requires intense analgesic care and provides ample opportunity for the utilization of specialized monitoring equipment and techniques. Towards this end Dr. Kaestner has written two chapters devoted to the anesthetic and analgesic care of the feline orthopedic patient. These chapters provide detailed and clinically applicable information regarding the clinical pharmacology, monitoring, and analgesic care of cats. Figures, tables, and boxes provide key background information. Anesthetic techniques, monitoring equipment, and common anesthetic problems and their therapy are discussed. A comprehensive list of analgesic drugs, drug dosages and analgesic techniques including local and regional analgesia are described and illustrated. Dr. Kaestner has provided the necessary basic applied information required to produce safe and effective anesthesia and analgesia in cats.

William Muir DVM, PhD, ACVA, ACVECC

Part 1
Clinical approach to the orthopedic patient

The independent and curious nature of the cat often places it in dangerous situations, making trauma the most common etiology of orthopedic problems. Motor vehicle accidents, falls from a height, or bite wounds are commonly encountered in cats and can cause severe and multiple injuries to the skeletal system and the soft tissues. The initial examination of the trauma patient concentrates on diagnosing and treating life-threatening disorders. Orthopedic injuries are addressed only after more severe soft-tissue injuries have been ruled out and the cat is in a stable condition. Fractures or joint injuries usually cause obvious clinical signs.

The lame cat without a history or signs of trauma can be a diagnostic challenge. First, the awareness of the clinician for orthopedic diseases in cats is often not as up to date as for dogs. This may be due to the smaller number of cats presenting for lameness and to the paucity of specific literature available addressing feline orthopedic patients. Second, both a thorough gait analysis and a complete orthopedic examination, necessary to detect subtle abnormalities, are often difficult to perform in the cat. Lastly, cats exhibit more discrete and distinct signs associated with orthopedic diseases than dogs, which may be missed or misinterpreted by owners and veterinarians. Awareness of specific feline orthopedic diseases and the clinical signs associated with them is helpful in making a correct diagnosis.

One should follow the same principles when examining a cat as one would in a dog, but with greater calm, and with more patience. Appropriate handling and restraint methods are the key for making cats cooperative and agreeable patients to work with. Commonly used diagnostic procedures for the feline orthopedic patient are described in the following sections. The authors have emphasized practical tips and peculiarities to the feline patient.

1 Patient assessment

K. Voss, F. Steffen

The complete patient assessment consists of the signalment, history, general, orthopedic, and neurological examination. A summary of the decision-making process for the feline orthopedic patient is shown in Figure 1-1. After the physical, orthopedic, and neurological examinations, the clinician should have a list of differential diagnoses in mind, which dictates the choice for further diagnostic procedures. Risks and benefits of these procedures should be assessed and discussed with the owners. The continuous analysis of information obtained at each step of the diagnostic examination and procedure has the goal of ruling out differential diagnoses, detecting concurrent diseases or conditions, obtaining a specific and accurate diagnosis, and finally making an appropriate treatment plan. Assessment of the severity of the disease process, presence of concurrent diseases, prognosis for return to function, morbidity associated with the treatment, cost, and the ability of the owners to provide necessary supportive care for their cat should also influence the choice of treatment.

1.1 History

The history obtained from the owner of a cat may not be as helpful as for other species. Mildly injured or ill cats

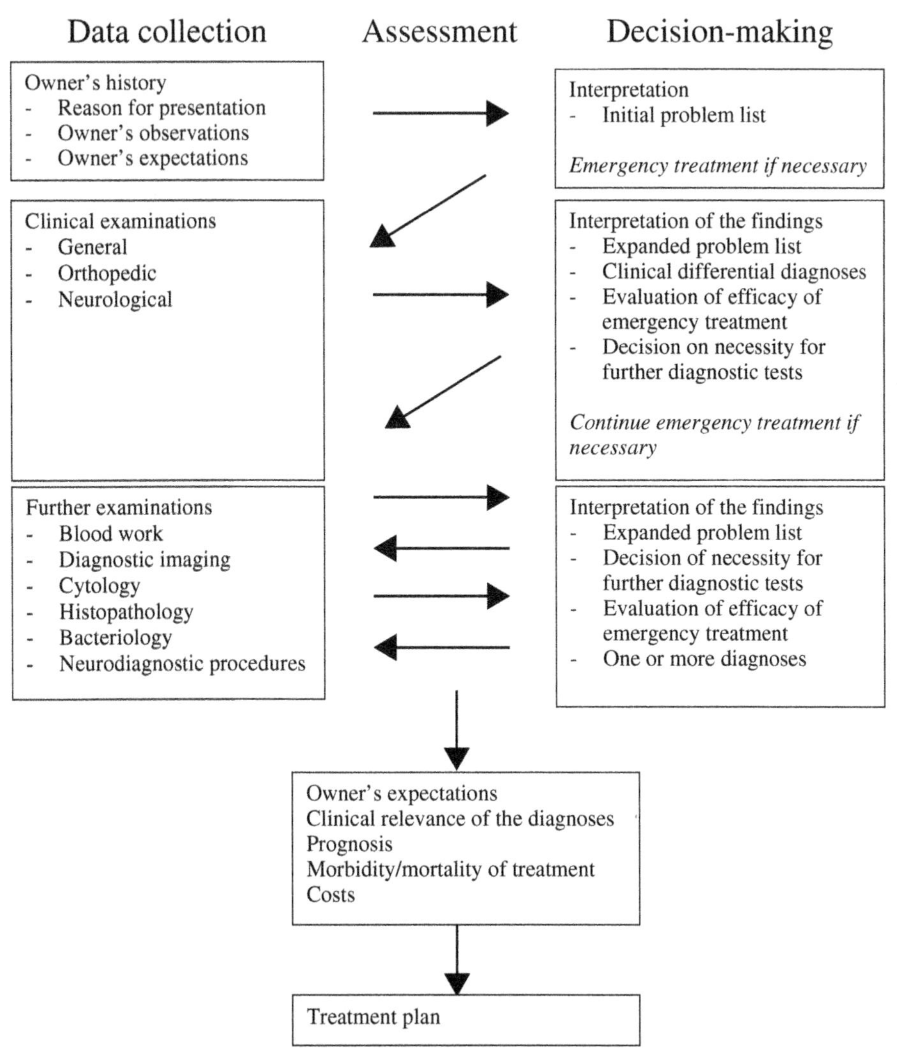

Figure 1-1 This flow diagram represents the process of data collection, continuous assessment of data, and decision-making in the feline orthopedic patient.

often do not exhibit obvious or specific clinical signs, and it may take longer for the owners to realize that something is wrong. Outdoor cats especially spend a large amount of time unobserved by their owners. General habits, like the ability to urinate or defecate, are observed occasionally at best. With trauma, the traumatic event itself is often not observed, and a common complaint relates to the cat coming home limping or injured. Despite these challenges, obtaining an accurate history is an important step in evaluating the feline patient. Because many cats are anxious in the hospital setting, it may be difficult for the clinician to detect behavioral changes efficiently or to assess general health, and the observation of the owners regarding the behavior of the cat at home gives important diagnostic and prognostic information.

The goals of taking the history are to ascertain whether there has been a possibility of trauma, and if so, to evaluate possible causes, to assess when a potential traumatic event or disease state occurred, to get an overview of the living habits and general health of the patient, and to localize the complaint to one or more body systems. Additionally the expectations of the owners regarding the treatment and its expected outcome, and their ability to care for the cat postoperatively, should be evaluated. Examples of questions that should be asked are listed in Table 1-1. The feline patient is left in its basket while the clinician talks to the owners to allow adjustment to the new surroundings.

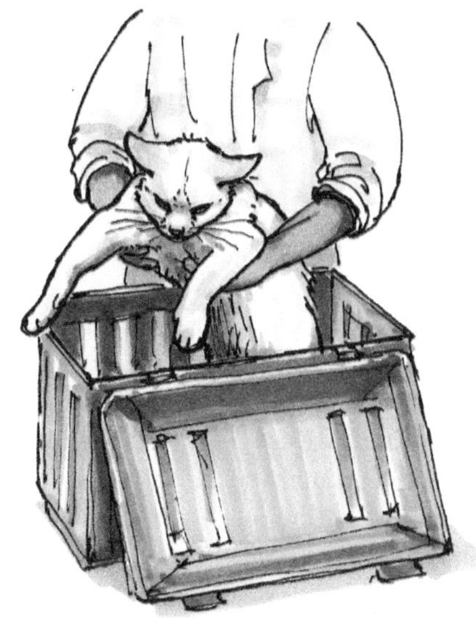

Figure 1-2 Transport boxes for cats should have a top construct designed to be opened or removable. Most cats can then be lifted out of the box by placing hands around their chest.

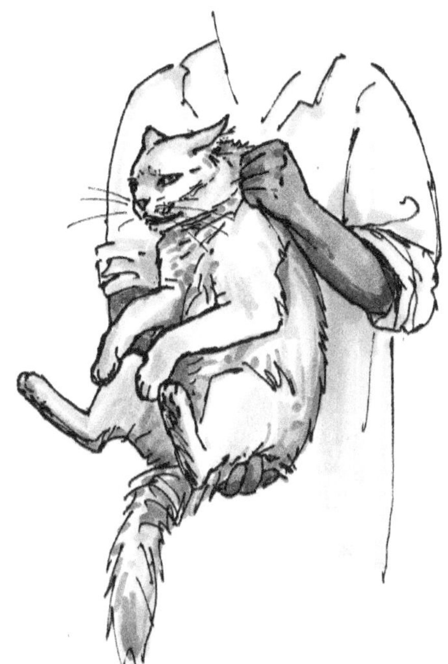

Figure 1-3 For scruffing or the neck grip, the loose skin on the dorsum of the neck is grasped with the whole hand. This is a painful maneuver, especially in older and heavier cats. The other hand is therefore used to support weight from the bottom.

1.2 Handling and restraint

Every veterinarian has encountered the fractious, scratching, and biting cat. This is not only a bad and even dangerous experience for owner, cat, and clinician, but also precludes a thorough examination and may alter clinical parameters, such as temperature, heart, and respiratory rate (1). Aggressiveness in cats may be induced by several mechanisms (2), but is often caused by fear, impossibility for escape, and pain during manipulations. Fear can be reduced by providing a quiet and calm environment, avoiding brisk movements and touch and loud voices. Ideally both the waiting room and the consultation room should be closed, quiet, and without dogs in the area. Successfully handling cats necessitates a feeling for the individual nature of the cat, and using minimal restraint (3). Over-restraining often leads to adverse reactions and can end with the cat immobilized from fear or too fractious to examine. Many cats will be cooperative patients when treated with patience and respect to their nature.

The cat is usually taken out of its basket by holding it around the chest (Fig. 1-2). Baskets in which the whole top can be removed are preferable. Before grasping the cat, it is gently stroked on the head and shoulders or the skin of the dorsum of the neck is gently tickled. The commonly used neck grip, scruffing (Fig. 1-3), should be avoided when possible (4). However scruffing controls the head movements of the cat and might have to be used in some cats during removal from a basket or cage to avoid scratching or biting. The cat should be immobilized with minimal force and pressure while examining it on the table. The clinician can hold the cat gently between body and one hand while the examinations

Question	Interpretation
Signalment (age, breed, and sex)	Gives first hint for diseases or injuries, which occur preferentially in certain breeds or age groups
Is the cat an outdoor or indoor cat?	Although indoor cats might have sustained an accident, the trauma is generally milder, and confined to one localization
Vaccination status?	Especially important in outdoor cats
Is there contact with other cats?	Evaluation for the possibility of bite wounds and infectious diseases
Was the onset of the complaint acute or progressive?	Trauma usually causes an acute onset of clinical signs, diseases usually a progressive course
If trauma is suspected or the cat has been missing, when was it last seen in a normal state?	Gives the time span when the trauma might have happened
How and when was the cat found? Is there progression of clinical signs since the trauma occurred?	Progression of clinical signs after trauma may indicate progression of shock, brain injury, injury to organs, or development of infection
Was the cat able to walk after the trauma? Did it use all limbs?	In cats unable to walk, multiple limb injuries, pelvic fractures, or spinal fractures/luxations should be suspected
Did the cat urinate since the trauma happened?	Urination does not rule out urinary tract injury, but lack of urination needs to be evaluated
Were any other signs observed, such as coughing, mouth-breathing, diarrhea?	Coughing and dyspnea may indicate thorax trauma or concurrent cardiac or respiratory diseases. General diseases can mimic orthopedic or neurological problems (for example, aortic thrombus formation with cardiomyopathy). Concurrent systemic diseases might have an influence on the treatment plan and the prognosis
Is the cat eating normally? Has it lost weight?	Weight loss with reduced food uptake usually indicates systemic diseases or painful conditions. Weight loss with increased food uptake may indicate feline hyperthyroidism
Is there a change in general behavior (activity, sleeping, grooming)?	Non-specific changes in behavior can be a sign of systemic disease or can be caused by pain
Was a limp or lameness noticed? If so, which leg?	Low-grade and intermittent lameness can be hard to detect in the clinic
Does the cat still jump on its favorite spots?	Reluctance to jump is a common sign of orthopedic and neurological problems in cats
Does the cat drink a lot?	This question should always be asked, because of the high frequency of kidney disease and diabetes mellitus in older cats
What is the cat fed?	An important question to rule out nutritional skeletal disorders
Is there a change in the cat's ability to urinate or defecate?	Urination or defecation outside the litter box may be a sign of skeletal pain or neurological dysfunction

Table 1-1. Examples of essential questions to be asked during history-taking, and their interpretation

are performed with the other hand (Fig. 1-4). Some cats relax by being groomed or stroked with a grooming mitt or brush, which can release endorphins.

Firm local grasping, especially at the lower back, tail, and feet, is avoided, as it often leads to defensive behavior. If more restraint is necessary for certain manipulations, the cat is held with flat hands around the neck, or chest and shoulders, or the pelvis. The handler should use minimal force, but must be ready to enhance the restraint quickly if the cat tries to scratch or bite. Cats should always be held by experienced staff and not by the owner. Although cats are usually affectionate with their owners, aggression can be directed against the owner in a stressful situation, leading to a scratch or bite.

Occasionally a cat will be encountered which cannot be handled at all without physical or medical restraint. Sedation may be preferable to mechanical restraint for lengthy procedures if the cat is well hydrated and in good body condition. Sedation is especially helpful if painful manipulations, for example, palpation of an unstable joint, are conducted. Mechanical restraint devices, such as a cat bag or a head and face mask, are available, and can be indicated in some instances. As much information as possible should be gained through history and observation of fractious or feral cats. Clinical and further examinations may then only be possible with the use of anesthesia. Intramuscular injection of narcotics or induction of general anesthesia can be performed with the help of restraint boxes. These devices, however, cause significant stress for the patient, do not allow appropriate monitoring, and should only be used for undomesticated or extremely aggressive cats.

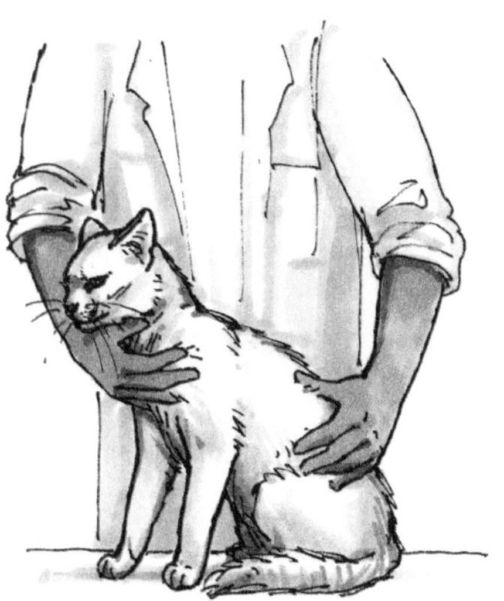

Figure 1-4 Minimal restraint is usually best. For non-painful and non-stressful manipulations the cat on the table is only supported with flat hands, with one hand around the patient's chest to prevent it from jumping away.

1.3 General physical examination

Goals of the general physical examination of an orthopedic patient are to assess the general health of the patient, to detect clinical signs indicating underlying disease processes, and to exclude concurrent problems. Older cats, especially, may suffer from systemic diseases. These diseases can cause or mimic orthopedic or neurological signs, or may be present concurrently with the actual orthopedic or neurological problem. The examination should include assessment of the general body condition, the vital parameters, and topographical examination of all body systems. Important features of the general physical examination of the orthopedic patient are described in the following section. The reader is referred to small animal textbooks for a complete description and interpretation of the general physical examination. When examining a traumatized patient, the complete physical examination is only performed after the cat has been stabilized. The diagnostic and therapeutic approach to the trauma patient is described in Chapter 10.

Overview and vital parameters

Evaluation of body condition, mental state, heart rate, respiratory rate and pattern, mucous membranes and capillary refill time, quality of femoral arterial pulse, and body temperature is performed at the beginning of the clinical examination. Normal values of vital parameters in cats (1, 4, 5) are listed in Table 1-2. Variability of the heart rate is high, depending on stress (1). Body weight is also recorded.

Table 1-2. Normal vital parameters in cats

Parameter	Normal values
Heart rate (1)	130 beats/min (± 19) at home 150 beats/min (± 23) at veterinary hospital 187 beats/min (± 25) under restraint
Respiratory rate	20–40 breaths/min
Body temperature	38–39°C
Pulse quality at femoral arteries	Easily palpable and regular
Mucous membranes	Light pink and moist
Capillary refill time	<1 second

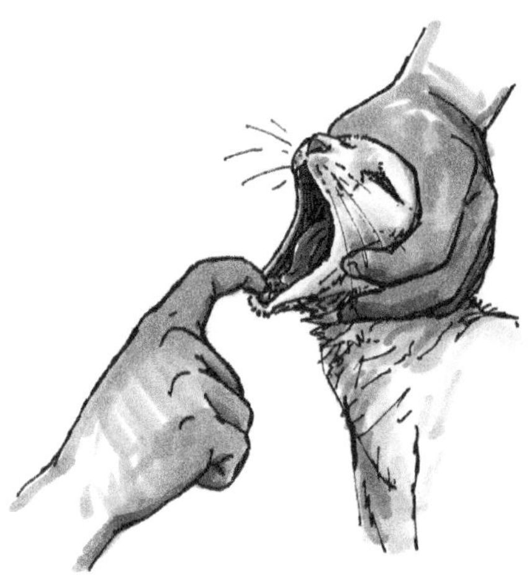

Figure 1-5 To open the mouth of a cat, one hand is placed over the top of head with the thumb and fingers under the zygomatic arches. The head is then gently tilted back. Pressure is applied on the lower incisors with one finger of the other hand until the mouth is opened.

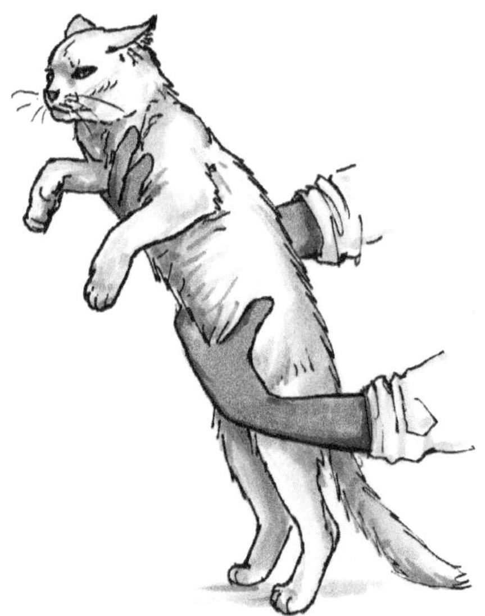

Figure 1-6 Palpation of the abdomen can be conducted while the cat is held upright with one hand under its chest, its back towards the examiner. Abdominal contents are then gently palpated with flat fingers. Firm sharp grasping or gripping is avoided, as this will cause pain and may even result in intra-abdominal injury.

Head and neck

Eyes, ears, nostrils, and the oral cavity are examined. Blood in the nostrils or the external ear canal may result from head trauma. Lacerations around the lips or nose also indicate head trauma and are commonly caused by falls from a height. The oral cavity is examined to evaluate dental occlusion and identify dental fractures, mandibular and/or maxillary fractures, cleft palate, masses, or other abnormalities. Special attention is made to check for mandibular symphyseal fractures and traumatic cleft palates in cats with a history of having fallen from a height. The correct way to open the mouth of a cat is shown in Figure 1-5 (5). The neck is gently moved through its range of motion and the cervical spine is palpated in order to detect spinal or muscular pain. Because of the high frequency of hyperthyroidism in older cats, the paratracheal region is carefully palpated from the larynx to the thoracic inlet for nodular masses, indicative of an enlarged thyroid gland.

Fur, skin, and lymph nodes

The quality and integrity of the fur are noted and the skin elasticity is checked in order to evaluate hydration status of the animal. The whole body is inspected for pain, swelling, and accumulation of blood or pus. The superficial lymph nodes, mandibular, prescapular, axillary, inguinal, and popliteal, are palpated for enlargement. The mammary glands are examined to detect masses.

Respiratory tract

Breathing pattern and the presence of respiratory noises are noted. Upper-airway obstruction results in stridor or stertor, and a deep and prolonged inspiratory phase with dyspnea. Open-mouth breathing can be secondary to airway obstruction, or stress and pain. Lung parenchymal disease, such as pulmonary contusion or edema, causes labored inspiration and expiration with elevation of the respiratory rate. Cats show rapid and shallow breathing, and a predominantly inspiratory distress with pleural space diseases, such as pneumothorax, pleural effusion, or diaphragmatic hernia. The thoracic wall is palpated for rib fractures and other structural changes. Auscultation of the lungs may reveal abnormal lung sounds, absence of normal lung sounds, and asymmetry between the right and left sides. The absence of normal lung sounds suggests pleural space diseases, such as pneumothorax, pleural effusion, or diaphragmatic hernia. Purring prevents proper auscultation and can be difficult to stop. Distracting the cat by running water from a tap can help.

Heart

Auscultation of the heart may reveal heart murmurs or arrhythmias. Gallop arrhythmias are common in cats with myocardial disease. Stress might cause previously subclinical heart disease to develop into heart failure. It can be difficult to differentiate between traumatic shock and cardiogenic shock in this situation. The presence of lung edema or pleural effusion, arterial thromboembolism, and jugular vein distension indicates heart failure. An inadequate response to the initial shock and dyspnea treatment should also alert the clinician to the possibility of the presence of underlying heart disease.

Abdomen

The abdomen is gently palpated, while the cat is standing or while it is held with the forelimbs off the table and one hand around the chest with the examiner standing behind the cat (Fig. 1-6). The normal stomach is not always palpable, especially when empty and located completely within the rib cage.

The small spleen and the edges of the liver may be located in non-obese cats. The small intestinal loops, a colon filled with feces, the kidneys and the urinary bladder should all be readily palpable, except in the obese animal. However, a palpable bladder does not rule out bladder rupture. Free abdominal fluid is palpable if present in a significant amount. It results in abdominal distension and ballottement.

Perineal region

The perineal region and the tail are inspected, mainly to diagnose the presence of injuries, abscesses, hematomas, and neurological deficiencies (Chapter 1–5). Bloody urine may be present around the vulva or penis in traumatized cats, and is generally due to injury to the urinary system.

Lameness grade	Description of lameness
Grade 1	Low-grade lameness: lameness hardly visible or no lameness is visible, but cat lifts foot when sitting (front limbs), or is unable to jump (from the history) (hindlimbs)
Grade 2	Medium-grade lameness: lameness clearly visible, but leg is used in most steps
Grade 3	High-grade lameness: cat is only toe-touching or not weight-bearing at all

Table 1-3. Proposal for scoring lameness in cats

1.4 Orthopedic examination

The orthopedic examination should include gait analysis, palpation of the cat in a standing position, and palpation and manipulation of every joint and bone on both sides with the cat in lateral recumbency.

1.4.1 Examination of gait

Gait examination can be difficult and often requires time and patience because cats generally cannot be led on a leash, and often tend to refuse to move around freely in a new environment.

The examination room door and windows should be closed at all times when a cat is unrestrained. Many cats tend to crouch on the floor and stay immobile initially, but motivating the cat to move around in a new environment is usually possible when the behavior of the cat is understood. Cats placed in the middle of a room usually look for a place to hide. If the cat is positioned near a corner, basket, or another place to hide, it will often move towards that area, allowing observation of a few steps at least. The place to hide should be organized in a way that it is possible to remove the cat from the area easily. The ability to jump can sometimes be assessed if the room has an elevated place, such as a table in a corner of the room. A closed room with a window can also be used to observe the gait from outside the room, after the cat has been allowed to get familiar with the room. Some cats can be motivated to play with the spotlight of a laser pointer. If a cat completely refuses to walk, and lameness cannot be assessed at the clinic, the observations of the owners have to be used to gather information. Another valuable method for gait evaluation in cats is to ask the owners to film their cat at home.

Although it is generally possible to observe a few steps, the cat usually cannot be seen moving at different gaits, and may only move in a crouched position. Despite the difficulties in gait examination, an effort is made to classify any lameness according to its severity in order to assess treatment success. A simple lameness classification score for cats is described in Table 1-3. Cats with low-grade lameness in the thoracic limbs sometimes appear to walk normally, but lift the foot off the ground when sitting.

Cats with bilateral orthopedic problems may not show a distinct lameness, but are inactive and reluctant to jump, sometimes standing or sitting with an abnormal posture, or walking with a crouched gait. Bilateral orthopedic conditions occur more frequently in the pelvic limbs, and can be confused with neurological disorders. Common bilateral pelvic limb problems include patellar luxation, bilateral cranial cruciate ligament disease, hip dysplasia, and coxarthrosis. Lumbar or lumbosacral degenerative disease and spondylosis may also cause pain and should be considered as differential diagnoses. Bilateral orthopedic diseases of the thoracic limbs are rarer, with degenerative disease of the elbow being the most common.

Orthopedic injuries of more than one limb, unstable pelvic fractures, and/or spinal fractures and luxations should be suspected in cats unable to stand and walk after trauma. A thorough orthopedic and neurological examination is performed after stabilization of the patient. Minor joint instability, and fracture or luxation of the proximal limbs such as femoral head and neck fractures, scapular fractures, and hip and shoulder luxations can initially easily be overlooked if the examination is not thorough, and concurrent more obvious injuries are present in other limbs.

1.4.2 Examination in a standing position

Palpation of the cat on the examination table in a standing position is conducted gently, and with the least amount of

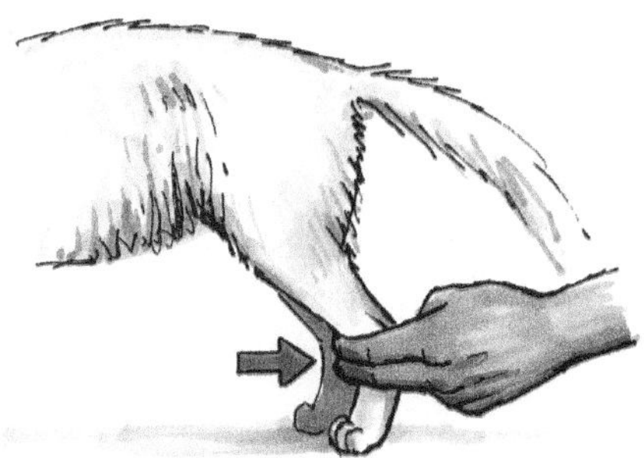

Figure 1-7 Comparison of weight-bearing asymmetry is only possible in cats standing symmetrically on the table, and is an additional method for detecting which of the paired limbs is loaded less. The amount of resistance before the leg is drawn back or lifted is compared between the two limbs.

restraint possible. Only non-painful manipulations are performed during this stage of the examination. The standing position allows direct comparison between paired limbs, and facilitates detection of asymmetry. One hand may have to be placed under the abdomen to lift the pelvic legs in order to keep the cat in a standing position. Another way to motivate cats to stand up is gentle scratching at the base of the tail.

Weight-bearing asymmetry can be compared between paired legs while the cat is standing. A gentle pull in a caudal direction with two fingers on the metatarsus will cause the cat to unload the limb (Fig. 1-7). The resistance to unload the limb will be greater in the unaffected side. A comparable test for the front limbs consists of pushing in the area of the accessory bone cranially, and assessing the difference in resistance to knuckling over.

The neck, back, thoracic limbs, and pelvic limbs are then gently palpated. Shoulder, back, pelvic, and thigh muscle hypotrophy or differences in muscle tone are noted. The bony protuberances on both sides are compared to each other to detect asymmetry, which is often present with pelvic fractures or hip joint luxations. Subtle changes in size or contour of joints and soft tissues are detected more easily if both sides are palpated simultaneously. The spine and back musculature is palpated gently, including the lumbosacral and sacrococcygeal area to reveal pain. Many cats dislike palpation of the lower back and adverse reactions should be interpreted with caution.

1.4.3 Examination in lateral recumbency

Cats have often become used to being touched after the standing examination and can then be put in lateral recumbency without anxiety. The cat should be held on the table with flat hands around the proximal thoracic and pelvic limbs (Fig. 1-8). All limbs are systematically examined, starting on the unaffected side and ending with the affected limb. It is not uncommon to find multiple limbs injured after trauma. The examination is started at the toes, working proximally, and includes palpation and manipulation of all joints and bones. Gentle palpation is performed first, and is used to detect axial deviation, temperature changes, changes in contour, and fluctuation. Manipulations are conducted after, and may reveal crepitation, joint hyper- or hypomobility, and pain. Any manipulations suspected to be painful are conducted at the end of the examination. Pain can also be elicited by deep palpation. The pain response in cats may be limited, and besides hissing and turning the head will also include subtle signs, such as changes in pupil size, breathing pattern, and positioning of the ears. Care is taken while examining the toes because many cats do not like manipulation of their feet.

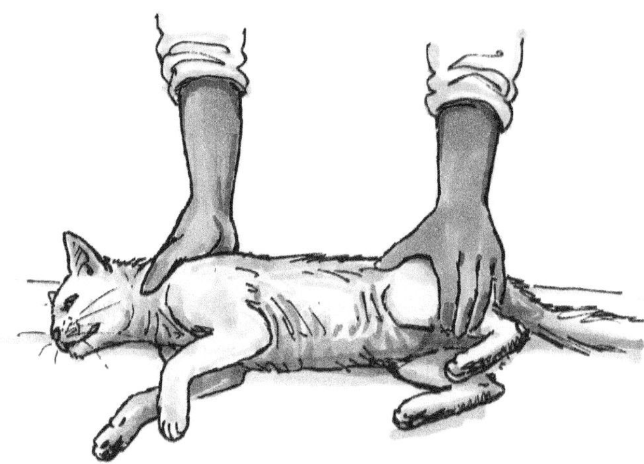

Figure 1-8 An assistant holds the cat gently on the table with flat hands for examination in lateral recumbency. One hand is positioned on the shoulders and around the neck to avoid turning of the head and biting. The other hand lies on the pelvis to prevent the cat from standing up. A cat held like this usually remains cooperative, allowing good assessment of pain responses.

Bones

Bones are palpated and manipulated to detect fractures, changes in contour, and pain. The toes, phalanges, and metacarpal or metatarsal bones are first palpated together, and then individually. Non-displaced metacarpal or metatarsal fractures can easily be missed, as they may only cause subtle soft-tissue swelling and pain. Every bone is then thoroughly palpated from distal to proximal to detect axial deviation, contour changes, crepitation, instability, and pain. Presence of abnormalities is usually caused by fractures in feline orthopedics. Neoplasia and other diseases of bone, with or without pathological fractures, are differential diagnoses.

Joints

Every joint is gently palpated to reveal periarticular swelling or joint effusion. Joint effusion is a non-specific sign, commonly encountered with traumatic hemarthrosis, degenerative joint disease, and arthritis. The joints are then moved throughout their range of motion to detect reduction in range of motion, joint instability, and/or crepitation. Instability or luxation may be detected secondary to traumatic ligament rupture. Knowledge of the anatomy of each articular ligamentous support is mandatory to perform adequate manipulations necessary to stress a specific ligament. Feline joints are more elastic than the canine joints. Comparing the range of motion of the joint to the contralateral side helps in diagnosing cases with minor instability. Clinically relevant collateral ligament sprain is always associated with periarticular swelling. Painful manipulations of injured joints are conducted at the end of the examination. Sometimes sedation or even a short general anesthetic is necessary to be able to diagnose the type and amount of instability accurately. Palpation and manipulation findings and their interpretation are summarized in Tables 1-4 and 1-5. Specific tests and types of diseases and injuries are further described in part 7 of the book.

Soft tissues

The skin, muscles, and tendons are also evaluated during the orthopedic examination. The claws, clawbeds, and the footpads are examined for pathological conditions (Chapter 7). The presence of several damaged and split nails is indicative of a traumatic event. Bite wounds are the most common cause for lameness in the cat, and should be suspected in every lame cat with reported contact to other cats. They often cause marked cellulitis with soft-tissue swelling and a severe pain response on palpation (Chapter 16). Muscles and muscle–tendon units are palpated for muscle hypotrophy or atrophy, swelling, and pain. Rupture of the tendon of the triceps muscle, the Achilles tendon, and the patellar tendon has been described. Please see part 7 of the book for further details.

1.5 Neurological examination

The neurological examination includes evaluation of posture, gait, mental status, cranial nerves, proprioception, spinal reflexes, and sensitivity of dermatomes and body areas (6–8). A standardized neurological examination should be performed in all patients before sedation. Tests requiring minimal manipulation such as cranial nerves and proprioceptive tests are performed first, followed by tests that include some degree of immobilization and discomfort like spinal reflexes, and palpation of the spine or other painful areas.

Table 1-4. A summary of specific findings on the major joints of the forelimbs and their interpretation

Joint	Findings	Interpretation
Carpus	Joint effusion	Arthritis, DJD, trauma
	Periarticular swelling	Ligament/capsule sprain, arthritis
	Crepitation during manipulation	Fracture, luxation, DJD
	Valgus or varus instability (with the carpus in extension)	Collateral ligament sprain
	Positive caudal drawer test	Medial collateral ligament rupture
	Palmar instability/ hyperextension	Rupture of palmar ligaments
Elbow	Joint effusion	DJD, arthritis, synovial cyst
	Periarticular swelling	Ligament/capsule sprain, synovial cyst, medial epicondylitis
	Crepitation during manipulation	Fracture, luxation, DJD
	Reduced range of motion in extension/flexion and supination/pronation	DJD, luxation, synostosis between radius and ulna
	Medial or lateral instability	Collateral ligament sprains
Shoulder	Crepitation during manipulation	Fracture, luxation, DJD, OC
	Reduced range of motion in flexion and extension	DJD, luxation, dysplasia, OC
	Mediolateral and craniocaudal instability (drawer tests)	Medial glenohumeral ligament rupture, subluxation, luxation, rupture of biceps tendon
	Positive biceps tendon test	Biceps tenosynovitis, rupture of the biceps tendon

DJD, degenerative joint disease; OC, osteochondrosis.

Table 1-5. A summary of specific findings on the hindlimbs and their interpretation

Joint	Findings	Interpretation
Tarsus	Joint effusion	Arthritis, DJD, trauma
	Periarticular swelling	Ligament/capsule sprain, arthritis
	Crepitation during manipulation	Fracture, instability, DJD
	Reduced range of motion in flexion/ extension	DJD, luxation
	Valgus or varus instability (with the joint held in extension/flexion)	Collateral ligament sprain, malleolar or distal fibular fracture
	Dorsal intertarsal or tarsometatarsal instability	Rupture of dorsal ligaments
	Plantar intertarsal or tarsometatarsal instability	Rupture of plantar ligaments
Stifle	Joint effusion	DJD, arthritis, OC, trauma
	Periarticular swelling	Capsule and collateral ligament sprain, disruption, DJD
	Crepitation during manipulation	Fractures, instability, DJD
	Reduced range of motion in flexion/extension	DJD
	Unstable patella	Patellar luxation
	Positive cranial and/or caudal drawer test	Cranial and/or caudal cruciate ligament rupture
	Valgus and varus instability (with stifle joint in extension)	Collateral ligament sprain, condylar fractures
Hip	Reduced range of motion in extension, flexion, circumduction, internal and external rotation, and abduction	Hip luxation or pain due to femoral head/neck fractures, DJD, femoral head/neck osteopathies
	Positive Ortolani test (not standardized in cats)	Hip joint instability, hip dysplasia
	Abnormal position of greater trochanter	Hip luxation, avulsion fracture of greater trochanter

DJD, degenerative joint disease; OC, osteochondrosis.

A neurological problem should be suspected when owners report gait abnormalities such as dragging of one or more limbs, swaying gait, legs sliding out from underneath or knuckling over. In addition, altered postures such as an arched back, low head carriage, or altered tail movement may indicate neurological disease. Behavioral changes also indicate potential neurological disorders. Aggression and fear, excessive or reduced appetite, loss of house training, and tail-chasing are the most common behavioral abnormalities in cats. Motor signs such as restless wandering, circling, and excessive vocalization also occur. Often, the signs cannot be attributed to one single anatomic location within the brain.

The feline nervous system is particularly susceptible to hypoglycemia, anoxia, liver malfunction, toxins and pharmacological agents. The major organ systems should therefore be carefully evaluated in every neurological cat.

1.5.1 Posture, gait, and mental status

The cat is observed for gait abnormalities, tendencies to drift to one side, head movements, and posture while the cat is moving. Abnormalities in posture include a head tilt, abnormal truncal posture, or a stiff or flaccid limb posture.

Although the gait pattern is not used as a sole criterion for the localization of a lesion, some gait abnormalities are characteristic. For example, vestibular ataxia is characterized by a head tilt, a broad-based stance, hypotonia of the muscles ipsilateral to the lesion, and hypertonia of the muscles contralateral to the lesion. During movement, affected animals drift or have a tendency to roll over to the weak side. Circling is usually not a localizing sign, except that tight circles are often associated with caudal brainstem lesions. Cerebellar lesions produce a gait characterized by hypermetria of all four limbs accompanied by loss of balance and tremor. Pacing

Degree	Description	Interpretation
Normal	Cat is awake and normal	Normal finding
Apathic	Cat is awake but shows decreased levels of reactions and activity	Non-specific sign caused by secondary or primary diseases of the nervous system
Stuporous	Cat is sleeping but can be awakened by strong mechanical or noisy stimuli	Occurs with lesions or disruptions between the cerebral cortex and the reticular formation
Comatose	Total absence of consciousness. Cat does not react to painful stimuli	Occurs in lesions that cause complete disruption between the brainstem and cerebral hemispheres

Table 1-6. Degrees of level of consciousness

is observed with cortical lesions, but infrequently lesions in the cervical spine may also result in this gait. Spinal cord lesions result in a wide variety of gait patterns and it is rarely possible to associate the gait abnormality with the site of the lesion. Lesions of major peripheral nerves may result in specific gait abnormalities, characteristic for the lesion.

The level of consciousness is mainly regulated by the reticular formation. This structure consists of a fine neuronal network that extends from the medulla oblongata to the diencephalon. Clinically, four degrees of level of consciousness can be differentiated (Table 1-6).

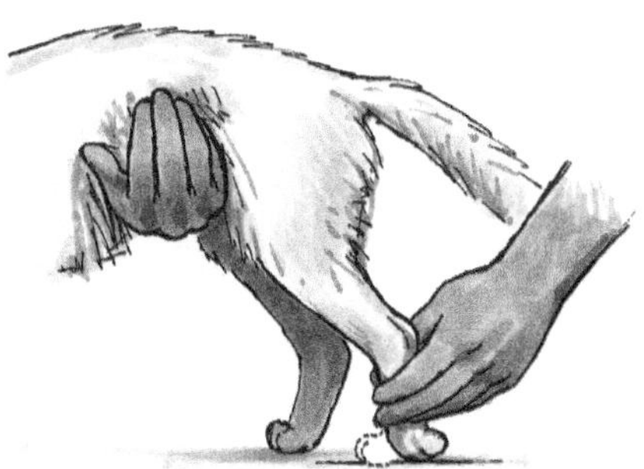

Figure 1-9 Knuckling over of the paw to test proprioception. The cat is supported under the abdomen to avoid a loss of balance when its foot is lifted.

1.5.2 Cranial nerve examination

Abnormalities of cranial nerve function are seen in various encephalopathies and neuromuscular diseases. Physiological function of cranial nerves, tests, and common causes of dysfunction are listed in Table 1-7. Cats with head trauma and possible brain injury are of special concern in view of the potential need for anesthesia and surgical treatment.

Initial assessment focuses on the level of consciousness, cranial nerve function, and motor activity/posture. Cranial nerve deficits in an otherwise alert and responsive cat indicate that the injury is outside the cranial vault. In general, the prognosis for recovery of a peripheral nerve injury is good, provided that neurotmesis has not occurred. Cranial nerve dysfunctions in apathic, stuporous or comatose cats are likely to be due to a central lesion. These patients need serial examinations, and therapeutic intervention may be required to decrease intracranial pressure. Special emphasis is given to the pupil size, symmetry, and reactivity, and presence of physiological nystagmus. A comatose cat with dilated, unresponsive pupils and absent physiological nystagmus is likely to have irreversible brainstem damage and carries the worst prognosis. Intact pupil reactivity, uni- or bilateral miosis, and intact deep pain perception indicate good chances for recovery of neurological function.

1.5.3 Proprioceptive testing

Proprioception means correct orientation of the body in the three-dimensional space during rest and locomotion. Proprioceptive tests include examination of ascending and descending tracts. They are very sensitive for detection of a neurological lesion, but are relatively non-specific for the neuroanatomic localization. Proprioceptive deficits may occur before motor dysfunction can be detected. Several neurological tests help to examine the proprioceptive function.

Proprioceptive positioning reaction

The simplest method of evaluation entails flexing the foot so that the dorsal surface is on the floor (Fig. 1-9). The normal response is immediate reposition of the foot into a normal position. Each limb is tested separately. Deficits may originate from lesions in the lower and upper motor neuron (UMN) system.

Cranial nerve	Function	Tests	Common causes for dysfunction
Olfactory nerve (CN I)	Sensory	Presentation of food, strong substances such as ether	Rhinitis, tumors of nose and cribriform plate, head trauma
Optic nerve (CN II)	Sensory (vision and pupillary light reflexes)	Menace reaction; visual placing; cotton-ball tracking test; pupillary light reaction (direct and indirect); dazzle reflex	Many encephalopathies affecting visual and pupillary light pathways
Oculomotor nerve (CN III)	Motor to extraocular muscles, parasympathetic to pupillary muscles	Observation for ventrolateral strabism, dilated pupil with absent pupillary light reflexes, eventually ptosis	Head trauma, increased intracranial pressure
Trochlear nerve (CN IV)	Motor to extraocular muscles	Observation for lateral rotation of the eyeball	Head trauma
Abducent nerve (CN VI)	Motor to extraocular muscles	Observation for medial strabismus; inability to retract the globe	Head trauma
Trigeminal nerve (CN V)	Motor to muscles of mastication and sensory to face and cornea	Palpebral reflex; corneal and facial sensitivity; jaw tone; palpation of masticatory muscles	Traumatic nerve injury, loss of facial sensitivity due to various encephalopathies and neuropathies
Facial nerve (CN VII)	Motor to facial muscles, sensory to tongue and palate, parasympathetic for nasal, salivary, and lacrimal glands (chorda tympani)	Palpebral reflex; muscle tone of ear, lips, and cheek; Schirmer tear test	Otitis interna, traumatic nerve injury; chorda tympani deficits are possible with middle-ear disease
Glossopharyngeal nerve (CN IX), vagal nerve (CN X)	Motor/sensory to laryngeal and pharyngeal muscles, parasympathetic for thoracic and abdominal organs (X)	Gag reflex; thoracic X-ray for megaesophagus; observation of vocal fold movement during light sedation	Brainstem diseases
Vestibulocochlear nerve (CN VIII)	Sensory	Vestibular dysfunction: head tilt; nystagmus; ventral strabismus, vestibular ataxia Cochlear dysfunction: brainstem auditory evoked potentials	Otitis interna, brainstem diseases
Accessory nerve (CN XI)	Motor to muscles of the neck	Muscle tone of cervical muscles	Thiamin deficiency (ventroflexion of the neck)
Hypoglossal nerve (CN XII)	Motor to the tongue	Observation of food intake and asymmetric tongue position/atrophy	Brainstem diseases

Table 1-7. Function, testing, and common etiologies of cranial nerve dysfunction

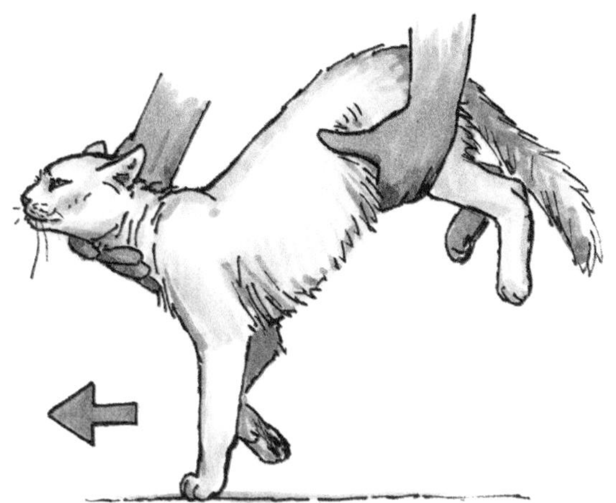

Figure 1-10 Wheelbarrowing with extended neck. While lifting hindlimbs off the floor and extending the neck, the cat is moved forward and movements of the front limbs are observed.

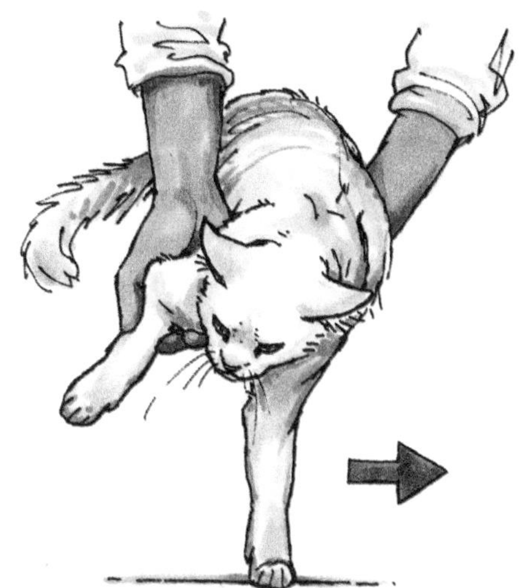

Figure 1-11 Hopping in the thoracic limb. The cat is supported under the abdomen and is moved to the side on a straight line. Hopping movements of the tested limb are observed for abnormalities such as delayed initiation or incorrect adaptation.

Wheelbarrowing reaction

The cat is supported under the abdomen, with all of its weight on the thoracic limbs. Normal animals can walk forward and sideways with coordinated movements (Fig. 1-10). The maneuver may be repeated by extending the head and neck with one hand. Visual control of movement is thus eliminated, making the animal mostly dependent on proprioceptive information. The cat should be observed for initiation of movement, paresis, and dysmetria. Deficits caused by a lesion in the cervical spinal cord, the brainstem, and cerebral cortex are detected with the aid of this test.

Hopping reaction

The test is performed with the cat supported under the abdomen, and one thoracic limb lifted from the ground so that the weight of the cat is supported by one limb. The patient is then moved medially, laterally, and forwards (Fig. 1-11). Poor initiation of the hopping reaction suggests sensory deficits, while poor follow-through suggests a motor system abnormality. Some neurologically intact cats have a tendency not to support their weight and exhibit a floppy behavior during the test. Thus, caution must be given to false-positive reactions.

Extensor postural thrust reaction

The cat is supported by the thorax caudal to the thoracic limbs and the pelvic limbs are lowered to the floor. When touching the floor, the limbs should move caudally in a symmetric walking movement. In addition, the limbs will be extended as they contact the floor. This is a vestibular reflex and absence of limb extension may indicate a lesion in the vestibular system.

Placing reaction

Visual placing is evaluated by supporting the cat under the thorax, and placing it near to the edge of a table. Normal animals will reach for the surface before the carpus touches the edge of the table. Tactile placing is performed in the same manner but the examiner covers the eyes of the patient with one hand. Immediately after contact with the edge of the table, the limbs should be placed on the surface and support weight. Normal tactile placing with absent visual placing indicates a lesion in the visual pathways. Normal visual placing with abnormal tactile placing suggests a sensory pathway lesion or a motor deficit in the cervical spinal cord, the brainstem, or cortex.

Tonic neck reaction

A cat about to jump on a table extends head, neck, and thoracic limbs, and flexes the pelvic limbs. If the head is extended manually, the same response of the limbs will be observed. A lesion in the cortex, brainstem, or cervical area will produce abnormal results.

Subtle proprioceptive and motor deficits may be detected in cats by observing them performing more demanding exercises such as landing. The way in which a cat lands from 1–2 foot (30–60 cm) off the ground can unmask a proprioceptive deficit, by showing weakness during landing, such as stumbling or abnormal limb positioning. Care is taken to ascertain first that the cat can support weight in order to avoid iatrogenic injury. Cats with orthopedic disease may land differently: a cat with bilateral elbow arthritis my land on its chin in preference to landing on its forelimbs.

1.5.4 Spinal reflexes

Spinal reflex testing examines the integrity of the sensory and motor components of the reflex arc, including the influence

Spinal nerve	Loss of sensation	Muscles affected
Suprascapular (C6–C7)	Medial aspect between elbow and shoulder	Supra- and infraspinatus
Musculocutaneus (C6–C8)	Dorsomedial side thoracic limb	Biceps and brachialis
Median, ulnar (C8–T2)	Ventral aspect of paw and forearm and the fifth digit	Flexor muscles of carpus and digits
Radial (C7–T2)	Dorsolateral forearm	Extensors of the forearm and carpus
Femoral (L4–L6)	Medial side of thigh and lower limb	Quadriceps group of muscles
Obturator (L4–L6)	–	Adductor, gracilis
Sciatic (peroneal and tibial branches)	Whole limb below stifle, except medial side	Flexors and extensors of the hock and digits
Peroneal nerve (L6–L7)	Dorsal leg and paw	Flexors of the hock, extensors of the digits
Tibial nerve (L6–S1)	Ventral leg and paw	Flexors of digits, extensors of the hock
Pudendal (S1–S3)	Perineum	Anal and exernal urinary sphincter
Caudal (Cc1–CcX)	Tail	Tail muscles

Table 1-8. Autonomous dermatomes and myotomes of spinal nerves

of the descending motor pathways on the reflex (Table 1-8). Absent or depressed reflexes indicate lower motor neuron (LMN) disease. Exaggerated reflexes indicate abnormality of the UMN system, or a deficit of the opposing muscle. Clonus may be observed during testing of extensor reflexes such as the patellar reflex. This is a repetitive contraction and relaxation of muscle in response to the reflex stimulus. It is a sign seen in chronic lesions of descending inhibitory pathways.

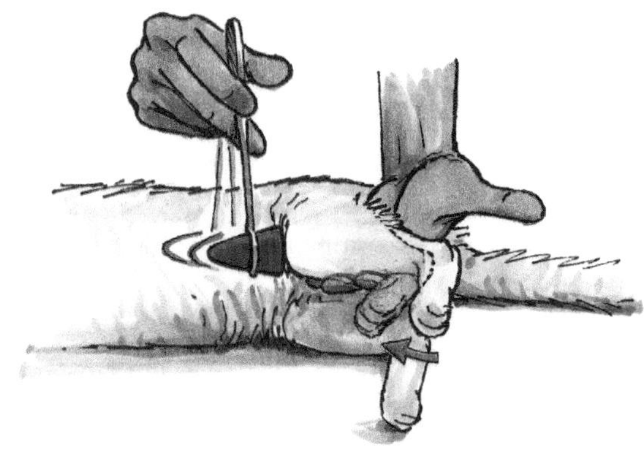

Figure 1-12 Patellar reflex testing. While the cat lies in a relaxed position the limb is supported with one hand. The patellar ligament is gently tapped with the pleximeter. The correct response is extension of the stifle joint.

Normal spinal reflexes

Quadriceps reflex (femoral nerve). The limb is supported in a relaxed position with the stifle in slight flexion. The patellar tendon is struck with the reflex hammer or pleximeter. In cats with a small patellar tendon it may be more accurate to place a finger on the ligament and tap the finger instead, thus indirectly stimulating the ligament. A normal knee jerk is a single, rapid extension of the stifle (Fig. 1-12). An absent or depressed patellar reflex indicates a lesion in the afferent or motor component of the reflex arc. An exaggerated reflex results from loss of descending inhibitory pathways or, alternatively, a deficit of opposing hamstring muscles or the sciatic nerve.

Cranial tibial reflex (peroneal nerve). With the hock held in a degree of extension, the belly of the cranial tibial muscle is struck with the pleximeter just below the stifle. The response is flexion of the hock. It can be difficult to elicit this reflex in normal cats and depressed responses should be interpreted with caution and always in combination with other neurological deficits.

Pelvic limb flexor reflex (sciatic nerve). This test can be performed by stimulating the dorsal surface of the foot, innervated by the peroneal nerve. Alternatively, the plantar surface of the foot is tested by stimulation of the tibial nerve. A noxious stimulus is applied to the foot with the cat in lateral recumbency. Squeezing the interdigital skin with two fingers is usually enough to elicit withdrawal of the limb. Pressure across the digits using a hemostat is applied if deep pain sensation needs to be assessed. The flexor reflex is divided in two components. Primarily, the segmental response occurs as a flexion of the entire limb. Secondarily, conscious perception of the noxious stimulus in the sensory cortex is proved if the cat shows a painful reaction such as hissing or orientation towards the stimulus. An exaggerated reflex may be mani-

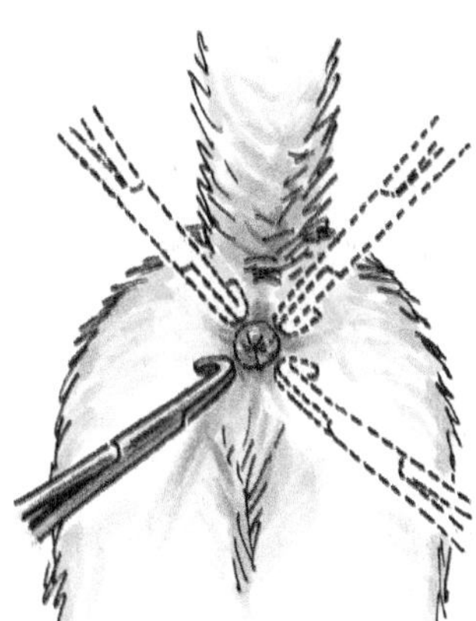

Figure 1-13 Stimulation of perineal area. The perineal area is mildly stimulated with an instrument to elicit contraction of the anal sphincter and flexion of the tail.

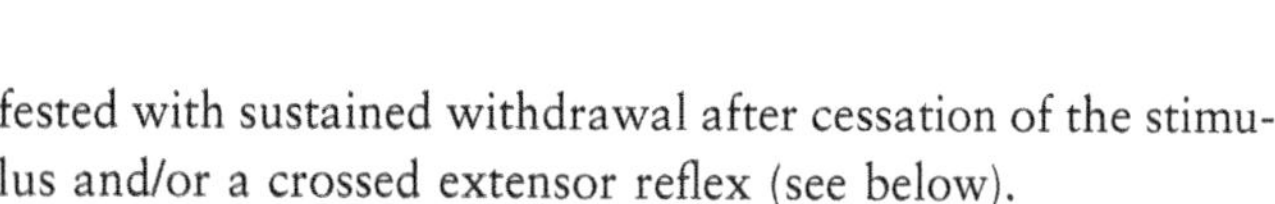

fested with sustained withdrawal after cessation of the stimulus and/or a crossed extensor reflex (see below).

Perineal reflex (pudendal nerve). Stimulation of the perineum with a hemostat elicits contraction of the anal sphincter and flexion of the tail (Fig. 1-13). Squeezing the penis or vulva causes a similar response (bulbocavernosus reflex). Absence or depression of the reflex indicates a pudendal nerve or sacral spinal cord lesion. Assessment of sacral reflexes is especially important in cats with sacrococcygeal fracture/luxation and urinary bladder dysfunction. An atonic anal sphincter and urinary incontinence are present in complete pudendal or sacral lesions.

Extensor carpi radialis reflex (radial nerve). This reflex is difficult to recognize in cats. With the animal in lateral recumbency, the forelimb is supported with the elbow and carpus in flexion. The extensor carpi radialis muscle is struck with the pleximeter just distal to the elbow. The response is a slight extension of the carpus (Fig. 1-14).

Thoracic limb flexor reflex (axillary, musculocutaneous, median, and ulnar nerves). The median palmar surface of the limb is innervated by the ulnar and median nerves, which originate from the spinal cord segments C8–T1. The lateral palmar surface and most of the lateral digit are innervated by branches of the ulnar nerve. For technique and interpretation of the response, see description under pelvic limb flexor reflex, above.

Abnormal spinal reflexes

Crossed extensor reflex. This reflex can be observed in the thoracic and pelvic limbs when the flexor is elicited. The opposite limb extends simultaneously with flexion of the stimulated limb. A crossed extensor reflex occurs with lesions of the UMN system. It is not an indicator of severity, but of chronicity of a lesion.

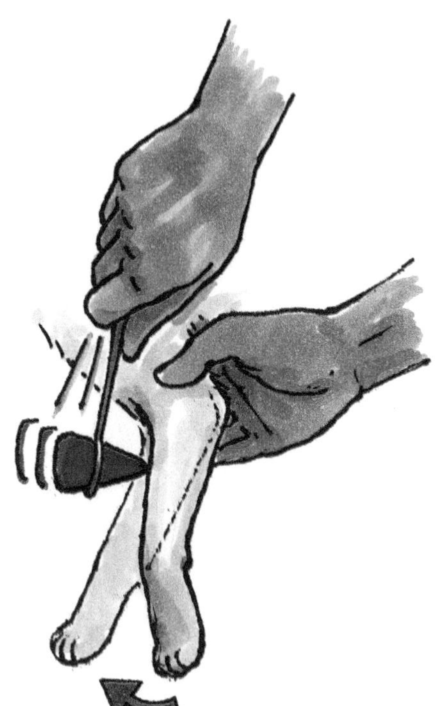

Figure 1-14 Extensor carpi radialis reflex. The limb must be supported in a relaxed position to obtain a response, and the muscle is tapped below the elbow at the craniolateral side of the forearm. The correct response is extension of the carpal joint.

Babinski (extensor toe) reflex. The reflex can be elicited in the pelvic limbs during stimulation of the caudolateral surface from the hock to the digits when the animal is in lateral recumbency and the limb is supported with the other hand. The abnormal response is an extension and fanning of the digits. Presence of this sign indicates a lesion of the UMN system. In most cases, clinical signs have been present for longer than 3 weeks.

Mass reflex. After eliciting a flexor reflex in a pelvic limb, flexion of the contralateral limb, flexion of the tail, contraction of the anal sphincter, and sometimes micturition and defecation, occur. This response is seen with complete spinal cord transections above the lumbar intumescence. Presence of a mass reflex carries a poor prognosis.

1.5.5 Sensitivity testing of peripheral nerves

Recognition of a sensory deficit is helpful in localizing specific nerve or nerve root dysfunction. Dermatomes are skin areas innervated by one or several nerves. They may be autonomous, i.e., innervated by a single nerve, or overlapping, i.e., innervated by several nerves. Sensitivity is best tested by pinching the skin with a surgical hemostat. Table 1-8 contains lists of the areas to which each peripheral nerve of clinical significance is sensory. The dermatomes are also depicted in Figure 1-15.

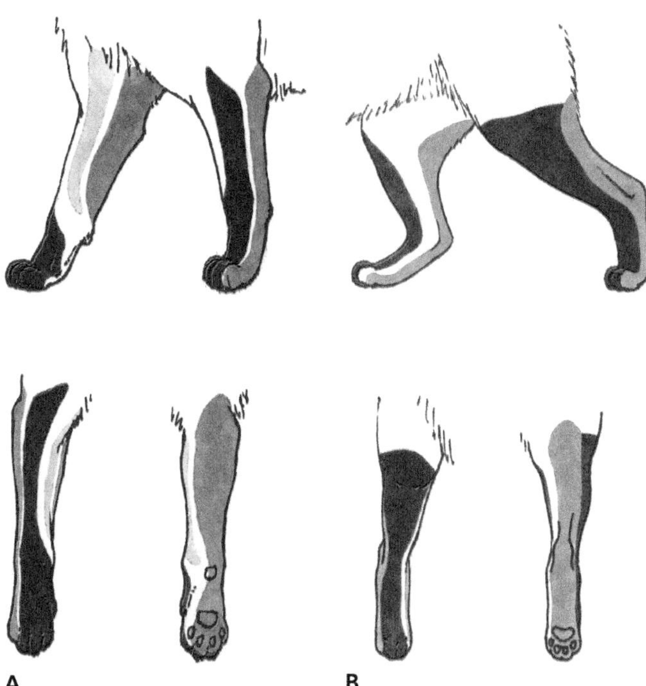

Figure 1-15 Dermatomes of the feline front and hindlimbs. Dermatomes may vary among individuals. (**A**) Dermatomes of the front limbs. Dark blue, radial nerve; mid-blue, ulnar nerve; turquoise, median nerve. (**B**) Dermatomes of the hindlimbs. Dark blue, peroneal nerve; mid-blue, tibial nerve; turquoise, saphenous nerve.

1.5.6 Localization within the nervous system

The nervous system can roughly be divided into the central nervous system (CNS) and peripheral nervous system (PNS). As a first approach, it may be helpful to attribute the neurological deficits to one of these divisions before the lesion is localized more accurately.

A generalized PNS lesion can be distinguished from a central lesion by assessment of the quality of the spinal reflexes. Generalized hyporeflexia in a mentally normal cat is an indicator of a generalized LMN problem. Other signs indicate a centrally located lesion.

If the problem is located in the CNS, it has to be further specified to a spinal cord or a brain lesion. Cranial nerve deficits and/or behavioral or mental abnormalities indicate the presence of a brain lesion, whereas absence of these signs indicates a spinal cord lesion (Fig. 1-16).

After the patient's problem has been attributed to one of the major divisions of the nervous system, PNS, spinal cord, or brain, a more detailed localization is warranted. Rudimentary knowledge of the anatomy and physiology of the divisions of the CNS is indispensable at this step. Clinically relevant features and main symptoms of the 10 clinically relevant localizations are briefly summarized in the following sections.

Peripheral nervous system

From a clinical point of view the PNS can be regarded as identical to the LMN, including the alpha-motor neuron in the ventral gray column of the spinal cord, the ventral and dorsal nerve roots, the peripheral nerve, the neuromuscular junction, and the muscle. A complete lesion to any one of the components results in flaccid paralysis of the affected limb, areflexia, atonia, and anesthesia. Incomplete lesions occur as different degrees of paresis and weakness, decreased postural reactions, hyporeflexia, and a decreased muscle volume and strength. Occasionally, an animal can have LMN weakness with normal reflexes, i.e., myopathy or myasthenia gravis. Monoparesis and monoplegia are most often the result of a traumatic, neoplastic, or vascular lesion. A generalized LMN lesion is generally caused by metabolic toxic, endocrine, inflammatory, degenerative, or inherited disease. Ventroflexion of the neck is seen in cats as a typical clinical feature in many disorders, i.e., hypokalemia, myasthenia gravis, or polymyositis.

Spinal cord: L4–S3 (Cx)

A lesion to this area entails various degrees of involvement of the nerves to the pelvic limbs, bladder, anal sphincter, and tail. Clinical signs range from flaccid weakness to paralysis of pelvic limbs, perianal myotomes, and tail. An identical clinical presentation can be seen with different lesions in the area affecting both spinal cord segments and the nerves of the cauda equina. In compressive lesions, pain is usually elicited with manipulation of the lower back and tail. The anal sphincter may be flaccid and dilated with fecal incontinence. In complete lesions, the bladder is atonic with urine retention and overflow incontinence. Sensory function of the different dermatomes may be reduced or absent depending on the severity of the lesion. This syndrome is commonly observed in cats with traumatic sacrococcygeal disruption.

Spinal cord: T3–L3

A thoracolumbar lesion results in different degrees of ataxia and paraparesis or paraplegia of the pelvic limbs. The dysfunction is of the UMN type. Urinary retention because of hypertonicity of the urinary sphincter or absence of the detrusor reflex is a common complication of this syndrome. The so-called Schiff–Sherrington phenomenon is unique to the dog and is not observed in cats. Increased sensitivity is found at the level of the lesion and decreased sensitivity behind the lesion.

Spinal cord: C6–T2

A lesion to these cord segments produces LMN signs in the thoracic limbs and UMN signs in the pelvic limbs. The degree

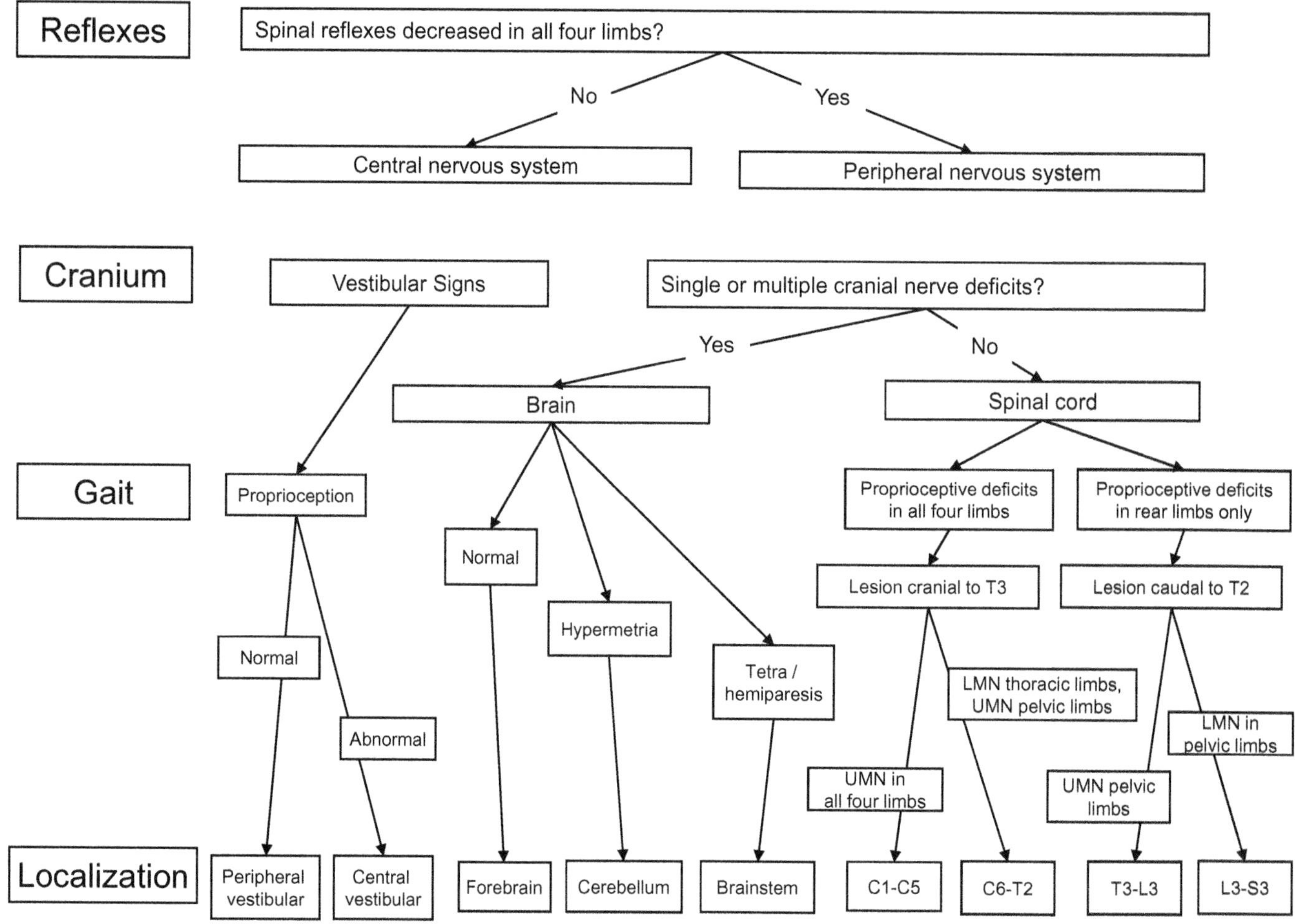

Figure 1-16 Algorithm for localization of neurological lesions. UMN, upper motor neuron; LMN, lower motor neuron; C, cervical; T, thoracic; L, lumbar; S, sacral spinal cord segments.

of gait abnormalities is broad and ranges from ataxia to tetraplegia with flaccid paralysis of the thoracic limbs. Hyporeflexia in one or both thoracic limbs is the most helpful clinical key to the localization. The panniculus reflex may be depressed unilaterally or bilaterally.

Spinal cord: C1–C5

A lesion to this area results in UMN signs to the thoracic and pelvic limbs, including different degrees of ataxia and spastic tetraparesis, proprioceptive deficits in all four limbs, and normal to increased reflexes. The neck is often painful and carried low with compressive or inflammatory lesions. In severe lesions, hypoventilation due to phrenic nerve deficits may occur.

Peripheral vestibular system

A lesion to this part of the system causes a head tilt ipsilateral to the lesion, and nystagmus with a horizontal or rotatory direction with the quick phase of the nystagmus away from the lesion. Vestibular ataxia has different degrees of severity consisting of falling or rolling towards the side of the lesion, hypotonia of the limb muscles ipsilateral to the lesion, and hypertonicity away from the lesion and/or a tendency to drift towards the side of the lesion. Proprioceptive deficits are typically not present in peripheral lesions. Horner's syndrome and facial paralysis frequently accompany peripheral vestibular syndrome due to their proximity in the middle and inner ear. Bilateral peripheral vestibular lesions are occasionally encountered in cats. They cause no head tilt but a characteristic swaying movement of the head, and a decreased extensor muscles tone resulting in a creeping gait. Vestibular eye movements are absent.

Central vestibular system

A central vestibular disorder results in similar deficits to a peripheral lesion. However, the neurological presentation differs in some key areas. Signs of paresis and/or proprioceptive deficits in association with a head tilt indicate a central lesion. The direction of the nystagmus is similar to that seen in peripheral lesions, but a positional or vertical nystagmus suggests the presence of a central lesion. Multiple cranial nerve dysfunctions are also strong indicators of a centrally located lesion. Paradoxical vestibular disease is defined as a vestibular deficit with the head tilt opposite to the side of the lesion. It is usually caused by a lesion near the cerebellar peduncles.

Brainstem

The syndrome is characterized by decreased mentation, obvious gait abnormalities such as tetraparesis, tetraplegia, hemiparesis and/or severe ataxia, and multiple cranial nerve deficits if the lesion is located in the pons or medulla oblongata, including cranial nerves V, VI, VII, VIII, IX, X, and XII. Respiratory function may be disturbed, resulting in altered patterns of breathing. Abnormal postures such as opisthotonus may be observed if the lesion is located in the cranial brainstem or midbrain. In unilateral lesions, the patient has a spastic hemiparesis on the opposite side. The animal may be stuporous or comatose with severe brainstem lesions. Oculomotor nerve (cranial nerve III) deficits with normal vision can be present.

Cerebellum

Cerebellar lesions result in a spastic, hypermetric gait of all four limbs, and the body may sway to one side or the other. Hypermetria is usually more pronounced in the thoracic limbs. The stance is broad-based and there is tremor of the head and body, especially when movement is initiated or during eating and drinking. Subtle oscillatory or pendulary eye movements may be observed. The menace response is decreased ipsilateral to the lesion without affected vision. Proprioceptive tests may show an exaggerated response with normal initiation. Cerebellar symptoms may be subtle in chronic or compensated cases. Severe lesions of the cerebellum may result in decerebellate rigidity with extension of the thoracic limbs and flexion of the pelvic limbs.

Cerebrum

A symmetric cerebral lesion causes various clinical signs in cats, ranging from apathy and depression to hyperexcitability, disorientation, aggression, and/or seizures. There is only a minimal ataxia with cortical lesions (i.e., pacing). But compulsive walking, restlessness, and head pressing may occur. In unilateral lesions, the cat circles usually to the side of the lesion or exhibits persistent sideward flexion of the head (pleurothotonus). Postural reactions are reduced in the contralateral limbs. Vision is impaired contralateral to the lesion but pupillary function is intact.

References and further reading

1. Abbott JA. Heart rate and heart rate variability of healthy cats in home and hospital environments. J Feline Med Surg 2005;7:195–202.
2. Beaver BV. Fractious cats and feline aggression. J Feline Med Surg 2004;6:13–18.
3. Martin SL. The domesticated cat. In: Sherding RG (ed.) The cat: diseases and clinical management, 2nd edn. New York: Churchill Livingstone; 1994: pp. 1–6.
4. Schmidtke HO. Klinische Allgemeinuntersuchung und Umgang mit der Katze. In: Horzinek MC, Schmidt V, Lutz H (eds) Krankheiten der Katze, 4th edn. Stuttgart: Enke Verlag; 2005: pp. 25–37.
5. Schaer M. The medical history, physical examination, and physical restraint. In: Sherding RG (ed.) The cat: diseases and clinical management, 2nd edn. New York: Churchill Livingstone; 1994: pp. 7–23.
6. Jaggy A, Tipold A. Die neurologische Untersuchung beim Kleintier und beim Pferd. Opuscula Veterinaria. Munich: Wak Verlag und Kunstberatung; 1999.
7. Glass EN, Kent M. The clinical examination for neuromuscular disease. Vet Clin North America Small Anim Pract 2002;32: 1–31.
8. Oliver JE, Lorenz MD, Kornegay JN. Neurologic history and examination. In: Handbook of veterinary neurology. Philadelphia: WB Saunders; 1997: pp. 3–46.

2 Further diagnostic procedures

S. Ohlerth, K. Voss, F. Steffen

Further diagnostic procedures are often required to confirm and further specify a clinical diagnosis, or to rule out a suspicion. It is tempting to use the wide range of sophisticated and interesting diagnostic tools available in many veterinary clinics nowadays, but the results obtained should always be interpreted in conjunction with the clinical findings.

Interpretation of the results from hematological and biochemical analysis of blood is important in systemically ill cats, and in the preanesthetic work-up. Basic knowledge of interpretation of blood parameters is well covered in several veterinary textbooks, and will not be discussed further here. The most important diagnostic tools for orthopedic surgeons are radiology and related diagnostic imaging methods. Further diagnostic tools in the orthopedic patient include cytological and bacteriological examination of synovial fluid, and cytological and histopathological interpretation of masses and bone lesions.

Diagnostic imaging of the traumatized and orthopedic feline patient, arthrocentesis, fine-needle aspiration, selected biopsy techniques, and neurodiagnostic procedures are described in this chapter.

2.1 Diagnostic imaging

Radiology represents the most fundamental diagnostic aid for the investigation of the lame or traumatized feline patient. It is used in conjunction with an accurate history, physical examination, and other diagnostic tests. Results of the radiographic examination may confirm or exclude a suspected diagnosis, reveal additional lesions, or indicate the need for further work-up. Computed tomography (CT), magnetic resonance imaging (MRI), and ultrasonography have also increased in importance for the investigation of feline skeletal diseases. The most important aspects of diagnostic imaging modalities in feline orthopedics are summarized in the text below. Veterinary radiology textbooks that may be of interest to the reader are listed in the reference section (1–7).

2.1.1 Radiographic technique

Radiographic quality

Radiographic quality is dependent on radiographic contrast, radiographic density, and radiographic detail. Good-quality radiographs are needed to be able to perceive radiographic details. Poor-quality radiographs may result in erroneous diagnoses.

Radiographic contrast. For a good-quality skeletal radiograph, moderate to high contrast is desirable that enables evaluation not only of bony structures, but also of soft tissues. A kVp technique in the range of 40–50 is chosen in the cat, which produces a moderately long scale of gray shades. Too high a contrast impedes assessment of soft tissues, and detection of mildly mineralized structures (e.g., periosteal reaction, osteophytes, enthesophytes, callus), subtle bone lysis, and gas.

Radiographic density. High radiographic density is required for sufficient blackness on the radiograph. The mAs is the primary factor affecting radiographic density, and varies with the X-ray machine.

Radiographic detail. Radiographic detail is a term used to describe image sharpness, which is dependent on various factors. Patient motion causes blurring of the image. A grid to remove scatter radiation is not required in feline orthopedic radiography since subject thickness does not usually exceed 12 cm. Instead, the cassette is placed on the table top. A slow-speed (100–200), detailed film–screen combination is used to improve radiographic detail. The appendicular and even the axial skeleton of the cat represents radiographic objects of low thickness. Therefore, a radiographic technique using a small focal spot size is indispensable. The X-ray beam should be collimated to the field of interest to reduce scatter.

Patient positioning

A radiograph represents a two-dimensional image of a three-dimensional object. Consequently, two orthogonal views should always be taken, as lesions may be missed due to superimposition on a single view. Sedation or anesthesia is recommended to avoid patient movement, and to decrease radiation exposure to the personnel.

Radiographic overview. In traumatized cats, a lateral and ventrodorsal overview is commonly used, including the thorax, the abdomen, and the spine (8). To enable assessment of the thorax within this overview film, radiographs are taken during maximum inspiration using exposure settings for an abdominal study (kVp 40–50, slightly higher than for a thoracic study). These radiographs are used for assessment of injuries to the thoracic or abdominal wall, diaphragmatic rupture, pneumothorax, pulmonary contusions, pleural, abdominal or retroperitoneal effusion, and fracture luxations of the spine or pelvis. However, overviews represent a technical compromise, and subtle lesions may be overlooked. Additional views focusing on the lesions or suspicious areas are highly recommended, because only then can the radiographic technique be optimized.

Appendicular skeleton. In general, two orthogonal views are taken, including a mediolateral and either a craniocaudal, caudocranial, dorsopalmar, or dorsoplantar view. To radiograph the manus or pes in the cat, the phalanges are taped on to the cassette to overcome the normal hyperflexed and hyperextended position of the interphalangeal joints. To assess a joint, the radiograph should be centered on the joint and collimated to include one-third of the adjacent long bones. To assess conditions of the long bones, collimation should include both joints adjacent to the affected bone. The beam is centered on the point of interest to avoid geometric distortion. The bone should be positioned parallel and close to the film. For postoperative fracture repair assessment and follow-up studies, superimposition of orthopedic fixation devices on the fracture site should be avoided to enable complete evaluation of fracture healing. For the assessment of fracture healing, four cortices should be visible on two orthogonal radiographs. If a plate was used for fixation, it should be positioned parallel to the X-ray beam to enable evaluation of the adjacent cortex, and detection of signs of implant loosening. The same exposure values and views are used for all follow-up radiographs of a fracture; they are only adjusted if thickness has markedly changed, for example due to loss of muscle mass.

Supplementary projections

Depending on the location of a lesion, oblique or skyline views may be necessary to avoid superimposition with surrounding structures. Additional radiographs of the opposite limb are especially useful in kittens, where incomplete ossification or open physes may mimic trauma or infection. Stress radiography of the appendicular skeleton is helpful in demonstrating joint instability due to ligament injury. To reduce radiation exposure to the personnel, tape, gauze, rope, and wedges should be used for positioning and stress application. Again, a comparison view of the opposite side may be helpful for the diagnosis. Mediolateral views of the carpus and tarsus in hyperflexion and hyperextension are generated to assess the dorsal and palmar or plantar ligament apparatus. With rupture of these ligaments, various degrees of subluxation or luxation are seen radiographically (Chapters 32 and 40).

Varus and valgus angulations are used on dorsopalmar and dorsoplantar radiographs for the evaluation of the collateral ligaments. With collateral ligament injuries, radiographs should be evaluated for widening of the medial or lateral joint spaces following application of stress. In dogs, it is recommended to perform varus and valgus stress radiographs of the talocrural joint in flexed and extended positions to evaluate both the short and long collateral ligaments. However the anatomy of the feline tarsal collateral ligaments is different (Chapter 40), and stressed radiographs are usually performed in extension (Fig. 2-1). Interpretation of valgus and varus stressed radiographs of the carpal joint, and anatomy of the radiocarpal ligament, is also different in cats when compared

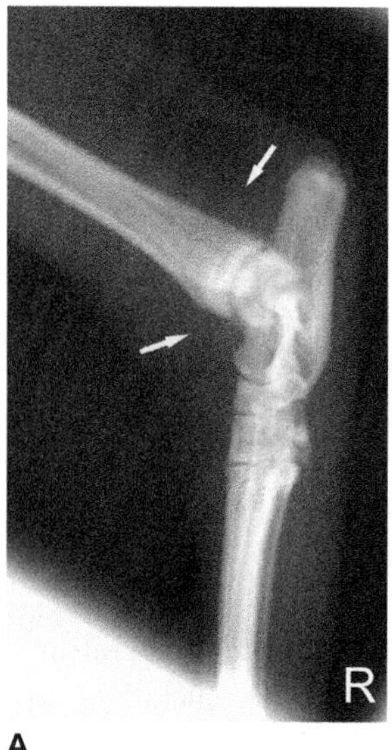

A

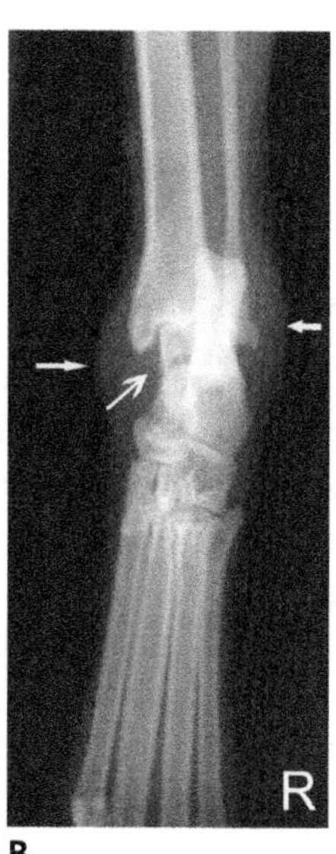

B

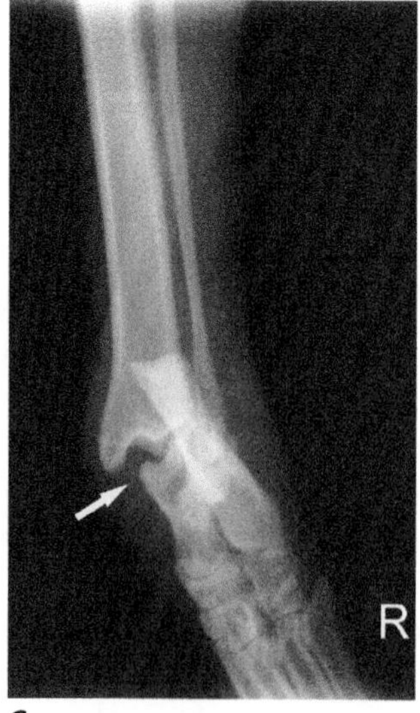

C

Figure 2-1 Mediolateral (**A**) and dorsoplantar (**B**) radiographs of the right tarsal joint of a cat with a history of trauma show marked soft-tissue swelling in the area of the talocrural joint (closed arrows), and a small linear structure of mineral opacity distal to the medial malleolus (open arrow). On the dorsoplantar valgus stress radiograph (**C**), marked widening of the talocrural joint space indicates medial joint instability. Findings are consistent with avulsion/rupture of the medial collateral ligament, and secondary joint effusion.

to dogs (9). The medial opening of the mediocarpal joint is less pronounced in valgus stress radiographs, and varus stress leads to palmar and medial displacement of the radial carpal bone (Chapter 32).

In the stifle, injury to the cranial or caudal cruciate ligament may be demonstrated on a mediolateral radiograph using shear maneuvers similar to a drawer sign.

2.1.2 Principles of radiographic interpretation

Radiographs should be evaluated in front of viewing boxes in a quiet, shaded room with the ceiling light turned off. For the assessment of bone diseases, a bright spotlight is indispensable for the illumination of subtle changes, such as periosteal reaction, soft-tissue mineralization, or lysis. The first step in interpreting radiographs is evaluation of the technique and quality. The veterinarian should be critical with film exposure, artifacts, and patient positioning; if not satisfactory, repeat radiographs should be attempted. Each radiograph is reviewed entirely and in the same way, using a systematic approach. To evaluate orthopedic diseases, several film-reading techniques may be used. One approach is system-based, which starts with the interpretation of the soft-tissue structures prior to reviewing the bony structures. Another approach would be to read a film systematically from proximal to distal (appendicular skeleton) or cranial to caudal (axial skeleton). Based on the radiographic description, a summary of radiographic findings is formulated, which may lead to a final diagnosis or a list of differentials.

Knowledge of normal radiographic anatomy in the immature and adult cat is crucial. In particular, skeletal features of the young growing animal are difficult to interpret, even for the experienced radiologist. Therefore, it is highly recommended to take radiographs of the contralateral limb for comparison. The authors refer to anatomic and radiographic textbooks to study normal anatomy (3, 4). Certain specific anatomic features are encountered in cats. Cats have a clavicle, which is mineralized at birth and located in the soft tissue craniomedial to the distal end of the scapula. It is slightly curved, about 2 mm thick and about 25 mm long in the adult cat. The feline acromion is unique in that it has a caudally directed suprahamate process that is visualized on some films. Cats lack the supratrochlear foramen in the distal humerus but they have a supracondylar foramen found in the medial cortex of the distal humerus, forming a passageway for the brachial artery and median nerve (Chapter 29). A sesamoid bone may be seen in the tendon of the origin of the supinator muscle articulating with the craniolateral aspect of the head of the radius (10). The medial sesamoid bone in the medial head of the gastrocnemius muscle may not be mineralized in some cats (11). Calcification at the cranial pole of the medial meniscus is a common finding, and can occur in both normal cats and secondary to joint trauma or cranial cruciate ligament rupture (11).

2.1.3 Patterns of soft-tissue and bone response

With the systematic process of reviewing skeletal radiographs, knowledge of basic soft-tissue and bone response patterns is essential. The clinician should note bone response patterns, their distribution within bones, and associated soft-tissue changes to formulate a correct radiographic diagnosis.

Soft-tissue changes

Soft-tissue changes may be primary pathologic changes or secondary to more serious bone disease. Fascial planes, tendons, and some portions of joint capsules may be seen because of fat within and around these structures. Fat is less radiopaque than muscle, skin, tendons, joint capsule, and synovial fluid. Soft-tissue structures should be evaluated for swelling, mineralization, and free gas. Swelling is usually caused by trauma, inflammation, infection, or neoplasia. Radiographic signs include focal or diffuse enlargement of soft-tissue opacity, displacement of fat around the joint capsule, e.g., the infrapatellar fat pad in the stifle joint, or around muscles and tendons. Soft-tissue mineralization may occur in conjunction with mineralization of hematoma, necrosis, inflammation, infection, calcinosis circumscripta, myositis ossificans, cancellous bone grafts, or neoplasia. Gas may be present in the soft tissues as a result of traumatic lacerations (open fracture), puncture wounds (cat bite), recent surgery, needle centesis, or gas-producing bacteria. Gas is less radiopaque than fat; calcification is more opaque than soft tissue. Adipose tissue and gas will only be recognized on skeletal radiographs if exposure values were appropriate, resulting in good contrast.

Periosteal reactions

The periosteum adheres to the external surface of bone, and contains many blood vessels that penetrate and supply the bone. It is capable of producing new bone. In the young growing animal, adhesion of the periosteum to bone is loose, and reaction to trauma is more pronounced and occurs faster than in the adult. Periosteal reactions are due to either trauma or a disease process, and they may be first seen radiographically after 7–10 days. There are different types of periosteal reaction, in order of increasing aggressiveness (Fig. 2-2): smooth, lamellar or onion skin, palisading, spiculated or sunburst, and amorphous. Smooth periosteal reaction is a non-aggressive type of new bone formation and is characterized by a solid, continuous (of pillar-like, longitudinal or undulating) appearance, but always with smooth contours. It is commonly seen with trauma (subperiosteal hematoma)

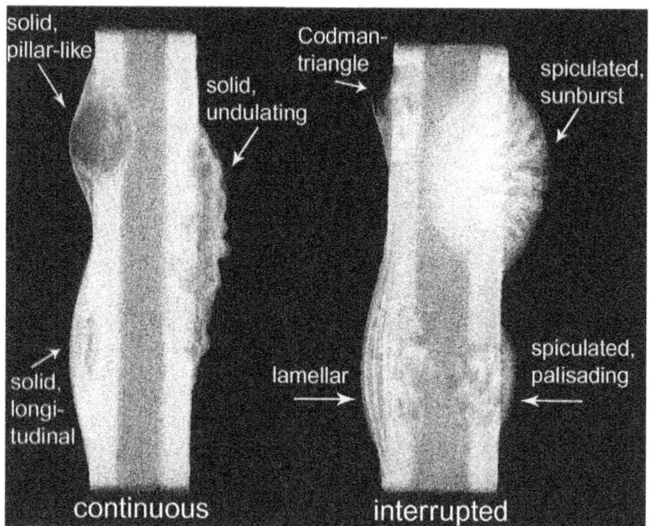

Figure 2-2 Radiographic characteristics of continuous and interrupted periosteal reactions.

or benign processes. The other types of periosteal reaction are included in the interrupted category, and are considered aggressive. Lamellar periosteal reaction represents multiple layers of new bone formation along a cortex and may be seen with trauma, infection or, less likely, neoplasia. With the spiculated type, new bone radiates from the cortex. This pattern may be associated with osteomyelitis, malignant tumor, or a healing fracture with motion present. Amorphous new bone is unorganized, non-functional bone laid down in the soft tissues next to a bone and may be seen with trauma, infection, or neoplasia. Although type of periosteal reaction can help to grade aggressive versus benign bone lesions, it should not be relied upon for diagnosis, as other features of the lesion are more reliable (see below).

Endosteal reaction and intramedullary new bone formation

Focal areas of smooth, homogeneous new bone formation along the inside of a cortex or medullary sclerosis are seen with trauma, bone infarct, or bone healing. With osteomyelitis or neoplasia, endosteal or intramedullary new bone formation becomes inhomogeneous, patchy, and irregular. Assessment of radiographs for endosteal reactions may be difficult due to superimposed periosteal reactions.

Cortical changes

Cortical bone surrounds the diaphysis and metaphysis of long bones. In the young growing animal, the outer surface of the metaphyseal cortex appears irregular due to remodeling, which is necessary to achieve the smaller diameter of the diaphysis. Cortical changes that can be identified radiographically consist of defects, erosion, lysis, and changes in thickness. Cortical defects are most commonly seen with fractures. In cats, they may also be found with bite wounds. Cortical defects must be differentiated from normal structures such as nutrient foramina and physeal lines. Sequestrum formation may also be associated with cortical defects. Cortical erosion may arise from the endosteal or periosteal surface. Erosions may be either smooth (pressure erosion, e.g., seen with a bone cyst) or irregular (infiltrative processes). Cortical lysis and irregular erosion are usually caused by infection or neoplasia. In general, 30–50% of bone per unit area must be destroyed before lysis is radiographically visible. Destruction of cortical bone is easier to detect than destruction of cancellous bone. Cortical lysis typically has a punctate pattern. Reduction of the cortical width in the absence of other bone changes may be the result of chronic decreased weight-bearing, poor fracture healing or other, for example metabolic causes of osteopenia.

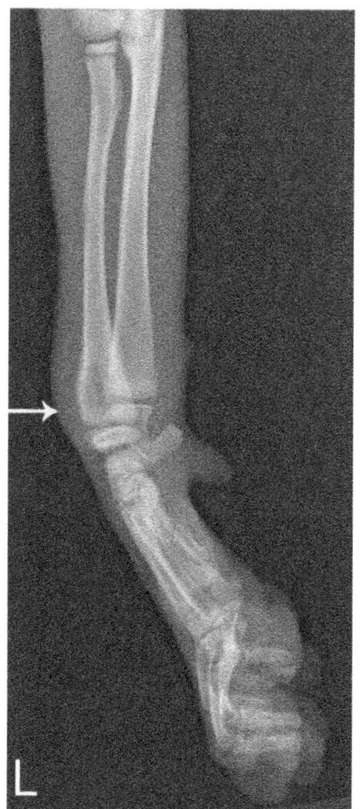

A

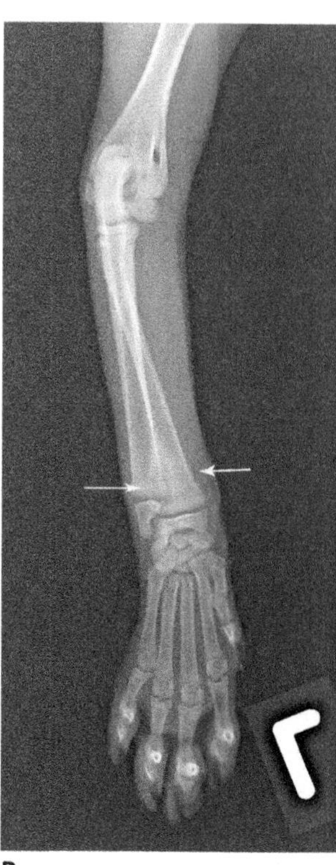

B

Figure 2-3 In the distal metaphysis of the radius in this kitten, geographic bone destruction is seen laterally (**B**) with a sclerotic rim proximally, smooth periosteal reactions dorsally (**A**), mild intramedullary new bone formation, and focal soft-tissue swelling. Surgically, a bone abscess was diagnosed.

Non-aggressive bone lesions

Non-aggressive or less aggressive bone lesions include bone cyst, bone abscess, or benign tumors such as osteoma, enchondroma, osteochondroma, or fibroma (Fig. 2-3). They

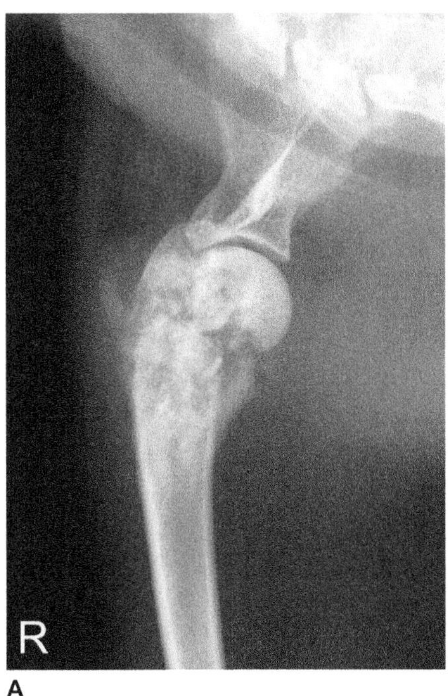

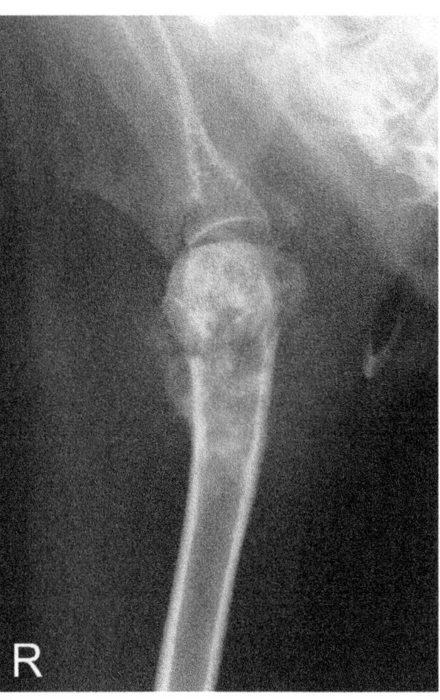

Figure 2-4 Mediolateral (**A**) and craniocaudal (**B**) radiographs of the proximal humerus of a cat with an aggressive bone lesion in the proximal metaphysis. An interrupted sunburst type of periosteal reactions is seen medially, laterally, and cranially, whereas a smoother type of periosteal reaction is seen caudally. Endosteal new bone formation, moth-eaten medullary lysis, and punctate cortical lysis, a pathological fracture at the level of the humeral neck, and marked soft-tissue swelling are also seen. An osteosarcoma was diagnosed histopathologically.

commonly show a well-defined smooth margin between normal and abnormal bone, a geographic pattern of bone destruction, possibly cortical thinning, but neither cortical lysis nor erosion, continuous and smooth periosteal reaction, homogeneous and smooth endosteal or intramedullary new bone formation, and little radiographic change over time. A single lesion or multiple confluent lytic bone lesions characterize geographic bone destruction. The lesions are usually large, with well-defined smooth margins and no changes in the adjacent bone. A sclerotic rim may be seen, denoting walling-off. Cortical thinning may occur due to pressure erosion.

Aggressive bone lesions

Many primary malignant bone neoplasms, metastases, and cases of osteomyelitis appear radiographically as aggressive bone lesions (Fig. 2-4). Primary bone tumors are usually solitary, whereas metastases and osteomyelitis may be found in multiple locations. Aggressive bone lesions typically change rapidly during radiographic follow-up examinations. The transition zone to normal bone is usually less distinct and irregular. Cortical destruction is commonly found. Irregular endosteal and intramedullary new bone formation may be seen. Interrupted periosteal reactions of a lamellated, spiculated, or amorphous type are seen. Moth-eaten or permeative patterns of bone destruction are recognized radiographically. Moth-eaten lesions are moderate in size, often poorly delineated, and cortical lysis or irregular cortical erosion is visible. Multiple very small lytic lesions involving the medulla and the cortex represent a permeative bone destruction pattern. This pattern is also characterized by a large transition zone to normal bone and is considered highly aggressive. Pathological fractures may occur with aggressive bone lesions. Differentiation between a malignant bone tumor and osteomyelitis, and differentiation of tumor types is not possible radiographically.

2.1.4 Radiographic evaluation of fractures

Radiology is the standard method to diagnose and classify a fracture, to evaluate fracture repair postoperatively, and to monitor fracture healing and associated complications (12).

Pre- and postoperative fracture evaluation

Radiographic assessment of fractures plays a crucial role in classifying a fracture, planning treatment, and estimating a prognosis. Again, systematic film reading including the following criteria is suggested (5, 7). Soft tissues, completeness, extent and location of the fracture are evaluated on preoperative radiographs. Classification of fractures is described in Chapter 13. Immediate postoperative radiographs are used to document the repair, detect potential problems, which may be corrected promptly by taking the patient back to surgery, and to provide a reference point for comparison with follow-up films. The immediate postoperative radiographs can be assessed using the "four A's": apposition, alignment, angulation, and apparatus (12). Orthopedic fixation devices are assessed for appropriateness of position, size, and length of implants. The fractured bone is evaluated for degree of apposition of the fracture surfaces (fracture reduction) and accuracy of alignment and angulation of fragments. Complications may be identified, such as intra-articular placement of devices, bridging of growth plates with implants, or fissures or fractures generated during the surgical procedure.

Evaluation of fracture healing

Follow-up radiographs for evaluation of fracture healing are taken every 3–6 weeks, depending on the age of the patient, and type and localization of the fracture. The healing rate of a fracture is very variable and determined by the age of the patient, severity of injury, location of the fracture, and accuracy of stabilization (Chapter 13). Follow-up radiographs should be compared with earlier studies to determine progression of bone healing. The same exposure values and positioning should be used to avoid misinterpretation. Follow-up radiographs are evaluated for fracture alignment, implant position, progression of fracture healing, changes in the adjacent joints and soft tissues, and complications.

Radiographically, uncomplicated secondary bone healing in the cat is similar to the dog, and happens according to the following scheme (Fig. 2-5):

5–10 days after reduction. The sharp ends of the fracture fragments become rounded and demineralized, which results in mild widening of the fracture gap.

10–20 days after reduction. Faintly mineralized internal and external callus formation is seen at a slight distance from the fracture gap. Callus formation is usually more obvious in young cats, in areas with a good blood supply, and in fracture fixation with only relative stability (Chapter 13).

30 days–3 months after reduction. The fracture lines gradually decrease and finally disappear. The opacity of the external callus increases and remodeling starts.

>3 months after reduction. Remodeling continues. The callus becomes smaller with smoother margins, and the cortex and medullary cavity are re-established.

Radiographically, a completely healed fracture shows absence of fracture lines, corticomedullary continuity, and restoration of the bone to its original form. A partially healed fracture shows a large callus, but cortical bone and the medullary cavity are not yet re-established. Original fracture lines may be faintly visible. However, a partially healed fracture may be strong enough to allow removal of the implants.

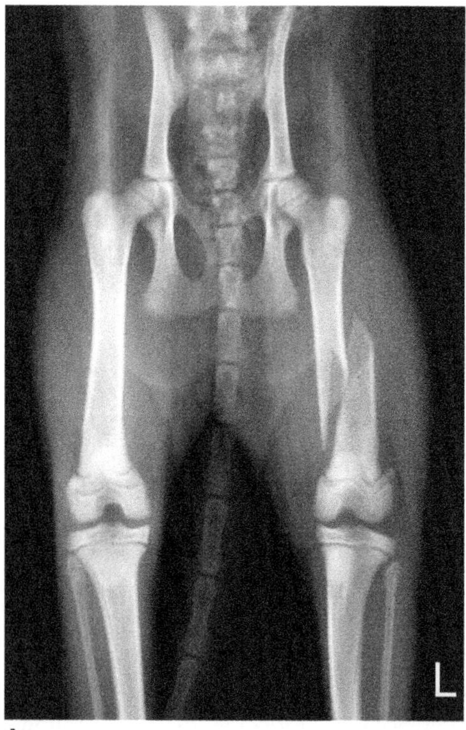

A

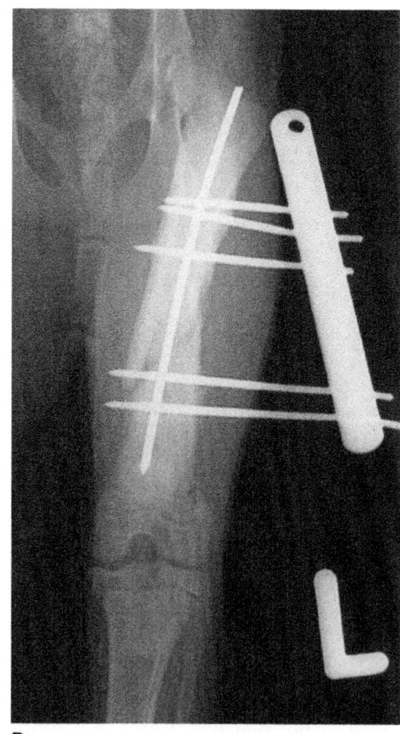

B

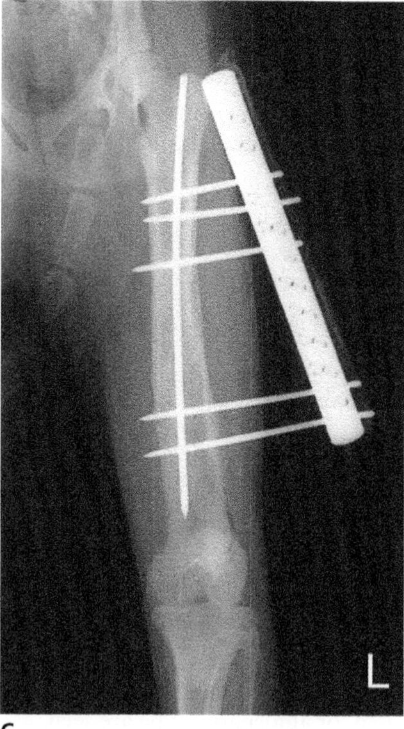

C

Figure 2-5 (**A**) Normal fracture healing in a 6-month-old cat with a closed spiral fracture of the left femoral diaphysis. (**B**) Three weeks after fixation with an intramedullary pin and external skeletal fixator, rounded ends of the fracture fragments are seen with external and internal callus formation at a slight distance from the fracture gap. The fixation devices appear stable. (**C**) Six weeks after reduction, the fracture line has disappeared due to bridging callus. Cortical bone is formed and the medullary cavity is re-established. The fracture has healed completely.

Estimation of healing time and removal of implants should be determined on an individual basis and according to the type of stabilization and fracture healing. Radiographic information is combined with clinical and historical information to determine clinical union, which is the time point in fracture healing at which fixation devices can be removed.

Complications of fracture healing

Implant loosening and failure. Implant loosening or failure may occur as a result of insufficient fixation, infection, and thermonecrosis due to high-speed drilling or recurrent injury. Radiographs should be checked for movement of implants, which would suggest loosening, and bending or breakage of orthopedic devices. Fracture alignment may be altered, resulting in instability. Initially, no bone abnormalities may be detected radiographically. Later, implants may be surrounded by a radiolucent zone, and by excessive or aggressive types of periosteal reaction.

Malunion. A malunion is a healed fracture that has not resumed its original form because of bone shortening, angulation, rotation, or synostosis. The fracture-healing process itself is normal.

Delayed union. Fractures that do not heal at the predicted rate are termed delayed unions (Fig. 2-6). Delayed unions may be caused by excessive distraction of fragments, instability, insufficient vascularity, or infection. Age of the patient and fracture type and site may play a role. Healing is slow but should eventually occur. Radiographically, fracture lines persist and callus formation may be either reduced (atrophic) or excessive (hypertrophic) but without bridging the fracture gap. If the underlying cause is severe and goes uncorrected a delayed union may progress to a non-union.

Non-union. Fractures with fragment ends that have not united are classed as non-unions. Hypertrophic non-unions are viable, indicating an adequate blood supply to the fracture and the most common reason for its development is instability/motion at the fracture site. Radiographically, non-bridging callus with a well-defined fracture gap and sclerotic, rounded fracture ends with a closed medullary cavity are seen. Bone ends may form a pseudoarthrosis (false joint). Atrophic non-unions (Fig. 2-7) have osteopenic tapered pencil-like fragment ends with a sclerotic marrow cavity, well-defined fracture gap, and minimal to no callus. This may be a sequel to avascular fracture sites, excessive motion, infection, or interposed tissue. Other factors significantly associated with development of a non-union in the cat include age, body weight, affected bone, fracture type, and fixation type. The tibia and proximal ulna appear to be the most common sites for non-unions (13).

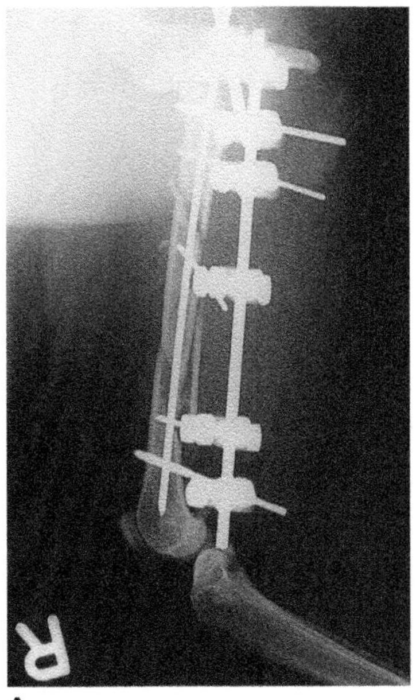

A

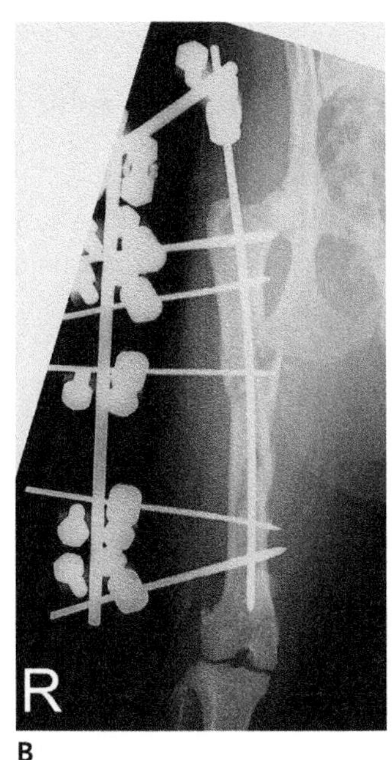

B

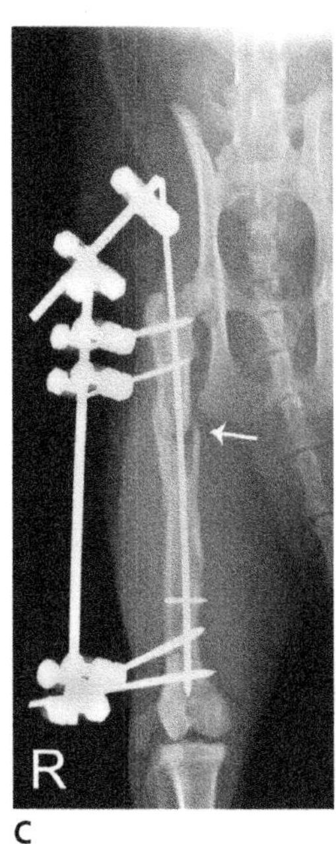

C

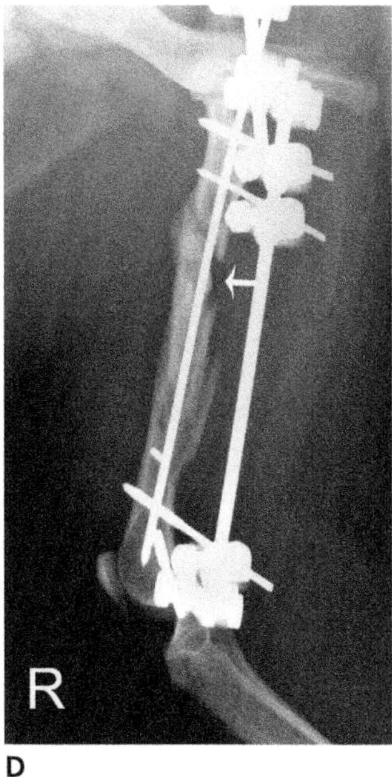

D

Figure 2-6 Delayed healing in a closed comminuted diaphyseal femoral fracture (**A**, **B**, postoperative radiographs). Four months after fracture fixation (**C**, **D**), partial healing has occurred distally. Proximally, the fracture line is still well visible; callus formation is seen on the cranial and lateral aspect of the fracture but is missing caudally and medially (arrows). Implants were stable, and the fracture went on to heal.

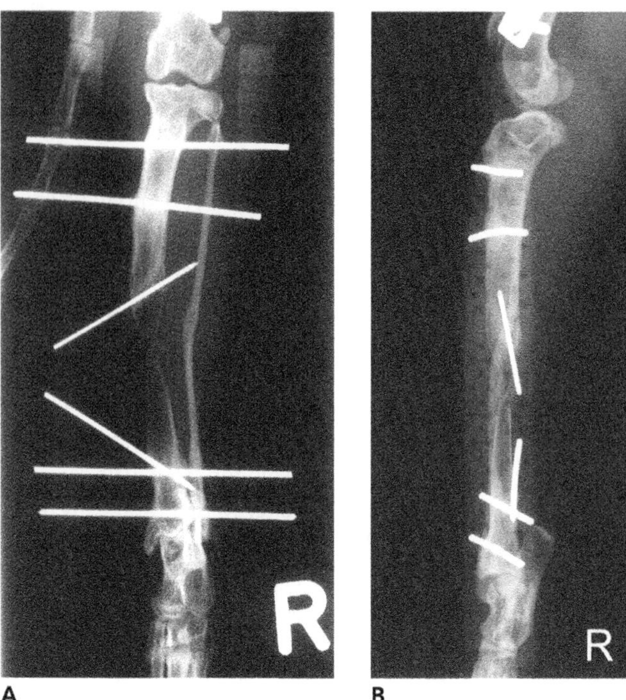

Figure 2-7 Atrophic non-union in an open oblique diaphyseal fracture of the tibia 8 months after fracture repair (**A**, **B**): osteopenic tapered fragment ends with a closed medullary cavity, and a well-defined fracture gap without callus is seen.

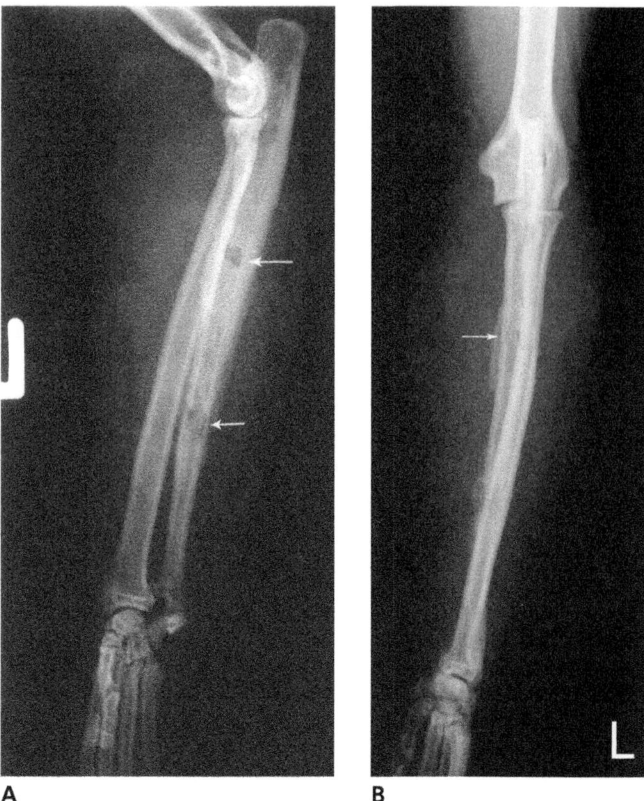

Figure 2-8 Osteomyelitis of the diaphysis of the ulna due to an infection with *Pasteurella* species after a cat bite (**A**, **B**): massive soft-tissue swelling is seen with extensive spiculated periosteal reaction, and corticomedullary lysis and sclerosis. The two focal lytic areas of a few millimeters in diameter represent the initial bite holes (arrows).

Osteomyelitis. Osteomyelitis as a complication in bone healing is usually due to a combination of local contamination with bacteria, inadequate blood supply to the fracture site, and instability. Clinical signs of osteomyelitis usually appear before radiographic changes are noted (Chapter 13). Radiographically, soft-tissue swelling, subcutaneous emphysema, generalized periosteal reaction of the aggressive type, corticomedullary osteosclerosis combined with osteolysis, and sequestrum formation are seen (Fig. 2-8).

Sequestrum. A sequestrum is a dead cortical fragment. Radiographically, it is more radiopaque than normal cortical bone and typically the fragment ends are sharp due to absence of resorption. In cases with concurrent infection, the sequestrum may be surrounded by a radiolucent zone in the parent bone, which in turn is surrounded by a sclerotic zone (involucrum). Occasionally, a draining tract (cloaca) is evident. In cases with a sterile sequestrum, changes in the parent bone are usually absent.

Joint complications. Degenerative joint disease may follow an intra-articular fracture or a changed load due to malunion or physeal growth deformities.

2.1.5 Radiographic evaluation of joint injury and diseases

Joint injury may be suspected alone or in combination with trauma to adjacent bones and soft tissues.

Soft-tissue changes

Extracapsular and/or articular soft-tissue swellings may be identified; however, they cannot always be differentiated radiographically. Intra-articular or extracapsular hemorrhage or edema is possible in a patient with acute trauma. Other differential diagnoses of articular or extracapsular soft-tissue swelling in the cat include abscess or cellulitis (cat bite), septic arthritis, soft-tissue neoplasia or, very rarely and most commonly in the elbow joint, synovial cysts (14).

Structures with the same radiolucency as gas within the joint represent air influx, indicating an open joint in a patient with acute injury, or can be seen immediately post surgery.

Intra-articular fractures and subluxation/luxation

Intra-articular fractures cause a roughened, irregular or incongruent articular surface, depending on the location and fragment displacement. A fracture line extending into the joint is usually visible.

Collateral ligament and joint capsule sprains may cause subluxation or luxation of a joint. Depending on the degree of separation of the articular surfaces the term subluxation (partial) or luxation (complete) is used (Chapter 14). Instability of a joint may be diagnosed radiographically on normal projections; however, joints most commonly appear normal and stress views are necessary (Fig. 2-1).

Osteoarthritis

Osteoarthritis commonly develops secondary to an intra-articular fracture or joint subluxation and luxation. Other acquired disorders and developmental diseases may also cause osteoarthritis in the cat. Primary osteoarthritis may also be found (Chapter 5). In general, radiographic signs include articular soft-tissue swelling, subchondral sclerosis, irregular articular surfaces, and development of osteophytes and enthesophytes (new bone formation at the insertion site of the capsule and ligaments), depending on the progression of the disease.

Septic arthritis

Septic arthritis may follow open joint injury or may represent a sequela to a surgical procedure. Radiographically, articular soft-tissue swelling is seen first. Later, subchondral lysis with irregular articular surfaces or even collapse of the joint space is identified. Collapse of the joint is best assessed in weight-bearing images. Osteophytes and enthesophytes develop rapidly, and appear very irregular.

2.1.6 Myelography

Myelography is a positive contrast procedure following the subarachnoid injection of iodinated contrast agent. Compressive lesions of the spinal cord and cauda equina as well as intramedullary swelling which may be caused by masses or myelomalacia can be identified. The procedure should only be performed by experienced clinicians, and if the possibility to proceed with surgery, depending on the results of myelography, exists. Survey radiographs should always precede myelography. Certain specific anatomic features of the feline spine have to be taken into account. Variations in the shape of the thoracic and abdominal spine are normal due to a higher flexibility. The epidural and the subarachnoid space in cats are small, with a relatively wide spinal cord. The spinal cord ends at the level of the sacrum.

Survey radiographs

Sedation or general anesthesia is required to reduce positional artifacts and motion. The area of interest should be placed parallel to the table top and in the center of the X-ray beam with adequate collimation. A small focal spot and exposure values similar to those for the appendicular skeleton should be used. Although the cat is a small animal, separate radiographs of the cervical, thoracic, thoracolumbar, and lumbar/lumbosacral regions should be made to reduce the artifacts caused by beam divergence at the film periphery. Studies of the spine include a laterolateral and a ventrodorsal view. Obliquity is prevented on the laterolateral view by using sponges to support the sternum, the midcervical, midlumbar, and skull regions and between the hind legs. For the ventrodorsal view of the spine and the pelvis, the cat may be placed in a trough. Additional views may be obtained in conjunction with myelography, where oblique ventrodorsal projections aid in evaluating localization and lateralization of a lesion.

Myelography

Myelography is always performed under aseptic conditions and general anesthesia. Non-ionic iodinated contrast media (monomers or dimers) are used. The dosage varies between 0.2 and 0.5 ml/kg body weight depending on the contrast agent (iodine concentration 200–300 mg/ml) and the study (regional versus full-spine myelography). A 22-gauge spinal needle with stylet should be used because of its short bevel, which is particularly important in the narrow subarachnoid space of the cat. The patient should never be moved while the needle is still in place.

For the investigation of cervical (C2–C7), caudal number (L4–L7) and lumbosacral lesions contrast medium is injected into the cerebellomedullary cistern through the atlanto-occipital space with the cat in lateral recumbency. The head is flexed ventrally and the needle is inserted on the midline just cranial to the center of a triangle formed by the external occipital protuberance and the cranial margins of the wings of the atlas. Advancement of the needle should be stopped frequently and the stylet removed to check for evidence of cerebrospinal fluid (CSF), to avoid inadvertent trauma to the cord. Penetration of the dura mater is usually felt as a slight popping sensation.

For the investigation of thoracolumbar, lumbar (L1–L4), and occasionally cranial cervical (C1–C2) lesions, contrast agent is injected into the dorsal or ventral subarachnoid space at the level of L6–L7, L5–L6, or occasionally L4–L5. The needle may be inserted in a median plane just cranial to the spinous process at a 90° angle with the cat in lateral recumbency. Alternatively, the needle may be inserted in a paramedian plane, from caudolateral to the spinous process and aiming cranioventrally at a 45° angle through the interarcuate space.

CSF may be collected before injection of the contrast agent. The latter should be done slowly and, when finished, the needle is withdrawn. Immediately afterwards, laterolateral, ventrodorsal, and oblique projections are made. Stress projections may be added if required. Flexion and extension as well as compression and distraction projections are used to assess dynamic instability and compressions. Stress views have to be taken with great care, or may be even contraindicated, with severe spinal compression or if spinal dislocation or fracture is suspected. The contrast media may be pooled to the region of interest by elevating or lowering the head or hindquarters.

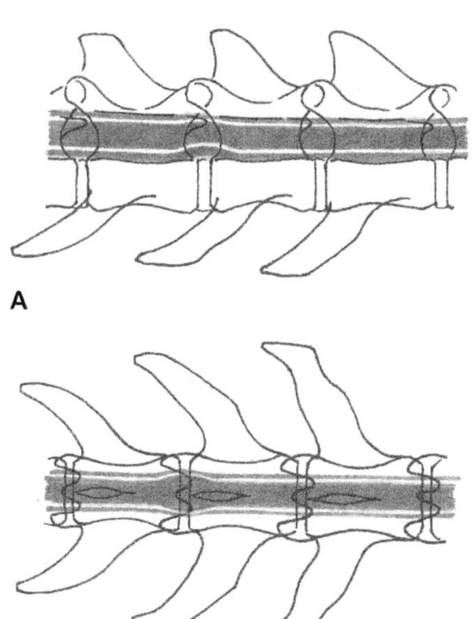

Figure 2-9 Schematic drawing of a ventral extradural lesion with myelography (lateral (**A**) and ventrodorsal (**B**) projection): there is displacement of the ventral contrast column away from the lesion in the lateral projection, whereas in the ventrodorsal projection, swelling of the spinal cord is seen with diverging thinned contrast columns.

Radiographic interpretation

Survey radiographs are evaluated for number, size, shape, alignment, and alterations to the radiopacity and margination of the vertebrae. Surrounding soft tissue and other bone structures should also be carefully assessed for signs of trauma, infection, or neoplasia. Radiographic signs of intervertebral disc disease include narrowing of the disc space, the dorsal intervertebral articular process joint space and the intervertebral foramen, extruded mineralized disc material, end-plate sclerosis, and spondylosis.

The clinician should be familiar with features of the normal myelogram, e.g., normal widening or thinning of the spinal cord and the contrast columns in certain locations. Common myelographic abnormalities include obstruction of contrast flow or changes in the size, shape, or location of the subarachnoid contrast medium columns and the spinal cord. Clinically significant subarachnoid filling defects are accompanied by thinning of the opposite contrast medium column or evidence of cord compression. Patterns are categorized into extramedullary (intradural or extradural) and intramedullary lesions. Extradural lesions are located outside the dura mater (Fig. 2-9). They cause thinning or absence of the contrast column and displacement away from the lesion in one projection, whereas in the second projection, perpendicular to the first, swelling of the spinal cord is seen with diverging thinned contrast columns. Differential diagnoses are disc protrusion, congenital or developmental malformations, ligament hypertrophy, hemorrhage, neoplasia, vertebral fracture or luxation. Intradural lesions (Fig. 2-10) are located within the subarachnoid space. Radiographically, the contrast column is widened focally with a filling defect that may resemble a "golf tee." In the orthogonal projection, the spinal cord may be widened and the contrast columns diverge, and are thinner. This pattern may be seen with primary or secondary neoplasia, hemorrhage, granuloma, or subarachnoid cysts. Intramedullary lesions (Fig. 2-11) are within the spinal cord. They produce widening of the spinal cord in both projections. The contrast columns may be thinned depending on the size of the lesion. Spinal cord neoplasia, edema, or hemorrhage following trauma or coagulopathy, and infectious or ischemic diseases may cause this myelographic pattern.

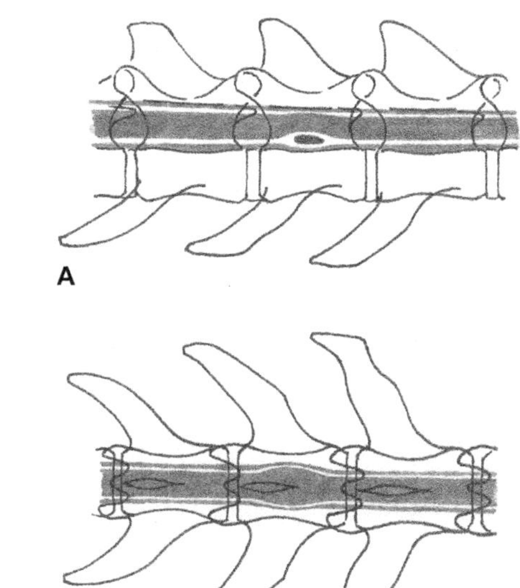

Figure 2-10 Schematic drawing of a ventral intradural lesion with myelography (lateral (**A**) and ventrodorsal (**B**) projection): in the lateral projection, the ventral contrast column is widened focally with a central filling defect that resembles a "golf tee" on both ends of the lesion. In the ventrodorsal projection, the spinal cord is widened and the contrast columns diverge and are thinner.

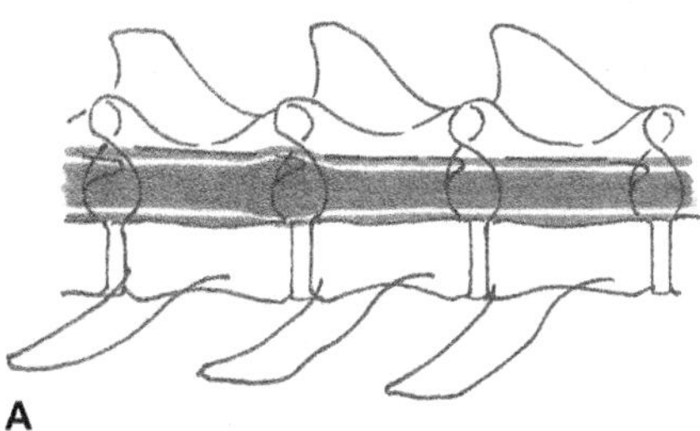

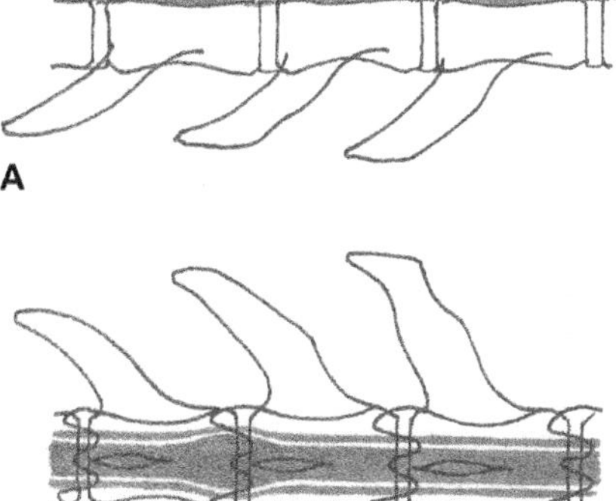

Figure 2-11 Schematic drawing of an intramedullary lesion with myelography (lateral (**A**) and ventrodorsal (**B**) projection): widening of the spinal cord is seen in both projections.

2.1.7 Ultrasonography

Ultrasound refers to sound waves of a high frequency, inaudible to humans. During their transmission through tissue, the ultrasound waves emitted by the ultrasound probe undergo absorption, reflection, scattering, and refraction at the interfaces between two different tissues. The reflected waves, called echo, are then received by the ultrasound probe and are used to produce the ultrasonographic image. The size, shape, location, and architecture of an organ can be assessed with ultrasonography. At bone surfaces, most waves are reflected or absorbed and little sound is available to image deeper structures; therefore, only the bone surface can be examined ultrasonographically. Although MRI is considered the method of choice to image diseases of soft tissue, ultrasonography is more accessible and cost-effective and often provides equivalent information. A thorough physical examination is required so that ultrasonographic findings may be correlated with the clinical information.

To examine superficial structures in the cat, e.g., the musculoskeletal apparatus, linear probes with high frequencies in the range of 8–15 MHz are used because they provide higher resolution in the near field. A standoff may be helpful. Muscular diseases, abscesses, hematomas, seromas, lipomas, cellulites, and neoplasia may be assessed. Foreign bodies in soft tissue may be identified. Tendons such as the calcaneal tendon (Fig. 2-12) can also be easily imaged ultrasonographically in the feline patient (15). Bicipital tenosynovitis was diagnosed in a cat using ultrasound, in combination with arthrography (16). However, ultrasonographic examination of most tendons and joints is limited in cats due to their small size. The surface of bones can be successfully examined for discrete changes like irregularities, discontinuities, periosteal reactions, fragments, and sequestra seen with trauma or infection. Every ultrasonographic evaluation of bone should be preceded by radiography.

2.1.8 Computed tomography

Similar to conventional radiography, the principle of CT is based on the absorption of X-rays by tissue. Whereas conventional radiography produces a summation image of a body region, CT as a cross-sectional imaging technique avoids superposition of adjacent structures by imaging a transverse slice of the patient in the range of 0.5–10 mm thickness. Thus, a series of two-dimensional images of a certain body region are produced. Three-dimensional images and images in different planes may be reconstructed on the basis of the digital data. In comparison to conventional radiography, contrast resolution of CT is higher. Within the five conventional radiopacities (gas, fat, soft tissue/fluid, bone, metal),

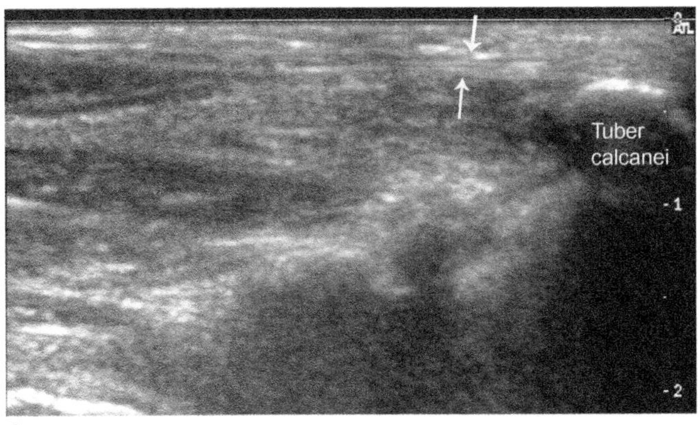

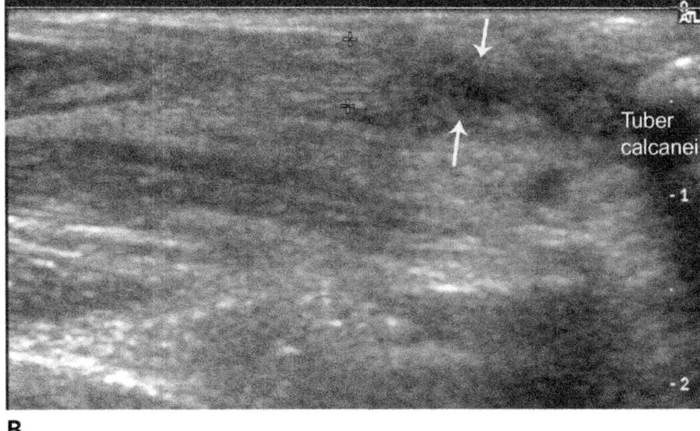

Figure 2-12 Longitudinal ultrasonographic images of a partial rupture of the right Achilles tendon in a cat: the superficial portion of the Achilles tendon (**A**) is intact (white arrows). The deeper medial portion (**B**) shows fiber alignment in the proximal part (calipers) but lacks longitudinal fibers in the distal part (white arrows). Instead, inhomogeneous hypoechoic tissue is seen in this region.

soft-tissue structures and fluid opacities may be further differentiated, e.g., muscles can be differentiated from tendons, and in the skull, the CSF differs from brain tissue and acute hemorrhage.

CT is more sensitive in detecting bone lysis or soft-tissue mineralization. This is of particular value for the assessment of neoplastic or infectious bone diseases (Fig. 2-13). In humans and animals with acute trauma in complex anatomic areas such as the head or spine, CT has been established as a standard method because of the advantage of being able to image fractures free of superimposition. Planning of surgical procedures or detection of small fragments or bone sequestra

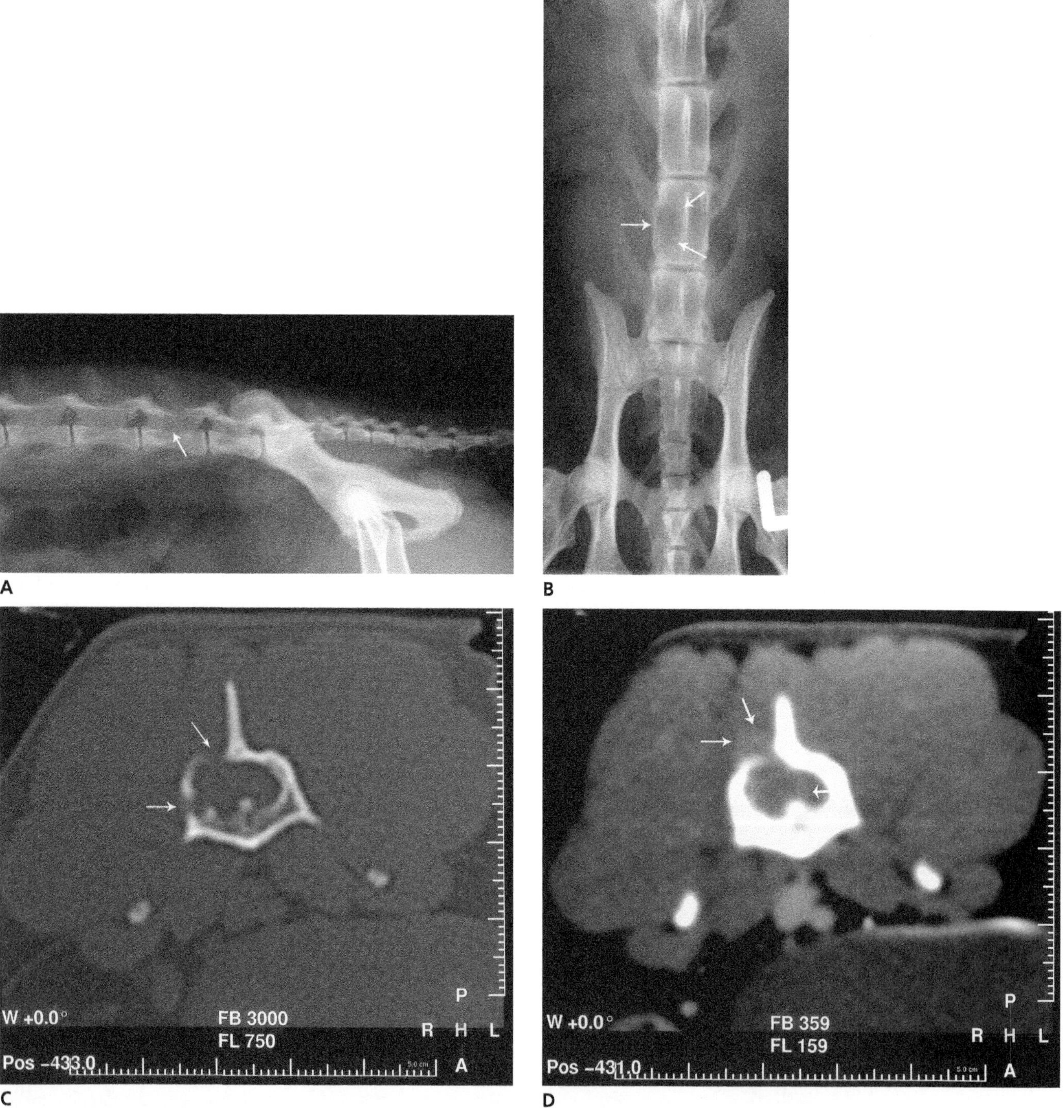

Figure 2-13 Osteosarcoma in the sixth lumbar vertebra: a lytic area (white arrows) is diagnosed in the right pedicle, which is well described in the ventrodorsal view (**B**) and less well delineable in the laterolateral view (**A**). On transverse computed tomography images (**C**, bone window), destruction of the right pedicle is well seen (white arrows) and the vertebral canal is widened. On postcontrast transverse images (**D**, soft-tissue window), a mildly enhancing soft-tissue mass is seen, occupying approximately 75% of the vertebral canal and expanding dorsally (white arrows).

is thus facilitated. In combination with myelography, CT aids in identifying compression of the spinal cord. For CT myelography a lower iodine concentration (approximately 100 mg/ml) of the agent is used, by diluting it with sterile saline. Newer CT technologies such as helical CT provide a dramatically increased spatial resolution, and with their increasing availability in veterinary medicine, new prospects may emerge.

2.1.9 Magnetic resonance imaging

With MRI, a patient is placed in a magnet and radiowaves are transmitted into the magnetic field. The transmitter is then turned off for a moment, and the patient re-emits the radiowaves, which are received and used for reconstruction of the image. The nuclei of hydrogen atoms in the magnetized tissue absorb and emit the radiofrequency energy. MRI is able to measure the hydrogen and protein content of tissue, and displays it as a shade of gray on the image. Like CT, MRI also represents a cross-sectional imaging technique. It avoids superimposition of adjacent structures by imaging a slice of the patient. In comparison to the radiographic techniques such as CT and conventional radiography, MRI provides excellent contrast resolution and is considered the imaging method of choice to examine soft tissue. MRI provides less bone detail because bone has a reduced signal due to its lower hydrogen density. Major indications for the use of MRI are for imaging diseases of the brain and spine, because definition between gray and white matter, CSF, spinal cord, epidural fat, and components of the intervertebral disc is possible. MRI of the appendicular skeleton in cats is limited due to their small size.

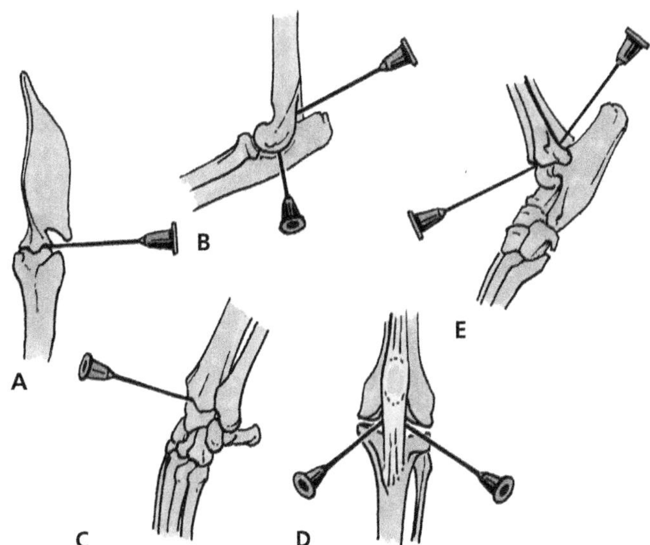

Figure 2-14 Recommended sites for arthrocentesis.
(**A**) Shoulder. The needle is inserted perpendicular to the skin surface slightly distal to the processus hamatus (acromion) of the scapula.
(**B**) Elbow. The needle can be introduced just medial to the lateral epicondyle and advanced along the olecranon into the olecranon fossa. Alternatively, the needle may be entered just caudolaterally to the condyle, while the leg is held in slight supination.
(**C**) Carpus. The needle is inserted into the radiocarpal joint from dorsally or dorsomedially while the joint is held in slight flexion.
(**D**) Stifle. The needle is inserted lateral to the patellar ligament and directed towards the lateral aspect of the medial femoral condyle through the infrapatellar fat pad. The same procedure can be performed from medial to the patellar ligament.
(**E**) Tarsus. The needle is inserted from dorsally into the talocrural joint in a slightly proximal direction. Digital pressure on the plantar joint sacs facilitates collection of synovial fluid. Alternatively, the lateroplantar joint space can be tapped by inserting the needle medially to the lateral malleolus with the joint in slight flexion.

2.2 Arthrocentesis and synovial fluid evaluation

Collection and laboratory evaluation of synovial fluid is an essential part of the diagnosis of arthropathies. The formation of abnormal synovial effusion can be initiated by cartilage damage and synovitis. Vasodilation in the subsynovial capillaries leads to increased vascular permeability and allows extravasation of fluid, protein, and inflammatory cells into the synovial fluid. Distinguishing the type and number of leukocytes can be used to differentiate between disease conditions.

2.2.1 Arthrocentesis

Synovial fluid can be obtained by needle arthrocentesis from all major joints of the limbs. Figure 2-14 shows the location for needle placement for arthrocentesis from the different joints. Only a small amount of synovial fluid is present in a normal feline joint. One drop to 0.25 ml can usually be retrieved from normal shoulder, stifle, and hip joints, and around 0.1 ml can be obtained from the carpal and tarsal joints (17). Joint effusion generally allows retrieval of sufficient synovial fluid for analysis. At least two, and preferably more joints should be tapped when investigating a case with possible polyarthritis.

Sedation or a short general anesthetic is necessary to perform the procedure in most cats. The hair is clipped over the region, and the skin is prepared aseptically as for surgery. Sterile gloves are worn. The joint is immobilized with one hand, and with the other hand a 22- or 25-gauge needle attached to a 2- or 3-ml syringe is inserted into the joint (17). Digital pressure on any joint distension opposite to the needle insertion site may help to place the needle inside the joint capsule. Once the needle is inside the joint cavity, gentle negative pressure is applied until some drops of synovial fluid have been obtained. If blood appears at the needle hub, the needle is retrieved, because contamination of the synovial fluid with blood alters the cell count. Slides are prepared immediately for cytological evaluation. If an adequate sample is obtained, the rest is placed in an ethylenediaminetetraacetic acid (EDTA) tube, which can be stored for 24 hours in the refrigerator. A sample for bacteriological culture is taken, and processed as described below.

2.2.2 Visual and cytological evaluation

The amount of synovial fluid obtained is noted, and the fluid is visually inspected. Normal synovial fluid is clear and colorless. Red-tinged fluid indicates hemorrhage due to trauma or inflammation, or iatrogenic contamination. Streaks of blood, rather than uniformly red or pink fluid, are observed with iatrogenic contamination. White or yellow turbid fluid is consistent with elevation of leukocytes due to inflammation or sepsis. Normal synovial fluid should form a 2–4-cm string due to its high viscosity.

A white blood cell (WBC) count below 3000 cells/µl, with more than 90% mononuclear cells, is considered normal in most laboratories (18). Synovial fluid obtained from healthy shoulder and stifle joints in cats contained 0–4535 red blood cells (mean 483), 2–1134 WBCs (mean 161), 0–39% neutrophils (mean 3.6%), and 61–100% mononuclear cells (mean 96.4%) (17). A positive correlation between body weight and WBC count was found. The findings suggest that cats have lower WBC counts compared to dogs, but with a similar cell distribution (17).

A slight elevation in total cell count with a normal or only minimally elevated percentage of neutrophils is often present in degenerative joint disease (Table 2-1). The presence of red blood cells may indicate hemorrhage due to trauma or inflammation, or hemorrhage as a result of arthrocentesis. Neutrophils enter the synovial fluid across the synovial membrane during inflammatory processes, both immune-mediated and infectious, and are then found in larger than normal numbers. Synovial fluid containing markedly more than 10% neutrophils is consistent with an inflammatory arthropathy. It is not always possible to differentiate between immune-mediated and infectious causes of arthritis based on cytological findings alone (Table 2-1). Although total cell count and percentage of neutrophils tend to be higher in infectious arthritis, immune-mediated arthritis can cause marked elevation of both total cell count and neutrophil percentage. The presence of degenerative neutrophils and intracellular bacteria indicates infection, but their absence does not rule out infection. Therefore, the results of synovial fluid analysis should be interpreted in conjunction with clinical and radiographical features, and bacteriological culture results.

2.2.3 Bacteriology

Synovial fluid should be cultured for aerobic and anaerobic bacterial and *Mycoplasma* growth. Synovial fluid simply placed on an aerobic culturette yields about 50% false-negative cultures (19). Contact with room air should be avoided to allow anaerobic culturing. Incubating synovial fluid on a blood culture medium for 24 hours before reculturing yields significantly more reliable results compared to direct aerobic culturing of synovial fluid and synovial membrane biopsy (19). Accordingly, it is recommended to place the synovial fluid both on an aerobic culturette and on a blood culture medium. The aerobic samples are cultured immediately to obtain rapid results, and the blood culture is recultured after 24 hours to achieve better accuracy (19). If a laboratory is available in-house or nearby, the sample is best left in the sterile syringe, and sent immediately for further processing. If an inadequate amount of synovial fluid was obtained for culture, the syringe can be rinsed with bacterial culture medium before placing it on the blood culture medium (20).

2.3 Selected biopsy techniques

Fine-needle aspiration or biopsies in the orthopedic patient are most commonly conducted for investigation of masses, soft-tissue swelling, or bony lesions. Cytology is generally used to differentiate inflammatory or infectious processes from neoplasia. Histopathological examination of biopsy

Fluid characteristics	Degenerative joint disease	Immune-mediated arthritis	Infectious arthritis (bacterial)
Viscosity	Normal to reduced	Reduced	Reduced
Clarity	Clear	Hazy to cloudy	Cloudy to opaque
Leukocyte count	<5000 cells/µl	4000–700 000 cells/µl	15 000–267 000 cells/µl
Percentage of neutrophils	<10%	25–99%	77–99%
			Degenerated neutrophils
			Intracellular bacteria

Table 2-1. Characteristics of synovial fluid in degenerative joint disease, and immune-mediated and infectious arthritis (18, 25)

samples is often a more sensitive diagnostic method, and is used if cytology was unrewarding. Histopathology is also needed to diagnose and classify tumors to determine treatment options and prognosis.

2.3.1 Fine-needle aspiration

Fine-needle aspiration and subsequent cytological examination is an easy-to-perform and non-invasive tool in the diagnosis of soft-tissue masses and swellings. Fine-needle aspiration of bone lesions is also possible in the presence of cortical lysis. Only loose cells are obtained through the needle, in contrast to a biopsy specimen. Depending on tumor type, a definitive diagnosis might not be possible. At the least, cytology often allows differentiation between inflammatory or infectious, and neoplastic processes.

Sedation or anesthesia is not usually necessary for fine-needle aspiration of superficial masses, and the skin is only prepared with an alcohol swab. Fine-needle aspiration of bone lesions requires sedation or even general anesthesia, and aseptic preparation of the overlying skin.

Two techniques can be used: the needle-off and the needle-on technique (21). The needle-off technique is preferred for vascular and small lesions, because it reduces the risk of blood contamination. It is described in Figure 2-15. For the needle-on technique, the needle is advanced into the tissue and suction is applied simultaneously with a syringe attached to the needle. The negative pressure helps to retrieve cells from tissues that do not exfoliate well. Suction is stopped and negative pressure released before the needle is withdrawn from the tissue. The needle is then temporarily removed from the syringe, the syringe filled with air, the needle replaced, and the cells in the needle are expelled on to glass slides.

Either a conventional smear technique or a squash technique for viscous material is used to prepare the glass slide for cytological examination. Inflammatory processes can normally be diagnosed, and based on the percentage of neutrophils versus mononuclear cells, the inflammation can be classified into acute, chronic active, and chronic or granulomatous (21). Diagnosis of neoplasia is made on nuclear, cytoplasmic, and structural characteristics (21). Tissue hyperplasia is often difficult to differentiate from neoplasia. Biopsies and histopathological examination are indicated when accuracy of the cytological diagnosis is questionable, and when the type of tumor necessitates histopathological grading for prognosis and treatment plan.

2.3.2 Bone biopsy

Bone biopsies are indicated in the presence of most lytic and/or proliferative bone lesions. Histopathological examination of the specimen usually allows differentiation between inflammatory and neoplastic processes, and diagnosis of tumor type. Prognosis and treatment plan depend largely on tumor type. The Jamshidi biopsy needle (Fig. 2-16) is better suited for cats when compared to Michel's trephine due to its smaller core diameter. Jamshidi needle biopsies had an accuracy rate of 92% for detecting neoplasia versus other disorders, and an accuracy rate of 82% for correctly diagnosing tumor subtype (22). A 14-gauge needle is used in cats (23). Bone biopsies are taken from the center of the lesion visible on radiographs, in order to avoid sampling the reactive bone on the periphery of the lesion (22). The skin incision and the biopsy tract are potentially subject to seeding by tumor cells.

A small skin incision is performed after clipping and surgical preparation of the biopsy field, and the Jamshidi biopsy needle is inserted with the stylet in place and advanced up to the bone surface. The stylet is then removed and the needle is further inserted into the bone with a corkscrew motion, hereby pressing a bone core into the needle. Penetration of the opposite cortex is avoided. Before removing the needle it is rotated 360° several times in the same direction, and/or gently rocked back and forth to break the base of the biopsy

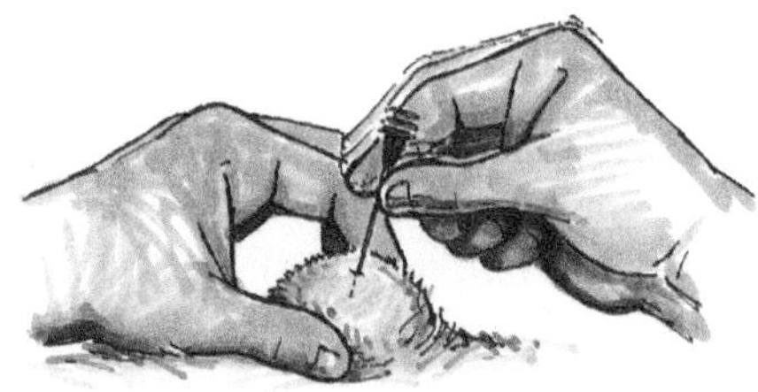

Figure 2-15 Fine-needle aspiration with the needle-off technique. The mass is held with one hand, and a 22- or 25-gauge needle is inserted into the mass with the other hand. The needle is then moved rapidly back and forth in different directions with a jabbing motion. The tip of the needle should not leave the deep margin of the mass in order to avoid retrieval of normal cells adjacent to the lesion, and to avoid seeding of tumor cells.

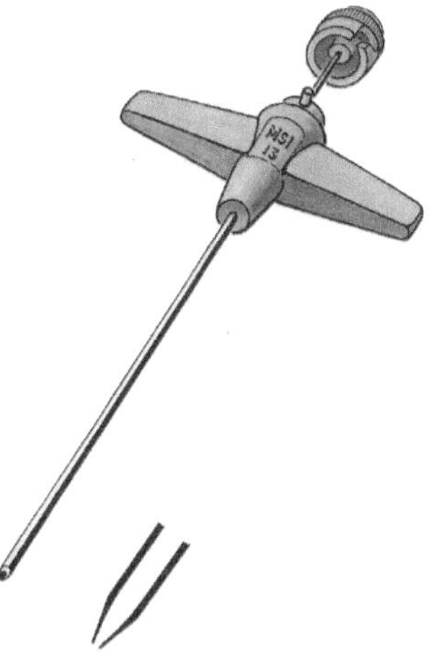

Figure 2-16 The Jamshidi bone biopsy needle has a tapered tip. The needle can therefore be withdrawn from the bone without losing the biopsy specimen. The piece of bone has to be retrograded with the help of the stylet through the tip of the needle for further processing.

specimen. The specimen is removed from the needle by pushing it out through the tip of the needle with the stylet or a small wire. The specimens should ideally have a length of at least 1 cm and if possible two or three biopsies are taken. The biopsy specimens are placed into 10% neutral buffered formalin for histopathological examination.

2.3.3 Synovial biopsy

A synovial biopsy and histopathological examination are indicated if synovial fluid cannot be obtained, if the cytological examination of the synovial fluid is not diagnostic, or if a tumor is suspected. Synovial biopsy is rarely pathognomonic of a disease, as the synovial membrane reacts similarly to many different types of injury (24). Histopathological changes associated with feline immune-mediated arthropathies have been described (25, 26). Inflammatory infiltrates, containing both mononuclear cells and neutrophils, are present during the first 1 or 2 months of the disease (26). The inflammation remains active as the disease progresses, but has more chronic characteristics, with mononuclear cells predominating over neutrophils. Granulation tissue and villous hypertrophy may also be present (26). Villous hypertrophy is a characteristic of rheumatoid arthritis in humans, and was described in conjunction with positive rheumatoid factor in cats (25). Histopathological examination of the joint capsule might also reveal infectious causes of arthritis or neoplasia.

The synovial biopsy can be obtained at the same locations as used for arthrocentesis or via arthroscopy (Chapter 25). Excisional biopsy is preferably performed in cats, as currently available biopsy needles are too large for the small feline joints. Excisional biopsy also has the advantage that the joint can be explored and a selected piece of synovial membrane may be taken. The joint capsule is incised in a longitudinal direction to prevent iatrogenic injury to ligaments. A full-thickness piece of the joint capsule is removed with a number 11 scalpel blade, and the capsular incision is closed with sutures.

2.4 Neurodiagnostic procedures

Neurodiagnostic procedures performed in feline patients include myelography, analysis of the CSF, and electrodiagnostic tests. Myelography is described in the section on diagnostic imaging in this chapter (Section 2.1).

2.4.1 Analysis of cerebrospinal fluid

CSF is collected from a cerebellomedullary or lumbar puncture site with the cat under general anesthesia. Lumbar puncture may provide more information in animals with spinal cord disease as CSF flows caudally. For technique and positioning of the patient, see the section on myelography. The quantity of collected fluid should not exceed 1–1.5 ml in adult cats. CSF should be stored in a plastic container as leukocytes adhere to glass. The sample must be analyzed within 30 minutes to avoid degradation of cells. Macroscopic examination provides limited information, but if the sample has increased turbidity, an increased cell count may be expected. Clots of fibrin or foam indicate marked elevation of protein. Artificial contamination with blood is frequently observed, especially in lumbar taps. Hemorrhage caused by puncture produces a red tinge to the fluid that disappears as the fluid continues to flow. Centrifugation should leave a colorless fluid. If xanthochromia is observed after centrifugation the cause is usually previous subarachnoidal hemorrhage. Prolonged icterus can also result in xanthochromia.

Quantitative measurement of CSF protein provides accurate information. Elevated protein levels are observed in inflammatory, neoplastic, and degenerative conditions. A poison or toxic insult that affects permeability of the blood–brain barrier, a lesion obstructing CSF flow, and necrosis of brain tissue may result in a high protein concentration. In healthy individuals the protein concentration should not exceed 25 mg/dl in cisternal samples. Total protein content in lumbar taps is considered normal up to a concentration of 45 mg/dl.

Total and differential WBC counts are the most important part of a CSF examination. Normal feline CSF contains 0–5 mononuclear cells/μl in cisternal taps. Total cell count is significantly elevated in inflammatory diseases. Minor increases may be observed in neoplastic, necrotizing, hemorrhagic, ischemic, or traumatic diseases. The more meninges and ependyma that are involved in the pathology, the more cells are expected. If the lesion is purely intraparenchymal, total cell count may be normal. The results of a differential cell count may vary within diseases depending on localization, chronicity, and severity. Thus, its results are rarely specific. Exceptions to this rule include identification of neoplastic cells or infectious organisms in a CSF specimen. A predominance of neutrophils is found in bacterial infections. However, neutrophils are also found in acute viral infections such as feline infectious peritonitis, meningiomas, and after myelography. Mononuclear cells are frequently found in CSF of patients with viral or autoimmune diseases, in compressive, degenerative, or neoplastic conditions.

Measurement of antibodies such as feline infectious peritonitis or toxoplasmosis from CSF can contribute significantly to a diagnosis. Results of these tests should be compared to the serum antibody titer. False-positive results can occur when the blood–brain barrier is impaired as migrating B cells may produce antibodies intrathecally without presence of the antigen in the central nervous system.

2.4.2 Electrodiagnostic testing

Electrodiagnostic testing is a mainstay in the diagnostic work-up of animals with neuromuscular disorders (27). Results of these tests disclose the distribution of the disease and may localize the lesion to the muscles, neuromuscular junction, the myelin, or the axon. Accurate nerve and muscle biopsies may be obtained based upon electrodiagnostic results. Electromyography (EMG) and peripheral nerve conduction studies are the most routinely performed tests. Sensory nerve conduction studies, repetitive nerve stimulation, F-wave examination, and single-fiber EMG may be performed in more thorough investigations.

EMG in veterinary patients is performed under general anesthesia, and is restricted to the assessment of spontaneous activity of the resting muscle and insertional activity elicited by insertion of the recording electrodes. Abnormal EMG findings include fibrillation potentials, positive sharp waves, complex repetitive discharges, and myotonic potentials. These pathological activities have to be distinguished from physiological discharges, specifically insertional activity, miniature end-plate potentials, end-plate spikes, and motor unit action potentials. Each of the listed EMG phenomena is accompanied by characteristic noises, which aid the experienced examiner in the interpretation of the EMG findings. Abnormal EMG activity is the result of a lesion of nerves and/or muscles that alter the physiological properties of cell membranes. It is important to note that abnormalities are not detected before 4–5 days after denervation in cats and they only reach their maximal changes after 8–10 days. Further limitations include the inability to distinguish between neuro- and myopathy, to infer clinical signs and neuropathic deficits, and to infer the underlying pathophysiological process. Although rarely specific, EMG can provide useful information about reinnervation and disease progression and regression. A significant decrease in the density of spontaneous activity often indicates successful reinnervation. The same finding may also indicate fibrosis. EMG is clinically useful in distinguishing between denervation and disuse atrophy. It has a high degree of sensitivity in detecting peripheral axonal loss, even when 95% of the axons are still intact. Thus, peripheral neuropathies may be diagnosed before clinical features such as hyporeflexia become evident.

Motor nerve conduction studies evaluate the function of motor and mixed nerves of thoracic, pelvic, and some cranial nerves. The nerve is stimulated at two different sites and a recording electrode is placed in an appropriate muscle. The result is a compound muscle action potential (CMAP). A number of measurements are considered for evaluation of the motor component of a peripheral nerve, including analysis of latency, amplitude, duration, shape, and area of the CMAP and assessment of the conduction velocity. The major abnormalities associated with motor nerve conduction studies center around altered CMAP amplitudes and conduction velocities. In general, axonopathies result in a decrease of CMAP amplitude and demyelination results in a decrease of the conduction velocity. A slowed conduction velocity without a significant decrease in CMAP amplitude is most indicative of demyelination in cats with diabetic neuropathy. In normal nerves, the conduction velocity should not be less than 50 m/s. Age has a significant influence on conduction velocity. Adult values in felines are not reached before 3 months of age.

Supramaximal repetitive nerve stimulation (SRNS) uses the principles of motor nerve conduction by stimulation of a peripheral nerve with a series of impulses and analysis of the evoked CMAPs. It is useful in evaluation of neuromuscular junctionopathies such as congenital and acquired myasthenia gravis and botulism.

Sensory nerve conduction studies assess function in sensory and mixed peripheral nerves. Clinically, sensory nerve conduction studies are more difficult to interpret than the results of motor nerve conduction as sensory nerve action potentials (SNAPs) are more prone to artifacts and results may vary from patient to patient and even between sides within the same animal. Calculation of the sensory conduction velocity provides information about demyelination and SNAP amplitude may indicate sensory axonal disease. It is important to note that sensory fibers only degenerate with a lesion to the dorsal root ganglion. Avulsion of the preganglionic nerve root and spinal cord results in degeneration of the associated sensory nerve distal to the ganglion, because the cell bodies are still connected to their sensory axons. Postganglionic injuries to the sensory nerve affect conduction velocity substantially.

References and further reading

1. Farr RF, Allisy-Roberts PJ. Physics for medical imaging. Edinburgh: WB Saunders; 1996.
2. Lavin LM. Radiography in veterinary technology, 2nd edn. Philadelphia: WB Saunders; 1999.
3. Farrow CS, Green R, Shively M. Radiology of the cat. St. Louis: Mosby; 1994.
4. Waibl H, et al. Atlas of radiographic anatomy of the cat. Stuttgart: Parey; 2004.
5. Morgan JP. Radiology of small animal fracture management. Philadelphia: WB Saunders; 1995.
6. Morgan JP. Radiology of veterinary orthopedics. Features of diagnosis, 2nd edn. Napa, California: Venture Press; 1999.
7. Thrall DE. Textbook of veterinary diagnostic radiology, 4th edn. Philadelphia: WB Saunders; 2002.
8. Zulauf D, et al. Radiographic examination and outcome in consecutive feline trauma patients. Vet Comp Orthop Traumatol 2008;21:36–40.
9. Voss K, et al. Antebrachiocarpal luxation in a cat. Vet Comp Orthop Traumatol 2003;4:266–270.

10. Wood AKW, et al. Anatomic and radiographic appearance of a sesamoid bone in the tendon of origin of the supinator muscle of the cat. Am J Vet Res 1995;56:736–738.
11. Mahoney PN, Lamb CR. Articular, periarticular and juxta-articular calcified bodies in the dog and cat: a radiologic review. Vet Radiol Ultrasound 1996;37:3–19.
12. Langley-Hobbs SJ. Biology and radiological assessment of fracture healing. In Practice 2003;1:26–35.
13. Nolte DM, et al. Incidence of and predisposing factors for non-union of fractures involving the appendicular skeleton in cats: 18 cases (1998–2002). J Am Vet Med Assoc 2005;226:77–82.
14. Stead AC, et al. Synovial cysts in cats. J Small Anim Pract 1995;36:450–454.
15. Kramer M, et al. Ultrasonographic examination of injuries to the Achilles tendon in dogs and cats. J Small Anim Pract 2001;42:531–535.
16. Scharf G, et al. Glenoid dysplasia and bicipital tenosynovitis in a Maine coon cat. J Small Anim Pract 2004;45:515–520.
17. Pacchiana PD, et al. Absolute and relative cell counts for synovial fluid from clinically normal shoulder and stifle joints in cats. J Am Vet Med Assoc 2004;225:1866–1870.
18. MacWilliams PS, Friedrichs KR. Laboratory evaluation and interpretation of synovial fluid. Vet Clin North Am Small Anim Pract 2003;33:153–178.
19. Montgomery RD, et al. Comparison of aerobic culturette, synovial membrane biopsy, and blood culture medium in detection of canine bacterial arthritis. Vet Surg 1989;18:300–303.
20. Johnson AL, Hulse, DA. Diseases of the joints. In: Fossum TW (ed.) Small animal surgery, 2nd edn. St. Louis: Mosby; 2002: pp. 1023–1157.
21. Ogilvie GK, Moore AS. Clinical cytology and neoplasia. In: Ogilvie GK, Moore AS (eds) Feline oncology. Trenton: Veterinary Learning Systems; 2001: pp. 42–48.
22. Powers BE, et al. Jamshidi needle biopsy for diagnosis of bone lesions in small animals. J Am Vet Med Assoc 1988;193: 205–210.
23. Ogilvie GK, Moore AS. Bone marrow aspiration and biopsy. In: Ogilvie GK, Moore AS (eds) Feline oncology. Trenton: Veterinary Learning Systems; 2001: pp. 26–29.
24. Hardy RM, Wallace LJ. Arthrocentesis and synovial membrane biopsy. Vet Clin North Am 1974;4:449–462.
25. Bennett D, Nash AS. Feline immune-based polyarthritis: a study of thirty-one cases. J Small Anim Pract 1988;29:501–523.
26. Pedersen NC, et al. Feline chronic progressive polyarthritis. Am J Vet Res 1980;41:522–535.
27. Cuddon PA. Electrophysiology in neuromuscular disease. Vet Clin North Am Small Anim 2002;32:31–62.

Part 2

Musculoskeletal diseases

Musculoskeletal diseases unrelated to trauma are infrequently diagnosed in daily feline practice. Whereas some of the diseases occurring in cats are indeed very rare, others occur more often, and are probably underdiagnosed. Recent studies have shown a surprisingly high radiographic incidence of degenerative joint disease, hip dysplasia, and patellar luxation in cats. Clinical signs associated with musculoskeletal diseases in cats tend to be less pronounced and often differ from those described in dogs. Musculoskeletal disease in cats therefore may go unnoticed by the owners, or may be attributed to the normal aging processes. The veterinarian's awareness of feline musculoskeletal diseases might also not be high enough to diagnose the problems. Additionally, the orthopedic examination and the interpretation of pain responses can be challenging in some cats.

Musculoskeletal diseases affect bones, joints, and muscles. Diseases of bones, with the exception of neoplasia, are infrequent. They are usually caused by hereditary metabolic, nutritional, or endocrine diseases, and are generalized. Miscellaneous localized conditions of bone such as bone cysts and diseases of the femoral head and neck have been described. Joint diseases may be degenerative in origin, inherited or developmental, or inflammatory. In the broader sense, neuromuscular diseases and certain conditions of the footpads and nails can also be included in the term musculoskeletal disease, as they may mimic orthopedic conditions by causing lameness and dysfunction. They are also covered in the following chapters.

3 Hereditary and congenital musculoskeletal diseases

M. Hubler, S. Arnold, S.J. Langley-Hobbs

Hereditary and congenital diseases of the musculoskeletal system usually cause clinical signs within days to months after birth, and therefore should be considered in the younger cat and kitten. This chapter covers hereditary metabolic diseases and congenital malformations of the skeletal system.

3.1 Hereditary metabolic diseases of the musculoskeletal system

Hereditary metabolic diseases of the musculoskeletal system include storage diseases, osteogenesis imperfecta, osteochondrodysplasia of Scottish Fold cats, congenital hypothyroidism, and hereditary rickets.

3.1.1 Storage diseases

Lysosomal storage diseases are rare disorders, mostly inherited in a simple autosomal-recessive pattern. They are caused by deficiency of one or more enzymes in the lysosomes of cells, or by deficiency of an activating enzyme or cofactor necessary for enzyme activity. The physiological catabolism of many macromolecules, in particular lipids, mucopolysaccharides (glycosaminoglycans, GAGs), glycogen, and glycoproteins, takes place within the lysosomes. This process is dependent upon the function and concentration of many enzymes and their corresponding cofactors. The failure of one step within the metabolic cascade results in the lysosomal storage of substrates of the deficient enzyme. Exceptions are chylomicronemia and glycogen storage disease type II and type IV, in which the glycan molecules accumulate within the cytoplasm. The various disorders are named after the accumulated substrate or the deficient enzyme or protein, as well as eponyms. In most storage diseases the macromolecules themselves are non-toxic, but the gradually increasing deposits interfere with normal cellular function and architecture and, in turn, cause the chronic progressive diseases.

There is a functional deficiency of a single enzyme in the majority of storage diseases (e.g., mucopolysaccharidosis (MPS) type I, VI, and VII, alpha-mannosidosis). Other storage diseases are caused by missing cofactors (e.g., GM1 and GM2 gangliosidosis) or deficiency of one of the enzymes responsible for targeting various enzymes to the lysosomes (e.g., I-cell disease).

Thirteen storage diseases have been described in cats. All have a common chronic progressive course, but there are considerable variations in the clinical signs. While cats with either MPS or I-cell disease mainly exhibit skeletal changes such as variable facial dysmorphism, the signs are mainly neurological in others. In some storage diseases, granules are seen within certain white blood cells. The presence of storage vacuoles within neutrophils is common for MPS and within lymphocytes for gangliosidosis GM2.

In the following section only the storage diseases with skeletal changes (Table 3-1) are included. These are alpha-mannosidosis, MPS type I, VI, and VII and mucolipidosis type II.

Alpha-mannosidosis

Alpha-mannosidosis is a chronic progressive disorder with a wide spectrum of clinical severity (1). Severe cerebellar dysfunction is a predominant feature common to all cases. The deficiency was associated with stillbirths and neonatal death in Persian cats, with no kitten surviving to 6 months of age (2). Clinical findings included hepatomegaly, corneal changes, and calvarial abnormalities. Neurological examination showed cerebellar signs (e.g., intention tremor, ataxia, and dysmetria). Other findings included bizarre behavior, dementia, apathy, and a diminished response to stimuli.

In a domestic short-haired kitten with alpha-mannosidosis, the presenting problem, at 4 months of age, was deformation of the forelimbs (3). The animal was represented to the veterinarian at 7 months of age because of a progressive loss of balance. Findings just before euthanasia at 9 months of age included hepatomegaly, lymph node enlargement, and radiographic abnormalities of the spine and long bones. The vertebrae had a moth-eaten appearance, which was especially noticeable in the lumbar region. The cortices of the long bones were thin with an uneven appearance. Ocular abnormalities included suture line cataracts and tapetal changes. Neurological findings included an intention tremor, ataxia, delayed righting reaction, and sluggish triceps and patellar reflexes.

The clinical course for a litter of domestic long-haired kittens was similar to the domestic short-haired kitten, but clinical signs were generally milder with a slower progression (1). Ataxia was the first abnormality observed. There were

Disease	Enzyme defect	Breed	Age at presentation	Presenting clinical signs	References
α-Mannosidosis	α-Mannosidase	Persian, DSH, DLH	2–4 months 6–12 months	Deformities of the limbs (Persian and DSH), generalized tremors, ataxia, head tremors, spastic paraplegia, opisthotonus	Vandevelde et al. (1982) (2) Blakemore 1986 (3) Cummings et al. (1988) (1)
Mucopolysaccharidosis I	α-L-iduronidase	Siam, DSH	4–12 months	Deformed skull, crouched gait, wheelbarrow posture, respiratory tract infection, corneal clouding	Thrall 2001 (4) Haskins et al. (2002) (5)
Mucopolysaccharidosis VI	Arylsulfatase B	Siam DSH	4–9 months	Dwarfism, deformed skull, abnormal gait, corneal clouding, ataxia, paraparesis	Thrall 2001 (4) Haskins et al. (2002) (5)
Mucopolysaccharidosis VII	β-Glucuronidase	DSH	2 months	Dwarfism, deformed skull, enlarged paws, deformed legs, abnormal gait, corneal clouding, ataxia, paraparesis	Gitzelmann et al. (1994) (6) Haskins et al. (2002) (5)
Mucolipidosis II I-cell disease	*N*-acetylglucosamine-1-phosphotransferase	DSH	At birth	Dwarfism, facial dysmorphismus, front-leg deformities (varus or valgus carpi)	Hubler 1996 (7) Mazrier et al. (2003) (8)

Table 3-1. Feline storage diseases causing skeletal changes
DSH, domestic short-hair; DLH, domestic long-hair.

	MPS I	MPS VI	MPS VII	ML II
Clinical feature				
Dwarfism	–	+	+	+
Large paws	–	+	+	+
Facial dysmorphism	+	+	+	+
Small ears	+	+	+	+
Corneal clouding	+	+	+	–
Retinal atrophy	–	+ (25%)	–	+
Thickened eyelid (drooping eyes)	–	(+)	–	+
Thickened skin	+ (neck)	+ (neck, head)	+ (paws)	+ (generalized)
Hepatomegaly	+	–	+	–
Gait abnormalities (hindlimbs)	+	+	+	+
Neurological deficits	+ (later stages)	+ (25%) (hindlimb paresis)	+	+
Laboratory findings				
Toluidine blue spot test for glycosaminoglycans	+	+	+	–
Decreased enzyme activity in peripheral leukocytes	+	+	+ (no activity)	+
Decreased enzyme activity in cultured fibroblasts	+	+ (no activity)	+	+ (no activity)
Light microscopy				
Excessive granulation in peripheral neutrophils	–	+	+	–
Electron microscopy				
Membrane-bound inclusions in peripheral leukocytes	+	+	+	–

*Severe form, genotype L476P/L476P.

Table 3-2. Clinical features and laboratory findings of mucopolysaccharidosis (MPS) type I, VI*, and VII and mucolipidosis (ML) type II (7)

no skeletal abnormalities, ocular abnormalities, or hepatomegaly as reported in the Persians and domestic short-haired kitten.

Mucopolysaccharidoses type I, VI, and VII and mucolipidosis type II

The MPS are characterized by the accumulation of GAGs, resulting from the impaired function of one of 11 enzymes required for normal GAG degradation. With the exception of the central nervous system, and cartilage and bone, the pathophysiology of these lysosomal storage disorders is predominantly related to increases in cell, tissue, and organ size. For example, in MPS the storage of GAGs within the cells of the heart valves causes these normally fusiform cells to become rounded. This change in turn causes valve leaflet and chordae tendinae to thicken, interfering with normal cardiac function and producing valvular stenosis, often with regurgitation (5).

In contrast, mucolipidosis type II (I-cell disease) results from a defect of one of the enzymes responsible for the post-translational phosphorylation of lysosomal hydrolases. The phosphorylation is necessary for targeting the enzymes (hydrolases) to the lysosomes. Thus, little enzyme reaches the lysosome, and large amounts are secreted extracellularly into the plasma. As a consequence, various macromolecules, not only GAGs as in MPS, accumulate in the lysosomes. These lysosomes are described as cellular inclusion bodies, leading to the term I-cell disease.

Storage of GAGs in MPS or variable macromolecules in mucolipidosis type II results in features common to most affected cats (Table 3-2). The radiographic findings of the

Radiography	MPS I	MPS VI	MPS VII	ML II
Pectus excavatum	+	+	+	–
Deformed vertebrae	+	+	+	+
Fusion of the cervical vertebrae	+	+	–	+
Bilateral coxofemoral subluxation	+	+	+	+
Shallow acetabulum and femoral head dysplasia	+	+	+	+
Epiphyseal dysplasia of the long bones	–	+	+	(+)

+, present; –, absent; (+), mild changes.
*Severe form, genotype L476P/ L476P.

Table 3-3. Radiographic findings of the skeleton in mucopolysaccharidosis (MPS) type I, VI*, VII, and mucolipidosis (ML) type II (7)

skeleton are summarized in Table 3-3. MPS VI is one of the most prevalent diseases in cats and is commonly found in those of Siamese ancestry. Two different mutations in the same gene, L476P and D520N, can result in three different phenotypes. The L476P mutation, when homozygous, results in a severe phenotype. The D520N mutation, when homozygous, has little clinical consequence and affected cats are most likely regarded as clinically normal. Investigations of experimental cat colonies revealed that only 1 of 18 cats homozygous for the D520N had mild degenerative joint disease of the shoulder (9). The compound form (L476P/D520N) results in cats that are normal in size and appearance. However, they are characterized by mild to severe degenerative joint disease of the shoulder (64% of the genotype) and stifle (20% of the genotype) (9). In cats having the genotype D520N/D520N or L476P/D520N, the only evidence of storage disease is the presence of neutrophil inclusion bodies.

The age at disease onset is variable and depends upon the severity of the underlying defect, but is usually before adulthood. It is progressive, with many animals surviving months or years. One, or a combination, of the following clinical signs may be indicative of a storage disease: dwarfism, facial dysmorphism, corneal clouding, deformity of the limbs, and neurological signs, especially progressive cerebellar deficits (7) (Fig. 3-1). Inclusion bodies in granulocytes, monocytes, or vacuolization of lymphocytes may be present on a blood smear. Organomegaly and skeletal deformities and/or degenerative joint disease may be demonstrated on radiographs (Figs 3-2 and 3-3).

All cats with MPS have a positive toluidine blue test that demonstrates excessive excretion of urinary GAGs (Table 3-2). In contrast to MPS, cats with I-cell disease do not excrete GAGs in the urine (Table 3-2). Screening tests for storage diseases are suitable for the localization of the biochemical defect, but are not specific for a single enzyme defect. In lysosomal storage diseases, simple urine spot-on tests are available for MPS (toluidine blue) and carbohydrates (Clinitest, Ketostix), as well as a one-dimensional paper chromatography for amino acids, organic acids, and carbohydrates. The final diagnosis of a specific enzyme defect, for example lack of a particular lysosomal hydrolase in the plasma or lack of activity of an enzyme in leukocytes or cultured fibroblasts from biopsies, is only performed in specialized laboratories.

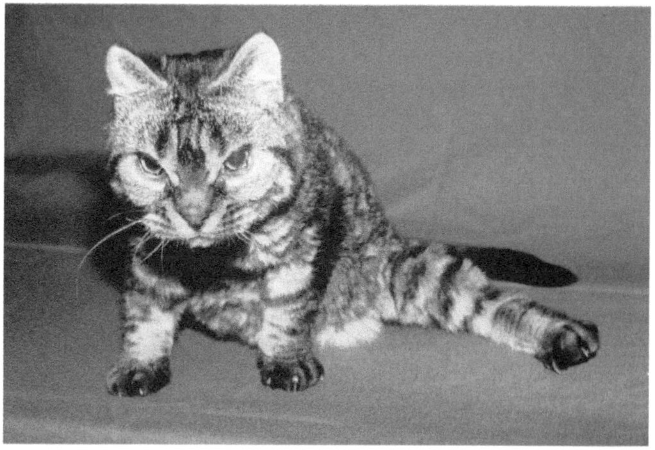

Figure 3-1. A cat with mucolipidosis type II. Note the broad flat face with hypertelorismus, frontal bossing, small ears, markedly thickened eyelids, and the large paws in relation to the body. (Reproduced from Hubler M, Haskins ME, Arnold S et al. Mucolipidosis type II in a domestic shorthair cat. J Small Animal Pract 1996;37:435–441, with permission from the *Journal of Small Animal Practice*.)

3.1.2 Osteogenesis imperfecta

Osteogenesis imperfecta is a disorder of bone that leads to spontaneous fractures. It is a well-known disease in humans where several types have been described. This heterogeneous syndrome can range from mild, subclinical disease to a lethal syndrome leading to stillbirth or neonatal death. In humans it has been shown that this group of diseases results from deranged metabolism of collagen. Depending on the collagen type and production, it may be accompanied by abnormal dentition, blue scleral hue, joint laxity, or growth deformities. The common features of all types of osteogenesis imperfecta

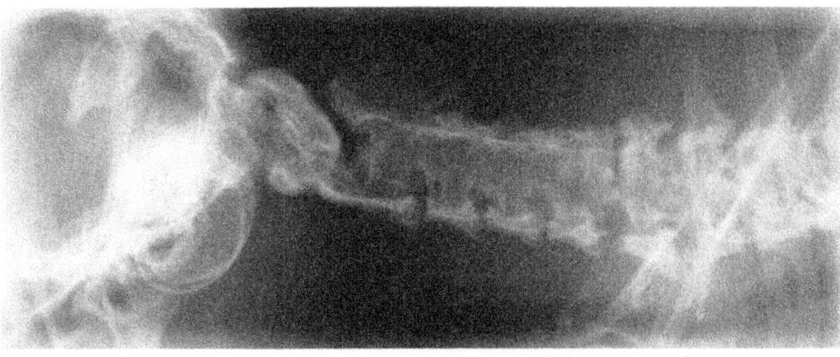

A

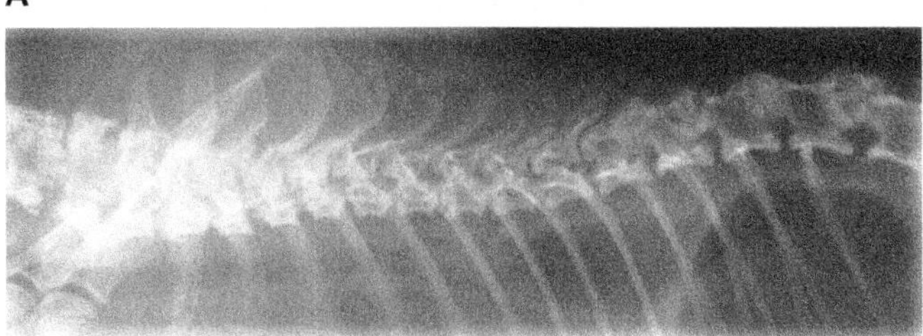

B

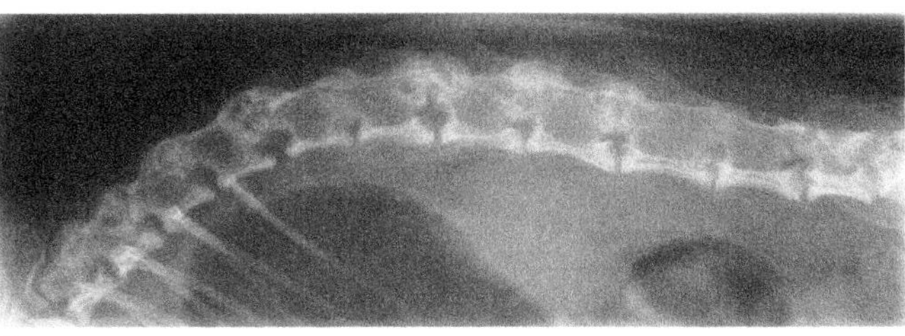

C

Figure 3-2. Lateral survey radiograph of the spinal column of a cat with mucolipidosis type II.
(**A**) Cervical spine: fusion of the vertebral arches and articular facets.
(**B**) Thoracic spine: small vertebral bodies and bowed, shortened spinous processes.
(**C**) Lumbar spine: fusion of the articular facets. (Reproduced from Hubler M, Haskins ME, Arnold S et al. Mucolipidosis type II in a domestic shorthair cat. J Small Animal Pract 1996;37:435–441, with permission from the *Journal of Small Animal Practice.*)

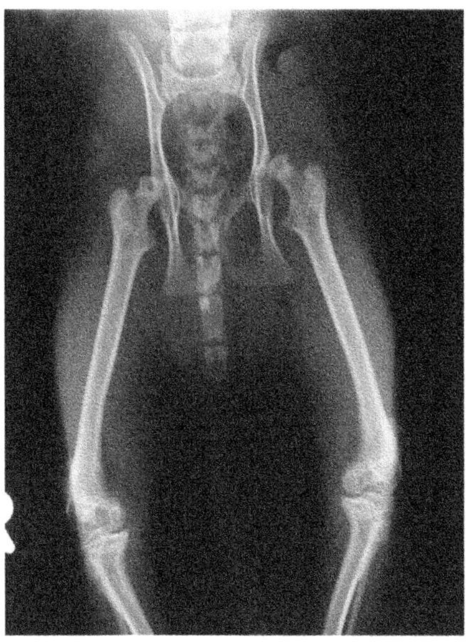

Figure 3-3. Ventrodorsal view of the pelvis and hindlimbs of the cat with mucolipidosis type II: bilateral hip dysplasia and hip luxation; mild malformation of the stifle joints. (Reproduced from Hubler M, Haskins ME, Arnold S et al. Mucolipidosis type II in a domestic shorthair cat. J Small Animal Pract 1996;37:435–441, with permission from the *Journal of Small Animal Practice.*)

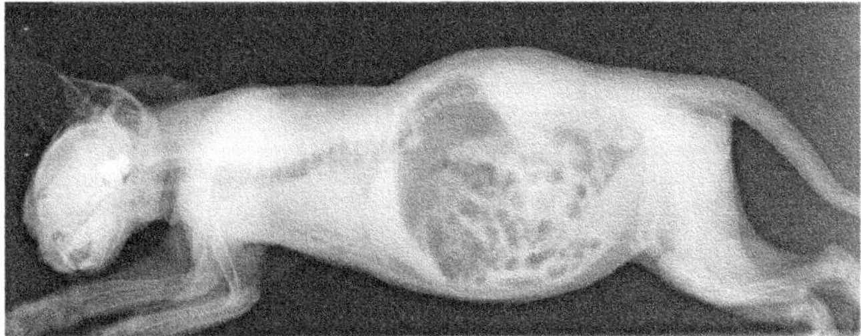

Figure 3-4. Laterolateral radiograph of a 4-month-old British Shorthair with osteogenesis imperfecta. Marked osteopenia of the skeleton is visible, except at the epiphyses and apophyses. Numerous spontaneous fractures of both femoral and tibial bones, the calcaneus, the pelvis, and the sixth lumbar vertebrae are present. Numerous bones including the thoracic spine are deformed.

are fragile bones that fracture spontaneously or in response to minimal trauma.

Osteogenesis imperfecta is a very rare disease in cats. Initially, feline nutritional secondary hyperparathyroidism was incorrectly referred to as a type of osteogenesis imperfecta. Gehring (10) reported on familial occurrences of osteogenesis imperfecta in Siamese and Persian cats, drawing the conclusion of a hereditary cause. This skeletal disease was recognized in young cats of both sexes, but was seen more often in males between 2 and 12 months of age. Affected cats showed lameness and pain in the pelvic region. They also walked very cautiously and avoided jumping on tables or other objects. If they did jump, even from a low height, they either did not walk at all afterwards, or only at a very slow and dragging pace, especially on their hindquarters. General condition of the cats, food intake, and digestion were normal until they suffered trauma. After a greenstick fracture, which appeared to be very painful, they had a reduced appetite, or become anorexic. They often avoided using the litter box for defecation, resulting in constipation. The regulation of defecation is very important, because in chronic cases intestinal paralysis may occur.

In cats with osteogenesis imperfecta, significant decrease in bone density can be documented radiographically. The compact substance of the bone is sometimes as thin as paper, especially in very young kittens, and the long bones often have kinks and deformities, resulting from greenstick fractures (Fig. 3-4). The pelvis has a lyrate shape on ventrodorsal radiographs, which is very typical in young animals. This malformation disappears with maturation of the skeleton. The long bones develop to a more or less normal density with increasing age and puberty. Deformities of the spine and thorax are often present, and may be so serious that, even after recovery from the skeletal disease, the life of the cat may be impaired (10).

In one report (10), affected cats did not respond to calcium or to vitamin therapies. The prevention of trauma is the most important measure, at least until the skeleton is sufficiently mineralized. A severe form of an osteogenesis imperfecta-like syndrome was reported in a 12-week-old kitten (11). In spite of prolonged cage rest there were multiple spontaneous fractures that subsequently necessitated euthanasia.

3.1.3 Osteochondrodysplasia in the Scottish Fold cat

The Scottish Fold is a purebred cat that originated in Scotland from the mating of a queen, affected with a spontaneous mutation, to local farm cats and British Shorthairs (12). Years earlier it was assumed that heterozygous cats have no skeletal changes, other than the folded ears, and that only homozygous cats develop progressive skeletal changes. Today it is accepted that the folded ear is an outward sign of generalized defective cartilage formation. The Rex Fold cat, which is a cross between the Devon Rex and Scottish Fold, is also affected by this osteochondrodysplasia (13). The mutation affects both bone growth and the formation of articular cartilage. Therefore, all Scottish Fold cats suffer from osteochondrodysplasia to some degree (14).

During growth, a disturbed osteochondral ossification leads to abnormal longitudinal growth of the skeleton, and in turn to shortened metatarsal and metacarpal bones and shorter and wider vertebrae of the proximal tail (14). In severe cases the extremities become deformed. The affected joints are abnormally stressed, resulting in degenerative joint disease and periarticular new bone formation at sites of ligamentous attachment to bone and joint capsules. This bone formation eventually leads to tarsometatarsal and intertarsal ankylosis (14).

There is considerable variation in the age of clinical manifestation, the severity of changes, and the rate of progression of osteochondrodysplasia in cats. Onset of clinical signs occurs between 5 months and 6 years of age (14). The affected cats show varying signs of skeletal disease, which may include lameness, reluctance to jump, or a stiff and stilted gait. Gait problems mainly originate from the tarsometatarsal and carpometacarpal joints, with the hind legs always being more severely affected. The joints have a reduced mobility and exostoses are often palpable. The tail can be shortened and thickened in the proximal area.

Radiographic changes are evident in all true joints of the spine and lower limbs. Splayed phalanges are commonly recognized. Affected joints have changes consistent with ankylosing polyarthropathy, with smoothly marginated and relatively homogeneous periosteal new bone proliferation around the carpal and tarsal bones. This bone growth leads to ankylosis in more severely affected joints. Signs of new bone formation may also be evident in soft tissues adjacent to joints, particularly at sites of ligamentous attachment to the bone. In cats with a short thick tail, the vertebrae are shorter and wider than normal and in severe cases an ossifying bridge may ankylose several caudal vertebrae (15).

Because the underlying disease is a genetic defect, therapy mainly aims at reducing the clinical signs and accompanying pain. Lameness and discomfort were reduced in some cats with the subcutaneous application of pentosan polysulfates or oral complex GAGs (14). Surgical approaches, which resolved lameness, included removal of the tarsal exostoses (16) or staged bilateral ostectomies and pantarsal arthrodesis of both hocks (17).

Recently, a novel therapeutic approach was described using palliative radiation therapy in a Scottish Fold cat (18). The cat had grossly thickened tarsi due to severe bilateral exostoses on the plantar aspect of the tarsus and metatarsus (Fig. 3-5). To decrease new bone formation, which eventually would lead to reactive inflammation and progressive ankylosing arthopathy, radiotherapy was initiated as a palliative treatment. The cat was irradiated in six fractions of 1.5 Gy each over 2 weeks. The cat experienced no side-effects of radiation therapy, and within 1 month it had no ambulatory problems and was again able to climb trees. No further signs of bony proliferation were visible on radiographs taken 28 months after therapy (18) (Fig. 3-6). Although the result of palliative radiotherapy was quite promising in this particular Scottish Fold cat, the continuation of this breed should be discouraged; the breed is already banned in the UK. Cats heterozygous for the folded-ear gene will also become affected by osteochondrodysplasia at some stage during their life (14).

3.1.4 Hypothyroidism

Congenital hypothyroidism leads to abnormal skeletal development. The effect of thyroid hormone on bone – more specifically on chondrocytes – is complex. Thyroid hormone displays a dual role in these tissues: it exerts anabolic as well as catabolic effects. While thyroid hormone promotes linear growth, it is equally important for bone remodeling, a process indispensable for normal bone maturation. During bone maturation, thyroid hormone promotes cartilage resorption, which is needed for normal bone formation. The catabolic activity of thyroid hormone may actually outstrip the ana-

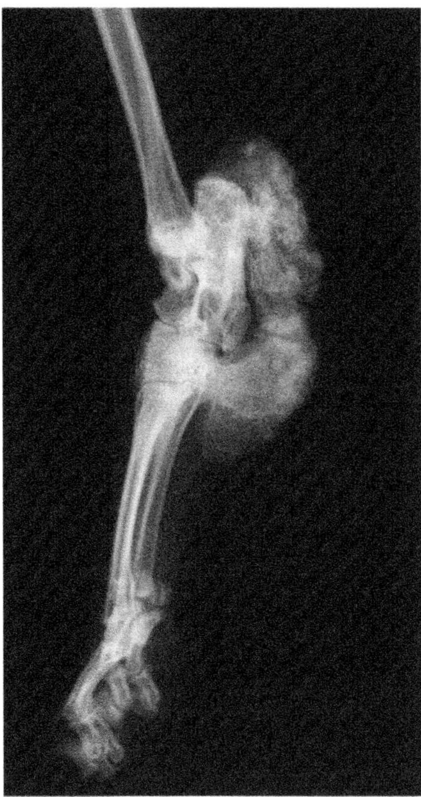

Figure 3-5. Mediolateral radiograph of the right tarsus of a cat with osteochondrodysplasia. New bone proliferation and osteophytes are present on the dorsal aspect of the tarsus, extending from the proximal talus to the proximal metatarsus. (Reproduced from Hubler M, Volkert M, Kaser-Hotz B et al. Palliative irradiation of Scottish Fold osteochondrodysplasia. Vet Radiol Ultrasound 2004;45:1–4, with permission from *Veterinary Radiology and Ultrasound*.)

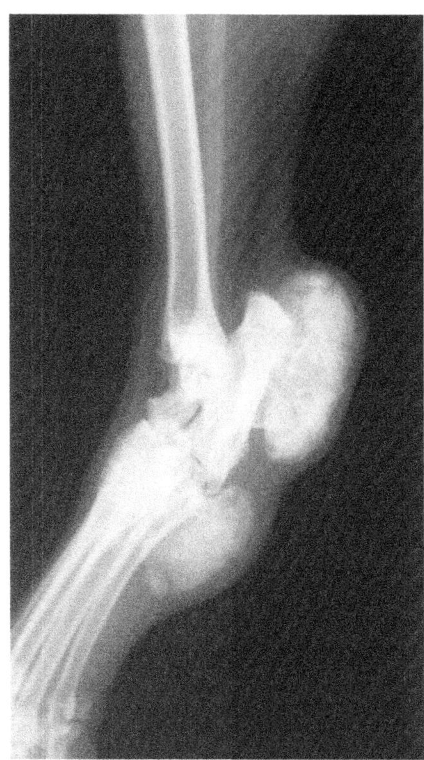

Figure 3-6. Radiograph of the right tarsus of the cat shown in Figure 3-5 28 months after radiation therapy. There are no signs of further bone proliferation. The exostoses have smooth surfaces and a less opaque, but more homogeneous, structure. The talocrural joint space is narrowed and the proximal intertarsal joint is nearly fused. Ankylosis is almost complete at the distal intertarsal and tarsometatarsal joints. (Reproduced from Hubler M, Volkert M, Kaser-Hotz B et al. Palliative irradiation of Scottish Fold osteochondrodysplasia. Vet Radiol Ultrasound 2004;45:1–4, with permission from *Veterinary Radiology and Ultrasound*.)

bolic activity it exerts on cartilage. Hypothyroidism during development, therefore, may cause both dwarfism and defective bone maturation. The diagnosis of congenital hypothyroidism is based on basal total thyroxine, total triiodothyronine and free thyroxine and the result of thyrotropin-releasing hormone and thyrotropin-stimulating hormone stimulation tests (19, 20).

Only a few sporadic cases of hypothyroidism in the cat are reported (21, 22). Familial occurrences are known in Japanese (19) and Abyssinian (20) cats. The first clinical sign of hypothyroidism is the stumpy shape, seen even before the retarded growth becomes obvious at the age of 3–4 weeks. Affected cats are characterized by a disproportionate dwarfism with a broad head, short neck and limbs, lethargy, mental dullness, juvenile hair coat, and hypothermia. Constipation was the cause for presentation in most affected kittens (23). In the Abyssinians (20), the hypothyroidism was due to abnormal or absent hormone production and the thyroid gland was also enlarged. In contrast, in Japanese cats (19), in which the hypothyroidism was due to a reduced response to TSH, the thyroid gland was hypoplastic. In both breeds the mutations were transmitted in an autosomal-recessive manner.

Marked epiphyseal dysgenesis is seen on radiographs in feline hypothyroidism. Long bones are typically shorter and wider than normal, with metaphyseal flaring, especially noticeable in the femur and sometimes with virtual absence of the ossification center in the distal femoral epiphysis (21). The vertebral bodies are malformed with a caudal beaking. Occasionally, the vertebral bodies are shortened and the end plates absent (21).

Based on the radiographic findings, in particular the vertebral changes, storage diseases must also be considered as a differential diagnosis. MPS type VI and VII, mucolipidosis, and sometimes alpha-mannosidosis may be accompanied by dwarfism (24). Cats affected by these storage diseases show no clinical signs until the age of 2–4 months (4). Clinical symptoms include growth retardation, corneal clouding (MPS VI and VII), and locomotion problems. Although neurological signs are present in these storage diseases, mental dullness is not a clinical feature. In MPS diseases granulation of the neutrophils and urinary excretion of GAGs are typical findings (4). Both are absent in congenital hypothyroidism.

3.1.5 Hereditary rickets

Rickets is a very rare disease, caused by chronic dietary deficiency of vitamin D or hereditary abnormalities. The dietary form is discussed in Chapter 4. Hereditary rickets in cats is either secondary to a defect in the vitamin D pathway (vitamin D-dependent rickets type 1, VDDR-1), the vitamin D receptors (VDDR-2), or renal tubular reabsorption of phosphate (25–28). Summaries of the different forms are listed in Table 3-4.

Inadequate levels of active vitamin D result in reduction of absorption of phosphorus and calcium from the intestine, and prevent mineralization of newly formed osteoid. The osteoid is highly stable and therefore uncalcifiable and difficult to resorb. In the young animal this results in cartilage cells that fail to degenerate and capillaries from the metaphysis are unable to penetrate the cartilage. Epiphyseal lines become thickened and irregular. In adults, osteomalacia occurs as vitamin D is needed for osteoclasts and osteocytes to respond to parathyroid hormone (parathormone), and allow bone resorption. The metabolic pathway for vitamin D is illustrated in Figure 3-7.

The main clinical features are disturbance of longitudinal growth of long bones, and skeletal demineralization. Affected animals are often young (less than 6 months), severely stunted, bowlegged, and plantigrade. Metaphyseal areas and costochondral junctions (the so-called rachitic rosary) are prominent. Signs can also be attributable to the systemic effects of hypocalcemia rather than the effects on bone. Thus, muscle weakness, tremors or seizures, vomiting, diarrhea and mydriasis, may be the predominant features (26).

Radiographically, the growth plates appear widened or cup shaped, due to the accumulation of cartilage at the epiphyses, and the metaphyses are irregularly mineralized (Fig. 3-8). Bone deformation and osteoporosis may also occur and, in adults, the bones can appear osteopenic and folding fractures may be present (25).

Type of rickets	Laboratory analysis	Treatment	References
Nutritional **Vitamin D deficiency –** diet deficient in vitamin D, calcium, and/or phosphate	Low $1,25(OH)_2D_3$ Hypophosphatemia and/or hypocalcemia Secondary hyperparathyroidism	Balanced diet, exposure to sunlight	
Hereditary **X-linked hypophosphatemic rickets** defect in renal tubular reabsorption of phosphate	Hypophosphatemia High urinary fractional clearance of P Normocalcemia Normal $25(OH)D_3$*(high 125) Normal to low $1,25(OH)_2D_3$ Secondary hyperparathyroidism	Calcifediol Phosphate salts	Henik et al. (1999) (25)
Vitamin D-dependent rickets type 1 (VDDR-1) defect in calcitriol production	Very low $1,25(OH)_2D_3$ Hypocalcemia Secondary hyperparathyroidism	Calcitriol supplementation	
Vitamin D-dependent rickets type 2 (VDDR-2) impaired responsiveness of target organs to calcitriol because of defects in vitamin D receptors	Normal $25(OH)D_3$ Elevated $1,25(OH)_2D_3$ Hypocalcemia Secondary hyperparathyroidism	Oral calcium supplementation Additional calcitriol, analgesics	Schreiner and Nagode (2003) (26) Godfrey et al. (2005) (27) Tanner and Langley-Hobbs (2005) (28)

Table 3-4. Summary of the different forms of rickets in cats

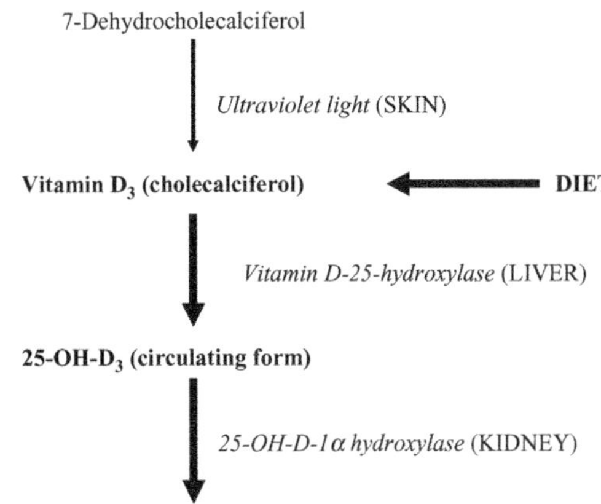

Figure 3-7. The metabolic pathway of vitamin D.

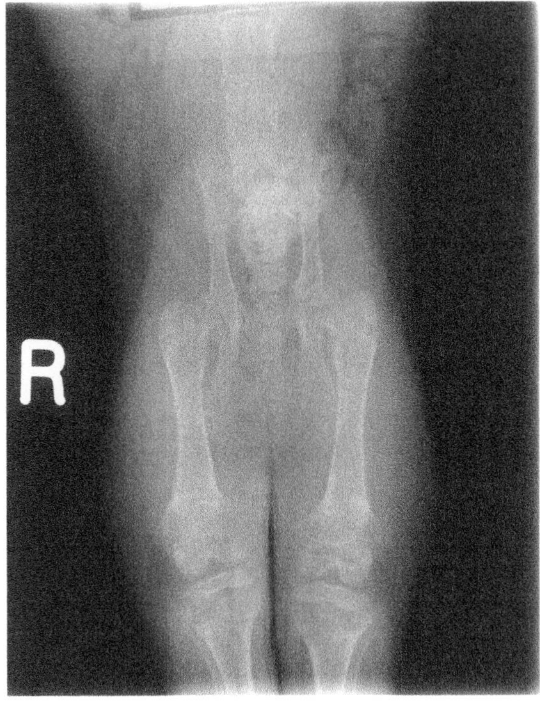

Figure 3-8. Ventrodorsal pelvic radiograph of a 4-month-old cat with vitamin D-dependent rickets type 2 (VDDR-2). There are characteristic radiographic changes, including generalized osteopenia, widened, cup-shaped epiphyses in the proximal and distal femur and proximal tibia, and stippled metaphyses.

Diagnosis of hereditary rickets is supported by elevations or decreases in vitamin D, parathormone, calcium, and phosphorus levels in blood. Table 3-4 summarizes the changes seen with the different hereditary forms of rickets.

In the two cases in the literature with VDDR-2 and characteristic skeletal changes (27, 28), treatment with calcium supplementation and various forms of vitamin D did not normalize the plasma calcium levels or reverse skeletal lesions. Schreiner and Nagode (26) were successful in their treatment of a VDDR-2 kitten by effectively doubling the recommended dosage of calcium together with a high dosage of calcitriol (50 ng/kg) to supersaturate the vitamin D receptors. This kitten had no skeletal changes and a milder form of VDDR-2 and it was able to maintain serum calcium concentrations within reference limits even when therapy was withdrawn at maturity.

3.2 Congenital skeletal malformations

The term congenital means a defect present at birth. For the breeder it is of interest to know if it is a congenital hereditary defect, or if teratogenic substances caused the deformity. In the case of a proven hereditary disease one or both parents should be excluded from breeding. Although many congenital defects are thought to be hereditary, some of them may also occur as a developmental defect or be triggered by a teratogenic substance during pregnancy. Often it is very difficult or almost impossible to establish an etiological diagnosis, for example in cleft palate. This can be a congenital defect that is hereditary, but it can also be a developmental defect, and it can be caused by griseofulvin treatment during pregnancy (29). The most frequent congenital defects are described in the following sections.

Dwarfism in cats is a rarely occurring disease with an autosomal-recessive heredity (30). Associated abnormalities include ascites, visceromegaly (liver, spleen, lymph nodes), and hepatic storage disease (31). Such cats die between 1 and 4 months of age.

Schistosoma is a rare lethal malformation that is characterized by a fissure of the abdomen, visceral herniation, and malformation or absence of the pelvic limbs (32). This developmental anomaly often causes dystocia (Fig. 3-9).

Siamese or conjoined twins is a rare malformation which is due to an incomplete splitting of the zygote during the early stages of pregnancy. Generally, the condition is named according to the sites of non-separation, i.e., thoracopagus if adhered at the chest, cephalopagus at the head, etc. As with *Schistosoma* kittens, dystocias are common in queens with conjoined twins.

3.2.1 Skull

Cleft palate is one of the most common defects. Defects of the lip and premaxilla are called a primary cleft palate, or harelip. Incomplete closure of the hard and soft palates is called a secondary cleft palate (Fig. 3-10). Surgery is needed in secondary cleft palates and large primary cleft palates to

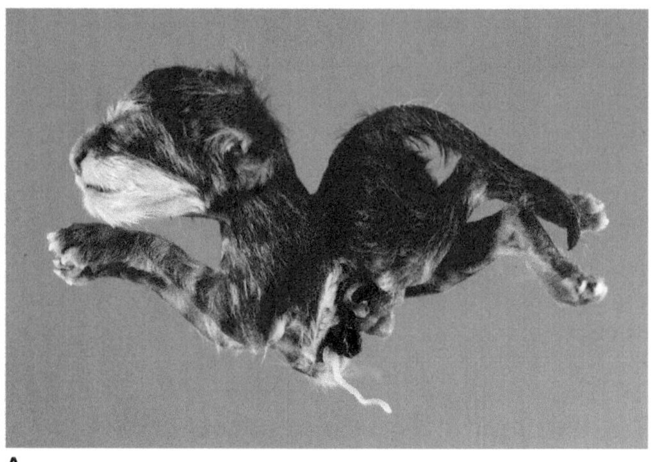

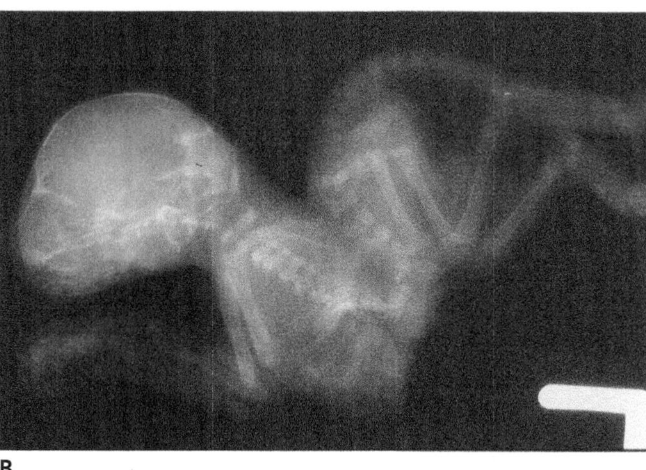

A B

Figure 3-9. (**A**) Macroscopic and (**B**) radiographic appearance of a newborn kitten with *Schistosoma reflexum*.

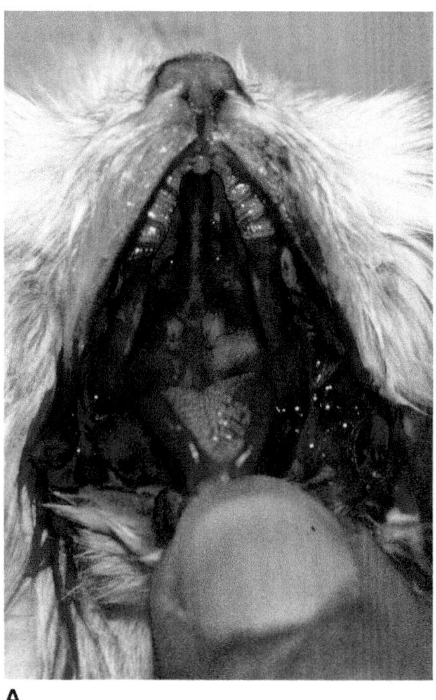

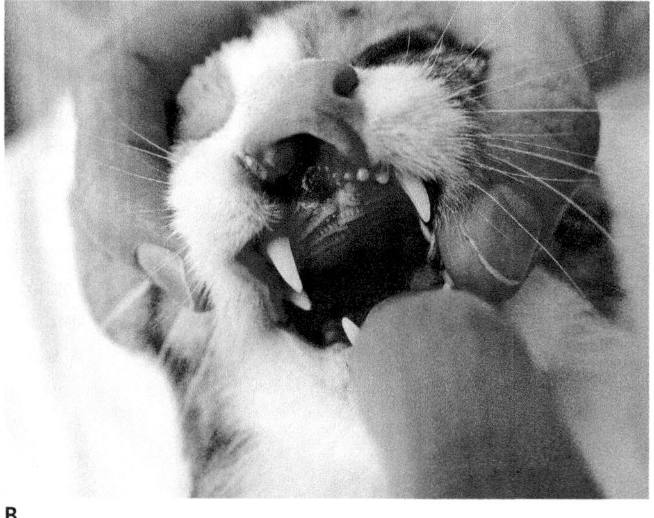

A B

Figure 3-10. Two examples of cats with cleft palates.
(**A**) A 2-day-old kitten with a large secondary cleft palate. The kitten was euthanized.
(**B**) A 4-month-old cat with a primary cleft palate, or harelip. The lesion was not treated, as the cat did not exhibit significant clinical problems.

restore the nasal floor in order to prevent aspiration pneumonia. Surgery is usually delayed until the patients are at least 2 months old. Cleft palate is hereditary in the Siamese breed. Based on the frequency of anomalous kittens among 10 litters an autosomal-recessive mode of inheritance was assumed (32). Cleft palate can also occur after treatment with vitamin A or griseofulvin during pregnancy (32).

Meningoencephalocele is herniation of the cerebrum through an opening in the skull. It is perinatally lethal, as it is usually associated with other severe malformations such as missing eye sockets and a cleft replacing the nostrils. Extensive hemorrhage and compression of the remaining brain in the skull are also present (32).

Brachycephaly results from a shortening of the maxilla and mandible and is characteristic of the Persian and Himalayan breeds. The condition is also called dish face and predisposes to respiratory, pharyngeal, and ocular disease (30).

Facial dysmorphism includes frontal bossing, depression of the nasal bridge, a short broad muzzle, and hypertelorism (excessive distance between the eyes). This is a common

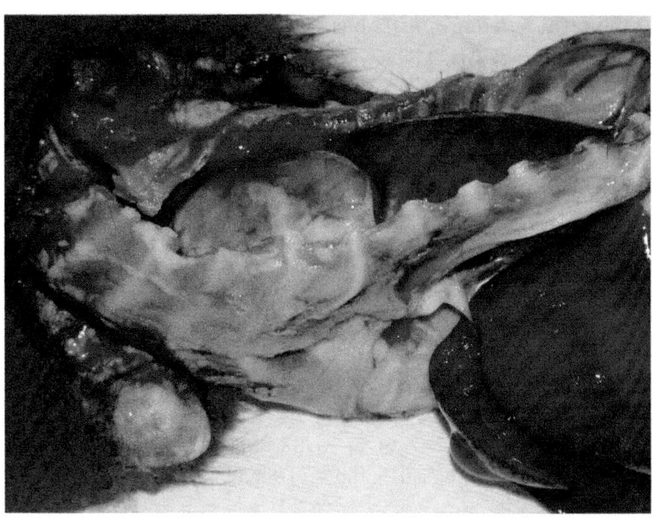

Figure 3-11. The thorax of the body of a domestic short-hair kitten with pectus excavatum. The marked depression of the sternum and the deformation of the rib cage resulted in clinically significant compression of the heart and the lung lobes.

feature of some storage diseases (MPS and mucolipidosis type II).

Craniofacial anomaly in the Burmese is an autosomal-dominant malformation with variable expression depending on modifying genes. This condition is characterized by exencephaly (a neural tube defect where the skull is incompletely fused, causing exposure or extrusion of the brain), lack of eyes or nose, mild to severe hydrocephalus, and a severely protruding jaw. Some affected individuals also exhibit a double set of whisker pads, cleft palate, and rotated pinnae (32).

3.2.2 Thorax

Pectus excavatum is a complete or partial depression of the sternum with an associated flattening of the chest, resulting in a reduction in the diameter of the thoracic cavity (Fig. 3-11). Siamese, Burmese, and related breeds are predisposed. The malformation can cause respiratory disease and compression of the heart, which can be life-threatening in severely affected kittens (29). Kittens with severe chest compression can be treated with traction sutures and casts (33). Mildly affected kittens often grow out of the condition.

Pectus excavatum has to be differentiated from the flat-chested kitten, or "swimmer" syndrome, where the dorsoventral flattening of the chest is secondary to the transient inability to walk.

3.2.3 Spine

Spinal dysraphism involves the failure of closure of part of the neural tube forming the vertebral canal. A milder form of abnormal closure is called *spina bifida,* which was described in a large number of kittens. The disorder is most common in the lumbar spine (Fig. 3-12). The defect is sometimes associated with protrusion of the spinal cord or meninges and/or spinal cord dysplasia. Depending on the severity, the defect may be surgically corrected. Spina bifida is most common in Manx cats, which have a genetic anomaly of the spinal cord (see later) (32). A double dorsal spinous process can be seen on radiography in some cases.

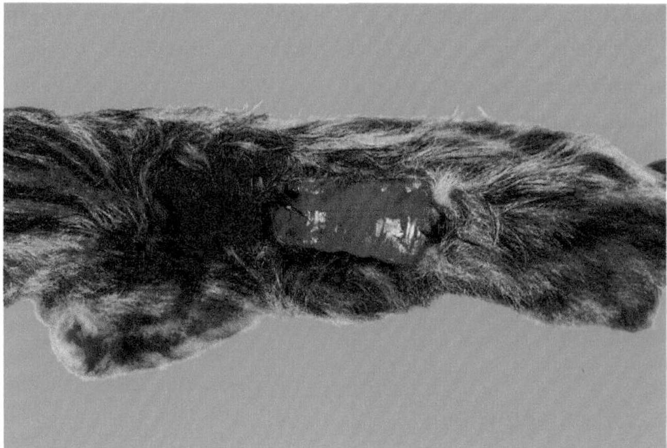

Figure 3-12. Stillborn kitten with spina bifida. The incomplete fusion of the vertebral arches can be seen under a thin layer of epaxial fascia and muscle. (Courtesy of F. Steffen.)

Vertebral body anomalies are common in cats and are usually of no clinical significance. The most common anomaly is the presence of a 14th thoracic, or transitional vertebrae. Although incomplete or fused vertebrae can be found anywhere throughout the spine, most are located in the thoracic and coccygeal spine (32).

Incomplete or fused vertebrae of the coccygeal spine may lead to a kinked tail. This deformity has to be differentiated from the hereditary form of the ***kinked tail,*** in which the vertebrae are normal, but an angular deformity is present at the intervertebral joint, namely at the connection of the annulus fibrosus to the bodies of the vertebrae. The defect is usually towards the end of the tail, but may be at any point. Corrective surgery is often ineffective (34). The kinked tail in Siamese cats is an anomaly with an autosomal-recessive mode of inheritance. In the same breed, an inherited shortening of the tail has also been described (32).

Absence of the tail is the primary characteristic of the Manx breed. The Manx gene is autosomal-dominant with incomplete penetrance (35). This means that a dominant gene, along with modifying genes, is responsible for variable tail length. The various tail types are generally classified into four groups: (1) no coccygeal vertebrae (rumpy); (2) several coccygeal vertebrae in upright position (rumpy-riser); or several coccygeal vertebrae with (3) a severe kink (stumpy), and (4) a normal-appearing tail (longy). Additional defects in some heterozygous Manx cats may affect the whole spine to some degree, but the major changes occur in the caudal part. These include small, deformed, fused vertebrae reduced in number in the thoracic, lumbar, sacral, and coccygeal region. In mild cases a stilted walk or hopping is apparent. In severe cases urinary and fecal incontinence may additionally occur. Kittens homozygous for the mutation die in utero (32).

See Chapter 6 for additional information on congenital spinal abnormalities.

3.2.4 Extremities

Agenesis of all or part of the digit (*ectrodactyly)* is an inherited malformation affecting the forepaws. *Polydactyly* (extra toes) is caused by a dominant gene with variable expressivity. It occurs predominantly in the forelimb. Amputation of extra digits is sometimes indicated if secondary complications occur, such as recurrent interdigital infections or traumatic injuries. *Syndactyly* is the term for fusion of toes. Paw changes in syndactyle cats can include abnormal or absent digits, abnormal shape, fusion or absence of digital pads, and abnormal shape or fusion of nails. Radiographic changes can include complete or incomplete fusion of phalanges and metatarsal or metacarpal bones. Feline complex syndactyly causes minimal to no discomfort and reported patients affected with this condition have presented without lameness (36). In the "kangaroo cat" the development of the long bone of the forelimbs is arrested, resulting in a forelimb *micromelia*. A female cat with micromelia has been described (37). Because some of the queen's progeny also had the deformity, a genetic trait was suspected. *Amelia* is lack of all limbs. *Peromelus ascelsus* is agenesis of the pelvic limbs only.

Two cases of bilateral *congenital elbow luxation* have been described in cats (38, 39). Affected cats can have good clinical limb function, and can then be treated conservatively. Surgical treatment is conducted if the lesion causes significant clinical problems. Arthrodesis of the elbow could be considered. See also Chapter 30.

Radial hemimelia is agenesis of the radius. Bilateral agenesis of the radius has been described in a Devon Rex cat (40).

Carpal agenesis of the right leg has been recently reported in a domestic short hair cat (41). Good leg function was achieved with pancarpal arthrodesis.

Proximal femoral dysplasia was recently described in two cats (42). One cat had bilateral agenesis of the femoral head and neck with hypoplasia of the acetabulum. The other cat had unilateral hypoplasia of the femoral neck and a grossly deformed femoral head. Treatment consisted of femoral head and neck excision if lameness was present.

Bilateral *patellar aplasia* has been described in two Siamese cat littermates (43). The condition was associated with deformity of the distal femur, the tibia and fibula, and the tail. The cats showed gait abnormalities, but were able to move around the house.

References and further reading

1. Cummings JF, et al. The clinical and pathologic heterogeneity of feline alpha-mannosidosis. J Vet Int Med 1988;2:163–170.
2. Vandevelde M, et al. Hereditary neurovisceral mannosidosis associated with alpha-mannosidase deficiency in a family of Persian cats. Acta Neuropathol (Berl) 1982;58:64–68.
3. Blakemore WF. A case of mannosidosis in the cat: clinical and histopathological findings. J Small Anim Pract 1986;27: 447–455.
4. Thrall MA. Mucopolysaccharidosis. In: August JR (ed.) Consultations in feline internal medicine 4. Philadelphia: WB Saunders; 2001: pp. 450–459.
5. Haskins M, et al. Animal models for mucopolysaccharidoses and their clinical relevance. Acta Paediatr Suppl 2002;439: 88–97.
6. Gitzelmann R, et al. Feline mucopolysaccharidosis VII due to beta-glucuronidase deficiency. Vet Pathol 1994;31:435–443.
7. Hubler M, et al. Mucolipidosis type II in a domestic shorthair cat. J Small Anim Pract 1996;37:435–441.
8. Mazrier H, et al. Inheritance, biochemical abnormalities, and clinical features of feline mucolipidosis II: the first animal model of human I-cell disease. J Hered 2003;94:363–373.
9. Crawley AC, et al. Two mutations within a feline mucopolysaccharidosis type VI colony cause three different clinical phenotypes. J Clin Invest 1998;101:109–119.
10. Gehring H. Osteogenesis imperfecta bei der Katze. Kleintierpraxis 1975;20:225–231.
11. Cohn LA, Meuten DJ. Bone fragility in a kitten: an osteogenesis imperfecta-like syndrome. J Am Vet Med Assoc 1990;197: 98–100.
12. Jackson OF. Congenital bone lesions in cats with fold-ears. Bull Fel Advis Bur 1975;14:2–4.
13. Schrey C, Gerlach KF. Osteochondrodysplasie bei Pudelkatzen (Rex Fold). Kleintierpraxis 2002;47:433–435.
14. Malik R, et al. Osteochondrodysplasia in Scottish Fold cats. Aust Vet J 1999;77:85–92.
15. Allan GS. Radiographic features of feline joint diseases. Vet Clin North Am Pract 2000;30:281–302.
16. Simon D. Osteochondrodysplasie bei einer Scottish-Fold Katze. Tierärztl Prax 2000;28:107–110.
17. Mathews KG, et al. Resolution of lameness associated with Scottish Fold osteodystrophy following bilateral ostectomies and pantarsal arthodesis: a case report. J Am Anim Hosp Assoc 1995;31:280–288.
18. Hubler M, et al. Palliative irradiation of Scottish Fold osteochondrodysplasia. Vet Radiol Ultrasound 2004;45:1–4.
19. Tanase H, et al. Inherited primary hypothyroidism with thyrotrophin resistance in Japanese cats. J Endocrinol 1991;129: 245–251.
20. Jones BR, et al. Preliminary studies on congenital hypothyroidism in a family of Abyssinian cats. Vet Rec 1992;15:145–148.
21. Arnold U, et al. Goitrous hypothyroidism and dwarfism in a kitten. J Am Anim Hosp Assoc 1984;20:753–758.

22. Peterson ME. Feline hypothyroidism. In: Kirk RW (ed.) Current veterinary therapy X. Philadelphia: WB Saunders; 1989: pp. 1000–1001.
23. Jezyk PF. Constitutional disorders of the skeleton in dogs and cats. In: Newton CD, Nunamaker DM (eds) Textbook of small animal orthopaedics. Philadelphia: Lippincott; 1985: pp. 637–654.
24. Haskins ME, Patterson DF. Inherited metabolic diseases. In: Holzworth J (ed.) Diseases of the cat: medicine and surgery. Philadelphia: WB Saunders; 1987: pp. 808–820.
25. Henik RA, et al. Rickets caused by excessive renal phosphate loss and apparent abnormal vitamin D metabolism in a cat. J Am Vet Med Assoc 1999;215:1644–1649.
26. Schreiner CA, Nagode LA. Vitamin D-dependent rickets type 2 in a four-month-old cat. J Am Vet Med Assoc 2003;222: 337–339.
27. Godfrey DR, et al. Vitamin D-dependent rickets type II in a cat. J Small Anim Pract 2005;46:440–444.
28. Tanner E, Langley-Hobbs SJ. Vitamin D-dependent rickets type 2 with characteristic radiographic changes in a 4-month-old kitten. J Feline Med Surg 2005;7:307–311.
29. Willoughby K. Paediatrics and inherited diseases. In: Chandler EA, Gaskell CJ, Gaskell RM (eds) Feline medicine and therapeutics, 3rd edn. Oxford: Blackwell; 2004: pp. 355–379.
30. Bennett D. The muculoskeletal system. In: Chandler EA, Gaskell CJ, Gaskell RM (eds) Feline medicine and therapeutics, 3rd edn. Oxford: Blackwell; 2004: pp. 173–233.
31. Schrader SC, Sherding RG. Disorders of the skeletal system. In: Sherding RG (ed.) The cat: diseases and clinical management, vol. 2. New York: Churchill Livingstone; 1989: pp. 1247–1292.
32. Robinson R, Pedersen NC. Normal genetics, genetic disorders, developmental anomalies and breeding programs. In: Pedersen NC (ed.) Feline husbandry. Diseases and management in the multiple-cat environment. Goleta, CA: American Veterinary Publications; 1991: pp. 61–129.
33. Shires PK, et al. Pectus excavatum in three kittens. J Am Anim Hosp Assoc 1988;24:203.
34. Saperstein G, et al. Congenital defects in domestic cats. Feline Pract 1976;6:18–43.
35. Wastlhuber J. History of domestic cats and cat breeds. In: Pedersen NC (ed.) Feline husbandry. Diseases and management in the multiple-cat environment. Goleta, CA: American Veterinary Publications; 1991: pp. 1-61.
36. Towle HA, et al. Syndactyly in a litter of cats. J Small Anim Pract 2007;48:292–296.
37. William-Jones BG. Arrested development of the long bones in a female cat. Vet Rec 1944;56:449.
38. Rossi F, et al. Bilateral elbow malformation in a cat caused by radio-ulnar synostosis. Vet Radiol Ultrasound 2003;44:283–286.
39. Valastro C, et al. Congenital elbow subluxation in a cat. Vet Radiol Ultrasound 2005;46:63–64.
40. O'Brien CR, et al. What is your diagnosis? Bilateral forelimb deformity and abnormal gait in a young Devon Rex. J Feline Med Surg 2004;4:112–113.
41. Gemmill TJ, et al. Carpal agenesis in a domestic short haired cat. Vet Comp Orthop Traumatol 2004;17:163–170.
42. Isola MB, et al. Radiographic features of two cases of feline proximal femoral dysplasia. J Small Anim Pract 2005;46: 597–599.
43. Milovancev M, Ralphs SC. Congenital patellar aplasia in a family of cats. Vet Comp Orthop Traumatol 2004;17:9–11.

4 Diseases of bone

K. Voss

Normal bone undergoes constant remodeling with a physiological balance between new bone formation and bone resorption. Osteoblasts and osteocytes are responsible for the formation of new bone, whereas osteoclasts dissolve mineralized bone substance. Bone remodeling is closely related to calcium homeostasis because bone is an important calcium reservoir. The activity of osteoblasts and osteoclasts is hormone-dependent. These hormones in turn respond to changes in serum calcium and phosphate levels. Important hormones participating in calcium homeostasis and bone remodeling are parathormone (PTH), vitamin D metabolites, and calcitonin (Table 4-1).

Chronic changes in hormone activity cause generalized bone disease. Nutritional and renal secondary hyperparathyroidism are the most common forms of clinically apparent acquired bone disease in cats. Other hormones, such as growth hormones, thyroid hormones, and sex hormones, also have a direct or indirect effect on calcium homeostasis and bone metabolism. Hyperthyroidism has been associated with decreases in ionized calcium, hyperphosphatemia, and elevation of serum PTH in up to 75% of cats in one study (1). The combined resorptive effects of thyroid hormone and PTH may reduce bone strength in these cats. Although the degree of osteoporosis does not seem to cause clinical disease, reduced bone strength should be expected in fracture repair of hyperthyroid cats. Sex hormones are important due to their effect on physeal closure and bone growth. Chronic vitamin D-deficiency and hypervitaminosis A also result in generalized skeletal abnormalities.

Localized bone disease is rare in cats, with the exception of neoplasia. Bone cysts, osteomyelitis, and disease of the bone of the femoral head and neck are examples of localized bone disease. Feline bone diseases are summarized in Table 4-2.

4.1 Secondary hyperparathyroidism

Secondary hyperparathyroidism occurs when there is chronic elevation of PTH in response to changes in serum calcium and phosphorus levels. Serum hypocalcemia and hyperphosphatemia induce PTH secretion. Hyperphosphatemia does not directly affect PTH secretion, but may depress calcium concentration by the interaction of calcium and phosphorus in the serum. Chronic elevation of PTH results in generalized osteoporosis due to absorption of calcium from bone (Table 4-1). Two clinical entities have been described: nutritional hyperparathyroidism and renal hyperparathyroidism. Nutritional hyperparathyroidism occurs most frequently in young cats secondary to inadequate dietary calcium intake, whereas renal hyperparathyroidism is a disease of older cats secondary to chronic increase of serum phosphorus concentration and relative hypocalcemia in cats with renal insufficiency.

4.1.1 Nutritional secondary hyperparathyroidism

Diets low in calcium and high in phosphorus cause a chronically low to normal serum calcium concentration. All-meat diets have an unfavorable calcium and phosphorus content,

Organs	Parathormone	Vitamin D metabolites	Calcitonin
Kidney	Increases calcium reabsorption Increases phosphate excretion Enhances synthesis of active vitamin D		
Intestine	Increases calcium absorption	Increases calcium absorption	
Bone	Enhances production and activity of osteoclasts	Enhances sensitivity of osteoclasts to parathormone	Reduces activity of osteoclasts
Overall effect on bone	Releases calcium from bone Osteoporosis	Stimulates release of calcium from bone Osteoporosis	Reduces absorption of calcium from bone

Table 4-1. Effects of parathormone, vitamin D, and calcitonin on calcium homeostasis and bone remodeling

Disease group	Diseases
Inherited (Chapter 3)	Storage diseases
	Osteogenesis imperfecta
	Osteochondrodysplasia in the Scottish Fold cat
	Hypothyroidism
	Hereditary rickets
Congenital (Chapter 3)	Several skeletal malformations described
Nutritional	Nutritional hyperparathyroidism
	Vitamin D deficiency (rickets)
	Hypervitaminosis A
Metabolic	Renal hyperparathyroidism
Miscellaneous	Cartilaginous exostoses
	Hypertrophic osteopathy
	Bone cysts
	Spontaneous femoral capital physeal fracture and femoral neck metaphyseal osteopathy (Chapter 36)
Infectious	Hematogenous osteomyelitis
Neoplastic (Chapter 8)	Primary bone tumor
	Metastatic bone tumor

Table 4-2. Bone diseases in cats

but hyperparathyroidism may also develop by feeding meat and rice or meat and vegetable diets (2). We have also observed mild clinical disease in cats fed a commercial diet from a non-scientific cat food supplier. Hypocalcemia causes an increase in PTH secretion and activation of vitamin D (calcitriol) in the kidneys. Both substances lead to calcium mobilization from bone. Intestinal calcium absorption and renal reabsorption are also enhanced. In very young cats it takes weeks, in older cats months, before clinically relevant osteoporosis occurs (3).

Initial clinical signs are inactivity, apathy, and generalized pain. Cats may also be presented with acute lameness or neurological symptoms after having suffered pathological fractures. Seizures, excitation, and muscle twitching, probably as a result of hypocalcemia, have also been described (2). Radiological features include generalized osteopenia, demineralization of the long bones and vertebrae, thinned cortices, and a widened medullary canal (Fig. 4-1). Pathological fractures commonly occur in cancellous bone, such as the metaphysis of the tibia or femur or humerus, and the vertebrae (2). The fractures tend to be minimally displaced and are also called compression or folding fractures. Additionally, deformation of the long bones, vertebral column, or the pelvis might be encountered.

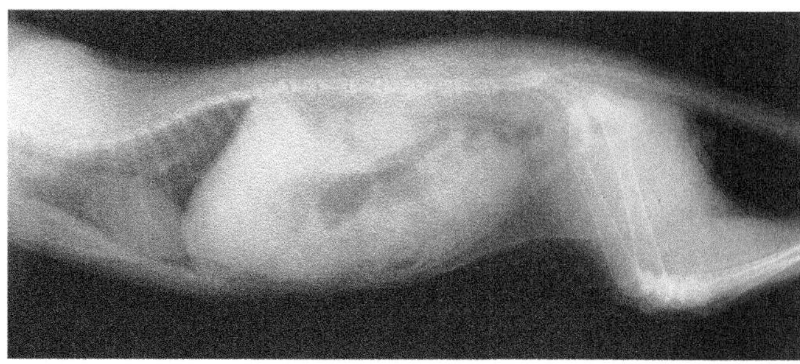

Figure 4.1 Laterolateral radiograph of a 3-month-old male domestic short-hair cat with nutritional hyperparathyroidism. The cat was fed with a meat-only diet. There is generalized osteopenia and demineralization of the whole skeleton and the cortices of the femurs and tibias are thin. A pathological folding fracture is visible in the proximal metaphysis of the femur.

A diagnosis of nutritional hyperparathyroidism should be suspected in cats or kittens with the signs described above, a history of an inappropriate diet, and the typical radiographical features. Total serum calcium is typically mildly reduced (2). Measurement of ionized calcium should be performed if available. Elevated PTH serum levels confirm the diagnosis. Serum PTH was markedly elevated in five of six cats with nutritional hyperparathyroidism in one study (2). Other common laboratory abnormalities include elevation of calcitriol and alkaline phosphatase.

Therapy consists of changing the diet to a high-quality commercial cat food, containing a balanced calcium:phosphorus ratio. Dietary correction results in rapid normalization of serum PTH levels, and normalized mineralization of bone occurs within 4–8 weeks (4). Cats need to be confined to a cage initially to prevent or treat pathological fractures. Pathological fractures of long bones often involve the metaphyseal regions and are not significantly displaced. They generally heal readily with an appropriate diet and cage rest alone. Surgical stabilization should be considered with severe fracture displacement or limb malalignment. Adequate implants, such as pins or internal or external fixators, must be used to stabilize the osteoporotic bone (Chapter 13). Surgical stabilization or corrective osteotomies can also be performed later in the treatment after establishment of more normal bone mineralization. Prognosis for cats with pathological spinal fractures depends on the degree of spinal cord compression, but is usually unfavorable.

4.1.2 Renal secondary hyperparathyroidism

Chronic renal failure is often associated with renal secondary hyperparathyroidism. Elevated serum PTH concentration was present in 84% of cats with chronic renal failure in one study (5). Renal phosphorus retention, resulting in increased serum phosphorus concentration and a subsequent relative

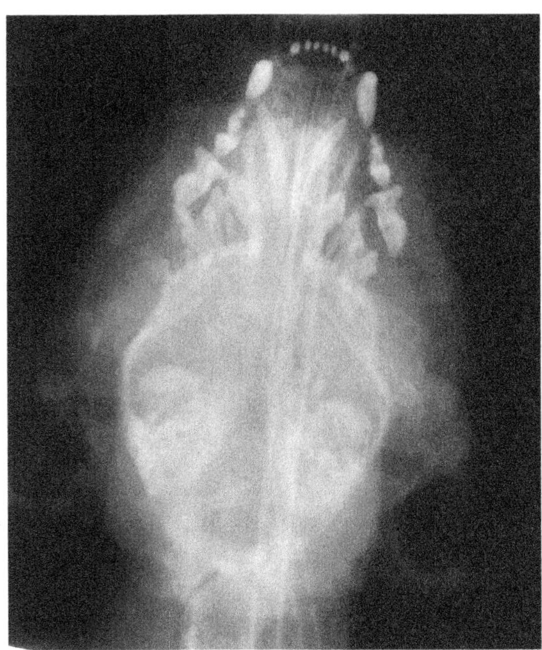

Figure 4.2 Radiograph of the skull of a 16-year-old cat with renal hyperparathyroidism. Marked osteopenia of the bones of the skull is visible. Osteopenia of the alveolar bone results in a "floating teeth" appearance.

decrease in ionized calcium concentration, plays an important role in the pathogenesis of renal hyperparathyroidism (5). Despite the presence of elevated serum PTH levels, most affected cats have low to normal calcium levels. Possible causes are reduction of active vitamin D production, and reduction of calcium reabsorption in the diseased kidneys (6).

Chronic renal hyperparathyroidism results in osteoporosis and metastatic calcium deposition in soft tissues (Chapter 8). The majority of cats with chronic renal failure have histological evidence of bone resorption (7). Although the bony changes are usually mild, some cats may exhibit clinical disease, such as bone pain, reluctance to move, osteolytic changes, or even pathological fractures (8). The bones of the skull are typically predominantly affected (Fig. 4-2).

Diagnosis of renal secondary hyperparathyroidism is based on laboratory findings consistent with chronic interstitial nephritis, and elevation of serum PTH. Therapy aims at reducing phosphorus and PTH concentrations. Within 5 months of feeding a diet restricted in phosphorus and protein, a significant fall in plasma phosphate and PTH concentrations was observed in cats with stable chronic renal failure (9). In cases where phosphorus and PTH levels do not return to normal, an intestinal phosphate-binding agent should also be used. Prognosis depends on maintenance of renal function. Pathological fractures are rare with renal secondary hyperparathyroidism, but carry a rather unfavorable prognosis due to the reduced bone quality.

4.2 Vitamin D deficiency (rickets)

Rickets is a very rare disease, caused by chronic dietary deficiency of vitamin D, or a hereditary defect in the vitamin D pathway or the vitamin D receptors, or renal tubular reabsorption of phosphate. Hereditary rickets is described in Chapter 3.

Cats do not synthesize cholecalciferol (pre-vitamin D_3) in their skin when exposed to sunlight, and therefore depend on dietary intake. Lean meat and vegetables contain low levels of vitamin D. Inadequate levels of active vitamin D result in reduction of absorption of phosphorus and calcium from the intestine, and prevent mineralization of newly formed osteoid. The main clinical features are disturbance of longitudinal growth of long bones, and skeletal demineralization. Radiographically, the growth plates appear widened and the metaphysis irregularly mineralized (10). Bone deformation and osteoporosis may also occur. Pathological fractures are rare. The diagnosis of nutritional rickets is supported if 25(OH)-vitamin D_3 and calcitriol serum levels are markedly reduced. Therapy consists of dietary supplementation of vitamin D and optimization of dietary calcium and phosphorus intake. Skeletal mineralization and appearance of metaphyses improve within 3 weeks (6).

4.3 Hypervitaminosis A

Hypervitaminosis A is a metabolic disorder caused by chronic excessive dietary vitamin A uptake over several months or years. Clinical disease has been observed both after feeding a diet rich in the liposoluble vitamin A, such as raw liver or fish, and after supplementation of a normal diet with vitamin A drops. The exact mechanisms of vitamin A toxicity on the skeletal system remain unclear, but enhanced susceptibility to periosteal trauma, individual predisposition for disturbances of vitamin A metabolism, and increased lability of membranes of osteoblasts and chondrocytes may play a role in the pathogenesis (11–13). The main feature of hypervitaminosis A is formation of bony exostoses close to joints, usually near attachment sites of tendons and ligament. The bony proliferations are mainly composed of chondroid tissue, surrounded by woven bone (11). The cervical spine is the classic location, but non-vertebral hypervitaminosis A (Fig. 4-3) has also been described, with the proximal appendicular joints most commonly affected (11).

Clinical signs are often first observed between 2 and 4 years of age (3). Depending on the site of skeletal involvement, clinical signs include lameness, reluctance to move, apathy, and weight loss. Hypersensitivity may be present to palpation of the cervical spine. Later in the disease process, fusion of cervical and thoracic vertebrae may limit range of neck motion. Thoracic limb lameness may be due to lesions around

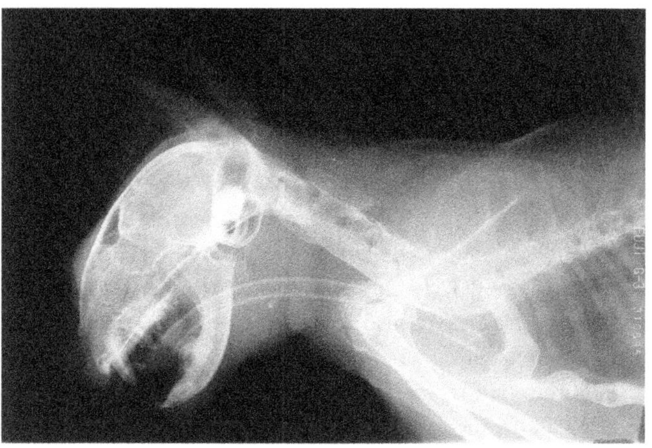

A

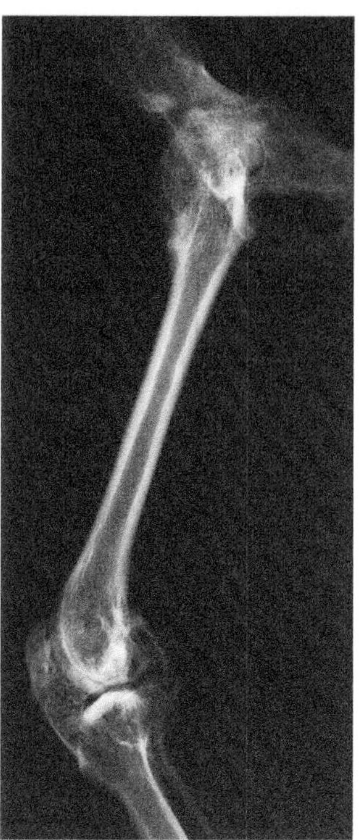

B

Figure 4.3 A 15-year-old cat with hypervitaminosis A, secondary to a liver-only diet. (**A**) Radiograph of the head, cervical spine, and thoracic inlet. The cervical spine is completely fused ventrally. Also note the bony exostoses around the shoulder joints, and the deformation of the sternebrae. (**B**) Also note the massive periarticular calcifications around the stifle and hip joint.

the shoulder or elbow joints, or due to entrapment of nerve roots or involvement of the brachial plexus (12). The first bony changes can be detected radiographically as early as 10 weeks after induction of the hypervitaminic diet (14), although cats are only usually presented after months of the abnormal diet. Initially, smoothly marginated enthesophytes develop in periarticular locations (14). They gradually grow, and with time, complete ankylosis of affected vertebrae or joints occurs.

Diagnosis is based on a history of feeding a diet rich in vitamin A, and the classic radiological signs. Serum vitamin A concentration may be elevated. Osteochondromas, feline osteochondromatosis, and synovial osteochondromatosis, and bone tumors are differential diagnoses to be considered.

Treatment consists of feeding a diet free of vitamin A. The diet can be home-made and includes rice, cooked chicken meat, corn oil, and iodinated salt (6). Analgesic therapy may improve overall well-being and reduce lameness. Although progression of the lesions stops with the appropriate diet, stiffness of joints and the spine remains. The clinical condition may be ameliorated in less severely affected cats, but prognosis is poor for severely affected cats.

4.4 Hematogenous osteomyelitis

Bacterial osteomyelitis is most often caused by inoculation of bacteria through a penetrating injury or a surgical incision. This is referred to as post-traumatic osteomyelitis and is described in Chapter 13. Cat bite wounds may result in osteomyelitis but the small skin lesions can be hard to detect, especially without clipping the hair. Bite wounds should be excluded by history and a thorough search for bite wounds or scars before hematogenous osteomyelitis is suspected.

Hematogenous osteomyelitis is a rare disease in cats and most often affects the metaphyses of long bones in young animals. Umbilical infections, pneumonia, and mastitis of the queen are possible sources of bacteremia in neonates. The vascular anatomy of the metaphyseal region in immature animals facilitates hematogenous seeding and lodging of bacteria. Abscesses in the metaphyseal region in children are referred to as Brodie's abscesses and staphylococcal species are responsible for the majority of these cases. Metaphyseal osteomyelitis has been described in the distal radial metaphysis of a young cat (15) (also see Chapter 2, Fig. 2-3). Hematogenous spread of bacteria into bone in adult cats rarely occurs but can be seen associated with distant infections (Fig. 4-4).

Affected cats are frequently systemically ill, and lesions can occur in multiple sites (3). Clinical signs include lameness, and swelling and pain over the area. Radiographs only reveal soft-tissue swelling for the first 2 or 3 weeks. Bone lysis and deformation within the metaphysis and/or epiphysis of long bones, and periosteal reaction appear later. Fine-needle aspiration of fluctuant areas or bone biopsies should be evaluated

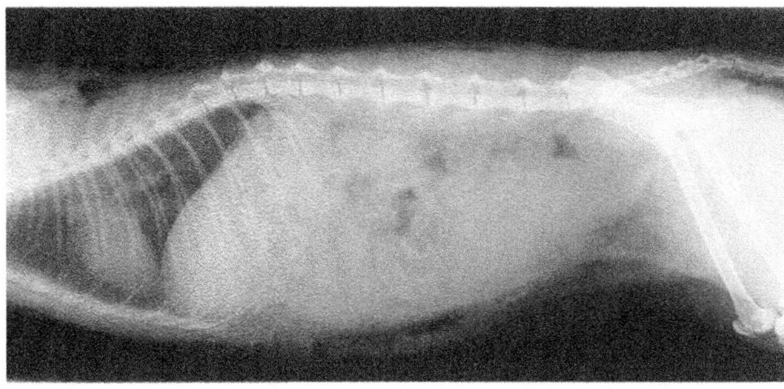

A

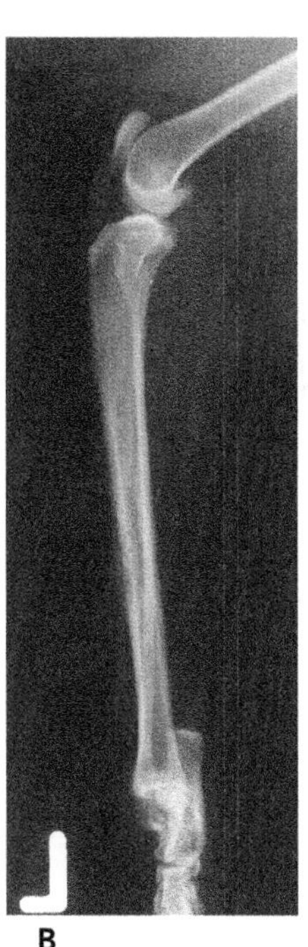

B

Figure 4.4 Radiographs of a cat which had suffered thoracic and abdominal dog bite wounds, and later developed hematogenous osteomyelitis in the tibia.
(**A**) Emphysema is seen around the thorax and the abdominal wall on the laterolateral radiographs taken 1 day after the bite injury, indicating perforating bite wounds.
(**B**) The cat was presented 6 weeks later with osteomyelitis in the tibia. The infection resolved with antimicrobial therapy.

cytologically or histopathologically, and samples should be cultured. Staphylococcal and streptococcal species are most likely to be isolated, but a *Salmonella* sp. was found in an older Persian cat with hematogenous osteomyelitis in the proximal tibia and distal radius (3).

Treatment includes antimicrobial therapy, curettage and drainage of the lesion, and bone grafting of the defect. A broad-spectrum antibiotic, such as cefazolin or amoxicillin/clavulanic acid, is administered intravenously initially. Further antibiotic treatment is selected according to culture and sensitivity results and must be administered for 4 weeks. Prognosis seems to be good if treated appropriately (3, 15). Destruction of growth plates in immature cats will result in growth abnormalities, requiring later correction when the cat is adult.

Fungal osteomyelitis occurs in the southern parts of the northern hemisphere. Histoplasmosis is a systemic fungal infection, usually originating in the lungs and then spreading to other regions, such as bone marrow. Affected cats may have clinical signs consistent with lung disease. Bony involvement causes lameness, pain, and swelling of the affected region. The distal bones of the appendicular skeleton are most commonly affected (16). Cats should be tested for feline leukemia virus (FeLV) and feline immunodeficiency virus (FIV), because dissemination of the disease is facilitated with immune deficiencies. The fungal organisms are often visible on cytology of the bone marrow. Histopathology may be a further diagnostic tool if cytology does not reveal organisms. Itraconazole orally (10 mg/kg per day) is considered the treatment of choice for feline histoplasmosis. It has to be administered for at least 2–4 months (17). Successful treatment has also been described with amphotericin B and ketoconazole administered for 4–6 months (16).

4.5 Bone cysts

Aneurysmal and solitary bone cysts have been described in cats. Bone cysts should be differentiated from neoplasia by histopathology.

Aneurysmal bone cysts are benign, locally expanding bone masses, containing numerous blood-filled spaces between bony trabeculae. They are thought to develop from disruption or shunting of intramedullary blood vessels, and tend to cause destruction of the inner cortical bone layers during expansion. Aneurysmal bone cysts occur predominantly in the flat bones of the axial skeleton. In cats, they have been described in the vertebrae, sacrum, ilium, scapula, and rib (3, 18, 19). Complete resection is the treatment of choice when possible, and carries a favorable prognosis (18). Other treatment options include surgical curettage with bone grafting, and radiation therapy.

Solitary bone cysts occur predominantly in long bones of young animals, most commonly in the distal radius and ulna. They are thought to develop after avascular necrosis of the metaphyseal cancellous bone. The cysts are lined with fibrous tissue and contain serosanguineous fluid. Elevated alkaline phosphatase level in the cystic fluid, compared to the serum, supports the diagnosis of a solitary bone cyst (20). Treatment involves curettage of the lesion and filling the defect with cancellous bone graft. Solitary bone cysts have been treated

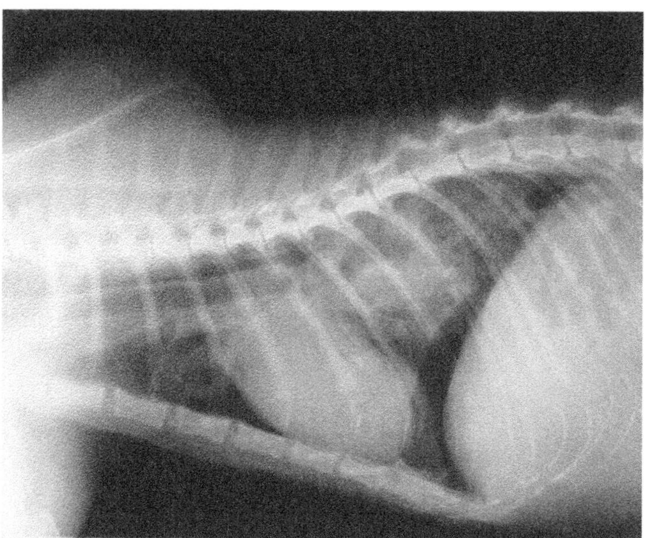

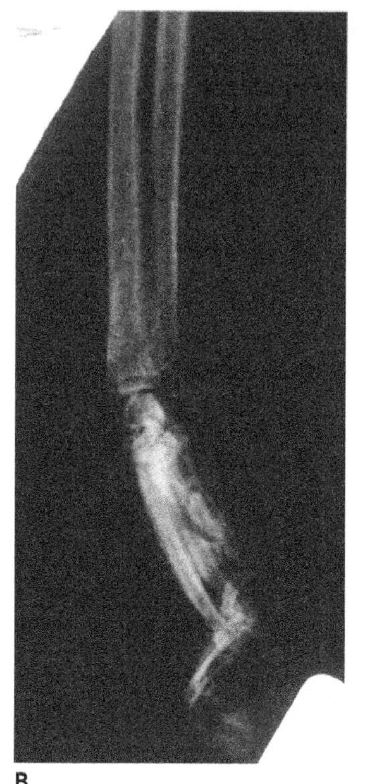

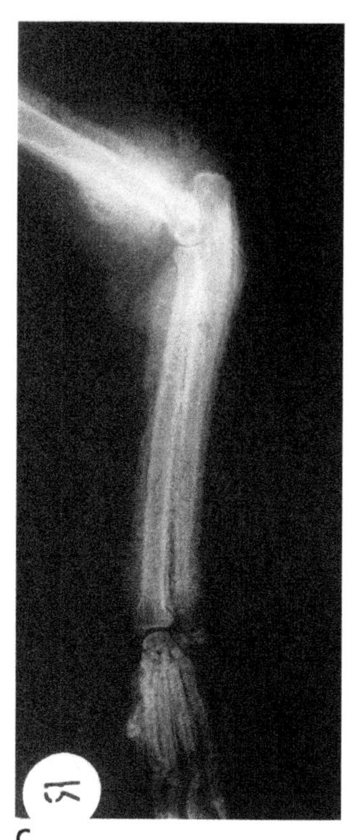

A B C

Figure 4.5 Radiographs of a cat with hypertrophic osteopathy secondary to a lung mass. The cat was presented with lameness of the right forelimb. (Courtesy of B. Haas.)
(**A**) Thoracic radiographs reveal a mass in the caudal lung lobes. The mass proved to be an adenocarcinoma.
(**B**) Radiographs of the right carpus at initial presentation. Periosteal bone proliferations are visible along the radial and ulnar diaphysis. Similar changes were present in all four limbs.
(**C**) Radiographs of the right forelimb 3 months later. Note the enormous progression of bone proliferation.

successfully with steroid injection directly into the cyst in humans. Recently, successful treatment of a solitary bone cyst in the distal ulna of a 9-month-old cat with repeated steroid injections was reported (20). Repeated needle drainage and injection of methylprednisolone acetate was performed every 3 weeks for 12 weeks. Remodeling of the bone occurred over 14 months without signs of recurrence.

4.6 Hypertrophic osteopathy

Hypertrophic osteopathy is characterized by periosteal new bone formation along the long bones of the fore- and/or hindlimbs, occurring secondary to a distant disease process, most commonly tumors in the thoracic cavity. Clinical features in early cases are warm and swollen distal limbs due to hyperemia, and lameness. Later in the disease process, limb hyperemia is less pronounced and periosteal new bone formation develops along the long bones (Fig. 4-5). The joints are not affected, but range of motion can be reduced due to periarticular new bone formation. The exact pathogenesis of the disease remains unclear, but periosteal bone formation, induced by changes in blood supply, caused by autonomic neurovascular reflexes, is suspected.

Hypertrophic osteopathy in cats has been described in a handful of case reports. One report describes a cat with hypertrophic osteopathy affecting predominantly the forelimbs secondary to a thymoma (21). Two cases of hypertrophic osteopathy were secondary to bronchogenic carcinoma (22, 23). Two more recent reports include cats with abdominal lesions, a renal papillary adenoma (24) and an adrenocortical carcinoma (25). The thoracic cavity of the latter two cats was normal.

Treatment and prognosis depend on the underlying disease, but prognosis is usually not favorable due to malignancy of the primary disease. Regression of the bony lesions has been described after successful removal of the mass (25, 26).

4.7 Osteocartilaginous exostoses

Osteocartilaginous exostoses are relative rapidly growing tumor-like masses growing on the bony surface (Fig. 4-6). A solitary form and a multiple form, also called feline osteochondromatosis, have been described. The solitary form tends to affect older, FeLV-negative cats, and the multiple form is more commonly seen in younger, FeLV-positive cats.

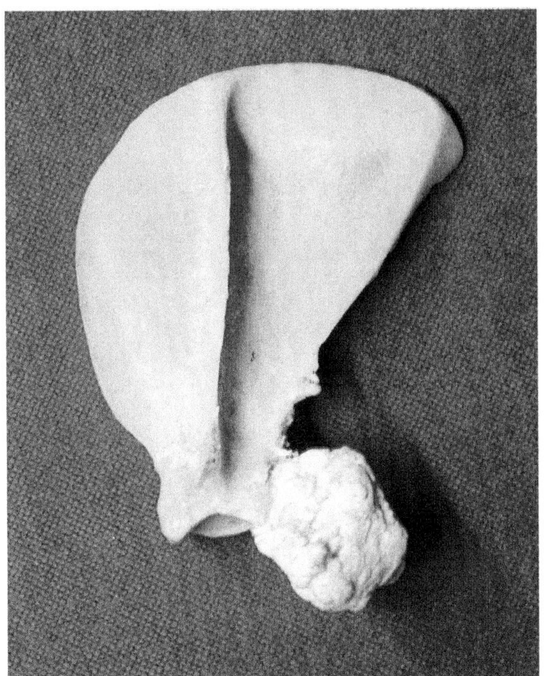

Figure 4.6 Bone specimen of a cat with a large solitary osteochondroma growing at the caudal aspect of the scapular neck.

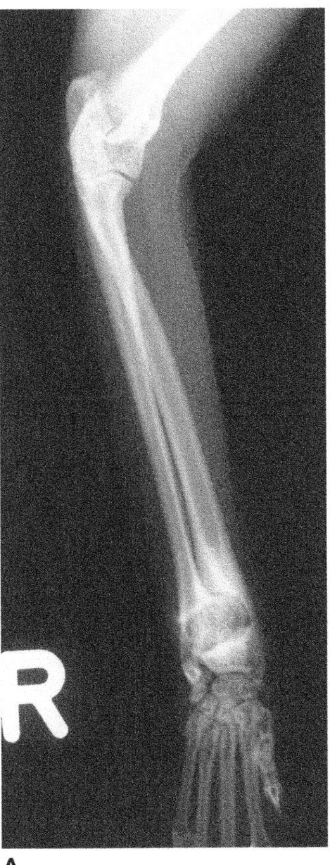

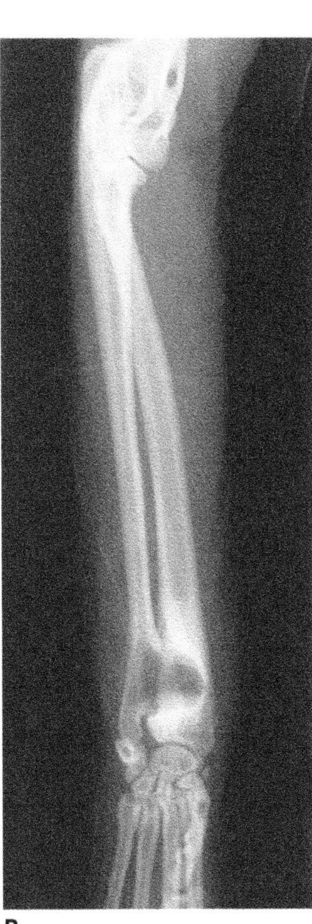

A B

Figure 4.7 Pre- and postoperative radiographs of the right radius and ulna of a 2-year old Persian cat with a solitary osteochondroma of the distal ulna.
(**A**) A smoothly marginated mass expands from the distal metaphysis of the ulna and deviates the distal radius. Histopathological examination revealed cartilaginous tissue, confluent with mature bone.
(**B**) The mass was locally excised with a partial distal ulnar ostectomy.

Siamese cats may be predisposed for both types. Malignant transformation of the lesions may occur.

4.7.1 Solitary osteochondromas

Solitary osteochondromas are exostoses consisting of cancellous bone, which grows from cartilaginous caps in the periosteum. They typically arise near growth plates. Whereas solitary osteochondromas cease growth after maturity in other species, they continue to grow in cats. The average age of cats with solitary osteochondromas was around 6 years in one survey (27). Solitary osteochondromas have been described to be localized in the spine, long bones, head, ribs, and pubis with decreasing frequency (28).

Clinical signs depend on the location and size of the mass, and include lameness, reluctance to move, joint stiffness due to impingement, and difficulty eating. Osteochondromas can reach large sizes. Radiologically, the lesions appear as broad-based, smoothly irregular masses with a clearly defined border (Fig. 4-7). Affected cats should be carefully screened for other bony lesions in order to rule out the multiple form of the disease, and a FeLV test should be performed. Hypervitaminosis A and synovial osteochondromas may be considered differential diagnoses in certain cases. Hypervitaminosis A is ruled out from the dietary history. Synovial osteochondromas (Chapter 5) also occur around joints, but these lesions do not originate from the bone itself (14). Definitive diagnosis is obtained by histopathological examination.

Treatment of choice is surgical excision (Fig. 4-7). Local regrowth is common, especially if the site of origin could not be excised completely. Regrowth usually occurs within months. Successful resection of a spinal osteochondroma was described (29). Radiation therapy or amputation may be other treatment options for masses where local resection is not possible (28, 30).

4.7.2 Feline osteochondromatosis

Osteochondromatous lesions are present at multiple sites in feline osteochondromatosis, The lesions are therefore also termed multiple cartilaginous exostoses (Chapter 8). Radiographically they appear similar to solitary osteochondromas, but differentiation is essential regarding treatment options and prognosis. Affected cats tend to be younger, with an average age of 2–3 years, than cats with the solitary form (28). The exact etiology of the disease is unclear, but may be associated with FeLV infection. Viral particles have been found in lesions (31), and several cats have tested positive for FeLV (27, 32). Histology is similar to the solitary form, but they may more resemble a sarcoma, rather than an osteochondroma.

Clinical signs depend on location of the masses and are similar as described for solitary osteochondromas. The lesions seem to have a predilection for flat and irregular bones and have been described to occur in the scapula, spine, ribs, pelvis, and long bones in decreasing frequency. The whole skeleton must be radiographed to detect all masses. The lesions continue to grow quite rapidly and no known treatment exists. Surgery or radiation therapy may be used as a palliative measure in selected cases.

References and further reading

1. Barber PJ, Elliott J. Study of calcium homeostasis in feline hyperthyroidism. J Small Anim Pract 1996;37:575–582.
2. Tomsa K, et al. Nutritional secondary hyperparathyroidism in six cats. J Small Anim Pract 1999;40:533–539.
3. Schrader SC, Sherding RG. Disorders of the skeletal system. In: Sherding RG (ed.) The cat: diseases and clinical management. New York: Churchill Livingstone; 1994: pp. 1599–1647.
4. Hazewinkel HAW. Nutrition in relation to skeletal growth deformities. J Small Anim Pract 1989;30:625–630.
5. Barber PJ, Elliot J. Feline chronic renal failure: calcium homeostasis in 80 cases diagnosed between 1992 and 1995. J Small Anim Pract 1998;39:108–116.
6. Hazewinkel HAW, Wiegand U. Generalisierte Skelettveränderungen. In: Horzinek MC, Schmidt V, Lutz H (eds) Krankheiten der Katze, 4th edn. Stuttgart: Enke Verlag; 2005: pp. 603–614.
7. Lucke VM. Renal disease in the domestic cat. J Pathol Bacteriol 1968;95:67–91.
8. Gnudi G, et al. Unusual hyperparathyroidism in a cat. Vet Radiol Ultrasound 2001;42:250–253.
9. Barber PJ, et al. Effect of dietary phosphate restriction on renal secondary hyperparathyroidism in the cat. J Small Anim Pract 1999;40:62–70.
10. Johnson KA, Watson ADJ. Skeletal diseases. In: Ettinger SJ, Feldman EC (eds) Textbook of veterinary internal medicine. Diseases of the dog and cat, 5th edn. Philadelphia: WB Saunders; 2000: pp. 1887–1919.
11. Franch J, et al. Back-scattered electron imaging of a nonvertebral case of hypervitaminosis A in a cat. J Feline Med Surg 2000;2:49–56.
12. Polizopoulou ZS, et al. Hypervitaminosis A in the cat: a case report and review of the literature. J Feline Med Surg 2005;7: 363–368.
13. Schmidt S, Geyer S. Hypervitaminosis A of the cat. Kleintierpraxis 1978;23:75–79.
14. Allan GS. Radiographic features of feline joint diseases. Vet Clin North Am Small Anim Pract 2000;30:281–302.
15. Bradley WA. Metaphyseal osteomyelitis in an immature Abyssinian cat. Aust Vet J 2003;81:608–611.
16. Wolf AM. Histoplasma capsulatum osteomyelitis in the cat. J Vet Intern Med 1987;1:158–162.
17. Taboada J. Systemic mycoses. In: Ettinger SJ, Feldman EC (eds) Textbook of veterinary internal medicine. Diseases of dogs and cats, 5th edn. Philadelphia: WB Saunders; 2000: pp. 453–476.
18. Biller DS, et al. Aneurysmal bone cyst in a rib of a cat. J Am Vet Med Assoc 1987;190:1193–1195.
19. Walker MA, et al. Aneurysmal bone cyst in a cat. J Am Vet Med Assoc 1975;167:933–934.
20. Miura N, et al. Steroid injection therapy in a feline solitary bone cyst. J Vet Med Sci 2003;65:523–525.
21. Richards CD. Hypertrophic osteoarthropathy in a cat. Feline Pract 1977;7:41–43.
22. Roberg J. Hypertrophic pulmonary osteoarthropathy. Feline Pract 1977;7:18–22.
23. Carr SH. Secondary pulmonary hypertrophic osteoarthropathy in a cat. Feline Pract 1971;1:25–26.
24. Nafe LA, et al. Hyerpertrophic osteopathy in a cat associated with renal papillary ademona. J Am Anim Hosp Assoc 1981;17:659–662.
25. Becker TJ, et al. Regression of hypertrophic osteopathy in a cat after surgical excision of an adrenocortical carcinoma. J Feline Med Surg 1999;35:499–505.
26. Brodey RS. Hypertrophic osteoarthropathy in the dog, a clinicopathologic survey of 60 cases. J Am Vet Med Assoc 1971; 159:1242.
27. Carpenter JL, et al. Tumors and tumor-like lesions. In: Holzworth J (ed.) Diseases of the cat. Medicine and surgery. Philadelphia: WB Saunders; 1987: pp. 407–596.
28. Moore AS, Ogilvie GK. Tumors of the skeletal system. In: Ogilvie GK, Moore AS (eds) Feline oncology. Trenton: Veterinary Learning Systems; 2001: pp. 233–250.
29. Reidarson TH, et al. Thoracic vertebral osteochondroma in a cat. J Am Vet Med Assoc 1988;192:1102–1104.
30. Wood BC, et al. What is your diagnosis? J Am Vet Med Assoc 2002;221:905–1080.
31. Pool RR, Harris JM. Feline osteochondromatosis. Feline Pract 1975;5:24–30.
32. Turrel JM, Pool RR. Primary bone tumors in the cat: a retrospective study of 15 cats and a literature review. Vet Radiol 1982;23:152–166.

5 Diseases of joints

K. Voss, S.J. Langley-Hobbs

Clinical degenerative joint disease is infrequently diagnosed in cats, whereas it is a common problem in dogs. In the last few years more attention has been focused on feline degenerative joint disease and the underlying joint pathologies in the veterinary literature. Recent studies have revealed a surprisingly high radiographic incidence of osteoarthritis in cats, but clinical relevance of the disease is likely to be underestimated. Improved awareness and diagnostic skills are required to obtain a clinical diagnosis of degenerative joint diseases in cats. Whereas degenerative joint disease is more often found in elderly cats, some of the underlying joint diseases may cause clinical signs earlier in life. These disease processes include hip dysplasia, patellar luxation, or osteochondrosis, which have hereditary components, but severity of clinical disease expression also depends on several other factors such as growth, nutrition, activity, and body weight.

Immune-mediated and infectious inflammatory joint diseases are well described in cats, but are encountered infrequently in daily feline practice. Both immune-mediated and infectious inflammatory arthritis have the potential for causing crippling arthropathies, and many of them carry a rather unfavorable long-term prognosis.

A summary of feline joint diseases is shown in Table 5-1. This chapter summarizes generalized joint diseases of cats. Diseases involving a specific joint, such as hip dysplasia, meniscal calcification, non-traumatic patellar fractures, or diseases of the elbow joint, are described in the corresponding chapters of part 7 of the book.

5.1 Degenerative joint disease

Degenerative joint disease can be classified into primary and secondary osteoarthritis. Primary or idiopathic osteoarthritis is considered to be due to wear and tear of the cartilage during the normal aging process. Secondary osteoarthritis is caused by an underlying joint pathology. Whereas osteoarthritis in dogs is especially common following joint dysplasia or osteochondrosis, inciting causes are rarely found in cats; potential causes were only identified in 11% of cats with radiographic osteoarthritis in one study (1). All joint patholo-

Disease group	Diseases
Inherited (Chapter 3)	Osteochondrodysplasia of the Scottish Fold cat Mucopolysaccharidosis
Congenital (Chapter 3)	Selected conditions of the skull, spine, thorax, and extremities
Inherited and developmental	Hip dysplasia (Chapter 36) Patellar luxation (Chapter 38) Osteochondrosis Elbow dysplasia (Chapter 30) Shoulder dysplasia (Chapter 28)
Degenerative	Primary and secondary degenerative joint disease
Nutritional (Chapter 4)	Hypervitaminosis A
Inflammatory	Erosive polyarthritis Non-erosive polyarthritis
Miscellaneous	Meniscal mineralization (Chapter 38) Non-traumatic patellar fractures (Chapter 38) Elbow epicondylitis (Chapter 30) Synovial osteochondromatosis Synovial cysts (Chapter 30)

Table 5-1. Joint diseases in cats. Some of the listed diseases, such as hypervitaminosis A and osteochondromas, arise from bone but result in secondary joint ankylosis

gies resulting in incongruity or instability have the potential to cause secondary osteoarthritis. Joint trauma and joint dysplasia are probably the most common inciting causes in cats.

Pathogenesis, pathophysiology, and treatment modalities for degenerative joint disease have been studied extensively in humans and dogs because of the high incidence in these species. The basic pathophysiological mechanisms of osteoarthritis are the same in the canine and feline patient, but results from experimental studies indicate that degenerative joint disease develops at a slower rate in cats than in dogs (2, 3). Pathological changes in a joint with osteoarthritis include cartilage fibrillation, erosion and clefts, subchondral bone sclerosis, formation of osteophytes and enthesophytes, fibrosis of the joint capsule, and variable degrees of synovitis. Osteoarthritis-associated pain is due to synovitis and changes in the subchondral bone, as the hyaline cartilage does not contain nerve endings.

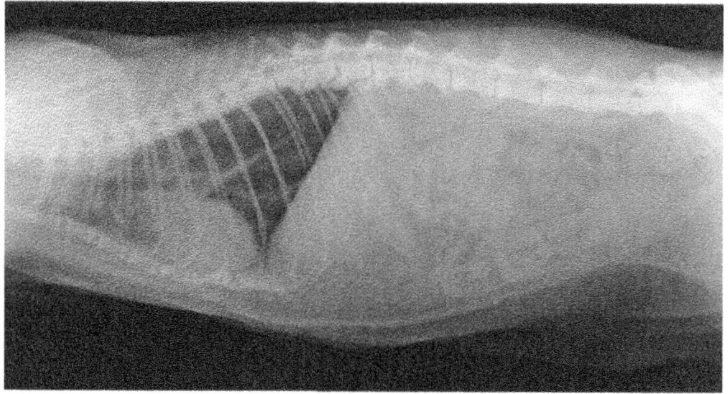

Figure 5-1 Laterolateral radiograph of a 15-year-old cat with degenerative disease of the thoracolumbar spine. Bridging spondylosis is the main radiographic finding. The cat showed no clinical signs associated with the lesions.

5.1.1 Incidence

Cats suffering from osteoarthritis are usually older (1). One study showed 34% of cats with a mean age of 6.5 years to have radiographic evidence of osteoarthritis (4). In cats older than 12 years, the radiographic incidence of osteoarthritis was reported to be as high as 90% (5). Despite these high numbers, the disease is rather infrequently diagnosed clinically. Only 33% of cats with radiographic osteoarthritis had clinically evident osteoarthritis in one study (1). This implies that cats are able to compensate for pain and functional deficits of minor joint diseases better than dogs, probably due to their agility and lighter body weights. Also, awareness of both owners and veterinarians for the disease is not as high as in canine patients, and the clinical signs may be misinterpreted or missed.

According to the literature, the spine was the most common site for degenerative joint disease in cats older than 12 years (5). Most of the spinal lesions were classified as low grade in this study, except for the lumbosacral articulation, where medium- or high-grade lesions were found. The elbow is the most commonly affected joint of the appendicular skeleton, followed by the hip joint (6). Severe elbow osteoarthritis was found in 17% of cats older than 12 years (5). In another report of 40 cats with osteoarthritis, the elbow joint was

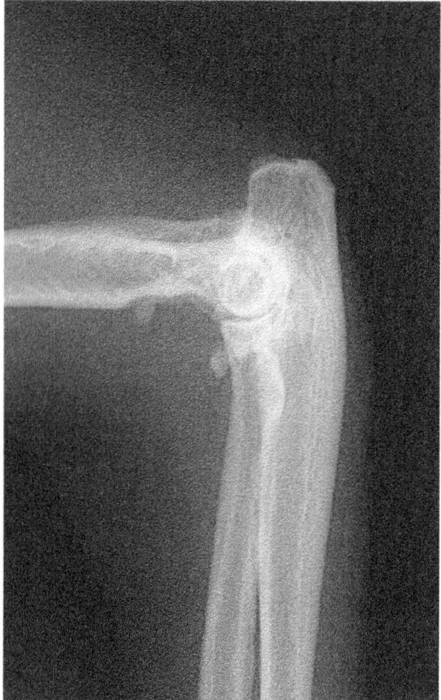

A

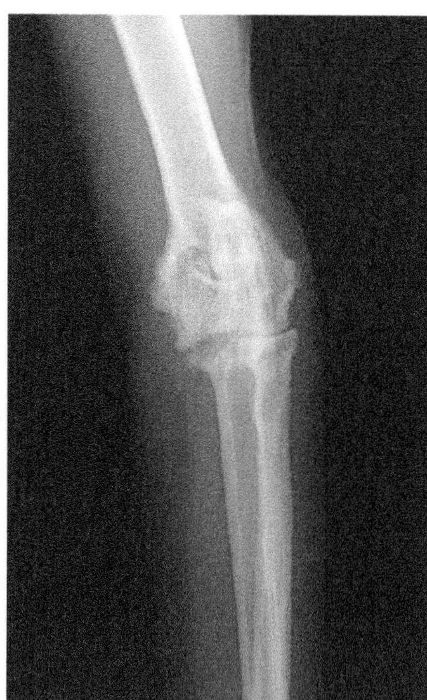

B

Figure 5-2 (**A**) Mediolateral and (**B**) craniocaudal radiographs of the elbow of a 14-year-old cat with elbow osteoarthritis, presented for intermittent forelimb lameness. Osteophytosis and soft-tissue mineralization are present, most evident at the cranial and medial aspect of the joint. The mineralization cranial to the radial head is most likely the sesamoid bone of the supinator muscle. Slight subchondral sclerosis is seen at the ulnar notch.

overrepresented by a factor of 4.3 (7). This high incidence of degenerative joint disease of the elbow raises the question if primary factors, such as elbow dysplasia or incongruity, could be inciting causes (Chapter 30). Osteoarthritis of the hip joint is often secondary to hip dysplasia (6). Gonarthrosis is also relatively common and is usually associated with rupture of the cranial cruciate ligament.

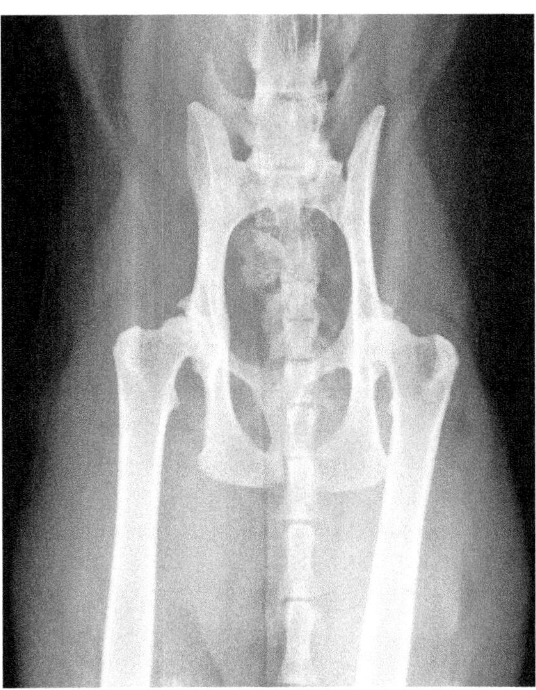

Figure 5-3 Ventrodorsal radiographs of a 10-year-old Persian cat with bilateral hip dysplasia and coxarthrosis. The acetabula are shallow, the femoral heads have an abnormal shape, and osteophytes are most evident at the cranial aspect of the acetabulum.

The limiting factor with these studies and figures on incidences is that they were mainly retrospective and involved looking at thoracic and abdominal radiographs where the hips, stifles, and elbows were often visible, but the carpi and tarsi were less commonly seen.

5.1.2 Diagnosis

The clinical manifestation of osteoarthritis is higher in obese cats than in cats with a normal body condition. Obese cats were three times as likely to be presented to a veterinarian for lameness (8). Clinical signs of degenerative joint disease in cats can be different from those in other species. Cats commonly show non-specific signs, such as changes in demeanor, inactivity or difficulty or reluctance to jump, and a stiff gait, rather than limping (6, 9). Owners may observe the cat hesitating before, or pausing during, activities such as climbing stairs. Pain can also change grooming habits, or can even lead to urination or defecation next to the litter box due to difficulties climbing into the box. Changes in behavior and activity in older cats are often attributed to advanced age, by both owners and clinicians.

Radiographic signs of osteoarthritis in cats are similar to those seen in dogs. Periarticular new-bone formation, subchondral bone sclerosis, changes in bone shape and density, thickening of the joint capsule, and calcified intra-articular bodies may be present (10, 11). Thickening of the joint capsule is usually less, and calcified intra-articular bodies are more commonly seen in cats than in dogs (11). Examples of radiographs of joints affected by osteoarthritis are shown in Figures 5-1 to 5-5. Please also see the chapters in part 7 of

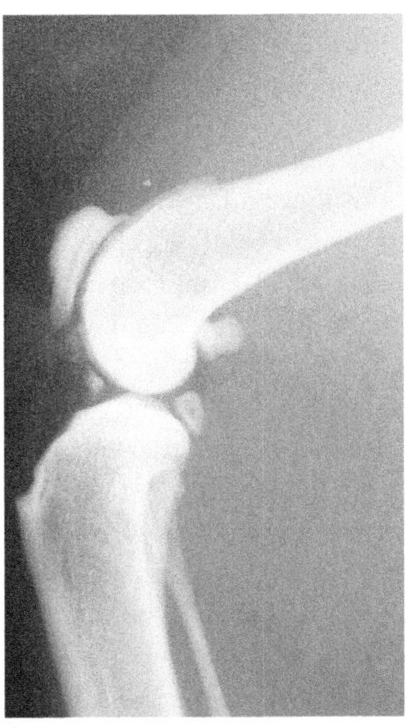

A

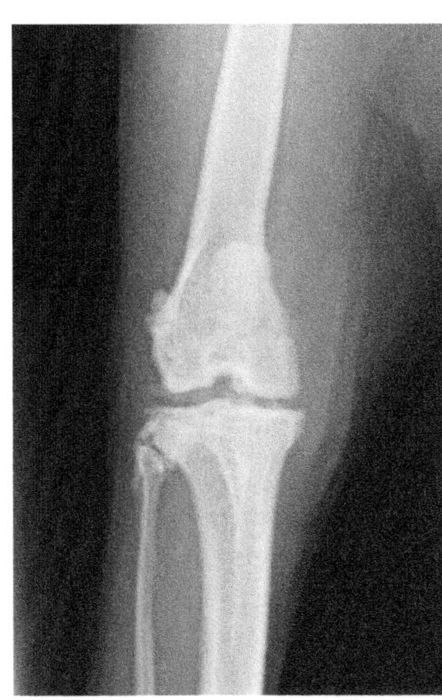

B

Figure 5-4 (**A**) Mediolateral and (**B**) caudocranial radiographs of a 15-year-old cat with osteoarthritis of the stifle joint. Osteophytes are present at the distal and proximal patella, along the proximal trochlear ridges, and at the dorsal borders of the tibia. Intra-articular mineralizations are seen, the distal one possibly associated with the medial meniscus.

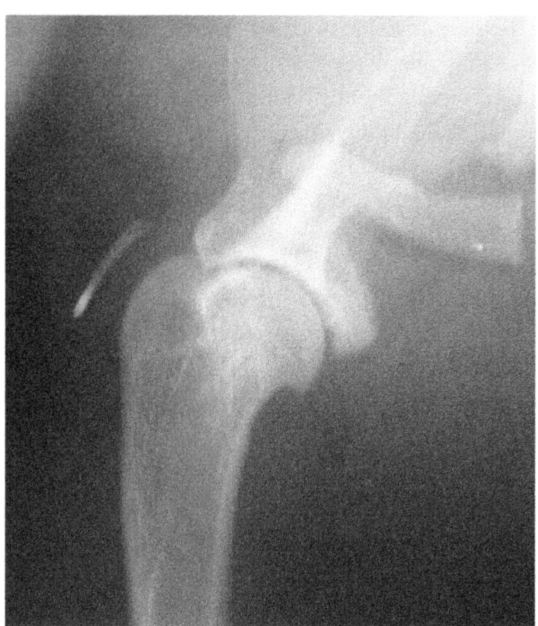

Figure 5-5 Mediolateral radiograph of an 11-year-old cat with shoulder osteoarthritis and intermittent lameness. Osteophyte formation is most evident at the caudal edge of the glenoid, resulting in a change of shape.

the book for more information on underlying causes and differential diagnoses in the specific joints.

Differential diagnoses for osteoarthritis in general include Scottish Fold osteochondrodysplasia, hypervitaminosis A, osteochondromas, synovial osteochondromatosis, and immune-mediated or infectious arthritis. The presence of bilateral joint pathology, especially with tarsal and carpal joint involvement, and concurrent systemic illness should alert the clinician to the possibility of inflammatory joint disease. Degenerative and inflammatory joint diseases can be differentiated by cytological examination of the synovial fluid (Chapter 2).

5.1.3 Treatment

Surgical treatment of osteoarthritis is reserved for cats with an inciting cause, such as joint instability, and is described in part 7 of the book. Most cases are treated conservatively.

Conservative management of osteoarthritis in cats involves environmental changes and physiotherapy, weight loss in obese cats, and pain control (10) (Box 5-1). Preferred feeding or sleeping spots should be made readily reachable for the cat, for example by building a ramp or dividing one large leap into smaller leaps with furniture or other objects. Moderate exercise is beneficial for osteoarthritic joints. As cats generally refuse to be led on a leash or to perform other types of exercise, the cat's daily routine has to be used to enhance activity. Gentle playing or taking the cat outdoors might enhance activity and overall well-being. The spotlight of a laser pointer motivates many cats to play and chase. Regular physiotherapy sessions with a physical therapist can also improve joint function and reduce pain (Chapter 21). Weight loss is an important factor in the management of osteoarthritis, as obese cats are more likely to suffer from clinical signs associated with degenerative joint disease. This point should be discussed thoroughly with the owners to enhance their motivation. Regular follow-up examinations are also helpful to improve compliance.

Meloxicam is currently the only non-steroidal anti-inflammatory drug (NSAID) licensed in Europe for long-term use in cats. Meloxicam has been shown to be an effective analgesic for feline locomotor diseases (12). Improvement of general demeanor, activity level, and ability to jump was observed after application of meloxicam for a 4–6-week period in clinical patients (6, 9), with 61% of owners feeling that their cat had markedly improved (6). Mild gastrointestinal side-effects did occur at the beginning of the treatment period in 18% of cats, when higher initial dosages were administered (6). Current dose recommendations are lower and are shown in Box 5-2. Meloxicam may also be administered with other analgesic substances if required (Chapter 18), but should never be combined with other NSAIDs or corticosteroids.

Box 5-1. Suggestions for conservative treatment of osteoarthritis

Weight reduction if necessary
Environmental changes (facilitated access to feeding, favorite sleeping spots, and litter box)
Physical therapy
Motivation for enhanced physical activity at home
Long-term application of slow-acting disease-modifying agents
Pain control (meloxicam)

Box 5-2. Meloxicam dosage for long-term application

Meloxicam (Metacam 0.5 mg/ml oral suspension for cats)
0.1 mg/kg on first day
Followed by 0.05 mg/kg SID
A lower dose of 0.025 mg/kg SID also has an effect, and may be tried

Other NSAIDs should be used very cautiously in the feline species. Cats have a reduced hepatic activity for glucuronide conjugation, which is necessary for metabolizing many drugs, including most of the NSAIDs. Therefore accumulation and toxicity might be encountered with drugs and dosages considered safe in other species. All NSAIDs are contraindicated in the presence of hypovolemia, dehydration, and kidney disease.

Chondroprotective slow-acting disease-modifying agents were shown to be efficient in the treatment of osteoarthritis in both dogs and humans (13, 14). Although similar studies are not available for cats, clinical impressions suggest that these agents may be beneficial in the treatment of feline osteoarthritis (9, 10). One commercial nutritional supplement available for cats contains chondroitin sulfate, glucosamine hydrochloride, and manganese ascorbate (Cosequin). These substances are precursors for synthesis of hyaline cartilage matrix. Additionally, glucosamine may have anti-inflammatory properties and stimulate the synthesis of hyaluronan by synovial cells. Chondroitin sulfate inhibits cartilage metalloproteinases. The overall effect of this combination of nutritional supplements is facilitation of synthesis of cartilage matrix and hyaluronan, reduction of cartilage degradation, and anti-inflammatory properties. The clinical response to those drugs only occurs gradually over several weeks.

5.2 Polyarthritis

Polyarthritis is a rare systemic inflammatory joint disease with a variety of different etiologies, involving at least two joints. The main feature of these diseases is marked inflammation of the synovial lining, and inflammatory cells migrating into the joint and synovial fluid. Smaller joints, such as the carpi and tarsi, are most commonly involved. Polyarthritis is grossly classified into erosive and non-erosive forms (Table 5-2).

5.2.1 Diagnosis

Cats with polyarthritis are usually systemically ill and reluctant to walk. Marked joint pain, joint effusion, and fever are detected on clinical examination. Pronounced swelling and edema of the overlying soft tissues may also be present (Fig. 5-6). Cats with chronic polyarthritis, especially with the erosive forms, often suffer from generalized muscle atrophy and weight loss, and can have a cachectic appearance.

Cytological examination of the synovial fluid is the single most important method for diagnosing polyarthritis, and it also may allow differentiation between immune-mediated and infectious arthritis (15). Neutrophil numbers are in the high range during the acute phase of immune-mediated polyarthritis (Fig. 5-7). Lymphocytes and plasma cells predominate later, with neutrophils still remaining above the top end of the normal range. With septic arthritis, degeneration of neutrophils and intracellular bacteria may be seen in addition to the high neutrophil count (Fig. 5-8). Bacteriological evaluation of the synovial fluid including sensitivity testing should also be performed, especially if cytology is suggestive for infectious arthritis. Some infectious agents are difficult to culture (see next section). Cytological and bacteriological

Form	General	Subclassification
Erosive	Feline chronic progressive polyarthritis (FCPP)	Periosteal proliferative form Destructive form/rheumatoid arthritis
	Septic polyarthritis	
Non-erosive	Immune-mediated non-erosive polyarthritis	Type 1: no underlying cause found Type 2: associated with systemic infection Type 3: associated with gastrointestinal disease Type 4: associated with malignancy
	Feline systemic lupus erythematosus	
	Drug-induced polyarthritis	Drugs (antibiotics) Vaccines
	Infectious	Calicivirus Lyme disease

Table 5-2. Classification of feline polyarthritis into erosive and non-erosive forms

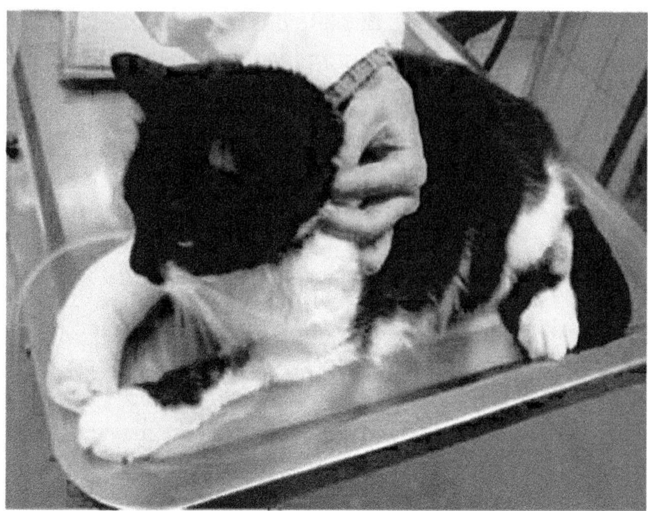

Figure 5-6 A 10-year-old cat with septic polyarthritis, presented with fever, apathy, and reluctance to walk. Note the swelling of the distal limbs. Culture of the synovial fluid revealed *Streptococcus canis*.

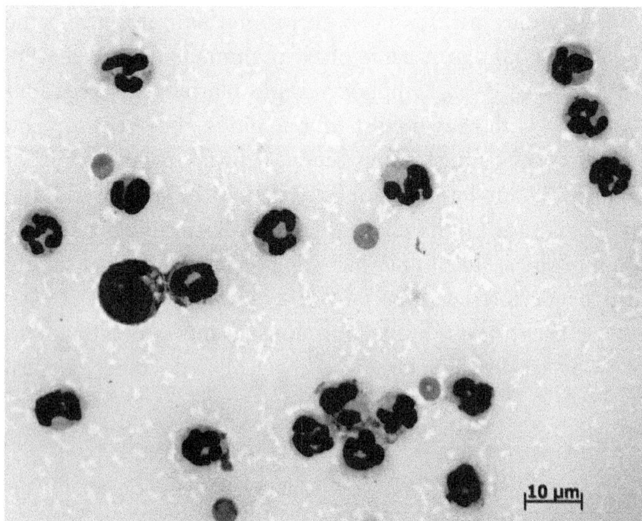

Figure 5-7 Cytology of the synovial fluid from the elbow of a 10-year-old cat with immune-mediated non-erosive polyarthritis. A large number of non-degenerate neutrophils were present in the joint fluid and culture was negative. The cat was feline leukemia virus (FeLV)-positive. (Courtesy of Veterinary Pathology, Zurich.)

examination of the synovial fluid is further described in Chapter 2.

Synovial biopsy may give additional information. Histopathological appearance of the synovium depends on the type and duration of disease. Exudative inflammation with a predominance of neutrophils is seen in the acute phases of immune-mediated polyarthritis. Cell types shift towards lymphocytes and plasma cells in chronic cases, and fibroplasia develops (16). Pyogranulomatous synovitis is present with septic arthritis (17).

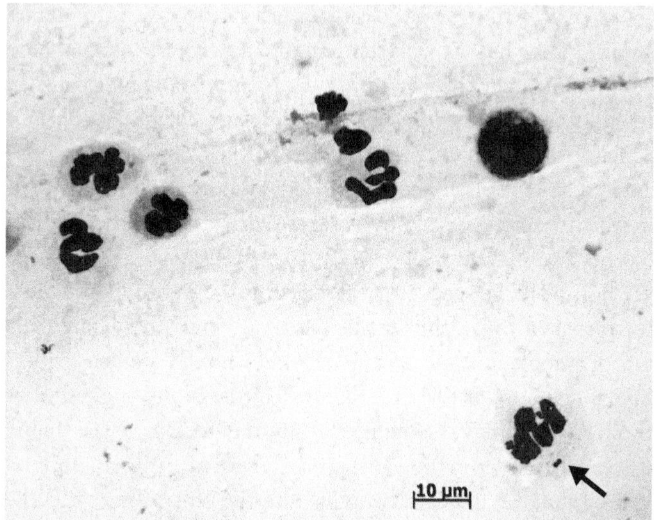

Figure 5-8 A smear of synovial fluid from the tarsus of a 10-year-old indoor cat with an acute hematogenous infectious arthritis. Intracellular cocci can be seen (arrow) but the neutrophils are non-degenerate. *Streptococcus canis* was cultured. (Courtesy of Veterinary Pathology, Zurich.)

Radiographs of affected joints help differentiate erosive from non-erosive forms of polyarthritis (Table 5-2). However, the bony changes seen on radiographs only develop with time, and lesions might not be apparent in the early disease process. Soft-tissue swelling is the only radiographic finding in cats with non-erosive polyarthritis.

Screening for general or malignant disease, feline leukemia virus (FeLV), and specific blood tests usually needs to be performed to find or rule out the inciting cause. Doxycycline can be given while awaiting the results of the diagnostic tests. It has antimicrobial properties against some of the infectious agents that could be causing the polyarthritis and its immune-modulating effects may improve clinical signs of cats with immune-mediated polyarthritis. Figure 5-9 shows a possible regime for the diagnostic and therapeutic approach in cats with polyarthritis.

5.2.2 Erosive polyarthritis

Erosive forms of polyarthritis are feline chronic progressive polyarthritis (FCPP) and septic arthritis.

Feline chronic progressive polyarthritis

Cats with FCPP are generally intact or neutered males, often between 1.5 and 5 years old (16). The tarsi and carpi are commonly affected. Around half of affected cats test positive for FeLV, and many cats are positive for feline syncytia-forming virus (FeSFV) (16, 18). Both viruses were also isolated from affected joints (16). The exact role of these viral infections in the disease mechanism is not clear yet. It was

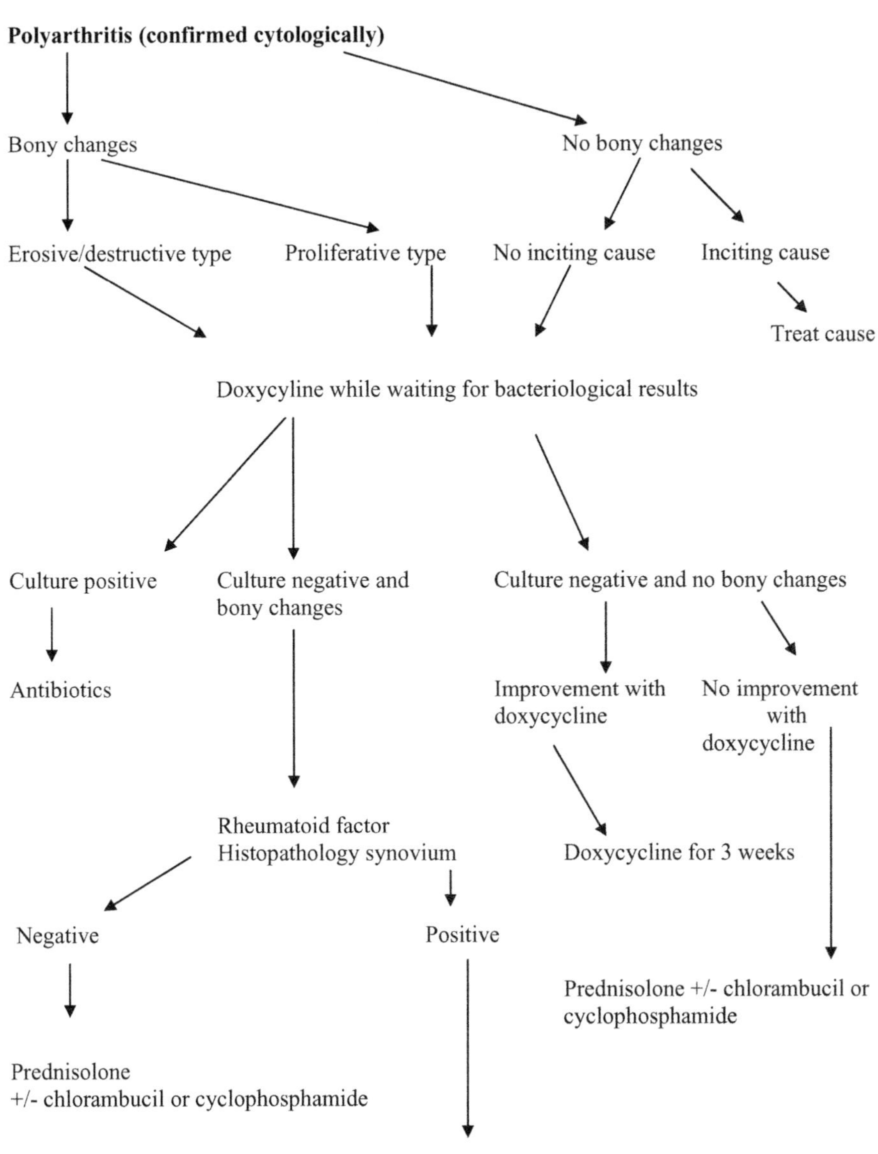

Figure 5-9 Diagram showing the diagnostic and therapeutic approach to feline polyarthritis.

suggested that immunosuppression caused by FeLV may allow FeSFV to multiply in the joints (16).

Two forms of FCPP have been described: the periosteal proliferative form, and the destructive form. The periosteal proliferative form is the more common of the two. Its main feature is progressive formation of periosteal new bone. Smaller areas of lysis and osteoporosis may also occur in the affected joints (Fig. 5-10). The destructive form of FCPP is less common, affected cats tend to be older, and the disease appears to be more chronic and insidious in onset (16, 19). Radiographic signs include areas of lysis, progressing later to marked joint destruction and instability. The disease has similarities to rheumatoid arthritis, but a positive rheumatoid factor or characteristic histological changes in the synovium must be present in addition to radiographic evidence of joint destruction in order to classify the disease as rheumatoid arthritis (18, 20). Siamese cats may be overrepresented (20).

A treatment trial with prednisolone is usually performed first. Prednisolone is administered at a dose of 2–4 mg/kg SID for 2 weeks, and is then slowly tapered to a dose of 0.25 mg/kg SID for a further 2–3 months. Treatment success is evaluated by assessment of the clinical response, and by repeating synovial fluid cell count and differentiation. Prednisolone therapy alone can improve clinical signs and slow down the processes of joint destruction. However, disease relapse is common, and many cats have to receive continuous therapy (16, 18). The addition of cytotoxic drugs, such as cyclophosphamide or chlorambucil, is indicated with lack of improvement with prednisolone alone. Azathioprine should not be

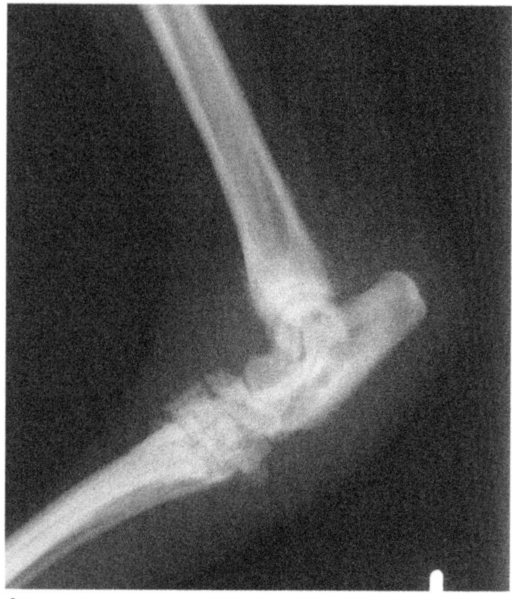

A

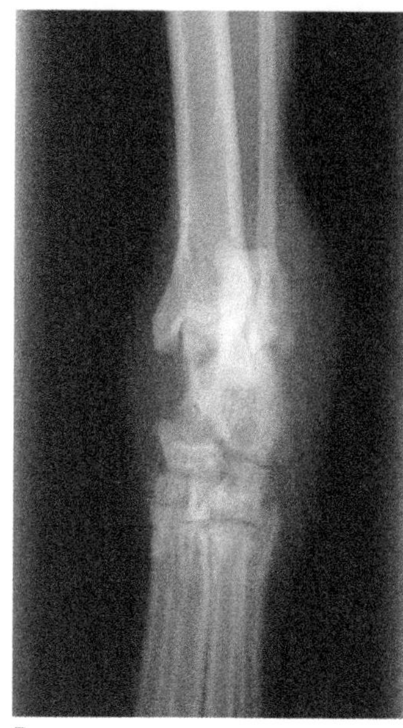

B

Figure 5-10 (**A**) Mediolateral and (**B**) dorsoplantar radiographs of the tarsal joint of a cat with the periosteal form of feline chronic progressive polyarthritis. Periosteal proliferative bone reactions are evident at the level of the distal tarsal bones, and on the lateral side of the tarsus. Also note the soft-tissue swelling around the joint.

used in cats due to severe and potentially fatal side-effects (16, 21). Cats receiving cytotoxic drugs should be monitored closely for side-effects. Complete blood counts are performed every 2–4 weeks to detect myelosuppression, requiring dose reduction or discontinuation of therapy. Cyclophosphamide may cause hemorrhagic cystitis, also necessitating discontinuation of therapy. Application of disease-modifying antirheumatic drugs (DMARDs) was described in 12 cats with rheumatoid arthritis and results appeared to be encouraging (20). Methotrexate and leflunomide given by the oral route resulted in marked improvement within 4 weeks in more than 50% of the cats. No serious toxic side-effects were encountered over the treatment period of 2–6 months (20). Drugs and dosages are summarized in Table 5-3.

Drugs	Dosages
Doxycycline	10 mg/kg SID
Prednisolone	2–4 mg/kg BW SID for 2 weeks, then gradually reduce to 0.25 mg/kg SID over 2–3 months
Cyclophosphamide	50 mg/m^2 on 4 consecutive days per week, max. 4 months (in combination with 0.25 mg/kg prednisolone)
Chlorambucil	0.1–0.2 mg/kg SID or on alternate days (in combination with 0.25 mg/kg prednisolone)
Methotrexate	2.5 mg at 0, 12, and 24 hours on the same day each week (total of 7.5 mg weekly) Decrease dose to 2.5 mg once a week after clinical improvement (20)
Leflunomide	10 mg daily (70 mg weekly) Decrease dose to 10 mg twice a week after clinical improvement (20)

Table 5-3. Drugs used in the treatment of immune-mediated polyarthritis

Septic polyarthritis

Bacteria can enter a joint via several routes: through a penetrating injury, during surgery, by extension from local infections, or via the hematogenous route. Penetrating wounds, especially cat bites, are the most common cause for septic monoarthritis in cats (Chapter 14). Hemotogenous spread of bacteria from a distant site of the body is less common in cats than in dogs (19). Kittens and cats with suppression of the immune system may be more susceptible to develop septic arthritis or polyarthritis. Several joints are usually involved, and the tarsi and carpi are most commonly affected. Diagnosis is based on the presence of degenerate neutrophils and intracellular bacteria in the synovial fluid (Fig. 5-8), and on positive bacteriology results.

Several bacteria have been isolated from cats with polyarthritis, including *Pasteurella* spp., *Streptococcus* spp., *Mycoplasma* spp., and L-form bacteria (17, 19, 22–25). Anaerobes, mycoplasma, and especially L-form bacteria are difficult to culture. L-form bacteria can grow on mycoplasma-specific culture medium, but differentiating between L-form bacteria and mycoplasma according to colony appearance is difficult

(19). Subcutaneous abscesses may precede bacterial L-form and mycoplasma polyarthritis (17), and the clinician should suspect these species in cats with subcutaneous abscesses and polyarthritis, and negative routine bacteriological cultures. Bacterial L-forms and mycoplasma are usually sensitive to tetracycline or doxycycline (Table 5-3). A positive response can be expected as early as 48 hours after initiation of therapy (19). Antibiotics are continued for several weeks if a positive response is seen. Repeating radiographs, cytology, and mycoplasma culture before cessation of therapy seems reasonable.

Antibiotic treatment is selected according to sensitivity testing if the bacterial culture reveals other organisms, such as *Pasteurella* or *Streptococcus*. Prognosis depends on the inciting cause of infection, the immunocompetence of the patient, and the duration of clinical signs but cats should respond well to long-term antimicrobial therapy.

5.2.3 Non-erosive polyarthritis

Non-erosive forms of polyarthritis include immune-mediated non-erosive polyarthritis, drug- and vaccine-induced polyarthritis, polyarthritis in association with systemic lupus erythematosus, viral-induced polyarthritis, and possibly Lyme disease.

Immune-mediated non-erosive polyarthritis

Immune-mediated non-erosive polyarthitis is caused by deposition of immune complexes in the synovial membrane, leading to subsequent inflammation. Several inciting causes might be responsible for activation of the immune system (Table 5-2). Systemic inflammatory or infectious diseases, diseases of the gastrointestinal, respiratory, and urinary tract, and neoplasia have been seen in association with non-erosive polyarthritis (Fig. 5-9) (18, 19). Myeloproliferative neoplasia was the most commonly diagnosed tumor (18). A bone marrow biopsy should therefore be performed if myeloproliferative disease is suspected from hematological results. An underlying cause is not found in many cats, and the polyarthritis is then classified as idiopathic, or type 1.

Therapy aims at removing the inciting cause, if possible. It may be difficult to differentiate immune-mediated non-erosive polyarthritis from other forms of non-erosive polyarthritis, such as drug-, vaccine-, or virus-induced arthritis, or Lyme disease. If in doubt an initial trial of doxycyline should be tried first (18). If a positive response is seen, doxycyline is administered for 2–3 weeks. Prednisolone therapy is started if the response is negative. Cytotoxic drugs may have to be administered in addition to prednisolone in cases with insufficient treatment response. Drugs and dosages are listed in Table 5-3.

Prognosis relates to the inciting cause. Three out of nine cats were euthanized due to persistent lameness or relapse in one study (19). The prognosis for cats with myeloproliferative tumors is poor.

Feline systemic lupus erythematosus

Systemic lupus erythematosus is a multisystemic disease occurring rarely in cats (18, 21). Affected cats may have autoimmune hemolytic anemia, thrombocytopenia, leukopenia, dermatitis, glomerulonephritis, polymyositis, and non-erosive polyarthritis. Antibodies against blood cells cause their alteration, and deposition of immune complexes results in dermatitis, myositis, and arthritis. The presence of circulating antinuclear antibodies supports the diagnosis, but antinuclear antibodies are not specific for systemic lupus erythematosus. Treatment is aimed at immunosuppression, using prednisolone in combination with other cytotoxic drugs, such as cyclophosphamide and chlorambucil (Table 5-3). Prognosis is guarded and becomes even more unfavorable if renal involvement occurs (21).

Drug-induced polyarthritis

Drugs or vaccinations may serve as antigenic sources for production of a hypersensitivity reaction in the synovial membrane. Antibiotics are known to be able to induce polyarthritis, especially sulfadiazine, erythromycin, and cephalosporins. Polyarthritis was observed in one cat after administration of trimethoprim–sulfadiazine for the treatment of cystitis (19). Drug-induced polyarthritis resolves if drug administration is discontinued.

Feline calicivirus vaccines can also induce polyarthritis in cats. Affected cats are generally younger than 6 months, and clinical signs often occurred within 1 week after the first vaccination (26). In a study of 123 cats with vaccine reactions or breakdowns after calicivirus vaccination, 80% of affected cats showed signs of inflammatory arthropathy, either alone or in conjunction with pyrexia and oral or upper respiratory disease (26). Vaccine-induced polyarthritis is self-limiting, and a specific treatment is not required.

Viral infections

Viral infections with FeLV, FeSFV, and feline calicivirus have been associated with polyarthritis and lameness in the cat. Polyarthritis seen with FeLV or FeSFV may rather be caused by the host's immunological reactions rather than by the virus itself.

Infection with feline calicivirus is able to cause respiratory and ocular disease, a febrile lameness syndrome with polyarthritis, or a combination of the two. Symptoms are most severe in cattery kittens, but older cats can also be affected

(26). Both field and vaccine strain of virus, and virus antigen could be isolated from joints in cats (27–29), but the presence of virus in the joint did not necessarily cause arthritis in every case (29). Lameness was more severe after exposure to a field strain of virus when compared to a vaccine strain in one study (29).

Treatment is usually not necessary, because the clinical signs resolve spontaneously after several days (21). NSAIDs can be used in severe cases to alleviate joint pain.

Lyme disease

Lyme disease is caused by the spirochete *Borrelia burgdorferi*, which is transmitted by ticks of the Ixodes group. The role of *Borrelia* in the pathogenesis of polyarthritis is unclear, but it seems to be able to cause a low-grade inflammatory arthropathy of one or several joints in dogs and cats (30, 31). In dogs, arthritis develops after an incubation period of around 2 months in joints closest to the tick bite (31). Systemic illness, such as fever or lymphadenopathy, may also be seen.

B. burgdorferi is difficult to culture, and serological testing is of questionable diagnostic value, as many clinically normal cats have positive titers. Approximately 5% of cats tested in the UK had antibodies against *B. burgdorferi* (32, 33). Antibodies develop consistently after experimental infection of cats with *B. burgdorferi*, but cats do not necessarily show clinical signs associated with the infection (30, 34).

Lyme disease could be considered a possible etiology of inflammatory non-erosive arthritis when no other causes are found, and when there is a history or possibility of tick infection, but it should be remembered that a positive *B. burgdorferi* antibody titer does not confirm the disease. Therapy in suspected cases of Lyme disease consists of administration of antibiotics, usually tetracyclines (Table 5-3).

5.3 Miscellaneous diseases

A few diseases of feline joints have been described in case reports or case series, but not much is known on incidence, cause, and treatment. These conditions are summarized below. Diseases involving a specific joint are described in the corresponding chapters of part 7 of the book.

5.3.1 Osteochondrosis

Osteochondrosis has been rarely documented in cats. It is a primary abnormality of endochondral ossification (35). Epiphyseal chondrocytes fail to mature normally and the extracellular cartilage matrix does not calcify. This failure results in local thickening of cartilage compared to normal areas. The increased thickness of the cartilage impedes nutrition of deeper layers, which eventually results in local necrosis and separation of a cartilage flap between the calcified and non-calcified layers. The loose flap may later dislodge and can become a free joint body. The disease is then called osteochondrosis dissecans. Synovitis and degenerative cartilage changes develop in the affected joint and sclerosis of the subchondral bone occurs around the area of the abnormal cartilage layer. The etiology of osteochondrosis in dogs remains unclear. Besides a hereditary component, factors such as diet, growth rate, trauma, changes in joint morphometry, and hormonal imbalance contribute to the expression of the disease.

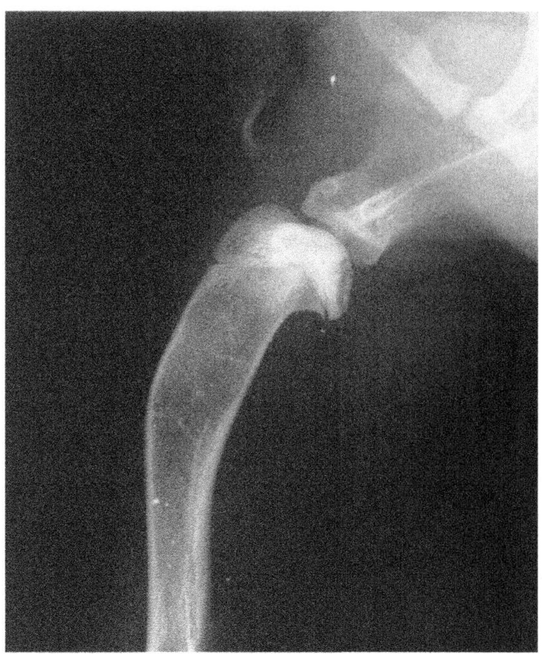

Figure 5-11 Mediolateral radiograph of the shoulder joint of a 10-month-old cat with an osteochondrosis-like lesion in the caudal humeral head. Deformation of the proximal humeral metaphysis is also present. The reason for these bony changes could not be determined. Similar changes were present in the contralateral shoulder. (Courtesy of J.C. Dubuis.)

Case reports suggest that osteochondrosis can also occur in the feline species. Three case reports describe osteochondrosis or osteochondrosis-like lesions in the shoulder and stifle joint (36–38). Affected cats were young and presented for lameness. Radiographic and intraoperative features of the cartilage flap were similar to those seen in dogs. Lesions were located on the caudal aspect of the humeral head (Fig. 5-11) and on the lateral femoral epicondyles. Histopathological analysis of the removed flap was performed in two of the described cases and appeared consistent with a dislodged osteochondrosis flap (37, 38).

Cats can be treated similarly to dogs, by an arthrotomy and removal of the loose cartilage flap. The area is curetted, until subchondral bone is exposed. Osteostixis creates vascular channels to facilitate healing of the defect. From the limited information available in the veterinary literature,

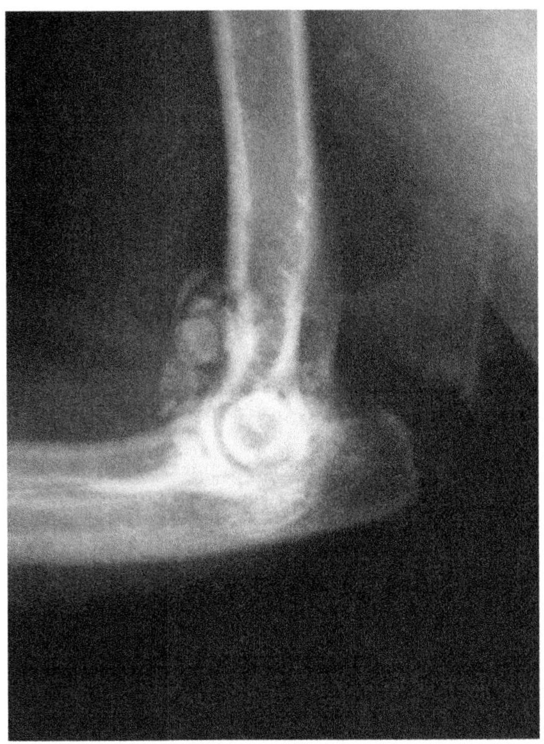

Figure 5-12 Radiograph of the elbow joint of a cat with suspected synovial osteochondromatosis. Several large rounded mineralized structures are seen at the cranial aspect of the joint, possibly located within the cranial joint capsule.

prognosis seems to be good, at least on a short- or medium-term basis (36, 37). The cat with bilateral stifle osteochondrosis returned to normal function (37).

5.3.2 Synovial osteochondromatosis

Ossified nodules located in joints may represent synovial osteochondromatosis, or synovial osteochondrometaplasia (Fig. 5-12). These nodules arise in the joint capsule from nodules of cartilage that are formed by synovial metaplasia. The cartilage nodules can ossify and are then visible on radiographs as rounded calcified structures in the vicinity of joints. In contrast to solitary osteochondromas or feline osteochondromatosis (Chapter 5), the calcifications seen in synovial osteochondromatosis do not seem to be attached to the bone, but the two conditions can look similar (39).

Synovial osteochondromatosis needs to be differentiated radiographically from other diseases causing periarticular calcification or ossification, such as feline osteochondromatosis (Chapter 4), hypervitaminosis A (Chapter 4), and fibrodysplasia ossificans or myositis ossificans (Chapter 7). A differential diagnosis for ossified bodies in the stifle joint is intra-articular calcification of the medial meniscus or cranial cruciate ligament (Chapter 38). Synovial osteochondromatosis of the elbow needs to be differentiated from severe elbow osteoarthritis, and from medial epicondylitis of the humerus (Chapter 30).

Synovial osteochondromatosis is usually treated conservatively, as the lesions are located within the joint capsule and are difficult to remove (40).

5.3.3 Synovial cysts

Synovial cysts are periarticular structures filled with synovial fluid. They originate from the synovium of joints, bursae, or tendon sheaths, and can grow to large sizes. Several cats with synovial cysts of the elbow joint have been described (41–43) (Chapter 30), but the cysts have also been seen in the shoulder and stifle joint (40). The cysts can cause pain when mechanically interfering with joint function. Repeated needle aspiration of the cyst is considered the treatment of choice, as the cysts tend to recur even after surgical resection (42).

References and further reading

1. Godfrey DR. Osteoarthritis in cats: a retrospective radiological study. J Small Anim Pract 2005;46:425–429.
2. Herzog W, et al. Hindlimb loading, morphology and biochemistry of articular cartilage in the ACL-deficient cat knee. Osteoarthritis Cartilage 1993;1:243–251.
3. Suter E, et al. One-year changes in hind limb kinematics, ground reaction forces and knee stability in an experimental model of osteoarthritis. J Biomechanics 1998;31:511–517.
4. Clarke SP, et al. Radiographic prevalence of degenerative joint disease in a hospital population of cats. Vet Rec 2005; 157:793–799.
5. Hardie EM, et al. Radiographic evidence of degenerative joint disease in geriatric cats: 100 cases (1994–1997). J Am Vet Med Assoc 2002;220:628–632.
6. Clarke SP, Bennett D. Feline osteoarthritis: a prospective study of 28 cases. J Small Anim Pract 2006;47:439–445.
7. Godfrey DR. Osteoarthritis in cats: a prospective series of 40 cases. BSAVA meeting 2003; Birmingham.
8. Scarlett JM, Donoghue S. Associations between body condition and disease in cats. J Am Vet Med Assoc 1998;212:1725–1731.
9. Bennett D, Clarke S. Feline osteoarthritis. ESVOT meeting 2004; Munich, Germany.
10. Hardie EM. Management of osteoarthritis in cats. Vet Clin North Am Small Anim Pract 1997;27:945–953.
11. Graeme SA. Radiographic features of feline joint disease. Vet Clin North Am Small Anim Pract 2000;30:281–302.
12. Lascelles BD, et al. Evaluation of the clinical efficacy of meloxicam in cats with painful locomotor disorders. J Small Anim Pract 2001;42:587–593.
13. Reginster JY, et al. Long-term effects of glucosamine sulfate on osteoarthritis progression: a randomized, placebo-controlled clinical trial. Lancet 2001;357:251.
14. Hulse D, et al. The effect of Cosequin in cranial cruciate deficient and reconstructed stifle joints in dogs. VOS 25th annual conference 1998; Snowmass, Colorado.
15. Hardy RM, Wallace LJ. Arthrocentesis and synovial membrane biopsy. Vet Clin North Am 1974;4:449–462.
16. Pedersen NC, et al. Feline chronic progressive polyarthritis. Am J Vet Res 1980;41:522–535.

17. Carro T, et al. Subcutaneous abscesses and arthritis caused by a probable bacterial L-form in cats. J Am Vet Med Assoc 1989;194:1583–1588.
18. Bennett D, Nash AS. Feline immune-based polyarthritis: a study of thirty-one cases. J Small Anim Pract 1988;29:501–523.
19. Carro T. Polyarthritis in cats. Compend Continuing Educ 1994;16:57–67.
20. Hanna FY. Disease modifying treatment for feline rheumatoid arthritis. Vet Comp Orthop Traumatol 2005;18:94–99.
21. Bennett D, May C. Joint diseases of dogs and cats. In: Ettinger SJ (ed.) Textbook of veterinary internal medicine, 4th edn. Philadelphia: WB Saunders; 1995: pp. 2032–2077.
22. Iglauer F, et al. *Streptococcus canis* arthritis in a cat breeding colony. J Exp Anim Sci 1991;34:59–65.
23. Stallings B, et al. Septicemia and septic arthritis caused by *Streptococcus pneumoniae* in a cat: possible transmission from a child. J Am Vet Med Assoc 1987;191:703–704.
24. Ernst S, Goggin JM. What is your diagnosis? Mycoplasma arthritis in a cat. J Am Vet Med Assoc 1999;215:19–20.
25. Moise NS, et al. *Mycoplasma gateae* arthritis and tenosynovitis in cats: case report and experimental reproduction of the disease. Am J Vet Res 1983;44:16–21.
26. Dawson S, et al. Investigation of vaccine reactions and breakdowns after feline calicivirus vaccination. Vet Rec 1993;132: 346–350.
27. Bennett D, et al. Detection of feline calicivirus antigens in the joints of infected cats. Vet Rec 1989;124:329–332.
28. Levy JK, Marsh A. Isolation of calicivirus from the joint of a kitten with arthritis. J Am Vet Med Assoc 1992;201:753–763.
29. Dawson S, et al. Acute arthritis of cats associated with feline calicivirus infection. Res Vet Sci 1994;56:133–143.
30. Gibson MD, et al. *Borrelia burgdorferi* infection of cats (letter). J Am Vet Med Assoc 1993;202:1786.
31. Straubinger RK, et al. Clinical manifestations, pathogenesis, and effect of antibiotic treatment on Lyme borreliosis in dogs. Wien Klin Wochenschr 1998;110:874–881.
32. May C, et al. *Borrelia burgdorferi* infection in cats in the UK. J Small Anim Pract 1994;35:517–520.
33. Magnarelli LA, et al. Tick parasitism and antibodies to *Borrelia burgdorferi* in cats. J Am Vet Med Assoc 1990;197:63–66.
34. Burgess EC. Experimentally induced infection of cats with *Borrelia burgdorferi*. Am J Vet Res 1992;53:1507–1511.
35. Olsson SE, Reiland S. The nature of osteochondrosis in animals. Summary and conclusions with comparative aspects on osteochondritis dissecans in man. Acta Radiol 1978;358:299.
36. Butcher R, Beasley K. Osteochondritis dissecans in a cat? Vet Rec 1986;118:646.
37. Ralphs SC. Bilateral stifle osteochondritis dissecans in a cat. J Am Anim Hosp Assoc 2005;41:78–80.
38. Petersen CJ. Osteochondritis dissecans of the humeral head of a cat. NZ Vet J 1984;32:115–116.
39. Hubler M, et al. Lesions resembling osteochondromatosis in two cats. J Small Anim Pract 1986;27:181–187.
40. Bennett D. The musculoskeletal system. In: Chandler EA, Gaskell CJ, Gaskell RM (eds) Feline medicine and therapeutics, 3rd edn. Oxford: Blackwell; 2004: pp. 173–233.
41. Prymak C, Goldschmidt MH. Synovial cysts in five dogs and one cat. J Am Anim Hosp Assoc 1991;27:151–154.
42. Stead AC, et al. Synovial cysts in cats. J Small Anim Pract 1995;36:450–454.
43. White JD, et al. What is your diagnosis? J Feline Med Surg 2004;6:339–344.

6 Diseases of the spine and nervous system

F. Steffen, F. Grünenfelder

The range of feline spinal cord and peripheral nerve diseases is wide. The historical information is often incomplete in cats and the clinical presentation for many spinal cord diseases and neuromyopathies is often similar. Thus, additional investigations, including examination of cerebrospinal fluid (CSF), plain and contrast radiography, computed tomography (CT), and magnetic resonance imaging (MRI) studies, and cytological and histopathological analysis, are mandatory to reach a diagnosis in most cases.

An overview of feline compressive and non-compressive spinal disorders is presented in Table 6-1. A selection of these diseases is discussed in more detail below. The most important feline neuromuscular diseases are also described in the following sections.

6.1 Compressive diseases of the spinal cord

The severity of damage associated with chronic compressive lesions and acute spinal trauma in cats can range from mild demyelination to total necrosis of both the white and gray matter. The underlying pathogenesis is different for the two types of spinal cord injury. The rate of development of the compressive force is the main factor that differs between the two entities. Two major forces have to be considered: the direct mechanical disruption of the cord tissue by the compressive lesion, and hypoxic changes resulting from pressure on the vascular system in the cord. In acute spinal trauma, these forces result in immediate functional deficits, which may be aggravated by a cascade of biochemical alterations that occur as a consequence of water and ionic changes, and spinal cord ischemia. With slowly progressive compressive disease processes there is remarkable attenuation of the soft, compressible tissue of the spinal cord without initial neurological signs. The chronic compression of the spinal cord leads to changes in the structure of blood vessels, loss of axons, and demyelination. Clinical signs occur when the cord can no longer compensate for the pathological changes.

Clinical signs of spinal cord compression are determined by their severity and neuroanatomic localization. Based on the degree of the deficits, spinal patients may be assigned to one of five groups (Table 6-2). In general, animals with grade V lesions carry a poor prognosis if decompression cannot be carried out within 48 hours.

Diseases causing compression of the spinal cord include intervertebral disc disease (IVDD), and tumors of the nerve roots, meninges, spinal cord, and vertebral column. Tumors of the nervous system are described in Chapter 8.

6.1.1 Intervertebral disc disease

Spontaneous IVDD is rarely encountered in cats when compared to dogs. One study reported an incidence of 0.12% in a feline hospital population (1). Both Hansen types I (disc extrusion) and II (disc protrusion) IVDD have been observed in the cat, with type II being more common in cats older than 8 years. This age predilection is analogous to that seen in non-chondrodystrophic dogs and in humans, where disc protrusion is the result of fibroid metaplasia of the disc with age. The presence of annular tears without changes of the nucleus pulposus in many older cats also suggests that these discs undergo similar changes as seen in non-chondrodystrophic dogs (2).

Although Hansen type II disc protrusions were seen more commonly in postmortem studies, Hansen type I disc extrusions were found in 8 out of 10 cats in a clinical study, and only 2 of the patients had Hansen type II protrusions (1). The apparent discrepancy between clinical and pathological findings may be explained by the slowly progressive nature of disc protrusions that do not necessarily result in clinically overt pain and dysfunction, as compared to disc extrusions. Chronic pain may easily be overlooked in cats.

The predilection sites of clinical IVDD are the thoracolumbar region and the mid to caudal lumbar spine, specifically the disc spaces of L4–L5 and L5–L6 (2). However, the highest incidence of disc protrusion has been found in the cervical spine in necropsied cats (3, 4). Interestingly, clinical reports of cervical disc disease are rare (5, 6). Similarly, lumbosacral disc disease occurs exceedingly rarely in cats (7).

Diagnosis

Plain radiography of the spine may reveal narrowed intervertebral disc spaces and mineralized intervertebral disc material in situ and/or within the spinal canal (Fig. 6-1A). But these are rather rare findings, and in general, plain radiographs are not as useful for identifying extruded discs in cats as they are in dogs. Myelography (Fig. 6-1B) or advanced imaging

Category	Diseases
Vascular	Infarct
	Focal malacia
Inflammatory/infectious	Feline infectious peritonitis
	Bacterial, viral, or fungal infections
	Toxoplasmosis
	Eosinophilic meningomyelitis
	Idiopathic poliomyelitis
Traumatic	Vertebral fracture/luxation (Chapters 15 and 34)
	Intervertebral disc disease
Congenital/inherited	Storage disease affecting spinal cord
	Syringohydromyelia
	Subarachnoid cyst
	Congenital malformations
Metabolic	Hypervitaminosis A
Neoplastic	Lymphosarcoma
	Vertebral column neoplasia
	Meningeal neoplasia
	Extradural neoplasia/metastasis
	Intramedullary tumors
Degenerative	Neuroaxonal dystrophy
	Degenerative myelopathy

Table 6-1. Feline spinal cord disorders

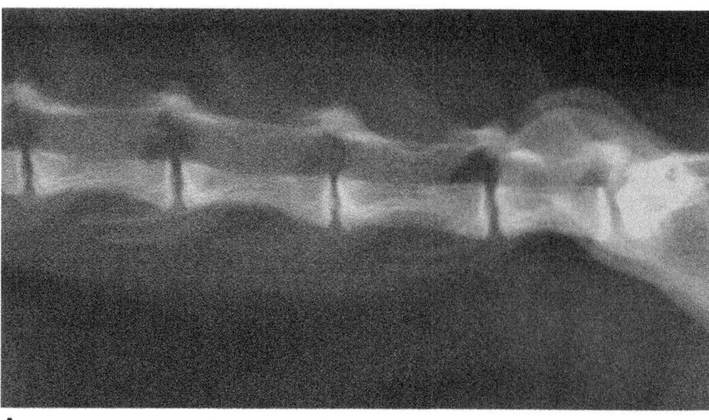

A

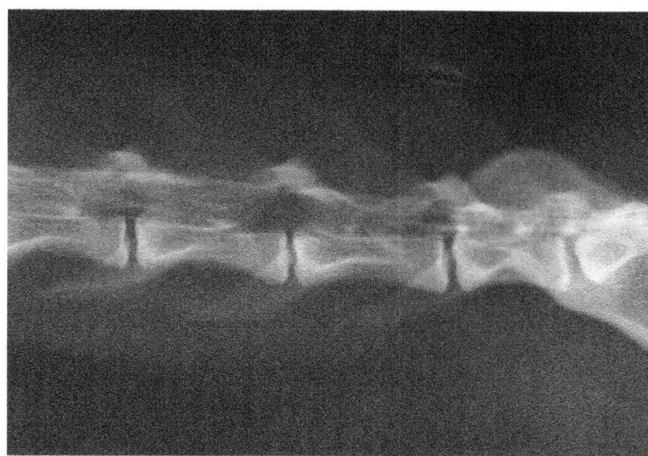

B

Figure 6-1 (**A**) Plain radiographs and lumbar myelogram (**B**) of a cat with a Hansen type I disc extrusion of the L5–L6 disc. (**A**) The L5–L6 disc space is narrowed and mineralized disc material is seen. (**B**) Myelography confirms extradural compression at the L5–L6 level.

Grade	Neurological signs
I	Back/neck pain only, no neurological deficits
II	Ambulatory paresis/ataxia, normal micturition
III	Ambulatory paresis/ataxia, urinary retention
IV	Non-ambulatory paresis/plegia, urinary retention, intact deep pain perception
V	Non-ambulatory plegia, urinary retention, absent deep pain perception

Table 6-2. Clinical degrees of spinal cord dysfunction

modalities, such as CT or MRI, are indispensable for exact diagnosis and localization of the disc herniation (8).

Non-surgical treatment

Non-surgical treatment is indicated in cats for the first episode of back pain without neurological deficits or in patients where surgery is declined for other reasons, such as financial constraints. Non-surgical treatment consists of strict confinement in a cage for 2–4 weeks. A gradual return to normal activity is difficult to achieve in cats, so they may require longer periods of cage rest. The use of steroids is controversial. Based upon the clinical observation that some ambulatory animals (grade I–III) improve significantly, a short course of prednisone (1–2 mg/kg SID for 2–4 days) is considered helpful by the authors. This effect may be attributed to reduction of spinal cord edema secondary to the compressive lesion. Prolonged glucocorticoid therapy for spinal injuries is discouraged. Non-steroidal anti-inflammatory drugs (NSAIDs) may be given for their anti-inflammatory and analgesic effects, but never concurrently with steroids. Opioids can be administered for analgesia together with either steroids or NSAIDs. The rationale behind non-surgical treatment is to allow time for healing a ruptured annulus and to limit the inflammatory response. Migrating herniated nucleus pulposus frequently showed a decrease in volume or even disappeared in some people in serial MRI studies of humans treated conservatively. In comparison, people with disc protrusions showed no or minimal changes in size of the protrusion over time (9). Similar studies have not been published in veterinary medicine.

More aggressive medical therapy should be instituted prior to surgery in a cat presented with paraplegia (grade IV and V). Experimental studies in cats have suggested that only soluble corticosteroids given within 1 hour of the trauma are beneficial (10). Methylprednisolone succinate given within 8 hours of spinal trauma was beneficial in humans (11). Application of methylprednisolone has been used as an initial bolus at a dose of 30 mg/kg IV, with additional doses of 15 mg/kg IV given at 2 and 6 hours after the initial dose in human studies. Ventral spinal cord trauma was simulated and methylprednisolone was administered following the protocol mentioned above in an experimental canine study. No significant benefit could be demonstrated. However, the degree of spinal trauma produced may not have been severe enough to allow for distinction between the treatment and control groups (12).

Success rates for conservative treatment of IVDD in cats are not yet available. Recovery rates for dogs with grade I–III deficits are reported to be 90%, and approximately 50% for those with grade IV lesions (13). In dogs with grade V lesions conservative treatment is ineffective in most cases.

Disadvantages of non-surgical treatment include slow or incomplete recovery, a relatively high risk for recurrence, persistence of pain, and neurological deterioration.

Surgical treatment

Decompressive surgery is the treatment of choice in any cat with recurrent back pain and/or neurological deficits of grade II or more. Depending on the location of the herniated disc, a hemilaminectomy or laminectomy may be performed in the cervical, thoracolumbar, and lumbar spine. Decompression of the cervical cord by a ventral slot procedure is technically more demanding in cats than in dogs. Principles of spinal surgery are described in Chapter 15, and decompression procedures in Chapter 34.

Outcome for surgically treated cats with IVDD in the thoracolumbar and lumbar spine is good to excellent for cats with intact deep pain perception (1, 14). Time to recovery is somewhat unpredictable, and may range from an immediate postoperative improvement to a slow improvement over weeks to months. Clinical studies documenting outcome for cats with loss of deep pain perception after disc herniation are not available. A recent study in dogs with loss of deep pain sensation showed that more than 50% regained deep pain sensation and the ability to walk within 4 weeks of decompressive surgery (15). The main long-term complication in animals with complete spinal cord injury is persistent urinary and fecal incontinence. Assessment of spinal cord integrity by durotomy in animals with loss of deep pain perception has been recommended. Presence of focal or extensive malacia of the cord has been associated with a hopeless outcome. However, it should be kept in mind that only 5–10% of intact axons are necessary for functional recovery. Identification of this small percentage of axons would be visually impossible at durotomy. Therefore, animals with malacia should only be euthanized if they develop ascending myelomalacia or show no improvement within a 4-week period.

Experimental studies in cats with complete spinal transection showed that 87% of the animals were able to walk unassisted on a treadmill 1 month after the injury. These cats received intensive physical rehabilitation consisting of 30 minutes of locomotor and proprioceptive exercises each day (16). In another study involving spinal cord transection no physical rehabilitation was given and only 30% of these cats regained full weight-bearing ability 4 weeks after transection (17). Fecal and urinary incontinence necessitated special nursing in these cats.

6.1.2 Spinal subarachnoid cysts

Spinal subarachnoid cysts represent a rare cause of myelopathy in cats (18, 19). Whether this condition is a developmental abnormality or a consequence of an acquired disease, such as spinal trauma or inflammation, is debatable. Proliferative lesions or arachnoid adhesions are thought to create a one-way valve that causes accumulation of the CSF. Alternatively, the diverticulum may result from herniation of the arachnoid membrane through a congenital defect in the dura. While the etiology remains unclear, the resulting neurological deficits can be explained by the compression of the underlying spinal cord, and extension of meningeal connective tissue along the spinal canal. Diagnostic imaging reveals a characteristic bulb-like dilatation of the dorsal contrast column (Fig. 6-2).

Surgical treatment consists of dural fenestration or excision of the cyst-like structure. The prognosis is usually good. Complications include recurrence of clinical signs due to reformation of arachnoid adhesions or incomplete recovery due to severe and irreversible spinal cord damage.

6.2 Non-compressive diseases of the spinal cord

The clinician offering a spinal surgery service should also be fully aware and up to date with the diagnosis and treatment of non-compressive disorders of the spinal cord. Diagnosis of these diseases can be challenging, and some disorders can easily be missed. New insights have been obtained with advanced diagnostic imaging, most notably MRI. Non-compressive diseases of the spinal cord include spinal cord infarction and the neurological form of feline infectious peritonitis (FIP). Many infectious diseases are also considered

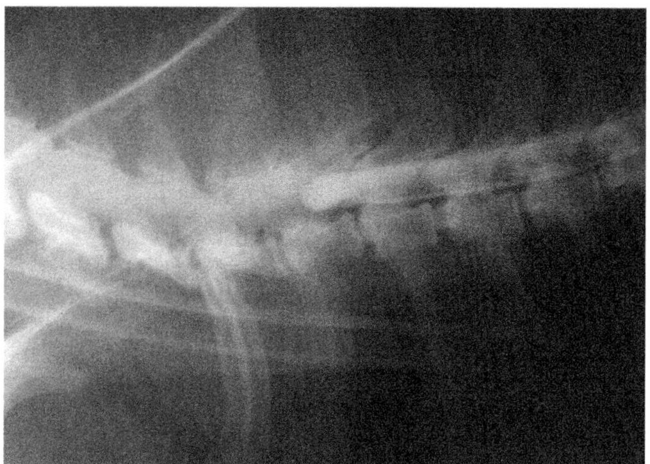

Figure 6-2 Lumbar myelogram of a 7-year-old cat with marked hindlimb ataxia of 4 months duration. The bulb-like dilation of the dorsal subarachnoid space at T2 is characteristic for a subarachnoid cyst. The cat was treated with dorsal laminectomy and marsupialization of the cyst after durotomy.

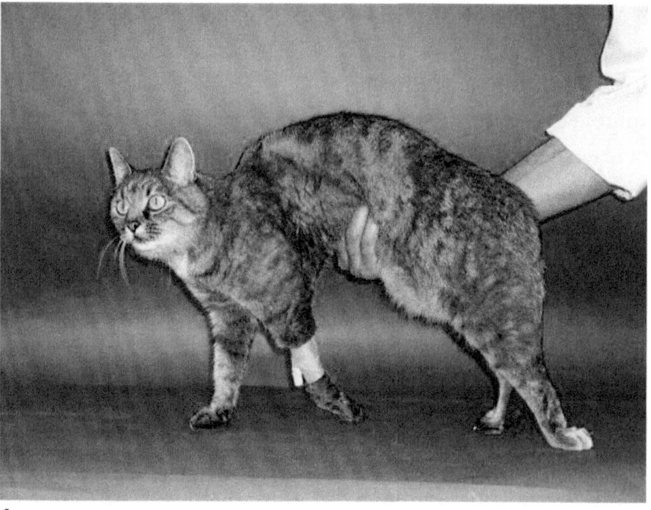

A

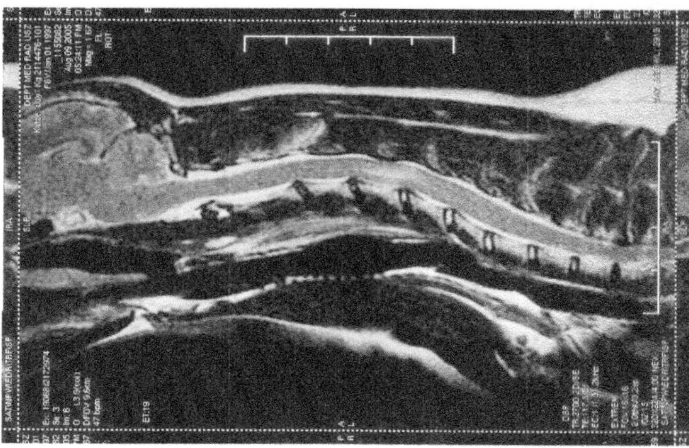

B

Figure 6-3 A feline patient with spinal cord infarction. (**A**) A 6-year-old cat with hemiparesis due to a spinal cord lesion between C1 and C5. The signs occurred acutely without associated trauma.
(**B**) T2-weighted sagittal magnetic resonance imaging of the cervical spine. Note the intramedullary, focal hyperintense signal between C4 and C5.

primarily non-compressive, although they may cause compression in rare cases.

6.2.1 Spinal cord infarction

Spinal cord infarction secondary to fibrocartilaginous embolization (FCE) of spinal vasculature is a rare entity in cats (20–22). However, it is an important differential diagnosis for non-painful myelopathies such as concussive spinal cord trauma or a low-volume/high-velocity disc extrusion. The cause of FCE in animal species is unknown. It is hypothesized that small pieces of intervertebral fibrocartilage enter the vasculature by direct penetration of vessels, arteriovenous communications, the vertebral sinus, or via herniation through the endplate or through an embryonic remnant vessel. One theory that could apply well to the outdoor free-roaming cat is the possibility of trauma to the intervertebral disc, causing a fragment of nucleus pulposus to enter the damaged venous system.

Onset of clinical signs is acute and the symptoms of spinal cord dysfunction are dependent on the area affected, but are usually asymmetrical (Fig. 6-3A). Typically, palpation and manipulation do not elicit painful reactions. Lower motor neuron signs or absence of deep pain perception usually indicate a hopeless prognosis for recovery. Plain radiography and myelography are normal. CSF analysis may show an elevated protein content. Magnetic resonance tomography may reveal high-signal intensities on T2-weighted images (Fig. 6-3B).

In one review of five cats with FCE, three of the cats were euthanized, and postmortem examination confirmed myelomalacia with intralesional FCE. Two cats survived and improved clinically within 3 weeks (22). Although FCE is rare in cats, it may be underdiagnosed because signs may only be transient when areas of the upper motor neuron are affected, and histopathological examination of the spinal cord is not routinely performed.

6.2.2 Feline infectious peritonitis

FIP is reported to be the most common infectious meningomyelitis in the cat and also the single most common cause of cord disease (23). The neurological form of FIP can be present despite normal results on physical and ophthalmological examination (24). Although the majority of cases will present with multifocal signs, with the brainstem being the most common site affected, focal spinal cord dysfunction has been described (25).

Antemortem diagnosis is challenging and will only be confirmed by histopathology in many cases. The clinical diagnosis of neurological FIP is based on results of the CSF analysis with a marked elevation of protein, and a mixed-population pleocytosis with a prevalence of neutrophils. It is not uncommon in cases of FIP that CSF cannot be obtained from subarachnoidal puncture due to its high viscosity. Hyperglobulinemia can often be demonstrated in the serum of affected cats. Absence of serum antibody titers against FIP virus does not rule out the disease. The prognosis is usually hopeless and steroids may only provide a temporary alleviation.

6.3 Infections of the spine and spinal cord

6.3.1 Discospondylitis

Discospondylitis is a bacterial infection of the intervertebral disc and adjacent vertebral bodies. The most common route of infection is by arterial spread of organisms from infected sites elsewhere in the body. The infection first localizes in the endplates, probably in the slowly flowing, tortuous venous sinuses of the subchondral area, and then spreads to the avascular disc by diffusing through the multiple nutrient foramina in the endplate. Primary sites of infection include the genitourinary system, skin, heart valves, and mouth. Immunosuppression may be a factor in the development of discospondylitis. Direct infection of the disc or vertebra occurs after penetrating wounds such as gunshot or bite, surgery or migrating foreign bodies such as grass awns (26).

Infection of the vertebral endplates results in inflammation and tissue necrosis with erosion of the endplates. Spinal pain and pyrexia are the first clinical signs at this stage. The course of infection may vary with the infecting organism and the patient's immune status. Neurological deficits develop when the spinal cord is compressed by proliferation of inflammatory tissue and exostosis. Occasionally, hypermobility of the infected vertebral segment occurs. Extension of the infection through the dura represents an occasional, but serious, sequela.

Diagnosis is usually possible with spinal radiographs taken at least 2 weeks after the onset of infection. The earliest radiographic change is a subtle irregularity of the endplates. The disc space may also be narrowed. Later, erosion of the endplates becomes more evident, and the disc space may widen because of lysis of adjacent bone. After a variable period of time, bone regeneration occurs with sclerosis and osteophyte production. Vertebral collapse and bony ankylosis represent the endstage appearance of discospondylitis. Scoliosis, fracture, and subluxation are possible complications of the disease.

Initial treatment of discospondylitis usually consists of antibiotics, cage rest, and analgesia. The antibiotic is ideally selected based on the results of culture and sensitivity testing of blood, urine, or material aspirated from the site of infection. If the infective agent is unknown, ampicillin, cephalosporin, or enrofloxacin may be used. The optimal duration of therapy has not been determined, but it is recommended that patients should be treated for at least 8 weeks in an attempt to clear the infection and to prevent recurrence.

There have been three reports of feline discospondylitis (27–29). In two animals, infection extended to the vertebral canal and meninges, resulting in paraparesis. The third case was presented with spinal pain without neurological deficits. Radiographic signs in all cats included osteolysis of adjacent vertebral endplates. The causative organism in one cat was *Streptococcus canis* and *Actinomyces* cultured from a paravertebral abscess. *Escherichia coli* was isolated in the second patient where hematogenous spread was suspected. The infective agent was not determined in the third case. The outcome was fatal in all three reported cases due to the advanced stage of the disease or lack of response to therapy (27–29).

6.3.2 Spinal empyema

Infection of the epidural space secondary to a penetrating wound or bite may represent a more common cause of infectious spinal cord disease in the cat than discospondylitis. Formation of an epidural abscess or empyema can result in spinal cord compression, accompanied by fever and pain. Reported cases of spinal empyema in cats were all associated with extradural granulomatous mass lesions. *Actinomyces* sp. was isolated from two cats, and *Fusobacterium* sp. and *Bacteroides* sp. from the other (30, 31). The infection occurred subsequent to a broken tail in one case, whereas cutaneous abscessation of the tail base was found in the other two. Diagnosis is best obtained by advanced diagnostic imaging, but exploratory surgery may be necessary for definitive diagnosis. Besides systemic antibiotics, surgical decompression, epidural lavage, and drainage may be necessary to treat this serious spinal disorder. Early recognition and surgical and antimicrobial treatment can result in a good outcome in dogs (32).

6.3.3 Fungal infections of the spinal cord

The most common systemic fungal infections in cats are cryptococcosis, histoplasmosis, coccidiomycosis, and blastomycosis. The geographic distribution of the four organisms is variable. Coccidiomycosis and blastomycosis most frequently appear in specific defined geographic locations, whereas cryptococcosis and histoplasmosis have a worldwide distribution. Cryptococcus is a saprophytic, yeast-like fungi, and pigeons are believed to be an important vector. However, outdoor cats are no more prone to infection than indoor cats. Feline leukemia virus (FeLV) and feline immunodeficiency virus (FIV) do not seem to have a significant influence on disease prevalence (33). Histoplasmosis is most frequently seen in regions with temperate and subtropical climates. Blastomycosis occurs in North America, Africa, and India, especially in regions with moist acidic soil. Coccidiomycosis is seen in sandy and dry regions of the American continent.

The major route of infection in all four groups is through the respiratory tract. Peroral infections in histoplasmosis, and percutanous infections in coccidiomycosis, are alternative pathways (33). Depending on the geographic location, cryptococcosis and histoplasmosis are fairly common associated with inflammatory central nervous system (CNS) disease. Spread from the respiratory tract to the spinal cord alone has been reported for both cryptococcosis and coccidiomycosis (23, 34). However, isolated cases of spinal cord infection are rare. Ocular involvement, especially retinal changes, can be seen with all four fungal species.

Thoracic radiography and rhinoscopy are helpful investigative procedures for establishing the diagnosis. Definitive diagnosis is normally obtained by identifying the organism in tracheal wash, CSF, urine, or cytology/biopsies of lesions. Culture of the organisms from the samples is helpful in determining the varieties and serotypes. Serological antibody screening can be used to narrow the tentative diagnosis, although false-negative results are common, especially with blastomycosis and histomycosis. A highly specific and sensitive latex agglutination test identifying cryptococcus capsule antigen in serum or CSF is commercially available (33). MRI is the recommended advanced diagnostic imaging modality for visualizing and evaluating CNS infection (35).

Amphotericin B, itraconazole, and fluconazole are commonly used therapeutic agents for all four fungal species. The main advantages of fluconazole are the relatively mild side-effects in the patient, and the good penetration into the CNS (36). Infected cats often have to be treated for several months to years, depending on clinical signs and serological course (33). Frequently, the organism cannot be completely eliminated, and the medical therapy has to be continued to prevent recurrence of the disease. Surgical treatment is only used to decompress compromised tissue. Since these are systemic diseases, the overall prognosis is guarded to poor.

6.4 Congenital abnormalities of the spine and spinal cord

Spinal cord and vertebral abnormalities can be divided into two major groups based on embryological origin. Aberrations may originate from tissues of mesodermal origin resulting in vertebral body and disc abnormalities. Those of ectodermal origin result in spinal cord and meningeal abnormalities. Deformity of the vertebral bodies and discs is rarely associated with primary clinical deficits, whereas malformation of the spinal cord is more likely to be associated with clinical signs.

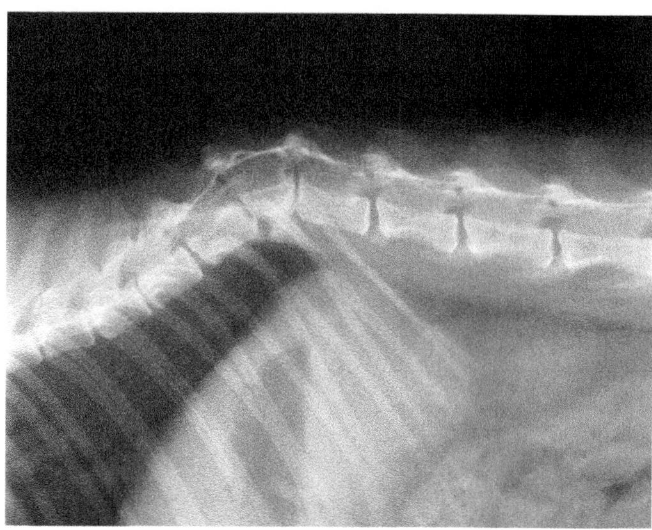

Figure 6-4 Radiograph of a 3-year-old cat with a hemivertebra at the thoracolumbar junction. This malformation was an incidental finding.

Malformations of the bony spine such as block vertebrae, butterfly vertebrae, hemivertebrae, or transitional vertebrae may be detected on routine plain radiographs (Fig. 6-4). It is imperative that compression of neural tissue be demonstrated before the clinical signs can be attributed to the radiological abnormality. Pain and pelvic limb weakness have been associated with an abnormal lumbosacral junction due to transitional vertebral segments with resulting compression of the cauda equina. Clinical signs were alleviated following dorsal laminectomy (37). Occipito-atlantoaxial malformation and atlantoaxial instability secondary to absence or malformation of the odontoid process have been described as a rare entity in cats (38). The condition was successfully treated by ventral cross-pin fixation and arthrodesis of the atlantoaxial articulation in one case. Congenital abnormalities of the spine are further described in Chapter 3.

Abnormalities of the spinal cord and vertebral arch are primarily influenced by neural tube development. Spina bifida is a combination of defects involving the vertebral column, spinal cord, and associated tissues. The defects may vary from incomplete fusion of vertebral arches to incomplete formation of the neural tube with or without protrusion and dysplasia of meninges, spinal cord, or both (Chapter 3). These related malformations are commonly encountered in the Manx breed. Absence of the tail is an autosomal-dominant trait in this breed, which provides the genetic basis for neural tube defects. Affected cats typically have a

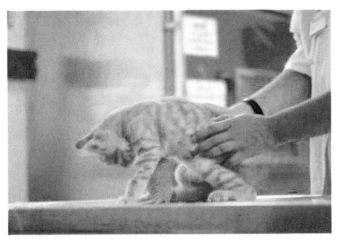

Figure 6-5 Four-month-old kitten with marked cervical ventroflexion due to hypokalemic polymyopathy. This sign is characteristic for neuromuscular weakness and can be caused by a variety of disorders.

bunny-hopping gait. More severe abnormalities include fecal and urinary incontinence, megacolon, and paraparesis. Signs may develop over weeks to months as the cat grows. This is likely due to failure of cranial migration of the spinal cord – so-called tethering. Tethering may result from attachment of the spinal cord at a specific level associated with a meningomyelocele. It is clinically relevant to distinguish the deficits associated with a tethered cord from those of cord dysgenesis, since untethering neurosurgical procedures may lead to significant improvement.

6.5 Peripheral nerve and muscle disorders

The neuromuscular diseases can be broadly divided into mono- and polyradiculo/neuropathies, myopathies, and neuromuscular junction diseases. The clinical sign common to all these disorders is muscle weakness. However, the expression of that weakness may vary considerably. Weak cats are prone to develop cervical ventroflexion because cats lack a nuchal ligament (Fig. 6-5). Other signs may include lower motor neuron signs, fatigability, and alterations in muscle size (hypotrophy, swelling), possibly accompanied by myalgia.

Accurate diagnosis of neuromuscular disorders in cats requires diagnostic tools which are selected according to the specific case. Useful tests include measurement of creatine kinase activity, viral and protozoal titers for FeLV, FIV, and toxoplasmosis, antiacetylcholine receptor antibodies, electrodiagnostic testing, and muscle and peripheral nerve biopsies. Muscle biopsies are usually evaluated using routine hemotoxylin and eosin staining together with histochemical analyses. Peripheral nerve fascicular biopsies are fixed in 2.5% glutaraldehyde and the plastic-embedded sections are stained with toluidine blue. Teased nerve fiber studies and electronic microscopy can be useful in reaching a final diagnosis. An

Disorder	Frequency
Ischemic neuromyopathy	Common
Polymyositis	Rare
Clostridial myositis	Rare
Masticatory myositis	Rare
Myositis ossificans	Rare
Feline immunodeficiency virus	Experimental
Acquired/congenital myasthenia gravis	Occasional
Hypokalemic myopathy	Common
Hyperkalemic myopathy	Occasional
Hypernatremic myopathy	Rare
Malignant hyperthermia	Rare
Feline X-linked muscular dystrophy	Rare
Myotonic myopathy	Rare
Nemaline rod myopathy	Rare
Glycogen storage disease type IV	Rare
Laminin alpha-2 (merosin) deficiency	Rare
Myopathy of Devon Rex cats	Rare
Inherited motor neuron disease/spinal muscular atrophy in Main Coon cats	Rare
Skeletal muscle tumors	Rare

Table 6-3. Feline neuromuscular disorders

overview of feline neuromuscular disease is presented in Tables 6-3 and 6-4. A selection of the most relevant disorders will be discussed below in detail.

6.5.1 Ischemic neuromyopathy

Ischemic neuromyopathy results from embolization or longstanding compression of arteries.

Ischemic neuromyopathy secondary to thrombus formation

Cardiomyopathy with thrombus formation occasionally occurs in cats. The emboli may be transported to any site within the arterial circulation, but the most common site of obstruction is the aortic trifurcation (90%). The internal and external iliac artery and the median sacral artery are obstructed, with resulting ischemia of the distal organs. Embolization of the brachial artery is very rarely observed.

The onset of clinical signs is acute. Painful paraparesis or paralysis occurs; asymmetric deficits are occasionally observed. The limbs are cool on palpation, there is absence of a femoral pulse, and the nail bed appears cyanotic. The gastrocnemius muscles are firm and painful. Pain sensation is often absent in the distal limbs. The ability to extend and flex the hip and stifle joints is usually preserved, and the

Disorder	Frequency
Ischemic neuromyopathy	Common
Idiopathic polyradiculoneuritis	Rare
Chronic inflammatory demyelinating polyneuropathy	Rare
Trigeminal neuritis	Rare
Tetanus	Occasional
Idiopathic self-mutilation (Siamese, Abyssinian, Himalayan)	Rare
Orofacial pain syndrome in Burmese cats	Rare
Traumatic neuropathy	Common
Toxic neuropathies	Rare
Thallium	
Organophosphate	Delayed
Salinomycin toxicity	
Irradiation (>15 Gy)	
Diabetic neuropathy	Common
Feline Niemann–Pick disease (sphingomyelinase deficiency)	Rare
Hyperchylomicronemia	Rare
Hyperoxaluria	Rare
Idiopathic facial paralysis	Common
Feline dysautonomia	Rare
Feline peripheral nerve tumors	Rare

Table 6-4. Feline peripheral nerve disorders

patellar reflex remains intact. Initially, the limbs may be held in extension because of ischemic muscle contraction.

Electrodiagnostic studies reveal decreased motor nerve conduction and absent or reduced evoked potentials from the interosseous and the cranial tibial muscles. The electromyogram may be isoelectric. Chest radiography and echocardiography often provide evidence of cardiac disease. The vascular occlusion may be demonstrated definitively with an abdominal ultrasound or an arteriogram.

The femoral pulse frequently returns within 1–2 weeks, and no specific treatment has been shown to result in an improved recovery rate. Surgical embolectomy does also not appear to be indicated, especially as these cats represent a high anesthetic risk. Thrombolytic agents await clinical trials. Pain may be managed by restricting movement, and by administering morphine sulfate (0.1 mg/kg SC every 4–6 hours for up to 2 days). For prevention of further episodes, lifelong administration of aspirin (25 mg/kg PO every third day) is recommended.

Most patients develop collateral circulation and recover to varying degrees within 6 weeks to 6 months. Deficits such as a plantigrade stance or weakness may persist lifelong.

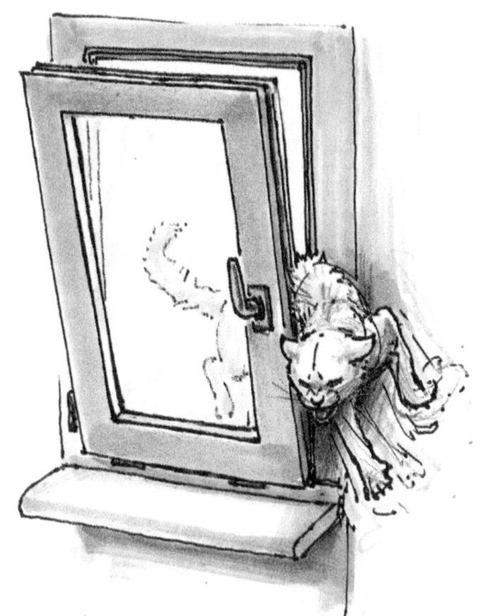

Figure 6-6 Cat trapped in a hung window. Ischemic neuromyopathy results from long-standing compression of blood vessels, muscles, and nerves.

Extensive tissue necrosis may necessitate limb amputation, but this is a rare complication.

The severity of cardiac disease usually determines the prognosis. In one retrospective study of cats with thromboembolic disease, all animals were dead 6 months after diagnosis. For cats with congestive heart failure, the prognosis is worse than for those without (39).

Ischemic neuromyopathy after entrapment in bottom-hung (hinged) windows

Cats getting caught in a bottom-hung or hinged window are commonly presented with signs of ischemic neuromyopathy (40). The resulting acute paralysis of the hindlimbs has been referred to as "window-cat syndrome." Affected cats are trapped in an open window, and while making useless attempts to free themselves, the abdominal area gets more and more compressed (Fig. 6-6). Damage to muscles, nerves, and occasionally abdominal organs and the spinal cord occurs as a consequence of ischemia. The neurological presentation is largely identical to cats with thromboembolic occlusion of the aortic trifurcation. Some cats are also in shock. The degree of neurological dysfunction and cardiovascular compromise is related to the time the cat is trapped in the window.

Diagnosis is straightforward as most cats are found in the window. However, pathophysiological events may be more complicated, as iatrogenic ligation of the abdominal aorta does not cause paraplegia (41). The presence of a thrombotic embolus seems essential to the pathogenesis and presence of ischemic neuromyopathy. The release of serotonin, thromboxane A_2, prostaglandins, and other vasoactive substances from thrombocytes causes constriction of collateral vessels and activates intravascular clotting.

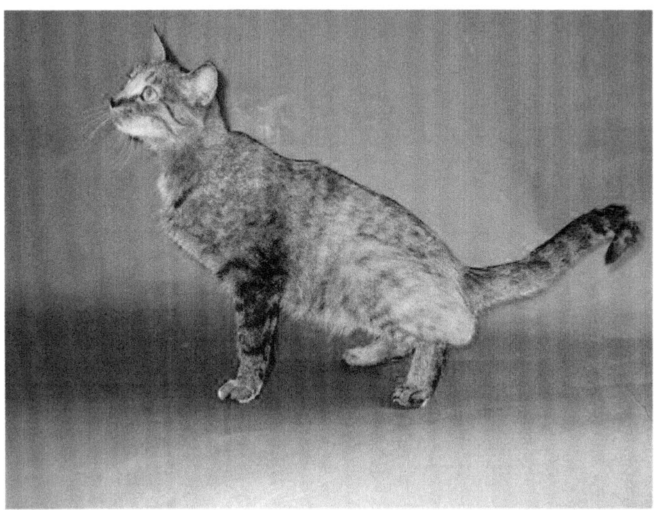

Figure 6-7 Typical posture of a cat in the recovery phase after paraplegia due to ischemic neuromyopathy from being caught in a hung window. Extension of the hindlimbs improves gradually over a period of days to weeks in most cases, even when deep pain sensation has been lost.

The levels of creatine kinase are usually massively elevated as a result of the damaged myocytes. However, this does not seem to be related to the prognosis. Azotemia and elevated alanine transaminase and aspartate aminotransferase reflect ischemic or direct traumatic damage of the kidneys and liver. Most laboratory values return to normal within a few days.

Survival was reported as 75% in a large retrospective study (40). Lethal complications include irreversible shock, and injury to the kidneys and intestines. Extensive necrosis of the limbs may complicate management and necessitate limb amputation in rare instances.

Intravenous fluid administration and the use of steroids such as dexamethasone, prednisolone, or methyprednisolone have been used in the acute stage. Pain may be controlled using the same regimen as in cats with thromboebolism due to cardiac disease. Physiotherapy has been suggested as being extremely useful in the rehabilitation of affected cats. Recovery of hindlimb paralysis occurs between 2 days and 1 month. Long-term prognosis is excellent, in contrast to ischemic neuromyopathy due to cardiomyopathy (Fig. 6-7).

6.5.2 Myositis

Infectious myositis is uncommon in cats. It is more likely to be one aspect of a multisystemic illness such as toxoplasmosis. Clinical signs include fever and apparent muscle pain. Diagnosis is based on demonstrating the presence of one of the following causative organisms in a cat with confirmed myositis.

Protozoal myositis occurs rarely. The cat with clinical toxoplasmosis typically has respiratory or gastrointestinal signs, and a purely muscular localization is unlikely. Clindamycin is the drug of choice for feline toxoplasmosis (25 mg BID). Naturally occurring *Neospora caninum* has never been reported in cats, although it has been shown to affect feline skeletal muscles in experimental settings.

Bacterial myositis secondary to *Clostridium chauvoei* and *C. septicum* has been reported in cats. Treatment consists of administration of penicillin.

Paraneoplastic myositis may occur secondary to malignant tumors, such as lymphoma. Animals with histopathologically confirmed non-infectious myositis that fails to respond to steroid treatment should be evaluated for underlying malignancies.

An acquired diffuse inflammatory myopathy, feline idiopathic myositis, has been described in cats. The disease may affect both young and old individuals, and is characterized by sudden weakness and cervical ventroflexion. Muscles are painful in some animals. Histopathology is the key to diagnosis, in addition to elevated creatine kinase and abnormal electromyographic findings. Muscle cells reveal mononuclear cell infiltration into non-necrotic fibers, a low degree of muscle fiber necrosis, and phagocytosis, myofiber regeneration, and variation in fiber size. Differentiation between cats with hypokalemic myopathy may be difficult, as some affected cats may also be hypokalemic. If correction of hypokalemia does not result in clinical amelioration and infectious causes have been ruled out, prednisolone is administered (4–6 mg/kg SID, then tapered over 8 weeks). The prognosis is generally good, but long-term administration of glucocorticosteroids may be necessary in some cats (42).

6.5.3 Diabetic neuropathy

Peripheral neuropathy is a well-recognized debilitating complication of diabetes mellitus in cats. Eight percent of diabetic cats are affected with neurological symptoms, but the incidence of subclinical disease is probably much higher. Signs are usually typical of a symmetric distal limb polyneuropathy, and include a plantigrade stance (Fig. 6-8) and paraparesis, distal limb muscular atrophy, and pelvic limb hyporeflexia. Involvement of the thoracic limbs is observed in rare cases. The most frequently observed signs of mild neurological dysfunction include difficulty jumping, abduction of the pelvic limbs, weakness when standing, and increased sensitivity to sensory stimuli applied to their feet.

Electrodiagnostic examinations show a reduced motor nerve conduction velocity in the distal portions of the nerves, and reflect prominent demyelination at all levels of the motor and sensory nerves. Inconsistently, mild increases in insertional and spontaneous activity in appendicular muscles are detected on electromyogram. This reflects the mild axonopathy associated with this neuropathy. The more severe the

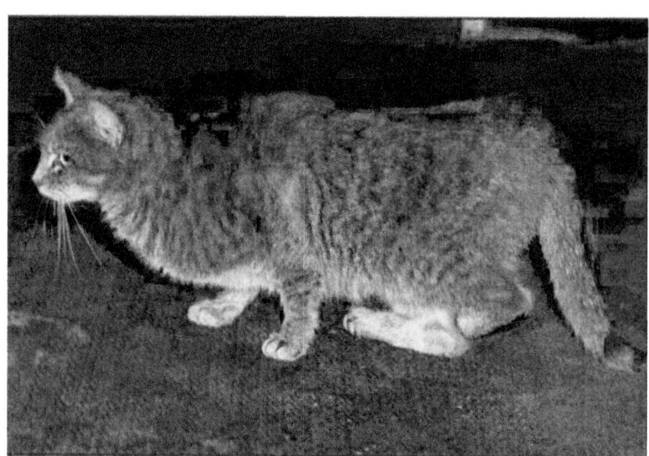

Figure 6-8 A 10-year-old cat with diabetes mellitus and associated neuropathy in the hindlimbs. Note the bilateral plantigrade stance, which is characteristic for a conduction block due to demyelination in the tibial nerves.

neurological signs, the more prominent the electrophysiological abnormalities.

Histological examination of nerve biopsies reveals multiple signs of Schwann cell injury with minimal axonal involvement. A combination of metabolic and vascular defects has been implicated in the pathogenesis of diabetic neuropathy (43–45).

Many cats continue to show some degree of clinical weakness and muscle atrophy, despite specific therapy with oral hypoglycemic agents or insulin. There is no specific treatment for this neuropathy as a full understanding of the pathogenesis and etiology of diabetic neuropathy is still lacking. Acetyl-L-carnitine has been used in a few cats with persistent neuropathy with subjectively good results (46). Alpha-liponic acid, a substance used for the treatment of human diabetic polyneuropathy, has also resulted in improvement of the neuropathy in a series of diabetic cats (unpublished personal results).

6.5.4 Hypokalemic myopathy

Hypokalemia may result in an acute onset of generalized weakness, muscular pain, and persistent ventroflexion of the head (Fig. 6-5). Affected cats show an exaggerated stilted, hypermetric gait in the forelimbs. Typical serum abnormalities include low or low/normal potassium and markedly elevated serum creatine kinase activity.

Renal loss of potassium associated with chronic renal failure is the most common cause. Other diseases resulting in hypokalemia include chronic vomiting or diarrhea, diuretic therapy, and hyperaldosteronism (47, 48).

Administration of oral potassium (initial dosage: 1–3 mEq/kg per day divided q8h, maintenance dose (when serum potassium normal): 1 mEq/kg per day q12h) and parenteral potassium (Table 6-5) leads to reversal of the polymyopathy, and creatine kinase activity returning to normal. Prognosis for recovery of the polymyopathy is favorable, but the long-term outcome is determined by the underlying cause of the hypokalemia.

Serum potassium (mmol/l)	Supplementation (mEq/l)
3.5–4.5	20
3.0–3.5	30
2.5–3.0	40
2.0–2.5	60
<2.0	80

Table 6-5. Supplementation of potassium according to serum potassium levels. Do not exceed an intravenous rate of 0.5 mEq/kg per hour

A different, probably hereditary form of hypokalemia has been described in Burmese cats aged 2–12 months (49). The inciting factor in the etiopathogenesis of this disease seems to be low potassium intake or increased renal loss. Affected cats can be normal between their episodes of weakness and neck ventroflexion. Specific dietary supplementation may reduce the problem in this breed.

6.5.5 Myasthenia gravis

Myasthenia gravis (MG) is a disorder of neuromuscular transmission resulting from either a deficiency or functional disorder of the nicotinic acetylcholine receptor (AChR). The most common cause in small animals is an autoimmune attack against AChRs, resulting in depletion of receptors (acquired MG). An increased risk for acquired MG was identified in Somali and Abyssinian cats when compared with the incidence in mixed-breed cats. Only a few cats have been reported with congenital MG (50).

Feline MG is less common than its canine counterpart, but MG should be considered in any cat that is presented with a recent onset of muscular weakness.

Typical signs include generalized weakness, megaesophagus, and dysphagia. Focal signs, including ventroflexion of the head, change of voice due to laryngeal paresis, absence of palpebral reflexes and dysphagia without generalized weakness, may occur. Thymomas have been found in a significant number of myasthenic cats; thoracic radiographs should be evaluated in all cats with confirmed or suspected MG. Acquired, drug-induced MG should be considered in hyperthyroid cats that become weak after initiation of treatment with methimazole (51).

Diagnosis is based upon clinical signs and demonstration of serum antibodies against AChR. Administration of edrophonium chloride (0.5–1 mg IV) may result in transient resolution of the clinical signs. The transmission disorder may be demonstrated by electromyelography with the aid of supramaximal repetitive nerve stimulation. This test is especially helpful for diagnosis of congenital MG, where AChR antibodies are not present.

Cats can be successfully treated with anticholinesterase drugs, such as pyridostigmine bromide (1–3 mg/kg BID–TID PO) or neostigmine bromide (2 mg/kg BID PO). However, immunosuppressive doses of corticosteroids (prednisolone 1–2 mg/kg SID–BID) may be necessary in most cases. Thymectomy is indicated if a thymoma is present. Long-term studies with serial AChR antibody titers are not available in cats; thus the natural course of the disease is not known and lifelong therapy might be indicated (52).

References and further reading

1. Munana KR, et al. Intervertebral disc disease in 10 cats. J Am Anim Hosp Assoc 2001;37:384–389.
2. Rayward RM. Feline intervertebral disc disease: a review of the literature. Vet Comp Orthop Traumatol 2002;15:137–144.
3. King AS, Smith RN. Protrusion of the intervertebral disc in the cat. Vet Rec 1958;70:509–512.
4. King AS, Smith RS. Disc protrusion in the cat: distribution of dorsal protrusions along the vertbral column. Vet Rec 1958; 70:509–515.
5. Heavener JE. Intervertebral disc syndrome in a cat. J Am Vet Med Assoc 1971;159:425–427.
6. Lu D, et al. Acute intervertebral disc extrusion in a cat: clinical and MRI findings. J Feline Med Surg 2002;4:65–68.
7. Jaeger GH, et al. Lumbosacral disc disease in a cat. Vet Comp Orthop Traumatol 2004;2:104–106.
8. Kneissl S, Schedlbauer B. Radiology corner. Sagittal computed tomography of the feline spine. Vet Radiol Ultrasound 1997; 38:282–283.
9. Komori H, et al. The natural history of herniated nucleus pulposus with radiculopathy. Spine 1996;21:225–229.
10. Braughler JM, Hall ED. Uptake and elimination of methyprednisolone from contused cat spinal cord following intravenous injection of the sodium succinate ester. J Neurosurg 1983; 58:538–542.
11. Bracken MB, et al. A randomized controlled study of methylprednisolone or naloxone in the treatment of acute spinal cord injury. N Engl J Med 1990;322:1405–1411.
12. Coates JR, et al. Clinicopathologic effects of a 21-aminosteroid compound (U74389G) and high-dose methyprednisolone on spinal cord function after simulated spinal cord trauma. Vet Surg 1995;24:128–139.
13. Coates JR. Intervertebral disc disease. Vet Clin North Am Small Anim Pract 2000;30:77–110.
14. Kathmann I, et al. Spontaneous lumbar intervertebral disc protrusions in cats: literature review and case presentation. J Feline Med Surg 2002;2:207–212.
15. Olby N, et al. Long-term functional outcome of dogs with severe injuries of the thoracolumbar spinal cord: 87 cases. J Am Vet Med Assoc 2003;222:762–769.
16. Lovely RG, et al. Effects of training on the recovery of full weight bearing stepping in the adult spinal cat. Exp Neurol 1990;92:206–218.
17. Giuliani CA, et al. Return of weight supported locomotion in adult spinal cats. Society for Neuroscience 1984, abstract 10:632.
18. Shamir MH, et al. Subarachnoid cyst in a cat. J Am Anim Hosp Assoc 1997;33:123–125.
19. Vignoli M, et al. Spinal subarachnoid cyst in a cat. Vet Radiol 1999;40:116–119.
20. Scott HW, O'Leary MT. Fibrocartilaginous embolism in a cat. J Small Anim Pract 1996;37:228–231.
21. Abramson CJ, et al. Tetraparesis in a cat with fibrocartilaginous emboli. J Am Anim Hosp Assoc 2002;28;153–156.
22. Mikszewski JS, et al. Fibrocartilaginous embolic myelopathy in five cats. J Am Anim Hosp Assoc 2006;42:226–233.
23. Marioni-Henry K, et al. Prevalence of diseases of the spinal cord of cats. J Vet Intern Med 2004;18:851–858.
24. Baroni M, Heynold Y. A review of the clinical diagnosis of feline infectious peritonitis viral meningoencephalomyelitis. Prog Vet Neurol 1995;3:88–94.
25. Legendre AM, Whitenack DL. Feline infectious peritonitis with spinal cord involvement in two cats. J Am Vet Med Assoc 1992;167:931–932.
26. Thomas WB. Discospondylitis and other vertebral infections. Vet Clin North Am Small Anim Pract 2000;30:169–182.
27. Norsworthy GD. Discospondylitis as a cause of posterior paralysis. Feline Pract 1979;9:39–41.
28. Malik R, et al. Bacterial discospondylitis in a cat. J Small Anim Pract 1990;31:404–408.
29. Watson E, Robertson RE. Discospondylitis in a cat. Vet Radiol 1993;34:397–399.
30. Bestetti G, et al. Paraplegia due to *Actinomyces viscosus* in a cat. Acta Neuropathol 1977;39:231–235.
31. Kraus H, et al. Paraparesis caused by epidural granuloma in a cat. J Am Anim Hosp Assoc 1998;194:789–790.
32. Lavely JA, et al. Spinal empyema in seven dogs. Vet Surg 2006; 35:176–185.
33. Kerl ME. Update on canine and feline fungal diseases. Vet Clin North Am Small Anim Pract 2003;33:749–758.
34. Foureman P, et al. Spinal cord granuloma due to *Coccidioides immitis* in a cat. J Vet Int Med 2005;19:373–376.
35. Lavely J, Lipsitz D. Fungal infections of the central nervous system in the dog and cat. Clin Tech Small Anim Pract 2005;20:212–219.
36. Wiebe V, Karriker M. Therapy of systemic fungal infections: a pharmalogic perspective. Clin Tech Small Anim Pract 2005;20: 250–257.
37. Colter SB. Congenital abnormalities of the spine. In: Bojrab MJ (ed.) Pathophysiology in small animal surgery. Philadelphia: Lea & Febiger; 1981: pp. 729–738.
38. Jaggy A, et al. Occipitoatlanto-axial malformation with atlantoaxial subluxation in a cat. J Small Animal Pract 1991;32: 366–372.
39. Atkins CE, et al. Risk factors, clinical signs, and survival in cats with a clinical diagnosis of idiopathic hypertrophic cardiomyopathy: 74 cases (1985–1989). J Am Vet Med Assoc 1992;201: 613–618.
40. Fischer I, et al. Akute traumatische Nachhandlähmung bei 30 Katzen. Tierärztl Prax (K) 2002;30:361–366.
41. Butler HC. An investigation into the relationship of an aortic embolus to posterior paralysis in the cat. J Small Anim Pract 1971;12:141–158.
42. Dickinson PJ, Lecouteur RA. Feline idiopathic inflammatory myopathy. Vet Clin North Am Small Anim Pract 2004;34: 1344–1345.

43. Kramek BA, et al. Neuropathy associated with diabetes mellitus in the cat. J Am Vet Med Assoc 1984;184:42–45.
44. Munana KA. Long term complications of diabetes mellitus, part I: retinopathy, nephropathy, neuropathy. Vet Clin North Am Small Anim Pract 1995;25:715–730.
45. Miszin AP, et al. Myelin splitting, Schwann cell injury and demyelination in feline diabetic neuropathy. Acta Neuropathol 1998;95:171–174.
46. Platt SR. Neuromuscular complications in endocrine and metabolic disorders. Vet Clin North Am Small Anim Pract 2002;32:125–143.
47. Dow SW, et al. Hypokalemia in cats: 186 cases (1984–87). J Am Vet Med Assoc 1989;194:1604–1608.
48. Jones BR. Hypokalemic myopathy in cats. In: Bonagura JD (ed.) Kirk's current veterinary therapy XIII: small animal practice. Philadelphia: WB Saunders; 2000: p. 958.
49. Lantinga E, et al. Periodic muscle weakness and neck ventroflexion caused by hypokalemia in a Burmese cat. Tijschr Diergeneeskd 1998;123:435–437.
50. Joseph RJ, et al. Myasthenia gravis in the cat. J Vet Intern Med 1988;2:753–768.
51. Shelton GD, et al. Risk factors for acquired myasthenia gravis in cats: 105 cases. J Am Vet Med Assoc 2000;216:55–57.
52. Shelton GD. Myasthenia gravis and disorders of neuromuscular transmission. Vet Clin North Am Small Anim Pract 2002; 32:189–206.

7 Diseases of soft tissues

C. Favrot, F. Gallorini, K. Voss, S.J. Langley-Hobbs

Diseases of the soft tissues of the locomotion system can result in gait disturbances and lameness. These include diseases of muscles and tendons, and disorders affecting the feet (Table 7-1). Diseases of tendons and diseases of muscles other than neuromuscular disorders are diagnosed infrequently in cats. They involve muscle contractures, fibrotic myopathy, and tendinopathies. Disorders involving the footpads, nail bed, and nails are more common. Examination of the nails and footpads is therefore an important part of the orthopedic examination in cats. This chapter covers non-neurological diseases of muscles, diseases of tendons, and diseases of the footpads, nailbeds, and nails. Neuromuscular disorders are described in Chapter 6.

7.1 Diseases of muscles

Most diseases of muscles encountered in cats are part of the neuromuscular disease complex. They can be inherited or acquired. Both inherited and acquired myopathies tend to cause systemic muscular weakness. Ventroflexion of the neck is a typical sign of myopathy in cats. Additional signs can include multisystemic illness, fever, and muscle pain. The most common feline neuromuscular diseases are described in Chapter 6.

Muscle contracture or fibrotic myopathy in cats has been described as occurring in the quadriceps muscle, the semitendinosus muscle, and the biceps muscle. Progressive ossifying fibrodysplasia (POF) is an unusual disease, characterized by generalized extensive periskeletal soft-tissue ossification.

7.1.1 Muscle contracture and fibrosis

Muscle contracture is a pathological shortening of the muscle which renders it unable to stretch. The condition is characterized by fibroplasia of muscular tissue. This replacement of muscle fibers by connective tissue results in a non-functional and taut muscle. Fibrotic myopathy is another term used to describe replacement of functional muscle tissue by connective tissue. Possible reasons for muscle contracture and fibrosis include external and exercise-induced trauma, neuropathy or myopathy, and muscle ischemia and necrosis. External trauma is likely to be the most common underlying cause in cats. Muscle contracture and fibrosis does not seem to be painful by itself, but irreversible loss of muscle function occurs. This can also impair function of adjacent joints, can lead to secondary joint pathology, and may result in a completely non-functional limb, depending on which muscle is affected. The condition usually affects one specific muscle, uni- or bilaterally. Muscle contracture and fibrosis occurs in various muscles in dogs, but seems to be rare in cats. The quadriceps muscle group is most commonly affected. Fibrotic myopathy of the semitendinosus muscle and contracture of the biceps muscle have also been described.

Contracture and fibrosis of the quadriceps muscle

Several cases of contracture of the quadriceps muscle secondary to femoral fractures (1–3) and one case of congenital quadriceps contracture (4) have been described. Adhesions between the muscle and femur and replacement of muscle fibers by fibrous tissue lead to contracture, inelasticity, and loss of quadriceps function. Quadriceps contracture limits motion of the stifle and tarsal joints, and the end stage of the disease is a stifle joint locked in full extension (Fig. 7-1). Initially, the condition may be partially reversible, but it rapidly becomes irreversible due to ongoing loss of muscle fibers, fibrosis, and degeneration, and ankylosis of the stifle joint. Adhesions or incorporation of the quadriceps muscle in the fracture callus is often present. It is unclear if adhesions

Affected tissue	Diseases
Muscles	Neuromuscular diseases (Chapter 6) Muscle contracture and fibrosis Progressive ossifying fibrodysplasia Localized myositis ossificans
Tendons	Biceps tenosynovitis (Chapter 28) Medial epicondylitis of the elbow (Chapter 30) Luxation of the superficial digital flexor tendon (Chapter 40)
Feet	Diseases of the nails and nail beds Diseases of the interdigital spaces Diseases of the foot pads

Table 7-1. Summary of diseases of soft tissues that can cause or mimic orthopedic problems

are a result of the contracture, or if they initiate immobilization and promote contracture (2).

Quadriceps contracture after internal fixation of femoral fractures in cats was reported to occur in 4 out of 22 cats (1). Most of these cats, including patients with comminuted fractures, were treated with intramedullary pins alone or in combination with cerclage wires. This kind of fracture repair often results in fracture instability and prolonged disuse of the leg, which may promote the development of quadriceps contracture. Sciatic nerve entrapment by the intramedullary pins and instability at the fracture site were identified in 3 of the 4 cases with quadriceps contracture in one series, and this was thought to have contributed to limb disuse (1). Although not statistically evaluated, mid-diaphyseal femoral fractures, fractures with moderate or severe displacement and shortening, fracture fixation more than 5 days after the injury, intramedullary pinning, and delayed use of the limb postoperatively were considered to be predisposing factors (1). Nowadays, the application of more stable fixation techniques results in a much lower incidence of quadriceps contracture.

Treatment of quadriceps contracture is unrewarding once the muscle is fibrotic and non-functional, and prevention is therefore most important. Early and stable fracture fixation, careful tissue handling, and postoperative physiotherapy allow early weight-bearing and limb use, which is crucial to maintain muscle function and joint mobility. Traumatic lesions of the quadriceps muscle are appropriately treated, as described in Chapter 16.

Treatment options include intensive physical therapy, surgical release of muscle adhesions, inclusion of a fat graft as an anatomical gliding plane, muscle-lengthening procedures, and application of a 90°–90° flexion splint or dynamic flexion apparatus. Each of these measures alone is not likely to result in a successful outcome and they must therefore be combined. Successful management of quadriceps contracture in a cat has been described with application of a dynamic flexion apparatus after surgical release of adhesions, stable fracture fixation, and physiotherapy (3, 5). The flexion apparatus consisted of an elastic band, anchored around transosseous pins in the pelvis and distal tibia, which held the stifle joint in flexion. The quadriceps muscle needs to be released sufficiently to allow flexion of the stifle joint prior to application of the flexion apparatus.

The authors have successfully treated two cats with quadriceps contracture secondary to femoral fracture by femoral ostectomy and plate osteosynthesis (Fig. 7-2). Shortening of the femur restores the relation between length of the contracted quadriceps muscle and the femur. The procedure is a promising one-step surgical method for treating cats with quadriceps contracture, provided that muscular fibrosis is not too extensive and some muscular function is left.

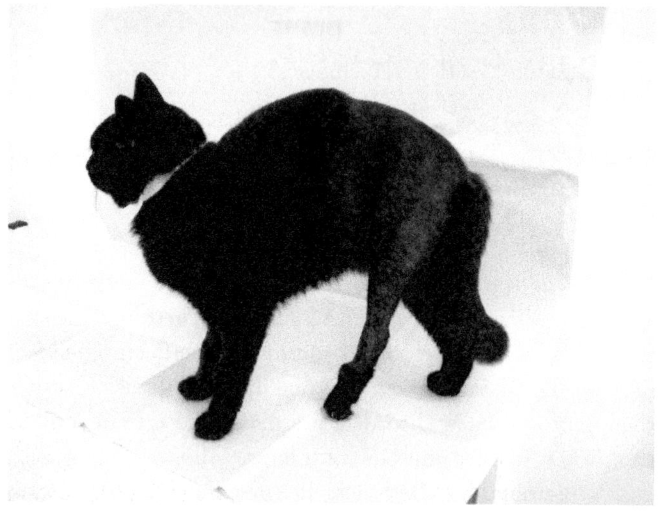

Figure 7-1 Photograph of a cat with quadriceps contracture of the left hindlimb, 4 weeks postoperative to a distal femoral fracture. Only approximately 10° of motion was left in the stifle joint, and the cat walked with the leg in extension.

Contracture and fibrosis of the semitendinosus muscle

Fibrotic myopathy of the semitendinosus muscle has been described in one cat (6). Gait abnormalities in this cat were consistent with inability to extend the stifle joint, flex the hip joint, and abduct the limb. A taut band could be palpated in the area of the semitendinosus muscle, as in dogs. Treatment of fibrotic myopathy of the semitendinosus muscle includes myotomy or myectomy, and muscle-lengthening procedures. Although surgery alleviates clinical signs in the short term, return to full function is unlikely. The fibrous band reformed during the healing phase, and clinical signs relapsed in the cat described (6). Best results are achieved with physiotherapy in dogs.

Contracture and fibrosis of the biceps muscle

Contracture and fibrosis of the biceps muscle was also described in one cat (7). Clinical signs were an inability to extend the elbow with resulting gait abnormality, and a taut muscle band was palpated over the craniolateral aspect of the brachium. Release of the fibrotic biceps muscle and sectioning of its tendon of insertion immediately alleviated clinical signs, but contracture occurred again after several months. A second surgery combined with physiotherapy resulted in a successful outcome.

7.1.2 Progressive ossifying fibrodysplasia (POF)

POF is an extremely rare genetic disease of the connective tissue characterized by a progressive heterotopic ossification of the tendons, ligaments, fasciae, and striated muscles. It is

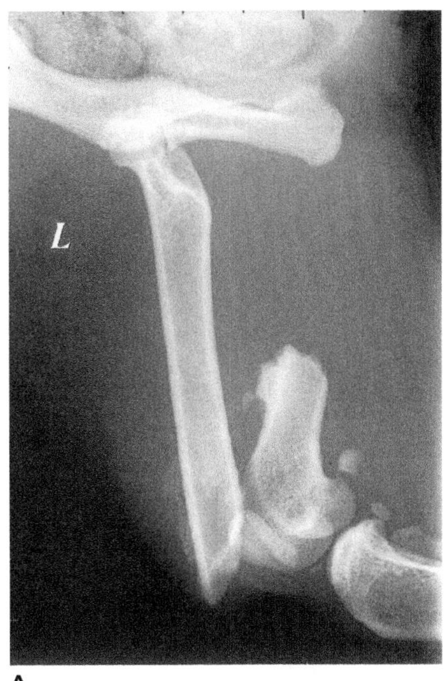

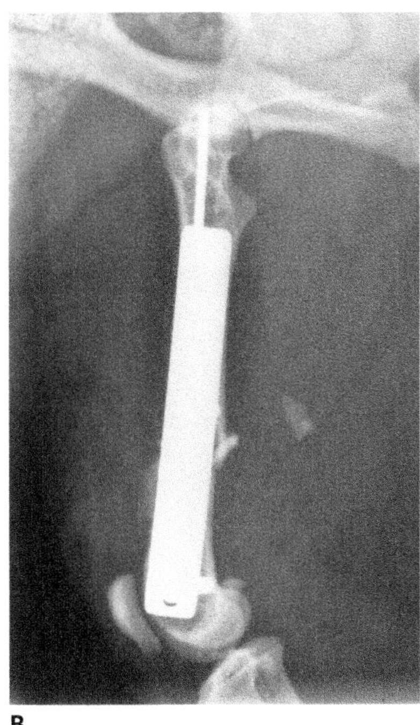

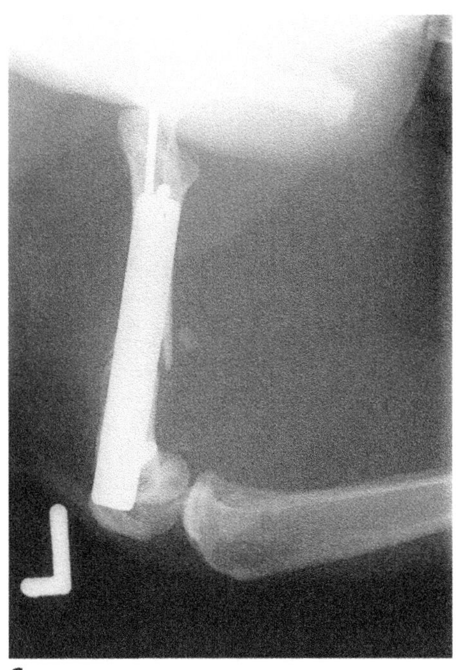

A B C

Figure 7-2 Radiographs of a cat with contracture of the quadriceps muscle.
(**A**) Preoperative mediolateral radiograph of the cat with a non-union of a distal diaphyseal femoral fracture, which had occurred 4 months ago.
(**B**) Postoperative radiograph of the cat. Because the fracture could not be reduced due to the tension exerted by the contracted and partially fibrosed quadriceps, a 2-cm ostectomy was performed prior to fracture stabilization. The stifle joint could be flexed 40° postoperatively.
(**C**) Two months after surgery the cat was using the leg well, and the stifle joint could be flexed 110°.

also called myositis ossificans, although it is not only muscle tissue that is affected. The condition can be generalized or localized.

The incidence of POF in humans is estimated to be 1 in 2 000 000, without sexual or racial predisposition (8). Clinical conditions, and radiographic or histological results similar to those observed in human POF, have been reported in cats (9, 10). The etiopathogenesis of the lesions in humans is linked to the excessive presence of bone morphogenetic protein-4 (BMP4) in the lymphocytes. Once activated at the tissue level, this cell population, both B and T types, produces a quantity of BMP4 without the normal biochemical regulatory mechanisms. This leads to the development of lesions, which in the early stages are of a highly vascularized, fibroproliferating type. These undergo a process of chondroid metaplasia, followed by endochondral ossification with formation of lamellae and medullary elements (11–13). The condition is genetically determined and is of the autosomal-dominant type linked to de novo genetic mutations (14).

The genetic means of transmission has not been demonstrated in cats at present, although the disease follows a similar clinical, radiological, and histological progression to that in humans. The disease occurs without sexual predisposition in young or middle-aged cats. The lesions appear in the early clinical stages as inflammatory-type lesions of the muscles, and sometimes effects on the overlying skin have been observed (10). In the later stages, the nidus takes on the appearance of swelling of the affected muscular groups with a hard bony consistency, that is not painful to the touch, and without perilesional edema or other signs of inflammation. The patient has a stiff, uncertain gait, with marked reduction in the range of motion of affected limbs and muscles (Fig. 7-3). There are usually no significant hematological or biochemical alterations, but fever and leukocytosis have been observed, linked to the inflammatory effects of the early lesions (10).

Diagnosis is made radiologically, based on the typical signs of heterotopic ossification. The areas of ossification have a trabecular appearance and clearly extend into the muscles, fasciae, and tendons (Figs 7-4 and 7-5). With the generalized form, the progression of the pathology is fairly rapid; death usually occurs within weeks to a few months after the manifestation of the first signs (10), but one cat was reported to be alive and well 18 months after initial presentation (15). Similarly to what occurs in human POF, any type of trauma, even of limited entity such as an intramuscular injection, can set off tissue reactions ending in ossifying lesions. Muscular biopsies and excisional surgery are contraindicated for this reason. Therapy based on selenium, vitamin E, and corticosteroids, followed by administration of sodium ethidronate, has been suggested for cats, but results are unsatisfactory (10).

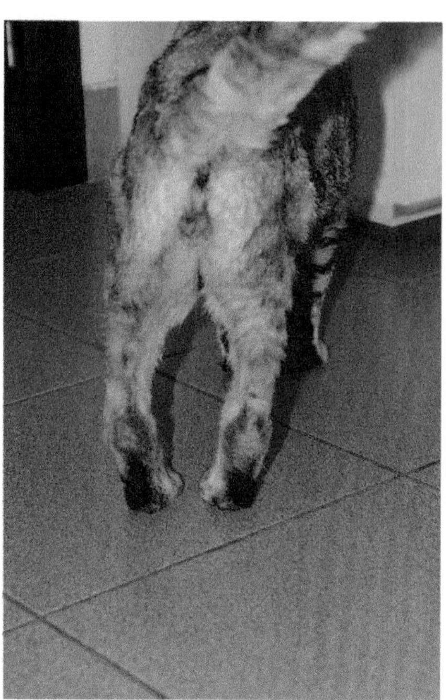

Figure 7-3 A 7-month-old cat with progressive ossifying fibrodysplasia, showing internal rotation of both hindfeet. The cat had a stiff and stilted gait. (Courtesy of F. Gallorini.)

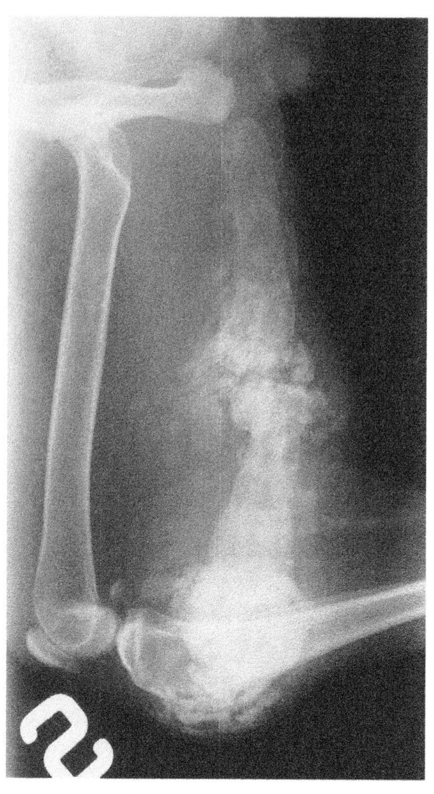

Figure 7-5 A close-up radiographic view of the tibia and the ossified lesions in the thigh. Note the trabecular structure of the soft-tissue ossification, almost resembling normal bone.

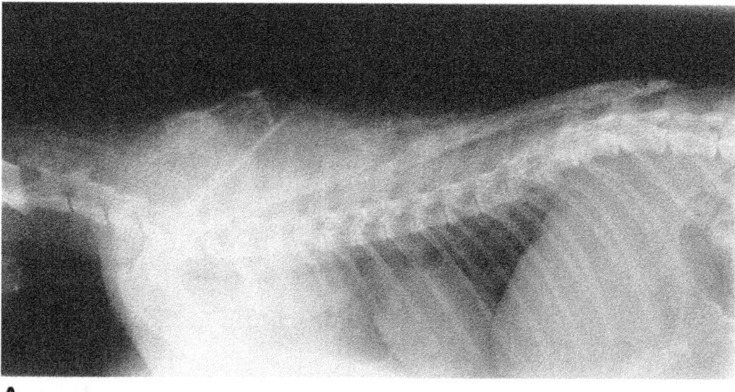

A

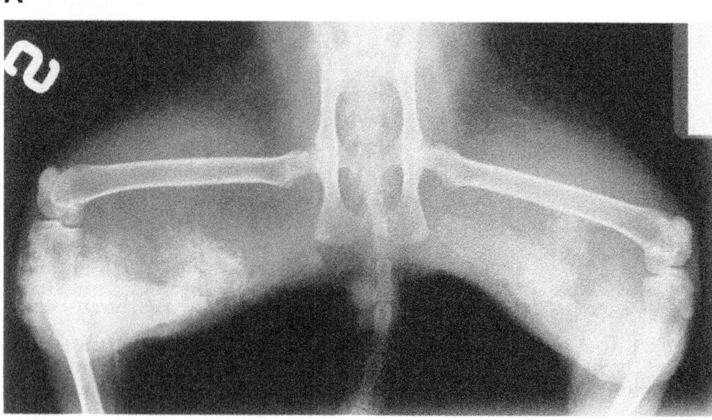

B

Figure 7-4 (**A**) Radiographs of the scapula and (**B**) the hindlimbs of the cat shown in Figure 7-3. Massive periskeletal ossification of the soft tissues is visible, predominantly affecting the thigh muscles. The scapular area has ossified lesions with a finer trabecular appearance.

7.1.3 Localized myositis ossificans

Care must be taken to differentiate the generalized muscle disease POF from the localized form of myositis ossificans, which has a much better and non-fatal prognosis. One of the authors has seen two cats with mineralization in the caudal thigh muscles. Both cats had gait abnormalities very similar to dogs with gracilis contracture, and similar to the gait abnormality reported for the cat with the semitendinosus contracture (6). In one cat the affected area of mineralization was resected and the condition recurred after about a year. In the other cat the condition was managed conservatively. It is possible that there is a relationship between fibrotic myopathy and localized myositis ossificans (7), as some dogs with gracilis contracture have areas of mineralization in the affected muscles.

7.2 Diseases of tendons

Diseases of tendons are extremely rare in cats, and only a handful of case reports exist on feline tendon diseases in the veterinary literature. These include biceps tenosynovitis, and luxation of the superficial digital flexor tendon from the calcaneus, although the latter might have been caused by trauma (16, 17) (Chapters 28 and 40). Also, rupture or strain of the Achilles tendon or triceps tendon is usually traumatic in origin, but cats occasionally present with bilateral tendon strains without a history of observed trauma. An underlying condition should be suspected if signs of chronicity, such as periosteal bone proliferation and soft-tissue calcification, exist, possibly resulting in weakness and pathological changes in the tendon. Some medical conditions, such as diabetes or hyperadrenocorticism, and certain drugs are known to promote tendon rupture. Exposure to quinolones and corticosteroids, for example, increases the risk for Achilles tendon rupture in humans (18). Such conditions have not yet been reported or identified in cats. Rupture of the Achilles tendon is described in Chapter 40, and rupture of the triceps tendon in Chapter 30.

7.3 Conditions of the feet

Pododermatitis or inflammatory conditions of the feet can induce discomfort, pain, and lameness in cats. These conditions may affect the nail, nail beds, the interdigital spaces, or the footpads. The most frequent pododermatitides are summarized below. Tumors affecting the feet are covered in Chapter 8.

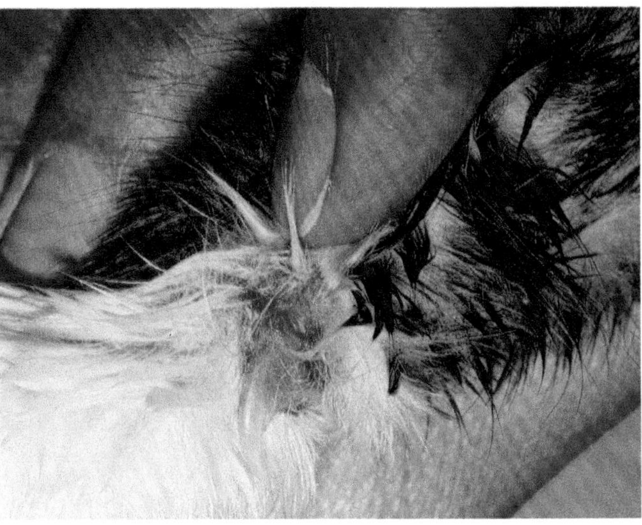

Figure 7-6 Bacterial paronychia. Note the inflammation of the nail bed with edema, erythema, and crusts.

7.3.1 Diseases of the nails and nail beds

Several diseases can affect the nail beds, all causing similar clinical signs. Diagnosis of the underlying cause is crucial for appropriate treatment. Bacterial paronychia is the most common condition affecting a single or a few nail beds. Bacterial paronychia in association with systemic disease, pemphigus foliaceus, onychomycosis, or nail chewing should be considered if several or all nail beds are affected.

Bacterial paronychia

Bacterial infection of the nail bed can occur secondary to local trauma, ingrowing nails, or it may be a complication after declawing. These causes are most likely if only one or two digits are affected, but neoplasia should be considered as a differential diagnosis (Chapter 8). Bacterial paronychia can also occur in association with systemic diseases and impairment of the immune system, such as feline leukemia virus (FeLV)/feline immunodeficiency virus (FIV) infection, diabetes mellitus, hyperadrenocorticism, glucocorticoid or hormonal treatments, and internal tumors (19–23). If several or all nail beds are affected, systemic disease, onychomycosis, and pemphigus foliaceus are the main differential diagnoses.

The nail beds are usually swollen, erythematous, and painful. Pus, crusts, and erosions are often present (Fig. 7-6). The affected digit can be thickened and very painful if the infection has caused osteomyelitis, or if a tumor is present.

The diagnostic work-up depends on whether the paronychia is localized or affecting several nail beds, but it can include skin scrapings, cytological examination, bacterial and fungal cultures, basic blood work, FeLV and FIV tests, radiographs, and skin and bone histological examination. As contamination is frequent, bacterial and fungal culture results should be interpreted with caution and always together with the history, cytological, and histological examination results (19–23). Histological diagnosis for immune-mediated diseases usually requires excisional biopsy of the third phalanx.

Cats with one or two adjacent nail beds affected can be given a treatment trial of antimicrobial therapy for 2–3 weeks prior to performing all the diagnostic tests. Possible antibiotics to use include cephalexin (25 mg/kg BID) or amoxicillin with clavulanic acid (12.5 mg/kg BID). Radiographs of the third phalanx and the thorax should be performed if a tumor is suspected (Chapter 8). It is not usually possible to differentiate between osteomyelitis and neoplasia based on radiological findings alone.

Prognosis for bacterial paronychia depends on the underlying cause. Most of the traumatically induced infections respond readily to systemic antibiotic therapy, as described above. If systemic disease is present, the prognosis depends on the ability to treat the disease itself.

Pemphigus foliaceus

Pemphigus foliaceus is the most frequent autoimmune disease in cats, and it can affect the nail beds. In such cases, pemphigus foliaceus may resemble bacterial paronychia (Fig. 7-7). However, the nail beds are not usually the only affected sites (19–23). Most cats with pemphigus foliaceus also present with symmetric and pustular dermatitis of the face and ears.

Cytological examination of the pus usually reveals numerous acantholytic cells. These cells may also be seen in association with bacterial or fungal infection, so histological, and bacterial and fungal cultures are always required. When

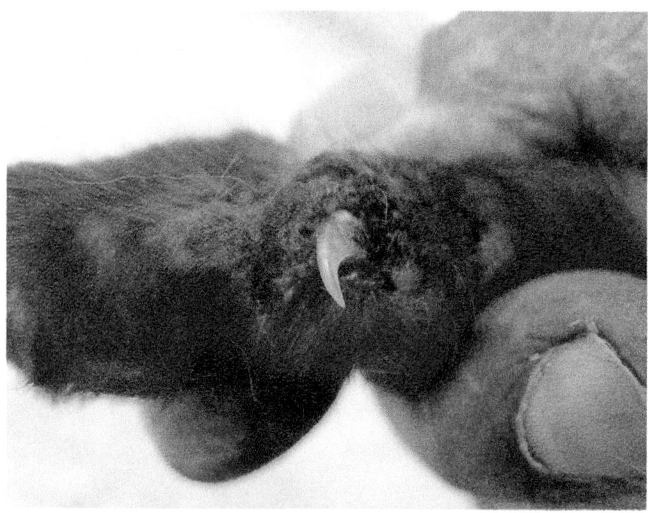

Figure 7-7 A cat with pemphigus foliaceus: erosions and purulent inflammation of the nail bed are visible.

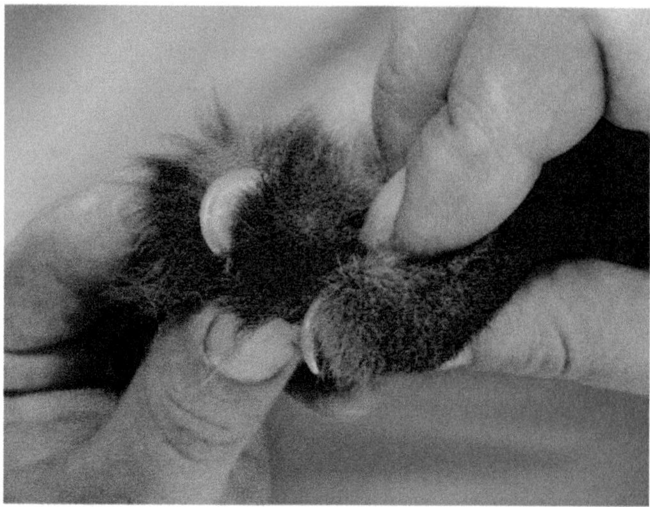

Figure 7-8 A cat with a long and abnormally grown nail, which has penetrated the skin and resulted in lameness.

nail beds are the only affected sites, definitive diagnosis requires excisional biopsy of the third phalanx. Treatment requires immunosuppressive doses of glucocorticoid (prednisolone 2–4 mg/kg daily) either alone or in association with other immunosuppressive drugs (chlorambucil 0.1 mg/kg daily).

Onychomycosis

Dermatophyte infections of the nail beds are rare in cats, and are often associated with impairment of the immune system (19–23).

These infections resemble other inflammatory conditions affecting the nail beds (see above). Work-up should include fungal culture, cytological examination of the exudate and evaluation of the immune system, including FeLV/FIV serology, and diagnostic screening for diabetes mellitus and hyperadrenocorticism. The prognosis depends on the underlying disease and both local and systemic treatments should be instituted. Local treatment can be carried out with enilconazole or miconazole solutions. Griseofulvin (ultramicrosized: 10 mg/kg daily) or itraconazole (5 mg/kg daily) are the best therapeutic options for systemic treatment.

Nail chewing

Behavioral disorders may be associated with nail chewing in cats (20). This condition is sometimes associated with secondary bacterial paronychia. History is mandatory to establish a proper diagnosis in such instances. Nail chewing can also be seen in cats recovering from neurotmesis, as sensation returns to the feet.

Idiopathic onychodystrophy

Idiopathic onychodystrophy results in abnormal growth of the nails (21–23). Abnormally long or shaped nails can penetrate the skin of the footpads, and thus cause lameness (Fig. 7-8). Several nails can be affected. The condition is most commonly seen in older cats whose ability to retract their claws seems to diminish with advancing years. Regular clipping of the nails is indicated to prevent injury to the skin of the footpads and lameness.

7.3.2 Diseases of the interdigital spaces

Compared to dogs, cats rarely suffer from diseases of the interdigital space. The main differential diagnoses include allergic conditions (eosinophilic plaques), and parasitic infections such as trombiculosis.

Eosinophilic plaques

Eosinophilic plaques can develop in the interdigital spaces and cause lameness (20). Cytological and/or histological examinations are usually necessary to obtain a specific diagnosis. Allergy work-up is mandatory to confirm or rule out allergic conditions such as food hypersensitivity or atopic dermatitis. Treatment with glucocorticoid (prednisolone 1–2 mg/kg daily) or cyclosporin A (5 mg/kg daily) is usually effective.

Trombiculosis (chiggers)

Chiggers (*Neotrombicula autumnalis*, North America: *Eutrombicula alfreddugesi*) larvae sometimes develop in the interdigital spaces of cats and may cause discomfort, pruritus, and lameness. *Trombicula autumnalis* infection is seasonal,

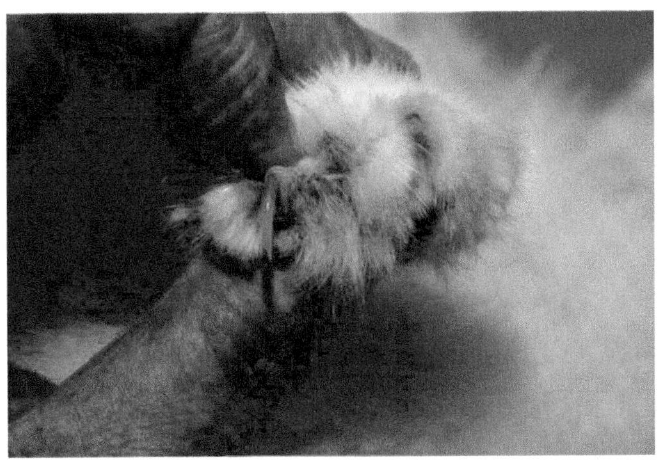

Figure 7-9 Cat with chiggers. The interdigital space is inflamed and the larvae are seen as small orange dots. (Courtesy of J. Declercq.)

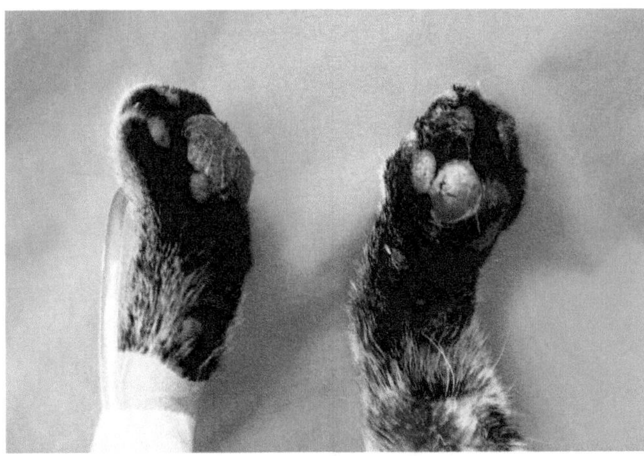

Figure 7-10 Footpads of the front limbs of a cat with plasmacytic pododermatitis. The pads are enlarged and softened. The main pad of the left front limb is ulcerated.

with most of the infections occurring in the late summer and early autumn. The larvae are seen as small orange dots between the toes, and often in Henry's pocket on the pinna (Fig. 7-9). The diagnosis is usually straightforward, and treatment requires parasite removal and acaricidal treatment.

7.3.3 Diseases of the footpads

Two conditions of the footpads secondary to systemic disease have been described in cats: plasma cell pododermatitis and metastatic calcifinosis of the paws.

Plasma cell pododermatitis

Feline plasmacytic pododermatitis is a rare disease of the footpads, characterized by soft and spongy swelling of multiple pads. Initially the disease does not seem to be painful, but pain, bleeding, and lameness occur if the pads ulcerate and become infected (Fig. 7-10). The pathogenesis of the disease is unknown, but histologically the lesions consist of an inflammatory infiltrate, mainly composed of mature plasma cells. This and the clinical response to immunosuppressive drugs suggests that it is an immune-mediated disease. Concurrent plasmacytic stomatitis and renal amyloidosis or glomerulonephritis have been reported (22, 23). One report suggested a link between plasma cell pododermatitis and FIV infection (24).

A tentative diagnosis can be made in the presence of the characteristic soft swelling of several footpads. Often all feet are involved, but the disease can also occur in only the front or only the hindfeet. The central pad is the most commonly affected. Definitive diagnosis requires histopathological confirmation of an inflammatory infiltrate of the dermis of the pads, containing mainly plasma cells. Neutrophil and macrophage numbers will increase if ulceration and infection are present.

Cats usually respond well to glucocorticoid therapy in immunosuppressive doses. Doxycycline, given for at least 3 weeks at a dose of 25 mg/kg BW orally every 24 hours, was also found to result in partial or complete remission in many cats (25). This effect is most likely due to the immunomodulatory properties of doxycycline. As doxycyline bears less risk for adverse side-effects compared to immunosuppressive drugs, a doxycycline trial for 3–4 weeks can be used before glucocorticoids are administered. Resolution has also been described after surgical resection of affected pads (26), but surgery should only be considered after failed conservative treatment, considering the invasiveness and morbidity associated with it.

Metastatic calcinosis of the paws

Metastatic calcinosis of soft tissues can be associated with any disease causing hypercalcemia and/or hyperphosphatemia. A solubility product of calcium and phosphorus of greater than 7 g/l is usually required for metastatic calcification to occur. Chronic renal failure in cats is frequently associated with hyperphosphatemia, which may be high enough to result in a solubility product greater than 7 g/l, despite normal serum calcium concentrations. Hyperparathyroidism also seems to play a role in the mechanism of calcification. Paw calcification as a manifestation of renal disease has been described in a small number of cats (27–29). Affected cats might be presented because of lameness. The calcifications appear as intact or ulcerated nodules involving multiple pads or the interdigital spaces (Fig. 7-11). The nodules are firm on palpation and appear whitish to gray. Laboratory results consistent with chronic renal failure, such as azotemia

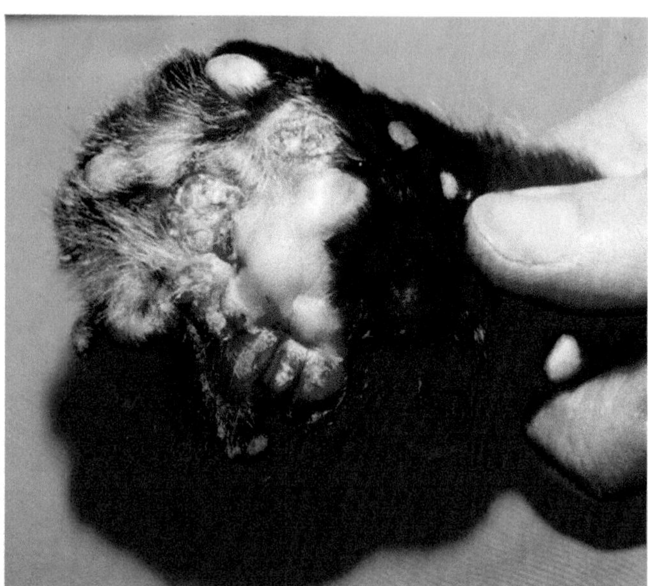

Figure 7-11 Photograph of a cat with renal failure, showing metastatic calcinosis of the foot. (Courtesy of J. Declercq.)

and hyperphosphatemia, are present. The paws are areas subject to trauma and therefore may be predisposed for deposition of calcium salts. Other soft tissues such as the aorta, stomach wall, and subcutaneous tissue, can also be affected (27, 29).

Diagnosis of calcinosis requires cytology and/or histopathology. Therapy consists of feeding a protein- and phosphorus-restricted diet. Intestinal phosphate-binding agents may be additionally prescribed. Paw calcification due to renal failure improved or regressed with a low-phosphorus/low-protein diet in some cases (27, 28).

Besides chronic renal failure, rare causes of hypercalcemia and/or hyperphosphatemia, such as hyperthyroidism, hypervitaminosis D, hypercalcemia of malignancy, or primary hyperparathyroidism, should be considered in the diagnostic work-up. Metastatic calcinosis of the paws associated with hyperthyroidism has recently been described in a cat (29). The lesions resolved after treatment with radioactive iodine.

Calicivirus infections

Calicivirus infections are sometimes associated, along with classical signs, with facial and/or pedal signs in young cats. Feet edema, pain, small crusts, and footpad ulceration may be noticed. Clinical signs usually regress within a few days. Antibiotic therapy is sometimes required to treat secondary bacterial infection.

Contact irritant dermatitis

Contact irritant dermatitis is rare in cats but may sometimes affect the footpads. Herbicides have, for example, been associated with such a condition (20). History is mandatory to make the diagnosis and rule out similar conditions such as plasma cell pododermatitis or calicivirus infection. Removal of the offending compound and local treatments are usually curative.

References and further reading

1. Fries SL, et al. Quadriceps contracture in four cats: a complication of internal fixation of femoral fractures. Vet Comp Orthop Traumatol 1988;2:91–96.
2. Carberry CA, Flanders JA. Quadriceps contracture in a cat. J Am Vet Med Assoc 1986;189:1329.
3. Liptak JM, Simpson DJ. Successful management of quadriceps contracture in a cat using a dynamic flexion apparatus. Vet Comp Orthop Traumatol 2000;13:44–48.
4. Leighton RL. Muscle contractures in the limbs of dogs and cats. Vet Surg 1981;10:132–135.
5. Wilkens BE, et al. Utilization of dynamic stifle flexion apparatus in preventing recurrence of quadriceps contracture: a clinical report. Vet Comp Orthop Traumatol 1993;6:219–223.
6. Lewis DD. Fibrotic myopathy of the semitendinosus muscle in a cat. J Am Vet Med Assoc 1988;193:240–241.
7. Taylor J, Tangner CH. Acquired muscle contractures in the dog and cat. A review of literature and case report. Vet Comp Orthop Traumatol 2007;20:79–85.
8. Mahboubi S, et al. Fibrodysplasia ossificans progressiva. Pediatr Radiol 2001;31:307–314.
9. Warren HB, Carpenter JL. Fibrodysplasia ossificans in three cats. Vet Pathol 1984;21:495–499.
10. Valentine BA, et al. Fibrodysplasia ossificans in the cat. A case report. J Vet Intern Med 1992;6:335–340.
11. Shafritz AB, et al. Overexpression of an osteogenic morphogen in fibrodysplasia ossificans progressiva. N Engl J Med 1996;335: 591–593.
12. Gannon FH, et al. Acute lymphocytic infiltration in an extremely early lesion of fibrodysplasia ossificans progressiva. Clin Orthop Relat Res 1998;346:19–25.
13. O'Connor P. Animal model of heterotropic ossification. Clin Orthop Relat Res 1998;346:71–80.
14. Delatycki M, Rogers RG. The genetics of fibrodysplasia ossificans progressiva. Clin Orthop Relat Res 1998;346:15–18.
15. Bradley WA. Fibrodysplasia ossificans in a Himalayan cat. Aust Vet Pract 1992;22:154–158.
16. Scharf G, et al. Glenoid dysplasia and bicipital tenosynovitis in a Maine coon cat. J Small Anim Pract 2004;45:515–520.
17. McNicholas WT, et al. Luxation of the superficial digital flexor tendon in a cat. J Am Anim Hosp Assoc 2000;36:174–176.
18. Van der Linden PD, et al. Increased risk of Achilles tendon rupture with quinolone antibacterial use, especially in elderly patients taking oral corticosteroids. Arch Intern Med 2003; 163:1801–1807.
19. Guaguère E, et al. Feline pododermatoses. Vet Dermatol 1992;3:1–12.
20. Guaguère E, et al. Diagnostic approach of feline pododermatoses. In: Guaguère P (ed.) A practical guide to feline dermatology. Lyon, France: Merial Eds; 2000: pp. 24.1–24.9.
21. Scott DW, Miller WH. Disorders of the claw and clawbed in cats. Compend Contin Educ 1992;14:449–455.
22. Scott DW. Feline dermatology 1979–72: introspective retrospections. J Am Anim Hosp Assoc 1984;20:537–564.
23. Scott DW. Feline dermatology 1983–85: the secret sits. J Am Anim Hosp Assoc 1987;23:255–257.

24. Simon M. Plasmacell pododermatitis in immunodeficiency virus-infected cats. Vet Pathol 1993;30:477.
25. Bettenay SV, et al. Prospective study of the treatment of feline plasmacytic pododermatitis with doxycycline. Vet Rec 2003; 152:564–566.
26. Yamamura Y. A surgically treated case of feline plasma cell pododermatitis. J Jpn Vet Med Assoc 1998;51:669–671.
27. Bertazzolo W, et al. Clinicopathological findings in five cats with paw calcification. J Feline Med Surg 2003;5:11–17.
28. Jackson HA, Barber PJ. Resolution of metastatic calcification in the paws of a cat with successful dietary management of renal hyperparathyroidism. J Small Anim Pract 1998;39:495–497.
29. Declercq J, Bhatti S. Calcinosis involving multiple paws in a cat with chronic renal failure and in a cat with hyperthyroidism. Vet Dermatol 2005;16:74–78.

8 Tumors of the musculoskeletal system

V.J. Poirier, F. Steffen

Tumors of the musculoskeletal system are uncommon in cats compared to dogs. The rarity of these tumors often makes their behavior and optimal treatment difficult to define. This chapter summarizes the knowledge and standard of care for cats with tumors involving the musculoskeletal system, based on the current data available in the literature. Table 8-1 lists the tumors covered in this chapter, and Table 8-2 outlines the characteristics, treatment, and prognosis of the most common tumors of the musculoskeletal system in cats.

8.1 Bone tumors

8.1.1 Incidence and risk

Primary bone tumors are uncommon in cats compared to dogs. The incidence of all bone tumors in cats is 4.9 per 100 000 (1). Osteosarcoma is by far the most common feline primary bone tumor, accounting for about 70% of primary bone tumors (2, 3). A multitude of other histopathological diagnoses have also been reported, including fibrosarcoma, chondrosarcoma, plasma cell tumor, hemangiosarcoma, and lymphosarcoma (4). Unfortunately, the behavior of most of these other feline bone tumors is unknown due to the rarity of the disease, and information must be extrapolated from what is known of the equivalent canine tumor.

8.1.2 Pathology and natural behavior

Histopathologically, feline osteosarcoma is characterized by neoplastic mesenchymal cells which produce osteoid (5) (Fig. 8-1). The production of osteoid is the hallmark of osteosarcoma. Multinucleated giant cells can be present. Different types of osteosarcoma have been reported, including osteosarcoma of medullary origin, parosteal osteosarcoma (6), fracture-associated osteosarcoma (7, 8), and extraskeletal osteosarcoma (2). Extraskeletal osteosarcoma is often seen at vaccination sites, and is classified in the same category as vaccine-associated sarcoma. This will be discussed in one of the following sections.

Skeletal osteosarcoma is much more common than extraskeletal osteosarcoma (2). The appendicular skeleton is affected more often than the axial skeleton, and the tumor occurs more frequently in the bones of the hindlimbs than the forelimbs (2, 3). Regardless of the primary site, feline skeletal osteosarcoma is considered locally invasive, with a low metastatic potential of only 5–10% (2, 3). This is an

Tumor localization	Tumor types
Primary bone tumors	Osteosarcoma, chondrosarcoma, multiple myeloma, hemangiosarcoma, fibrosarcoma
Soft-tissue sarcomas	Vaccine-associated sarcoma, undifferentiated sarcoma, hemangiosarcoma, fibrosarcoma, malignant fibrous histiocytoma, rhabdomyosarcoma
Oral tumors	Squamous cell carcinoma, fibrosarcoma
Tumors of the nervous system	**Vertebral bodies**
	Osteosarcoma, chondroma, chondrosarcoma, fibrosarcoma
	Spinal cord and meninges
	Lymphoma, meningioma, meningeal sarcoma, glioma, astrocytoma
	Peripheral nerve tumors
	Schwannoma, fibrosarcoma, lymphoma
Miscellaneous	Multiple cartilaginous exostosis
	Metastatic digital carcinoma
	Synovial cell sarcoma, synovioma

Table 8-1. Tumors involving the feline musculoskeletal system. Osteosarcoma, vaccine-associated sarcoma, and spinal lymphoma are the most common

Tumor type	Characteristics	Treatment options	Prognosis
Osteosarcoma	Hindlimbs more commonly affected	Amputation	Reasonable chance of cure, 10% risk of metastasis
Vaccine-associated sarcoma	Found at vaccine sites, highly invasive, moderate metastatic potential	Surgery	Time to recurrence: 3 months for marginal excision, 9 months for radical excision
		Surgery combined with radiation therapy (treatment of choice)	Time to recurrence: 18 months
		Surgery and chemotherapy	Time to recurrence: 12 months
Spinal lymphoma	Many cats feline leukemia virus-positive, often becomes systemic	Radiation for local tumor Chemotherapy for generalized disease	Poor

Table 8-2. Characteristics, treatment, and prognosis of the most common musculoskeletal tumors of cats

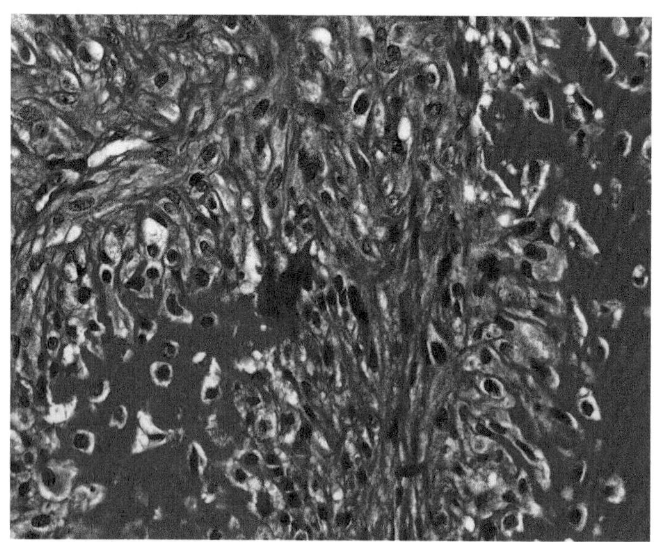

Figure 8-1 Bone biopsy histology of a lytic lesion of the right distal radius. Presence of neoplastic mesenchymal cells with osteoid production (extracellular matrix) indicates osteosarcoma. (Courtesy of Veterinary Pathology, Vetsuisse Faculty, University of Zurich.)

important difference to the disease in dogs, where more than 90% of patients will have metastases.

Plasma cell tumor involving bone in cats is a rare entity and it can be a presentation of the systemic form of the plasma cell tumor, multiple myeloma (9–11). Little is known about the biological behavior of the other feline primary bone tumors but metastases have been seen with chondrosarcoma and hemangiosarcoma (4, 12, 13).

8.1.3 History and clinical signs

Middle-aged to older cats are usually affected, but a wide age range from 3 months to 20 years is reported (2, 3). Cats with bone tumors usually present for lameness or deformity, depending on the location of the tumor. Pathological fractures may also occur.

8.1.4 Diagnostic work-up

Local radiographs and thoracic radiographs are recommended to define the primary lesion and rule out gross metastasis. Feline bone tumors are usually characterized by bone lysis, cortical disruption with an indistinct zone of transition, and variable periosteal reaction on local radiographs of the affected bone (Fig. 8-2). The pattern of lysis is either moth-eaten or permeative (Chapter 2). Most primary bone tumors are located in the metaphyseal region of long bones, whereas bone metastases are often in the diaphyseal region of the bone. Multiple myeloma is typically associated with multiple, purely lytic lesions.

Metastases on thoracic radiographs can be challenging to diagnose, because they have a different pattern in the cat when compared to dogs, where most of the metastasis is nodular in nature. Lung metastases in cats are more often seen as a diffuse pattern, or as ill-defined nodules.

A definitive diagnosis can be made on bone cytology and/or biopsy, and it is important to rule out benign bone diseases, such as cartilaginous exostoses (Chapter 4). The technique for bone biopsy using a Jamshidi bone biopsy needle is described in Chapter 2. Hematology, blood chemistry, and urinalysis are recommended to rule out concurrent disease. If a plasma cell tumor is suspected, survey skeletal radiographs, serum electrophoresis, and a bone marrow aspirate should be performed to rule out multiple myeloma. For tumors of the axial skeleton, a computed tomography (CT) scan can be performed to evaluate the extent of the tumor and for planning surgery.

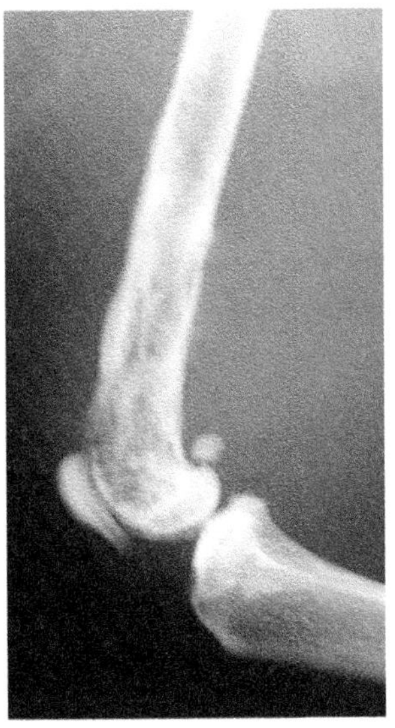
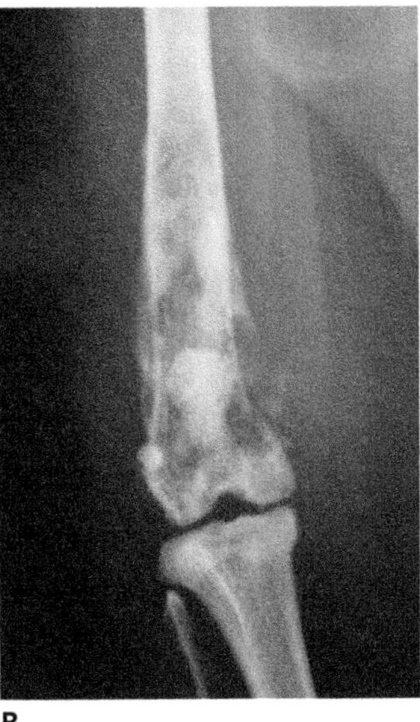

A B

Figure 8-2 (**A**) Mediolateral and (**B**) craniocaudal radiographs of a distal femoral osteosarcoma in a cat.

8.1.5 Therapy and prognosis

Limb amputation is the treatment of choice if the bone tumor is located in the bones of the appendicular skeleton. Palliative radiation therapy can also be used to manage pain in cases where the owner will not consider amputation, or the cat is not a suitable candidate for amputation (14). Aggressive resection is recommended for tumors of the axial skeleton. Radiation therapy can be considered if complete resection is impossible, although no studies are available to confirm the efficacy of this treatment. No adjuvant therapy is known to be efficacious. However, in cases of primary bone hemangiosarcoma without evidence of metastases, a course of doxorubicin chemotherapy is recommended. A course of melphalan and prednisone can be used in cases of multiple myeloma (15–17).

The prognosis for appendicular osteosarcoma treated by amputation is good (Table 8.2). Amputation is often curative. A median survival of 24–44 months has been reported for appendicular osteosarcoma with amputation as the sole treatment (2, 3). No adjuvant chemotherapy is recommended at this point due to the low metastasis potential of the appendicular osteosarcoma in cats.

A median survival of only 6 months has been reported for axial osteosarcoma. It is however unclear if axial osteosarcoma truly has a poorer prognosis than its appendicular counterpart, or if it is related to whether the tumor can be completely removed by surgery. It is important to understand that the prognosis for axial osteosarcoma is dependent on its invasiveness (2, 3). If clean surgical margins can be obtained, the cat is likely to be cured.

The prognosis for cats with multiple myeloma is poor, with a median survival of 2–3 months (9–11), although some cats can survive longer than 1 year. The prognosis for other feline primary bone tumors is unknown.

8.2 Soft-tissue tumors

8.2.1 Incidence and risk

Epidemiological studies have found a strong association between the administration of inactivated feline vaccines and subsequent soft-tissue sarcoma development at sites where vaccination was performed (15, 16). The prevalence of soft-tissue sarcoma development at sites of vaccination has been reported as 1–3.6 cases/10 000 vaccines administered (17). It is now believed that vaccines are not the only cause of sarcomas seen at injection sites, but that anything that produces local inflammation may be responsible for injection site sarcoma in susceptible cats. Inflammation remains the most accepted hypothesis in the pathogenesis of vaccine-associated sarcomas. Another reported syndrome is the development of ocular sarcomas in cats due to trauma and foreign bodies (18).

8.2.2 Pathology and natural behavior

The tumors that develop at vaccine sites are typically mesenchymal in origin, and include fibrosarcomas, malignant fibrous histiocytomas, osteosarcomas, chondrosarcomas, undifferentiated sarcomas, and rhabdomyosarcomas (19, 20). They usually have an increased amount of inflammation and necrosis when compared to non-vaccine-associated sarcomas (21). Vaccine-associated sarcomas are characterized by local invasion (Fig. 8-3), and when compared to non-vaccine-associated sarcomas, they have a higher metastatic potential, reportedly as high as 23% (22).

8.2.3 Diagnostic work-up

Primary work-up should consist of thoracic radiographs to rule out metastases, and performing hematology, biochemistry, and urinalysis to rule out concomitant disease. An incisional biopsy is taken to confirm the diagnosis. Excisional biopsy for suspected vaccine-associated sarcoma is not recommended. If the diagnosis of vaccine-associated sarcoma is confirmed, a CT scan or magnetic resonance imaging (MRI) is a very useful imaging adjunct for evaluation of the tumor extent, and for planning surgery (Fig. 8-3).

8.2.4 Therapy and prognosis

Aggressive surgical resection is the mainstream therapy for vaccine-associated sarcoma. Marginal excision must be

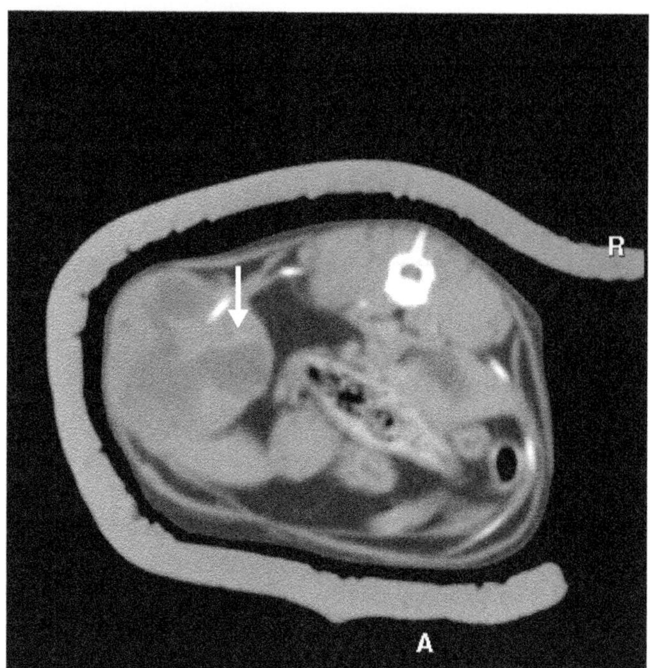

Figure 8-3 Contrast computed tomography scan of a cat with a vaccine-associated sarcoma. Note the invasion of the tumor inside the abdomen (arrow).

avoided since it is seldom curative, and it makes further attempts at more aggressive surgery more difficult. A study reported a median time to first recurrence of 79 days for cats with marginal excision versus 325 days for cats with radical excision. Unfortunately, only 13.8% of the cats treated with surgery alone had long-term (>2 years) survival (22). In another study, the cats with complete surgical margins had a median tumor-free interval of 16 months versus 4 months for incompletely excised tumor. Importantly, more than 50% of the cats with complete excision, based on histopathological analysis of margins, had tumor recurrence (23), which means that even with clean margins only 50% of cats were cured.

Due to the high recurrence rate of vaccine-associated sarcoma, when treated with surgery alone, radiation therapy has been used to try to achieve better local control. Radiation therapy has been used pre- and postsurgery. In a report of 78 cats treated with postoperative radiation therapy, the median disease-free interval was 405 days, which means that the tumor either recurred or metastasized in more than half of the cats after 13 months. Factors with a negative influence on prognosis included cats having more than one surgery performed prior to radiation therapy, and a large primary tumor (24). The median disease-free survival was 584 days in another report of 92 cats treated with preoperative radiation therapy. When tumor margins were clean, postradiation therapy, the median disease-free survival was 986 days versus 292 days for incompletely excised tumor (25). It is now believed that the chance of a cure increases with the use of a combination of aggressive surgery and radiation therapy. Whenever possible, radiation therapy should be recommended even in cats with clean margins.

Several chemotherapeutic agents have been shown to have efficacy against vaccine-associated sarcoma. Doxorubicin and carboplatin are most commonly used. Both have a reported response rate in the macroscopic disease setting of around 40%, but all those responses were short-lived with a median time to progression of 2–3 months. In a report of 67 cats that received chemotherapy (doxorubicin or doxil) following surgical excision, when compared to a historical control group treated with surgery alone, those that received chemotherapy had a longer time to first recurrence versus those treated with surgery alone (415 versus 87 days) (26). Interestingly, adding chemotherapy to the combination of surgery and radiation does not seem to bring benefit, but further information is required on this subject.

8.2.5 Prevention

The National Feline Vaccine-Associated Sarcoma Task Force recommends that no vaccine be given in the interscapular space. Instead, vaccines should be injected into the distal aspect of the rear leg. It is also recommended that any vaccine lump present after 3 months of vaccination, or with a diameter greater than 2 cm, be removed after a biopsy. Other recommendations concerning vaccination frequency and which vaccines to use are available on the National Feline Vaccine-Associated Sarcoma Task Force website at http://www.avma.org/vafstf/default.asp.

8.3 Oral tumors

Oral tumors account for 3% of all feline tumors (27). Most cats will present with facial deformity or inappetence. Seventy percent of feline oral tumors are squamous cell carcinoma and 20% are fibrosarcoma (28). Squamous cell carcinomas are usually located in the bone of the maxilla or mandible or under the tongue, whereas fibrosarcomas usually derive from the gingiva. Recommended investigations should include local and thoracic radiographs, cytology of the regional lymph nodes, and incisional biopsy of the primary tumor. A CT scan can be performed to evaluate further the extent of the disease if the tumor is potentially amenable for surgical resection (Fig. 8-4).

Unfortunately, treatment is often unrewarding due to the local extent of these tumors. Survival is poor, with fewer then 10% of the cats living to 1 year, regardless of whether surgery alone (29), surgery and radiation therapy (30, 31), and additional chemotherapy (32, 33) is performed.

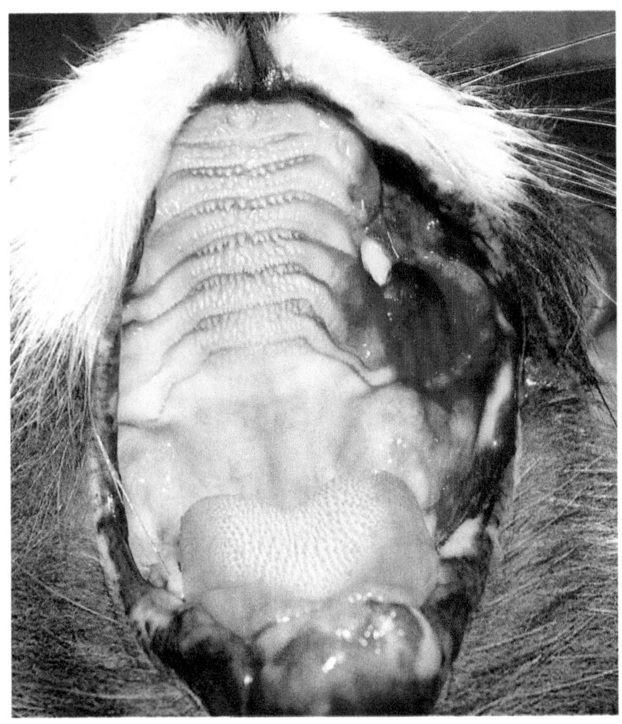

A

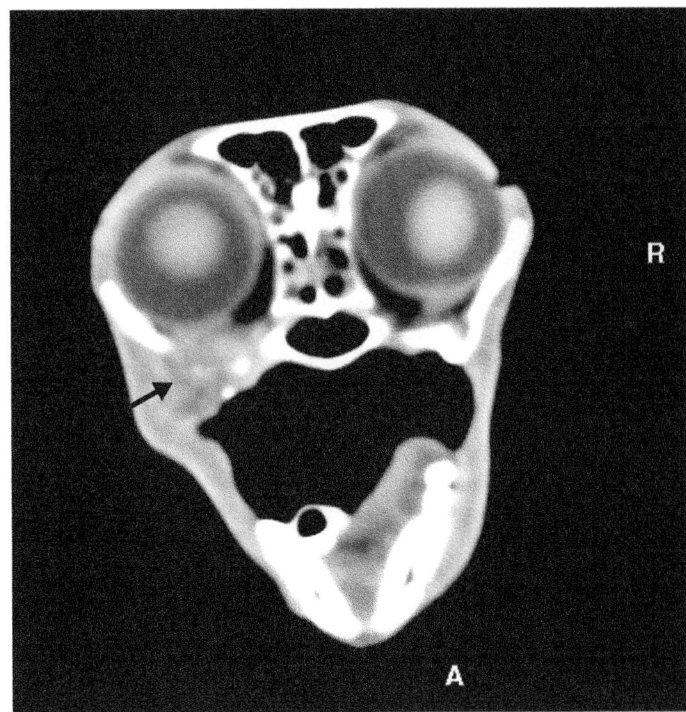

B

Figure 8-4 Cat with oral squamous cell carcinoma.
(**A**) Typical appearance of a squamous cell carcinoma of the left caudal maxilla.
(**B**) Contrast computed tomography scan of the cat in the picture. Note the invasion of the tumor into the orbit, and the lysis of the maxilla, (arrows).

8.4 Tumors of the nervous system

8.4.1 Tumors of the vertebral bodies and spinal cord

Neoplasia of the spinal cord and vertebral column accounts for up to 50% of all spinal lesions in cats. Associated myelopathies typically progress from initial asymmetric presentation to para- or tetraparesis. The onset may be insidious or acute.

The most common neoplasm affecting the spinal cord of cats is lymphosarcoma (34). In many cases, lymphosarcoma has multifocal localization within the central nervous system and other organ systems. Cats with vertebral canal lymphosarcoma are usually feline leukemia virus (FeLV)-positive, and have bone marrow involvement. Cerebrospinal fluid often contains malignant lymphocytes. Cats with vertebral canal lymphoma may initially respond to corticosteroid treatment and chemotherapy. However, long-term prognosis is unfavorable because of the propensity of multifocal involvement, local recurrence, and the development of systemic FeLV-related disease (34).

Several non-lymphoid tumors affecting the spinal cord have been reported (35) (Fig. 8-5). The most common vertebral tumor was osteosarcoma, followed by fibrosarcoma in a large pathology-based study (36). Extradural non-lymphoid tumors in cats include lipoma and plasma cell tumors. Tumors with a meningeal origin include meningioma, meningeal sarcoma, and neoplasia of histiocytic origin. The epidural space is a favored place for tumor metastasis. Intramedullary tumors may be of glial or neuroectodermal origin. Gliomas and astrocytomas have been reported.

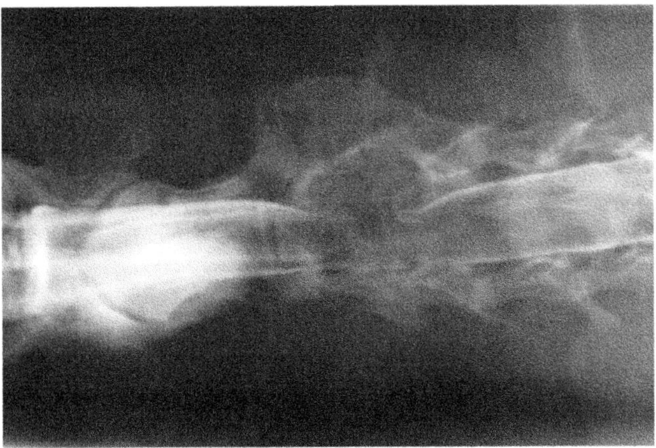

Figure 8-5 Ventrodorsal myelogram of a 1-year-old cat with neoplasia affecting the third and fourth cervical vertebral bodies. The tumor has expanded medially, causing dramatic compression of the cervical spinal cord. Based upon the radiological appearance, cartilaginous exostosis has to be considered as a differential diagnosis to neoplasia, especially if the cat is young. Bone biopsy is necessary for a definitive diagnosis.

Results suggest that contemporary neurosurgical techniques commonly result in incomplete excision of feline non-lymphoid vertebral and spinal cord tumors, but are efficacious at palliation of clinical signs of spinal cord dysfunction (37). Benign non-lymphoid vertebral canal tumors in cats, such as meningiomas, that undergo surgery can have a fair to good prognosis. The median survival time for cats was 518 days for cats with benign tumours (37). Thus, more in-depth investigations such as advanced diagnostic imaging, biopsy, and exploratory surgery may be justified. Bone tumors and intramedullary neoplasia however carry a poor prognosis despite aggressive surgical and medical therapy, with a median survival time of 110.5 days after surgical debulking (37).

8.4.2 Peripheral nerve tumors

Primary nerve sheath tumors, originating from Schwann cells, perineural fibroblasts, or a combination of the two, are rare in cats (38). They may present as cutaneous tumors of adult to aged animals. They are usually poorly circumscribed and locally invasive with a tendency to recur. Various sites have been reported, including the perineum, limbs, thorax, vertebral canal, neck, and head, with a greater frequency reported for the limbs and head (39). Invasion of bone is uncommon, but can result in compression of underlying neural structures. Intradural expansion may cause resorption and enlargement of adjacent intervertebral foramina as well as compression of the spinal cord (40).

Lymphoma is considered to be the most common secondary tumor of the peripheral nerves. Based upon the small number of reported cases, it is not possible to determine predilection sites but the incidence of brachial plexus lymphoma seems to be higher than involvement of nerves at other sites (41).

Diagnosis of peripheral nerve tumors is based upon the presence of neurological deficits, atrophy of affected myotomes, palpation of a mass, electromyography, and ultrasonography. MRI is a very sensitive tool for diagnosis of the extent of a peripheral nerve tumor (Fig. 8-6).

Treatment consists of resection of the affected nerve, and eventually amputation of the affected limb if major nerve plexuses are affected. Care is taken to try and resect the nerve beyond the neoplastic portion. A hemilaminectomy and a durotomy may be necessary to remove all the affected parts if nerve roots are affected. The optimal treatment for cats with lymphoma involving the peripheral nerves and plexuses has not been established. Chemotherapy and radiotherapy are effective treatment modalities for feline lymphoma, but surgical resection might be necessary if nerve function is impaired irreversibly (42). Recurrence of lymphoma at other sites has been reported despite aggressive therapy of the tumor at the primary site.

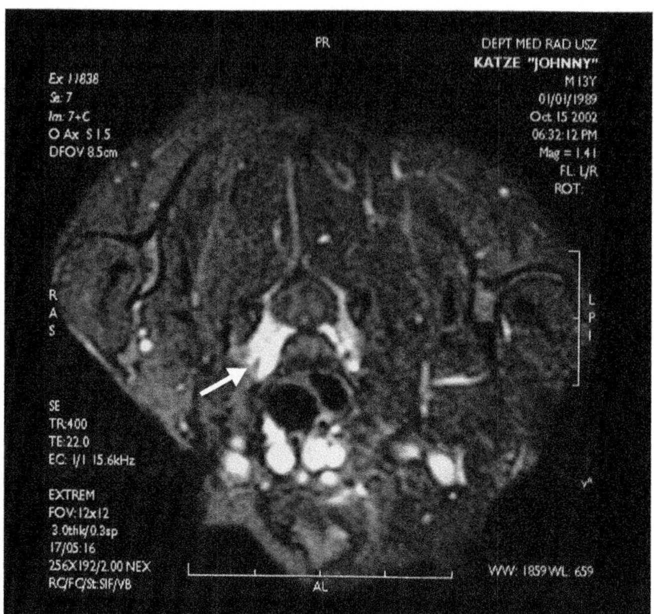

Figure 8-6 Magnetic resonance image (T1-weighted, postcontrast) at the level of the seventh cervical vertebra in a 8-year-old cat with a schwannoma of the right nerve root. There is marked contrast enhancement of the affected nerve root (arrow), and subtle enlargement of the right intervertebral foramen.

8.5 Miscellaneous tumors

8.5.1 Multiple cartilaginous exostoses

Multiple cartilaginous exostosis (osteochondromatosis) is a tumor-like disease that mostly affects the axial skeleton. It is seen in younger, FeLV-positive cats (43, 44). In contrast to dogs, multiple cartilaginous exostosis does not seem to be familial in origin, is often asymmetric, and the lesion occurs after the closure of the growth plate. The condition is often seen in the scapula, vertebrae, and mandibula, although any bone can be affected. Radiologically, the lesions are characterized by sessile or pedunculated protuberances from bone surfaces, with indistinct borders with normal bone. Cats often present with rapidly progressing hard swellings over the affected area causing pain and loss of function. Multiple cartilaginous exostosis has an aggressive natural behavior. Surgery or radiation therapy has been used to palliate the clinical signs but no effective treatment exists at this time (45).

Multiple cartilaginous exostosis must be differentiated from solitary osteochondromas, because prognosis and treatment differ (Chapter 4).

8.5.2 Metastatic digital carcinoma

Metastasis of primary pulmonary neoplasia, usually bronchial or pulmonary carcinoma, to the digits is a well-described

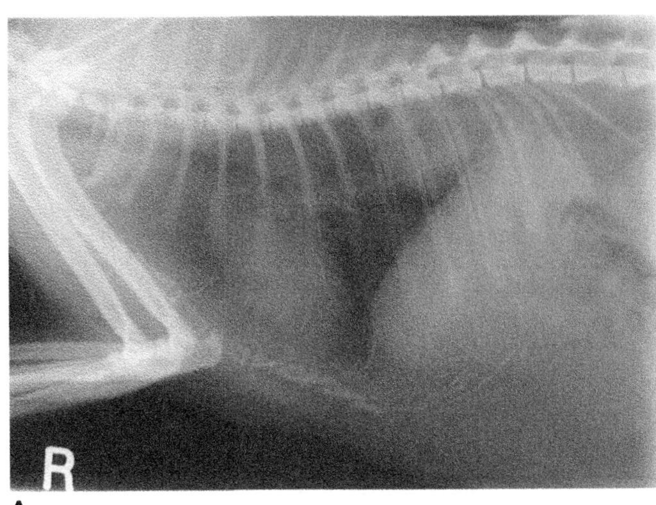

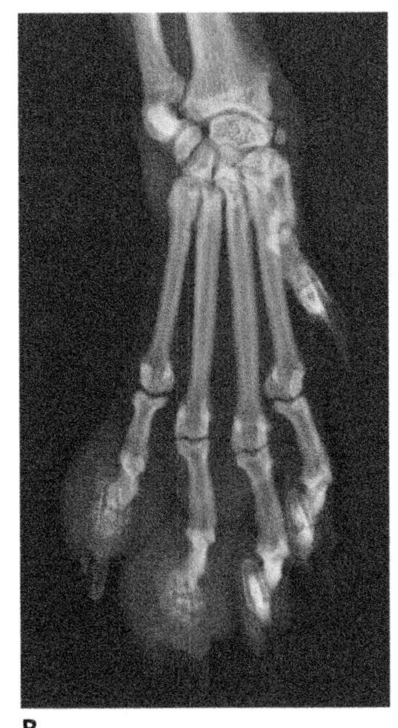

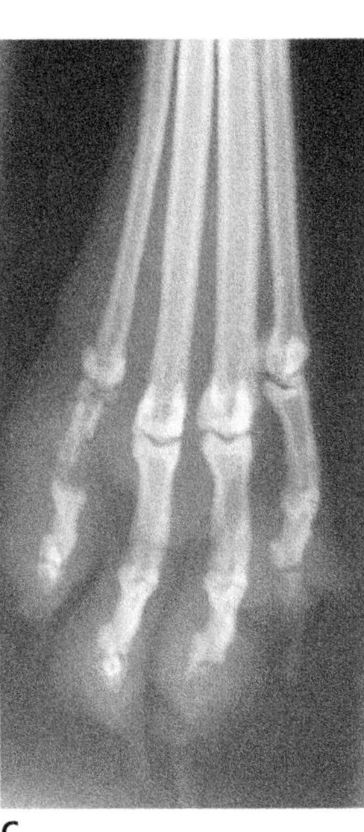

A B C

Figure 8-7 This 14-year-old cat presented with chronic lameness associated with multiple swollen digits. (**A**) A thoracic radiograph shows a radiodense area in one of the caudal lung lobes. (**B**, **C**) Radiographs of the feet show lysis of several phalangeal bones and soft-tissue swelling around the toes. These changes are characteristic of a pulmonary carcinoma with digital metastases.

syndrome in cats (46). It is typically characterized by swelling of several digits. A single lung mass is usually seen on thoracic radiographs (Fig. 8-7). A recent study of primary and metastatic carcinomas in the digits of cats concluded that 87.5% of digital carcinomas were metastases of a primary pulmonary carcinoma. Treatment is unrewarding since multiple digits on multiple limbs are usually affected. The prognosis is poor with a median survival time of 4.9 weeks, compared to 29.5 weeks for cats with primary digital squamous cell carcinoma (47).

8.5.3 Synovial cell tumors

Synovial cell sarcoma is a rare tumor in cats, but it is believed to be the most common primary joint tumor (48). Affected cats present with a soft-tissue mass in the vicinity of a joint. Described cases have involved the elbow and carpal joint (48–51). Lameness is usually, but not necessarily, present (50). A diagnosis of synovial cell sarcoma is suspected based on radiographic evidence of bone lysis with or without periosteal new bone formation, affecting the epiphyses of the bones proximal and distal to a joint. Biopsy is required to obtain the diagnosis. A report documented two cats with metastasis to the regional lymph nodes. Both were treated by amputation and adjuvant doxorubicin, and had survival times or 444 and 41 days, respectively (51).

Synoviomas are benign joint tumors, and have mainly involved joints, tendon sheaths, and the distal limbs (52–54). Although synoviomas do not metastasize, they usually recur after local resection, so amputation is recommended.

References and further reading

1. Dorn CR, et al. Survey of animal neoplasms in Alameda and Contra Costa Counties, California II: cancer morbidity in dogs and cats from Alameda County. J Natl Cancer Inst 1968;40: 307–318.
2. Hellmann E, et al. Feline osteosarcoma: 145 cases (1990–1995). J Am Anim Hosp Assoc 2000;36:518–521.
3. Bitetto WV, et al. Osteosarcoma in cats: 22 cases (1974–1984). J Am Vet Med Assoc 1987;190:91–93.
4. Quigley PJ, Leedale AH. Tumor involving bone in the domestic cat: a review of fifty-eight cases. Vet Pathol 1983;20:670–686.
5. Lui S, et al. Primary and secondary bone tumours in the cat. J Small Anim Pract 1974;15:141–156.
6. Banks WC. Parosteal osteosarcoma in a dog and a cat. J Am Vet Med Assoc 1971;158:1412-1415.
7. Fry PD, Jukes HF. Fracture-associated sarcoma in the cat. J Small Anim Pract 1995;36:124-126.
8. Bennett D, et al. Osteosarcoma associated with healed fractures. J Small Anim Pract 1979;20:13–18.
9. Patel RT, et al. Multiple myeloma in 16 cats: a retrospective study. Vet Clin Pathol 2005;34:341-352.
10. Weber NA, Tebeau CS. An unusual presentation of multiple myeloma in two cats. J Am Anim Hosp Assoc 1998;34:477–483.
11. Hanna F. Multiple myelomas in cats. J Feline Med Surg 2005;7:275–287.
12. Turrel JM, Pool RR. Primary bone tumors in the cat: a retrospective study of 15 cats and a literature review. Vet Radiol 1982;23:152–166.

13. Berman E, Wright JF. What is your diagnosis? (osteosarcoma of tibia and hemangiosarcoma of femur metastatic to lungs in irradiated cat). J Am Vet Med Assoc 1973;162:1065–1066.
14. McEntee MC. Radiation therapy in the management of bone tumors. Vet Clin North Am Small Anim Pract 1997;27:131–138.
15. Hendricks MJ, et al. Postvaccinal sarcomas in the cat: epidemiology and electron probe microanalytical identification of aluminium. Cancer Res 1992;52:5391–5394.
16. Kass PH, et al. Epidemiologic evidence for a causal relation between vaccination and fibrosarcoma tumorigenesis in cats. J Am Vet Med Assoc 1993;203:396–405.
17. Coyne MJ, et al. Estimated prevalence of injection sarcomas in cats during 1992. J Am Vet Med Assoc 1997;210:249–251.
18. Dubielzig RR, et al. Clinical and morphological features of post-traumatic ocular sarcomas in cats. Vet Pathol 1990;27:62–65.
19. Couto SS, et al. Feline vaccine-associated fibrosarcoma: morphologic distinctions. Vet Pathol 2002;39:33–41.
20. Hendricks MJ, Brooks JJ. Postvaccinal sarcomas in the cat: histology and immunohistochemistry. Vet Pathol 1994;31:126–129.
21. Hendrick MJ, et al. Comparison of fibrosarcomas that developed at vaccine sites and at nonvaccination sites in cats: 239 cases (1991–1992). J Am Vet Med Assoc 1994;205:1425–1429.
22. Hershey AE, et al. Prognosis for presumed feline vaccine-associated sarcoma after excision: 61 cases (1986–1996). J Am Vet Med Assoc 2000;216:58–61.
23. Davidson EB, et al. Surgical excision of soft tissue fibrosarcomas in cats. Vet Surg 1997;26:265–269.
24. Cohen M, et al. Use of surgery and electron beam irradiation, with or without chemotherapy, for treatment of vaccine-associated sarcoma in cats: 78 cases (1996–2000). J Am Vet Med Assoc 2001;219:1582–1589.
25. Kobayashi T, et al. Preoperative radiotherapy for vaccine-associated sarcoma in 92 cats. Vet Radiol Ultrasound 2002;43:473–479.
26. Poirier VJ, et al. Liposome-encapsulated doxorubicin (Doxil) and doxorubicin in the treatment of vaccine-associated sarcoma in cats. J Vet Intern Med 2002;16:726–731.
27. Stebbins KE, et al. Feline oral neoplasia: a ten year survey. Vet Pathol 1989;26:121–128.
28. Withrow SJ. Cancer of the gastrointestinal tract. In: Withrow SJ, MacEwen EG (eds) Small animal clinical oncology, 3rd edn. Philadelphia: WB Saunders; 2001: pp. 261–279.
29. Postorino Reeves NC, et al. Oral squamous cell carcinoma in the cat. J Am Anim Hosp Assoc 1993;29:438–441.
30. Hutson CA, et al. Treatment of mandibular squamous cell carcinoma in cats by use of mandibulectomy and radiotherapy: seven cases (1987–1989). J Am Vet Med Assoc 1992;201: 777–781.
31. Bregazzi VS, et al. Response of feline oral squamous cell carcinoma to palliative radiation therapy. Vet Rad Ultrasound 2001;42:77–79.
32. LaRue SM, et al. Shrinking-field radiation therapy in combination with mitoxantrone chemotherapy for the treatment of oral squamous cell carcinoma in the cat. Proceedings of the 11th Annual Vet Cancer Society Conference, Minneapolis, 1991.
33. Jones PD, et al. Gemcitabine as a radiosensitizer for nonresectable feline oral squamous cell carcinoma. J Am Anim Hosp Assoc 2003;39:463–467.
34. Spodnick GJ, et al. Spinal lymphoma in cats: 21 cases (1976–1989). J Am Vet Med Assoc 1992;373–376.
35. Levy MS, et al. Nonlymphoid vertebral canal tumors in cats: 11 cases (1987–1995). J Am Vet Med Assoc 1997;210:663–664.
36. Marioni-Henry K, et al. Prevalence of disease of the spinal cord of cats. J Vet Intern Med 2004;18:851–858.
37. Rossmeisl Jr, H, et al. Surgical cytoreduction for the treatment of non-lymphoid vertebral and spinal cord neoplasms in cats: retrospective evaluation of 26 cases (1990–2005). Vet Comp Oncol 2006;4:41–50.
38. Hayes HM, et al. Occurrence of nervous tissue tumors in cattle, horses, cats and dogs. Int J Cancer 1975;15:39–47.
39. Jones BR, et al. Nerve sheath tumors in the dog and cat. NZ Vet J 1995;43:190–196.
40. LeCouteur RA. Tumors of the nervous system. In: Witrow SJ, MacEwen EG (eds). Small animal oncology, 3rd edn. Philadelphia: WB Saunders; 2001: pp. 500–531.
41. Mellanby RJ, et al. Magnetic resonance imaging in the diagnosis of lymphoma involving the brachial plexus in a cat. Vet Radiol Ultrasound 2003;44:522–525.
42. Elmslie RE, et al. Radiotherapy with and without chemotherapy for localized lymphoma in 10 cats. Vet Radiol 1991;32:277–280.
43. Carpenter JL, et al. Tumors and tumor-like lesions. In: Holzworth J (ed.) Disease of the cats: medicine and surgery. Philadelphia: WB Saunders; 1987: pp. 406–596.
44. Riddle WEJ, Leighton RL. Osteochondromatosis in a cat. Vet Pathol 1972;9:350–359.
45. Hubler M, et al. Palliative irradiation of Scottish Fold osteochondrodysplasia. Vet Radiol Ultrasound 2004;45:582–585.
46. Gottfried SD, et al. Metastatic digital carcinoma in the cat: a retrospective study of 36 cats (1992–1998). J Am Anim Hosp Assoc 2000;36:501–509.
47. Van der Linde-Sipman JS, Van den Ingh TS. Primary and metastatic carcinomas in the digits of cats. Vet Q 2000;22:141–145.
48. Silva-Krott IU, et al. Synovial sarcoma in a cat. J Am Vet Med Assoc 1993;203:1430–1431.
49. Borenstein, N, et al. What is your diagnosis? (Synovial sarcoma.) J Small Anim Pract 1999;40:236–237.
50. Ireifej SJ, et al. What is your diagnosis? (Synovial sarcoma.) J Am Vet Med Assoc 2007;230:1305–1306.
51. Liptak JM, et al. Metastatic synovial cell sarcoma in two cats. Vet Comp Orthop Traumatol 2004;2:164–170.
52. Hulse, EV. A benign giant cell synovioma in a cat. J Pathol 1966;91:269–271.
53. Davies JD, Little NR. Synovioma in a cat. J Small Anim Pract 1972;13:127–133.
54. Thoday KL, Evans JG. Synovioma in a cat. J Small Anim Pract 1972;13:399–401.

Part 3
Polytrauma

The majority of orthopedic problems encountered in feline practice are due to trauma. Frequent causes of trauma include motor vehicle accidents, falls from a height, bite wounds, and gunshot injury. Traumatized cats often sustain injuries to multiple body systems, including potentially life-threatening injuries of the thorax, abdomen, and head. These injuries have to be recognized and treated appropriately, before addressing concurrent orthopedic injuries. Mortality rates of traumatized cats presented at a veterinary clinic have been reported to be around 20–25% (1–3). Thoracic, abdominal, or brain injuries are usually the cause of death in these cats (3), emphasizing the importance of a complete and thorough assessment and appropriate emergency management of the feline trauma patient.

The following part of the book addresses the initial assessment and emergency treatment procedures for the polytraumatized feline patient. Additionally, basic diagnostic and therapeutic features of commonly encountered soft-tissue and neurological injuries are summarized. This book focuses on orthopedic surgery, and does not cover a complete description of the pathophysiology of trauma, critical care techniques, and soft-tissue surgery. For a detailed description of these topics the reader is referred to specialized textbooks.

9 Etiology and severity of polytrauma

K. Voss

The definition of polytrauma is the presence of injuries to several body regions or organs. Polytrauma is more common in cats than in dogs. Different studies suggest that multiple injuries occur in around 30–60% of traumatized cats (1–4), and the presence of more than three concurrent injuries is not unusual (Fig. 9-1). Several reasons may account for the high frequency of polytrauma in cats. Cats usually tend to sustain high-impact trauma, such as road traffic accidents and falls from a height. Due to their small body size, less body mass is available to absorb the energy generated during the accident, and the cat's organs are less protected as compared to larger animals (5).

The severity and distribution of the injuries vary with the cause of trauma. Table 9-1 summarizes results from different studies (1, 2, 6, 7). Road traffic accidents and falls from a height often result in injury to the extremities, head and neck, pelvis, and thorax. Injuries due to encounters with lawnmowers and harvesting machinery usually result in extensive soft-tissue injuries or traumatic amputations, especially of the distal limbs. Dog bites may cause severe intra-abdominal or thoracic injuries.

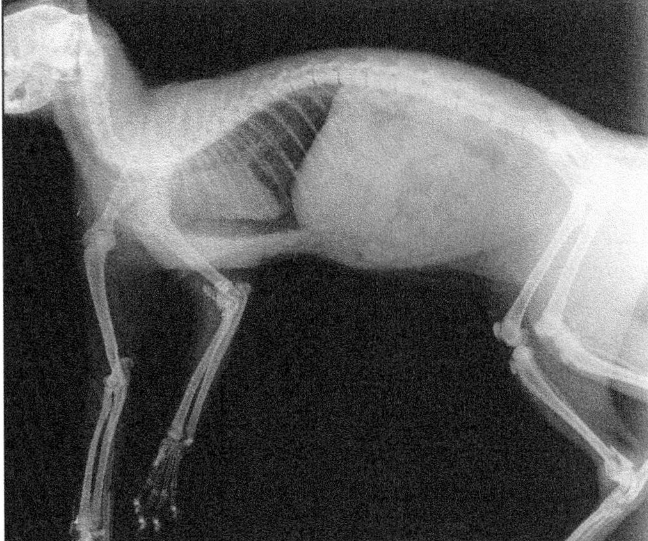

Figure 9-1 A lateral radiograph of a polytraumatized cat that presented in shock, with dyspnea, and injuries to multiple limbs. Film taken after fluid resuscitation and thoracocentesis with aspiration of air. Injuries visible on the radiograph are pneumothorax, loss of abdominal detail, a distal articular humeral fracture, a distal articular tibial fracture, and a non-displaced fracture of the fourth lumbar vertebral body.

The severity of injuries can be rated with the help of scoring systems. An example is shown in Table 9-2 (8). Scoring systems help in roughly predicting prognosis for survival and in estimating treatment costs. It should be remembered, however, that clinical signs of certain injuries such as urinary tract trauma might not be evident at the time of initial presentation. Owners should therefore be informed that additional injuries might only be diagnosed during the course of treatment, and their presence may influence morbidity, mortality, prognosis, and treatment costs. In one study, evaluating correlations between radiographic diagnosis and epidemiological factors in 100 consecutive traumatized cats, negative correlations were found between survival and older age, between survival and spinal trauma, and between survival and abdominal trauma (3).

9.1 Road traffic accidents

Road traffic accidents often result in blunt trauma, causing any variation of thoracic, orthopedic, neurological, and abdominal injury. An epidemiological study performed in the UK showed that younger cats, male cats, and non-pedigree cats had a higher risk of being hit by a motor vehicle (9). Cats between 7 months and 2 years had the highest risk of being in a road traffic accident, and the odds decreased by 16% for every 1-year increase in age (10). Older cats may be less at risk because they are more experienced and therefore better able to deal with dangerous situations, and they may alter their behavior by staying closer to home and spending less time outside. Accidents were evenly distributed throughout the year, but tended to happen more often at night (10). Wearing reflective collars did not seem to prevent road traffic accidents (10).

Distribution and severity of injuries depend on the velocity of the car and the body area hit. Injuries of the head, the extremities, pelvic fractures, and thoracic injuries were most commonly diagnosed (1, 2). The hindlimbs were affected more often than the front limbs. Many of the injuries sustained after road traffic accidents are severe and need to be treated surgically. In one study, 50% of cats had to be treated surgically (2), and approximately half of these cats then required a second surgery (2). The second surgery was neces-

Features	Motor vehicle accident	Fall from a height	Gunshot injury	Dog bite wounds
Mortality	16–24%	10%	Unknown	Unknown
Most common localization of injuries	Extremities (hindlimbs more often than forelimbs) Head and neck Pelvis	Thorax Head Extremities (forelimbs more often than hindlimbs)	Humerus Spine	Abdominal wall Intra-abdominal organs

Table 9-1. The mortality of cats after different trauma and the most common sites of injury

Grade	Grade description	Types of injuries
0	No definable injury	No physically or radiographically definable injury
1	Minor	Small skin lacerations or abrasions Undisplaced pelvic fractures Simple metacarpal or metatarsal fracture
2	Moderate	Extensive or deep lacerations or abrasions Skull or spinal fractures without neurological signs Joint luxations and ligament ruptures Simple fractures of long bones, ribs, or pelvis
3	Severe, not life-threatening	Multiple extensive deep lacerations or abrasions Skull or spinal fractures with minimal neurological deficits Pneumothorax, hemothorax or lung contusion with minimal respiratory compromise Multiple pelvic or long-bone fractures
4	Severe, life-threatening	Multiple extensive lacerations with shock Skull and spinal fractures with major neurological deficits Thoracic trauma with respiratory compromise Abdominal trauma with signs of shock Ruptured urinary bladder or hemoperitoneum Major pelvic fractures with extensive soft-tissue trauma Multiple open long-bone fractures with shock

Table 9-2. An example of a scoring system for trauma patients, ranging from minor to severe and life-threatening (adapted from Kolata (8)). Severe injuries occur in around 50% of traumatized cats

sary either as a continuation of treatment, for previously undetected injuries, or because the initial surgery had failed. Mortality rates of cats treated in a hospital after a road traffic accident are relatively high, ranging from 16% to 24% in the literature (1, 2). These numbers do not include cats that were killed immediately after the accident or those that died during transportation to the hospital.

9.2 High-rise syndrome

The term high-rise syndrome represents a variety of possible injuries resulting from falling from a height equivalent to the second storey or higher. Cats have the unique capability of being able to turn themselves during a fall and landing on their feet, and therefore sometimes suffering only surprisingly mild injuries. However, severe injuries do occur, and the mortality rate is reported to be around 10% (6, 7).

Type and severity of injury depend on the height of the fall, and the type of ground the cat lands on (6). Thoracic trauma occurs in up to 90% of cats with high-rise syndrome (6). Lung contusion and pneumothorax are most common, and are often the reason for death in these patients. The incidence of thoracic injuries however does not seem to depend on the height of the fall (7). Facial trauma, including hard palate fractures, and injuries of the extremities also occur frequently. Injuries of the forelimbs are present more often after falls from a height than after road traffic accidents, and tend to be localized distal to the elbow. Distal femoral fractures seem to be the most commonly encountered injuries of the hindlimbs. Impalement injuries have been described after falling on to sharp objects, such as metal railings (11).

The number or rate of injuries is related to the force of impact on the ground, which in turn depends on the velocity with which the cat reaches the ground. Cats spread out horizontally during falling, and reach their terminal velocity (60 mph, 97 km/h) after a distance matching approximately the height of a fifth storey (6). According to this assumption, the rate of injuries increased in a linear fashion up to a height of approximately seven storeys in one study (6). Falls from higher than seven storeys resulted in a decrease of total injuries and fractures (6). The decrease in the number of fractures after falls from more than seven storeys is explained by the fact that, after having reached terminal velocity, the vestibular system is no longer stimulated by acceleration. The cat may then relax and orient its legs more horizontally. This positioning possibly allows for a better distribution of the impact force and a reduction in the incidence of fractures (6).

9.3 Gunshot injury

Cats with gunshot injuries are encountered infrequently, and information in the veterinary literature is mainly based on findings in dogs (12). Due to the small body size of cats, most gunshot injuries involve the proximal body parts, such as the thorax, spine, abdomen, and proximal limbs. Around 50% of gunshot injuries to the limbs are associated with fractures (12). Fractures caused by gunshot injury are always severe, because the sudden release of high energy results in fracture comminution and significant soft-tissue trauma. The injuries are therefore always classified as grade 3 open fractures (Chapter 13). The humerus and the spine are most commonly affected in the author's experience.

Animals with gunshot injuries of the thorax or the limbs have a better prognosis than animals with abdominal or spinal injuries (12). The prognosis for vertebral column injuries is poor if there is loss of deep pain sensation and severely comminuted and displaced vertebral fractures/luxations suggestive of transection of the spinal cord. Spinal concussion may result in reversible neurological deficits in rare cases. Spinal concussion should be suspected if radiological evidence of severe spinal injury is missing, and if neurological deficits show some improvement within a few hours.

9.4 Dog bite wounds

Dog bite wounds are far less common than cat bite wounds, but they may cause severe trauma. Cat bite wounds do not usually result in polytrauma because the lesions are confined to a small area. They are described in Chapter 16.

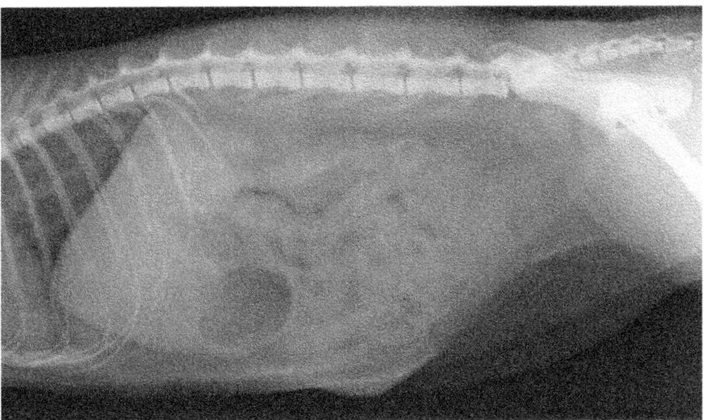

Figure 9-2 Laterolateral abdominal radiograph of a cat, which was bitten by two dogs 1 hour previously. The overlying skin was intact, but there is swelling and discontinuity of the ventral abdominal wall. Exploratory celiotomy revealed an abdominal wall rupture, a perforated small intestinal loop, and a splenic laceration.

Shearing, tensile, and compressive forces are involved in dog bite wounds, of which tensile and compressive forces are the most devastating. Tensile forces result in avulsion of the skin from underlying tissue, compromising blood supply and promoting infection due to creation of dead space. Compressive forces may cause crushing of underlying tissue, possibly resulting in fractures, body wall lacerations, and injury to intrathoracic or abdominal organs. These severe injuries occur below the skin, and are likely to be present even if the skin lesions do not appear to be serious. Cats with dog bite wounds are also at risk for developing systemic inflammatory response syndrome and/or sepsis due to widespread tissue destruction and development of infection.

In a survey addressing bite wounds in dogs and cats the limbs were the most frequently affected, followed by the head and neck, and the regions overlying the thoracic and abdominal cavity (13). In the author's experience most dog bite wounds in cats affect the abdominal area, causing abdominal hernias and/or injury to abdominal organs (Fig. 9-2). Forty percent of abdominal hernias in cats were due to bite wounds in one study (14). Exploratory celiotomy is often indicated to rule out injuries to intra-abdominal organs. Chest wall injuries and open or closed pneumothorax can occur after dog bites in the thoracic region. Fractures and joint injuries may also be encountered.

9.5 Trauma by entrapment in bottom-hung windows

Trauma by entrapment in a hinged bottom-hung window occurs if a cat gets stuck in the V-shaped opening of the window, while climbing through it. Cats usually get caught between the ribs and the pelvis, and slide down the V-shaped opening even further in an attempt to free themselves. This results in a time-dependent development of ischemic injury to several organs. Ischemic neuromyopathy, damage to abdominal organs, such as the kidneys, bladder, and colon, and spinal cord ischemia are possible consequences. Shock develops after some time. Pathophysiology, signs, treatment options, and prognosis for the window-cat syndrome are described in Chapter 6.

References and further reading

1. Kolata RJ, et al. Patterns of trauma in urban dogs and cats: a study of 1000 cases. J Am Vet Med Assoc 1974;164:499–502.
2. Rochlitz I. Clinical study of cats injured and killed in road traffic accidents in Cambridgeshire. J Small Anim Pract 2004;45:390–394.
3. Zulauf D, et al. Radiographic examination and outcome in consecutive feline trauma patients. Vet Comp Orthop Traumatol 2008;21:36–40.
4. Griffon D, et al. Thoracic injuries in cats with traumatic fractures. Vet Comp Orthop Traumatol 1994;7:98–100.
5. Oechtering G, et al. Polytrauma. In: Horzinek MC, Schmidt, V, Lutz H (eds) Krankheiten der Katze, 4th edn. Stuttgart: Enke Verlag; 2005: pp. 649–665.
6. Whitney WO, Mehlhaff CJ. High-rise syndrome in cats. J Am Vet Med Assoc 1987;191:1399–1403.
7. Vnuk D, et al. Feline high-rise syndrome: 119 cases (1998–2001). J Feline Med Surg 2004;6:305–312.
8. Kolata RJ. Trauma in dogs and cats: an overview. Vet Clin North Am Small Anim Pract 1980;10:515–522.
9. Rochlitz I. Study of factors that may predispose domestic cats to road traffic accidents: part 1. Vet Rec 2003;153:549–553.
10. Rochlitz I. Study of factors that may predispose domestic cats to road traffic accidents: part 2. Vet Rec 2003;153:585–588.
11. Pratschke KM, Kirby BM. High rise syndrome with impalement in three cats. J Small Anim Pract 2002;43:261–264.
12. Fullington RJ, Otto CM. Characteristics and management of gunshot wounds in dogs and cats: 84 cases (1986–1995). J Am Vet Med Assoc 1997;210:658–662.
13. Holt DE, Griffin G. Bite wounds in dogs and cats. Vet Clin North Am Small Anim Pract 2000;30:669–679.
14. Shaw SR, et al. Traumatic body wall herniation in 36 dogs and cats. J Am Anim Hosp Assoc 2003;39:35–46.

10 General approach to the trauma patient

K. Voss

The approach to a traumatized cat should be efficient, systematic, and complete. The approach described here is a guideline, but may need to be adjusted, depending on the individual case. It involves the initial general examination of the patient, emergency treatment, reassessment of the patient during emergency treatment, the complete clinical, orthopedic, and neurological examination, and further diagnostic tests (Fig. 10-1).

The initial clinical examination and assessment of a traumatized patient focus on rapid evaluation of life-threatening respiratory, circulatory, and neurological conditions. This first look includes assessment of mental state, respiratory rate and pattern, heart rate, mucous membrane color and capillary refill time, and measurement of body temperature. Treatment is initiated immediately in cats with respiratory compromise, cats in shock, or cats with brain trauma (Chapter 11). Oxygen supplementation and thoracocentesis are performed first if respiratory compromise is predominant. If shock is considered the main problem, fluid resuscitation is initiated as a first step. The patient is re-evaluated every 10–15 minutes during resuscitation to assess response to treatment.

Once the animal is considered stable and can be handled safely, a thorough general physical, orthopedic, and neurological examination is performed. This second look is aimed at diagnosing or excluding injuries, and obtaining additional findings, which suggest the need for further diagnostic tests. It should be possible to give a rough estimation of the severity of injuries to the owners and to discuss further measures with them after the complete physical examination, and the response seen to the emergency treatment.

Routine blood analysis and thoracic and abdominal radiographs should be obtained from all traumatized cats. Blood is taken as soon as possible in order to have baseline values

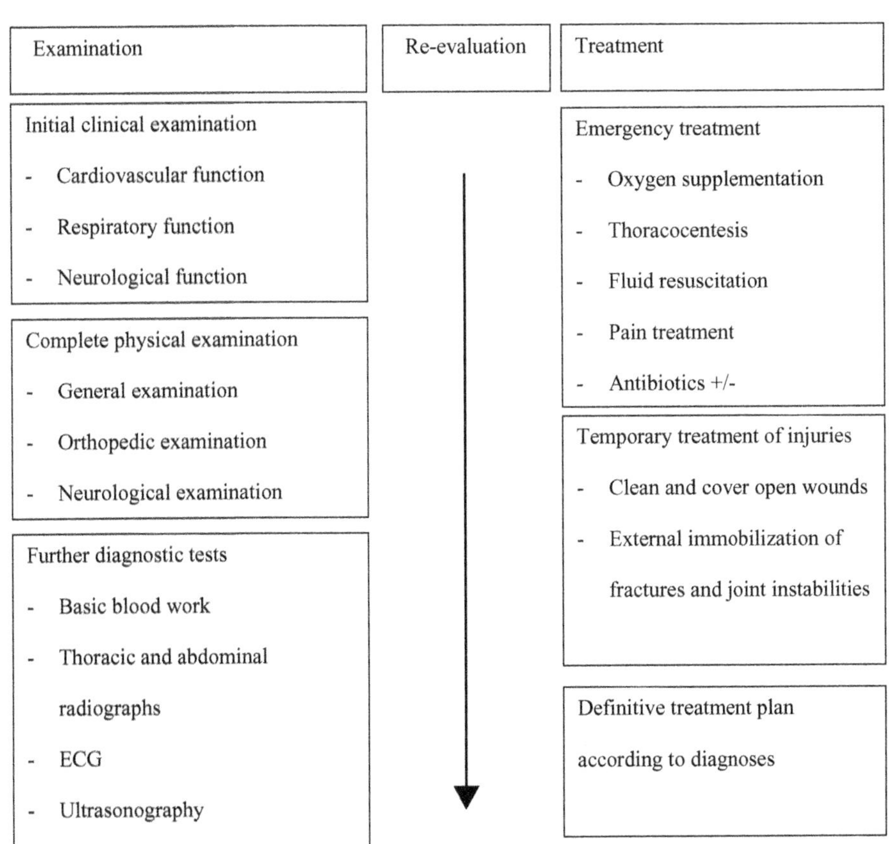

Figure 10-1 General approach to the trauma patient. ECG, electrocardiogram.

Percentage of cats	Body system affected	Types of injuries (in decreasing frequency)
53%	Thorax	Pneumothorax Lung contusion Pleural effusion Rib fractures Diaphragmatic hernia
39%	Abdomen	Loss of abdominal detail Loss of retroperitoneal detail Abdominal wall trauma
34%	Pelvis	Fractures Sacroiliac fracture luxations
26%	Spine	Sacrococcygeal fracture/luxations Thoracolumbar fracture/luxations
18%	Surrounding soft tissue	Swelling Subcutaneous emphysema

Table 10-1. Radiological findings of whole-body radiographs from 100 consecutive traumatized cats from an urban area. Trauma types included unknown trauma (32%), hit by car (30%), falls from a height (25%), bite wounds (7%), and others (6%). Because the limbs are usually not included on the whole-body radiographs, only injuries to the trunk were evaluated

for later comparison. Thoracic and abdominal radiographs are used to confirm and to specify the clinical diagnosis and to detect additional abnormalities missed on physical examination. Only stable cats should be radiographed. See Chapter 12 for the emergency treatment of specific injuries.

Due to the small body size of cats, it is possible to radiograph both the thorax and the abdomen on the same film. This does not lead to perfectly centered radiographs, but gives a good overview of all body systems. In a study evaluating 100 consecutive whole-body radiographs of traumatized cats in an urban area, injuries were found in 96% of cases (1). A summation of the findings of this study is depicted in Table 10-1. Not all of the injuries recognized need treatment, but recognizing them may help in the decision process and estimation of prognosis.

Further diagnostic tests may be indicated according to clinical or radiological findings. Electrocardiography is performed in order to detect arrhythmias due to traumatic myocarditis or underlying heart disease. Ultrasonography may be necessary to evaluate further intra-abdominal or intrathoracic injuries.

Pain medication should be provided as soon as possible after presentation. Pain causes peripheral vasoconstriction and decreases peripheral circulation. Pain also restricts respiratory movements in patients with painful thoracic wall or diaphragmatic injuries, thus contributing to hypoventilation. Opioids, like morphine, fentanyl or buprenorphine, are appropriate analgesics in most patients (Chapter 18). No official guidelines exist on the need for antimicrobial therapy in feline trauma patients, but it seems reasonable to administer antibiotics to patients with decompensated shock, and to those with severe lung contusions. Antimicrobial therapy should always be instituted in cats with contaminated or infected open wounds, including open fractures or joint injuries.

Orthopedic and neurological injuries are treated when the animal is considered stable for anesthesia and surgery. The animals must be hemodynamically and metabolically stable, pulmonary function should not be compromised, packed cell volume should exceed 20%, and albumin should exceed 20 g/l. With some injuries, such as spinal fractures and luxations, open fractures and joint injuries, and femoral and physeal fractures in immature cats, the prognosis for functional outcome is time-dependent. In these cases the cats are taken to surgery as soon as possible.

Reference and further reading

1. Zulauf D, et al. Radiographic examination and outcome in consecutive feline trauma patients. Vet Comp Orthop Traumatol 2008;21:36–40.

11 Traumatic hemorrhagic shock

K. Voss

Shock is defined as an inadequate delivery of oxygen to tissues to maintain their metabolic requirements. Traumatic hemorrhagic shock results from a combination of blood loss and tissue trauma, and is frequently encountered in traumatized cats. Acute external or internal bleeding reduces circulating blood volume and causes direct hypovolemia. Patients with an acute blood loss of more than 20% require aggressive fluid substitution, and blood loss exceeding 50% usually results in death of the patient (1). The normal blood volume of cats is 66 ml/kg body weight (2).

Tissue trauma contributes to hemorrhagic shock by redistribution of blood flow at the capillary level, initiated by neurogenic mechanisms and pain-induced vasoconstriction. This causes indirect hypovolemia. Inadequate blood supply and oxygen delivery to the kidneys, gastrointestinal tract, and pancreas in the later stages of shock is responsible for initiation of pathophysiological mechanisms, which can lead to the development of multiorgan failure and death.

11.1 Stages of shock

Three phases of shock are described: the compensatory stage, the early decompensatory stage, and the terminal decompensatory stage. The compensatory mechanisms are a life-saving measure taken by the organism to protect itself.

The compensatory stage of shock is essentially characterized by release of catecholamines, resulting in increased cardiac output and systemic vascular resistance. The animal is in a hypermetabolic state, and the main clinical feature is tachycardia. Arterial blood pressure can be normal or elevated, mucous membrane color is normal or reddish, and capillary refill time may be normal or slowed. Prognosis is usually excellent with volume replacement.

The early decompensatory stage of shock is characterized by redistribution of blood flow to the heart and brain, and initiation of tissue hypoxia. Tissue hypoxia causes the cells to change from aerobic to anaerobic metabolism, resulting in lactic acidosis. Cytokines are released from different cells and tissues, causing hypotension, activation of inflammation and coagulation, tachycardia, tachypnea, and catabolism. Clinical signs of early decompensatory shock include hypothermia, cool limbs and skin, pale mucous membranes, prolonged capillary refill time, mental depression, and tachycardia. Cats do not always exhibit tachycardia, as compared with dogs (3). Aggressive fluid resuscitation is life-saving in many animals, but deterioration and reperfusion injury may be encountered.

In the terminal decompensatory stage, the compensatory mechanisms fail to provide sufficient tissue oxygenation, and the heart and brain begin to fail. Heart rate slows, vasodilation, blood pooling, and profound hypotension occur, and respiration is depressed. Clinical signs include bradycardia, severe hypotension, pale or cyanotic mucous membranes, absent capillary refill, weak or absent pulses, hypothermia, anuric renal failure, and pulmonary edema. Terminal shock is frequently unresponsive, even to aggressive fluid therapy.

11.2 Signs of shock in cats

Clinical signs of shock in cats differ from those in other species (Box 11-1). The mean heart rate of normal cats measured in a veterinary hospital environment was around 150–180 beats/min (4). Cats in shock may present with normal heart rates or even bradycardia, despite the presence of hypotension (3). One explanation for this is that cats may lack the initial compensation for shock by elevation of the heart rate, as seen in other species (3). It may therefore be difficult in the feline patient to differentiate between early and late decompensatory shock, because cats in both stages can present with bradycardia and hypotension. Other common signs of shock in the feline patient are mental depression and severe hypothermia. Hypothermia may be worsened by bradycardia and low cardiac output. In contrast, hypothermia contributes to bradycardia by depressing the sinus node (3).

Box 11-1. Signs of shock in cats

Clinical parameters indicating shock
Mental depression
Hypothermia (<98°F or 37°C)
Elevated, normal, or reduced heart rate
Weak or non-palpable peripheral pulse
Mucous membranes gray or white
Capillary refill time delayed or absent

Fluid type	Rate
Isotonic crystalloid solution alone	Up to 50 ml/kg per hour
Hetastarch/HAES (6% or 10%)	Resuscitation: 10 ml/kg over 20 minutes (crystalloids at 20 ml/kg per hour) Maintenance: 10–20 ml/kg per day
Hypertonic saline (7.5%)	3–5 ml/kg over 5–10 minutes (crystalloids at 20 ml/kg per hour)
Fresh whole blood and packed red cells	5–10 ml/kg per hour (until PCV > 15–20%) Volume to be transfused (ml) = kg × 66 × [(desired PCV – recipient PCV)/donor PCV]
Fresh frozen plasma	10–15 ml/kg (at maintenance rate)
Hemoglobin-based oxygen carriers	1–2 ml/kg per hour with a maximum volume of 5–10 ml/kg

PCV, packed cell volume.

Table 11-1. Rate and dosage of fluid administration in cats with traumatic hemorrhagic shock

11.3 Fluid resuscitation

Treatment of shock includes fluid resuscitation, active warming of the cat in the presence of hypothermia, and oxygen therapy. Although rapid fluid resuscitation is needed to treat shock, it should be performed more cautiously in cats than in dogs. Cats are more prone to develop lung edema with volume overload, and this may be fatal, especially in the presence of concurrent intrathoracic injuries. Careful monitoring of the patient during fluid therapy is therefore essential.

11.3.1 Crystalloid and colloid resuscitation

Placement of a peripheral intravenous catheter can be difficult in cats with severe shock as the veins collapse. A cut-down procedure to improve visibility of the peripheral vein, placement of a central venous catheter, or temporary intraosseous fluid administration in immature cats may be used to gain vascular access in such cases.

Rapid volume loading with isotonic crystalloid solutions is the mainstay of shock treatment, but crystalloid fluid starts shifting into the interstitial space after 30–60 minutes. Cats are susceptible to develop pulmonary and pleural fluid accumulation if large volumes of crystalloid solutions are administered rapidly. Simultaneous administration of crystalloids and colloids is the preferred treatment of choice for shock in cats (3). The addition of colloids (hetastarch) or hypertonic saline in dextran (7.5% saline in dextran 70) helps retain fluids in the intravascular space. This is especially important when large amounts of fluid have to be administered, and in patients with brain trauma or lung contusions. Colloids are usually given as a bolus, which may be repeated in cases with an inadequate response. The bolus must be given slowly, as rapid infusion of colloids can cause hypotension and vomiting. Initial fluid doses are listed in Table 11-1.

The doses listed in Table 11-1 are not necessarily given during the whole hour. Cardiovascular function, respiratory function, body temperature, and mental state should be re-evaluated every 10 minutes while intravenous fluids are being administered rapidly. Fluid rates are reduced as these clinical parameters return towards normal. Mean systemic arterial blood pressure should ideally reach 60–80 mmHg, and central venous pressure 6–8 cm H_2O. In cats with ongoing hemorrhage, mean arterial blood pressure should be kept lower than normal, around 50–60 mmHg, to reduce the risk of continuous bleeding. Perfusion parameters indicating an adequate response to fluid therapy are listed in Table 11-2 (5).

Cats must be carefully monitored for development of lung edema, and/or pleural effusion. If volume overload occurs, infusions are markedly reduced or stopped, and furosemide at 2–4 mg/kg is administered intravenously.

11.3.2 Transfusion of blood products

Transfusion of blood products is not usually indicated in the initial treatment of shock, but may be necessary in the later stage of treatment. An exception to the rule is the presence of significant bleeding, where fresh whole blood may be advantageous for fluid resuscitation.

Fresh whole blood and packed red blood cells

Cats have three major blood types: A, B, and AB (6). Group A is the most common type, especially in non-pedigree cats, followed by type B, which tends to be more common in some pedigree cats (7). Type AB is very rare. There are no universal

Parameter	Desired endpoint goals
Heart rate	160–200 beats/min
Body temperature	100–102.5°F 38–39°C
Mucous membrane color	Light pink (may remain pale in the presence of blood loss, despite adequate volume substitution)
Capillary refill time	1–2 seconds
Peripheral pulses	Femoral artery pulse easily palpable
Mean arterial pressure	60–80 mmHg
Central venous pressure	5 cm H_2O

Table 11-2. Parameters indicating adequate response to shock treatment

blood donors in cats, as cats with type A blood have anti-type B antibodies, and vice versa (8). Fatal transfusion reactions are likely to occur when a cat with type B blood receives type A blood (9), but also cats with type A blood may develop mild reactions after receiving type B blood. Therefore both the donor and the recipient blood must be blood-typed (RapidVet H Feline; dms laboratories, Flemington, NJ, USA) and cross-matched before transfusion. Cats with type AB blood should be transfused with type-specific blood, or, if not available, type A blood (8). Transfusion reactions are rare with adequate donor selection and compatibility testing (10).

A healthy cat with a body weight of 4 kg can donate between 40 and 50 ml (absolute maximum) of blood (20% of total blood volume), provided that fluid is administered intravenously during collection of blood (11). Two or three times the volume of blood taken should be substituted with crystalloid solutions. The packed cell volume (PCV) of the donor cats is always measured before blood is taken. Cats usually have to be sedated for the procedure.

Fresh whole blood is the transfusion of choice in the presence of severe acute bleeding, when multiple blood components are required. Volume overload may be a problem if treating chronic anemia and the administration of packed red blood cells is therefore preferred in this situation. The PCV of packed red blood cell infusions is around 45–65% in cats (8). The goal of administering fresh whole blood or packed red cells is to maintain or achieve a PCV of more than 20%, especially if the patient has to undergo surgery. Cats seem to be more tolerant to anemia than dogs (12), and a PCV as low as 15% is often well tolerated in cats that do not require surgery. The formula for calculating the amount of blood necessary to achieve the desired PCV is shown in Table 11-1. As a rough guideline, 2 ml/kg of whole blood raises the recipient's PCV by 1%, or 1 ml/kg of packed red blood cells raises the PCV by 1%. Blood products are administered through a 170-µm filter into a dedicated fluid line. The line is flushed with 0.9% saline after the infusion, because saline contains no calcium and therefore should reduce the risk of clotting.

Hemoglobin-based oxygen carriers

Hemoglobin-based oxygen carriers (HBOCs) contain bovine hemoglobin and are used to augment oxygen delivery to tissue. HBOCs lack cell surface antigens and are universally compatible blood products. Currently the solution is not registered for use in cats, but dosage recommendations are 5 ml/kg per hour at a maximal dose of 5–10 ml/kg (8). HBOCs have profound colloidal effects and patients should be carefully monitored to prevent volume overload.

Fresh frozen plasma

Fresh frozen plasma contains clotting factors, albumin and other serum proteins, and plasma protease inhibitors. The most common indication for administration of fresh frozen plasma to traumatized animals is the prevention or treatment of disseminated intravascular coagulopathy by providing clotting factors. Fresh frozen plasma is not ideal to treat hypoproteinemia, because it does not significantly raise albumin concentrations. A dose of 45 ml/kg would be required to elevate albumin concentration by 10 g/l (which would cause volume overload). Hypoproteinemic cats may benefit from a mild increase in albumin in the short term. Cats with albumin concentrations less than 20 g/l should receive hetastarch at a maintenance rate to maintain colloid pressures.

Fresh frozen plasma is slowly warmed to 37°C and administered through a 170-µm filter and a dedicated fluid line. Once warmed, it should be used within 4 hours, because the clotting factors do not remain stable after that time.

References and further reading

1. Day TK. Shock: pathophysiology, diagnosis, and treatment. In: Slatter D (ed.) Textbook of small animal surgery, 3rd edn. Philadelphia: Saunders; 2004: pp. 1–17.

2. Turnwald GH, Pichler ME. Blood transfusion in dogs and cats. Part II. Administration, adverse effects and component therapy. Compend Continuing Educ 1985;7:115–122.
3. Kirby R, et al. Cats are not dogs in critical care. In: Bonagura JD (ed.) Kirk's current veterinary therapy XIII. Philadelphia: WB Saunders; 2000.
4. Abbott JA. Heart rate and heart rate variability of healthy cats in home and hospital environments. J Feline Med Surg 2005;7: 195–202.
5. Rudloff E, Kirby R. Colloid and crystalloid resuscitation. Vet Clin North Am 2001;31:1207–1229.
6. Griot-Wenk ME, Giger U. Feline transfusion medicine. Blood types and their clinical importance. Vet Clin North Am Small Anim Pract 1995;25:1305–1322.
7. Knottenbelt CM. The feline AB blood group system and its importance in transfusion medicine. J Feline Med Surg 2002; 4:69–76.
8. Haldane S, et al. Transfusion medicine. Compend Continuing Educ 2004;26:502–518.
9. Auer L, Bell K. The AB blood group system in cats. Animal Blood Groups, Biochem Genet 1981;12:287–297.
10. Weingart C, et al. Whole blood transfusions in 91 cats: a clinical evaluation. J Feline Med Surg 2004;6:139–148.
11. Knottenbelt C, Mackin, A. Blood transfusions in the dog and cat. Part 1. Blood collection techniques. In Pract 1998;20: 110–114.
12. Knottenbelt C, Mackin A. Blood transfusion in the dog and cat. Part 2: Indications and safe administration. In Pract 1998;20: 191–199.

12 Specific injuries in the polytraumatized cat

K. Voss

Thoracic, abdominal, and neurological injuries are often present in the feline trauma patient. Injuries to these organs are frequently more severe and more important for survival and prognosis than concurrent orthopedic injuries. Initial management of the most common problems and injuries is summarized in this chapter.

12.1 Thoracic trauma

Thoracic trauma is common in fracture patients. Around 40% of cats with fractures have radiographic evidence of thoracic injuries (1). Patients with fractures of the head and thoracic limbs are significantly more likely to have sustained thoracic injuries, compared to patients with fractures of the pelvis and pelvic limbs (1). The thoracic injuries most commonly encountered are lung contusions, pneumothorax, rib fractures, and diaphragmatic hernia. Intrathoracic tracheal avulsion has also been described in cats after trauma (2). Respiratory compromise induces an elevated respiratory rate and abnormal breathing patterns. The type of breathing pattern varies with different conditions. Pleural space disease generally causes rapid shallow breathing with a predominantly inspiratory distress. Pulmonary parenchymal disease causes labored inspiration and expiration. Severe and life-threatening respiratory compromise is associated with open-mouth breathing, postural changes, and paradoxical motion of the chest and abdomen. Cyanosis corresponds with a PaO_2 of less than 40 mmHg and is a sign of extreme hypoxemia.

The initial treatment of traumatized cats with dyspnea is aimed at enhancing oxygen intake and reducing oxygen demand (Table 12-1). Oxygen should be supplied immediately to all trauma patients with respiratory distress. A flow-by method or a face mask may be used during emergency examination and vascular access procedures. The flow-by method is better tolerated by most cats, but smaller fractions of oxygen are achieved than with the face mask. An oxygen cage is preferable for cats requiring prolonged oxygen supplementation. A flow rate of 2 l/min into a closed oxygen cage will result in a fraction of inspired oxygen of 40–50%, which is safe for long-term application. The ambient temperature and humidity within the cage should be monitored and regulated. Ideally, oxygen saturation should be maintained

Measure	Pharmaceutical agent/treatment	Dosage/rate	Indication
Oxygen	Flow-by	6–8 l/min	All patients with dyspnea
	Face mask	6–10 l/min	
	Oxygen cage	2 l/min	
Analgesia	Buprenorphine	0.01–0.03 mg/kg IV/IM/SC	All patients with dyspnea
	or:		
	Morphine	0.1–0.3 mg/kg IM	
	or:		
	Butorphanol	0.2–0.4 mg/kg IV/IM	
Fluid therapy	Crystalloid solution	10 (–50) ml/kg per hour	All patients in shock
	Colloid solution (hetastarch)	10 ml/kg over 20 minutes	Add collloids if large volume is required (and reduce crystalloid rates)
Thoracocentesis			All patients with continuing dyspnea despite initial treatment
Sedation	Acepromazine	0.01–0.02 mg/kg IV/IM	In very excited cats or those difficult to handle
Anti-inflammatory	Dexamethasone	0.02 mg/kg IV	Upper-airway obstruction

Table 12-1. Initial therapy of traumatized cats with dyspnea. Oxygen, analgesia, and fluids are administered to every patient. Further measures or medications depend on the severity of dyspnea, and the underlying cause

at >94% and the PaO_2 should reach values of > 80 mmHg. Artificial ventilation is indicated if severe hypoxemia (PaO_2 < 60 mmHg) persists despite appropriate oxygen supplementation.

Open-mouth breathing and tachypnea may be solely due to stress and pain in some feline trauma patients. Early administration of analgesics during assessment and initial treatment should markedly improve respiration in these patients (Table 12-1). Pain medication will also reduce oxygen demands. Rarely, mild sedation is indicated in very stressed cats, with the goal of reducing oxygen demand due to excitement. Upper-airway obstruction may be seen with sublingual, laryngeal, or pharyngeal swelling in cats with head trauma. These patients may benefit from a single injection of dexamethasone to reduce swelling. A tracheotomy is necessary in cases with upper-airway obstruction not responding to conservative treatment.

Thoracocentesis is performed in any dyspneic trauma patient before obtaining radiographs. Thoracocentesis is both diagnostic and therapeutic if fluid or air can be retrieved from the thoracic cavity. In one study, air was retrieved in more than 50% of cats with dyspnea (3). If the condition of the cat allows, the hair is clipped, and the puncture site is aseptically prepared. Sterile gloves should be worn during the procedure. Thoracocentesis is described in Figure 12-1. If no air or fluid can be retrieved from one side, the other side is tapped as well.

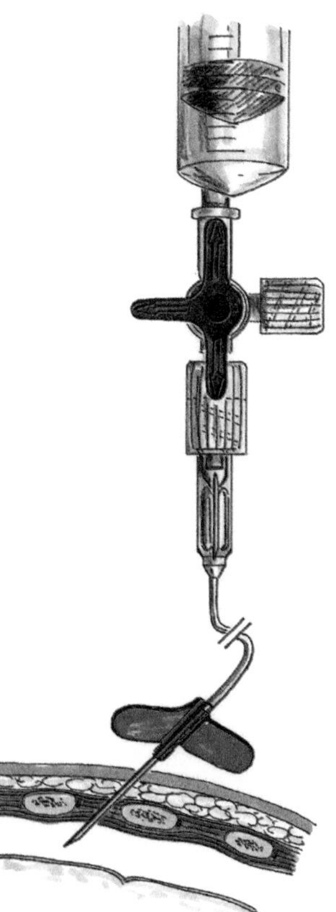

Figure 12-1 Thoracocentesis. An 18–22-gauge butterfly needle is attached to an extension set, three-way tap, and a 20-ml syringe to provide a closed suction system. The needle is inserted between the seventh and ninth intercostal space, just cranial to the rib to preserve the intercostal artery. The most dorsal area of the thorax, with respect to the patient position, is tapped if pneumothorax is suspected. If fluid is suspected, the ventral aspect of the thorax is tapped. Care has to be taken not to injure the internal thoracic artery, which courses ventrally parallel to the sternum.

Radiographs of the thorax are obtained from every traumatized patient. Not all thoracic injuries cause clinical signs of respiratory distress and some would go undiagnosed without radiographs. This is especially true for diaphragmatic ruptures without herniation of a large amount or number of organs. Cats with respiratory distress need to be stabilized before taking them to radiology. The stress caused from obtaining the radiographs will elevate the patient's oxygen demand to a level that will possibly exceed maximal uptake capacities, causing hypoxemia and even death. In rare instances, a patient may show progressively worsening respiratory distress, despite medical stabilization and negative thoracic taps. Radiographs have to be obtained despite dyspnea in such patients, especially to rule out or diagnose diaphragmatic hernia. A laterolateral radiograph is sufficient for this purpose, or a horizontal beam view may be preferable for the cat whose dyspnea worsens when it is laid on its side. Oxygenation should be provided during radiography.

12.1.1 Pneumothorax

Rupture of the thoracic wall, bronchi, and pulmonary parenchyma may cause accumulation of air in the intrapleural and/or mediastinal space. The most common injury is pulmonary parenchymal tears after blunt thoracic trauma with accumulation of air in the intrapleural space, leading to loss of negative intrapleural pressure and collapse of lung lobes. A radiograph of a cat with pneumothorax is shown in Figure 12-2. Tension pneumothorax develops if the site of leakage acts as a one-way valve, resulting in rapid accumulation of air, progressive increase in intrapleural pressure, and rapid deterioration of the patient. As described above, thoracocentesis (Fig. 12-1) is the most important diagnostic and thera-

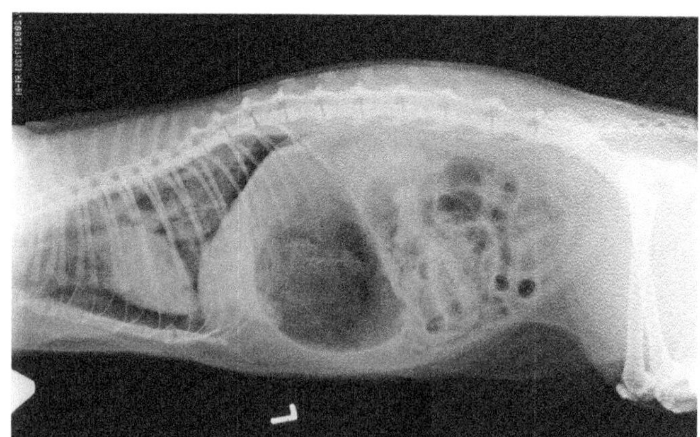

Figure 12-2 Cat with traumatic pneumothorax. The heart base is elevated from the sternum and free gas is present between the caudal lung lobes and the diaphragm. The caudal lung lobes are consolidated. The gas-filled stomach is due to aerophagia secondary to dyspnea, and impairs diaphragmatic excursions.

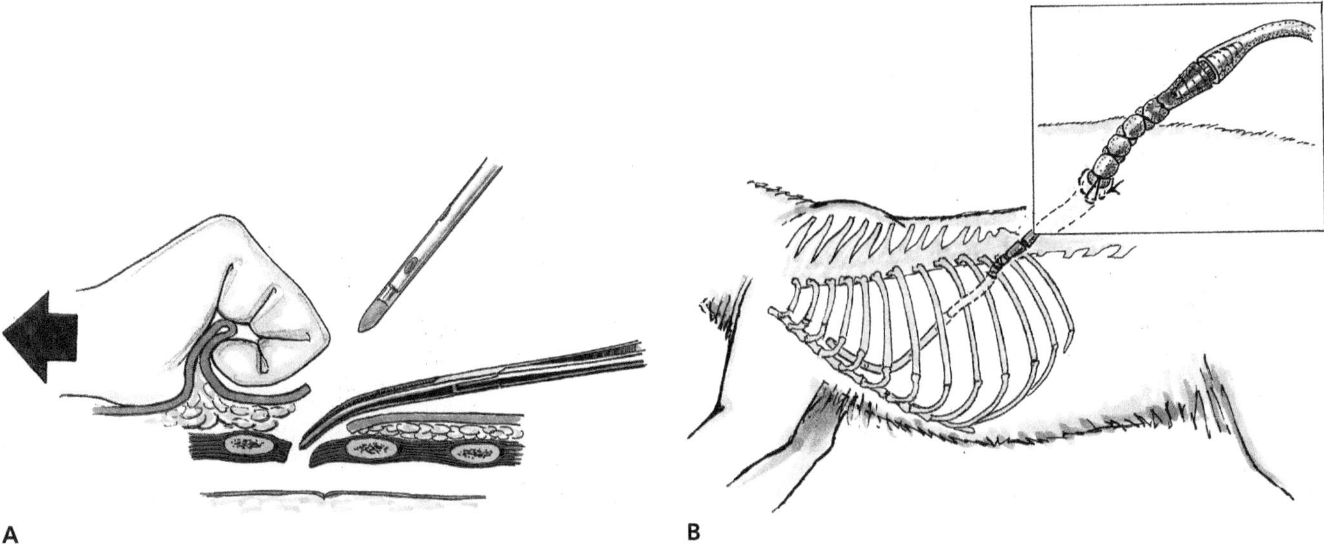

Figure 12-3 Insertion of a thoracic drain. Although commercially available chest tubes with a metal stylet inside could be inserted bluntly, the following insertion technique minimizes the risk of lung perforation. A small skin incision is made in the dorsal third of the thorax over the 11th rib. (**A**) The skin is pulled cranially until the incision is located over the eighth intercostal space. A curved hemostat is used to penetrate the thoracic wall bluntly, before the chest tube is inserted. (**B**) The tube is advanced along the inner thoracic wall in a cranioventral direction. Correct positioning of the chest tube is shown. Air or fluid is retrieved as soon as the tube is placed. The tube is then closed or connected to a suction system, and secured to the skin with a Chinese finger-trap suture to prevent dislodgement. The entrance site is covered with a small bandage.

peutic measure if pneumothorax is suspected. The taps are repeated if respiratory distress persists or relapses due to continuing air accumulation.

Most pulmonary parenchymal tears seal after several hours and no further therapy is needed. If pneumothorax persists after several taps or if tension pneumothorax develops, a thoracic drain should be placed (Fig. 12-3), which allows intermittent or continuous suction with a three-bottle system. Exploratory thoracotomy is rarely indicated at that time, but should be considered if air leakage does not subside after 3 days of continuous suction. Surgery for orthopedic conditions should be delayed until pneumothorax has resolved. Care has to be taken during anesthesia to prevent re-rupture of the sealed leakage site with excessive ventilation pressure.

12.1.2 Pulmonary contusion

Pulmonary contusions represent pulmonary hemorrhage and may occur alone or in addition to other thoracic injuries. They are the most commonly diagnosed thoracic injury. Dyspnea or tachypnea occurs if functional capacity of the lung is reduced due to large areas of lung parenchyma obstructed by hemorrhage. Radiographs taken soon after the accident may underestimate the degree of contusion, because radiographic changes are only fully visible after some hours (Fig. 12-4). Treatment of lung contusions is supportive and consists of oxygen supplementation, cautious fluid therapy, analgesia, especially in the presence of rib fractures, and minimizing stress. Antibiotics may be administered in the more severe cases to reduce the risk of development of pneumonia. Intubation and mechanical ventilation should be instituted if the animal cannot be stabilized with oxygen therapy and supportive care and PaO_2 drops below 60 mmHg.

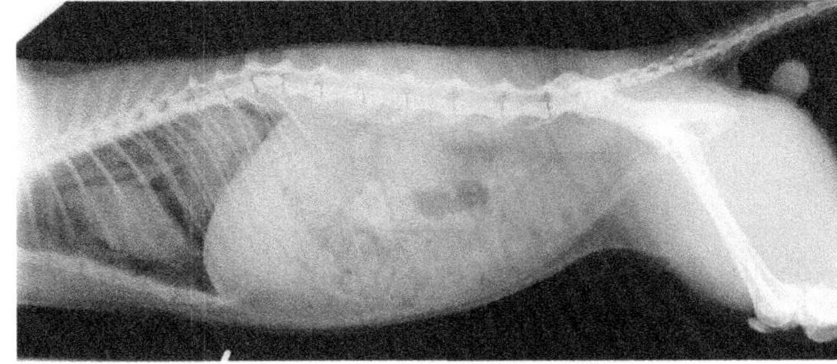

Figure 12-4 Cat with contusion of the caudal lung lobes. Also note aerophagia secondary to dyspnea.

12.1.3 Thoracic wall injury

Rib fractures are most often due to injuries caused by interaction with other animals or due to motor vehicle accidents (4). Nearly all cats with rib fractures have concurrent pulmonary contusions (4). Displaced rib fragments may cause rupture of lung parenchyma and pneumothorax. The respiratory distress seen in patients with rib fractures probably results from concurrent lung contusions or intrapleural disease rather than from the unstable rib cage. However, pain caused by the rib fractures may cause reluctance to expand the thoracic wall and can also impair ventilation. A survival rate of 78% of cats with rib fractures has been described (4). Cats with concurrent pleural effusion, diaphragmatic hernia, and flail chest were more likely to die than cats without these injuries (4). A flail chest is the most severe form of rib fracture and occurs when several consecutive ribs are fractured segmentally. The resulting free segment of the chest wall then moves paradoxically during respiration. Flail chest is accompanied by pulmonary contusions, pneumothorax, and subcutaneous emphysema in most cases (5).

Rib fractures in cats can generally be treated conservatively. The adequate treatment of concurrent intrathoracic injuries, such as pneumothorax and lung contusions, is most important for survival. Adequate pain medication is also important to facilitate breathing. If a flail chest is present, the cat is positioned with the free segment downwards in order to reduce movement of the free segment. Traditionally, stabilization of the flail segment has been suggested in order to reduce the paradoxical movement of the segment and its negative effects on ventilation. More recently the need to stabilize the flail segment has been questioned, as respiratory compromise is more likely to be caused by intrathoracic injuries (5). Comparison of conservative and surgical management of flail chest in dogs and cats revealed survival rates of 66.7% for surgically managed cases and 93.3% for conservatively managed cases (5). However, these results may be biased by patient selection.

Penetrating thoracic wounds can be caused by dog bite wounds or by impalement, for example after falls on sharp objects. Concurrent rib fractures, intercostal muscle disruption, subcutaneous emphysema, and pneumothorax are usually visible on radiographs (Fig. 12-5). The open wound is immediately covered with sterile and airtight bandages. Thoracocentesis is performed to evacuate intrapleural air if present. Wound management and exploration of the thorax are usually necessary after stabilization of the patient.

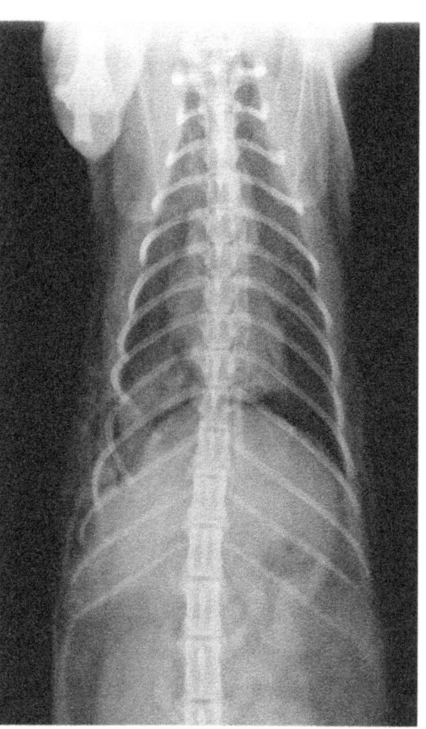

Figure 12-5 Ventrodorsal radiograph of a cat with a right-sided open chest injury after a fall on to a sharp object. The thoracic wall is disrupted in the area of the eighth and ninth rib, and subcutaneous emphysema, pneumothorax, and contusion of the right lung lobe are visible. Exploratory lateral thoracotomy, lobectomy of the lacerated lung lobe, and repair of the thoracic wall were performed.

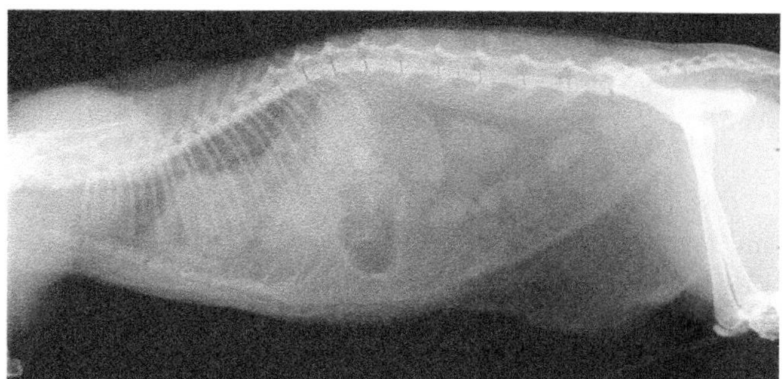

Figure 12-6 Cat with traumatic diaphragmatic hernia. The normal contour of the diaphragm is not visible. Most of the small intestine and probably parts of the liver are displaced through the defect into the thoracic cavity. The abdominal cavity has an empty appearance.

12.1.4 Diaphragmatic hernia

Rupture of the diaphragm occurs with acute intra-abdominal pressure elevation caused by blunt abdominal trauma when the glottis is open simultaneously. The pressure wave then continues in a cranial direction and may lead to rupture of the diaphragm. Diaphragmatic ruptures occur more commonly after road traffic accidents than after falls from a height (3). Abdominal organs usually dislodge into the thoracic cavity during the accident, but with small diaphragmatic tears, organ displacement may occur at a later date. Liver lobes, spleen, omentum, stomach, and small intestines are displaced most frequently (Fig. 12-6). The amount of organs displaced dictates the degree of respiratory compromise. Clinical symptoms are tachypnea, muffled heart sounds, and vomiting (6). Cardiovascular stabilization and oxygen supplementation should be performed prior to surgery.

Many patients with diaphragmatic hernias do not have to be rushed into surgery, allowing time for preoperative cardiovascular stabilization. In rare instances, ventilation and oxygenation do not improve with the stabilization procedures. These cats often have significant amounts or numbers of organs displaced into the thoracic cavity, preventing adequate lung expansion, and should be operated immediately. Herniation of a bloated stomach is another indication for immediate surgery, but is rare in cats. The bloated stomach can be tapped percutaneously during preparation for surgery in order to reduce its volume. Elevating the chest of the cat, ideally with the use of a tilting table, may also help to facilitate ventilation.

Surgery involves careful repositioning of herniated abdominal organs and herniorrhaphy. The surgeon may encounter circular or radial tears, or a combination of these. The defect is closed from dorsal to ventral in a continuous pattern. Care is taken not to obstruct the caudal vena cava by placing sutures too close. In rare cases, for example chronic defects, diaphragmatic tissue may be missing, preventing primary closure. Small intestinal submucosa grafts can then be used to fill the defect.

The mortality rate in cats with diaphragmatic hernias has been reported to be 17.6% in one study (6). The duration of the hernia prior to surgery had no effect on mortality, but cats were more likely to die in the presence of concurrent injuries or diseases, such as abdominal wall hernia or cardiomyopathy (6).

12.1.5 Intrathoracic tracheal avulsion

Intrathoracic tracheal avulsion is a rare injury, which has been described in several case reports and in a study of nine cats (2). Intrathoracic tracheal avulsion is thought to be caused by overstretching of the trachea during hyperextension injury of the neck. The avulsion usually occurs just cranial to the bifurcation. The airway lumen usually remains patent because a pseudomembrane surrounds the defect (Fig. 12-7). These cats are often only presented 1–3 weeks after the trauma due to dyspnea and respiratory distress. The development of respiratory symptoms is associated with stenosis of the avulsed tracheal ends. Acute symptoms may occur in rare cases if air leaks into the mediastinum (2). Treatment consists of end-to-end anastomosis of the trachea for which a right lateral thoracotomy may be used (2). Prognosis is good with careful anesthetic and surgical technique (2).

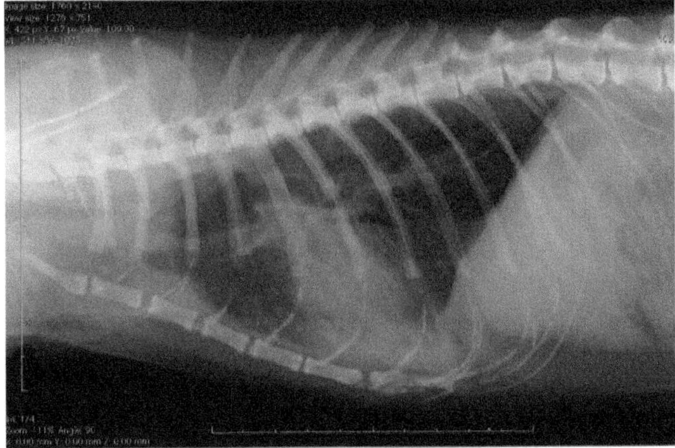

Figure 12-7 Radiograph of a cat with intrathoracic avulsion of the trachea. Loss of continuity of the cranial thoracic trachea is seen. The dilated space between the tracheal ends is surrounded by a pseudomembrane, and is air-filled.

12.2 Abdominal trauma

Abdominal trauma has been reported to occur in 7–39% of traumatized cats (3, 7, 8). Abdominal trauma is generally not acutely life-threatening but may become so if underdiagnosed or missed. Diagnosis is often delayed for hours or even days, because symptoms are rather non-specific, and are often only detected during the course of treatment. There should be a high index of suspicion of abdominal trauma, especially in animals with pelvic fractures or other significant injuries of the caudal half of the body. Urinary tract injuries, abdominal wall hernias, and intra-abdominal bleeding are most common. Rupture of the gallbladder or common bile duct, traumatic pancreatitis, or perforation or necrosis of the intestinal tract may be encountered on rare occasions.

Once the patient has been stabilized and can be handled safely, the abdomen is thoroughly and gently palpated, with special emphasis on the integrity of the abdominal wall and urinary bladder shape and filling. Abdominal pain, bruising and hematoma formation, vomiting, and urinary tract symptoms should alert the clinician to the possibility of abdominal injury.

Abdominal radiographs should be obtained from all traumatized cats with moderate and severe injuries (8). Loss of integrity of the abdominal wall, displacement of organs, loss of abdominal detail, or loss of detail and widening of the retroperitoneal space are common findings. Abdominal ultrasonography is usually performed if intra-abdominal abnormalities are detected on radiographs. Ultrasonography is useful in detecting small amounts of free abdominal fluid, guiding needle aspiration of the fluid, and to detect structural abnormalities of intra-abdominal organs.

Abdominocentesis is a quick and easy method to retrieve free abdominal fluid for cytology, and biochemical and bacteriological tests, although around 5–6 ml/kg of free abdominal fluid must be present to avoid false-negative results with blind abdominocentesis (9). Ultrasound-guided abdominocentesis is a sensitive and non-invasive method for controlled aspiration of small or localized fluid accumulations (10). Diagnostic peritoneal lavage is another reliable technique for retrieval of abdominal fluid but usually necessitates sedation, which is often not recommended in traumatized animals. Any abdominal fluid collected is analyzed in order to diagnose its origin. Smears are prepared for cytology, abdominal fluid is preserved for biochemical tests, and a bacteriology sample is taken. Biochemical testing includes creatinine, potassium, bilirubin, and glucose levels. Possible types of free abdominal fluid and their characteristics are summarized in Table 12-2. Free intra-abdominal blood is found most commonly after

Table 12-2. Types of free abdominal fluid and their distinguishing characteristics

Type of free abdominal fluid	Fluid characteristics
Blood	Packed cell volume and total protein are similar to blood levels
Urine	Creatinine and potassium exceed blood levels
Bile	Yellow color; bilirubin exceeds blood levels
Septic effusion	Degenerate neutrophils, intracellular bacteria, food particles Glucose less than 50 mg/dl Blood-to-abdominal fluid glucose difference >20 mg/dl (21)

trauma, followed by urine (10). Leakage of bile and septic peritonitis are uncommon findings in trauma patients.

Exploratory celiotomy is indicated in the presence of intra-abdominal urine accumulation, presence of septic abdominal fluid, and accumulation of bile. Open abdominal injuries can be caused by gunshot injury, bite wounds, and stab wounds. Damage to intra-abdominal organs occurs frequently with these types of injury, and early exploration of the abdominal cavity is indicated to exclude, diagnose, and possibly treat sustained trauma to organs.

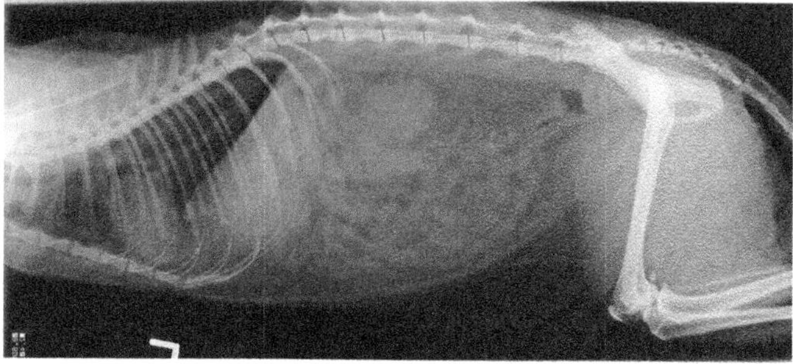

Figure 12-8 Retroperitoneal fluid accumulation. Radiographs demonstrate loss of retroperitoneal detail and ventral displacement of abdominal organs. Rupture of a ureter was later diagnosed by excretory urography in this cat.

12.2.1 Urinary tract injuries

Urinary tract injuries are often due to blunt abdominal trauma, such as motor vehicle accidents. They are less commonly encountered with high-rise syndrome (3). Leakage of urine into the abdominal cavity results in uroabdomen. Following trauma, rupture of the urinary bladder is the reason for uroabdomen in more than 80% of cases (11). Injuries of the kidney and ureters classically result in retroperitoneal urine accumulation, but urine can still flow into the abdominal cavity due to concurrent rupture of the thin retroperitoneal fascia. Rupture of the urethra may result in uroabdomen or subcutaneous urine accumulation in the perineal region and hindlimbs, depending on the site of the lesion.

Hematuria is a frequent finding in traumatized cats. Hematuria does not necessarily indicate severe urinary tract injury. It may result from kidney trauma or partial-thickness lesions of the urinary bladder mucosa, and usually subsides in 1–2 days. Hematuria may be severe enough to cause anemia, and packed cell volume should be checked on a regular basis. Diagnosis of urinary tract injury is often delayed due to the non-specific nature and latency of onset of the clinical signs. Urinary tract injury should particularly be suspected in patients with orthopedic injuries of the pelvic limbs and spine. The most common clinical symptoms with uroabdomen are anuria, dysuria, lethargy, and vomiting (11). Small bladder ruptures may seal if the bladder is empty; therefore the ability to void does not exclude bladder rupture. A distended abdomen and fluid waves are only palpable if large amounts of urine have leaked into the abdominal cavity. Bradycardia may be caused by severe hyperkalemia or may be associated with shock (Chapter 11). Hematological abnormalities include azotemia in nearly all cases, and hyperkalemia and hyperphosphatemia in around 50% of cases (11). Abdominal radiographs and ultrasound are used to detect abdominal or retroperitoneal fluid accumulation (Fig. 12-8). The presence of urine in the abdominal cavity is confirmed if potassium and creatinine in the abdominal fluid exceed blood levels (Table 12-2). Because urea diffuses back into circulation more rapidly than creatinine, it is a less reliable parameter. Bacteriological cultures can be positive (11).

The site of urinary leakage is diagnosed by retrograde positive contrast cystourethrography and/or by excretory urography. Retrograde positive contrast cystourethrography is indicated if rupture of the urinary bladder or urethra is suspected (Fig. 12-9). Excretory urography is used if radiographs reveal accumulation of retroperitoneal fluid suggestive of urine. If retroperitoneal fluid accumulation is due to bleeding, it will resorb with time. If it is due to urine leakage, the amount of fluid will increase. Patients need to be well hydrated before conducting excretory urography in order to prevent renal damage by the contrast media.

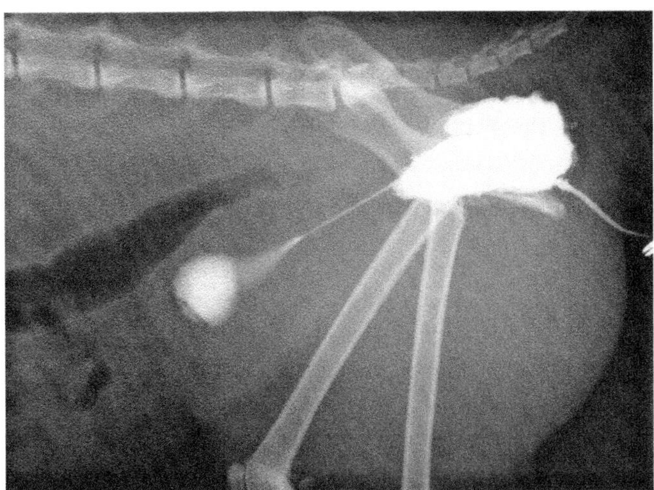

Figure 12-9 Retrograde positive contrast cystourethrography demonstrates intrapelvic rupture of the urethra. The cat had suffered a road traffic accident and also had a proximal femoral physeal fracture.

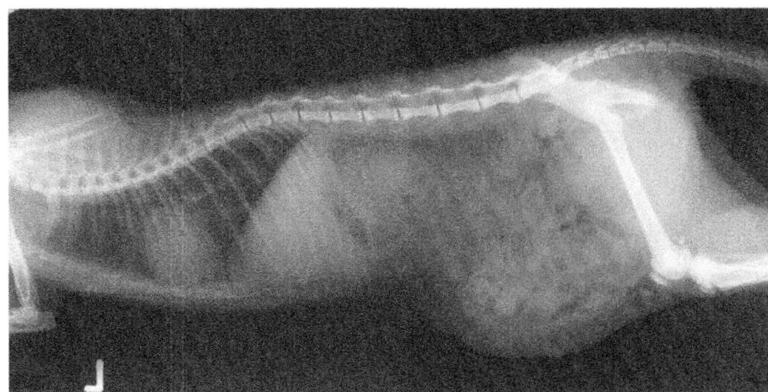

Figure 12-10 Radiograph of a polytraumatized cat. A fracture of the ilium and a caudal abdominal wall hernia are visible. The contour of the caudal abdominal wall is disrupted and small intestinal loops and the colon are herniated through the defect.

Initial stabilization of the patient includes fluid resuscitation, correction of serum potassium levels, and drainage of urine from the abdominal cavity if necessary. Patients with hyperkalemia are infused with a 0.9% saline solution to dilute serum potassium and to enhance glomerular filtration rate. If potassium levels are high enough to cause clinically significant bradycardia, calcium gluconate (50–100 mg/kg) is infused slowly (12). Calcium is cardioprotective by improving cardiac conduction until potassium concentrations are lowered by other therapeutic measures. Patients with uroabdomen require drainage of urine from the urinary bladder and abdominal cavity if surgery has to be delayed.

Surgery is performed as soon as the patient is considered hemodynamically and metabolically stable, and the site of urine leakage has been determined. A midline exploratory celiotomy and abdominal exploration are performed. Tears in the urinary bladder wall are sutured. Devitalized tissue has to be debrided beforehand. Urethral tears can be more difficult to repair. Sharp non-circumferential lacerations may be sutured although they can also heal with conservative management using an indwelling catheter for around 2 weeks. Complete disruption of the urethra has to be treated by urethral anastomosis or urethrostomy, depending on the location of the lesion. Ureteral avulsion from the renal pelvis and midureter lacerations are probably best treated with ureteronephrectomy if the contralateral kidney and ureter are intact and functional. Suturing or anastomosis of ureters is technically difficult in cats, and stricture formation is a common complication (13). Distal ureteral lesions may be treated by ureteronephrectomy or ureteroneocystotomy.

Postoperatively, a soft urinary catheter, connected to a closed suction system, may be left in place for some days. The closed suction system helps to prevent distension of the urinary bladder, and allows assessment of the amount of urine produced. An indwelling catheter is usually not necessary after adequate repair of urinary bladder tears, but is indicated if the bladder wall is markedly inflamed and thickened, or if concurrent neurological deficits prevent normal detrusor function. A urethral catheter is also indicated after repair of urethral lesions, because stricture formation may be reduced by avoiding contact of the lesion with urine (13). Azotemia should resolve in 1–2 days following surgery. Morbidity and mortality largely depend on the preoperative status, severity of the lesion, associated injuries, and delay of therapy. Cats die after 47–90 hours in an experimental setting if uroabdomen is left untreated, but death may occur sooner in clinical cases (14).

12.2.2 Abdominal wall hernias

Traumatic abdominal wall hernias are most commonly caused by road traffic accidents and dog bite wounds (15, 16). Blunt abdominal trauma results in tearing of abdominal muscles or avulsion of muscle attachments, sparing the more elastic skin. Dog bite wounds cause crushing and tearing of tissue and the abdominal wall injury may be associated with penetrating injuries of the skin. Traumatic abdominal wall hernias can occur at any location, but they are found more frequently in the paralumbar region, the femoral region, the area of attachment of the cranial pubic tendon, the ventral abdominal wall, and the paracostal region (15, 17). The organs most commonly herniated through caudal body wall defect are the omentum, small intestines, and the urinary bladder (Fig. 12-10).

Herniation of abdominal organs is usually diagnosed by abdominal palpation. Clinical diagnosis of caudal abdominal hernias can be difficult in obese cats, and in the presence of cellulitis or necrosis of subcutaneous fat. Radiographic diagnosis is straightforward if intra-abdominal organs are herniated. Herniation of omentum or intra-abdominal fat may not be readily visible on radiographs, and ultrasonography can add information in unclear cases.

Traumatic abdominal wall hernias are repaired surgically in order to restore continuity of the body wall and prevent incarceration of abdominal organs. Surgery is performed once the animal is considered stable. Emergency surgery is only indicated in cases where the urinary bladder or small intestinal loops are incarcerated and at risk of avascular necrosis. A midline celiotomy and abdominal exploration are preferable to a local approach, as the incidence of concurrent intra-abdominal injuries is nearly 30% (15). The defect is sutured with slowly absorbable or non-absorbable suture material using interrupted mattress or cruciate sutures. If the abdominal muscles are avulsed from the pubic floor, small holes drilled into the cranial rim of the pubic floor may serve to anchor the sutures. Postoperatively, cage rest should be provided.

Prognosis is usually favorable for smaller defects. Large abdominal wall hernias associated with massive soft-tissue trauma may induce systemic inflammatory response syndrome or sepsis. The survival rate for cats with traumatic abdominal wall hernias has been reported as 80% (15).

12.2.3 Intra-abdominal bleeding

Intra-abdominal bleeding may occur after blunt abdominal trauma, and the liver and spleen are the most likely sources. Intra-abdominal hemorrhage often subsides spontaneously and may go unnoticed if only a small volume of blood is lost. If significant intra-abdominal hemorrhage occurs, affected cats are presented in hypovolemic shock, and blood accumulation may be large enough to cause abdominal distension. Radiographs show loss of abdominal detail. A packed cell volume and total protein content of the abdominal fluid that is similar to blood levels is consistent with intra-abdominal bleeding (Table 12-2).

Initial treatment consists of fluid resuscitation (Chapter 11). Hypotensive resuscitation should be used, because bleeding is more likely to stop with lower than normal arterial blood pressures (Chapter 11). Whole blood or packed red cell transfusions are necessary if the packed cell volume drops markedly below 20%. An abdominal wrap may help stop the bleeding by elevating intra-abdominal pressure.

Surgical hemostasis is rarely necessary. Concrete clinical guidelines do not exist to help in the decision for the need of surgical management. A lack of response to conservative management, deterioriation of the patient during fluid therapy, an increase in the amount of free abdominal fluid, and continuous dropping of the packed cell volume in both the abdominal cavity and peripheral blood are signs of continuous hemorrhage (18). Surgical exploration is recommended in humans when transfusion requirements exceed 20 ml/kg (18). Immediate blood transfusions and exploratory celiotomy are performed if ongoing bleeding is suspected, based on the mentioned parameters.

12.2.4 Injuries to other abdominal organs

Injuries to abdominal organs other than the urinary tract, liver, or spleen are rare. Intestinal perforation or crushing may occur after dog bite wounds or penetrating trauma, such as gunshot or impalement injuries. Exploratory celiotomy is indicated in any cat with penetrating abdominal trauma. Waiting for a diagnosis of septic peritonitis leads to delay in treatment and enhances morbidity and mortality. Other rare intra-abdominal injuries include intestinal necrosis resulting from vascular damage, rupture of the gallbladder or ducts, traumatic pancreatitis, and avulsion or tearing of the uterus.

12.3 Brain injury

Head and brain injuries are a common sequel in cats after motor vehicle accidents. Brain trauma may cause primary damage to the nervous tissue that may not be influenced by therapeutic measurements. Secondary pathophysiological mechanisms result in hypoxia, ischemia, edema, and elevation of intracranial pressure (ICP) minutes to days after the injury. Treatment is aimed at reducing these secondary complications and preventing irreversible lesions of neurons and axons. Stabilization of respiratory and cardiovascular function has major priority in the treatment of head-injury patients. Close monitoring of patients with head trauma is essential: worsening of mental status, pupil size, and reactivity should lead to more aggressive treatment.

Subcutaneous hematomas, and hemorrhage from the nose or the ears may be a sign of skull fracture. Initial neurological dysfunction is related to the site of injury (Chapter 1). Patients with injury to the brainstem usually carry a worse prognosis than patients with injuries to the brain hemispheres. When deterioration of neurological function occurs during the course of treatment, brain edema and elevation of ICP should be suspected. Common clinical signs for an elevation of ICP include deterioration of mental state, loss of cranial nerve function, especially pupil size and responsiveness to light, loss of body posture, and changes in breathing pattern. Elevation of ICP may also result in bradycardia due to the Cushing reflex. Skull fractures and intracranial hematomas are best diagnosed by computed tomography. However, anesthesia, which is necessary for computed tomography, should only be performed once the patient has been stabilized. Therefore treatment is usually initiated based on clinical findings only.

Treatment is aimed at reducing cerebral edema and ICP and at preservation of cerebral blood flow and oxygen levels. Fluid is administered cautiously in order to avoid overloading. Mean arterial blood pressure should be maintained between 70 and 110 mmHg, because cerebral trauma can result in loss of the autoregulatory processes within the brain, and both reduction and elevation of arterial blood pressure disturb cerebral blood flow. Hypertonic saline can be added to crystalloid solutions in order to draw fluid back into the vessels (Chapter 11).

Hypoxia is a common reason for death, and therefore, hyperoxygenation is indicated in most patients (oxygen cage, intubation, and ventilation in comatose cats). Hyperventilation decreases ICP by reducing cerebral blood flow and mean arterial CO_2 pressure. The head of the patient is elevated 30° without obstructing the jugular veins to facilitate venous outflow. The jugular veins should not be used for obtaining blood. Mannitol is the most effective drug to decrease ICP rapidly and its effect lasts 2–4 hours. It is indicated if the patient shows deterioration in neurological function during treatment. A dose of 0.5–1 g/kg body weight is administered over 20 minutes. Recently, the administration of methylprednisolone was shown to enhance mortality in human patients with brain trauma (19). Corticosteroids are therefore not recommended for patients with head trauma. In cats that are presented in an excitatory state or status epilepticus, intravenously or rectally applied diazepam may be used. Phenobarbital is necessary in some cases to control seizure activity. Phenobarbital may also lower the metabolic demands of neurons and reduce cerebral arterial pressure. Pentobarbital may be indicated to achieve rapid cessation of seizure activity, as phenobarbital can take up to 30 minutes to show an effect.

Surgical intervention is indicated if neurological function continues to deteriorate despite appropriate medical and supportive therapy or if compressive lesions, such as bone fragments or a sizeable blood clot, are identified on computed tomography, or suspected on clinical and radiological examination. A craniotomy and durotomy allow the brain tissue to expand and therefore help to reduce ICP. Intracranial hematomas can be reached by a lateral craniotomy in 75% of cats (20). Prognosis is favorable if patients with minor neurological dysfunctions are treated adequately. Severe neurological dysfunction, such as stupor or coma, dilated unresponsive pupils, and loss of deep pain perception, has a guarded or grave prognosis, especially when occurring immediately after the accident.

References and further reading

1. Griffon D, et al. Thoracic injuries in cats with traumatic fractures. Vet Comp Orthop Traumatol 1994;7:98–100.
2. White RN, Burton CA. Surgical management of intrathoracic tracheal avulsion in cats: long-term results in 9 consecutive cases. Vet Surg 2000;29:430–435.
3. Whitney WO, Mehlhaff CJ. High-rise syndrome in cats. J Am Vet Med Assoc 1987;191:1399–1403.
4. Kraje BJ, et al. Intrathoracic and concurrent orthopedic injury associated with traumatic rib fracture in cats: 75 cases (1980–1998). J Am Vet Med Assoc 2000;216:51–54.
5. Olsen D, et al. Clinical management of flail chest in dogs and cats: a retrospective study of 24 cases (1989–1999). J Am Anim Hosp Assoc 2002;38:315–320.
6. Schmiedt CW, et al. Traumatic diaphragmatic hernia in cats: 34 cases (1991–2001). J Am Vet Med Assoc 2003;222: 1237–1240.
7. Kolata RJ, et al. Patterns of trauma in urban dogs and cats: a study of 1000 cases. J Am Vet Med Assoc 1974;164:499–502.
8. Zulauf D, et al. Radiographic examination and outcome in consecutive feline trauma patients. Vet Comp Orthop Traumatol 2008;21:36–40.
9. Walters MJ. Abdominal paracentesis and diagnostic peritoneal lavage. Clin Tech Small Anim Pract 2003;18:32–38.
10. Boyson SR, et al. Focused abdominal sonogram fro trauma (FAST) in 100 dogs. In: Proc Intern Vet Emerg Crit Care Symp 2003; p. 765.
11. Aumann M, et al. Uroperitoneum in cats: 26 cases (1986–1995). J Am Anim Hosp Assoc 1998;34:315–324.
12. Syring RS, Drobatz KJ. Preoperative evaluation and management of the emergency surgical small animal patient. Vet Clin North Am Small Anim Pract 2000;30:473–489.
13. Gannon K, Moses L. Uroabdomen in dogs and cats. Compend Continuing Educ 2002;24:604–611.
14. Burrows CF, Bovee KC. Metabolic changes due to experimentally induced rupture of the canine urinary bladder. Am J Vet Res 1974;35:1083–1088.
15. Shaw SR, et al. Traumatic body wall herniation in 36 dogs and cats. J Am Anim Hosp Assoc 2003;39:35–46.
16. Waldron DR, et al. Abdominal hernias in dogs and cats. J Am Anim Hosp Assoc 1986;22:817–823.
17. Friend EJ, White RA. Rupture of the cranial pubic tendon in the cat. J Small Anim Pract 2002;43:522–525.
18. Vinayak A, Krahwinkel DJ. Managing blunt trauma-induced hemoperitoneum in dogs and cats. Compend Continuing Educ 2004;26:276–290.
19. Sauerland S, Maegele M. Effects of intravenous corticosteroids on death within 14 days in 10008 adults with clinically significant head injury (MRC CRASH trial): randomized placebo-controlled trial. Lancet 2004;364:1321–1328.
20. Dewey CW. Emergency management of the head trauma patient. Principles and practice. Vet Clin North Am Small Anim Pract 2000;30:207–225.
21. Bonczynski JJ, et al. Comparison of peritoneal fluid and peripheral blood pH, bicarbonate, glucose, and lactate concentration as a diagnostic tool for septic peritonitis in dogs and cats. Vet Surg 2003;32:161–166.

Part 4
Introduction to musculoskeletal injuries

Injury to the musculoskeletal system is by far the most common reason for orthopedic problems in the feline patient. Trauma to the pelvic limbs is encountered more frequently than trauma to the thoracic limbs. Musculoskeletal injuries in cats are often caused by major trauma, such as motor vehicle accidents or falls from a height. These cats commonly suffer from concurrent and more severe injuries of vital organs, which have to be diagnosed and treated prior to addressing orthopedic problems (Chapters 9–12). Occasionally, cats may also sustain indoor trauma, such as being shut in a door, being stepped on, or having something fall on them. Trauma sustained indoors is usually minor compared to trauma sustained outdoors.

Orthopedic injuries in cats tend to be severe, with associated soft-tissue and vascular compromise, and multiple orthopedic injuries are common. Atraumatic surgical technique is important to minimize further tissue damage. The following chapters review the basic knowledge necessary for treatment of feline fractures, joint injuries, injuries of the spine and spinal cord, and soft-tissue injuries. Postoperative treatment and rehabilitation therapy of injured patients are described in Chapters 20 and 21, respectively. Part 7 of this book provides surgical anatomy, a description of specific conditions of the different anatomical areas, and technical details for surgeries.

13 Fractures

K. Voss, P.M. Montavon

The basic principles of fracture repair and treatment of joint injuries are the same for cats and dogs, but there are some clinically important differences between the species. The bones of cats are straighter and more slender than dog bones, and there is little variation in size among different breeds. This uniformity leads to less variation in implant sizes and types necessary to treat feline fractures. The old saying that when two pieces of a cat's bone are put together in one room they will heal is of course not true. Although most feline fractures seem to heal readily based on clinical impressions, complications and pitfalls do occur, and adhering to the principles of osteosynthesis is as important in cats as in other species to treat fractures successfully. Compared to dogs, the surgeon has slightly less need to be concerned about the absolute stability of the implants or fixation due to the lighter body weight of cats, their quieter behavior, and the increased ease of restricting activity during the recovery period. On the other hand the small size of feline bones limits the choice of implant size and strength, and meticulous technique is required when working with small bone fragments. The basic knowledge of this chapter should help the clinician with the decision for selecting the optimal treatment option for a specific fracture. Implants and their application are described in part 6 of this book.

According to most authors around 50% of fractures in cats involve the long bones (1). The incidence of fractures of specific bones in cats presented to the Clinic for Small Animal Surgery of the Vetsuisse Faculty of the University of Zurich is shown in Figure 13-1.

13.1 Fracture biomechanics

Understanding the biomechanical behavior of bone in response to external forces and the differences in bone quality at different locations helps to choose appropriate treatment methods. Bone deformation occurs in response to increasing external forces. Initially elastic deformation occurs, meaning that after the force is removed, the bone returns to its original structure. Internal damage starts to occur if the load is increased beyond this elastic property of bone, resulting in plastic deformation. Plastic deformation is characterized by microfractures and cracks, resulting in a permanent change in shape. The point at which plastic deformation occurs is called the yield point. If bone is loaded beyond, it will ultimately fracture. Cortical and cancellous bone have different mechanical properties (2). Cortical bone has a lower porosity, and is stronger and more brittle than cancellous bone. Cancellous bone has a higher porosity, is weaker, more elastic, and has greater capability for plastic deformation before it ultimately fails. The differences in porosity between cortical and cancellous bone also have an influence on the bone-holding power of implants. Implant anchorage is stronger in cortical than in cancellous bone. Cortical bone in adult cats tends to be more brittle than in dogs and might fissure more easily (3).

Four principal forces act on a bone: axial compression, bending, torsion, and axial tension (Fig. 13-2). Local internal stresses and strains build up inside the bone if it is subject to these external forces, and a fracture can occur along the area of the largest internal stresses. The direction and energy of the applied external forces are responsible for the development of different fracture configurations and types (Fig. 13-2). Axial compression of a bone results in an oblique fracture. Bending forces cause transverse fractures. A small fragment, called a wedge or butterfly fragment, might be created at the compression side of the fracture. Torsional forces create spiral fractures. Tensile forces cause transverse fractures, usually seen as avulsion fractures.

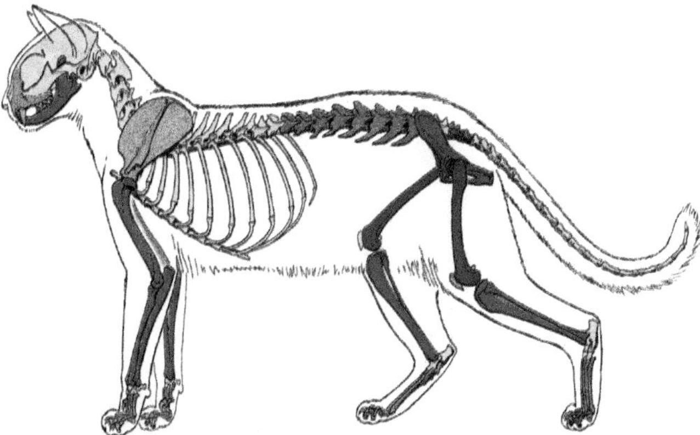

Figure 13-1 Between 1990 and 1999, 1853 cats with fractures were admitted to the Clinic for Small Animal Surgery of the University of Zurich. Shades of red represent the frequency of fracture occurrence. Fractures of the pelvic limbs, including pelvic fractures, were present in 60% of cases. Fractures of the thoracic limbs were encountered in 19% of cases. Mandibular and maxillary fractures accounted for 14%, and fractures of the spine for 6%.

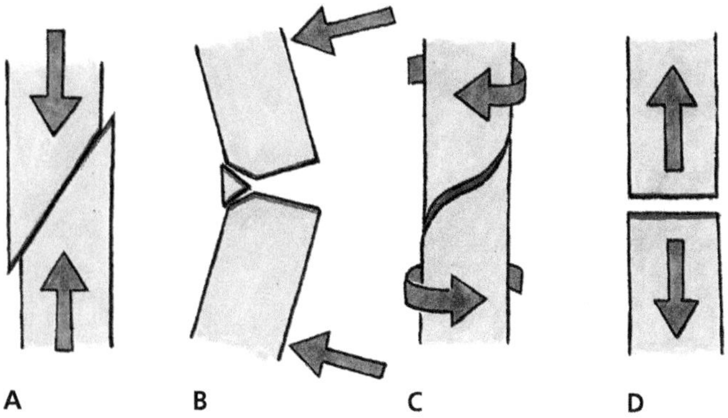

A B C D

Figure 13-2 The four principal forces acting on bone are (A) axial compression; (B) bending; (C) torsion; and (D) axial tension. They influence the resulting fracture configuration. Axial compression causes oblique fractures. Bending forces result in transverse fractures. A wedge or butterfly fragment may be present at the compressive side of the fracture. Torsional forces cause spiral fractures. Axial tension results in fractures perpendicular to the direction of the force, usually seen as avulsion fractures of attachment sites of ligaments or tendons.

The velocity of the applied load also has an influence on fracture pattern. With rapidly occurring loads, such as gunshots and motor vehicle accidents, both stiffness and ultimate strength of the bone increase, and more energy is absorbed by the bone and then released into the surrounding tissues. Rapid loading of a bone therefore causes more comminution and soft-tissue trauma than the same load applied at a slower rate. Many of the fractures encountered in cats are due to high-velocity trauma and high fracture comminution and severe soft-tissue injury is common. Quality of bone also has an influence on the degree on comminution. Whereas immature cats with soft bones usually sustain simple fractures, fractures in older cats with stiffer bones tend to be comminuted. An example of a low-energy fracture in a young cat is the spiral tibial fracture with an intact fibula.

13.2 Fracture classification systems

Fracture classification systems help assess the severity of a fracture, improve communication between clinicians, and allow categorization of the fracture with regard to treatment options and prognosis. Classifications have been developed for long-bone fractures, sacral fractures, and pelvic fractures in small animals. The whole system is based on an alphanumerical code. The first digit represents the anatomic site of the fracture within the whole-body system. Numbers 1–4 have been assigned to the long bones, number 5 can be used for the sacrum, and number 6 the pelvis.

13.2.1 Classification of long-bone fractures

The Arbeitsgemeinschaft für Osteosynthesefragen/Association for the Study of Internal Fixation (AO/ASIF) classification system for long-bone fractures is based on the assessment of over 1000 fractures in both cats and dogs (4). It includes the methodological description of the affected bone, the fracture localization in the bone, the fracture type, and the fracture morphology. The humerus is assigned number 1, radius/ulna number 2, the femur number 3, and the tibia/fibula number 4. Each bone is divided into a proximal (1), middle (2), and distal (3) segment. Fracture morphology is classified according to severity and inherent fracture stability and is described by the letters A, B, and C. The classification system is explained in a simplified form in Figure 13-3.

13.2.2 Classification of sacral fractures

The sacrum has been assigned number 5. Sacral fracture in small animals can be classified into five categories (5) (Fig. 13-4). Type I fractures are associated with sacroiliac luxation. Type I and type III fractures are most common in cats. Type IV fractures are avulsions of the sacrotuberal ligament, and do not occur in cats because they do not have a sacrotuberal ligament.

13.2.3 Classification of pelvic fractures

A classification system for pelvic fractures has been developed from the AO/ASIF system for pelvic fractures in humans. Modifications were made because of the unique features of pelvic fractures in small animals, based on a review of 556 dogs and cats with pelvic fractures (6). The system takes into account the severity of the fracture, with the higher numbers and letters indicating increasing fracture severity. The pelvis is assigned number 6. The second digit 1, 2, or 3, describes involvement of the weight-bearing parts of the pelvis, which include the acetabulum, the ilial body, and the sacroiliac joint. The third digit (A–C) indicates the localization of the most significant fracture (Table 13-1).

13.2.4 Classification of physeal fractures

The classification system for physeal fractures in animals has been adapted from the Salter and Harris classification in children (7, 8). Physeal fractures can be assigned to one of six possible types (Fig. 13-5). In humans, higher numbers indicate a greater possibility of development of growth abnormalities. Salter and Harris type I fractures run through the physis. Salter and Harris type II fractures run through the physis and metaphysis. The small metaphyseal fragment is known as the Thurston–Holland sign. Salter and Harris type III fractures run through the physis and epiphyis and are therefore articular fractures. Salter and Harris type IV fractures run through the metaphysis, across the physis, and into the epiphysis, and are also articular fractures. Healing of type

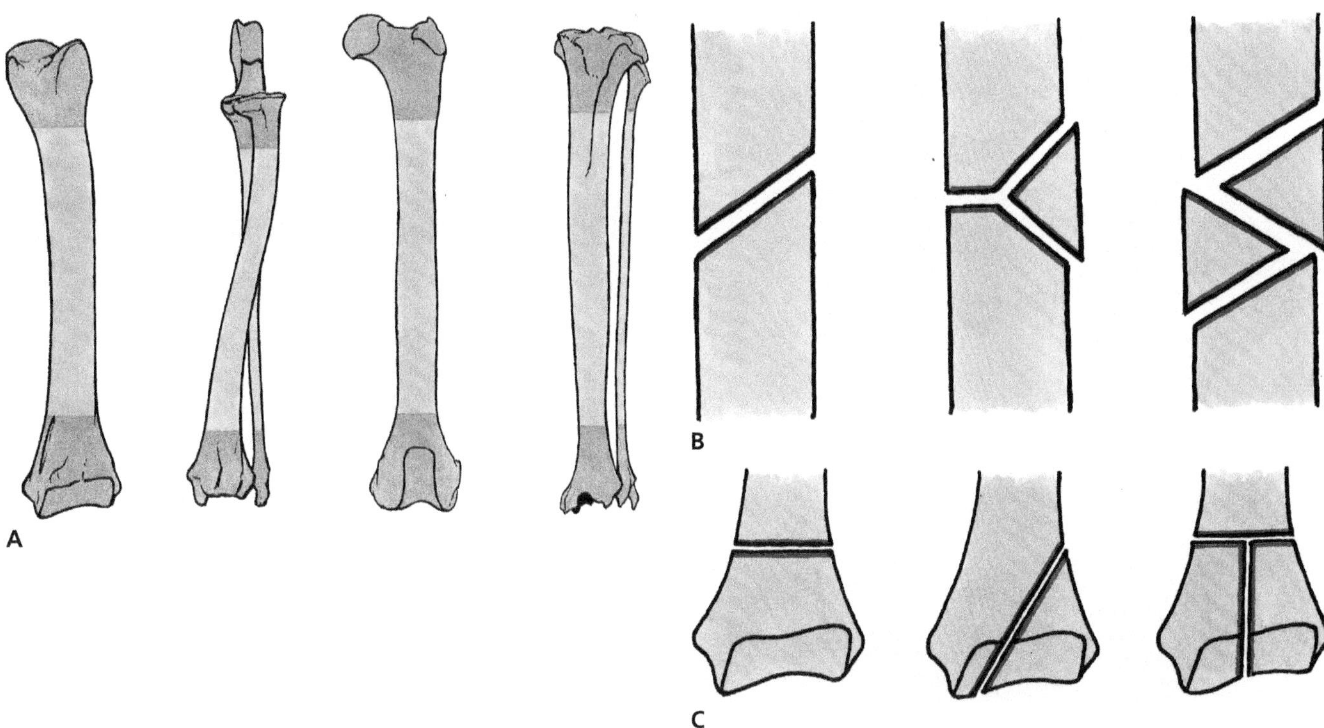

Figure 13-3 Classification of long-bone fractures. (A) Fractures of long bones can involve the proximal epiphysis and metaphysis (green), the diaphysis (yellow), or the distal epiphysis and metaphysis (green). (B) Diaphyseal fractures can be simple-reducible (left), have one or two reducible large fragments (middle), or can be comminuted, non-reducible (right). (C) Fractures of the distal or proximal bone segment can be metaphyseal or supracondylar (left), involve the lateral or medial portion of the condyle, also called unicondylar (middle), or can be supra- and intracondylar, also called bicondylar (right).

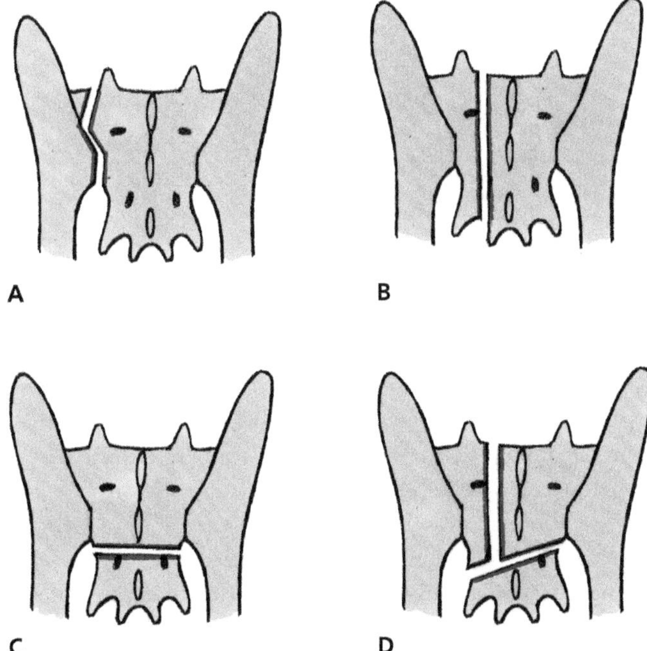

Figure 13-4 Classification of sacral fractures. Type I and type III sacral fractures are most common. (A) Alar fractures are classified as type I. These are associated with luxation of the sacroiliac joint. (B) Foraminal fractures are classified as type II. (C) Transverse fractures are classified as type III. (D) Comminuted fractures are classified as type V.

III and IV fractures may lead to formation of a bridging callus, preventing further growth. Salter and Harris type V fractures are compression injuries of the physis. They are not visible on initial radiographs, but may result in symmetrical physeal closure. Salter and Harris type VI fractures are partial compression injuries resulting in asymmetrical closure of one portion of the physis.

13.2.5 Classification of open fractures

Open fractures are classified according to the extent of soft-tissue injury, and origin of the fracture (9, 10). Higher numbers indicate more severe soft-tissue defects and infection, resulting in more complex treatment and a higher likelihood for development of complications (Table 13-2). Grade 1 fractures are caused by bone penetrating the skin from the inside, causing a small puncture wound. The chance for development of infection is low, when appropriately treated. Grade 2 fractures are characterized by moderate soft-tissue injury and higher fracture comminution. These have a moderate risk for becoming infected. Grade 3 open fractures are caused by high-energy injuries, such as gunshots, and they have high fracture comminution, exposure of bone, and extensive soft-tissue injury. Infection is present or likely to

Pelvis	Weight-bearing elements		Most significant fracture	
6 (Pelvis)	6 1	No involvement of weight-bearing elements	6 1 A	Fractures of the pelvic margin
			6 1 B	Fractures of the pelvic floor
			6 1 C	Fractures of the ischial body
	6 2	Unilateral involvement of weight-bearing elements	6 2 A	Unilateral sacroiliac luxation
			6 2 B	Unilateral fracture of the ilial body
			6 2 C	Unilateral fracture of the acetabulum
	6 3	Bilateral involvement of weight-bearing elements	6 3 A	Bilateral sacroiliac luxation
			6 3 B	Bilateral involvement of weight-bearing elements, including a fracture of the ilial body
			6 3 C	Bilateral involvement of weight-bearing elements, including a fracture of the acetabulum

Table 13-1. Classification of pelvic fractures

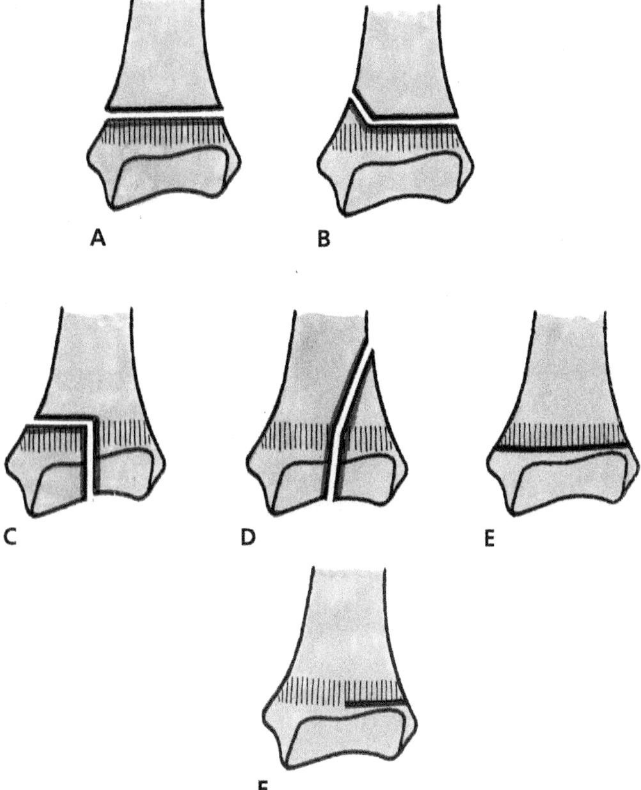

Figure 13-5 Salter and Harris classification of physeal fractures. (**A**) Salter and Harris type I fracture. (**B**) Salter and Harris type II fracture. (**C**) Salter and Harris type III fracture. (**D**) Salter and Harris type IV fracture. (**E**) Salter and Harris type V fracture. (**F**) Salter and Harris type VI fracture.

Fracture classification	Description of fracture
Grade 1	Small skin laceration (< 1 cm) Bone has penetrated skin from within Usually simple fracture
Grade 2	Larger skin laceration (> 1 cm) Wound communicates directly with bone Usually minimally comminuted fracture Moderate soft-tissue trauma
Grade 3	Extensive soft-tissue trauma Loss of skin and/or bone Comminuted fractures Significant neurovascular damage possible

Table 13-2. Classification of open fractures

develop. Grade 3 open fractures can be further subclassified according to skin loss and arterial blood supply.

13.3 Fracture healing

Rate and quality of bone healing largely depend on adequate blood supply to the fracture region, and on fracture stability.

In adult animals, around two-thirds of diaphyseal bone thickness is supplied by the intraosseous artery, and the outer third is supplied by the extraosseous blood supply. Abundant extraosseous blood supply is derived from the thick periosteum in immature animals, whereas only one-third of the thickness of the diaphyseal bone is supplied through the intraosseous artery. The metaphysis and epiphysis of long bones have a rich blood supply (Fig. 13-6).

The intraosseous blood vessels are often disrupted after a fracture has occurred, and a temporary extraosseous blood supply is instituted (Fig. 13-7). These extraosseous vessels supplying the fracture region are derived from surrounding soft tissues, such as muscle attachments. Soft-tissue attachments to the bone should therefore be preserved during surgery.

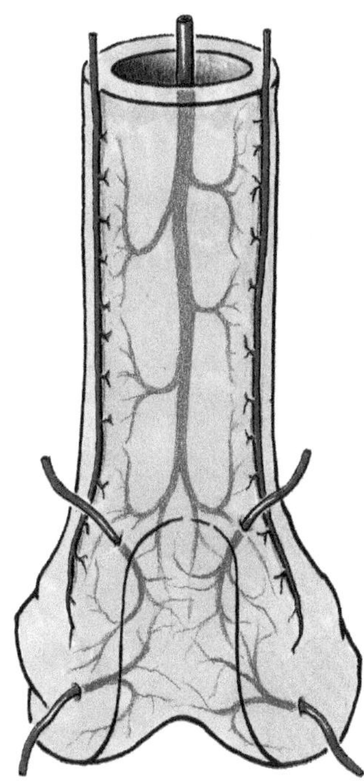

Figure 13-6 Blood is supplied to the diaphysis of the long bones via intraosseous arteries and periosteal blood vessels. In adult animals, the inner two-thirds of the cortex are supplied by the intraosseous artery. In immature cats, periosteal blood supply is more important. Blood supply to the metaphysis and epiphysis is derived from direct arteries.

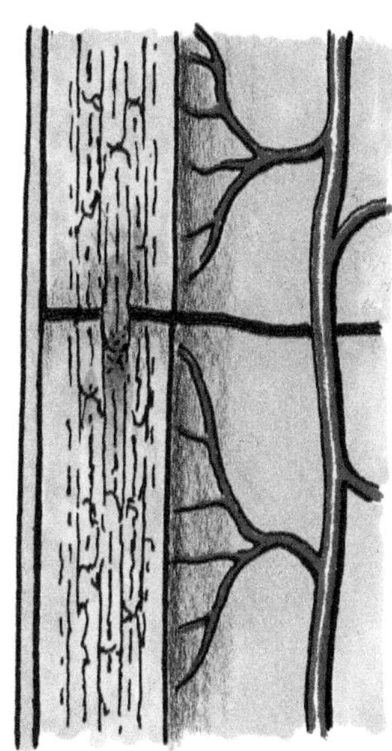

Figure 13-8 Primary bone healing is characterized by direct bridging of the fracture site by osteons. Primary bone healing is only possible if the fracture has been anatomically reduced and rigidly stabilized under interfragmentary compression.

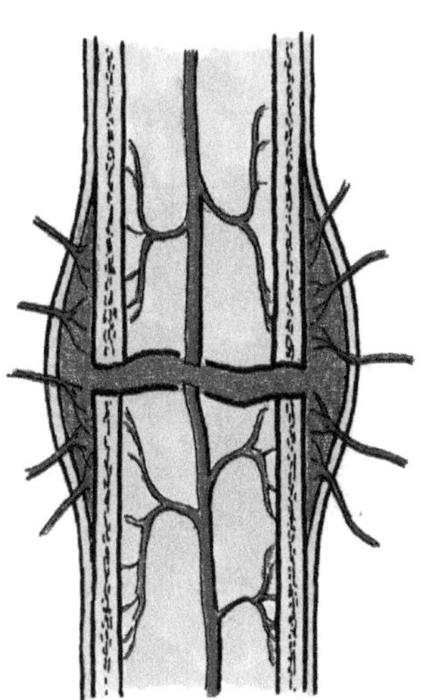

Figure 13-7 The intraosseous artery is often disrupted after a fracture. The blood supply for fracture healing then derives initially from extraosseous blood vessels, located in the soft-tissue attachments to the bone.

13.3.1 Healing of cortical bone

Healing of cortical bone is classified as primary (direct) and secondary (indirect) bone healing. Primary bone healing is characterized by direct osteonal remodeling and bridging of the fracture gap, usually in the absence of an extraosseous callus (Fig. 13-8). Contact healing and gap healing are subgroups of primary bone healing. Perfect alignment of fracture ends and absolute stability are necessary for primary bone healing to occur.

Most fractures will heal by secondary bone healing in a clinical situation. Secondary bone healing is characterized by the formation of bone through transformation of precursor tissues (Fig. 13-9). The first tissue present in a fracture gap is the fracture hematoma. Granulation tissue then forms, which is slowly replaced by fibrocartilage. Mineralization of this so-called soft callus and endochondral ossification of the fibrocartilage marks the beginning of the bony callus, which becomes visible on radiographs. The bony callus is built in and around the fracture gap. The last step is remodeling of the initially unorganized bone into lamellar bone, a process that takes several months.

The objective of this stepwise transformation of tissues into bone is gradually to enhance stability in the fracture region. The different tissues are able to survive different interfragmentary strains. Granulation tissue can withstand 100%, fibrous tissue and cartilage 10%, and bone only 2% interfragmentary strain. Multiple fracture gaps share the displacement of fragments and are therefore more tolerant to instability than single fracture gaps. If motion at a fracture site exceeds the tolerance for building osseous tissue, two main mechanisms exist to reduce interfragmentary strain. First, the fracture ends are absorbed by osteoclasts in order to enlarge the fracture gap and therefore reduce interfragmentary strain. This will mainly happen in simple fractures. Second, the formation of callus through the above steps is activated by minimal amounts of movement at the fracture site (11). The bony callus increases the cross-sectional diameter of the bone and therefore increases stability in the area. An intact or re-established extraosseous blood supply is essential for callus development.

13.3.2 Healing of cancellous bone

Fracture healing is different in areas with predominantly cancellous bone, such as the metaphysis and epiphysis of long

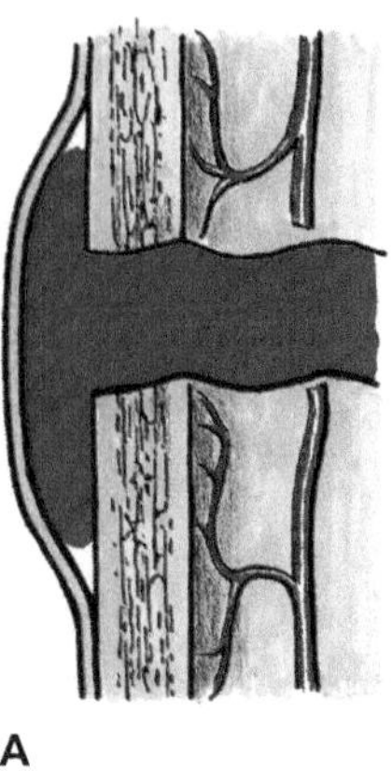

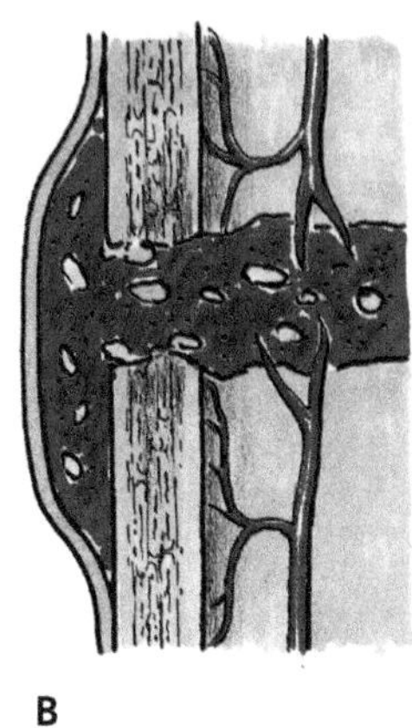

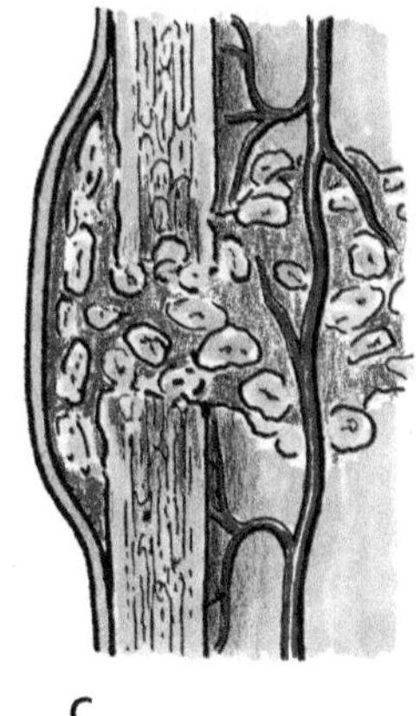

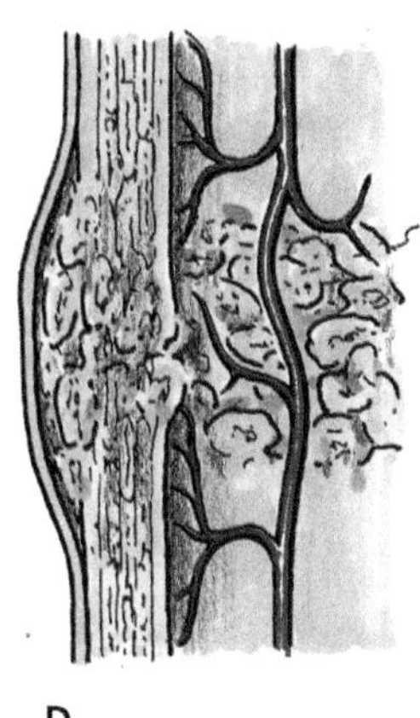

Figure 13-9 Secondary bone healing is characterized by transformation of precursor tissues into bone. It occurs in the presence of a fracture gap and micromotion. The fracture hematoma (**A**) is transformed into granulation tissue first, followed by fibrocartilage (**B**). A bony callus is formed if the fracture strain is reduced to less than 2% (**C**). Restoration of the cylindrical shape occurs through remodeling of the bony callus (**D**).

bones, flat bones of the pelvis, maxilla, and mandibula, and vertebral bodies. Healing of cancellous bone usually proceeds at a faster rate than that of cortical bone. Osteoblasts are responsible for new bone deposition in the fracture gap. New bone is laid on to the existing bone trabeculae, and along fibrous tissue fibers. Healing of the thin cortical shell lags behind cancellous bone healing, and an extraosseous callus is usually absent (12) (Fig. 13-10). The appearance of an extraosseous callus may be seen with gross instability or displacement (12).

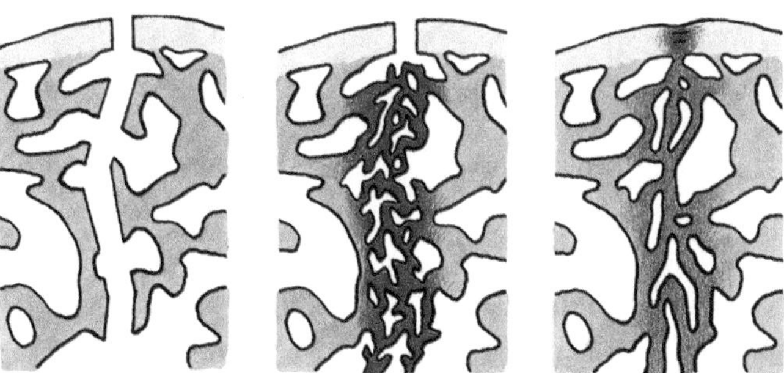

Figure 13-10 Healing of cancellous bone occurs through new bone formation along fibrous tissue in the fracture gap. Cancellous bone heals at a faster rate than cortical bone.

13.3.3 Clinical factors influencing bone healing

Clinical union of a fracture is a term used to describe the time when fracture healing is considered stable enough to remove the implants. Healing times vary with factors such as age of the animal, type, severity, and location of the fracture, and technique and implants used. Published times to fracture healing in studies on feline fractures are summarized in Table 13-3. Overall, the fractures had healed in mean times ranging from 1 to 3 months. Subjectively, cats seem to have less and smaller callus formation than dogs with similar fractures.

Few data exist on clinical or epidemiological factors influencing bone healing in the feline patient. A study of feline fractures stabilized with external fixators has shown age of the patient to be the only factor influencing healing time; fractures healed faster in immature cats than in older cats, regardless of fracture type (1). In another study of feline tibia fractures repaired by different methods, severely comminuted and displaced fractures and open fractures took longer to heal, regardless of patient age (13). A further study has shown that the incidence of non-union is significantly greater in tibial and proximal ulnar fractures (14). Results of the same study indicate that older cats and obese cats have a higher risk of developing non-unions. Results of those studies (13, 15–18) are summarized in Table 13-4.

13.4 Decision-making in fracture treatment

The main goal of fracture repair is early weight-bearing, and complete restoration of limb function. Early postoperative use of the limb improves vascularity in the fracture region, reduces muscle atrophy and fibrosis, reduces osteoporosis, and improves function of adjacent joints. Many implant types are suitable for fracture repair, and each of them has its own indications, advantages, and disadvantages. Careful preoperative planning of a fracture repair is vital to reduce surgery time, achieve the goal of early limb function, and avoid complications. Decision-making depends on the biomechanical

Number of cats	Bone	Fixation method	Time to fracture union
13 cats (Langley-Hobbs et al. 1997 (16))	Humerus	External skeletal fixation	5.5 weeks (mildly comminuted) 10.5 weeks (severely comminuted)
48 cats (Richardson & Thacher 1993 (13))	Tibia	External coaptation	4.5 weeks
		Intramedullary pin	8 weeks
		External skeletal fixation (closed reduction)	7 weeks
		External skeletal fixation (open reduction)	12 weeks
		Bone plate	12.5 weeks
34 cats (Langley-Hobbs et al. 1996 (15))	Femur	External skeletal fixation	8.5 weeks (to implant removal)
7 cats (Haas et al. 2003 (18))	Radius/ulna (distal)	External skeletal fixation	12 weeks (to implant removal)
12 cats (Gemmill et al. 2004 (17))	Radius/ulna and tibia	External skeletal fixation	9.5 weeks

Table 13-3. Reported times for fracture healing and removal of external skeletal fixators, for diaphyseal long-bone fractures in cats

Factors	Influence on fracture healing
Comminuted fractures	Higher incidence of non-union
Open fractures	Higher incidence of non-union and osteomyelitis
Tibial fractures and proximal ulnar fractures	Higher incidence of non-union
Age	Faster healing in young cats Higher incidence of non-union in older cats
Obesity	Higher incidence of non-union

Table 13-4. Factors influencing fracture healing in cats

evaluation of the fracture, severity of concurrent soft-tissue trauma, estimated time to healing, and on individual patient factors, such as age, general health, temperament of the cat, or number of limbs injured. Cats with injuries to several limbs, for example, are forced to bear weight on at least one of the operated limbs immediately postoperatively, and fixation stability therefore should be accordingly high.

13.4.1 Diaphyseal long-bone fractures

Repair of diaphyseal fractures of long bones has evolved in recent years from the classical concept of anatomic reduction and absolute stable fracture fixation towards a more biological approach (11). This approach involves less rigid fracture stabilization, thereby promoting early callus formation through minimal movement at the fracture site. Care is taken to preserve the blood supply to the fracture region by indirect fracture reduction, minimal surgical approach, and implant selection and positioning (11). The more flexible fracture fixation should not compromise early and complete return to function, which is still the main goal of fracture repair. It should rather create an ideal environment for fracture healing.

Micromotion at the fracture site promotes early callus formation, which in turn results in early stability. The amount of instability tolerated and warranted is difficult to assess in the clinical situation, and depends on fracture type and configuration, fracture healing time, activity of the animal, and concurrent orthopedic injuries. With the same load applied, interfragmentary strains are higher in small fracture gaps compared to large or multiple fracture gaps. Fixation of simple fractures therefore must be more stable to keep the interfragmentary strain low enough for fracture healing, compared to that required for comminuted fractures.

Two important criteria should be considered before a long-bone fracture is repaired: first, is the fracture reducible? Second, does reduction add to fixation stability? If both questions can be answered with yes, anatomic reduction and rigid fixation are usually performed. This is mainly the case in simple fractures. Bone plates are often used in this situation. The application of a plate in compression function (Chapter 24) causes axial compression across the fracture line, and adds additional stability by allowing the bony column to carry a significant part of the load. Ideally, the plate is placed on the tension side of the bone. Long oblique fractures may be primarily aligned and compressed with lag screws or cerclage wires. A plate is additionally applied in neutralization function (Chapter 24), protecting the initial fixation. Both the bone and the plate then share the loads.

If one of the answers to the above questions is no, it is better not to attempt anatomic reduction, and thereby preserve soft-tissue attachments and vascularity at the fracture site. This is the case with comminuted fractures. The implants, plates, or internal and external fixators are applied in buttress function (Chapter 24). Because all loads are conducted across the implant, it should be strong and durable enough to withstand the forces until the fracture has healed. An intramedullary pin may be inserted additionally to compensate for the lack of bone buttress and to increase bending stability. Preservation of blood supply usually results in rapid callus formation, and in early stability (Figs 13-11 and 13-12).

Bone necrosis can occur as a consequence of reduced blood supply to the bone and carries the risk for sequestra formation and infection. A problem sometimes encountered after fracture repair is porosity of bone below the implants. Whereas this phenomenon was earlier attributed to stress shielding due to too rigid implants, current thinking is that bone necrosis and subsequent internal bone remodeling are more likely to be caused by vascular damage in the contact area of the implant to the bone (11, 19). Bone porosity is occasionally encountered after fracture repair in cats, possibly due to the large plates applied on a small bone. Internal or external fixators do not require an extensive surgical approach with stripping or damaging of the periosteum, and

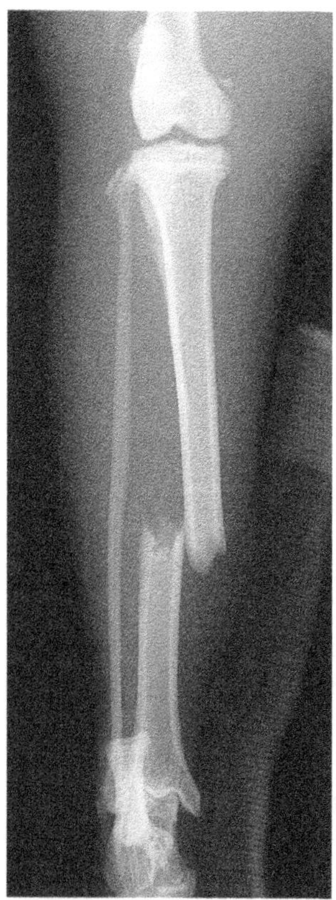
A

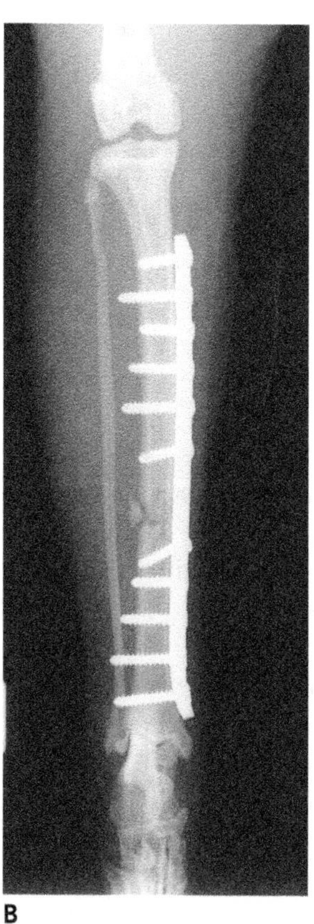
B

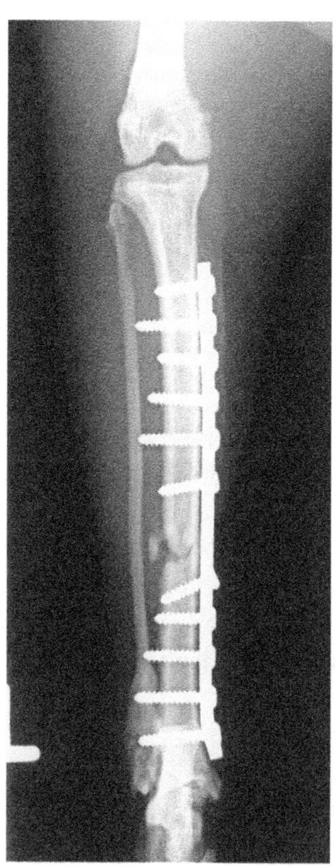
C

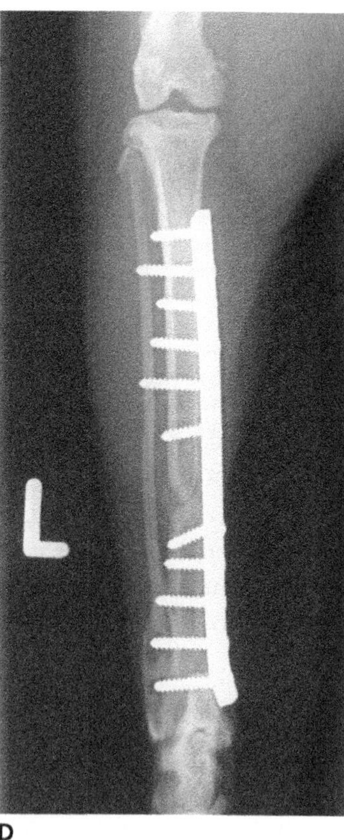

D

Figure 13-11 (**A**) Preoperative, (**B**) immediate postoperative, and follow-up radiographs at (**C**) 4 and (**D**) 10 weeks of a cat with a diaphyseal fracture of the left tibia, treated by open reduction and plate osteosynthesis. Please compare with Figure 13-12.

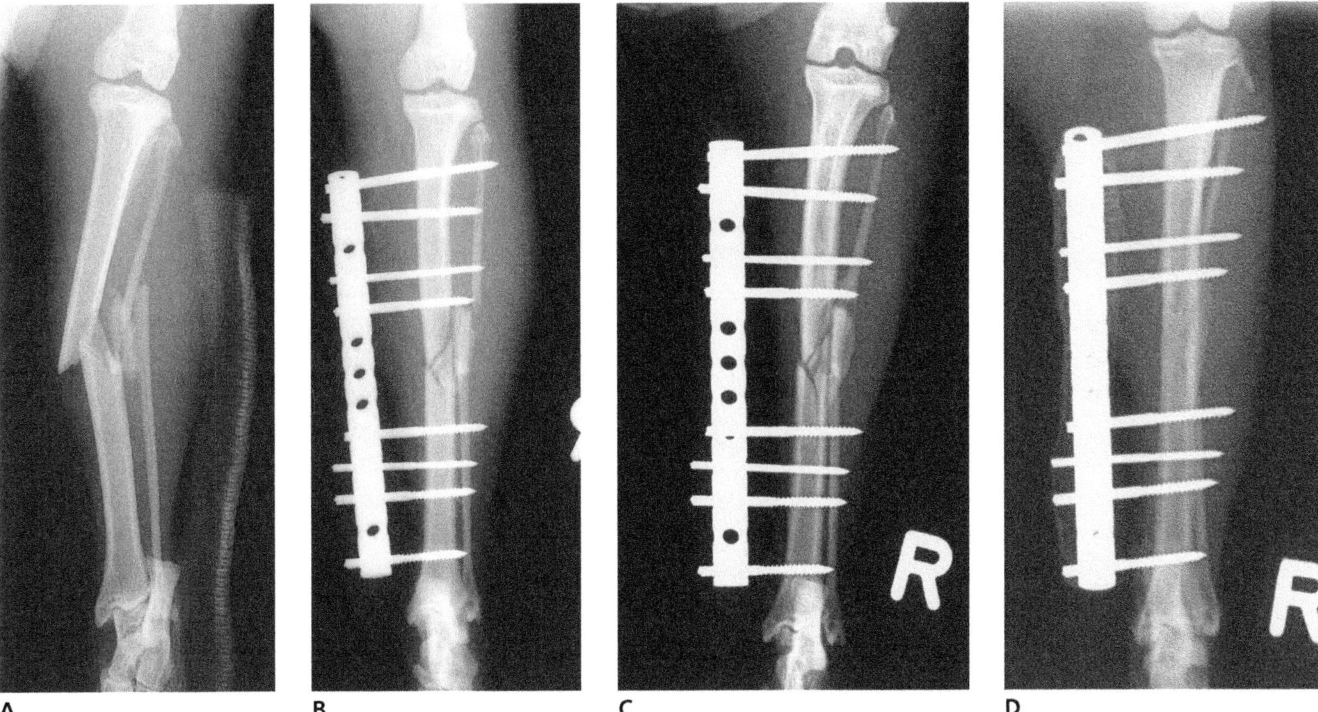

Figure 13-12 (**A**) Preoperative, (**B**) immediate postoperative, and follow-up radiographs at (**C**) 4 and (**D**) 10 weeks of a diaphyseal fracture of the right tibia of the cat in Figure 13-11. Both fractures were sustained and repaired at the same time. This fracture was treated by closed reduction and external skeletal fixation. Fracture healing in the right leg was more obvious at 4 weeks postoperatively, and more complete at 10 weeks, compared to the left leg (Fig. 13-11).

the implants are not pressed on to the bone surface. They are ideal for preserving extraosseous blood supply.

Table 13-5 provides general suggestions for treatment of different types of long-bone fractures.

13.4.2 Metaphyseal long-bone fractures

Metaphyseal fractures are characterized by rapid bone healing due to adequate vascularity and cancellous bone quality in this region. The main problem the surgeon encounters is the limited amount of bone stock to anchor the implants. Internal fixators, miniplates, screws, threaded pins, and external fixators are therefore most appropriate (Table 13-6). Holding power of implants is not as good as in bone areas with a thick cortical shell. Due to the close vicinity to joints, anatomic fracture reduction is attempted to maintain physiological joint motion.

13.4.3 Joint fractures

Joint fractures should always be perfectly reduced, and rigidly stabilized under compression in order to restore congruity of the joint surface. Less than anatomic reduction or fracture instability will invariably lead to severe degenerative joint disease and chronic pain. Fractures of the lateral or medial portion of a condyle, or intracondylar fractures, are usually stabilized by lag screw fixation, combined with an antirotational pin, and metaphyseal plating if indicated (Table 13-6). Fractures of the glenoid of the scapula and the acetabulum are commonly repaired with small bone plates. A meticulous surgical approach to the joint must be performed to avoid iatrogenic damage to periarticular structures.

13.4.4 Fractures of flat bones

Treatment of fractures of flat bones of the pelvis and skull follows the same basic principles as for long-bone fractures. Bone healing is good in flat bones, because they are surrounded by abundant soft-tissue mass and the bone is predominantly cancellous. Holding power of implants is not as good as in long bones, not only due to the thin cortical shell but also because the flat shape often only allows for insertion of small and short implants. It is therefore important to place the implants on the tension side of the bone. Flat bones often have curved shapes, making adequate contouring of plates more difficult. Reconstruction plates are commonly used, because they allow plate contouring in all directions (Chapter 24).

Fracture type	Fracture location	Reduction possible?	Age of cat	Stabilization methods
Simple transverse or short oblique fracture	Distal to elbow or stifle joint	Closed reduction possible	Young	External fixator Cast
			Old	External fixator (± IM pin in tibia or ulna) Interlocking nail (tibia) Cast
		Closed reduction not possible	Young	External fixator (± IM pin in tibia or ulna) Internal fixator Interlocking nail (tibia)
			Old	Compression plate Internal fixator External fixator (± IM pin in tibia or ulna)
	Proximal to elbow or stifle joint		Young	Internal fixator External fixator (± IM pin) Interlocking nail
			Old	Compression plate Internal fixator External fixator (± IM pin) Interlocking nail
Simple long oblique fracture	Any long bone		Young	External fixator (+ IM pin, except for radius) Internal fixator Interlocking nail (except radius)
			Old	Lag screw and plate Internal fixator External fixator (+ IM pin, except for radius) Interlocking nail (except for radius) IM pin and hemi-/cerclage (except for radius)
Multifragment fracture	Any long bone	Anatomic reduction possible	Young	Internal fixator External fixator (+ IM pin, except for radius) Interlocking nail (except for radius)
			Old	Lag screw and plate Internal fixator External fixator (+ IM pin, except for radius) Interlocking nail (except for radius)
	Distal to elbow or stifle joint	Anatomic reduction not possible	Young and old	Closed reduction and: External fixator (± IM pin in tibia) Interlocking nail (tibia) Open reduction and: External fixator (+ IM pin in tibia) Internal fixator Plate (± IM pin in tibia) Interlocking nail (tibia)
	Proximal to elbow or stifle joint		Young and old	Plate and rod External fixator (+ IM pin) Internal fixator Interlocking nail

Table 13-5. A summary of selected treatment options for diaphyseal long-bone fractures
IM pin, intramedullary pin.

Table 13-6. Treatment suggestions for metaphyseal and epiphyseal fractures in cats

Fracture type	Growth plates	Stabilization methods
Metaphyseal and supracondylar fractures	Open	Internal fixator External fixator (± IM pin, except for radius) Interlocking nail *Avoid bridging of growth plates!*
	Closed	Internal fixator Plate(s) (± IM pin, except for radius) External fixator (± IM pin, except for radius) Miniplate, T-/L-plate Interlocking nail
Lateral or medial portion of the condyle (unicondylar fracture)	Open or closed	Lag screw and antirotational Kirschner wire
Intracondylar and supracondylar (bicondylar fracture)	Open	Lag screw to stabilize condyle + Cross pins or rush pins
	Closed	Lag screw to stabilize condyle + Internal fixator(s) + Plate(s) + External fixator + Cross pins or rush pins

IM pin, intramedullary pin.

13.4.5 Fractures in immature animals

Treatment of fractures in immature animals differs from treatment of fractures in adult animals for the main reasons of differences in bone quality and blood supply. Immature animals have an abundant extraosseous blood supply deriving from the thick periosteum. This blood supply allows for faster fracture healing provided that the periosteum is not damaged during the initial trauma or surgery. The strong periosteum may even prevent fracture displacement and add to stability, when it remains intact around a fractured bone. These fractures are called greenstick fractures, and are ideal fractures for conservative treatment (Fig. 13-13). Holding power of implants is not as good as in adult animals due to the soft bone quality. Intramedullary nails and internal or external fixators are ideal implants for repair of diaphyseal long-bone fractures in immature animals. These implants preserve the extraosseous blood supply, and implant stability does not rely as much on holding power of the implants in the bone as it does with conventional plates.

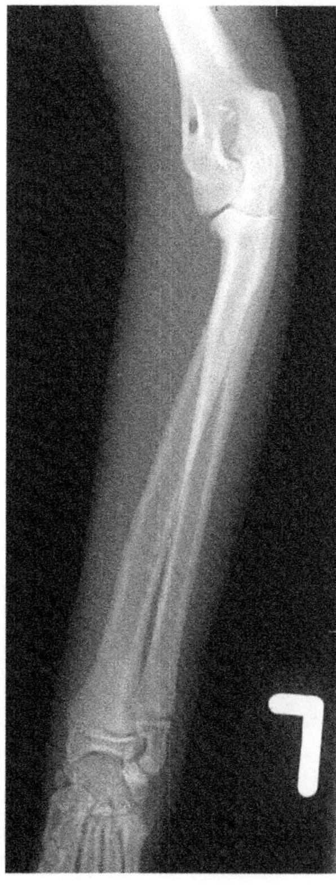

Figure 13-13 Greenstick fracture of the radius and ulna in a 9-month-old cat.

Open growth plates of growing animals are a weak area, and physeal fractures are common. Physeal fractures in growing animals always carry the risk for premature physeal closure and symmetrical or asymmetrical cessation of growth. Histologically, the growth plates contain several distinct zones (Fig. 13-14). The cells of the proliferating zone are rapidly dividing and are responsible for the growth potential. Hence, if the proliferating zone is damaged, cell division and bone growth subside or cease. The Salter and Harris classification (Fig. 13-5) was originally thought to provide a prognostic indicator for premature closure of the physis, with type I fractures bearing the lowest, and type V and VI fractures bearing the highest risk for growth disturbances. Although Salter and Harris type I and II fractures predominantly involve the hypertrophic zone, a clinical study has shown that type I and type II fractures also commonly deviate into the proliferative zone, potentially causing premature physeal closure (20). The classification is therefore not very useful in prognosticating the outcome in small animals. Instead each injury should be evaluated individually, and a guarded prognosis given until evidence for continued growth is seen radiographically.

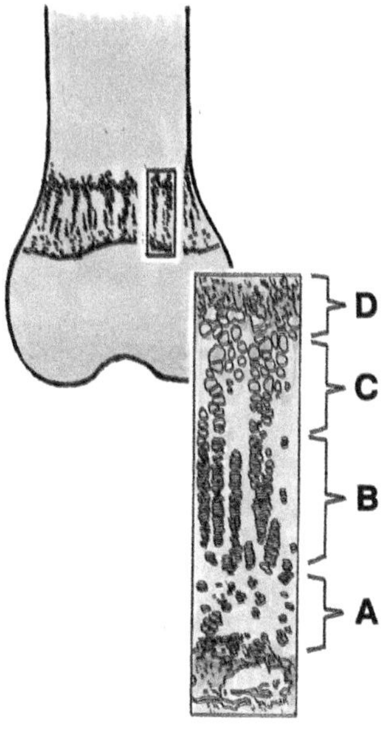

Figure 13-14 Histological zones of a growth plate. (A) The reserve zone is located immediately adjacent to the epiphyseal bone. (B) The proliferative zone contains dividing chondrocytes, oriented in columns. (C) The chondrocytes enlarge in the hypertrophic zone, and the amount of matrix decreases in between them. (D) Calcification of the matrix occurs in the provisional calcification zone.

The different growth plates close at different times during skeletal growth. They can be classified into an early group, a middle group, and a late group according to the time they close (21) (Table 13-7). Neutering has been shown to delay physeal closure in cats, especially of the later-closing growth plates (22–24). Open growth plates may be diagnosed in male castrated cats up to an age of 3–4 years, but physeal fractures do not cause growth disturbances in adult cats.

Type I and II physeal fractures are the most common physeal fractures in cats and they are stabilized with cross or

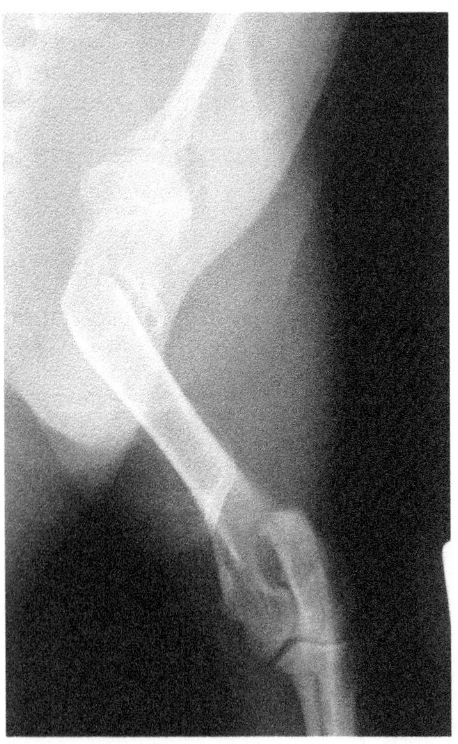

A

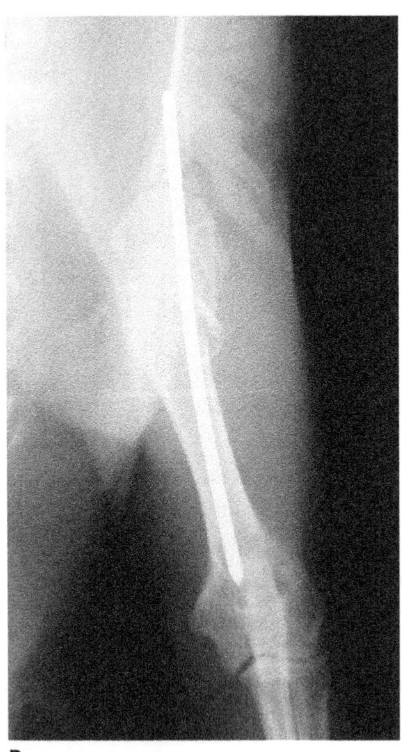

B

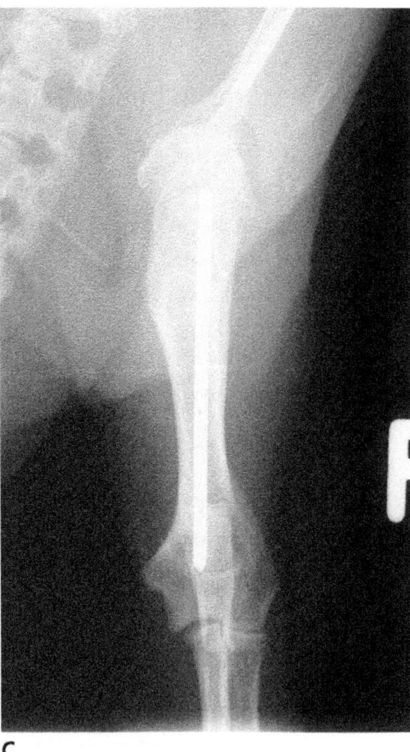

C

Figure 13-15 (**A**) Preoperative, (**B**) postoperative, and (**C**) 4-week follow-up radiographs of a 7-month-old cat with a pathological humeral fracture secondary to nutritional hyperparathyroidism. The fracture was stabilized with an intramedullary pin, because marked axial deviation was present. Fracture healing was rapid after the cat was fed a balanced diet.

Closure	Approximate age at closure	Physes
Early	4–8 months	Phalanx
		Scapula
		Distal humerus
		Proximal radius
		Ilioischial physis
Middle	8–14 months	Proximal femur
		Distal tibia and fibula
		Metacarpus, metatarsus
		Proximal ulna
Late	14–20 months	Proximal tibia and fibula
		Distal femur
		Proximal humerus
		Distal radius
		Distal ulna
		Spine

Table 13-7. Growth plates may be classified into an early-, middle-, or late-closing group (21). The time frames for physeal closure are derived from intact cats

parallel pinning. Smooth pins are used if further growth is expected. In fractures involving the joints, type III and IV, anatomical reconstruction and rigid stabilization of the joint surface are performed using a lag screw. Any physeal injury in growing animals should be rechecked radiographically after 2–3 weeks to be able to detect premature closure, and plan an intervention if necessary.

13.4.6 Open fractures

Open fractures are probably more common in cats than in dogs, although most of the literature is based on findings in dogs. They usually occur distal to the elbow and stifle joint, where the bone is surrounded by little soft tissue.

Open fractures are considered orthopedic emergencies, although concomitant life-threatening injuries may necessitate delaying treatment. Bacteria isolated before treatment are the causative agents for later infection in 66% of cases (9). Contamination after initial trauma is also common and referring veterinarians should be advised to cover the wound for transportation with a sterile dressing and a splinted bandage.

The goal of first-line treatment of open fractures is prevention of additional contamination and reduction of bacterial numbers. Tissue samples are obtained for aerobic and anaerobic cultures and sensitivity testing before treatment is started. Early administration of intravenous antibiotics has been shown to decrease infection rates (25). A first-generation cephalosporin or amoxicillin-clavulanate penetrate well into bone and are effective against most commonly encountered bacteria. In older wounds and in the presence of necrosis and avascularity anaerobic infection is likely. Clindamycin or metronidazole in combination with amoxicillin-clavulanate should be considered in these cases. The wound is cleaned and debrided as soon as the patient is considered stable for anesthesia. Wound debridement is performed under aseptic technique to avoid nosocomial infection. The wound is covered with a sterile water-soluble gel during clipping of hair to prevent hair entering the wound. Copious flushing of the wound with isotonic fluid removes debris and reduces bacterial contamination. Tissue is only surgically removed if obviously devitalized and necrotic. Severe soft-tissue wounds might have to be sequentially debrided over several days as the true extent of the necrosis becomes obvious.

If the patient is stable for a prolonged anesthetic, it is advantageous to stabilize the fracture at the same time as debridement and culture. Early stabilization not only enhances bone healing but also facilitates establishment of new soft-tissue vascularization. Open fractures are considered infected if they have existed for longer than 6–8 hours before treatment (25). Grade 1 fractures, which are less than 8 hours old and adequately managed, can be treated as closed fractures and the wound can usually be closed after fracture repair. Grade 1 fractures older than this and grade 2 and grade 3 fractures carry a higher risk for infection and delayed union or non-union. Open wound treatment and fracture stabilization with an external skeletal fixator is then the treatment of choice. Open wounds are bandaged with wet to dry dressings until healthy granulation tissue covers the bone. The cat is closely monitored for signs of sepsis until demarcation of necrotic tissue is obvious and a decision can be made regarding further treatment, if viability of the distal limb is questionable.

Bone grafting promotes fracture healing and is advantageous to use in all open fractures. It is mandatory in cases with bone loss from the fracture itself or after necrosis of bone fragments. Its application is delayed when the wound is extensive and/or dirty, until a healthy granulation bed has been formed and the wound can be secondarily closed.

Antibiotic therapy is based on results from aerobic and anaerobic cultures. Cultures are repeated, with special attention to the presence of anaerobic infection, if clinical signs of infection persist despite adequate treatment and antibiotic therapy. Duration of antibiotic therapy depends on the initial grade of contamination or infection, on the clinical appearance of the wound, and on the radiological assessment of fracture healing. A 10-day course is sufficient in uncomplicated cases with appropriate wound management. If the wound is infected, or if osteomyelitis is present, 4–6 weeks of antibiotic treatment is necessary.

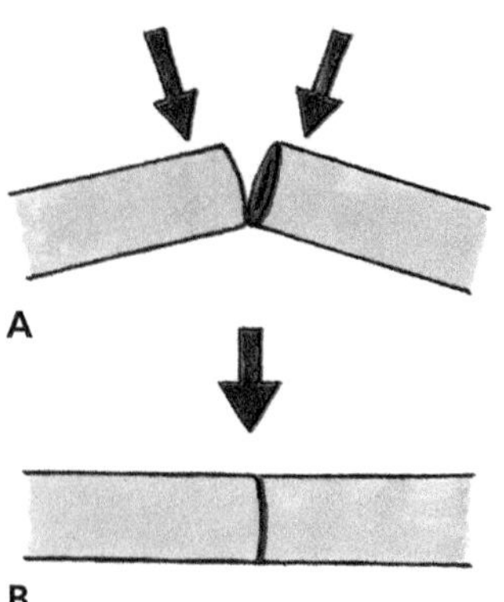

Figure 13-16 Direct reduction of a simple transverse fracture (toggling). (**A**) The bone segments are elevated until the bone ends are in direct contact. (**B**) The bone is then gradually and carefully straightened by applying digital pressure while bone contact is maintained.

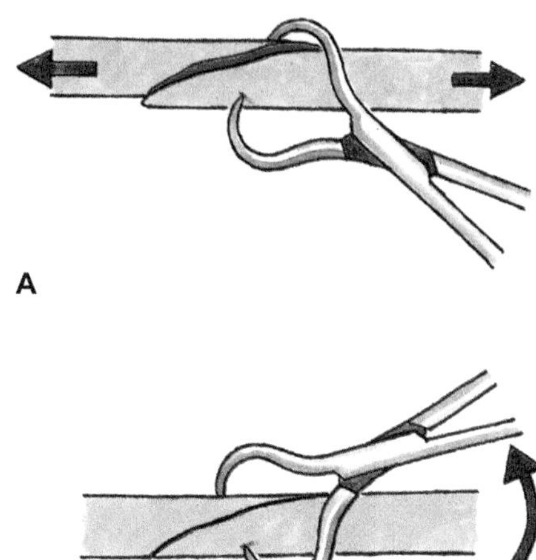

Figure 13-17 Reduction of a long oblique fracture. (**A**) The bone segments are distracted with the help of self-retaining bone reduction forceps. Once the fracture line is close to apposition, a pair of pointed bone reduction forceps is placed at an angle to the fracture line. (**B**) As the instrument is slowly closed, the fracture should glide into the correct position. The forceps are used to maintain reduction temporarily until the fracture is stabilized. They must be carefully positioned so they will not interfere with the subsequent placement of implants.

13.4.7 Pathological fractures

Pathological fractures occur in weakened osteopenic bone during normal activities. They are often localized to areas with predominantly cancellous bone, such as the metaphyseal regions of long bones and the spine, and they typically have the appearance of a folding fracture (Fig. 13-15). Thorough investigations should be made to find underlying bone disease (Chapters 4 and 8). Bone tumors and hyperparathyroidism are the most common diseases resulting in pathological fractures.

Treatment is aimed at eliminating the primary disease, if possible. Undisplaced fractures can be treated with cage rest alone and tend to heal well if the underlying disease can be treated, for example in cases with nutritional hyperparathyroidism (Chapter 4). Surgical stabilization should be considered for displaced fractures or multiple-limb involvement (Fig. 13-15). Intramedullary pins or internal and external skeletal fixators are commonly used because implant holding power is markedly reduced in osteoporotic bone.

13.5 Fracture reduction techniques

Fracture reduction is often the most challenging and time-consuming part of osteosynthesis. Manipulation of the fracture fragments needs to be performed carefully to avoid inadvertent damage to soft tissues. Feline bones tend to fissure easily if excessive force is applied during reduction and application of bone holders.

Fracture reduction can be performed by direct and indirect techniques. Direct techniques are used if anatomic reduction is the aim. Indirect reduction is used if biological osteosynthesis is to be performed. It may be conducted in a closed manner, or by using a minimally invasive approach.

Direct fracture reduction is mainly indicated for simple transverse and oblique fractures. Simple transverse fractures can be reduced by elevating the bone ends through the incision, placing them in contact to each other, and then applying digital pressure to achieve alignment – a process called toggling (Fig. 13-16). Alternatively, a slim instrument, such as a pediatric Hohmann retractor, can be used to lever the fracture ends into the correct position, without creating fissures. Simple long oblique fractures are reduced by applying traction with the help of self-retaining bone reduction forceps placed on both segments. Once the fracture fragments are nearly apposed, reduction is facilitated by placing a pair of pointed bone reduction forceps obliquely across the fracture line. Careful and slow compression of the fracture site will cause the fracture fragments to glide into position (Fig. 13-17). A pointed dental hook is ideal for reducing and holding small fracture fragments, such as small periarticular avulsion fragments (Fig. 13-18).

Indirect fracture reduction is used in comminuted fractures. Only the main fracture segments are manipulated in order to achieve physiological limb length and spatial alignment of adjacent joints. By applying traction across the fracture site, the small fracture fragments are realigned by tension in the surrounding soft tissues. Pointed bone-holding forceps or transosseous pins for external skeletal fixators can be used to hold and manipulate the main fracture segments (Fig. 13-19). Alternatively, insertion of an intramedullary pin prior to definitive fracture repair with an external skeletal fixator or a plate can be used to distract and align the main fragments. A correctly prebent plate can also serve as a reduction tool. The plate is anchored to the proximal fragment in the first

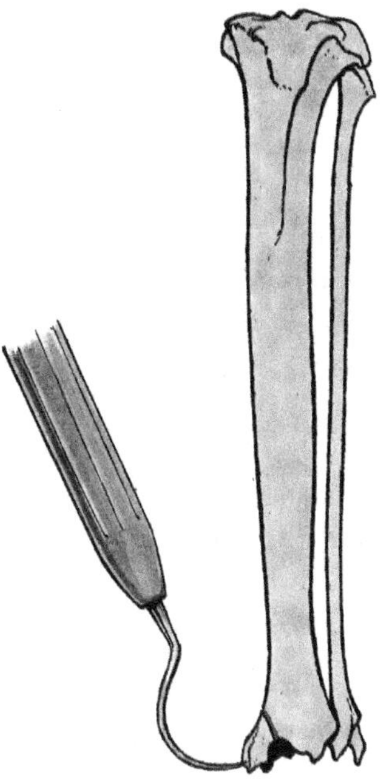

Figure 13-18 Reduction of an avulsion fracture with a dental hook. Small avulsion fractures, for example the medial malleolus, are difficult to manipulate with large bone forceps. A dental hook can be used to reduce the fragment and apply compression across the fracture line while inserting the implants.

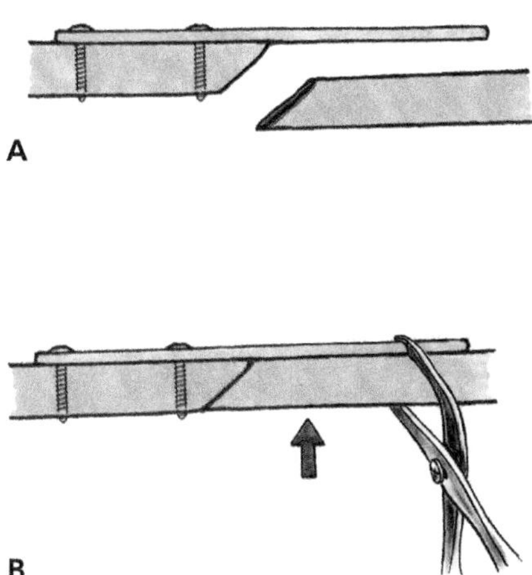

Figure 13-20 Fracture reduction with the help of a precontoured plate. The plate is fixed to the larger fragment with two screws (**A**), and is then used to pull the smaller, usually the distal metaphyseal, fragment, towards the plate. The reduced fragment is secured to the plate with the help of a Verbrugge bone clamp before insertion of the screws (**B**).

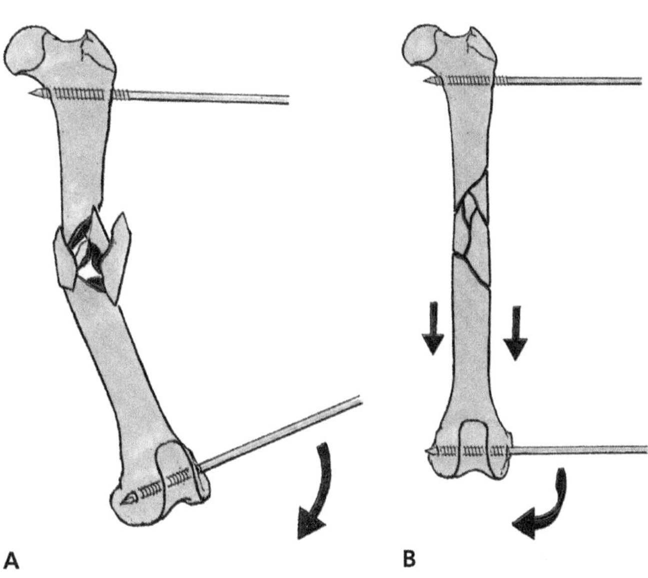

Figure 13-19 Indirect reduction of a comminuted fracture with transosseous pins. Pointed reduction forceps can be used as an alternative to transosseous pins. (**A**) The distal fragment is manipulated to achieve distraction and spatial alignment. Overdistraction must be avoided, especially in the tibia. (**B**) Fracture reduction is slightly exaggerated towards varus and internal rotation to avoid valgus and external rotation.

step, before the distal fragment is pulled towards it (Fig. 13-20).

Overdistraction of the fracture site must be avoided, because it allows invasion of soft tissues into the fracture gap, possibly resulting in delayed healing, and the increased axial tension created may predispose to fracture collapse and implant pull-out. Emphasis must also be paid to correction of valgus–varus, rotational, and craniocaudal alignment. Fractures of the extremities tend to orient themselves with a lateral or valgus malpositioning and external rotation. This tendency must be counteracted by slightly exaggerating reduction towards varus and internal rotation.

13.6 Complications in fracture repair

Fracture complications include fracture union disorders, osteomyelitis, and fracture disease. Fracture union disorders include delayed union, non-union, and malunion.

Although complications cannot be avoided completely, they often occur as a result of inadequate fracture treatment. Many complications can be treated, and a good outcome achieved, if recognized early enough. Fractures of growth plates in immature animals carry the risk for growth abnormalities. Growth abnormalities are described later in this chapter.

13.6.1 Delayed union and non-union

Delayed union is a term used to describe slower than expected bone healing. Delayed union is a subjective diagnosis, because healing times vary and depend on many factors, such as age of the cat, bone, type of trauma and fracture, and fixation method. All the biological and mechanical factors present must be considered when evaluating healing time. Fractures in immature animals can be expected to heal within 2–6 weeks. Fractures in adult animals usually heal within 1–2.5 months (Table 13-3), but longer healing times may still be normal for heavily comminuted fractures, in situations without much soft-tissue coverage, and in old cats.

If delayed union is suspected, but the implants are considered stable, the healing progress is followed on serial radiographs, generally taken every 3–4 weeks. Delayed union is usually due to inadequate blood supply in the presence of stable implants. Surgical revision is necessary if the implants are unstable, or if fracture healing ceases to progress.

A non-union is diagnosed if visible healing processes have ceased. The diagnosis is made from the typical radiographic features (Chapter 2), and if serial radiographs do not show ongoing healing. The possible causes of non-union are multifactorial. Impaired blood supply, fracture instability, large fracture gaps, interposition of soft tissue in the fracture gap, and infection may delay or prevent fracture healing. Non-unions are classified into viable and non-viable, according to the presence of radiographic signs of biological activity at the fracture site. Viable non-unions have a blood supply and evidence of new bone formation at the fracture site, but they fail to heal, mainly due to instability at the fracture site (Fig. 13-21). Non-viable non-unions have a poor or absent blood supply to one or both fracture ends, resulting in absence of new bone formation and fracture bridging. Avascular and necrotic bone segments may be present (Fig. 13-22). Cats often tend to have less callus formation than dogs, and differentiation of viable and non-viable non-union should be based not only on the presence of callus but also on the appearance of the fracture ends. Avascular bone is sclerotic and appears radiodense.

The incidence of non-union after fracture treatment of the appendicular skeleton has been reported as 4.3% in cats (14). In this retrospective clinical study of 344 cats with fractures of the appendicular skeleton, several predisposing factors were found for the development of non-union (14): the tibia and the proximal ulna were the most common sites of non-union. Approximately 15% of cats with tibial fractures developed non-union. The reduced vascularity and poor soft-tissue cover of the tibia may explain this high incidence. Open and comminuted fractures were also associated with an increased risk for non-union. Additional predisposing factors were older age and greater body weight of the cats, and fracture stabilization with type II external fixation. External fixation is commonly used to treat fracture types predisposed to non-union, which can explain the higher incidence of non-unions with type II external fixation seen in this particular study. Bone defects have been evaluated as a model for non-union in cats (26). Tibial defects greater than 1.25 times the diaphyseal diameter, stabilized with a 2.7 dynamic compression plate, were unable to heal in 12 weeks. Histologically, the fracture gap was mainly filled with fibrous tissue and striated muscle.

Treatment of viable non-unions is not usually problematic. Replacement of unstable implants with either a plate or an external fixator, removal of soft tissues from the fracture gap, and placement of cancellous bone graft will allow healing in most cases. Non-viable non-unions are a therapeutic challenge. All necrotic bone pieces are removed, and the medul-

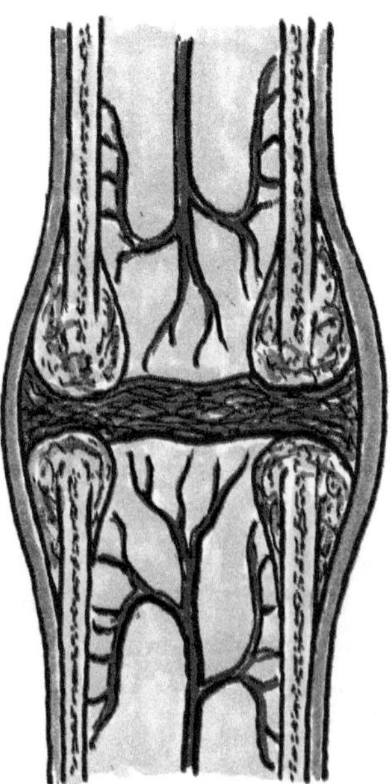

Figure 13-21 Viable non-union. A bony callus has been formed around the fracture site, indicating an adequate blood supply, but the fracture ends are sclerotic and the fracture gap is not filled with new bone.

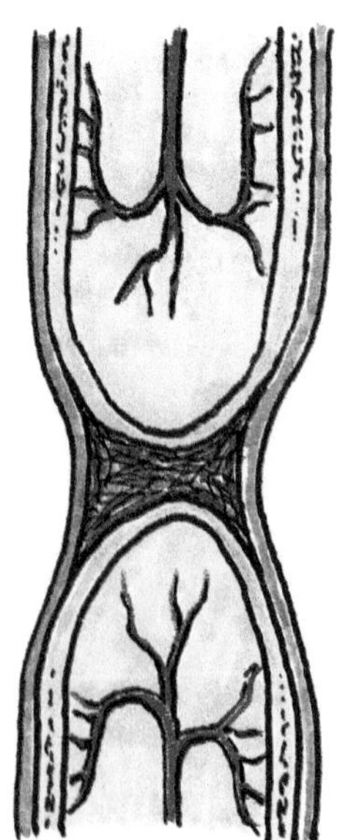

Figure 13-22 Non-viable non-union. Absence of a bony callus may indicate insufficient blood supply. The bone ends are sclerotic and often appear rounded and atrophied.

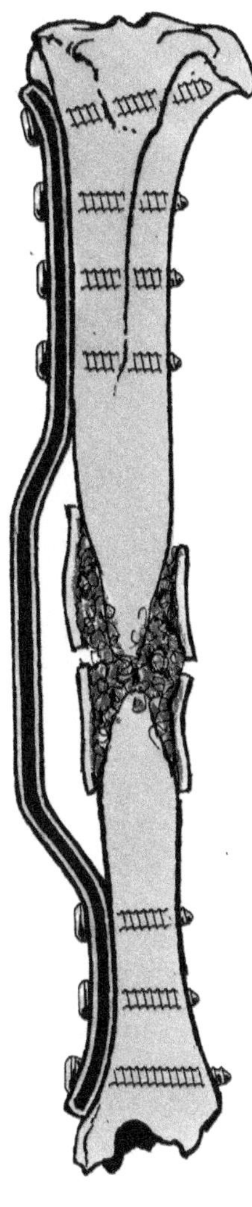

Figure 13-23 Wave plate treatment of a non-union fracture. The plate is contoured around the fracture region to allow placement of an adequate amount of bone graft in and around the defect, and facilitate vascular ingrowth from the surrounding soft tissues. The wave plate increases the functional diameter of the non-union site, and improves stability.

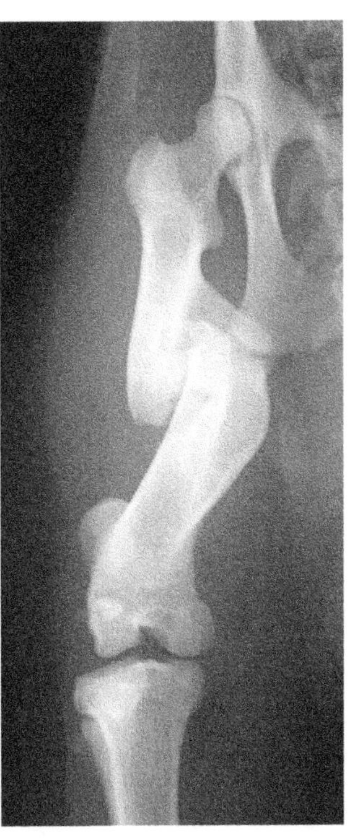

Figure 13-24 Malunion of a femoral diaphyseal fracture. Malunion often causes dysfunction of muscles and adjacent joints. Patellar luxation may occur after malunion of a femoral fracture.

lary cavity is opened by drilling holes in the sclerotic ends of the fracture segments. This should allow intraosseous vessels to reach the fracture gap. The fracture gap is packed with cancellous bone graft. Corticocancellous chips may be placed around the defect. The fracture is best stabilized using a wave plate technique (Fig. 13-23) or with an internal fixator.

A technique has been described for treatment of non-viable non-unions, which involves a segmental ostectomy of the necrotized fracture ends, followed by compression plating (27). This technique might be used if the fracture ends cannot be stabilized under compression due to large gaps or atrophy. A maximum of 15–20% of bone length can be removed. Most non-unions can be induced to heal with adequate treatment.

13.6.2 Malunion

Malunion is fracture healing in a non-physiological position. Malunion occurs if a fracture is not stabilized, if it is inadequately reduced, or if implants bend or loosen before healing is complete. Malunions in cats are most commonly seen after untreated pelvic and femoral fractures, the latter resulting in shortening of the total femoral length (Fig. 13-24). Deviations from the physiological axis of less than 5–10° are usually acceptable, and cause no clinical problems. Larger axial deviations change limb biomechanics and lead to functional deficits and degenerative changes of adjacent joints and muscles. Clinically significant malunions are treated with corrective osteotomies. Irreversible muscle or joint changes are often present in chronic cases, precluding normal limb function even after correction of the bone axis (see also fracture disease, below).

Prevention of malunion is much easier than its treatment, and revision of the repair should therefore be undertaken immediately if postoperative radiographs have revealed significant axis deviation.

13.6.3 Post-traumatic osteomyelitis

Post-traumatic osteomyelitis is relatively rare in cats. The most common reasons for osteomyelitis are extension from soft-tissue infections and open fractures (28) (Fig. 13-25). Bone necrosis, ischemia, instability, foreign bodies, and the presence of implants promote infection after open fractures. The most common bacteria isolated from cats and dogs with osteomyelitis are β-lactamase-resistant staphylococci, especially *Staphylococcus intermedius* (29). Polymicrobial

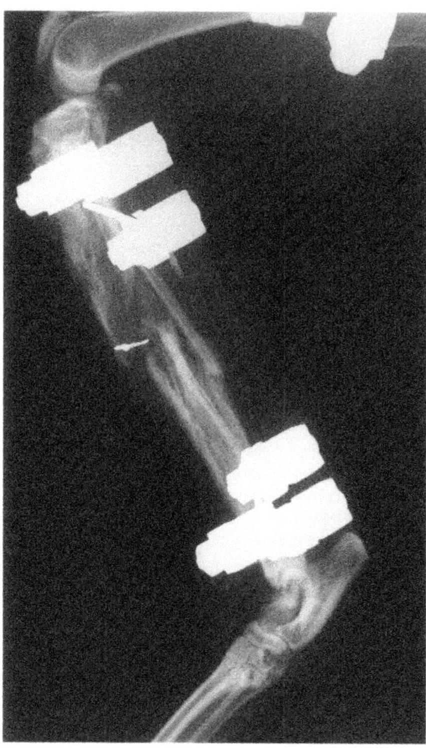

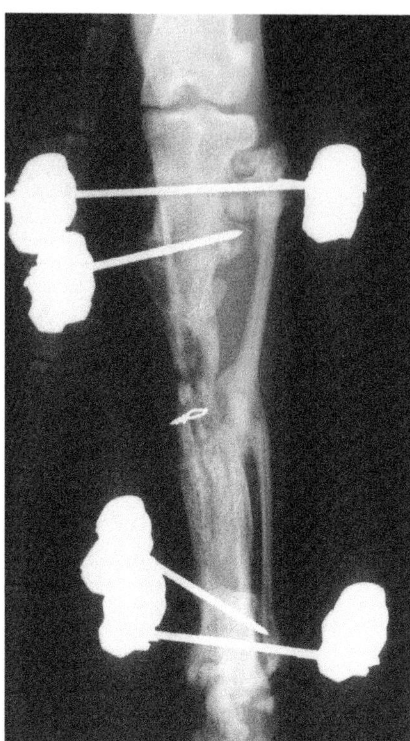

Figure 13-25 (**A**) Mediolateral and (**B**) caudocranial radiographs of a cat with tibial osteomyelitis, 2 months after having sustained an open comminuted fracture. Bone lysis, cortical sclerosis, periosteal reaction, and a non-viable healing disorder are evident. Also note lysis around the proximal transosseus pins (**B**), indicating pin loosening. Revision of this situation requires removal of the hemicerclage wire and bone sequestrae, replacement of the external fixator, open wound treatment until the area is clean, and bone grafting.

infection often includes *Streptococcus* spp., and aerobic Gram-negative bacteria, such as *Pseudomonas* spp., *Escherichia coli*, and others. Anaerobic bacteria may be encountered in up to 70% of osteomyelitis cases (30). Anaerobes and *Pseudomonas* spp. are normally present in the mouth and might cause infection after bite wounds.

Acute osteomyelitis causes local soft-tissue swelling, pain, and fever a few days after the injury or surgery. It can usually be treated with appropriate antibiotics and wound management, if fracture fixation is stable. Chronic osteomyelitis is characterized by sequestrum formation, development of draining tracts, and delayed union or non-union. Radiographic signs include periosteal new bone formation, resorption of cortex and fracture ends, and sequestration (Fig. 13-25). Treatment requires wound debridement, removal of all devitalized tissue and sequestra, and opening of all infected cavities. Internal implants are removed and the fracture is stabilized with an external fixator. A suitably stable configuration should be chosen, because fracture union may be delayed. Tissue samples, such as the sequestrum and purulent material, are submitted for both aerobic and anaerobic culturing and sensitivity testing. Specimens for anaerobic culture should not be exposed to room air and oxygen for longer than a few minutes. The wound area is flushed copiously. Often open wound treatment with wet-to-dry bandages is necessary to allow further drainage. Once the wound is filled with granulation tissue and is ready for closure, any bone defects are filled with cancellous bone graft. External fixators may be replaced by a plate or internal fixator at this stage.

Antibiotics are given for 4–6 weeks, according to bacteriological results and sensitivity testing. Amoxicillin-clavulanate or cefazolin are usually effective against most of the involved aerobic bacteria (29). Amoxicillin-clavulanate is also effective against many anaerobes, but some might be resistant. Clindamycin and metronidazole are good choices for anaerobic infection. If Gram-negative organisms are involved, quinolone antibiotics, such as enrofloxacin, may be given. Antibiotics may have to be combined for polymicrobial infections.

13.6.4 Fracture disease

Fracture disease is a term used for fracture-related secondary changes of bone, joints, and muscles. Maltreated fractures prevent limb use after surgery. Prolonged disuse of a limb may cause muscle atrophy and contractures, bone atrophy, and loss of joint range of motion due to capsular fibrosis and cartilage degeneration. At worst, the entire limb is rendered non-functional. Probably the most common form of fracture disease encountered in cats is quadriceps contracture (Chapter 7). Treatment of advanced fracture disease is often not possible and the affected limb often has to be amputated. Prevention of fracture disease is achieved by adhering to the correct principles of osteosynthesis, using gentle tissue handling and

Type of graft	Osteogenesis	Osteoinduction	Osteoconduction
Cancellous autograft	+++	++	+++
Cancellous allograft		++	+++
Demineralized bone matrix		+++	+

Table 13-8. Functions of bone grafts graded from + to +++

fasciotomy of swollen muscle groups and encouraging the early postoperative use of the limb.

13.7 Bone grafting

Bone grafts are used to enhance fracture healing. Their use is indicated for repair of fractures with low healing potential, such as heavily comminuted fractures, fractures with large fracture gaps, and open fractures. Bone grafting is an important part of the treatment of delayed union or non-union fractures and post-traumatic osteomyelitis, and is used to enhance healing of arthrodeses. Both autografts and allografts can be used in the feline patient.

Bone grafting accelerates bone formation by three general functions (31) (Table 13-8). Osteogenesis is new bone formation by transplanted viable cells. Osteoconduction is provided by the structure of the graft, which acts as a framework for vascular and bony ingrowth of surrounding tissue. Osteoinduction, probably the most important attribute, is the transformation of undifferentiated cells into osteoblasts by growth factors. Live cells are only provided by autogenous bone graft. Allografts lack the osteogenic function. In one study using a feline non-union model evaluating the effects of both fresh autogenous and deep-frozen allogenic cortical chips, both types of graft effectively promoted bone healing, but a more rapid and consistent response was observed with the autogenous graft (32). These differences are most probably due to the lack of osteogenic potential, reduced osteoinductive potential, and antigenicity of allografts. Antigenicity of banked allografts is reduced due to processing, but not completely eliminated, and an immunological response may lead to excessive graft resorption and lack of new bone formation in some cases.

Autogenous cancellous bone graft is the gold standard for bone grafting. Its disadvantages are the increased surgery time and additional morbidity associated with the harvest site. The proximal humerus, the ilial wing, and to a lesser extent the proximal and distal femur can be used as harvest sites. The graft is usually collected at the beginning of the surgery, and separate draping and instruments are used in order to prevent spreading of infection between donor and recipient site. The cortical bone is opened with a burr, large Kirschner wire, or drill bit. The opening needs to be large enough to be able to insert and handle a sharp bone curette without risking iatrogenic fracture. Cancellous bone is then harvested with the curette (Fig. 13-26). The graft obtained is kept moist with blood until it is used. The syringe plunger cavities might offer a better storage solution than a sponge as the small fragments can become entwined with the threads of the surgical sponge. Especially in older cats, it can be impossible to obtain an adequate amount of cancellous bone, and an allograft might have to be added to it. Alternatively, corticocancellous morsels can be obtained from the dorsal ilial wing. These are obtained by making a dorsal surgical approach to the iliac crest, and nibbling off pieces of bone with a small pair of rongeurs. Morsels should be 2 mm or less in size to avoid sequestra formation.

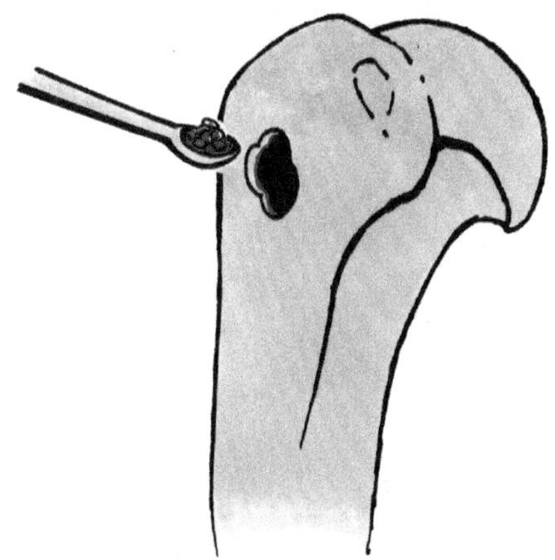

Figure 13-26 Cancellous autograft can be harvested from the proximal humerus. The cortical access hole must be large enough to allow easy passage and manipulation of the bone curette in order to avoid iatrogenic fractures during levering. The cancellous bone is harvested from the subchondral area, without disturbing the nutrient artery, which is located more distally.

Autogenous corticocancellous strips can be used to enhance healing of arthrodeses or large cortical defects. The strips are also obtained from the lateral side of the wing of the ilium (Fig. 13-27). The strips are placed around the fracture site with the cancellous side towards the bone. Corticocancellous strips have the same properties as cancellous graft, but additionally provide some mechanical strength and more bone stock.

Allografts lack an osteogenic potential due to the processing, but they can be stored, and are readily available without extending surgery time and causing additional morbidity to

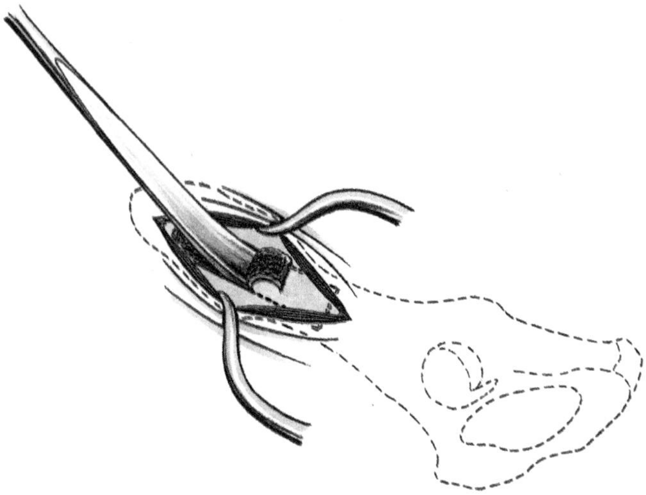

Figure 13-27 Corticocancellous bone strips can be obtained from the lateral side of the ilium. The strips are harvested with the help of a Slocum gauge or a smaller bone gauge after splitting the gluteus medius muscle.

the patient. The beneficial effect of cancellous allograft on bone healing in cats has been proven in experimental settings, although bone union occurred less rapidly and consistently when compared to fresh autogenous cancellous graft (32). Allografts may be preferable in patients with enhanced anesthetic risk, for old cats, or when large amounts of graft are needed. Feline allograft is commercially available (Veterinary Transplant Services). It is freeze-dried and can be stored at room temperature for 12 months. Cancellous allograft should be mixed with bone marrow or cancellous autograft to provide progenitor cells or osteoblasts. For the filling of small defects, 0.5 ml is usually adequate. Filling of large defects may require 1.0 ml.

13.8 Growth deformities

Growth deformities occur secondary to premature closure of growth plates in immature animals. They are rare in cats, and not much is known on incidence or risk factors. Premature closure of growth plates can be secondary to traumatic or infectious damage to the proliferating cells of the physis. Resulting clinical appearance and limb deformities may not be as pronounced as in dogs due to the smaller growth potential of the feline patient. Thorough evaluation of the limb and its radiographs, comparison to the unaffected side, and careful planning of surgery are essential for successful treatment.

13.8.1 Compensatory bone overgrowth

Compensatory bone overgrowth of both adjacent bones in the limb and the same bone after fracture is a well-recognized and reported phenomenon in dogs (33), and can compensate for smaller disparities of bone length.

Age in months	Femoral length in mm		Tibial length in mm	
	Right	Left	Right	Left
3.5	84	–	88	–
5	86	92	96	92
9	90	106	111	109
12.5	92	110	115	114
17	93	113	118	117
27	93	113	118	117

Table 13-9. Serial femoral and tibial length measurements of a cat with a distal comminuted supracondylar fracture of the right femur, sustained at 3.5 months of age. Shortening of the right femur occurred. The right tibia showed temporary compensatory overgrowth (Study of Stergior Vlachopoulas.)

Compensatory overgrowth of the tibia has been seen in a 14-week-old male cat with an intracondylar fracture of the femoral condyle with supracondylar comminution, repaired with a transcondylar screw and two dynamic intramedullary pins (Stergios Vlachopoulos, personal communication). Mediolateral radiographs taken 6 weeks postoperatively, prior to implant removal, showed mild shortening of the right femur (6 mm) and elongation of the right tibia (4 mm) when compared with the opposite leg. Interestingly, as the cat matured, the discrepancy between the lengths of the tibias decreased, indicating that after an initial phase of overgrowth a phase of undergrowth of the left tibia followed, starting from an initial discrepancy in tibial length of 4.35% at 6 weeks postoperatively to 0.85% 1 year postoperatively. The right femur remained shortened (Table 13-9).

13.8.2 Principles of correction of limb deformities

Several problems may be encountered with limb deformities caused by growth disturbances, including loss of bone length, bone deformation, and incongruity of adjacent joints. Treatment of clinically apparent limb deformities requires an osteotomy for angular and rotational realignment of the limb. An opening wedge or closing wedge osteotomy are the most practical to correct angular limb deformities in cats due to the small bone sizes (Fig. 13-28). The osteotomy can be stabilized with an external fixator, an internal fixator, or a bone plate after alignment.

Besides restoration of angular limb deformity, restoration of limb length may be necessary. Loss of bone length is considered clinically significant if exceeding 15–20%, compared to the contralateral unaffected side. Distraction osteogenesis can be performed in cats, using small linear or circular distraction devices. Uncomplicated new bone formation was achieved without encountering muscle contraction with a distraction rate of 0.7 mm/day (34) (Fig. 13-29).

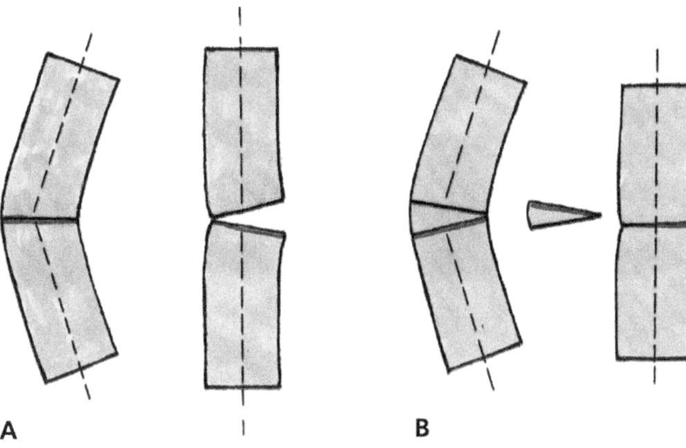

Figure 13-28 (**A**) Opening and (**B**) closing wedge osteotomies. (**A**) Opening wedge osteotomy has the advantage of gaining bone length. Its disadvantage is that the osteotomy ends are stabilized without contact. (**B**) Closing wedge osteotomy has the advantage of good bone contact after fixation, but it reduces bone length.

13.8.3 Premature physeal closure of the distal radial physis

The most common site for premature physeal closure in dogs is the distal ulnar physis, which is predisposed to compressive injury due to its conical shape. The distal ulnar physis in cats is oriented perpendicular to the long axis of the radius and is therefore less susceptible to premature physeal closure.

Premature closure of the distal radial physis can be caused by distal radial physeal fractures, but may also occur after other injuries to the distal antebrachium and paw. Trauma to the distal antebrachium can cause compressive lesions of the physis, not visible on initial radiographs. Control radiographs after 2–3 weeks should be suggested to owners after any kind of trauma to the distal antebrachium in immature cats. Cats falling from a height, and cats with fractures of the ulnar styloid process, may be predisposed to premature closure of the distal radial physis (34). Growth cessation of the distal radial physis results in short-radius syndrome. In contrast to dogs, antebrachiocarpal incongruity seems to develop from continued ulnar growth, rather than elbow incongruity (34) (Fig. 13-30).

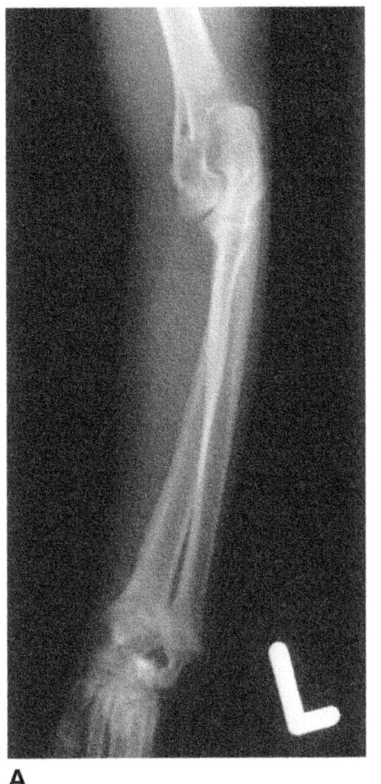

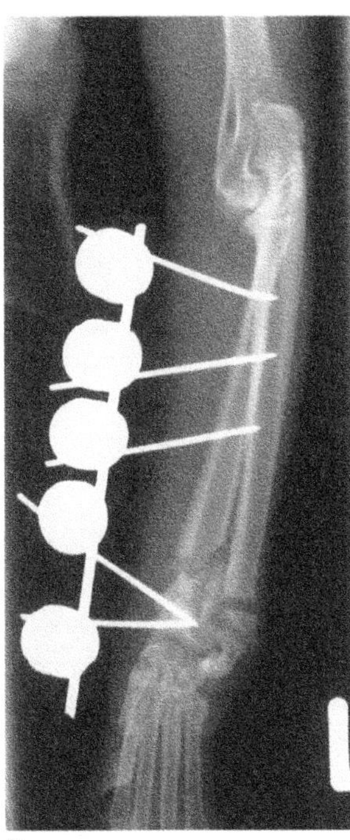

Figure 13-30 A 6-month-old cat with premature closure of the distal radial physis after having sustained a Salter and Harris fracture of the distal radial physis. (**A**) Preoperative radiographs. The distal radial physis is closed, the ulnar physis is still open. A large gap is present on the lateral aspect of the radiocarpal joint. (**B**) Radiographs after radial and ulnar osteotomies. Realignment of the distal radius resulted in improved carpal congruity. (Reproduced with permission from: Voss K, Lieskovsky J. Trauma-induced growth abnormalities of the distal radius in three cats. J Feline Med Surg 2007;9:117–123.)

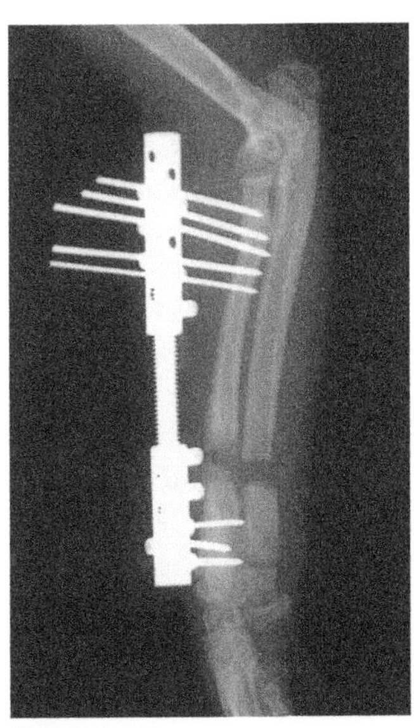

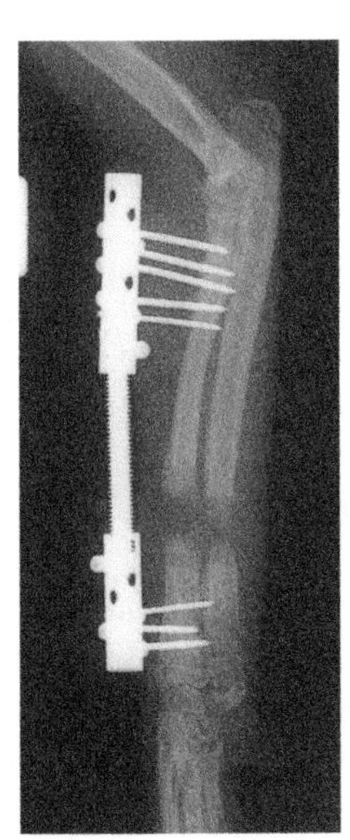

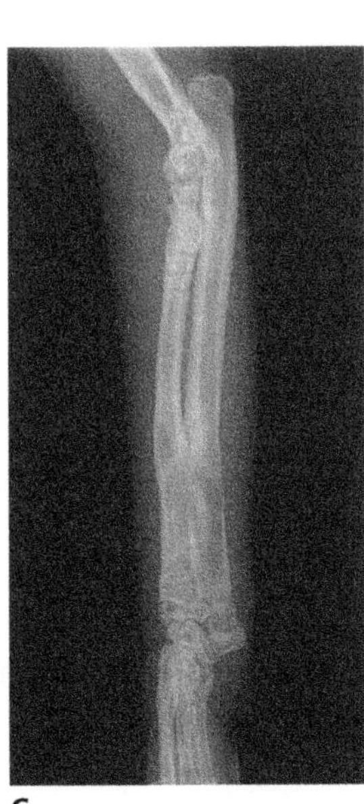

Figure 13-29 Distraction osteogenesis of a 4.5-month-old cat with radius brevis. (**A**) Radiograph taken after 10 days of distraction. (**B**) Radiograph taken after 2.5 weeks of distraction when it was stopped. Uncomplicated new bone formation was achieved with a distraction rate of 0.35 mm twice daily. (**C**) Radiograph after healing of the osteotomies and removal of the external skeletal fixator 5 weeks later. (Reproduced with permission from: Voss K, Lieskovsky J. Trauma-induced growth abnormalities of the distal radius in three cats. J Feline Med Surg 2007;9:117–123.)

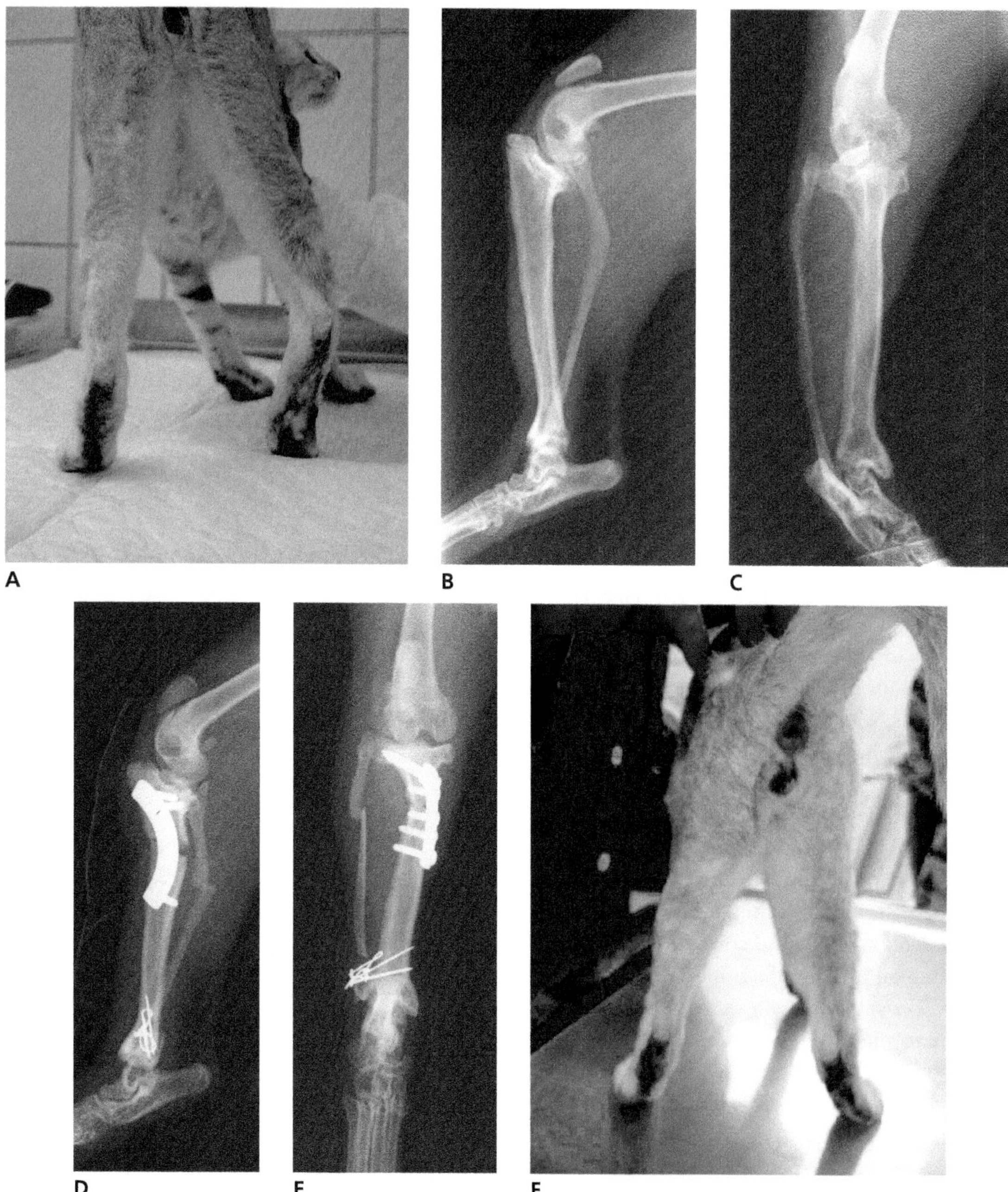

Figure 13-31 A case example of a 1-year-old cat with a hindlimb deformity secondary to premature physeal closure of the proximal tibial physis. (**A**) Preoperative appearance of the right hindlimb of the cat, with a marked varus deformity at the level of the tarsal joint. (**B**, **C**) Preoperative radiographs of the tibia. The tibia was shortened and the tibial plateau deformed (**B**). The varus deformity at the tarsal level was mainly caused by continuous growth of the fibula, pushing the tarsus into varus and internal rotation (**C**). (**D**, **E**) Postoperative radiographs. An opening wedge osteotomy of the proximal tibia was performed to correct the slope of the tibial plateau (**D**). Proximal and distal fibular ostectomies and stabilization of the lateral malleolus in a more proximal position ameliorated tarsal deformity (**E**). (**F**) Appearance and function of the limb were excellent after 4 months, although the tibia was markedly shorter than on the contralateral side.

Treatment varies according to age of the patient, and progression of limb deformity. Osteotomy and realignment of the radius are performed to correct angular deformity (Fig. 13-30). If carpal incongruity is mainly due to excessive length of the distal ulna in comparison to the radius, a distal ulnar ostectomy is performed, allowing the distal part of the ulna to migrate proximally. Cats younger than 4 months of age at the time of injury can be expected to have a clinically relevant loss of antebrachial length when fully grown, and distraction osteogenesis of the radius should be considered (Fig. 13-29). Satisfactory clinical function was achieved in three cats with premature closure of the distal radial growth plate, although the range of motion in flexion of the carpal joint remained reduced (34).

Table 13-10. Indications for implant removal after healing has been achieved

Implant type	Indications for removal
External fixator	Always
Pins	Loose and migrating
	Interfering with joint function
Intramedullary pin	Loose and migrating
	Interfering with soft tissue (e.g., sciatic nerve)
Plates or internal fixators	Causing soft-tissue or skin irritation
	Interfering with joint function
	Causing osteoporosis (temporary stabilization with external fixator might be necessary)
	Causing thermic conduction (e.g., tibia, radius)
All internal implants	After infections
	After open fractures

13.8.4 Premature closure of the proximal tibial physis

Premature closure of growth plates other than the radial physis is rare, but deformity of the proximal tibia has been described (35), and the authors have seen one affected cat. The cat presented with a shortened tibia, marked varus deformity of the tarsus, and a caudally tilted tibial plateau (Fig. 13-31). Historically, the cat had an episode of fever and lameness at a younger age, which resolved after a short course of antibiotics. The reason for premature closure might have been hematogenous metaphyseal osteomyelitis based on the owner's history. The varus deformity of the tarsus improved impressively after distal ostectomy of the fibula. Additionally, osteotomy and realignment of the tibial plateau were performed (Fig. 13-31). Distraction osteogenesis would have been indicated to lengthen the tibia, but was declined by the owner. Functional outcome was good.

The cat reported in the literature, with an excessive tibial plateau angle and a cranial cruciate ligament rupture, was successfully treated by a combination of tibial plateau-leveling osteotomy and cranial closing wedge osteotomy (35).

13.9 Implant removal

Implants have no function after fracture healing is completed. Routine implant removal is a matter of preference of the surgeon in many cases. The fear that implants may cause bone tumors is not substantiated by the literature. Only a few case reports on fracture- or implant-related tumors exist, including sarcoma (36), fibrosarcoma (37), and osteosarcoma (38). Definitive reasons for plate removal in dogs and cats include fixation instability, infection, soft-tissue irritation, thermic conduction, and chronic lameness (39). Besides implant loosening and infection, soft-tissue irritation is probably the most common reason for implant removal in cats. Bone plates are often relatively oversized in the feline patient. Skin irritation occurs in areas where the plates are located directly under the skin and may include lick granulomas, repetitive skin damage, and skin necrosis. Implants positioned near joints may interfere with joint motion and cause swelling and fibrosis. All implants must be removed in the presence of infection, as the glycocalyx surrounding the implants prevents clearance of bacteria by host immune mechanisms and antibiotics. Bacterial growth can even be found in routinely removed metallic implants (40). Indications for implant removal are summarized in Table 13-10. Radiographs are obtained after removal of the implants, and the cat is kept confined to a crate for 2 weeks and to the house for a further 2 weeks to prevent fracture through implant holes.

References and further reading

1. Harari J. Treatment for feline long bone fractures. Vet Clin North Am Small Anim Pract 2002;32:927–947.
2. Carter DR, Spengler DM. Biomechanics of fracture. In: Sumner-Smith G (ed.) Bone in clinical orthopedics, 2nd edn. Dübendorf: AO Publishing; 2002: pp. 261–285.
3. Schrader SC. Orthopedic surgery. In: Sherding RG (ed.) The cat: diseases and clinical management. New York: Churchill Livingstone; 1994: pp. 1649–1709.
4. Unger M, et al. Classification of fractures of long bones in the dog and cat: introduction and clinical application. Vet Comp Orthop Traumatol 1990;3:41–50.
5. Anderson A, Coughlan AR. Sacral fractures in dogs and cats: a classification scheme and review of 51 cases. J Small Anim Pract 1997;38:404–409.
6. Messmer M, Montavon PM. Pelvic fractures in the dog and cat: a classification system and review of 556 cases. Vet Comp Orthop Traumatol 2004;4:167–173.
7. Salter RB, Harris WR. Injuries involving the epiphyseal plate. J Bone Joint Surg Br 1963;45:487–622.
8. Piermattei DL, Flo GL. Fractures in growing animals. In: Brinker WO, Piermatei DL, Flo GL (eds) Handbook of small animal

orthopedics and fracture repair, 3rd edn. Philadelphia: WB Saunders; 1997: pp. 676–685.
9. Tillson DM. Open fracture management. Vet Clin North Am Small Anim Pract 1995;25:1093–1110.
10. Grant GR, Olds RB. Treatment of open fractures. In: Slatter D (ed.) Textbook of small animal surgery, 3rd edn. Philadelphia: WB Saunders; 2003: pp. 1793–1798.
11. Perren SM. Evolution of the internal fixation of long bone fractures. The scientific basis of biological internal fixation: choosing a new balance between stability and biology. J Bone Joint Surg Br 2002;84:1093–1110.
12. Uhthoff HK, Rahn BA. Healing patterns of metaphyseal fractures. Clin Orthop Relat Res 1981;160:295–303.
13. Richardson EF, Thacher CW. Tibial fractures in cats. Comp Continuing Educ 1993;15:383–394.
14. Nolte DM, et al. Incidence of and predisposing factors for nonunion of fractures involving the appendicular skeleton in cats: 18 cases (1998–2002). J Am Vet Med Assoc 2005;226: 77–82.
15. Langley-Hobbs SJ, et al. Use of external skeletal fixators in the repair of femoral fractures in cats. J Small Anim Pract 1996;37:95–101.
16. Langley-Hobbs SJ, et al. External skeletal fixation for stabilisation of comminuted humeral fractures in cats. J Small Anim Pract 1997;38:280–285.
17. Gemmill TJ, et al. Treatment of canine and feline diaphyseal radial and tibial fractures with low-stiffness external skeletal fixation. J Small Anim Pract 2004;45:85–91.
18. Haas B, et al. Use of the tubular external fixator in the treatment of distal radial and ulnar fractures in small dogs and cats. Vet Comp Orthop Traumatol 2003;16:132–137.
19. Gautier E, et al. Porosity and remodelling of plated bone after internal fixation: result of stress shielding or vascular damage. In: Ducheyne P, Van der Perre G, Aubert AE (eds) Biomaterials and biomechanics. Amsterdam: Elsevier Science; 1984: pp. 195–200.
20. Johnson JM, et al. Histological appearance of naturally occurring canine physeal fractures. Vet Surg 1994;23:81–86.
21. Smith RN. Fusion of ossification centres in the cat. J Small Anim Pract 1969;10:523–530.
22. May C, et al. Delayed physeal closure associated with castration in cats. J Small Anim Pract 1991;32:326–328.
23. Root MV, et al. The effect of prepubertal and postpubertal gonadectomy on radial physeal closure in male and female domestic cats. Vet Radiol Ultrasound 1997;38:42–47.
24. Houlton JEF, McGlennon NJ. Castration and physeal closure in the cat. Vet Rec 1992;131:466–467.
25. Popovitch CA, Nannos AJ. Emergency management of open fractures and luxations. Vet Clin North Am Small Anim Pract 2000;30:645–655.
26. Toombs JP, et al. Evaluation of Key's hypothesis in the feline tibia: an experimental model for augmented bone healing studies. Am J Vet Res 1985;46:513–518.
27. Blaeser LL, et al. Treatment of biologically inactive nonunions by a limited en bloc ostectomy and compression plate fixation: a review of 17 cases. Vet Surg 2003;32:91–100.
28. Griffiths GL, Bellenger CR. A retrospective study of osteomyelitis in dogs and cats. Aust Vet J 1979;55:587–591.
29. Johnson KA. Osteomyelitis in dogs and cats. J Am Vet Med Assoc 1994;12:1882–1887.
30. Muir P, Johnson KA. Anaerobic bacteria isolated from osteomyelitis in dogs and cats. Vet Surg 1992;21:463–466.
31. Fitch R, et al. Bone autografts and allografts in dogs. Comp Continuing Educ 1997;19:558–575.
32. Toombs JP, Wallace LJ. Evaluation of autogeneic and allogeneic cortical chip grafting in a feline tibial nonunion model. Am J Vet Res 1985;46:519–528.
33. Schaefer SL, et al. Compensatory tibial overgrowth following healing of closed femoral fracture in young dogs. Vet Comp Orthop Traumatol 1995;8:159–162.
34. Voss K, Lieskovsky J. Trauma-induced growth abnormalities of the distal radius in three cats. J Feline Med Surg 2007;9: 117–123.
35. Hoots EA, Petersen SW. Tibial plateau leveling osteotomy and cranial closing wedge ostectomy in a cat with cranial cruciate ligament rupture. J Am Anim Hosp Assoc 2005;41:395–399.
36. Fry PD, Jukes HF. Fracture associated sarcoma in the cat. J Small Anim Pract 1995;36:124–126.
37. Sinibaldi K, et al. Osteomyelitis and neoplasia associated with use of the Jones intramedullary splint in small animals. J Am Vet Med Assoc 1982;181:885–890.
38. Bennett D, et al. Osteosarcoma associated with healed fractures. J Small Anim Pract 1979;20:13–18.
39. Emmerson TD, Muir P. Bone plate removal in dogs and cats. Vet Comp Orthop Traumatol 1999;12:74–77.
40. Smith MM, et al. Bacterial growth associated with metallic implants in dogs. J Am Vet Med Assoc 1989;195:765–767.

14 Joint injuries

K. Voss, P.M. Montavon

Joint injuries in cats frequently occur after motor vehicle accidents and falls from a height. The pelvic limbs are involved more often than the thoracic limbs, and the hip and tarsus are the most commonly affected joints. The incidence of joint injuries in cats presented at the Clinic for Small Animal Surgery of the University of Zurich is shown in Figure 14-1. Injuries of joints can be classified into ligament sprains, joint luxations, joint fractures, and open joint injuries. Regardless of the type of injury, disruption of normal joint alignment and stability results in development of painful osteoarthritis and functional deficits. Treatment is therefore aimed at restoring joint surfaces and joint stability to minimize osteoarthritic changes and maintain joint function. Structure and function of joints, healing of joint injuries, surgical principles, treatment of complications such as post-traumatic septic arthritis, and principles of arthrodesis are described in this chapter. Joint fractures are covered in Chapter 13.

14.1 Structure and function of joints

Normal joint function allows a pain-free and full range of motion, while providing stability during weight-bearing. Synovial joints consist of a joint cavity, a joint capsule, the synovial fluid, the articular cartilage, and the subchondral bone. The synoviocytes of the inner synovial membrane of the joint capsule produce the synovial fluid. Synoviocytes are also capable of phagocytosis. The outer fibrous layer of the joint capsule provides some stability to the joint, but the main joint stabilizers are the collateral and intra-articular ligaments. The capsule contains nerves and vessels.

Synovial fluid is a dialysate of blood, enriched with glycosaminoglycans (GAGs). The main GAG in the synovial fluid is hyaluronic acid. Synovial fluid has two functions: lubrication and nutrition of the articular cartilage. Lubrication is necessary to decrease friction between the joint surfaces to reduce wear and tear of the articular cartilage. Synovial fluid has a viscous consistency, which is important for the adhesion between the two articular surfaces. The articular cartilage is nourished by diffusion from synovial fluid into the cartilage layers.

Articular cartilage allows gliding of two joint surfaces on each other, and acts as a buffer during weight-bearing. Articular cartilage lacks blood and lymphatic vessels, and nerves. It consists of approximately 80% water, 10% collagen, and 10% proteoglycans. Proteoglycans and collagen are synthesized by the chondrocytes. The collagen fiber network in the cartilage is mainly responsible for resisting shear forces, which occur when the cartilage is compressed during weight-bearing. Proteoglycans are stiff macromolecules, consisting of a hyaluronic acid backbone and several core proteins to which GAGs are attached. Proteoglycans are capable of binding water, and form most of the cartilage matrix.

14.2 Healing of joint injuries

Trauma to joints can result in laceration or abrasion of cartilage, and/or rupture of the joint capsule and associated ligaments. Trauma additionally initiates an inflammatory response, causing synovitis and joint effusion. Regenerative and degenerative processes occur simultaneously during the healing phase of joint injuries.

Cartilage is an avascular tissue with very limited healing capacities, and inflammatory cells and blood vessels have no access to superficial cartilage defects. The healing response therefore depends on synthesis of new matrix from chondrocytes surrounding the defect. This matrix is usually insufficient to fill larger defects. Inflammatory cells and blood vessels can enter the defect from the bone if the lesion reaches

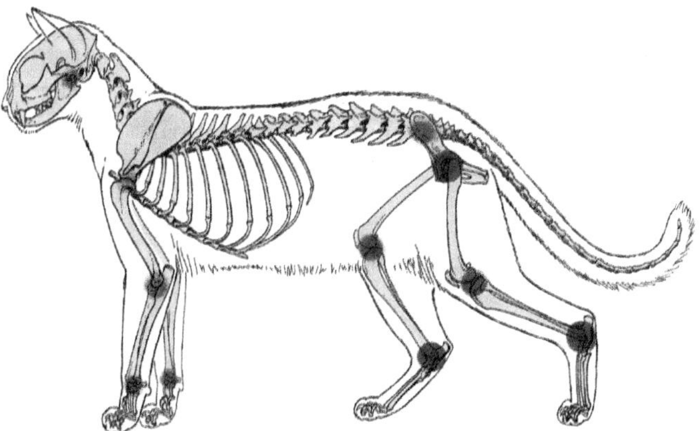

Figure 14-1 Distribution of joint injuries in 531 cats presented at the Clinic for Small Animal Surgery of the University of Zurich. Shades of red represent the incidence of injury. A total of 467 injuries (88%) involved the joints of the pelvic limb, and 64 injuries (12%) involved joints of the thoracic limb. The hip joint, tarsal joint, and stifle joint were most commonly affected. Of the joints of the thoracic limbs, the carpus was the most frequently injured.

down to the subchondral bone. The defect is then initially filled with a fibrin clot, which is replaced by fibroblast-like cells and collagen fibers. These fibroblast-like cells differentiate into chondroblasts after about 2 weeks, and are capable of synthesizing cartilage matrix. The new cartilage does not have the same quality, thickness, and mechanical properties as normal hyaline cartilage, and is prone to fibrillation and erosion.

Healing of joint capsule and collateral ligament ruptures occurs through invasion of the defect with blood vessels, inflammatory cells, and fibroblasts from the surrounding tissues. The defect is filled with granulation tissue during the first 2 weeks of the healing phase. This tissue is still weak, and it takes another 2–4 weeks until fibrous scar tissue which is strong enough to withstand tensile forces has formed. Remodeling of the scar tissue involves longitudinal orientation of the collagen fibers to improve tensile strength. This process requires a controlled amount of tensile stress across the wound.

Intra-articular ligaments, such as the cruciate ligaments of the stifle joint, do not heal, because they lack sufficient intrinsic vascular supply, and the possibility of cell migration from surrounding tissue. Periarticular fibrosis and thickening of the joint capsule are the body's attempt to stabilize the affected joint. Excessive periarticular fibrosis is undesirable because it reduces range of motion.

Joint injuries always initiate some degree of degenerative changes in the affected joint by several mechanisms. Articular cartilage can undergo further degeneration, because injury may induce loss of proteoglycans and water, which in turn reduces resilience of the articular cartilage, and makes it susceptible to mechanical damage. Prolonged immobilization of joints in the postoperative period also causes thinning and softening of the articular cartilage (1). The soft cartilage is easily damaged in the period of remobilization. Changes in amount and quality of synovial fluid reduce lubrication of cartilage and increase friction between the joint surfaces. Continuous instability may result in abnormal force transmission and enhanced wear of the cartilage. Osteophytosis often develops after joint injuries, and is probably an attempt by the body to stabilize the affected joint, in conjunction with fibrosis of the joint capsule.

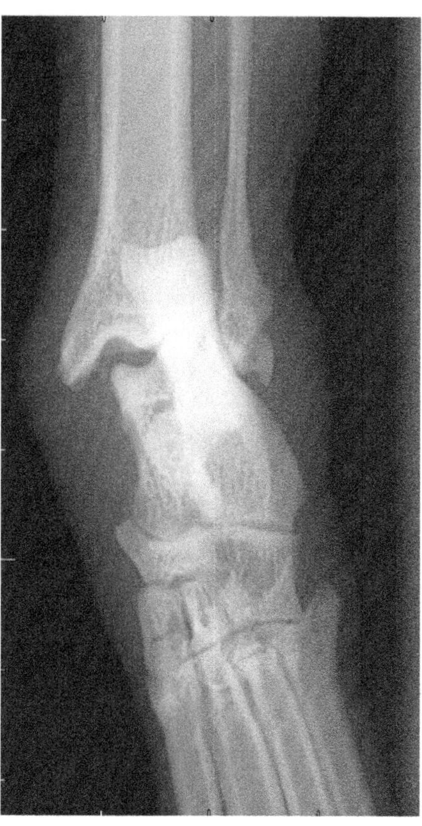

Figure 14-2 Example of a cat with tibiotarsal instability/ subluxation. Valgus stress radiographs result in opening of the tibiotarsal joint space medially, indicating rupture, or grade III sprain, of the medial collateral ligament.

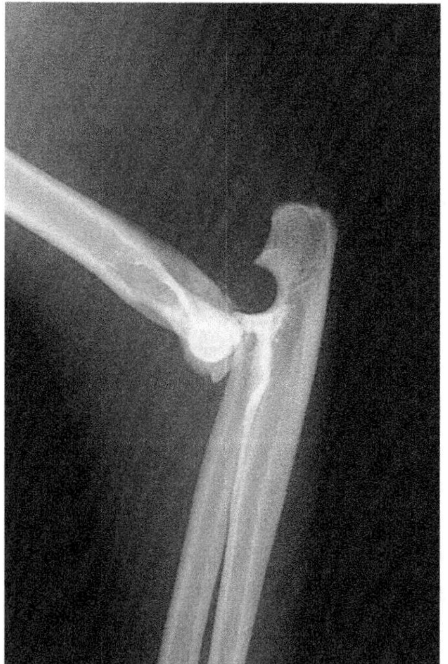

Figure 14-3 Example of a cat with caudal elbow luxation. The humeroulnar and humeroradial joint surfaces are completely dislocated. The sesamoid bone of the tendon of the supinator muscle is seen cranial to the radial head.

14.3 Diagnosis of joint injury

Joint instability and subluxation are usually caused by sprain or rupture of one of the joint ligaments, and the joint capsule (Fig. 14-2). Joint luxation is defined as complete loss of contact between the adjacent joint surfaces, and occurs if several ligaments and the joint capsule are disrupted (Fig. 14-3).

Ligament sprains are classified into three categories (Table 14-1) (2). Grade I collateral ligament sprains cause relatively mild clinical signs, which are usually self-limiting. Grade II and III sprains result in more obvious clinical signs, including marked pain on palpation, periarticular swelling, and joint

Sprain	Characteristics	Clinical findings	Radiographic findings
Grade I	Parenchymal hematoma/edema Only few fibers torn	Mild lameness Mild local swelling and pain	Mild soft-tissue swelling No bony lesions or instability on stress radiographs
Grade II	Partial tear of ligament Functional deficits but ligament grossly intact	Obvious lameness Obvious swelling Obvious pain on palpation/ manipulation	Obvious soft-tissue swelling Mild instability on stress radiographs
Grade III	Complete rupture of the ligament Complete loss of function	Severe lameness Obvious swelling and pain on palpation/manipulation Crepitation Abnormal mobility	Soft-tissue swelling Avulsion fractures possible Subluxation possible Marked instability on stress radiographs

Table 14-1. Classification and clinical findings in sprain injuries

instability. These often require surgical intervention. Joint injuries in cats are often due to severe trauma, such as motor vehicle accidents and falls from a height. The high energy released with these types of injury often causes grade II or III sprains. Grade I sprains are rarely diagnosed in feline patients.

Diagnosis of joint instability or subluxation requires precise knowledge of the regional anatomy and normal range of joint motion. The joint is carefully palpated to detect pain, joint effusion, and periarticular swelling. Crepitation may be felt during manipulation. Range of motion is tested, and the joint is manipulated in order to stress the individual ligaments. The anatomy and specific tests for the individual joints are described in part 7 of this book. Routine radiographs are performed to rule out articular fractures. Stress radiographs confirm the diagnosis, and help to document the site of instability (Chapter 2) (Fig. 14-2). They are especially useful in the diagnosis of ligament sprains in joints with several joint levels, such as the carpus and tarsus. The definitive diagnosis may only be obtained at surgery.

Joint luxations are easy to diagnose as they cause marked limb deformity, swelling, pain, crepitation, changes in range of motion, and dislocations of the palpable bony prominences. Radiographs are used to confirm the diagnosis, and to rule out fractures.

A common reason for open joint trauma in cats is degloving injuries, most often seen at the tarsal and carpal joints. They may cause various degrees of collateral ligament and joint capsule damage, and cartilage and bone loss. Diagnosis of degloving injuries is obvious, but stress radiographs should be used to evaluate the exact site and degree of instability. Another common reason for open joint injuries is cat bite wounds, which often result in less obvious signs of an open joint injury. Affected cats are often only presented several days after the incident, and the small skin punctures may be difficult to detect. Instability is not usually present, but septic arthritis will cause marked pain, swelling, and joint effusion.

14.4 Principles of joint surgery

The goal of joint surgery is to restore congruity and stability of an injured joint, necessary for a normal range of motion and prevention of abnormal wear and tear. Surgery should be performed as soon as possible after injury to avoid the development of permanent changes. Knowledge of the regional anatomy, a correct diagnosis, and meticulous surgical technique are vital for success. Postoperative management is also important to achieve a good outcome after joint surgery.

14.4.1 Arthrotomy

An arthrotomy is a surgical exploration of a joint, which should include inspection of the cartilage, intra-articular structures, joint capsule, and ligaments. The incision through the joint capsule is generally performed in a longitudinal direction in order to avoid damage to the periarticular structures, particularly the ligaments. The capsular incision is started with a stab incision using a number 11 scalpel blade, taking care not to injure the underlying intra-articular structures. The incision is then elongated with scissors under visual control. Finger-held retractors such as small Meyerding, Hohmann, and Senn retractors or mini self-retaining retractors such as Gelpi's are suitable for retraction of the joint capsule, and distraction of the articular surfaces, which is necessary for adequate exposure and exploration.

Frequent irrigation of the cartilage with Ringer's solution is performed because the superficial cartilage layers are rapidly damaged when exposed to room air (3). Loose cartilage flaps and small bone fragments are removed as they do not heal and may dislodge and become free joint bodies. Meticulous hemostasis, removal of intra-articular blood clots, and flushing of the joint before closure are beneficial for postoperative healing, because the presence of blood in a joint can induce cartilage damage (4). Osteophytes or ossified bodies in the joint capsule are only removed when they seem to interfere mechanically with joint function or if they cause regional synovial inflammation. Osteophytes rapidly reform after removal. Free ossified bodies, or joint mice, are removed if possible. Partial synovectomy of a hypertrophied synovial membrane may be beneficial by reducing inflammation and pain (2).

The joint capsule is closed with fine absorbable monofilament suture material in a cruciate or continuous suture pattern. Care should be taken to place the sutures in the fibrous part of the capsule, remaining protected by the synovium, to avoid abrasion of cartilage.

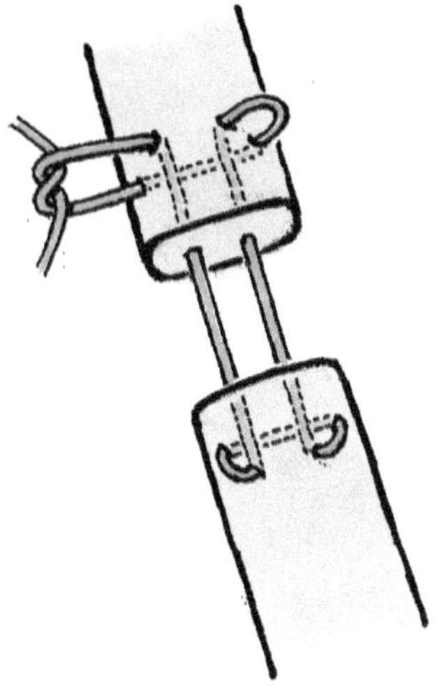

Figure 14-4 The locking-loop suture, or modified Kessler suture, is the most appropriate tension suture for repair of the small feline ligaments.

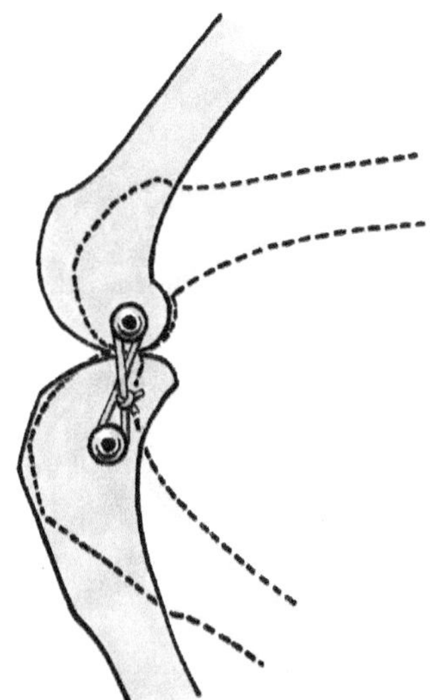

Figure 14-5 A collateral ligament prosthesis is applied to protect the ligament suture. Care has to be taken to position the screws at the anatomical attachment sites of the ligament to respect the center of motion of the joint. If the center of motion is not respected premature suture breakage is likely.

14.4.2 Treatment of ligament sprains

Grade I, or stable grade II ligament sprains can be treated conservatively. Restriction of activity is all that is needed for grade I sprains. Application of a splinted bandage for 2–3 weeks is often sufficient for minimally unstable grade II sprains. Grade II and III ligament sprains resulting in marked joint instability should be surgically stabilized in small animals, because conservative management cannot be monitored or planned as precisely as in humans, and most animals start weight-bearing soon after the injury. Although fibrous healing will ultimately result in a stable joint in most cases, prolonged joint instability would promote degenerative joint changes. Collateral ligaments are repaired primarily if possible. Intra-articular ligaments, such as the cruciate ligaments, have low healing capabilities. Their function is therefore imitated by performing extracapsular stabilization techniques. Depending on the joint involved and the stability obtained with the repair, additional postoperative immobilization may be indicated for 2–3 weeks. Fibrous healing of a ruptured ligament takes 2–3 months, and activity should be restricted during that time period.

The shredded collateral ligament ends are apposed with sutures if possible. A fine monofilament slowly absorbable suture material is usually used. The small size of the collateral ligaments in cats and frayed ligament ends may render placement of a stable suture difficult. The modified locking-loop suture pattern is most appropriate in cats (Fig. 14-4). In most cases, a collateral ligament prosthesis is also required to protect the ligament suture in the postoperative period. The ligament prosthesis consists of a figure-of-eight suture anchored between two screws, suture anchors, or bone biters (Chapter 24). Non-absorbable multifilament suture materials have good tensile resistance and knot security; they activate capsular fibrosis, but are at risk of becoming infected. They are never used in open wounds. Non-absorbable or slowly absorbable monofilament suture material usually provides sufficient stability in cats. The screws have to be placed at the anatomical insertion sites of the ligament in order to respect the center of motion of the joint (Fig. 14-5). The ligament prosthesis is subject to abnormal loads and is at risk for early breakage if it is not applied in the correct anatomical position.

Intra-articular ligaments, and the palmar and plantar ligaments of the carpus and tarsus, are not repaired primarily in cats. Function of intra-articular ligaments has to be restored by extracapsular stabilizing procedures. The short palmar and plantar ligaments of the carpus and tarsus are subject to

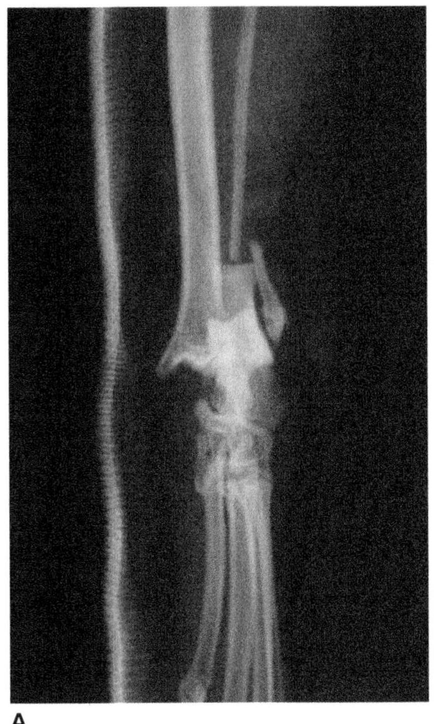

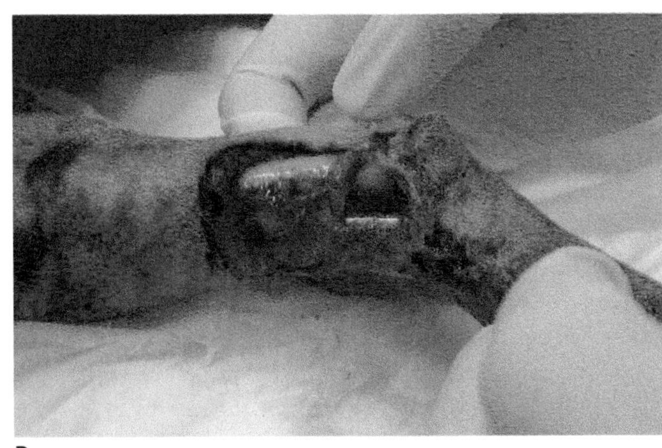

A B

Figure 14-6 A cat with an open tibiotarsal luxation.
(**A**) Radiograph of the tarsus of the cat, showing a lateral tibiotarsal luxation.
(**B**) Photograph of the tarsal area after reduction of the luxation. Skin loss, dirt and hair in the wound, and the soft-tissue defect make development of septic arthritis possible. Early and aggressive treatment can save the joint, but osteoarthritis and functional deficits are likely to develop.

large tensile forces. Primary repair and healing of these ligaments do not result in adequate stability to resist these tensile forces; therefore partial or panarthrodesis of the affected joint levels is necessary.

14.4.3 Treatment of joint luxations

Joint luxations occur if several of the joint stabilizers are disrupted, allowing complete dislocation of the adjacent articular surfaces. Two general treatment options exist: closed reduction and external immobilization, and closed or open reduction and surgical stabilization. Closed reduction and external immobilization is a possible treatment option for temporomandibular, shoulder, elbow, and hip joint luxations. All of these joints may have sufficient stability after closed reduction. The temporomandibular joint and the elbow joint have a stable bony configuration and the shoulder and hip joint have strong secondary joint stabilizers, such as tendons and muscles. Reduction is attempted as soon as possible after luxation to reduce the risk of ongoing cartilage damage due to ongoing injury and malnutrition. General anesthesia is necessary for closed reduction to achieve muscle relaxation and reduce pain.

Joints that largely depend on ligamentous support for stability have to be surgically stabilized after reduction. These include the carpal, stifle, and tarsal joints. Shoulder, elbow, or hip joint luxations may also have to be treated surgically. General indications for joint luxation surgery are unsuccessful closed reduction, immediate or delayed re-luxation, marked instability after closed reduction, and the presence of articular bone fragments or fractures. Surgical stabilization involves suturing of joint capsule tears, and repairing collateral ligaments as described above. Avulsion fractures are reattached with small Kirschner wires, or with screws if the fragments are large enough. In some cases, a transarticular external skeletal fixator or a temporary transarticular pin is inserted for postoperative immobilization. Transarticular external skeletal fixators can be applied across the elbow, carpus, stifle, and tarsus. Temporary transarticular pinning is mainly used for the stifle and hip.

14.4.4 Treatment of open joint injuries

Open joint injuries are relatively common in cats, with the tarsus being most frequently involved. Many open joint injuries in cats are caused by degloving trauma, and are heavily contaminated with hair, dirt, and commensal bacteria from the skin or intestine (Fig. 14-6). Open joint injuries are surgical emergencies. There is a high incidence of development of septic arthritis if these injuries are not treated appropriately.

Septic arthritis is a devastating condition, resulting in degeneration and even total destruction of the articular cartilage. As with open fractures, wound debridement and lavage of open joint injuries are best performed within 6–8 hours of the injury occurring. Anesthesia is usually necessary for wound debridement, and the patient should be stabilized beforehand.

Wound debridement is performed under aseptic conditions to avoid introduction of additional bacteria. The hair around the injury is clipped while the wound is protected with a sterile lubricating jelly. Obvious avascular or necrotic tissue is excised. The joint is explored, and foreign bodies and blood and fibrin clots are removed. Samples for bacterial culture and sensitivity testing are obtained. The joint is copiously lavaged with sterile Ringer's solution. It is not reported how much lavage is needed, but we suggest flushing the joints with around 0.5–1 liter. The joint is left open and a sterile wet-to-dry bandage is then applied. The bandage may either be splinted for stabilization, or a transarticular external skeletal fixator can be applied. The wound is allowed to heal by second intention. Sterile bandage changes are performed daily initially, with decreasing frequency after granulation tissue has been formed. Further flushing of the joint can also be necessary, depending on signs of persisting infection with synovial fluid cytology.

When stabilization procedures are necessary they are delayed until the whole wound is covered with a healthy-looking granulation bed. Monofilament absorbable suture material is used instead of multifilament material for collateral ligament repair in open injuries to reduce the risk of bacterial contamination. Synovial fluid cytology and bacteriology should be repeated at the time of surgery.

Prognosis largely depends on type and severity of the injury, contamination grade at admission, and development of septic arthritis. A surprisingly high level of joint function can often be achieved with adequate and aggressive treatment, although postoperative osteoarthritis will develop to different degrees in all patients.

14.5 Postoperative management of joint injuries

In contrast to fractures, postoperative immobilization is required after reconstruction of unstable joints in order to protect the surgical repair and to allow healing of periarticular tissues. Joint immobilization can be achieved with a splinted bandage, transarticular external skeletal fixator, or temporary transarticular pin, depending on the joint involved and the severity of injury. The duration of immobilization is selected according to the grade of instability, and the negative effects of postoperative immobilization on joint function have to be weighed against their positive effects of providing stability. Immobilization for a time period of 2 weeks is usually sufficient for cases with minor joint instability; 3–4 weeks may be required in severely unstable lesions. General aspects on postoperative treatment of joint injuries are provided in Chapter 20. Physiotherapy is an important adjunct to the treatment of joint injuries and is described in Chapter 21.

14.6 Complications of joint surgery

Complications after joint surgery include the development of septic arthritis and severe postoperative osteoarthritis. A certain degree of degenerative joint disease will develop after any type of severe joint trauma. Fortunately, cats are often able to compensate for mild to medium-grade osteoarthritis clinically, but severe postoperative osteoarthritis causes lameness, inactivity, reduction of range of motion, and chronic pain.

14.6.1 Post-traumatic osteoarthritis

The incidence of post-traumatic osteoarthritis is not known, but some degree of degenerative joint disease is likely to develop in most cases. Osteoarthritis can be induced by direct damage of the cartilage, by causing joint instability, and by initiating inflammatory responses in the joint. Post-traumatic osteoarthritis is characterized by cartilage degeneration and loss, joint capsule fibrosis and thickening, joint effusion, osteophyte formation, and subchondral sclerosis. Clinical signs include lameness, pain, thickening of the joint, and reduced range of motion. Cats may show marked radiographic changes with relatively few associated clinical signs. The integrity of the articular cartilage of the joint surface and the degree of capsular fibrosis are probably more important for joint function than the periarticular osteophytosis. Assessment of severity of post-traumatic osteoarthritis should therefore not be based on the radiographic changes alone.

Even after major joint trauma, the severity of post-traumatic osteoarthritis can usually be minimized to an extent, allowing good to satisfactory limb function, if the initial treatment of the traumatized joint was appropriate. Not many treatment options exist for post-traumatic osteoarthritis. Conservative management of degenerative joint disease may improve the clinical condition of the cat and is described in Chapter 5. Salvage procedures include excision arthroplasty or arthrodesis in selected cases that do not respond to medical and physical therapy. Current limb function, and morbidity and expected limb function after the salvage procedures, must be taken into account when deciding on the appropriate treatment.

14.6.2 Post-traumatic septic arthritis

Septic arthritis is a bacterial infection of joints. Hematogenous osteomyelitis is rarely encountered in cats, and is described in Chapter 5. More commonly bacteria enter the joint during trauma, surgical procedures, or possibly after arthrocentesis. Specific literature on feline post-traumatic septic arthritis is not available. The most commonly isolated organism in dogs with septic arthritis is *Staphylococcus* spp. (5), but other aerobic and anaerobic bacteria are also encountered. Infection causes rapid degradation and loss of cartilage within 1 week, fibrin deposition on cartilage surfaces, synovial inflammation, release of lysosomal enzymes, and joint instability due to infection of the joint capsule and ligamentous structures (6). The infection may ultimately invade the subchondral bones, resulting in osteomyelitis.

Animals with septic arthritis usually have marked or non-weight-bearing lameness. Affected joints are warm, swollen, and very painful. A history of recent trauma or surgery should alert the clinician to the presence of septic arthritis. If there is no history of trauma, the area around the affected joint should be carefully checked for cat bite wounds, as this is a very common cause of septic arthritis in felines (Fig. 14-7). Diagnosis is mainly based on cytological and bacteriological examination of the synovial fluid (Chapter 2). Radiological changes other than soft-tissue swelling are only seen in more chronic infections, and include subchondral bone lysis and sclerosis, periosteal new bone formation, and joint surface irregularities.

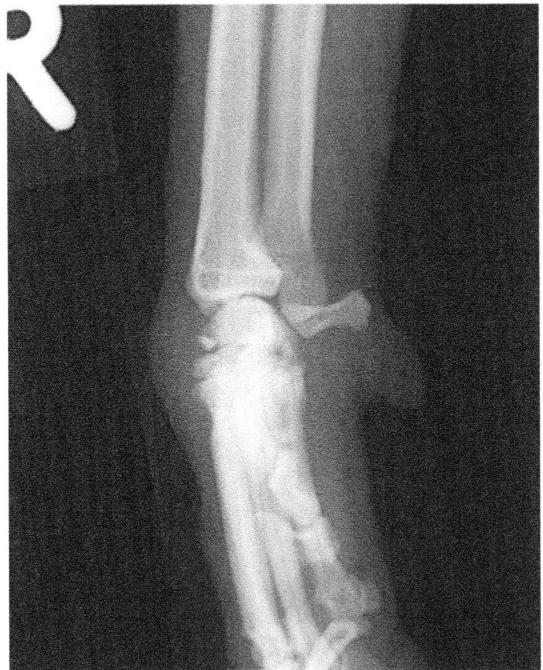

Figure 14-7 Mediolateral radiograph of the carpus of a cat with septic arthritis of the radiocarpal joint after having been bitten by another cat. There is soft-tissue swelling in the carpal area. A small radiodense structure is seen dorsal to the radial carpal bone; this proved to be a small piece of tooth at surgery.

Post-traumatic septic arthritis should be considered an orthopedic emergency. Immediate treatment is instituted, as the degree of joint destruction and the prognosis largely depend on the duration of infection. Broad-spectrum antibiotics, such as the combination of amoxicillin and clavulanic acid, or cephalosporins, are administered intravenously immediately after the sample for bacteriological testing has been taken. Aggressive joint lavage is the most important part of the treatment, and has the goal of reducing bacterial numbers in the joint (7). Joints with septic arthritis following injuries or surgical procedures usually need to be opened and explored. Blood clots, foreign bodies, and fibrin layers are removed. The joint is then copiously flushed, preferably with sterile Ringer's solution. The joint capsule is usually closed, but it may be left open for drainage in severe cases or if tissue is missing.

Especially joints with more chronic infections often need to be flushed several times. This is usually performed every second day until the infection has cleared. Repeated arthroscopic flushing with large amounts of Ringer's solution is currently considered the best treatment in human medicine (8), but is often not instituted in cats due to the small size of joints or lack of arthroscopic equipment. Instead, the joint can be flushed using large-diameter needles, or an ingress–egress drainage system can be instituted. Lavage can then be performed continuously, or 2–3 times daily. Once the synovial fluid seems more normal from visual assessment, cytology and bacteriology are repeated. Flushing is stopped when these tests indicate resolution of infection. Oral antibiotics are selected according to the bacteriological results and sensitivity and are administered for a time period of 4–6 weeks.

Prognosis depends on the amount of cartilage destruction. In a study of dogs with septic arthritis, most responded well to treatment, and were free of septic arthritis at follow-up (5). Such information is not available for cats, but based on clinical experience most articular infections resolve with aggressive joint lavage and appropriate antimicrobial treatment. Prognosis for joint function is variable, and depends on the duration of infection and the degree of cartilage destruction (7).

14.7 Principles of arthrodesis

Arthrodesis is a permanent surgically induced fusion of a joint. It is a salvage procedure and is only performed if other treatments do not result in pain relief or joint stability. Indications for arthrodesis may include comminuted joint fractures, open joint luxations with traumatic destruction of cartilage, severe disabling degenerative joint disease, selected ligamentous injuries, and some neurological dysfunctions. Arthrodesis is not commonly performed in cats, but has been described for the elbow joint, carpal joint, and tarsal joint (9–12). In joints with several joint levels, such as the carpal and tarsal joint, either panarthrodesis or partial arthrodesis can be performed. Partial arthrodesis preserves most joint motion but is a treatment option only if the antebrachiocarpal, or the tarsocrural joint, is intact.

The goal of arthrodesis is to fuse a joint at a physiological angle and to prepare the joint to achieve rapid fusion. The implants are subject to cycling and may break prematurely if fusion progresses too slowly. It is also beneficial to apply the implants on the tension side, if anatomically possible, to reduce the risk of implant breakage.

Before surgery, the standing angle of the joint is measured on the contralateral limb. Joints are fused at an angle slightly more flexed than physiological to facilitate ambulation. All of the joint cartilage has to be debrided, using a burr or a small bone curette. Osteostixis is performed with a small drill bit to create vascular channels through the subchondral bone. Cancellous or corticocancellous bone graft (Chapter 13) is placed into the joint spaces. The two bones are then rigidly stabilized, ideally under compression. Long-enough implants should be used in order to prevent iatrogenic fractures at the end of the implants. Plates are used in most circumstances, but arthrodesis with Kirschner wires, transarticular screws, and external fixators has also been described (10, 13). External skeletal fixators are a good option in the presence of open wounds. Additional cancellous or corticocancellous bone graft is placed around the joint before closure of the wound.

A splinted bandage is applied postoperatively for 4–6 weeks. Bony fusion can be expected after 3–4 months. It seems beneficial to remove plates after fusion is completed to reduce the risk of fractures at the plate ends and because low-grade infection may be present. Outcome depends on the joint involved. Cats ambulate relatively well after carpal and tarsal arthrodeses, although a slight gait abnormality is usually noted (11, 12). Most successful outcome after elbow arthrodesis seems to depend on the flexion angle (10). Complications include failure to fuse, premature implant loosening or breakage, angular and rotational deformities due to incorrect positioning of the joint, and infection. Failure to fuse is often due to inadequate debridement of the joint surfaces. The incidence of complications after stifle arthrodesis in four cats was also high, with a tibial fracture and a femoral fracture occurring in two cases (Langley-Hobbs, unpublished data). Amputation may be a preferable option to arthrodesis in the elbow and stifle, high-motion joints, giving cats a more functional outcome.

References and further reading

1. Vanwanseele B. et al. The effects of immobilization on the characteristics of articular cartilage: current concepts and future directions. Osteoarthritis Cartilage 2002;10:408–419.
2. Piermattei DL, Flo GL. Principles of joint surgery. In: Piermattei DL, Flo GL (eds) Small animal orthopedics and fracture repair, 3rd edn. Philadelphia: WB Saunders; 1997: pp. 201–217.
3. Mitchell N, Shepard N. The deleterious effects of drying on articular cartilage. J Bone Joint Surg Br 1989;71:89–95.
4. Roosendaal G. et al. Blood-induced joint damage: a canine in vivo study. Arthritis Rheum 1999;42:1033–1039.
5. Marchevsky AM, Read RA. Bacterial septic arthritis in 19 dogs. Aust Vet J 1999;77:233–237.
6. Roy S, Bhawan J. Ultrastructure of articular cartilage in pyogenic arthritis. Arch Pathol 1975;99:44–47.
7. Bubenik LR. Infections of the skeletal system. Vet Clin North Am Small Anim Pract 2005;35:1093–1109.
8. Bonnaire F, et al. Bakterielle Gelenkinfektion. OP J 2005; 21:232–239.
9. DeCamp C, et al. Pantarsal arthrodesis in dogs and a cat: 11 cases. J Am Vet Med Assoc 1993;203:1705–1707.
10. Moak PC, et al. Arthrodesis of the elbow in three cats. Vet Comp Orthop Traumatol 2000;13:149–153.
11. Vannini R. Tarsal panarthrodesis. In: Proceedings of the BSAVA Meeting, Birmingham, 1998.
12. Simpson D, Goldsmid S. Pancarpal arthrodesis in a cat: a case report and anatomical study. Vet Comp Orthop Traumatol 1994;7:45–50.
13. Willer RL, et al. Partial carpal arthrodesis for third degree carpal sprains – a review of 45 carpi. Vet Surg 1990;19:334–340.

15 Injuries of the spine, spinal cord, and peripheral nerves

K. Voss, F. Steffen

Neurological injuries occur relatively frequently in the cat. Spinal fractures and luxations account for 6% of all fractures at the Vetsuisse Faculty of the University of Zurich. Half of the lesions are localized at the sacrococcygeal spine. Spinal cord injury may also be caused by traumatic disc extrusion. Although less frequent than spinal cord injury, trauma to the peripheral nerves is also seen, and may occur with or without concurrent orthopedic lesions.

General considerations and principles of spinal trauma and surgery are covered in the following chapter. The most common peripheral nerve injuries are also described. Diseases of the spine or spinal cord and neuromuscular diseases are important differential diagnoses in cats with neurological dysfunction, because the traumatic incident is often not directly observed. Neurological diseases are described in Chapter 6.

15.1 Injuries of the spine and spinal cord

Injuries of the spinal column include spinal fractures, luxations, and traumatic disc extrusion. The resulting neurological deficits allow clinical localization of the lesion, and are the most important prognostic factors. An understanding of both the pathophysiological events that occur after acute spinal cord trauma and the biomechanics of the spinal column is important for making treatment decisions and estimating the prognosis for return to function.

15.1.1 Structure and function of the spine and spinal cord

The spinal cord consists of eight cervical, 13 thoracic, seven lumbar, three sacral, and approximately seven coccygeal segments. Dorsal and ventral nerve roots emerge from each spinal cord segment, leaving the vertebral canal at their corresponding vertebral foramen after having fused to form a segmental spinal nerve. Clinically, the most important nerve roots are the ones that form the brachial and pelvic plexuses. The nerves of the brachial plexus supply the front limbs, and the nerves of the pelvic plexus the hindlimbs, the bladder, the rectum, and the perineal region (Chapter 1). The medullary cone of the spinal cord extends more caudally in cats than in dogs, terminating at the level of the vertebral body of S1 in most cats (1, 2).

The normal feline spine allows for a high degree of dorsiflexion, ventroflexion, and torsion. Lateral bending is possible to a lesser degree. The upper thoracic and cervical vertebrae have the highest degree of dorsiflexion, enabling extensive movement of the head and neck, particularly important in grooming behavior and hunting (3). The lower thoracic and lumbar spine is particularly designed for ventroflexion (3). Ventroflexion of the thoracolumbar spine is caused by contraction of the ventrally located psoas minor, iliopsoas, and quadratus lumborum muscles, and is important for sitting, locomotion, and jumping. The physiological range of motion of the feline spine in torsion is large, reaching almost 180° at the mid-thoracic region (3).

Intervening soft-tissue structures allow high motion in the spine while both the soft-tissue and osseous structures are responsible for spinal stability. The anulus fibrosus is highly resistant against tensile forces, and prevents excessive bending and torsional movements. The intervertebral discs have been shown to be the most important stabilizers against torsion in vitro (4). The articular facets with their joint capsule provide rotational stability on the dorsal side of the spine. Traumatic or iatrogenic disruption of the anulus fibrosus, together with fractures or luxations of the articular facets, therefore causes significant rotational instability. The supra- and interspinous ligaments are important in preventing hyperflexion (5). Hyperflexion is also restricted by the vertebral bodies, which act as a ventral buttress. The dorsal and ventral longitudinal ligaments and the ligamentum flavum contribute to spinal stability to a lesser degree.

15.1.2 Pathophysiology of acute spinal cord injury

Acute extradural spinal cord compression and injury occur after spinal fractures and luxations, and with traumatic disc extrusions. Trauma to the spinal cord results in both direct and indirect injury mechanisms (6). Direct injury involves contusion, tearing, or crushing of nervous tissue. Trauma and compression further initiate a cascade of secondary injury mechanisms, including ischemia of the spinal cord, raised intraneuronal calcium, and free radical-induced lipid peroxidation, resulting in alterations in spinal cord blood flow and swelling of the spinal cord (6). These secondary injury mechanisms happen within a short time of the injury, and eventually cause additional irreversible damage to the nervous tissue. Progressive myelomalacia is an ascending necrosis of the spinal cord and is the most severe form of the secondary injury mechanisms.

Differentiation between irreversible and reversible damage to the spinal cord is not always possible with the clinical examination and diagnostic imaging techniques available. It is important to realize that many of the neurological deficits due to secondary injury mechanisms are reversible, if decompression of the spinal cord is conducted early enough in the disease process. Stabilization of vertebral body fractures is also necessary to prevent further damage to the spinal cord. In contrast, neurological deficits caused by direct injury and disruption of the nervous tissue are irreversible. Vertebral fractures and luxations tend to cause more direct damage to the spinal cord than do other forms of extradural spinal cord compression that occur more slowly and with less energy.

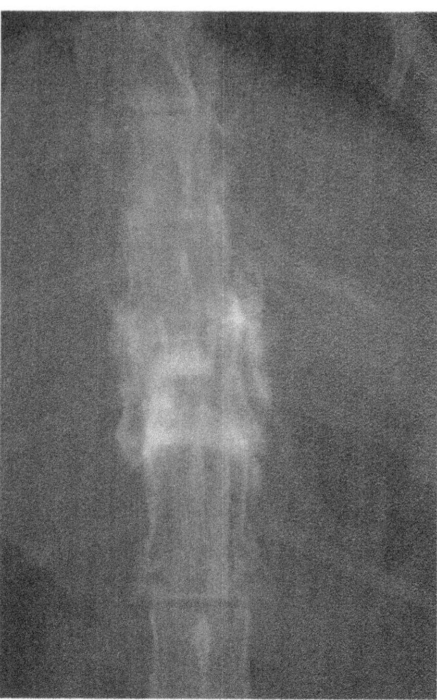

Figure 15-1 Myelography of a cat with a comminuted vertebral body fracture of T12. Leakage of the contrast medium from the intradural space indicates disruption of the dura mater. These patients can be expected to have sustained severe, irreversible spinal cord damage.

15.1.3 Diagnosis of spinal and spinal cord injuries

The mainstay of diagnosis is the clinical neurological examination (Chapter 1). The goals of the neurological examination are localization of the lesion, and assessment of the severity of the injury. A grading system for extramedullary spinal cord compression, based on severity of the neurological deficits, is listed in Table 6-2 (Chapter 6). Cats with suspected fractures or luxations of the spine should be manipulated as little as possible during examination to prevent further injury to the spinal cord by dislodging unstable vertebral segments during manipulation.

Radiographs are obtained after clinical localization of the lesion. Spinal radiography usually requires general anesthesia to enable correct positioning of the patient. However general anesthesia reduces muscle tone, and may increase spinal instability. Therefore, cats with suspected spinal instability should be manipulated as carefully as possible while positioning for radiography. Both a laterolateral and ventrodorsal view should be obtained. Consideration should be made to taking horizontal beam views if there are concerns about turning the patient for taking ventrodorsal radiographs. Spinal fractures and luxations are usually readily visible on radiographs, but some lesions are only displaced minimally and diagnosis requires careful examination of each vertebra and orthogonal radiographs. Traumatic disc herniation is suspected in the presence of narrowing of an intervertebral space or subluxation of vertebrae.

It is important to note that the vertebral displacement visible on radiographs is not of prognostic value. The correlation between vertebral displacement and the neurological state of the patient has been reported as poor (7). Radiographs only provide a static record of the position of the vertebrae and fragments, and the grade of dislocation sustained during injury is likely to be underestimated on radiographs. The severity of a spinal fracture and luxation should therefore be assessed based on the grade of neurological deficits present.

Additional diagnostic imaging procedures useful for assessment of spinal injuries include myelography, magnetic resonance imaging (MRI), or computed tomography (Chapter 2). Myelography or MRI is indicated in the diagnostic work-up of suspected traumatic disc extrusions. These imaging modalities can also be used to obtain further information for spinal fractures where the radiographic findings do not match the clinical localization of the lesion or its severity, if multiple lesions are seen on radiographs and their clinical significance is not clear, and if additional information is necessary for planning a surgical procedure. Myelography and MRI may also give additional information regarding the prognosis by demonstrating disruption of the dura mater and spinal cord in cases with severe neurological deficits (Fig. 15-1). A computed tomography scan can provide further information on exact fracture configuration.

15.1.4 Spinal fractures and luxations

Spinal fractures and luxations occur after motor vehicle accidents, and falls from a height in most cats. Cats with spinal fractures and luxations frequently sustain concurrent injuries. A thorough clinical examination and full-body radiographs should therefore be performed in every cat with a spinal fracture or luxation.

Hyperflexion, axial compression, rotation, and hyperextension are the principal forces causing a spinal fracture or luxation. A combination of these forces is usually present in clinical cases (Fig. 15-2). Fracture/luxation configuration is a result of the type and direction of the forces applied during the trauma. Understanding the biomechanics of spinal fractures and luxations helps to assess the spinal instability radiologically.

Endplate fractures are the most common spinal fracture type in cats (8) (Fig. 15-3). These simple fractures of the vertebral bodies can be relatively stable injuries, but if simultaneous trauma to the dorsal compartment is present, the lesions should be considered unstable. Concurrent injuries to the dorsal compartment include rupture of the supra- and interspinal ligaments, and/or fractures of the articular facets. Concurrent trauma to the articular facets is common, although not always detectable on radiographs (9). Endplate fractures with vertebral subluxation are likely to have been caused by rotational and ventral bending forces.

Fractures through the vertebral bodies are not as common in cats. They result from ventral bending and/or axial compression forces, and can be simple or comminuted. Varying degrees of concurrent dorsal compartment injury may occur (Fig. 15-4). The lack of a ventral buttress results in ventral bending instability. These injuries should be stabilized surgically.

Vertebral subluxations and luxations occur after disruption of the anulus fibrosus of the intervertebral disc, and fractures and/or luxations of the articular facets (Fig. 15-5). These

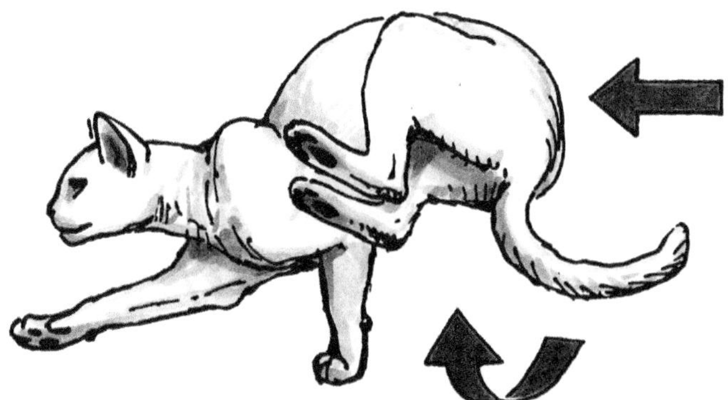

Figure 15-2 Vertebral fractures are commonly caused by a combination of external forces, such as hyperflexion, axial compression, and rotation of the spine.

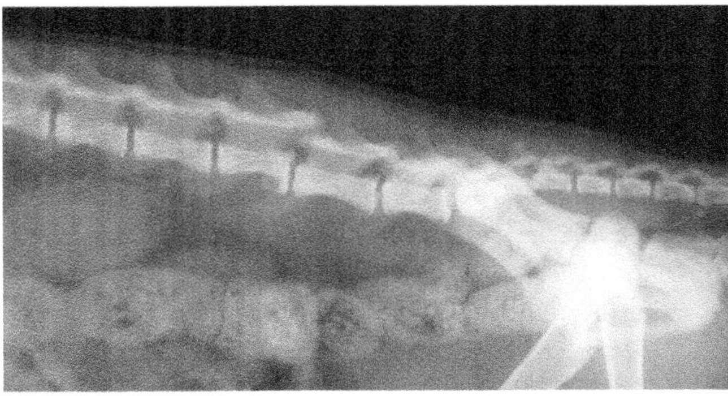

A

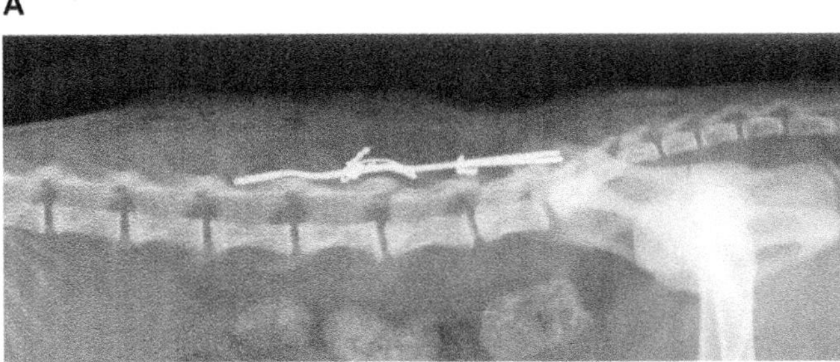

B

Figure 15-3 Cat with an endplate fracture of L5.
(**A**) Laterolateral radiograph shows an endplate fracture of L5 with L5/L6 subluxation. A fragment is visible in the dorsal aspect of the spinal canal, possibly an avulsion fracture of the facet joints. The facet joint space is enlarged. This injury should be considered unstable because both the dorsal and ventral compartment is affected.
(**B**) Postoperative radiograph showing reduction and stabilization of the L5/L6 lesion using a dorsal tension band technique.

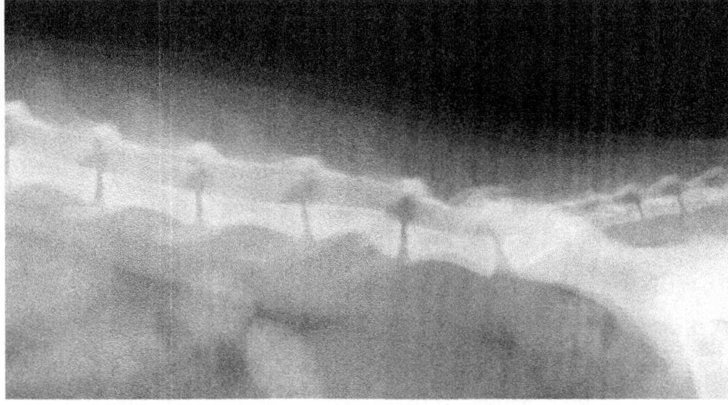

A

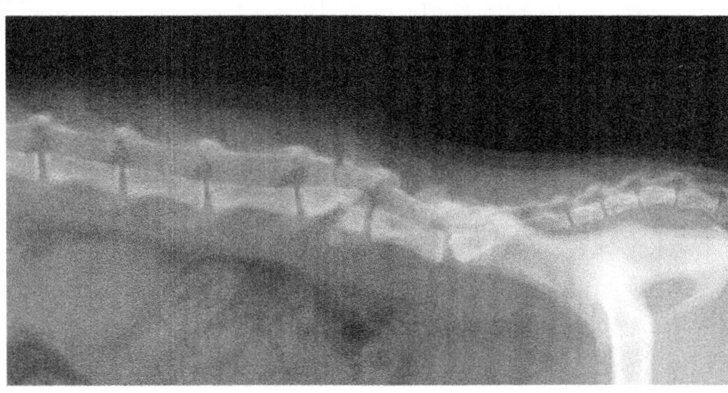

B

Figure 15-4 Cat with an oblique fracture through the vertebral body of C6 with concurrent fracture of the dorsal spinous process and dorsal lamina.
(**A**) Laterolateral radiograph taken at admission. Because the fracture was only minimally displaced, conservative therapy was chosen.
(**B**) Laterolateral radiograph 3 weeks after the injury. The neurological status of the cat had not improved, and radiographs show further displacement of the fragments, and callus formation. This unstable lesion should have been stabilized surgically.

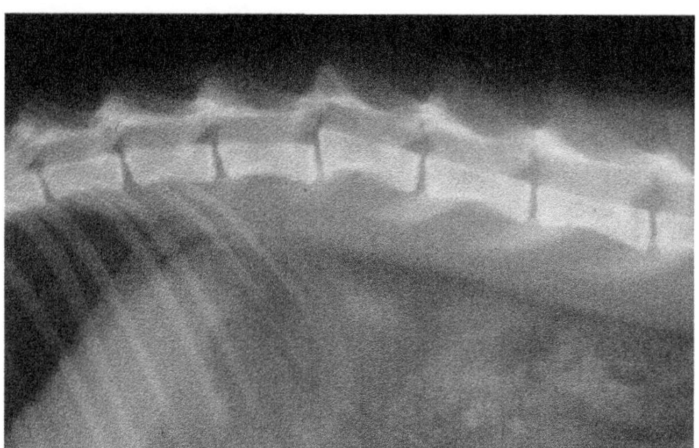

Figure 15-5 Cat with a vertebral luxation between L1 and L2. The lumen of the spinal canal is occluded by approximately 50%. Open reduction and internal stabilization are required.

injuries are predominantly caused by rotational forces, and should be considered rotationally unstable.

Isolated injuries of the dorsal compartment are rare, but could result from hyperextension injury, or from direct trauma, such as dog bite wounds. Isolated dorsal compartment fractures are usually stable injuries, but may cause dorsal compression of the spinal cord.

Although successful conservative management of spinal fractures and luxations has been described (8, 10), surgical stabilization of a spinal fracture/luxation is indicated in all cats exhibiting marked neurological deficits and/or unstable lesions in the authors' opinion. Conservative treatment of unstable lesions is likely to result in delayed healing and a prolonged period of pain, and carries the risk of further displacement of the fragments (Fig. 15-4). Additionally, excessive callus formation may result in secondary spinal cord compression. In one study only 18% of cats with grade 3 neurological deficits treated conservatively recovered neurologically, versus 71% of surgically treated cases (11).

The severity of neurological deficits may influence the treatment decision. In general, the prognosis is excellent in cats with sustained motor function, and good to moderate in paraplegic cats without loss of deep pain sensation. The prognosis for patients with loss of deep pain sensation is grave in the presence of fractures or luxations, because loss of deep pain is usually due to direct irreversible spinal cord damage. Such patients should be euthanized. Myelography, MRI, or exploratory hemilaminectomy with durotomy may reveal spinal cord transection or myelomalacia, and can aid in the decision process in unclear or borderline cases (Fig. 15-1).

15.1.5 Traumatic disc extrusion

Acute disc herniations may occur spontaneously (Chapter 6) or secondary to trauma. Traumatic disc extrusion involves rupture of the anulus fibrosus secondary to external injury, allowing the normal nucleus pulposus to herniate into the spinal canal. The nucleus tends to extrude explosively in traumatic cases, resulting in significant spinal cord contusion and myelomalacia (8).

Traumatic disc extrusion can accompany other spinal injuries or may occur as a single problem. It should be suspected in cats with a history or likelihood of trauma that show neurological deficits in the absence of radiologically visible fractures or luxations. The main findings on myelography are intramedullary swelling or epidural contrast medium leakage (12). Extradural compression is usually not visible, as the extruded disc material is soft and unmineralized, and it tends to spread out within the medullary canal. An MRI helps in obtaining the diagnosis. Definitive diagnosis and differentiation between spontaneous and traumatic disc herniation are sometimes only possible intraoperatively. Rupture of the anulus fibrosus, hematoma formation in the area, and the presence of non-degenerate nucleus pulposus in the spinal canal are compatible with a diagnosis of traumatic disc extrusion.

Surgical exploration of the spinal canal and decompression of the spinal cord are indicated if traumatic disc herniation is suspected. Large ruptures of the anulus fibrosus may result in spinal instability. Rotational instability is a particular concern, even more so in the presence of concurrent fractures or luxation of the articular facets, or if the articular facets are removed during decompression procedures. Unstable segments should be stabilized. Cats with grade IV or V neurological deficits may benefit from concurrent medical treatment (Chapter 6). The prognosis for traumatic disc extrusions is good to excellent if deep pain sensation is present (8). Prognosis for patients with disc extrusions and loss of deep pain sensation is questionable, but there is a fair chance for recovery if treatment is instituted within the first hours after the onset of clinical signs.

15.2 Principles of spinal surgery

The two main goals of spinal surgery are decompression of the spinal cord and stabilization of the spinal column. Treatment decision-making and principles of decompressive surgery and stabilization procedures are summarized in the following section.

15.2.1 Decompression

Neurosurgery in cats requires meticulous surgical technique. The spinal cord diameter is relatively large compared to the diameter of the spinal canal, leaving little epidural space to work in. Good lighting is necessary, and the use of magnification is also beneficial. Bipolar electrocautery should be used.

Instruments used for performing spinal surgery in cats include small Gelpi self-retaining retractors, a Freer periosteal elevator, blunt and pointed scrapers and nerve hooks, curettes, and fine rongeurs.

Hemilaminectomies and pediculectomies can both be performed with an electric or pneumatic burr, or with fine rongeurs, such as micro-Friedman, small Kerrison, and/or synovectomy rongeurs. The rongeurs must be used very carefully in order to prevent iatrogenic spinal cord damage during insertion of the instrument into the narrow epidural space. Manipulation of fracture fragments or disc material within the spinal canal can be performed with fine blunt or pointed nerve hooks or scrapers, or with the tip of small Halsted hemostatic forceps. Care is taken not to injure the venous plexus with the instruments, because significant bleeding may result. Several methods for hemostasis can be used if bleeding occurs: a small piece of muscle can be excised and placed in the area of bleeding, commercially available hemostyptic products such as surgical cellulose can be used, or an ice-cold isotonic solution can be poured into the surgical wound. Ice-cold solutions work well, but it is crucial to monitor body temperature and keep the cat warm.

Decompression is not required for all spinal fractures/luxations, because in many cases indirect decompression occurs with reduction of the fractures or luxations. The different decompression techniques are described in more detail in Chapter 34.

15.2.2 Stabilization

Surgical stabilization of the spine is indicated for all unstable spinal fractures and luxations. Assessment of stability based on radiographic findings is difficult because soft-tissue stabilizers, such as the supra- and interspinous ligaments, and the anulus fibrosus are not visible. However, the type of fracture and the degree of displacement do allow some assessment to be made of the stability of the lesion (see sections above). Fracture reduction and stabilization will restore integrity and width of the spinal canal, prevent further spinal cord injury, allow faster healing without excessive callus formation, reduce pain, and permit a faster return to function.

The small size of the feline vertebrae and the thin lamina and spinous processes limit the implants that can be used for repair to small, relatively flexible implants that are appropriate to the bone size and strength. Most thoracolumbar fractures and luxations can be stabilized with dorsal stapling techniques, using small-diameter Kirschner wires and orthopedic wire. The dorsal tension band fixation, a modification of spinal stapling, was shown to be a suitable technique for most thoracolumbar fractures in cats (Fig. 15-3) (9). The use of other implants, such as internal fixators, or pins and polymethylmethacrylate, may be necessary in cervical or certain caudal lumbar fractures. Techniques for stabilization of specific spinal fractures and luxations are described in Chapter 34.

15.3 Traumatic neuropathy

Peripheral neuropathy of traumatic origin is the most common cause of peripheral nerve damage in small animals. Injury results from mechanical blows, fractures, pressure, gunshot wounds, surgical injury/implants, and stretching (13). Mechanical injury can induce temporary or permanent motor and sensory deficits, depending on the site of the lesion and likelihood of functional repair (Chapter 1). Three fundamental types of nerve injuries can be identified but, in most spontaneous injuries, a combination of these should be expected.

A localized conduction block without structural damage is present in neuropraxia. Recovery occurs within days to weeks. The axon is severed but the endoneural sheath is preserved in axonotmesis. Recovery occurs after weeks to months. The nerve is completely transected and spontaneous recovery is unlikely to occur in neurotmesis. Axonal regeneration occurs at a rate of 1–4 mm/day, depending on the specific nature of the nerve. Axonal regrowth is limited to a period of 4 months. This equals an approximate distance of 10–15 cm that can be bridged within this time. If reinnervation of a muscle has not occurred within this period of time or the distance to the target muscle is longer than 10–15 cm, recovery is unlikely (14). Additionally, irreversible damage to the receptors at the denervated muscles occurs after 6–9 months (15). The majority of peripheral nerve injuries are associated with pelvic fractures. Injury to other nerves such as the radial nerve with humeral fractures is less common.

15.3.1 Brachial plexus avulsion

This type of traumatic nerve lesion is common in cats. It results from severe abduction and/or traction of the thoracic limb. Avulsion of the ventral nerve roots is the most common form of brachial plexus injury, probably due to a lack of a perineurium at this site. The sensory nerve roots seem to be more resistant to traction, and therefore there may be some inconsistency in the patterns of motor and sensory deficits. In acute, complete avulsions of the brachial plexus, the clinical picture includes monoplegia with dragging of the foot, a dropped elbow, and absence of spinal reflexes and deep pain response in all dermatomes. If the nerve roots of C8–T3 are involved there may be an ipsilateral Horner's syndrome and lack of a cutaneous trunci reflex (Fig. 15-6). Proprioceptive deficits may be present in the ipsilateral rear limb in cases where the nerve roots are torn out of the spinal cord. In chronic cases, the affected forelimb can become rigid

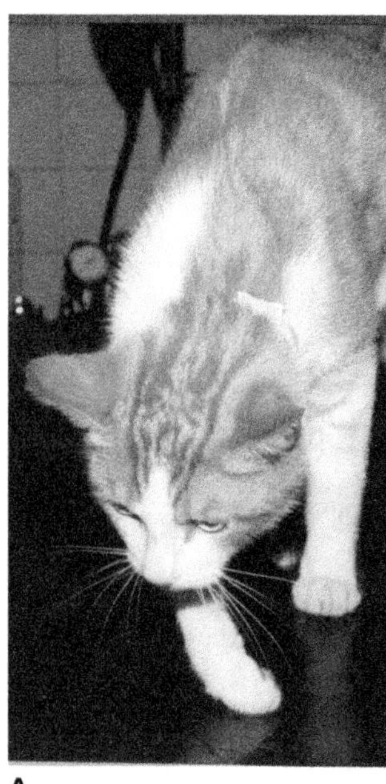
A

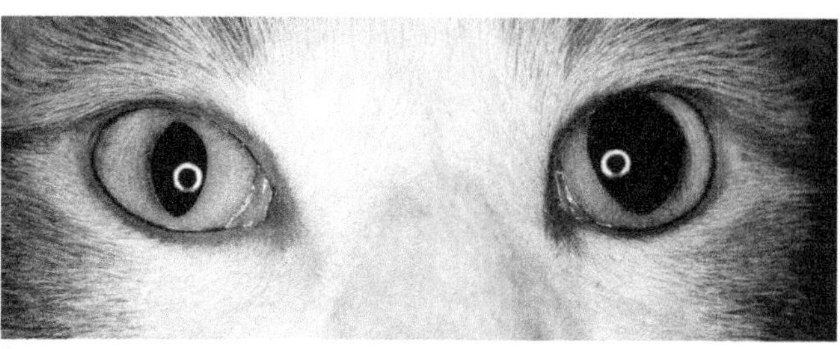
B

Figure 15-6 (**A**) Cat with traumatic avulsion of the nerve roots of the brachial plexus, resulting in lower motor neuron monoparesis of the right forelimb. (**B**) Also note signs of ipsilateral Horner's syndrome: miosis, ptosis, and protrusion of the third eyelid.

due to muscle fibrosis and immobile elbow and carpal joints.

In incomplete lesions of nerve roots, motor and sensory function may be retained in some myo- and dermatomes. Weight-bearing function of the limb is preserved if only the cranial nerve roots are involved in the avulsion. Further diagnostic procedures should include electrophysiological testing. The use of electromyelography (EMG) to confirm the diagnosis is very useful if performed at least 7 days after the injury (Chapter 2). Serial nerve conduction studies of the radial nerve can provide valuable prognostic information.

In general, the prognosis for brachial plexus injury is poor for functional return of the limb. If the nerve roots are avulsed there is no chance of improvement, but some degree of recovery may occur if the roots are still intact. Resorption of hematomas and edema may contribute to restoration of axonal function in the nerve roots. In animals that show no improvement within a 1–2-month period, the prognosis is considered to be hopeless for recovery of limb function.

The main complications of brachial plexus injuries include contracture of joints due to muscle fibrosis, abrasions of the foot, trophic ulcers, and paresthesias and resultant self-mutilation. Attempts to lessen the effects of the injury include tendon relocation directed at providing extension of the elbow and carpus, and carpal arthrodesis. However, the success of these techniques is questionable. Surgical reinnervation of avulsed and reimplanted ventral rootlets in the cervical spinal cord, and reinnervation by nerve transfers was successful in experimental settings (16, 17), but limb amputation is often the most practical course of action for severe injuries.

15.3.2 Injury to the lumbosacral plexus

Nerve structures lying close to the pelvis are the most common sites for serious nerve injury. These nerves include the ventral branches of nerve roots L6, L7, and S1, and the lumbosacral trunk, including the intrapelvic portion of the sciatic nerve. The sciatic nerve has been reported to be injured in 11% of cats with pelvic fractures (18). Craniomedial displacement of ilial fractures and cranial displacement of sacroiliac luxations are most likely to cause nerve trauma (19) (Fig. 15-7).

Clinically, the signs of injury to these structures can be largely identical but vary with severity of injury. Paralysis and hyporeflexia resulting in knuckling and dragging of the limb are the most obvious features. Neurogenic loss of muscle mass occurs within a few days of denervation. EMG mapping of muscle denervation helps to confirm the level of the injury in cats with a sciatic-type deficit due to pelvic fractures (Chapter 2). If the lesion involves the L6 spinal nerve and the lumbosacral trunk (gluteal and obturator nerves), denervation will occur in muscles supplied by both nerves. In a lesion affecting the extrapelvic portion of the sciatic nerve, pathological EMG activity will be observed only in the sciatic myotomes distal to the lesion.

Recommendations as to whether to perform internal fixation of pelvic fractures and sacroiliac joint fracture/luxations should be followed according to orthopedic principles and guidelines (Chapter 35). Cats with pelvic fractures and sciatic nerve deficits should undergo exploratory surgery and fracture stabilization. The sciatic nerve roots course ventromedial to the sacroiliac joint, and they may become entrapped or damaged with sacroiliac fracture/luxations. The nerve roots

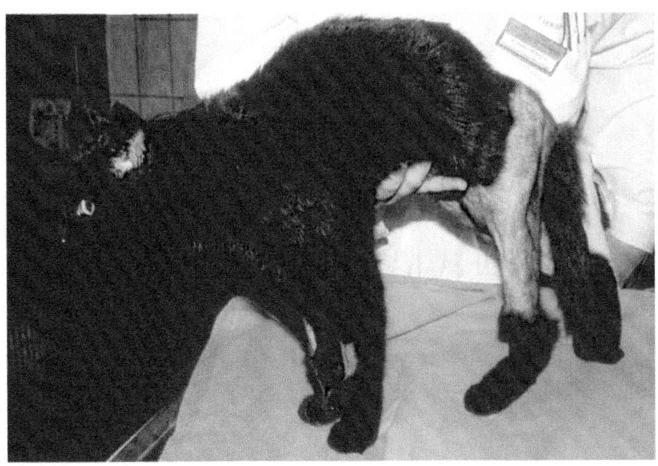

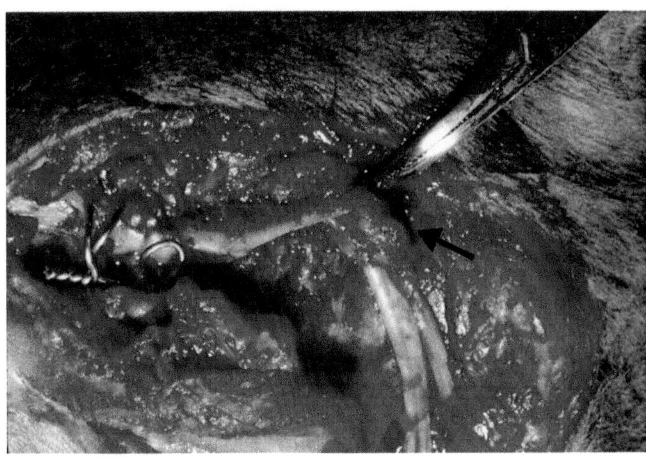

A B

Figure 15-7 Cat with sciatic nerve damage after failed surgical correction of a fractured ilial shaft.
(**A**) Note hypotrophy of the hamstring muscles and the plantigrade stance of the left hindlimb, indicating sciatic nerve deficits.
(**B**) Postmortem examination of the sciatic nerve. The sharp edge of the fractured ilial shaft has injured the sciatic nerve after failure of an inadequate fracture fixation with pin and wires. Note the extensive formation of fibrous tissue around the nerve (arrow). Extension of fibroblasts into the nerve is associated with conduction block and questionable functional recovery even after surgical release.

are best explored using an abdominal approach but a lateral approach to the pelvis is preferable if sciatic nerve trauma is suspected to result from an ilial or ischial fracture. Surgery will allow visualization of the injured nerve, but simple anastomosis is not feasible in crush or traction injuries. Successful use of a saphenous nerve graft was described for the treatment of sciatic neurotmesis in a dog (20). Overall, 81% of 34 dogs and cats had an excellent or good recovery of neurological deficits following pelvic fractures (19). Limb amputation is indicated in cases with permanent paralysis to prevent morbidity caused by muscle contractures, abrasion and ulcers on the feet, and paresthesia.

References and further reading

1. Kot W, et al. Anatomical survey of the cat's lumbosacral spinal cord. Prog Vet Neurol 1994;5:162–166.
2. Frewein J, Vollmerhaus, B. Anatomie von Hund und Katze. Berlin: Blackwell; 1994.
3. Macpherson JM, Ye Y. The cat vertebral column: stance configuration and range of motion. Exp Brain Res 1998;119:324–332.
4. Shires PK, et al. A biomechanical study of rotational instability in unaltered and surgically altered canine thoracolumbar vertebral motion units. Prog Vet Neurol 1991;2:6–14.
5. Smith GK, Walter MC. Spinal decompressive procedures and dorsal compartment injuries: comparative biomechanical study in canine cadavers. Am J Vet Res 1988;49:266–273.
6. Caughlan AR. Secondary injury mechanisms in acute spinal cord trauma. J Small Anim Pract 1993;34:117–122.
7. McKee WM. Spinal trauma in dogs and cats: a review of 51 cases. Vet Rec 1990;126:285–289.
8. Grasmueck S, Steffen F. Survival rates and outcomes in cats with thoracic and lumbar spinal cord injuries due to external trauma. J Small Anim Pract 2004;45:284–288.
9. Voss K, Montavon PM. Tension band stabilization of fractures and luxations of the thoracolumbar spine in dogs and cats: 38 cases (1993–2002). J Am Vet Med Assoc 2004;225:78–83.
10. Selcer RR, et al. Management of vertebral column fractures in dogs and cats: 211 cases (1977–1985). J Am Vet Med Assoc 1991;198:1965–1968.
11. Besalti O, et al. Management of spinal trauma in 69 cats. Dtsch Tierarztl Wochenschr 2002;109:315–320.
12. Montavon PM, et al. What is your diagnosis? Swelling of spinal cord associated with dural tear between segments T13 and L1. J Am Vet Med Assoc 1990;196:783–784.
13. Forterre F, et al. Periphere Nervenerkrankungen: Teil I Monoparese, -plegie bei Hund und Katze: Retrospektive Studie über 94 Fälle. Kleintierpraxis 2003;48:125–184.
14. Welch JA. Peripheral nerve injury. Semin Vet Med Surg 1996;11:273–284.
15. Chrisman CL. Peripheral neuropathies. In: Bojrab MJ (ed.) Disease mechanisms in small animal surgery. Philadelphia: Lea & Febiger; 1993: pp. 1158–1173.
16. Hoffmann CF, et al. Reinnervation of avulsed and reimplanted ventral rootlets in the cervical spinal cord of the cat. J Neurosurg 1996;84:234–243.
17. Moissonnier P, et al. Restoration of elbow flexion by performing contralateral lateral thoracic and thoracodorsal nerve transfers after experimental musculocutaneous nerve transection. J Neurosurg 2005;103:70–78.
18. Bookbinder PF, Flanders JA. Characteristics of pelvic fracture in the cat. Vet Comp Orthop Traumatol 1992;5:122–127.
19. Jacobson A, Schrader SC. Peripheral nerve injury associated with fracture or fracture-dislocation of the pelvis in dogs and cats: 34 cases (1978–1982). J Am Vet Med Assoc 1987;190: 569–572.
20. Granger N, et al. Cutaneous saphenous nerve graft for the treatment of sciatic neurotmesis in a dog. J Am Vet Med Assoc 2006;229:82–86.

16 Soft-tissue injuries

K. Voss

While injuries to the deeper soft tissues, including muscle and tendons, are relatively infrequent in cats, skin wounds are common. Skin wounds are classified by etiology into abrasion, avulsion, incision, laceration, and puncture wounds (1). Abrasion injury of the skin frequently accompanies orthopedic trauma in cats, especially trauma of the distal limbs, and has been termed degloving injury. Cat bite wounds are also commonly encountered in feline practice. They are usually puncture wounds with a high incidence of infection, resulting in subcutaneous abscesses, cellulitis, or infection of deeper structures. Diagnosis and treatment of injuries to muscles, tendons, and skin are described in this chapter.

16.1 Muscle injuries

Muscle injury may be due to contusion, strain, or laceration and is usually associated with fractures and, less commonly, with blunt trauma. Severe or mistreated muscle injury can result in irreversible muscle contracture and fibrosis (Chapter 7).

16.1.1 Muscle contusion, strain, and laceration

Muscle contusion resulting from blunt trauma is characterized by hemorrhage, edema, inflammation, pain, ischemia, and possibly necrosis. Muscle strain or rupture is caused by eccentric contraction and stretching of a muscle. Human quadriceps strains have been categorized into four grades (2). Grades 1 and 2 involve tearing of a few muscle fibers and hematoma formation; the muscle fascia is still intact. In grade 3 strains a larger number of muscle fibers and the fascia are ruptured. Complete muscle rupture is categorized as grade 4. Clinical signs of both muscle contusion and strain include pain, swelling, bruising, hematoma, and muscle spasm. Serum creatine phosphokinase activity in the serum may be elevated.

Clinically apparent muscle injuries in cats are usually associated with fractures. The commonest injuries seen are contusion and laceration of muscle by sharp fracture fragments. Hematoma, ischemia, denervation, and rupture may occur subsequently. Much of the energy released during trauma is absorbed by the surrounding soft tissues. Muscle damage is therefore often approximately proportional to fracture severity.

Marked pressure elevation due to hematoma and edema formation in a muscle compartment may cause necrosis of muscle fibers. This is called compartment syndrome. Four susceptible muscle compartments have been identified in the dog: the femoral, craniolateral crus, caudal crus, and the caudal antebrachial compartment. Although compartment syndrome has not been described in the feline literature, intracompartmental pressure elevation should be suspected if one of the listed compartments is very firm, swollen, and painful. Muscle fibrosis and contracture may be the final result of compartment syndrome if ischemia and necrosis have been present for more than a few hours. Pressure within a muscle compartment can be measured, with values above 30 mmHg being of concern in dogs (3, 4), but no reference data exist for cats.

Diagnoses of muscle strains unassociated with fractures are rare in cats. Clinically, the serratus ventralis muscle and the abdominal wall muscles are most commonly affected. Rupture of the serratus ventralis muscle causes laxity and dorsal displacement of the scapula (Chapter 27). Muscles of the abdominal wall are subject to strain and rupture after blunt abdominal trauma. Herniation of intra-abdominal organs can occur through full-thickness lacerations of the abdominal wall (Chapter 12).

16.1.2 Treatment of muscle injuries

Muscle injuries heal through the sequential stages of inflammation, repair, and remodeling. The final stage of healing is either muscle fiber regeneration or scar tissue formation, dependent both on the size of the original defect and other injury factors. Regeneration is desirable because healing by scar tissue reduces the muscle's ability to produce tension. A source of myoblasts, extracellular matrix, vascularization, and innervation is required for regeneration to occur. Vascular ingrowth occurs slowly, and prolonged ischemia results in death of muscle fibers. Large gaps therefore heal by scar formation (5, 6). In the remodeling phase of healing, some stress is necessary to allow remodeling and longitudinal orientation of muscle fibers.

Conservative treatment of muscle contusion and lower-grade strains is aimed at minimizing the initial inflammatory processes. Cage rest and systemic non-steroidal anti-inflammatory drugs are administered. Local ice packs can be applied for the first 1–2 days if the cat cooperates. Later on, warm packs may facilitate resorption of hematoma and promote vascularization. Grade 3 and 4 strains are best treated surgically with debridement of damaged or necrotized tissue, and apposition of muscle tissue by suturing the muscle fascia. Cruciate sutures or mattress suture patterns with fine monofilament suture material may be used. If muscle lacerations are encountered during fracture repair, hematomas and devitalized tissue are debrided, and significant lacerations are sutured. The fascia is left unsutured or is only loosely apposed if swollen muscle is identified at surgery. Small fascial incisions should be made to relieve intracompartmental pressure if pressure elevation is suspected in a muscle compartment, or if a large hematoma is seen under the intact fascia.

Postoperatively, cold packs and non-steroidal anti-inflammatory drugs may be administered for 1–2 days if marked swelling and inflammation are present. Patients with severe contusions, large lacerations or high-grade strains are cage-rested for 3 weeks to reduce and control activity. Gentle physical therapy helps to prevent contracture (Chapter 21).

16.2 Tendon injuries

Tendon injury may be caused by both direct and indirect trauma. Direct trauma with sharp objects causes tendon laceration. Degloving injury may cause partial or complete loss of tendons. Indirect trauma by excessive eccentric loading leads to tendon sprain or rupture.

Healing of a tendon defect is a slow process. In tendons without a tendon sheath, it follows the same basic mechanisms as healing of extra-articular ligaments (Chapter 14). If a small gap is present between the tendon ends, blood vessels and fibroblasts from the surrounding tissue enter the gap, and form granulation tissue. A fibrous scar forms in the first 3 weeks, which then starts to reorganize in a way that the tendon fibers regain a longitudinal orientation. The longitudinal orientation requires limited tensile forces across the lesion. The whole process of remodeling takes several months. Tendons regain approximately 50% of their normal strength 6 weeks after surgery, which is sufficient to withstand the forces exerted during active motion (7). Tendon strength returns to around 80% of normal after 1 year (7). Tendons in tendon sheaths have the disadvantage of poorer blood supply and healing, and the potential for adhesions between the tendon and the tendon sheath.

Anatomically and surgically important tendons in cats include the Achilles tendon complex, the patellar tendon, the tendon of the deep gluteal muscle, the tendon of the deltoid muscle, and the tendon of the triceps muscle. The tendons of the deep and middle gluteal, deltoid, and triceps muscle are sutured if tenotomy is performed during surgical approaches to the hip joint, shoulder joint, and elbow joint, respectively. The Achilles tendon (Chapter 40), patellar tendon, and triceps muscle tendon (Chapter 30) usually need repair after traumatic rupture (8, 9).

Reapposition of the tendon ends and immobilization during the initial phases of healing are necessary. The common feature of all tendon and ligament suture patterns is one or more transverse bites through the tissue. Because the collagen fibers in a tendon are mainly oriented longitudinally, sutures tend to slip along the fibers and tear out of the tissue. The transverse part of the tendon suture patterns compresses the longitudinal fibers when the suture is tightened, and thus prevents the suture from tearing out of the tissue. Non-absorbable monofilament suture materials are usually used. Braided composite sutures may be taken if greater suture strength is required. Frayed and necrotic tissue at the stump of the severed tendon is sharply resected before the tendon ends are apposed. The locking-loop suture is a simple suture pattern to apply, which is adequate for small and flat tendons (Chapter 14, Fig. 14-4). The three-loop pulley suture pattern was shown to have a superior tensile strength than the locking-loop pattern (10). It is used for larger round tendons, such as the tendons of the Achilles mechanism (Fig. 16-1). Flat tendons, such as the deep gluteal tendon, can be sutured with a continuous suture pattern (Fig. 16-2).

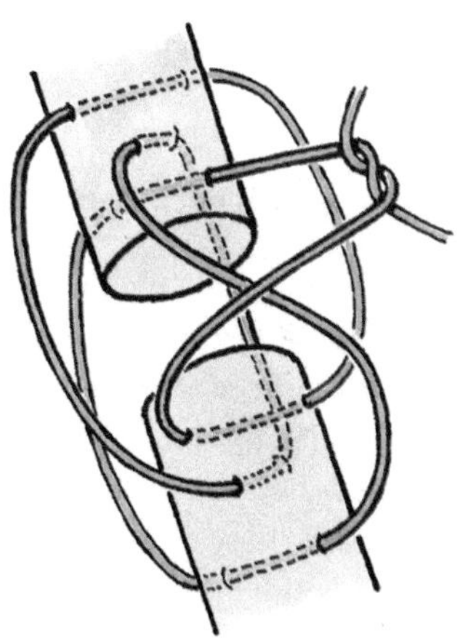

Figure 16-1 Three-loop pulley suture pattern for repair of large tendons.

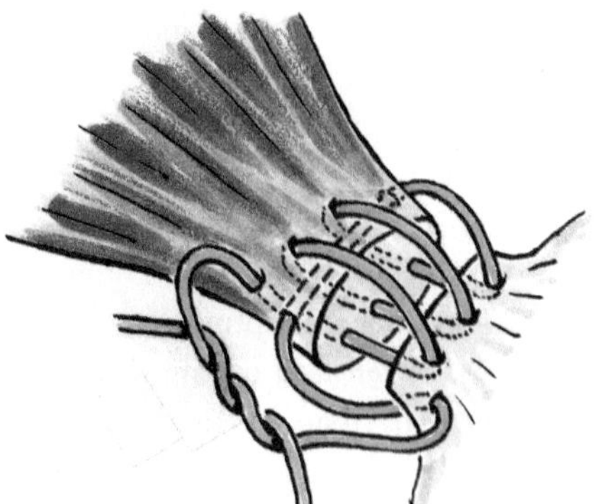

Figure 16-2 Continuous suture pattern for repair of flat tendons (recommended by Ken Bruecker).

A 3-week period of complete immobilization is usually recommended postoperatively, followed by another 3 weeks of less immobilization with a gradual increase in tensile loads (5, 6). Practically, this can be achieved for example with a transarticular external skeletal fixator applied across the affected joint for the first 3 weeks, followed by a splinted bandage, and then by a modified Robert Jones bandage (Chapter 22).

16.3 Degloving injuries

Degloving injuries occur most commonly during motor vehicle accidents. It has been proposed that they happen when the brakes are applied with the car wheel positioned on the limb, causing the limb to shear along the ground surface. In dogs, the distal limbs are affected more commonly than the proximal limbs, the rear limbs are affected more commonly than the front limbs, and the medial tarsal area is the most commonly affected area overall (11). No large studies have been performed in cats but the distribution of degloving injuries seems to be similar to that in the dog. In most cases not only skin but also deeper tissue layers are lost, resulting in bone or joint exposure (11). Prognosis depends on the location and amount of tissue lost. Patients without bone and joint exposure usually have an excellent prognosis (11). Dogs with shearing injuries of the limbs with either bone or joint exposure had an excellent outcome in approximately 55%, a good outcome in about 30%, and a poor outcome in 15% of cases (11). No similar studies have been performed in cats, but our clinical impression is that many cats have a good prognosis despite severe loss of tissue, joint exposure, and joint instability if treated appropriately. Degenerative joint disease and intermittent lameness may develop in some cases. Shearing injuries of the medial tarsus with loss of a substantial part of the medial malleolus may result in persistent joint instability despite treatment. These injuries carry a poorer prognosis.

Treatment consists of wound debridement and care, as described in detail below. Treatment is usually costly and time-consuming. Patients frequently need more than one surgical wound debridement, daily bandage changes, and potentially additional surgeries for stabilization procedures, skin grafting, or arthrodesis.

16.3.1 Initial treatment of the wound

Most degloving wounds are left to heal by second-intention healing, because they are grossly contaminated, and lack of skin precludes tension-free closure. The first step in treatment of a degloving injury is wound cleaning and debridement, with the goal of reducing bacterial numbers, and creating an environment for undisturbed healing. Wound cleaning and debridement are performed under aseptic conditions to prevent the introduction of nosocomial bacteria. The wound is protected with a sterile water-soluble gel or with sterile sponges, while the hair is clipped. Hair around the wound edges is removed with clippers or scissors. Foreign bodies in the wound, such as hair and dirt, are also removed.

Surgical wound debridement involves sharp excision of obviously devitalized tissue with a scalpel blade. Overzealous debridement is avoided initially, and tissue with questionable viability is initially left. After approximately 3 days, demarcation results in changes in skin color and consistency, which facilitates assessment of tissue viability. Nerves, vessels, and tendons are spared whenever possible.

The wound is copiously lavaged. Wound irrigation should be performed with some pressure to reduce bacterial numbers effectively. Adequate pressure can be generated with a 35-ml syringe and a 19-gauge needle (1). Several solutions may be used as irrigants, including tap water, sterile saline solution, and Ringer's solution. Ringer's solution may be preferred, because it has been shown to cause less cell damage and lower cell mortality than tap water or saline solution (12). Wounds older than 12 hours are always considered infected, and the addition of an antiseptic to the initial lavage solution may additionally help decrease bacterial numbers. The antiseptics have to be diluted to avoid tissue inflammation and cell damage. Chlorhexidine diacetate as a 0.05% solution and povidone-iodine as a 1% solution may be used. Antiseptics should not be added to the irrigation solution in the presence of open joint injuries, as they may cause cartilage damage.

Degloving injuries are left to heal by second-intention healing after wound cleaning and debridement. Second-intention wound healing is characterized by formation of granulation tissue, wound contraction, and epithelialization from the wound edges. The goal of treatment is to promote the development of granulation tissue and to prevent infection. Adherent wound dressings are chosen in the initial inflammatory stages of wound healing; these result in superficial mechanical debridement during bandage changes. Wet-to-dry bandages are an easy and effective method to achieve this goal. The initial layer consists of a sterile gauze sponge, moistened with sterile Ringer's solution and covered with a second absorptive layer of dressing material. Evaporation of fluid results in hypertonicity of the fluid in the dressing, causing fluid from the wound to be drawn into the dressing. Wet-to-dry bandages are usually changed once a day, and wound debris is therefore removed with the dressing from the wound surface. Once granulation tissue has been formed over the entire wound bed, the wound dressing is changed to a non-adherent type (Chapter 22) to allow undisturbed maturation, contraction, and epithelialization of the wound. The mean healing time for degloving injuries left to heal by second intention

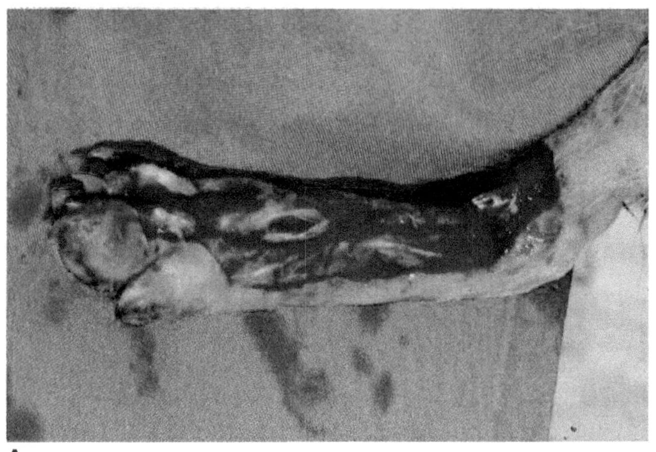

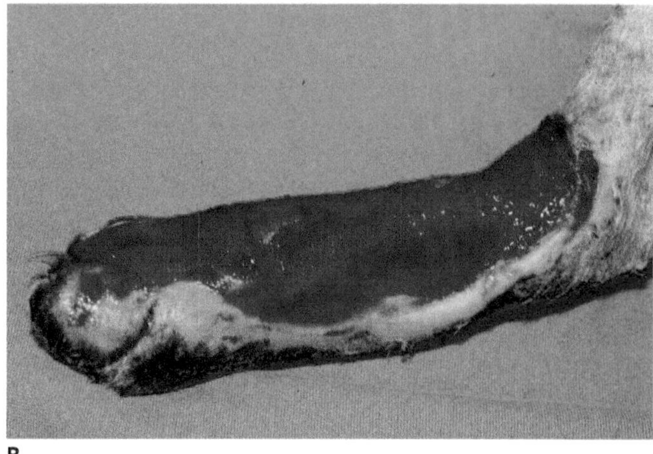

Figure 16-3 (**A**) The paw of a cat with a large degloving injury of the tarsus and metatarsus, 5 days after trauma. (**B**) The injury was treated with wet-to-dry bandages for 2.5 weeks until granulation tissue had covered the wound. The wound bed is now ready to accept a skin graft.

was 6.7 weeks in dogs (11), but this is of course dependent on the size of the defect. Second-intention wound healing has recently been demonstrated to be slower in cats than in dogs (13).

Systemic antibiotics are usually used both prophylactically and therapeutically, but they are not a substitute for proper wound management. Most superficial wound infections are caused by staphylococcal species, and either cephalosporins or amoxicillin-clavulanate may be efficacious to use while awaiting culture and sensitivity results. However, continued therapeutic use of systemic antibiotics should be based on culture and sensitivity testing. Antimicrobial therapy is discontinued once granulation tissue has been formed, because the highly vascularized granulation tissue is very resistant to infection.

16.3.2 Skin grafting

A wound devoid of skin will close by contraction and epithelialization. Contraction starts from the wound edges and is slow during the first week after wounding, but then accelerates in the following 2 weeks (13). Excessive wound contraction in areas over joint surfaces may cause reduction in range of motion of a joint. Additionally, large wounds tend to be only covered by a thin epithelial layer centrally, which has suboptimal mechanical strength, and is at risk for repetitive injury. Large wounds on the distal limbs, which have not healed after approximately 2 weeks, should therefore be covered by a skin graft. Different methods of skin grafting exist, but a full-thickness mesh graft is easy to apply in cats, allows future hair growth, has a good resistance to mechanical damage, and results in a good cosmetic appearance. A 90–100% graft take can be expected for skin grafting of distal limb wounds in cats (14).

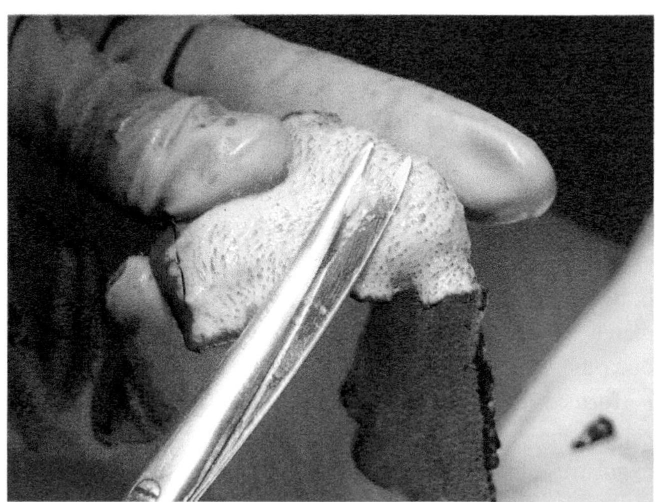

Figure 16-4 Preparation of a full-thickness mesh graft. First, all subcutaneous fat is meticulously removed with curved Metzenbaum scissors, until the graft has a granular appearance. Before the graft is sutured to the wound bed, small longitudinal incisions are performed all over the graft. These allow drainage of wound secretions and prevent seroma formation between recipient site and graft.

The graft can be applied as soon as the whole wound is covered by healthy granulation tissue (Fig. 16-3). An appropriate-sized skin graft is harvested from the lateral thoracic or abdominal wall. Color of hair and direction of hair growth should be considered when choosing the harvest site. The retrieved piece of skin is spread on a sterile piece of cardboard with needles. All the subcutaneous fat is removed with scissors until the bases of the hair follicles are clearly visible (Fig. 16-4). The graft then has a granulated appearance. The graft is meshed with a number 15 scalpel blade, and is kept moist until used. The epithelial line at the wound edges of the recipient site is carefully removed with a scalpel blade and

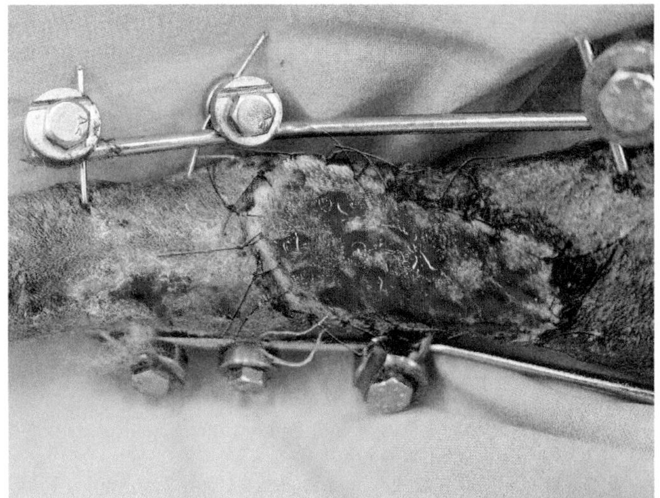
A

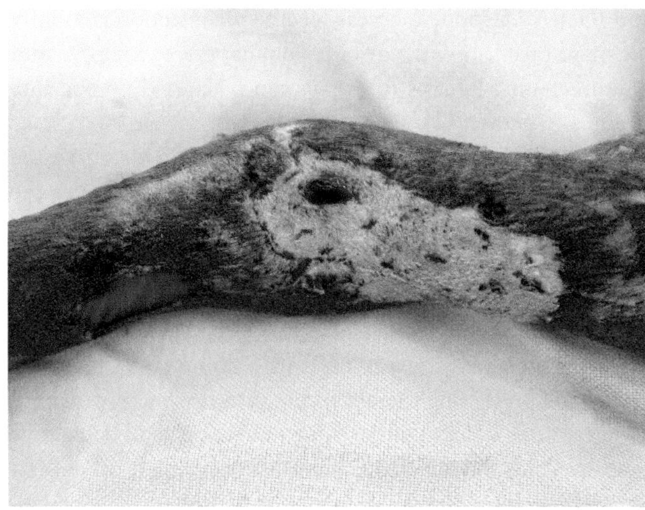
B

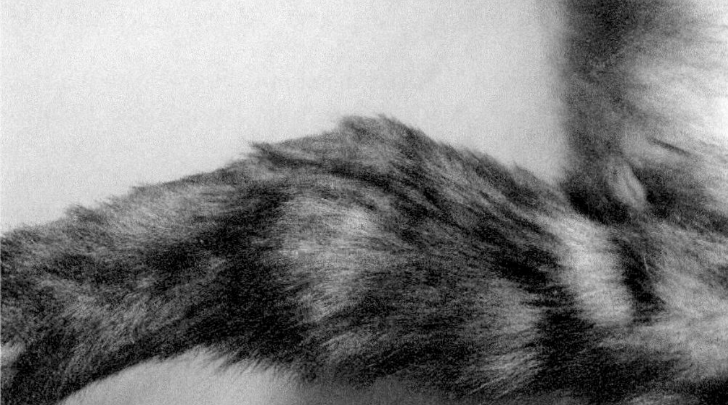
C

Figure 16-5 Appearance of a full-thickness mesh graft on the dorsum of the tarsus after 4 days, 2.5 weeks, and 4 months.
(**A**) After 4 days the graft is attached to the wound bed and is pink and well vascularized. Fluid is able to drain through the mesh incisions.
(**B**) The graft has taken completely after 2.5 weeks and new hair growth is already visible. The bandage and external skeletal fixator were removed at this time.
(**C**) Appearance of the leg 4 months postoperatively. The hair has fully regrown.

any residual debris in the graft bed is removed with sponges. Bleeding is controlled by digital pressure before the graft is applied. The graft is sutured to the wound edges with simple interrupted sutures, again considering the direction of hair growth. The graft should have maximal contact with the wound bed and the mesh incisions should be slightly open.

A non-adherent wound dressing is then applied and the leg is immobilized in a splinted bandage. The timing of the first bandage change is controversial. We usually perform it on the fourth or fifth day after surgery, because any motion between graft and wound bed before that time may interfere with graft take. We prefer to keep the cats hospitalized to ensure proper cage rest and frequent bandage checks. At the first bandage change the wound dressing has to be removed carefully, so the fragile connection between graft and wound bed is not disturbed; a cat that is likely to struggle is therefore best anesthetized. After 5 days the graft should ideally have a slightly reddish or cyanotic appearance (Fig. 16-5), but even pale areas may still survive. Another bandage is applied at this stage, and is replaced every 4–5 days. Graft take is usually complete after 3 weeks (Fig. 16-5). The bandage can be removed if there is presence of new hair growth, but excessive licking at the graft site should be prevented for another 2–3 weeks.

16.4 Cat bite wounds

Territorial fights between cats often result in bite wounds. Cat bites were reported to contribute to 4.3% of all visits made by cats to veterinarians (15), and a cat bite wound is one of the most common causes of acute lameness in the feline patient. The limbs, head, and lower back and perineum are most frequently affected. Bite wounds can cause lacerations, crushing, avulsion of skin, and puncture wounds (16). The sharp canine teeth of cats tend to cause predominantly deep puncture wounds. Bite wounds are always considered infected, due to proliferation of bacteria from the cat's normal oral flora, such as *Pasteurella*, beta-hemolytic *Streptococcus*, and *Bacteroides* spp. Whereas local tissue infection is usually the main problem with cat bite wounds, more extensive and life-threatening injuries to organs can be caused by dog bite wounds (Chapter 12).

The small skin puncture lesions often go unnoticed by the owners, and cats may only be presented 1–2 days after the injury, when cellulitis is already present. Common reasons for presentation are fever, depression, anorexia, and lameness if the limbs are involved. Careful palpation of the cat for local swelling, pain, and small scabs, and clipping of hair in the suspected area may reveal the small skin lesions. Another reason for presenting the cat to the veterinarian is when the owner notices a fluctuant swelling indicating a subcutaneous abscess. Once the infected tissue has been walled off and an abscess has developed, cats are usually free of general systemic signs. However, the lesion can be very painful and may induce behavioral changes, such as aggression or hiding.

Antibiotic therapy with β-lactamase penicillins is usually sufficient to resolve the infection in the early stages when cellulitis is present. Care must be taken not to miss a joint infection if the bite wound is located close to a joint (Chapter 14). Radiographs, arthrocentesis, and evaluation of the synovial fluid, or surgical exploration is conducted if joint involvement is suspected.

Small abscess cavities should be opened with a scalpel blade and debrided. The incision is left open for second-intention healing. Large abscess cavities may have to be drained for a couple of days to prevent healing of the skin incision before the infection has resolved. Large abscesses at the tail base sometimes result in areas of skin necrosis due to undermining and reduced blood supply of the skin. Systemic antimicrobial treatment is not necessarily required when an abscess cavity has been drained, but antibiotics should be given in the presence of systemic signs of infection, and if cellulitis is present in the tissues surrounding the abscess.

Viral diseases, such as rabies, feline leukemia virus (FeLV), and feline immunodeficiency virus (FIV), can be transmitted through bite wounds. Serological testing of cats for FeLV and FIV may be performed 6 months after the bite wound if there is a concern about potential infection (16). The measures taken against potential transmission of rabies after a bite depend on the vaccination status of the cat, whether rabies is endemic, and the specific guidelines for each country.

References and further reading

1. Waldron DR, Zimmerman-Pope N. Superficial skin wounds. In: Slatter D (ed.) Textbook of small animal surgery. Philadelphia: WB Saunders; 2002: pp. 259–273.
2. Ryan A. Quadriceps strain, rupture and charlie horse. Med Sci Sports 1969;1:106–111.
3. Hargens AR, et al. Quantification of skeletal-muscle necrosis in a model compartment syndrome. J Bone Joint Surg Am 1981;63: 631–636.
4. Basinger RR, et al. Osteofacial compartment syndrome in the dog. Vet Surg 1987;16:427–434.
5. Fitch RB, et al. Muscle injuries in dogs. Comp Continuing Educ Pract Vet 1997;19:947–958.
6. Fahie, MA. Healing, diagnosis, repair, and rehabilitation of tendon conditions. Vet Clin Small Anim Pract 2005;35: 1195–1211.
7. Dueland R, Quenin J. Triceps tenotomy: biomechanical assessment of healing strength. J Am Anim Hosp Assoc 1980;16: 507–512.
8. Brunnberg L, et al. Injury to the patella and the patella ligaments in dogs and cats II: rupture of the patellar ligament. Eur J Comp Anim Pract 1993;3:69–73.
9. Liehmann L, Lorinson D. Traumatic triceps tendon avulsion in a cat. J Small Anim Pract 2005;47:94–97.
10. Moores AP, et al. Biomechanical and clinical evaluation of a modified 3-loop pulley pattern for reattachment of canine tendons to bone. Vet Surg 2004;33:391–397.
11. Beardsley SL, Schrader SC. Treatment of dogs with wounds of the limbs caused by shearing forces: 98 cases (1975–1993). J Am Vet Med Assoc 1995;207:1071–1075.
12. Buffa E, et al. The effects of wound lavage solutions on canine fibroblasts: an in vitro study. Vet Surg 1997;26:460–466.
13. Bohling MW, et al. Cutaneous wound healing in the cat: a macroscopic description and comparison with cutaneous wound healing in the dog. Vet Surg 2004;33:579–587.
14. Siegfried R, et al. Treatment of large distal extremity skin wounds with autogenous full-thickness mesh skin grafts in 5 cats. Schweiz Arch Tierheilkd 2004;146:277–283.
15. Leonard CA, Tillson M. Feline lameness. Vet Clin North Am Small Anim Pract 2001;31:143–163.
16. Holt DE, Griffin G. Bite wounds in dogs and cats. Vet Clin North Am Small Anim Pract 2000;30:669–679.

Part 5
The surgical patient

Complicated and invasive surgical procedures are now frequently performed in cats, thereby increasing the demand for appropriate surgical preparation, effective and safe anesthesia, pain management, and postoperative care. Peri- and postoperative analgesia have previously been neglected in cats, probably due to lack of recognition of pain in the feline patient and fear of side-effects from the analgesic drugs. Only in recent years has feline analgesia gained more attention in the literature, and effective and safe protocols have been instituted. Anesthesia and perioperative analgesia for the feline patient are described in Chapters 17 and 18, respectively

Preparation of the patient for surgery includes aseptic preparation of the surgical field, the surgical team, and the instruments, and is aimed at reducing the risk of surgical infection. These measures are the same for both cats and dogs. The most important features are summarized in Chapter 19 and the reader is referred to other textbooks for more information. Postoperative management of traumatized or orthopedic patients, such as general postoperative care, nutritional support, and physical therapy, is often as important as the surgical procedure itself. Benefits include a shortened recovery time and improvement in overall well-being and outcome. Postoperative care of the traumatized and orthopedic patient and rehabilitation therapy are described in Chapters 20 and 21, respectively.

17 Anesthesia

S. Kaestner

Every surgical procedure bears a risk. For evaluation of the surgical risk many individual factors should be considered, such as anesthetic risk, preoperative health status, postoperative morbidity, risk of infection, risk of surgery-related complications, and the long-term prognosis for functional recovery and quality of life.

Overall anesthetic-related mortality in cats is reported to be between 0.1% and 0.42%, whereas serious anesthetic complications occur in 1.3–11% of cats (1–3). In a recent study in the UK, the incidence of anesthetic-related mortality in healthy cats was 0.11%, and 1.4% in sick cats (4). Preoperative assessment of the physical status according to the American Society of Anesthesiologists (ASA) is useful for evaluating the anesthetic risk for the cat (Table 17-1). Cats with an ASA status of 3 or higher are four times or more at risk for serious perianesthetic complications, including cardiac arrest, as compared to cats with an ASA status of 1 or 2 (2, 3). Age alone does not necessarily increase the anesthetic risk (3), but older cats might have a higher incidence of specific disease conditions.

Surgical risk factors have been evaluated in several studies on cats and dogs and these are summarized in Box 17-1. Many orthopedic feline patients have sustained trauma and injuries to multiple body systems, thus markedly enhancing anesthetic risk. Appropriate stabilization of the patient before surgery, a balanced anesthesia, pain management, prevention and treatment of infections, correct surgical techniques, and intensive postoperative care all reduce the surgical risk.

ASA grade	Physical status
ASA 1	Healthy patient – elective surgery not required for the patient's well-being
ASA 2	Mild systemic disease, no functional limitations – routine necessary surgery that would not cause any added risk
ASA 3	Severe systemic disease limiting activity but not incapacitating
ASA 4	Incapacitating systemic disease that is a constant threat to life
ASA 5	Moribund; not expected to live 24 hours with or without surgery
E	Emergency anesthesia

Table 17-1. American Society of Anesthesiologists (ASA) patient physical status assessment

17.1 Preoperative assessment of the surgical patient

Preanesthetic assessment involves obtaining an owner's history, and performing a physical examination according to standard procedures. The cardiovascular and the respiratory system are the most important body systems to assess, followed by renal and hepatic function, and electrolyte status. True resting values (Table 17-2) are often difficult to obtain in cats in a foreign environment, such as the veterinary hospital. Heart rates up to 240 beats/min and body temperatures up to 40.5°C can occur in stressed but otherwise healthy cats.

Blood work has little impact on anesthetic management in the apparently healthy young cat. However, after the physical examination, minimal screening of hematocrit, plasma total solids, and blood urea nitrogen will help to rule out subclinical problems such as mild dehydration, anemia, or renal disease, which will influence the response to and consequences of administration of anesthetics. More intensive lab work,

Box 17-1. Factors influencing surgical risk. The factors at the top of the list have the greatest impact on surgical risk

- Physical status according to the American Society of Anesthesiologists (ASA)
- Emergency surgical procedures
- Hypoalbuminemia (albumin < 21 g/l)
- Anemia (packed cell volume < 20%)
- Renal uremia
- Liver dysfunction
- Coagulation disorders
- Dyspnea
- Age
- Weight loss
- Risk for infection
- Complexity and duration of surgery

Parameter	Normal range
Heart rate	100–240 beats/min, mean true resting 128 beats/min
Respiratory rate	20–40 breaths/min
Body temperature	36–39°C
Packed cell volume	33–45%
Hemoglobin	11.3–15.5 g/dl
Erythrocytes	7.0–10.7 × 10^6/μl
Mean corpuscular hemoglobin	14–17 pg
Mean corpuscular hemoglobin concentration	33–36 g/dl
Mean corpuscular volume	41–49 fl
Leukocytes	4.6–12.8 × 10^3/μl
Band neutrophils	0–123/μl
Segmented neutrophils	2315–10 000/μl
Lymphocytes	1050–6000/μl
Monocytes	46–678/μl
Eosinophils	100–600/μl
Basophils	0–143/μl
Platelets	180–680 × 10^3/μl
Total solids	64–80 g/l
Albumin	30–40 g/l
Bilirubin (total)	1.7–7.2 μmol/l
Glucose	4–9 mmol/l
Blood urea nitrogen	7.4–12.6 μmol/l
Creatinine	98–163 μmol/l
Aspartate aminotransferase	19–44 U/l
Alanine transaminase	34–98 U/l
Lipase	8–26 U/l
Sodium	158–165 mmol/l
Potassium	3.8–5.4 mmol/l
Chloride	121–131 mmol/l
Calcium	2.4–2.8 mmol/l
Phosphate	0.9–1.8 mmol/l

Table 17-2. Normal values for heart rate, respiratory rate, body temperature, and clinical chemistry and hematology in domestic felines

including clinical chemistry and hematology, is indicated in geriatric cats older than 8 years, because of increasing incidence of compensated disease processes with age, and in traumatized patients.

Further diagnostic procedures should be centered round abnormal findings. Cardiac as well as respiratory abnormalities warrant chest radiographs and/or echocardiographic examination. Chest radiographs will also help to rule out lung metastases in cats with tumors. Elective surgical procedures may need to be delayed if there are significant abnormal findings (e.g., respiratory infections, untreated diabetes mellitus). Patients with debilitating disease (ASA 3 and higher) should be stabilized prior to anesthesia, and possible complications related to the specific disease condition should be recognized and preparations made for intervention (i.e., blood transfusion, ventilatory management).

Traumatized cats need to be stabilized before anesthetic induction. Aggressive fluid therapy up to 50 ml/kg per hour is required (Chapter 11), and at least 50% of the fluid deficit should be replaced before anesthesia can be considered. Chest and abdominal radiographs should be obtained from every traumatized cat, to rule out clinically unapparent internal injuries (Chapter 12).

A complete clinical examination is not always possible in uncooperative cats without risking injury to personnel or excessive stress to the cat. After obtaining a complete history and health status of the patient from the owners, these unapproachable animals may have to be anesthetized to allow handling. The safest, least depressive, and easiest to eliminate or reversible sedative or anesthetic should be given. A basic physical examination and blood samples can then be performed after induction of anesthesia or sedation, taking the drug effects into account when evaluating the results (e.g., changes in packed cell volume).

17.2 Preparation for anesthesia

After the physical examination, diagnostics, and appropriate preanesthetic therapy, the owners should be informed of the risks associated with the planned procedure. They can be asked to sign a written informed consent to perform anesthesia and surgery. This procedure will assure proper client communication in the light of increasing numbers of liability trials. The results of the preanesthetic assessment and ASA classification should also be documented in combination with an anesthetic record (Fig. 17-1). Undocumented measures are considered non-existent in cases of litigation. The protocol should document the type of premedication, anesthetic induction, and anesthetic maintenance, including time of administration, drugs used, and route of administration.

Food should be withheld for 8–12 hours in adult cats in preparation for scheduled surgical procedures. Fasting time is reduced to 1–2 hours in animals younger than 5 weeks, and suckling kittens are left with the queen to reduce the risk of hypoglycemia. Fasting will reduce the chance of pre- and intraoperative vomiting and possible aspiration of gastric contents and reflux esophagitis. A full stomach will also impair ventilation and cardiac filling by compression of the lung and the caudal vena cava. Water should be available until induction of anesthesia to avoid disturbance of the fluid balance. The exact body weight of the cat is determined for calculation of doses for sedatives, anesthetics, and fluid rates.

17.3 Venous access

Venous access is necessary for safe and effective administration for the majority of anesthetics, and for fluid administration during anesthesia. Accessible veins in the cat include the cephalic, saphenous, femoral, and recurrent tarsal vein. For blood sampling the external jugular vein is easily accessible and it can also be used for placement of central venous catheters.

Indwelling catheters using the over-the-needle technique with sizes 20 and 22G and a length of 1.5 cm are suitable for the peripheral veins in cats (Fig. 17-2). In uncastrated males with very thick skin, perforation of the skin with a hypodermic needle is sometimes necessary to avoid damage to the catheter tip. A cut-down to the vein might be required in very small animals or dehydrated or hypovolemic cats. Preparation of the skin with EMLA cream (euthetic lidocaine/prilocaine mixture, Astra) to provide skin anesthesia has been described (5), but catheter placement is successful in only 40% of unsedated cats.

Catheters up to size 18G can be used for the jugular vein. Short catheters will easily dislodge from the jugular vein because of the flexibility of the neck, and a length of at least 6 cm is therefore recommended. Conventional over-the-needle catheters of this length can be difficult to introduce in the neck area of cats and a through-the-needle technique might be necessary for insertion of a jugular catheter after induction of anesthesia. For placement of a central venous catheter intended for long-term use, commercial human pediatric catheter kits are suitable. Catheter lengths should not exceed 12 cm in the average-sized cat to avoid placement of the catheter tip into the right atrium.

Preparation of the catheter area depends on the type of catheter used and intended duration of catheter placement. The hair should be clipped around the vessel to be catheterized, and the clipped area prepared with an antiseptic solution. The area is surgically draped and sterile gloves are worn when using a cut-down technique or inserting long catheters using guidewires (Seldinger technique).

The catheter is fixed by tape to the limb, or is sutured to the skin of the neck. It is flushed with heparinized saline (2 units heparin/ml) or an intravenous fluid infusion to avoid clotting and obstruction of the catheter. To avoid accidental extraction of the catheter, the infusion line should also be secured to the body of the animal. A variety of different catheter types and connectors are available to provide unrestricted access to the vein with concurrent fluid administration. The catheter is protected with a bandage, is inspected and redressed every 24 hours, and is removed if there are signs of inflammation (fever, thrombophlebitis).

17.4 Premedication

Preanesthetic medication serves several purposes, including reduction of stress and decreasing anesthetic drug requirements. The choice of drugs used can have a significant influence on the induction and maintenance of anesthesia, and the recovery phase.

17.4.1 Sedation

Excitement or stress induces high levels of circulating catecholamines, which results in increased anesthetic requirements, and consequently more severe cardiovascular depression. Catecholamines also contribute to arrhythmia formation in combination with certain anesthetics (i.e., thiopental, halothane). Therefore, preanesthetic calming of the cat not only makes handling easier but also makes anesthesia

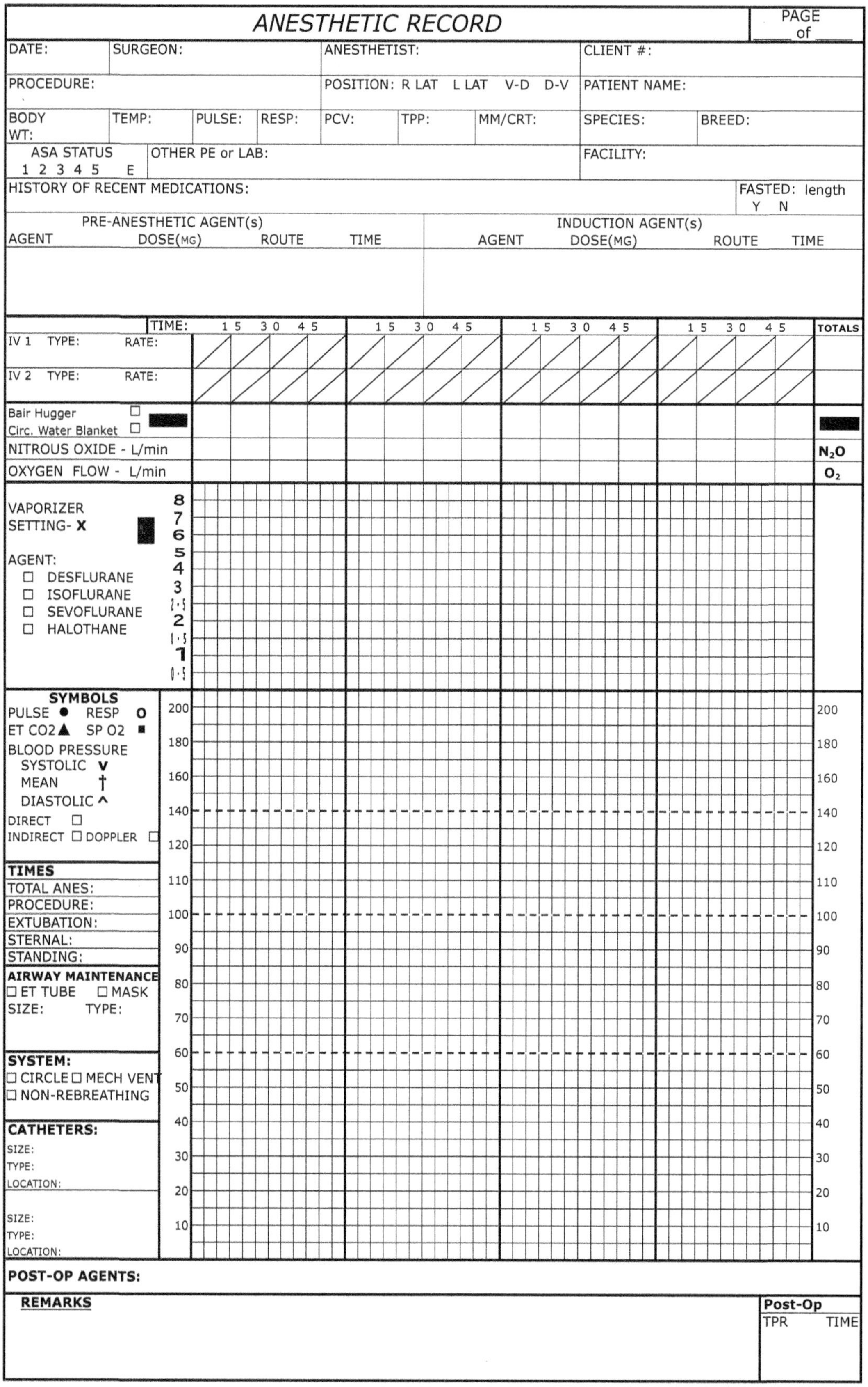

ANESTHETIC RECORD

PAGE ___ of ___

DATE:	SURGEON:	ANESTHETIST:	CLIENT #:
PROCEDURE:		POSITION: R LAT L LAT V-D D-V	PATIENT NAME:

BODY WT:	TEMP:	PULSE:	RESP:	PCV:	TPP:	MM/CRT:	SPECIES:	BREED:

ASA STATUS 1 2 3 4 5 E	OTHER PE or LAB:	FACILITY:

HISTORY OF RECENT MEDICATIONS:	FASTED: length Y N

PRE-ANESTHETIC AGENT(s)				INDUCTION AGENT(s)			
AGENT	DOSE(MG)	ROUTE	TIME	AGENT	DOSE(MG)	ROUTE	TIME

TIME:	15 30 45	15 30 45	15 30 45	15 30 45	TOTALS
IV 1 TYPE: RATE:					
IV 2 TYPE: RATE:					
Bair Hugger ☐ Circ. Water Blanket ☐					
NITROUS OXIDE - L/min					N_2O
OXYGEN FLOW - L/min					O_2

VAPORIZER SETTING- **X**

8, 7, 6, 5, 4, 3, 2.5, 2, 1.5, 1, 0.5

AGENT:
- ☐ DESFLURANE
- ☐ ISOFLURANE
- ☐ SEVOFLURANE
- ☐ HALOTHANE

SYMBOLS
PULSE ● RESP **O**
ET CO2▲ SP O2 ■
BLOOD PRESSURE
SYSTOLIC **V**
MEAN †
DIASTOLIC **^**
DIRECT ☐
INDIRECT ☐ DOPPLER ☐

200, 180, 160, 140, 120, 110, 100, 90, 80, 70, 60, 50, 40, 30, 20, 10

TIMES
TOTAL ANES:
PROCEDURE:
EXTUBATION:
STERNAL:
STANDING:

AIRWAY MAINTENANCE
☐ ET TUBE ☐ MASK
SIZE: TYPE:

SYSTEM:
☐ CIRCLE ☐ MECH VENT
☐ NON-REBREATHING

CATHETERS:
SIZE:
TYPE:
LOCATION:

SIZE:
TYPE:
LOCATION:

POST-OP AGENTS:

REMARKS	**Post-Op** TPR TIME

Figure 17-1 Anesthesia record for documentation of the preanesthetic evaluation, anesthetic protocol, and monitoring.

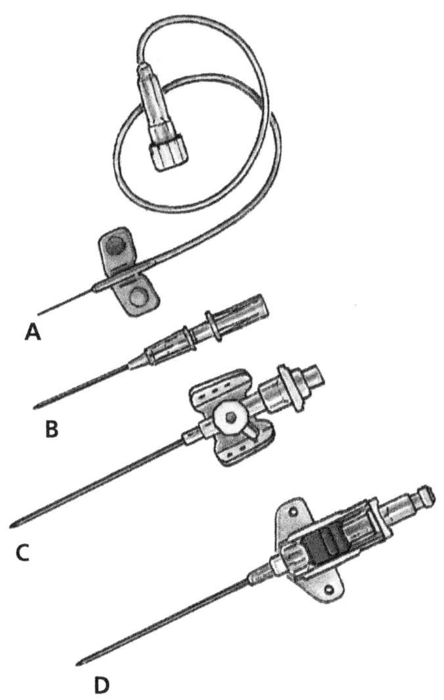

Figure 17-2 Different styles of catheters suitable for cats. (**A**) Butterfly needle with extension; (**B**) plain over-the-needle catheter; (**C**) catheter with side-port; (**D**) catheter with flow-switch mechanism.

safer. In cats there is often no clear differentiation between sedative premedication, induction of anesthesia, and total intravenous anesthesia (TIVA). The same drugs or drug combinations are often used and the overall effect is mainly dose-dependent. Drug dosages and drug combinations are summarized in Tables 17-3 and 17-4.

Phenothiazines

The most widely used member of this class of neuroleptics is acepromazine. Other examples include chlorpromazine and promazine. Their mechanism of action depends on antagonism at excitatory dopamine receptors and at alpha$_1$ adrenergic receptors. Acepromazine induces muscle relaxation and reduction of spontaneous activity. The degree of sedation with acepromazine can be very variable, and higher doses only prolong the duration of action. Acepromazine exerts antiemetic effects and this makes it a useful premedicant in combination with opioids. Hypothalamic thermoregulation is depressed, predisposing the cat to hypothermia or hyperthermia, so body temperature should be monitored.

High doses of chlorpromazine were found to lower the threshold for seizures (6), and it is not recommended to use acepromazine in known epileptics, head trauma patients, and prior to myelography. Acepromazine also lowers systemic blood pressure by reducing vascular tone, and it reduces the packed cell volume.

Acepromazine lacks analgesic effects and for most indications it is combined with an opioid or with ketamine to deepen sedation and provide analgesia. In contrast to thiopental, the induction dose of propofol was not reduced by acepromazine in cats (7). Dilution (1 : 10) of the commercial 1% solution of acepromazine is suggested to improve proper dosing in cats. Acepromazine has no specific antagonist and in cases of overdose and severe hypotension palliative treatment with intravenous fluid therapy for volume replacement should be instituted immediately.

Benzodiazepines

Benzodiazepines bind to gamma-aminobutyric acid (GABA) receptors and stimulate inhibitory neurons in the brain and spinal internuncial neurons. They have anticonvulsant, anxiolytic, and muscle relaxant activities, and they produce sedation and amnesia in humans with minimal cardiovascular and respiratory depression and with a wide safety margin. The calming effects are unreliable in healthy adult cats, and a state of abnormal behavior and euphoria occurs quite frequently. Therefore, benzodiazepines are rarely used alone in healthy cats. Benzodiazepines are often administered in conjunction with ketamine to prevent seizures and muscle rigidity. Low doses of benzodiazepines have been used to stimulate appetite in anorexic cats.

Diazepam exists in two different formulations. It is either dissolved in propylene glycol, known as Valium (Roche), or it is available as an emulsion with soya bean oil, and known as Diazemuls (Roche). The formulation with propylene glycol (Valium) is more stable and an open vial can be used over several days; however, the propylene glycol can cause thrombophlebitis, pain on intravenous injection, and cardiovascular depression when used in high doses. The oily or emulsion formulation (Diazemuls) is not suitable for intramuscular injection, and it should not be mixed with other drugs prior to injection. Diazepam is also available for rectal administration, which can be useful in seizuring cats without venous access.

Midazolam is a water-soluble benzodiazepine with a rapid elimination half-life. It can be administered via either the intramuscular (IM) or the intravenous (IV) route. It has a rapid onset of action and is rapidly absorbed after IM injection in cats (7, 8). About 50% of awake cats responded with euphoric behavior after various doses of midazolam given IV or IM (8). The combination of ketamine and midazolam is well tolerated for IM injection.

Benzodiazepine antagonists

It is not usually necessary to antagonize the benzodiazepine effects in cats, but it can be useful to use an antagonist in the case of an inadvertent overdose resulting in central nervous system and respiratory depression or excessive euphoria/

Drug	Dose (mg/kg)	Route	Comments
Acepromazine	1–3 0.02–0.2	PO IM/IV SC unreliable	Reduction of spontaneous activity, dose-dependent mild to deep sedation, non-painful procedures, travel sickness Onset: 15–20 minutes, duration: 3–4 (6) hours Contraindications: hypovolemia, seizure activity, severe anemia
Diazepam	0.1–0.5	IV	Unreliable sedation, potent muscle relaxation, combine with ketamine or butorphanol, give immediately prior to induction of anesthesia
Midazolam	0.1–0.5	SC/IM/IV	
Climazolam	0.1–0.5	SC/IM/IV	
Xylazine	0.2–0.5 (1.0)	SC/IM	Dose-dependent mild to deep sedation, analgesia
Medetomidine/ Dexmedetomidine	0.03–0.08 0.02–0.04	SC/IM	Dose-dependent mild to deep sedation, analgesia
Romifidine	0.1–0.2	IM	Dose-dependent mild to deep sedation, analgesia
Acepromazine + Buprenorphine	0.02–0.03 0.012	IM	Dose-dependent mild to moderate sedation, analgesia
Acepromazine + L-methadone	0.02–0.03 0.1–0.3	IM	Dose-dependent mild to moderate sedation, analgesia
Acepromazine + Ketamine	0.03 10	IM	Moderate to deep sedation, sometimes lack of muscle relaxation
Midazolam + Ketamine	0.2 5–10	IM/IV	Moderate to deep sedation, transition to anesthesia
Midazolam + Butorphanol	0.2 0.2	IM/IV	Mild to moderate sedation
Xylazine + Ketamine	0.5 5–(10)	IM	Moderate to deep sedation, transition to anesthesia
Medetomidine + Ketamine	0.05 5	IM	Moderate to deep sedation, transition to anesthesia
Romifidine + Ketamine	0.1 5	IM	Moderate to deep sedation, transition to anesthesia

Table 17-3. Drugs and drug combinations used for premedication and sedation in cats; PO, peroral; SC, subcutaneous; IM, intramuscular; IV, intravenous.

excitation. The available antagonists are non-competitive antagonists at the GABA receptor.

Flumazenil has a rapid onset of action within 2–4 minutes, and in humans the elimination half-life is similar to midazolam. Redosing might be necessary to antagonize a large dose of benzodiazepines. No data are available on antagonist/agonist ratios for cats. In dogs it is 26:1 for diazepam and 13:1 for midazolam (9). Titration to effect might be necessary in a cat with severe central nervous system depression.

Sarmazenil has similar properties to flumazenil but with a longer duration of action. This makes it more suitable to antagonize the long-lasting effects of high doses of benzodiazepines without necessity for repeat dosing. An agonist/antagonist dose ratio of 10:1 has been used clinically with success.

Alpha$_2$ agonists

Alpha$_2$ agonists act on central and peripheral alpha$_2$ adrenoreceptors and partially, with low affinity, on alpha$_1$ adrenoreceptors. Their central effects mediate analgesia, sedation, and muscle relaxation with minimal respiratory depression. Unfortunately, dose-dependent cardiovascular depression, including bradycardia and bradyarrhythmias, is associated with the use of alpha$_2$ agonists. These is most prominent after intravenous injection. Administration by the IM route is therefore preferred. Other effects include stimulation of the chemoreceptor trigger zone that can induce vomiting. Alpha$_2$ agonists have the characteristic that their sedative effects reach a plateau, so a very high dose will only prolong the duration of action. Other side-effects of alpha$_2$ agonists to consider in compromised cats are hyperglycemia and diuresis.

Table 17-4. Injectable anesthetic protocols for induction and/or maintenance of anesthesia in the cat

Anesthetics	Dose	Route	Purpose	Comments
Acepromazine + Ketamine + Buprenorphine or Butorphanol	0.05 mg/kg 20–30 mg/kg 0.01 mg/kg 0.2–0.4 mg/kg	IM	Short surgical procedures (30–40 minutes)	All ketamine protocols: Long recoveries Possible dysphoric recoveries Contraindicated with head trauma
Xylazine + Ketamine	1 mg/kg 20 mg/kg	IM	Short surgical procedures (20–30 minutes)	Avoid with hypertrophic cardiomyopathy Alpha$_2$ agonist and ketamine combination not recommended for concurrent IV injection, because of massive vasoconstriction
Medetomidine + Ketamine	0.05–0.08 mg/kg 5 mg/kg	IM	Short surgical procedures (30–40 minutes)	
Romifidine + Ketamine	0.2 mg/kg 5–(10) mg/kg	IM	Short surgical procedures (30–40 minutes)	
Diazepam + Ketamine	0.2–0.5 mg/kg 5 mg/kg	IV	Induction of anesthesia	
Midazolam + Ketamine	0.2 mg/kg 5 mg/kg	IV	Induction of anesthesia	
Midazolam + Ketamine	0.2 mg/kg 10–20 mg/kg	IM	Short minor procedures	
Thiopental	10 mg/kg (1–1.25% solution) dose to effect	IV	Induction of anesthesia	Always use with premedication (acepromazine, benzodiazepines) Can cause tachyarrhythmia Do not use in hypovolemic states and with cardiac disease
Propofol	2–6 mg/kg 0.2–0.5 mg/kg/min dose to effect	IV CRI	Induction of anesthesia TIVA maintenance	Use with premedication and analgesic Dose reduction depending on premedication Toxic effects with prolonged and repeated use Do not use in hypovolemia Oxygen supplementation and intubation recommended for repeated dosing
Alphaxalone/ alphadolone	Without premed 3–9–(12) mg/kg Redose 2–6 mg/kg	IV	Induction TIVA	Possible histamine release, with paw, laryngeal or tongue swelling Possible excitation during recovery
Alphaxalene	3–5 mg/kg 0.1–0.15 mg/kg/min	IV CRI		
Etomidate	0.5–2 mg/kg 50–150 µg/kg per minute	IV CRI	Induction TIVA maintenance	Not recommended without premedication because of muscle rigidity Minimal cardiovascular depression Adrenal suppression
Diazepam + Fentanyl + Etomidate	0.25 mg/kg 0.01 mg/kg 0.25–1 mg/kg	IV	Induction	Can also be used without fentanyl Minimal cardiovascular suppression High-risk patients

TIVA, total intravenous anesthesia; CRI, constant rate infusion; IM, intramuscular; IV, intravenous.

When using alpha$_2$ agonists with or before general anesthesia their potent anesthetic-sparing effects need to be taken into account. They are powerful drugs which have to be used with due consideration to exploit their advantages. Alpha$_2$ agonists should not be used in animals with cardiac disease, hypovolemia (shock), and endotoxemia.

Xylazine is the least potent alpha$_2$ agonist used in veterinary medicine, meaning that a higher dose rate is required to obtain the same effect than with a more potent drug. After IM and SC administration the incidence of vomiting in cats is high.

Romifidine has higher alpha$_2$/alpha$_1$ selectivity than xylazine, it has a longer duration of action, and produces less muscle relaxation when compared to xylazine at equipotent doses.

Medetomidine is the most selective alpha$_2$ agonist in clinical use. It is a racemic mixture, with the D-isomer being the active ingredient. Dexmedetomidine represents the purified D-isomer of medetomidine and it is twice as potent as the racemic mixture. Dexmedetomidine, particularly, seems to be suitable as an anesthetic and analgesic adjunct, and as an analgesic given by low-dose infusion to minimize cardiovascular and sedative effects.

Alpha$_2$ antagonists

An often-cited advantage of alpha$_2$ agonists is that they are true competitive antagonists available to be used in case of an emergency or to shorten recovery. However, it should be noted that in a healthy animal without anesthetic complications antagonizing the sedative and analgesic effects will often have no advantage, and might leave an overstimulated or painful animal. The dose required to antagonize a specific alpha$_2$ agonist depends on species, dose of agonist used, time of administration, and degree of desired antagonism. Intravenous administration of an antagonist can lead to tachycardia, hypertension, defecation, vomiting, and hyperexcitability. The only licensed alpha$_2$ antagonist for use in cats is atipamezole (Antisedan, Orion). Atipamezole has high alpha$_2$/alpha$_1$ selectivity and is highly specific with no activity at other receptors. To antagonize medetomidine sedation, 2–4 times the preceding dose of medetomidine is required. The current recommendation in cats is to give a volume equivalent to half of the medetomidine dose. The recommended route of administration is IM or SC and sedation will be antagonized within 5–10 minutes after injection. Documented alpha$_2$ antagonist doses for cats (10) are listed in Table 17-5.

Alpha$_2$ antagonist	Dose
Atipamezole after medetomidine:	80–600 μg/kg SC/IM
Atipamezole after xylazine:	200 μg/kg SC/IM
Yohimbine after medetomidine:	500 μg/kg IV
Yohimbine after xylazine:	100–200 μg/kg IV
Tolazoline after xylazine:	2 mg/kg IV

Table 17-5. Documented alpha$_2$ antagonist doses for cats

17.4.2 Analgesia

Analgesics given as part of the premedication serve several purposes. They will improve sedation, reduce requirements for general anesthetics, and help to obtain a smooth and pain-free recovery. Pre-emptive analgesia will improve analgesic effectiveness by counteracting peripheral and central sensitization. The most important class of drugs used perioperatively are the opioids, followed by the non-steroidal anti-inflammatory drugs (NSAIDs). A detailed description of perioperative analgesia is given in Chapter 18.

17.4.3 Anticholinergics

Anticholinergics block acetylcholine at muscarinic sites, and therefore block parasympathetic transmission at postganglionic nerve terminals. This leads to a decrease in oral, gastric, and respiratory secretions, reduction of bronchial tone and gastrointestinal motility, an increase in heart rate by reduction of the vagal influence on the heart, and mydriasis by central activity. The routine use of anticholinergic premedication is not necessary, but can be indicated in some instances. It reduces disease or drug (i.e., ketamine)-related salivation, or increased bronchial secretions to avoid airway obstruction. It can also be beneficial in surgical procedures, which might elicit vagal reflexes (surgery in the head and neck area).

A controversial issue is the use of concurrent administration of anticholinergics to prevent bradycardia induced by alpha$_2$ agonists. Bradycardia might be resolved by this approach and heart rates improve, but cardiac work can be massively increased when the heart has to pump against a high vascular resistance during the hypertensive phase.

Atropine can be given by the SC/IM and IV route. After IV injection an initial increase in vagal tone can occur; therefore IM injection is recommended when used in a therapeutic manner. Atropine crosses the blood–brain barrier readily and induces mydriasis by central actions, and it can also induce tachycardia. Recommended doses are 0.02 mg/kg IV or 0.04–0.1 mg/kg SC/IM. High doses can cause central excitation. Contraindications are glaucoma and predisposition for tachyarrhythmias (i.e., hyperthyroidism).

Glycopyrrolate is a large polar molecule with a quarternary ammonium structure that does not readily cross the blood–brain barrier and the placenta. This lack of permeability means it does not induce mydriasis and is suitable for pregnant cats. It can be given by the SC/IM/IV route with an onset of action within 1 minute after IV injection. The duration of action is longer than with atropine (3–4 hours). Glycopyrrolate is less likely to induce tachycardia than atropine but initial arrhythmias can occur immediately after injection. Recommended doses are 0.01 mg/kg IV or 0.02 mg/kg IM/SC.

17.5 Injectable anesthetics

Injectable anesthetics can be used for induction followed by inhalational anesthesia, or as the sole anesthetic used to maintain general anesthesia (TIVA; total intravenous anesthesia). There is a dose-dependent transition from sedation to general anesthesia for some injectable anesthetics. Dose rates required for induction and maintenance of anesthesia depend on the premedication given and individual sensitivity. Fragmented dosing of the calculated amount of anesthetic helps to prevent overdosing.

17.5.1 Barbiturates

Short-acting barbiturates have been the classic injectable anesthetics used in veterinary medicine for more than 60 years. Barbiturates produce hypnosis with no analgesia, and high doses are required to produce surgical anesthesia. Barbiturates can cause tissue necrosis when perivascular injection occurs.

Pentobarbital has been used widely in cats in veterinary practice. Approximately 2 hours of surgical anesthesia result from one IV injection of 25 mg/kg pentobarbital. Pentobarbital, however, has a narrow safety margin and doses three times the anesthetic dose (72 mg/kg) are lethal in cats. Recovery from pentobarbital anesthesia is very prolonged, and as such it is no longer recommended for clinical anesthesia in cats. Its main use in veterinary medicine is as a euthanatizing agent, causing very rapid loss of consciousness.

Thiopental (thiopentone) as the sole anesthetic agent requires doses up to 20 mg/kg when given slowly. Rapid injection of a lower dose (5–6 mg/kg) results in about 10 minutes of anesthesia, which is usually sufficient to enable endotracheal intubation and maintenance under gaseous anesthesia. Thiopental has no analgesic effects, and causes dose-dependent cardiovascular and respiratory depression as well as arrhythmias (11). Thiopental is therefore best used with an acepromazine/opioid premedication to reduce the required dose (5–10 mg/kg). Thiopental should be used as a dilute solution of 1–1.25% to avoid venous irritation. The distribution/redistribution kinetics of thiopental into different body tissues result in rapid recovery after a single dose, but prolonged recoveries occur after multiple injections or infusions.

17.5.2 Propofol

Propofol is a rapidly acting alkylphenol producing a short duration of anesthesia with rapid recovery, even after multiple doses. Propofol is currently formulated as a white oil-in-water emulsion. This emulsion is an ideal culture medium for bacteria. Open vials should therefore be refrigerated and should not be used once they have been opened for more than 24 hours. Special disinfection procedures to avoid contamination have been used to prolong usability of open vials.

Intramuscular injection does not induce anesthesia and inadvertent perivascular injection is not irritating. Too rapid an injection of propofol can lead to apnea, so an injection time of 2 minutes is recommended for induction doses, to be able to titrate to effect and to avoid apnea. In contrast to dogs, the induction dose of propofol is not reduced to a significant extent by acepromazine premedication (12), but opioids and alpha$_2$ agonists reduce propofol requirements in cats significantly.

The most prominent cardiorespiratory effects are moderate hypotension, which can cause problems in hypovolemic cats, and its use should be avoided in shock patients. Respiratory depression with hypercapnea and a drop in arterial oxygenation occur after repeated or continuous propofol dosing. Oxygen supplementation is therefore advisable during prolonged propofol administration. Cats have a relative deficiency of glucuronide conjugation, which is required for metabolism of phenolic compounds, and feline hemoglobin is prone to oxidative injury by phenolic compounds. Repeated propofol anesthesia on consecutive days or prolonged infusions will result in significant Heinz body formation, anorexia, diarrhea, facial edema, depression, and prolonged recovery from anesthesia (13). When propofol is used for induction and maintenance it should be titrated to effect similar to an inhalant anesthetic because of the variable influence of premedicants, concurrent analgesics, and surgical stimulation. The maintenance rate for TIVA ranges from 0.2 to 0.5 mg/kg per minute (or 2 mg/kg every 5 minutes).

17.5.3 Dissociatives

The phencyclidine derivatives ketamine and tiletamine differ from the classic anesthetic substances. These agents produce dissociative anesthesia by functional dissociation, characterized by somatic analgesia with very superficial sleep. They induce a state of catalepsy, an akinetic state with loss of orthostatic reflexes. The tone of the muscles is increased and visceral analgesia is insufficient. Therefore dissociatives alone cannot produce a state of surgical anesthesia. They have to be combined with a muscle relaxant and analgesic to prevent muscle stiffness and convulsions.

Ketamine is a water-soluble agent, with a standard concentration of 10% (100 mg/ml) for veterinary use. Racemic ketamine is a scheduled drug in the USA because of possible abuse by humans. Ketamine is effective after SC, IM, and IV administration, and also by transmucutaneous uptake from the oral mucous membranes. This flexibility makes ketamine suitable for use in cats that are difficult to handle. Intramuscular injection of ketamine is painful and often resented by cats. Laryngeal and pharyngeal reflexes are retained after administration, but salivation is often profuse in cats, and airway patency has to be monitored closely. Spontaneous, athetotic (writhing or jerky) movements may occur unrelated to surgical stimulation or lightening of anesthesia. Ketamine exerts indirect sympathomimetic effects resulting in cardiovascular stimulation with increased heart rates and blood pressures similar to awake blood pressures in the healthy animal. But it has also direct negative inotropic effects on the myocardium, which might predominate in the compromised animal. Ketamine-induced respiratory depression is minimal at clinical doses but it induces an apneustic breathing rhythm (periods of rapid breathing alternating with apnea), and overdosing causes apnea. Ketamine increases cerebral blood flow and intracranial pressure and therefore should be avoided in patients with suspected head trauma. It is also avoided in cats with hypertrophic cardiomyopathy because it increases myocardial oxygen consumption. Domestic cats excrete the majority of ketamine unchanged via the kidney so recovery after large doses or repeated doses of ketamine can be prolonged in cats with renal dysfunction.

Recovery from ketamine anesthesia can be associated with increased sensitivity to external stimuli and increased motor activity, so cats should be allowed to recover in a quiet room.

17.5.4 Alphaxalone/alphadolone

Neuroactive steroids induce hypnosis and muscle relaxation via $GABA_A$ receptors enhancing the inhibitory effects of GABA. A combination of alphaxalone/alphadolone in Cremophor EL was marketed as Saffan. Saffan administered intravenously can induce histamine release which is related to the Cremophor EL. Transient hyperemia, and facial and paw edema, occur in approximately 25% of cats treated with Saffan. Saffan has therefore been taken off the market. Alphaxalone (Alfaxan; Jurox, Australia) has recently been introduced for anesthesia induction in dogs and cats, although it has been used for some years in Australia and New Zealand. The alphaxalone molecule is solubilized in the Alfaxan formulation using 2α-hydroxypropyl beta cyclodextrin (HPBCD). Cyclodextrins are complex polysaccharides derived from starch that have a hydrophobic center for lipophilic drugs like alphaxalone. Unlike Cremophor EL, HPBCD does not cause histamine release in dogs and cats. Alfaxan provides smooth inductions and less excitement during recovery, and has a shorter duration of action.

17.5.5 Etomidate

Etomidate is an imidazole derivative inducing hypnosis without analgesia. Etomidate induces very little cardiovascular and respiratory depression and is well suited for use in high-risk patients. It induces myoclonus without premedication. Etomidate is rapidly hydrolyzed and has little cumulative effects, making it suitable for constant-rate infusion. However, etomidate suppresses adrenal steroidogenesis and is therefore not recommended for long-term use. A single injection can inhibit adrenal function for several hours but this lack of stress response after a single injection is well tolerated. Etomidate is available as a solution with 35% propylene glycol and similar to propofol as an emulsion in soya bean oil, egg lecithin (Lipuro, Braun, Germany). The emulsion requires aseptic handling procedures and an open vial should not be used after it has been open for more than 24 hours. Acute hemolysis has been reported after etomidate injection in cats, which is related to the osmolality changes induced by rapid injection of the propylene glycol-containing solution. Rapid IV injection can also be painful and perivascular injection can cause phlebitis.

17.6 Inhalation anesthesia

Inhalation anesthesia is the preferred technique for maintaining general anesthesia for surgical procedures, because the depth of anesthesia can easily be altered and drug accumulation is not a problem with modern inhalation anesthetics. Administration of inhalation anesthetics requires specialized equipment, and an understanding of basic principles is necessary. The focus of this chapter is on the volatile anesthetics currently in clinical use, including nitrous oxide (N_2O), halothane, isoflurane, and sevoflurane. Desflurane has also been used in cats (14), but the costs of maintenance requirements for the sophisticated vaporizer make routine use in veterinary practice very unlikely. The central nervous system depression defined as general anesthesia is directly related to the partial pressure of the anesthetic in the brain, and depth of anesthesia varies with changes in this partial pressure and not with changes in concentration or total amount of the anesthetic in the brain tissue.

The minimum alveolar concentration (MAC) of an inhaled anesthetic is the major index of anesthetic potency. It can be described as the medium effective dose (ED_{50}) of an inhalation anesthetic, where 50% of animals respond and 50% do not respond with purposeful movements to a standard supramaximal stimulus (i.e., tail clamp). MAC values are determined in healthy animals, and anesthetic requirements may vary with disease and individual cat. MAC can be lowered by N_2O, analgesics and sedatives, hypothermia, and pregnancy, whereas central stimulation (i.e., atropine), hyperthermia, and hypernatremia will increase MAC. MAC-sparing measures are highly desirable because cardiovascular depression will be reduced by lower concentrations of volatile anesthetics.

17.6.1 Pharmacological characteristics of volatile anesthetics

The relatively non-specific central depression exerted by the volatile anesthetics is always accompanied by cardiovascular and respiratory depression.

N_2O is an odorless gas at room temperature and is provided as compressed gas in tanks. N_2O can be characterized as a rapidly acting anesthetic with a very low potency in cats. At atmospheric pressure N_2O cannot be used as the sole anesthetic agent; however, as an adjunctive anesthetic with other anesthetics it has several advantages. N_2O has good analgesic effects with only minimal cardiovascular and respiratory depression contributing to MAC reduction of other volatile anesthetics. N_2O has to be used in high concentration to achieve an analyesic effect. Nitrogen in air-filled spaces has lower blood solubility than N_2O; thus more N_2O will be available for exchange than N_2 will leave, and volume extension will occur. Therefore, N_2O is contraindicated in intestinal obstructions and pneumothorax.

At the end of anesthesia, large amounts of N_2O diffuse into the lungs and can displace oxygen (diffusion hypoxia). This effect can be prevented by keeping the cat on high oxygen flow rates for at least 5 minutes after the N_2O has been turned off. The use of N_2O (at least 50% is required to achieve analgesia) limits the amount of oxygen that can be delivered to the patient, and at least 30% oxygen should be contained in the inspired gases. To insure appropriate oxygen delivery to the tissues in patients requiring higher fractions of inspired oxygen (anemia, shock), N_2O is contraindicated. A similar problem can occur with the use of N_2O in low-flow anesthesia systems (see later). Because the oxygen is metabolized by the patient, N_2O can accumulate, and hypoxia can occur. Oxygen concentrations are always monitored when using N_2O in low-flow systems.

Halothane was introduced in the 1950s and is still widely used in veterinary anesthesia. Halothane has a fairly rapid action with a moderate potency. It is best delivered by a precision vaporizer. Halothane depresses respiration and chemoreceptor sensitivity in a dose-dependent manner with decreased responses to hypoxia and hypercapnea. It also seems to reduce bronchial tone, which might be an advantage in asthmatic cats. Cardiovascular function is depressed dose-dependently with reduction of cardiac output, stroke volume, and arterial pressures. Heart rates remain stable within a clinical dose range but cardiac output is reduced by reduction in myocardial contractility. Halothane predisposes the heart to premature ventricular contractions in the presence of catecholamines. Halothane increases cerebral blood flow with a concurrent increase in intracranial pressure, and it depresses autoregulation of cerebral blood flow. Its use should therefore be avoided in head trauma patients. Liver function is reduced both by direct effects of halothane and by reduction of liver blood flow during anesthesia, thus prolonging the effects of concurrently used drugs. Halothane should not be used in animals with compromise of liver function. Transient increase in liver enzymes can occur after anesthesia; however, severe liver damage is a very rare event. Halothane can trigger malignant hyperthermia in sensitive animals but this effect is extremely rare in cats.

Isoflurane is a halogenated ether, allowing rapid induction and rapid changes in anesthetic depths. Therefore, isoflurane seems to be suited for mask or chamber induction, but it has a pungent smell and cats can become agitated or hold their breath during mask induction. Isoflurane has a similar vapor pressure to halothane so halothane vaporizers can be adapted to be used with isoflurane after recalibration. Alveolar ventilation is depressed in a dose-dependent manner, with relative constancy in respiratory frequency but decreased tidal volume. Cardiac output is better maintained with isoflurane than with halothane at the same anesthetic depths, and with isoflurane the myocardium is not sensitized to catecholamine-induced arrhythmias. A dose-related decrease in arterial blood pressure caused by vasodilation can be quite pronounced in cats. With isoflurane, cerebral blood flow and intracranial pressure are increased at doses above 1.2 MAC but autoregulation of cerebral blood flow in response to changes in systemic blood pressure seems to be maintained. Isoflurane can therefore be used in patients with head trauma.

Sevoflurane is a fluorinated ether, allowing very rapid induction of anesthesia and changes in anesthetic depth. The lack of pungency and the aromatic smell make it well tolerated for mask or chamber induction in cats. Sevoflurane has shown dose-dependent cardiovascular depression in cats, which is mainly attributable to myocardial depression. In one study, heart rates and systemic vascular resistance remained stable whereas stroke volume and mean arterial blood pressures decreased (15). Sevoflurane does not sensitize the myocardium to the arrhythmogenic effects of catcholamines. Respiratory depression is also dose-dependent and seems comparable to isoflurane. Cerebral blood flow and intracranial pressure are minimally increased at clinical doses. Recovery when sevoflurane is used alone is very rapid but can be associated with excitement and paddling. This recovery period can be influenced by premedication or concurrently used drugs.

17.6.2 Equipment

The administration of inhalational anesthetics requires a carrier gas including oxygen, an anesthetic vaporizing device, and a patient breathing system. In-depth information on the construction of anesthetic machines, vaporizers, and breathing systems is not covered in this text and the reader is referred to other sources on this subject (16, 17).

Anesthetic machine

A variety of different commercial veterinary and human anesthetic machines are available, from the very basic apparatus to sophisticated electronically regulated all-in-one anesthetic and monitoring systems. The basic components of all these machines are the same. A source of oxygen and N_2O, a gas-regulating and measuring device, and a vaporizer to control vaporization of the liquid anesthetic (Fig. 17-3) must be present.

In the low-pressure system of the anesthetic machine the gas first passes through the flowmeter. By using the flowmeter the amount of gas (l/min) delivered to the patient can be altered. For each gas a calibrated flowmeter is present. The flowmeter control knobs are color- and often touch-coded to avoid oxygen and N_2O being confused. Within the flowmeter cylinder a ball or a rotor indicates the gas flow rate. The flow level is read from the center of the ball or the top of the rotor. As the gas passes through the flowmeters, the pressure is further reduced to allow safe passage of gas into the patient's airways.

A vaporizer converts a liquid anesthetic to the vapor state, and adds a controlled amount of vapor to the carrier gas. Vaporizers can be positioned within the breathing system (VIC) or after the flowmeter, outside the breathing system (VOC). Modern volatile anesthetics are most safely delivered by precision vaporizers in a VOC position. Vaporizer output is very stable over a range of commonly used fresh gas flows until very low flow rates (<250 ml/min). Vaporizer performance and calibration should be tested at least once a year. Adaptation of halothane vaporizers to use with isoflurane (similar vapor pressure) is possible; however, this requires cleaning and recalibration of the vaporizer by specialized companies. Otherwise cross-agent use is dangerous and strongly discouraged.

Most anesthetic machines have an oxygen flush which allows the oxygen to bypass the vaporizer via a separate line, directly to the common gas outlet. Pure oxygen is delivered at high flow rates. This is useful in emergency situations, and can also be used to dilute the anesthetic concentration in the breathing system at the end of anesthesia. The oxygen flush has to be used with caution in combination with non-rebreathing systems, because the high flow rates produced by the flush are directly transferred into the patient and can easily damage the lung of the cat.

Before using any anesthetic machine or breathing system in an animal a short function check should become routine. The pressure relief valve should be closed and the machine and the breathing system should be pressurized with oxygen to

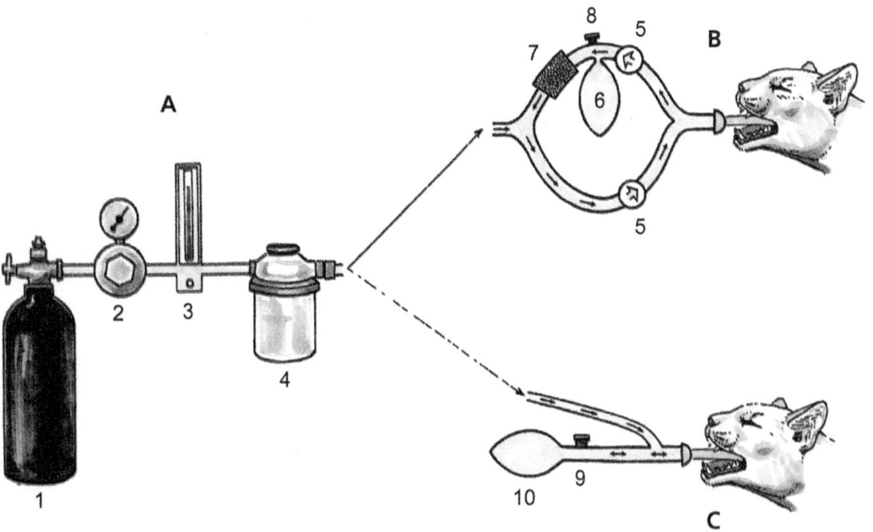

Figure 17-3 Diagram illustrating the basic elements of an anesthetic machine and the different breathing systems. (**A**) The anesthetic machine has an oxygen source (1), pressure regulator (2), flowmeter (3), and vaporizer (4). (**B**) Rebreathing (circle) system with unidirectional valves (5), reservoir bag (6), soda lime canister (7), and pressure relief valve (8) (**C**) Non-rebreathing system with pressure relief valve (9) and reservoir bag (10).

30 cmH_2O (mbar). This pressure should remain for 20–30 seconds without further gas supply. Any leak present can be measured by the amount of oxygen needed to maintain this pressure (flowmeter setting). The leak should not exceed 300 ml/min. It should also be ensured that enough oxygen is available and the vaporizer is filled with the proper anesthetic.

Breathing systems

The breathing system carries the anesthetic gas mixture to the patient and draws off expired gases. An important feature of the breathing system is the removal of expired carbon dioxide (CO_2). There are two major ways of removing CO_2: first, absorption of CO_2 via a chemical reaction with soda lime in combination with rebreathing systems; and second, elution of CO_2 in non-rebreathing systems.

Rebreathing systems

Rebreathing systems allow partial or complete rebreathing of exhaled gases. Circle systems are most commonly used. The gas flow in this system is unidirectional. A circle system contains unidirectional valves, a reservoir bag, a pressure relief valve, CO_2 absorber (soda lime canister), a pressure manometer, and breathing hoses connected by a Y-piece (Fig. 17-3). Circle breathing systems have many advantages: they allow economic use of anesthetic gases when operated in a low-flow fashion, and preserve airway moisture and body heat by recycling exhaled gases. These are factors of particular concern in small patients like cats. However, the large volume of this system, the valves, and the CO_2 absorber pose a significant resistance to breathing in cats. Some modern pediatric circle breathing systems with small-volume absorber and small-diameter breathing hoses have a low resistance to breathing, but most cats in a surgical plane of anesthesia require mechanical ventilation to move the gas volume and avoid rebreathing of CO_2-containing gas when using a circle system.

Circle breathing systems can be used in different ways. A low-flow approach facilitates the advantages of partial rebreathing of respired gases. With this mode, the system is not totally closed, and some gas leaves the circle via the pressure relief valve (semi-closed). Low-flow anesthesia in cats can be performed with gas flows of 25–50 ml/kg per minute with special anesthetic machines (flowmeter calibration, vaporizer output). However, with the commonly used anesthetic machines, fresh gas flows should reach 200–300 ml/kg per minute to allow safe inhalational anesthesia. In a low-flow system N_2O can accumulate, and oxygen flows have to be 100–150 ml/kg per minute to avoid hypoxic oxygen concentrations (<30%) in the inspired gas, when N_2O is used in combination with oxygen (Table 17-6). Gas concentrations are most predictable in a high-flow system (400–500 ml/kg per minute for a cat). However, with this mode of operation the advantages of rebreathing humidified and warm gas will be abolished.

Systems	Gas flow rates
Induction	
Chamber induction	5 l/min
Mask induction	300 ml/kg per minute or 1–3 l/min per cat
After intravenous induction	200–500 ml/kg per minute
Maintenance	
Rebreathing system	25–500 ml/kg per minute
Bain system	200 ml/kg per minute
Other non-rebreathing systems	200–300 ml/kg per minute

Table 17.6. Recommended gas flow rates

Fresh gas flow rates will vary during induction and maintenance phases. During induction higher flow rates are used than during maintenance. This is necessary to saturate the anesthetic circuit with anesthetic gas and to wash out the nitrogen from the lung and bloodstream of the patient. The chosen carrier gas flow rate will affect the amount of anesthetic received by the animal. Low fresh gas flow rates result in more rebreathing of expired gas, which contains lower anesthetic concentrations. The lower the fresh gas flow rate, the lower the anesthetic concentration with the same vaporizer setting. Therefore, precision vaporizer settings have to be increased when a low-flow approach has been chosen. In addition, low flows will make a system less dynamic, meaning that changes in vaporizer settings will only change anesthetic concentrations in the system very slowly. If a more rapid change is desired, gas flow rates have to be increased (Table 17-6).

Non-rebreathing systems

For most non-rebreathing systems, flow rates of at least 300 ml/kg per minute are required to function properly. These systems have the advantage of a low resistance to breathing. They come in many different designs, but basically they all fit in the original Mapleson classification (Fig. 17-4). The systems differ in the position of the fresh gas inlet, the reservoir bag, and where the exhalation valve is positioned: this determines the required gas flow rates. In the valve-less non-rebreathing systems the high gas flow rate ensures CO_2 elution. Light-weight systems with the exhalation valve distant from the patient's head (Mapleson D and E) are advantageous for cats (Ayres T-piece, Kuhn system, Bain system). The coaxial Bain system (Mapleson D) (Fig. 17-5) is a special design with two concentric tubes. The inner tube

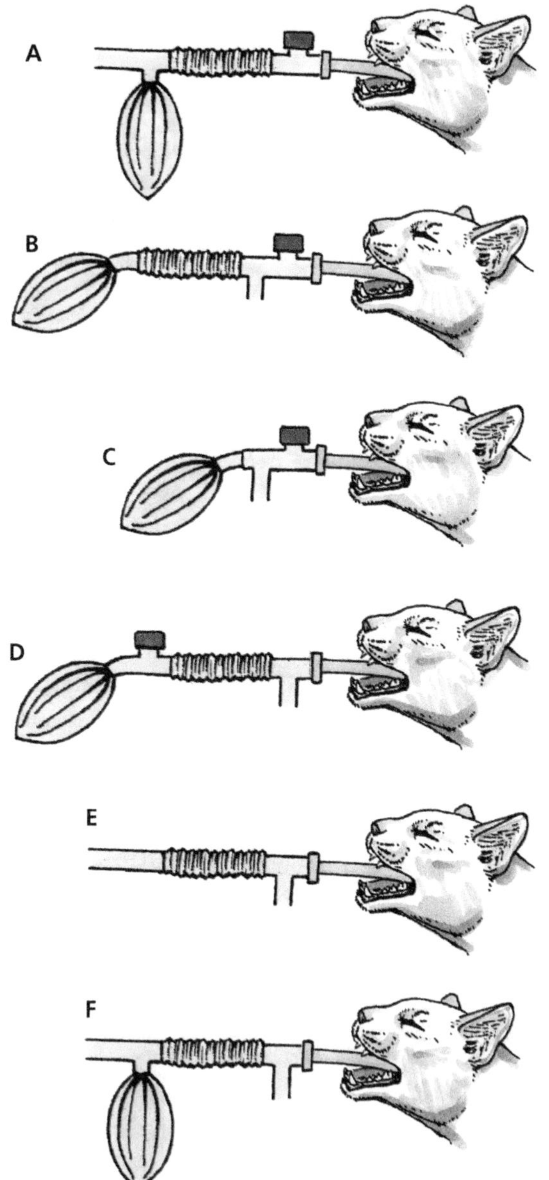

Figure 17-4 Classification of non-rebreathing systems according to Mapleson (**A–F**) vary in placement of the reservoir and pressure relief valve. Systems **D** (Kuhn system, coaxial Bain system) and **E** (Ayres T-piece) are most commonly used in cats.

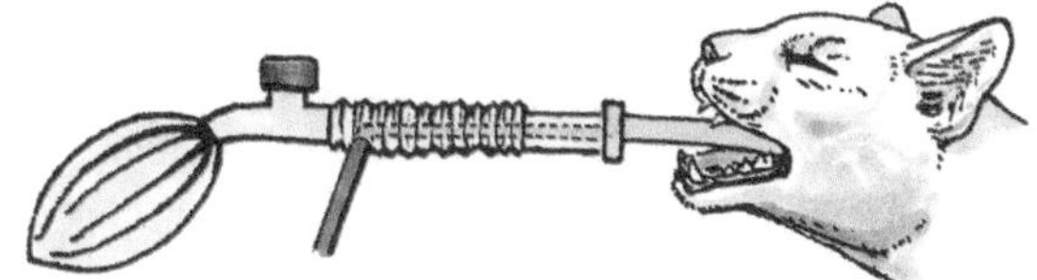

Figure 17-5 Coaxial Bain system. Fresh gas flow is supplied via the inner tube. Expired gas is transported within the outer tube.

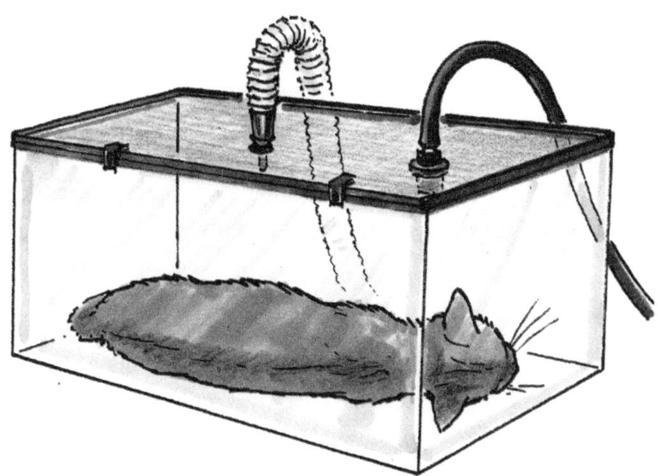

Figure 17-6 Induction chamber with connectors to fresh gas flow from the anesthetic machine and to the scavenging system.

carries the fresh gas and exhalation occurs via the outer tube, thereby warming the fresh gas slightly. Special care has to be taken that the inner tube is not detached from the tube connector to avoid rebreathing of CO_2. The Bain system can be operated with flow rates of 200 ml/kg per minute. Commercial light-weight pediatric non-rebreathing systems are available and well suited for the cat.

17.6.3 Chamber and mask induction

Inhalation anesthesia is usually used for maintenance after induction with an intravenous anesthetic, but chamber and mask induction are alternatives. Induction in a see-through or transparent chamber using a rapidly acting inhalational anesthetic like sevoflurane might be less stressful than restraint in a crush or squeeze cage in uncooperative cats (Fig. 17-6). The drawback to chamber induction is that monitoring of the animal's vital signs in the chamber can be difficult.

Mask induction with a tight-fitting face mask and isoflurane or sevoflurane in oxygen or in an oxygen/N_2O mixture can be used for induction of anesthesia, followed by intubation or by maintenance by mask for short procedures such as blood sampling or radiography. When available, sevoflurane is preferred over isoflurane for mask induction because of a more rapid onset of action and lack of pungency compared to isoflurane. For mask induction in healthy cats, vaporizer settings of 7–8% sevoflurane or 4–5% isoflurane are combined with gas flows of 3 l/min in a non-rebreathing system. As soon as the cat can be positioned in lateral recumbency (1–3 minutes) vaporizer settings are reduced. Lower initial concentrations are recommended in debilitated patients, and adapted to the individual patient (18).

17.6.4 Endotracheal intubation

The upper airway of a cat is very delicate and easily damaged or blocked by secretions. Endotracheal intubation is the only way to achieve complete control of the airways during general anesthesia. It allows direct oxygen supplementation and mechanical ventilation and protects the airways from aspiration of gastric reflux, blood, and debris. Intubation in cats can be associated with specific problems. The larynx is very small and the protective reflexes are very well developed. Rough treatment of the larynx can lead to swelling and laryngeal spasm, which might cause problems during intubation, and also later in the recovery phase. Endotracheal intubation is only possible when the laryngeal reflexes are suppressed. This requires either very deep planes of anesthesia, which is not without risk, or decreasing the sensitivity of the larynx by superficial application of local anesthesia with lidocaine. Most commercial lidocaine sprays contain high concentrations of lidocaine (10% = 100 mg/ml) and excessive spraying should be avoided.

Cats can be intubated in the lateral, prone, or supine position. The prone position with the head extended and the tongue pulled forward is the easiest way and allows good visualization of the larynx facilitated by a laryngoscope with a small blade (Fig. 17-7). The blade should only be used to depress the base of the tongue and should not touch or depress the epiglottis, because this action alone can cause laryngeal spasm. Attempts to intubate are only made once the larynx opens. Some time has to be allowed for the topical lidocaine to exert its effect.

Different styles of cuffed and uncuffed endotracheal tubes are available for cats (Fig. 17-8). The commercial products made for human or veterinary anesthesia are usually too long so the tube should be cut at the adapter side to avoid inadvertent endobronchial intubation or increased equipment dead space. The endotracheal tube connector should be at the level of the incisors. Tube sizes between 3.0 and 5.0 internal diameter are suitable for adult cats. Some types of tubes are very flexible and intubation is made easier by using a stylet to stiffen the tube, but the stylet should not protrude over the tip of the tube to avoid laceration of the trachea. The cuff should lie in the cervical part of the trachea. Overinflation of endotracheal tube cuffs can result in tracheal rupture and consecutive strictures at the site of the cuff, regardless of cuff type. The longest ruptures were associated with the use of high-volume, low-pressure tubes (19). Therefore, cuffs should be filled with care using a 2-ml syringe with the lowest possible volume necessary to obtain a seal. For clinically normal adult cats the average volume to obtain an airtight seal was 1.6 ml (19).

The endotracheal tube is securely tied around the head of the cat with a gauze bandage to prevent inadvertent extraction. As cats produce high amounts of saliva and mucus and the endotracheal tubes are small, the tubes can easily become blocked in cats. Patency of the tube has to be regularly checked and excessive saliva should be removed with a suction catheter.

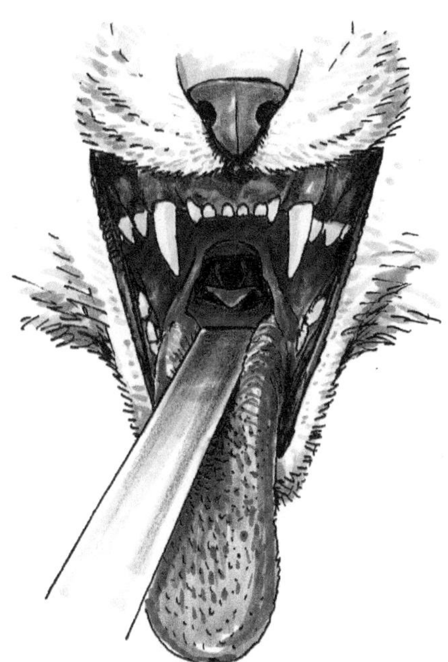

Figure 17-7 A small blade laryngoscope is used for endotracheal intubation in the cat. The blade is used to depress the tongue and should not touch the larynx.

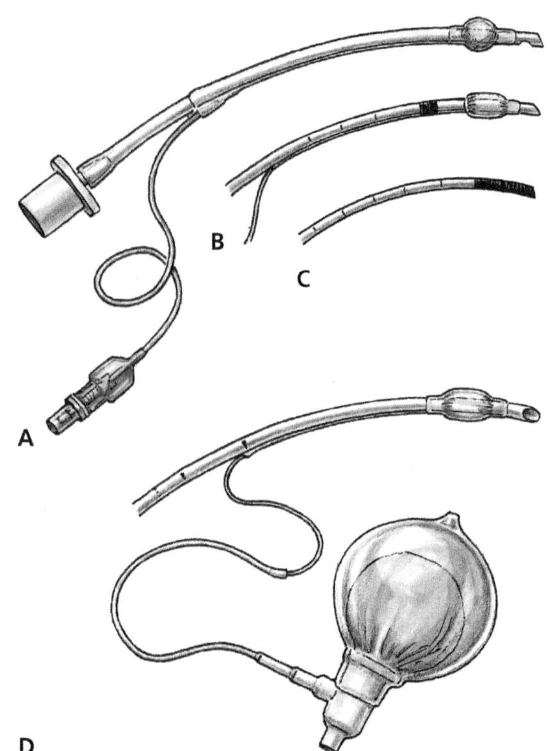

Figure 17-8 Different styles of cuffed and uncuffed endotracheal tubes suitable for use in the cat. (**A**) Low-volume, high-pressure cuff; (**B**) high-volume, low-pressure cuff; (**C**) uncuffed for very small animals. Note the different shapes of the inflated cuffs, resulting in differences in contact area with the tracheal mucosa. (**D**) Special design of the pilot balloon (Lanz pressure-regulating valve) prevents pressure increase in the cuff during anesthesia with nitrous oxide.

Ventilator	Settings
Tidal volume	5–20 ml/kg
Respiratory rate	12–20 breaths/min
Minute volume	400–600 ml
Peak inspiratory pressure	20 cm H_2O
Inspiratory to expiratory time ratio	1:2 to 1:3

Table 17-7. Suggested ventilator settings in cats

17.6.5 Ventilation

Anesthesia can usually be well maintained in cats under spontaneous respiration. In circumstances where mechanical respiration is necessary, the reservoir bag is replaced with a ventilator. Ventilators suitable for use in cats (human pediatric, small-animal ventilators) come in varying designs depending on the cycling mechanism and the mechanism producing the inspiratory phase (pressure or flow generator). However, for safe use in cats, independent of the working principles, the ventilator should be able to deliver small tidal volumes (20–200 ml) at a safe working pressure (10–60 cm H_2O) to avoid barotrauma to the lungs. Ventilator settings (Table 17-7) have to be adapted to the individual animal's ability to maintain eucapnia (30–35 mmHg) based on partial pressures of CO_2 in expired gas (end-tidal CO_2) or arterial blood ($Paco_2$).

17.7 Monitoring

Monitoring of a patient undergoing general anesthesia begins at induction of anesthesia, and continues during anesthesia (at least every 10 minutes) and also after surgery until complete recovery (20). Observation should be instituted after premedication in certain situations looking for vomiting, respiratory depression or excessive sedation for example. A recent study of perioperative fatalities in small animals revealed that 62% of anesthetic-related deaths in cats occurred in the immediate postoperative period (0–3 h), probably related to no or reduced monitoring during that period (21).

Acceptable ranges of important parameters of cats under general anesthesia are summarized in Table 17-8.

17.7.1 Physical monitoring

Basic monitoring for all anesthetized cats should include assessment of depth of anesthesia by testing palpebral reflexes, eyeball position, and jaw tone. With inhalation anesthetics, thiopental, and propofol, the eyeballs rotate rostroventrally during light and moderate planes of anesthesia (Fig. 17-9), and return to a central position with dilated pupils in deep

Parameter	Values
Heart rate	80–160 beats/min
Respiratory rate	15–30 breaths/min
Tidal volume	15–20 ml/kg
Capillary refill time	<2 seconds
Mean arterial blood pressure	60–120 mmHg
Central venous pressure	0–5 cm H_2O
Body temperature	35.0–40°C
Spo_2	95–100%
Pao_2	>60 mmHg
End-tidal CO_2	25–50 mmHg
$Paco_2$	25–60 mmHg
FIo_2	>30%
Arterial pH	7.30–7.45

Table 17-8. Range of acceptable parameters in cats under general anesthesia

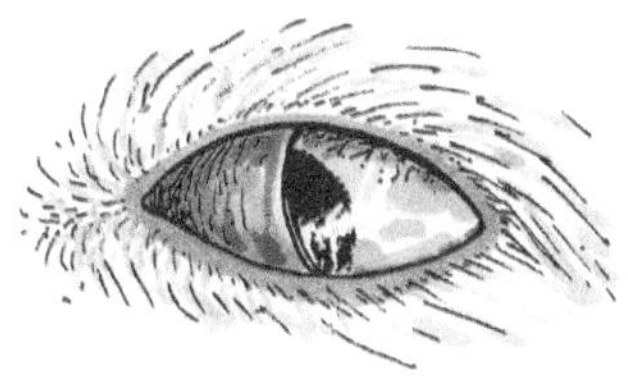

Figure 17-9 Eyeballs rotated rostroventrally with mild dilation of the pupils during light and moderate planes of anesthesia.

anesthesia. The presence of the palpebral reflex and high tone of the jaw muscles indicate a very light plane of anesthesia in the cat. With ketamine anesthesia, muscle tone is not reduced and the eyeball remains in a central position with brisk palpebral reflexes; therefore these signs cannot be used to judge depth of anesthesia.

Ventilation can be assessed by counting the respiratory rate, observation of chest excursions, or movement of the reservoir bag. Information on oxygenation is obtained from mucous membrane color. Heart rate, pulse strength, and capillary refill time will give information on circulation. In general, cardiovascular and respiratory depression will increase with an increasing depth of anesthesia. However, these signs can be unreliable in indicating depth of anesthesia as they may vary with the different combinations of anesthetics and analgesics used.

17.7.2 Cardiovascular monitors

Esophageal stethoscope

A simple device for monitoring heart rate and rhythm is an esophageal stethoscope. The stethoscope is introduced into the esophagus until the balloon at the end lies at the base of the heart. This position can easily be checked and controlled by auscultation via the stethoscope.

Electrocardiogram

Information on the electrical rhythm and rate of the heart is obtained from an electrocardiogram using standard limb leads. Clip or adhesive electrodes are taped on the paws of the cat. Placement of the electrodes should not interfere with the surgical intervention or cause artifacts by movement of the electrodes (i.e., breathing).

Arterial blood pressure monitoring

Usually arterial blood pressures during general anesthesia are lower than those in the awake state. Protocols using ketamine, tiletamine, or high doses of $alpha_2$ agonists might increase systemic arterial pressures. Decreased blood pressure can be related to decreased cardiac output or peripheral vasodilation or a combination of both. Arterial blood pressure can be determined by direct methods requiring catheterization of an artery or indirect methods using Doppler ultrasound or oscillometric techniques.

The Doppler ultrasound probe can be placed over the metatarsal or metacarpal artery, on the plantar or palmar surface of the paw just proximal to the main footpad, or the coccygeal artery on the ventral surface of the tail. An inflatable cuff is placed around the limb or the tail proximal to the transducer (Fig. 17-10). The appropriate cuff size, with cuff widths being between 40 and 60% of the circumference of the limb, has to be selected for accurate results. Cuffs made for human newborns (size 1 and 2) are suitable in the cat. The cuff is inflated above systolic pressure and slowly released again. Theoretically, the pressure on the aneroid manometer where the first pulse sounds are heard is the systolic pressure. The specific sounds indicating diastolic pressure cannot be heard in many cats. A cuff placed too loosely or too tightly will result in overestimation or underestimation of blood pressure. Comparison of the Doppler method with direct femoral artery pressures showed that it underestimated direct systolic pressures by 14–25 mmHg (22, 23). The conclusion is that the Doppler method seems to be more indicative for mean arterial blood pressure than for systolic blood pressure in cats.

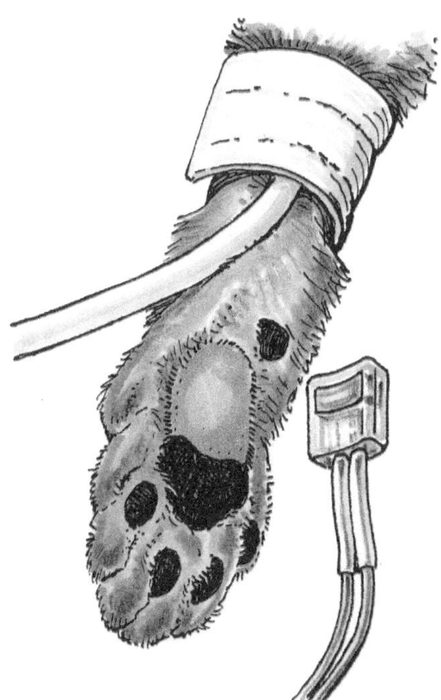

Figure 17-10 Doppler ultrasound probe placed over the metacarpal artery on the palmar surface of the paw just proximal to the footpad. Metacarpal (front leg) measurements give the best results in the cat.

Systems using the oscillometric method function with self-inflating cuffs. Systolic, diastolic, and mean arterial pressure as well as heart rate are displayed on the monitors. The median artery (thoracic limb) gives the best results for indirect blood pressure measurements when using this method. There are a variety of oscillometric systems made for human anesthesia that do not accurately reflect blood pressures in cats; however, devices specifically made for veterinary medicine (i.e., Dinamap) can give good results. Often no measurements are obtained when using the oscillometric method in low-pressure states.

The most accurate method of assessing blood pressure is by invasive measurement. Direct measurement of arterial blood pressure in the cat requires catheterization of the femoral artery. The cranial tibial, coccygeal, or dorsal pedal artery may also be accessible with a 24-gauge catheter in large cats. Over-the-needle-type catheters can be used for arterial catheterization. Catheters employing the Seldinger technique with insertion of a thin flexible guidewire make catheterization of small cat arteries easier. A simple method to measure arterial pressure is by use of an aneroid manometer connected via extension tubing and three-way taps to the catheter, and a syringe filled with heparinized saline. Care has to be taken to avoid saline entering the manometer by leaving an air gap that needs to be at the zero reference level (right atrium). Mean arterial pressure is measured when the manometer is open to the artery. Continuous-pressure waveforms are obtained with an electrical pressure transducer placed at the level of the heart and the zero calibration open to ambient air pressure. The pressure transducer is ideally connected to the catheter by short, non-compliant tubing completely filled with heparinized saline. The waveform is displayed on an anesthetic monitor.

Central venous pressure

Central venous pressure is used to assess adequacy of blood volume. A long catheter is advanced via the jugular vein into the cranial vena cava. The pressure is measured by venous manometers, fluid-filled tubing, and a ruler or an electrical pressure transducer. The zero reference level is the right atrium, which is approximated by the sternal manubrium. Central venous pressure is usually reported as cm H_2O (1 cm H_2O = 0.736 mmHg). Normal central venous pressure ranges from 0 to 5 cm H_2O. Pressures above 12 cm H_2O might indicate hypervolemia or cardiac failure.

17.7.3 Respiratory system monitors

Apnea alarm

Apnea alarms record respiratory rate and give an alarm when apnea occurs. The signal is created by a thermistor registering temperature changes caused by the gas flow.

Tidal volume monitors

Tidal volume or minute volume can be determined by volumeters or flowmeters based on different measurement principles. The routinely used Wright's respirometer is not sensitive enough for the small volumes produced by cats. Pediatric adapters for the Datex spirometry system (D-lite) included in anesthesia monitors are suitable for clinical anesthesia in cats.

Pulse oximetry

Pulse oximetry is a non-invasive method for determination of hemoglobin oxygen saturation and pulse rate. The measurement principle is based on the different light absorption spectra of oxyhemoglobin and reduced hemoglobin. The pulsatile flow of arterial blood is displayed by some monitors as a plethysmogram. The pulse oximetry clip probe is usually placed on the tongue during anesthesia. For some pulse oximeter brands rectal probes are available. Pulse oximeters are useful tools to detect states of inadequate oxygenation; however, their signal is very sensitive to noise, and measurement artifacts may occur. In case of doubt the pulse rate displayed by the monitor should be compared to the actual pulse rate. Sometimes clip pressure can decrease blood flow, resulting in artificially low measurements, which requires changing probe position. Many different brands for human and veterinary medicine are available with varying accuracy and signal stability.

Capnography

Capnography measures the concentration of CO_2 in expired gas. In healthy animals it can be used as a non-invasive continuous estimate of the arterial CO_2 tension ($PaCO_2$). Capnometers give a numerical value on a breath-by-breath basis, whereas capnographs display a CO_2 waveform. Capnography is a useful tool for diagnosing circulatory and respiratory problems, as well as mechanical equipment failure (Box 17-2). It will guide ventilator settings in mechanically ventilated animals.

Box 17-2. List of possible problems indicated by changes in the capnogram readings

High end-tidal CO_2
Hypoventilation
Malignant hyperthermia

Low end-tidal CO_2
Hyperventilation
Hypothermia
Deep anesthesia (low cardiac output)
Cardiac arrest
Sampling line broken
Tube cuff deflated

Inspiratory concentration above zero = rebreathing of CO_2
Large technical dead space
Soda lime exhausted
Expiratory valve malfunction
Panting (rapid, shallow breathing)

Flat curve slopes
Lung disease (bronchoconstriction, obstruction)
Slow inspiratory time
Leak in breathing circuit
Leak in sampling line
Gas sampling slow

Side-stream capnographs aspirate a gas sample from the Y-piece or endotracheal tube and measure CO_2 in a remote infrared analyzer. Mainstream capnographs are inserted between the endotracheal tube and the breathing system, and the CO_2 concentration is measured in the immediate expired gas flow. The adapter of mainstream capnographs can significantly increase equipment dead space, whereas high gas sampling rates of side-stream monitors can dilute the gas sample with fresh gas, which gives erroneously low values. The given end-tidal concentration only truly represents alveolar gas in equilibration with arterial blood when there is a plateau phase present on the capnogram. Pneumothorax, open-chest surgery, and lung disease increase the end-tidal arterial CO_2 difference, and capnographic readings will not represent arterial CO_2 tension. Arterial blood gas sampling is indicated in such situations.

Blood gas analysis

Definitive information on oxygenation and ventilation can only be gained from the analysis of arterial blood gases. Samples should be drawn anaerobically (no air bubbles) from an arterial catheter or by percutaneous puncture of an accessible artery. The blood is collected into a heparinized syringe or capillary tube. Information on rectal or esophageal temperature of the cat is required for temperature correction of the blood gases.

17.7.4 Anesthetic gas analyzers

Anesthetic gas analyzers measure the concentration of the volatile anesthetic, oxygen, N_2O, and CO_2 in inspired and expired gas. End-tidal anesthetic concentration will represent alveolar concentration and is compared to the MAC value of the respective volatile anesthetic. The MAC values given by most commercial monitors are MAC values for adult humans. End-tidal anesthetic concentration during surgery has to be 1.2–1.5 MAC to prevent movement during monoanesthesia with an inhalant. Premedication, concurrent administration of analgesics, or local analgesic techniques will reduce end-tidal anesthetic concentrations below MAC values.

Side-stream monitors aspirate gas from the endotracheal tube adapter with rates up to 150 ml/min, which can cause a problem when using a low-flow technique in cats. Special makes of side-stream monitors for very small laboratory animals, with low gas sampling rates, are available. The exhaust from the monitor should be returned into the breathing or the scavenging system to avoid environmental contamination.

17.7.5 Temperature monitoring

Monitoring of the body temperature is crucial in a small patient like the cat. Hypothermia occurs quickly during general anesthesia, in particular when using non-rebreathing systems. Rectal temperature or esophageal temperature can be monitored continuously with flexible thermistor probes or at intervals with a conventional thermometer. Prolonged hypothermia during anesthesia will interfere with immune system function and wound healing and will cause central nervous system depression with prolonged recoveries. Monitoring of body temperature should continue until complete recovery of the cat.

17.8 Supportive care during anesthesia

17.8.1 Fluid administration

During inhalational anesthesia a significant amount of fluids are lost via the respiratory tract, open wounds, or hemorrhage. In addition, with most anesthetics vascular tone is reduced, and intravascular volume has to be replaced to maintain an adequate perfusion pressure.

For all procedures with a duration exceeding 30 minutes it should be routine to administer IV fluids. In a systemically healthy patient any isotonic crystalloid solution (i.e., lactated Ringer's solution, saline) can be used at a rate of 5–10 ml/kg per hour. Dehydrated, hypovolemic, and shock patients have to be stabilized prior to induction of anesthesia (Chapter 11). Fluid therapy is continued during anesthesia according to the patient's needs with colloids, isotonic or hypertonic crystalloids, or blood.

17.8.2 Temperature control

Hypothermia due to decreased heat production and increased heat loss can occur quickly during anesthesia in cats, with detrimental effects on recovery and surgical success. The greatest decrease usually occurs during surgical preparation. Prevention of hypothermia is easier than rewarming, and every effort should be taken to avoid a decrease in body temperature. Heat loss can be minimized by warm environmental temperatures, placing the cat on or between two circulating warm water pads or on a self-heating pad, placing warmed gel packs around the cat, or wrapping parts of the cat with plastic bubble sheets or an aluminum rescue blanket. The most effective way of warming a small animal is with forced warm-air blankets (i.e., Bair Hugger) placed around the cat underneath the surgical drapes. Intravenous fluids should be warmed by commercial IV fluid-warming systems, coiling the infusion line through warm-water baths, on the heating pad or underneath forced warm-air blankets.

Active heating should be continued during recovery until physiological body temperature is reached. This can be done by infrared heating lamps placed outside the cage to avoid skin burns, or by using hair dryers or forced warm-air blankets. Heated cage floors are usually not enough to raise body temperature again.

Hyperthermia can occur occasionally in cats. It can be due to excessive heating underneath the surgical drapes, hot and humid environment, and a thick haircoat. Malignant hyperthermia is extremely rare in cats. After a triggering event (i.e., halothane), body temperature increases rapidly concurrent with a massive increase in CO_2 production. The use of high doses of opioids, such as hydromorphone, morphine sulfate, or fentanyl, can also be associated with a transient increase in body temperature above 40°C.

Turning off the heating devices and cooling the cat with fluids or alcohol may be necessary to bring the temperature into physiological ranges. In cases of malignant hyperthermia the inhalant is stopped immediately, and hypercarbia is

Box 17-3. Emergency support (ABCD system)

- Airway: Establish patent airway by intubation or checking the endotracheal tube for obstruction if already present
- Breathing: Start ventilation (intermittent positive-pressure ventilation) with highest possible oxygen concentration (breathing system, self-inflating Ambu bag or mouth-to-tube ventilation) at a rate of 8–12 breaths/min. All anesthetics are turned off immediately if arrest occurs during anesthesia
- Circulation: Start external cardiac massage with the cat in lateral recumbency, and compress the thorax between the thumb and the opposing fingers of one hand at a rate of about 100 compressions per minute. Compression and release have the same lengths. Effectiveness of cardiac massage (i.e., producing a cardiac output) is ideally monitored with a capnograph indicating return of CO_2 from the tissues. At this stage of resuscitation, an electrocardiogram is established to check electrical activity of the heart
- Drugs: Prolonged life support begins with IV fluid and drug treatment. Repeated doses of epinephrine (every 5 minutes) for cardiac stimulation and redistribution of blood flow to vital organs, and atropine to reduce vagal tone followed by volume replacement are the first measures to take. Further drugs are selected according to the existing problem. Drugs can be given with a long urinary catheter through the endotracheal tube into a bronchus to reach the resorptive alveoli in the lung if no venous access can be established. Blind intracardial injection is discouraged as coronary vessels can be damaged and epinephrine injection into the myocardium can cause refractory ventricular fibrillation and local necrosis

treated by aggressive ventilation. Dantrolene at 3 mg/kg IV has been recommended as specific treatment for malignant hyperthermia in different species.

17.9 Cardiopulmonary resuscitation

Rapid action is necessary in cats with apnea and cardiac arrest. Loss of cardiac pump function can be related to cardiac arrest, ventricular fibrillation, or electromechanical dissociation. The chances of regaining spontaneous circulation are increased with early intervention and a systematic approach. All equipment and drugs for emergency intervention should be ready to use on a so-called crash cart or in an emergency kit. Emergency drugs should be prepared in a ready-to-use fashion and required doses in ml/kg should be available on a self-explanatory list, because in an emergency situation there is no time and too much pressure to calculate doses. A well-trained team following a set algorithm (Box 17-3) will have the best results.

External cardiac massage can provide effective cardiac output in cats. Internal cardiac massage has no major advantages in this species. A precordial "thump" might help to restart myocardial contraction in case of electromechanical dissociation (maintained electrical activity without or ineffective myocardial contractions). Ventricular fibrillation should be treated as early as possible by electrical conversion with an electrical defibrillator for best success. External paddles are best used on either side of the chest in cats. Energy output is set at 1 J/cat and defibrillation is attempted repeatedly or until success (sinus rhythm). Cardiac massage should be resumed between defibrillation attempts. For more information the reader is referred to other texts (24).

References and further reading

1. Gaynor JS, et al. Complications and mortality associated with anesthesia in dogs and cats. J Am Anim Hosp Assoc 1999;35: 13–17.
2. Dyson DH, et al. Morbidity and mortality associated with anesthetic management in small animal veterinary practice in Ontario. J Am Anim Hosp Assoc 1998;34:325–335.
3. Hosgood G, Scholl DT. Evaluation of age and American Society of Anesthesiologists (ASA) physical status as risk factors for perianesthetic morbidity and mortality in the cat. J Vet Emerg Crit Care 2002;12:9–16.
4. Brodbelt DC, et al. Anesthetic-related mortality risks in small animals in the UK. Proceedings of the AVA spring meeting 2005, Rimini, Italy, p. 68.
5. Flecknell PA, et al. The use of lignocaine-prilocaine local anaesthetic cream for pain-free venepuncture in laboratory animals. Lab Anim 1990;24:142–146.
6. Hedges D, et al. Antipsychotic medication and seizures: a review. Drugs Today 2003;39:551–557.
7. Ilkiw JE, et al. The behaviour of healthy awake cats following intravenous and intramuscular administration of midazolam. J Vet Pharmacol Ther 1996;19:205–216.
8. Ilkiw JE, et al. The optimal intravenous dose of midazolam after intravenous ketamine in healthy awake cats. J Vet Pharmacol Ther 1998;21:54–61.
9. Tranquilli WJ, et al. Flumazenil efficacy in reversing diazepam or midazolam overdose in dogs. J Vet Anaesth 1992;19: 65–68.
10. Thurmon J, Tranquilli WJ, Benson GW. Lumb & Jones' veterinary anesthesia, 3rd edn. Baltimore: Williams & Wilkins; 1996.
11. Middleton D, et al. Physiological effects of thiopentone, ketamine and CT1341 in cats. Res Vet Sci 1982;32:157–162.
12. Brearley JC, et al. Propofol anesthesia in cats. J Small Anim Pract 1988;29:315–322.
13. Andress JL, et al. The effects of consecutive day propofol anesthesia on feline red blood cells. Vet Surg 1995;24:277–282.

14. McMurphy RM, Hodgson DS. The minimum alveolar concentration of desflurane in cats. Vet Surg 1995;24:435.
15. Pypendop BH, Ilkiw JE. Hemodynamic effects of sevoflurane in cats. Am J Vet Res 2004;65:20–25.
16. Dorsch JA, Dorsch SE. Understanding anesthesia equipment, 4th edn. Baltimore: Williams & Wilkins; 1999.
17. Moyle JTB, Davey A, Ward C. Ward's anaesthetic equipment, 4th edn. London: WB Saunders; 1998.
18. Tzannes S, et al. The use of sevoflurane in 2:1 mixture of nitrous oxide and oxygen for rapid mask induction of anesthesia in the cat. J Feline Med Surg 2000;2:83–90.
19. Hardie EM, et al. Tracheal rupture in cats: 16 cases (1983–1998). J Am Vet Med Assoc 1999;214:508–512.
20. ACVA Suggestions for monitoring anesthetized veterinary patients. J Am Vet Med Assoc 1995;206:936–937.
21. Brodbelt DC. Update results from the enquiry into perioperative small animal fatalities. Proceedings of the AVA spring meeting 2006, Liverpool, UK, pp. 119–121.
22. Grandy JL, et al. Evaluation of the Doppler ultrasonic method of measuring systolic arterial blood pressure in cats. Am J Vet Res 1992;53:1166–1169.
23. Caulkett NA, et al. A comparison of indirect blood pressure monitoring techniques in the anesthetized cat. Vet Surg 1998; 27:370–377.
24. Plunkett SJ, McMichael M. Cardiopulmonary resuscitation in small animal medicine: an update. J Vet Intern Med 2008;22: 9–25.

18 Perioperative analgesia

S. Kaestner

The term perioperative encompasses the preoperative, intraoperative, and postoperative periods. The importance of preemptive analgesic treatment is well recognized with the knowledge that the administration of analgesics before and during the surgical procedure will reduce postoperative pain. This is achieved by several mechanisms, with peripheral and central sensitization of the nociceptive system as well as wind-up mechanisms being reduced by pre-emptive analgesia. The use of analgesia preoperatively reduces the required doses or minimum alveolar concentration (MAC) of anesthetic drugs, and analgesics given early will have developed their full effect by the time of recovery from anesthesia, so breakthrough of severe pain is avoided. Local anesthetics, opioids, and non-steroidal anti-inflammatory drugs (NSAIDs) are the main options for perioperative analgesia. The choice of the specific drugs to be used depends on the degree of pain expected from a specific procedure and the response of the animal to the therapy. A multimodal approach using different classes of drugs acting at peripheral and central sites of the nociceptive system is advantageous. Some examples of multimodal therapy are illustrated in Box 18-1.

18.1 Local anesthetics

Local anesthetics are used for specific nerve blocks, local infiltration, regional blocks, brachial plexus blocks, or in epi/subdural anesthesia (Table 18-1). Interpleural infusion of bupivacaine diluted in 5 ml saline infused into the interpleural space via a chest tube provides good analgesia after thoracotomy (Table 18-1).

Lidocaine, and the long-acting substance bupivacaine, are the most commonly used local anesthetics in cats. Toxic side-effects include cardiovascular depression, bradycardia, bradyarrhythmia, salivation, and seizures, so total applicable doses are limited to 4 mg/kg lidocaine and 2 mg/kg bupivacaine. Ropivacaine has a lower toxicity than bupivacaine, but safe dose rates are not available for cats.

18.1.1 Brachial plexus block

Brachial plexus blocks provide analgesia for surgical procedures on the thoracic limb within or distal to the elbow. The block is performed with the cat under general anesthesia. A 22G, 5-cm needle is inserted medial to the shoulder joint, advanced parallel to the spine, and directed towards the costochondral junction of the ribs. If no blood can be aspirated, lidocaine or bupivacaine, diluted to a volume of 5 ml to facilitate spread, is injected during withdrawal to reach the ulnar, radial, median, musculocutaneous, and axillary nerves. The use of a nerve stimulator to locate the nerves and to give more specific dosages improves the results.

Additional analgesia for amputation of a thoracic limb can be achieved by a splash block. The nerves of the brachial plexus are prepared by splashing lidocaine or bupivacaine (longer action) directly on them, prior to severing them with a sharp scalpel blade.

18.1.2 Epidural/spinal anesthesia

Epidural anesthesia in the cat is performed under deep sedation or general anesthesia in the lumbosacral space, between

Box 18-1. Examples of multimodal perioperative analgesia

Mild pain expected

Buprenorphine premedication
One preoperative dose of carprofen or meloxicam
Buprenorphine every 6–8 hours for 2 days

Moderate pain expected

Buprenorphine premedication
Local blocks (plexus block, epidural/spinal)
Meloxicam pre- and postoperative
Buprenorphine every 6–8 hours for 3 days

Severe pain expected

Morphine premedication
Fentanyl patch
Local blocks (plexus block, epidural/spinal)
Intraoperative fentanyl constant-rate infusion
Postoperative fentanyl constant-rate infusion or morphine until the fentanyl patch is effective (approx. 7–10 hours)
Meloxicam pre- and postoperative
Consider ketamine constant-rate infusion as adjunct

Table 18-1. Dosages and concentrations of local anesthetics used for perioperative analgesia in cats

Drug	Type of block	Dosage/concentration	Onset/duration
Lidocaine	Local infiltration	1–2%, do not exceed 4 mg/kg	10 minutes/1 hour
	Nerve block	1–2%, do not exceed 4 mg/kg	10 minutes/1 hour
	Epidural	1–2%, do not exceed 4 mg/kg	1.5 hour
Bupivacaine	Nerve block	0.5%, do not exceed 2 mg/kg	20 minutes/6–(8) hours
	Epidural	1 mg/kg (0.25–0.5%)	20 minutes/6 hours
	Spinal	0.5 mg/kg (0.25–0.5%)	Shorter than epidural
	Interpleural	1.5 mg/kg (0.5%) in 5 ml	6–8 hours
Morphine/ bupivacaine	Epidural	0.1 mg/kg morphine	20 minutes/6–12 hours
	Spinal	1 mg/kg Half epidural dose	

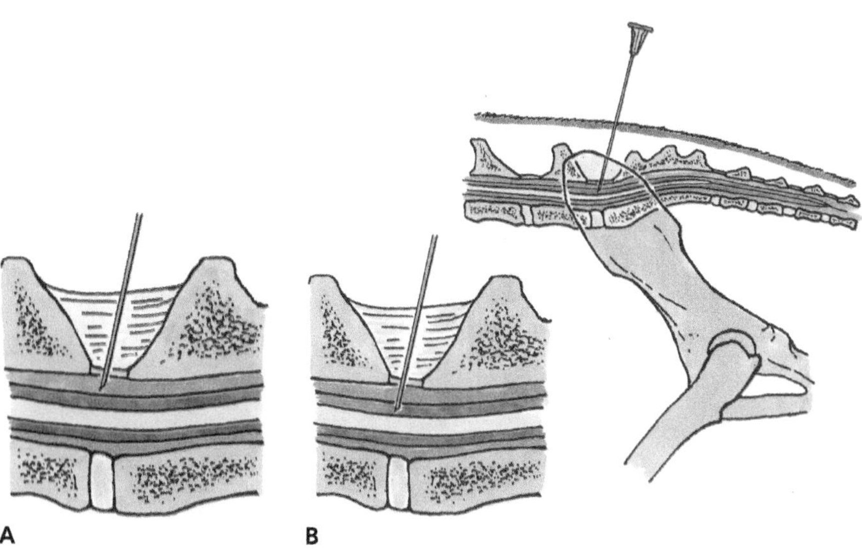

Figure 18-1 Needle placement between the last lumbar (L7) and first sacral (S1) vertebrae for epidural/subdural (spinal) anesthesia. In the cat the spinal cord ends at the level of the sacral vertebrae and subarachnoid puncture occurs quite frequently. (**A**) Epidural needle placement; (**B**) subdural needle placement.

L7 and S1. The cat is placed in lateral or sternal recumbency with the hind legs flexed forward (frog position) and the lumbosacral space is localized dorsally between the iliac wings. Palpation of the craniodorsal iliac crests with thumb and middle finger and placing the index finger on L7 will facilitate orientation. The area is prepared aseptically. A 22G, 2.5-cm spinal needle is inserted in the midline at two-thirds of the distance between the dorsal spinal processes of L7 and S1, and is advanced until the interarcuate ligament is penetrated, creating a popping feeling. This popping feeling is less obvious in cats than in dogs. Injection of a small volume of air or saline with a glass syringe or low-resistance syringe without encountering resistance, or the "hanging drop" technique, verifies placement of the needle tip in the epidural space (Fig. 18-1). Careful inspection of the needle for cerebrospinal fluid (CSF) or blood before injection of the anesthetic is necessary. When blood flows back, the needle is removed without injection. Backflow of CSF indicates subarachnoid puncture, which occurs quite often in cats because the spinal cord ends at the level of the sacral vertebrae. The spinal needle can be withdrawn minimally, or one-half of the calculated dose of the anesthetic is injected for spinal anesthesia (Fig. 18-1).

Epidural anesthesia/analgesia can be performed via single injections or via placement of an epidural catheter with intermittent injections or continuous infusions. Commercial pediatric epidural catheter kits containing a 20G, 5-cm epidural needle and a 24G, 7.5-cm catheter including a bacterial filter are suitable for cats. Proper placement in the epidural space requires radiographic verification.

The volume of the injected anesthetic/analgesic determines the spread of the block and the concentration of a local anesthetic determines the degree of motor block: 1 ml/5 kg will produce a block up to L1 (pelvic limb) and 1 ml/3.5 kg will produce analgesia up to T4 (abdominal). With low concentrations of local anesthetics less motor dysfunction occurs. Epidural use of morphine will induce analgesia up to the cervical spine without motor block (Box 18-1).

Contraindications for epidural anesthesia are septicemia, coagulation disorders, hypovolemic shock, skin infections at the puncture site, and deformation due to fractures or luxations of the spine or pelvis. Possible complications include local skin infection, meningitis, and trauma to the spinal cord.

18.2 Opioids

Opioids exert their effects via opiate receptors. Opiate receptors are mainly located in the central nervous system in the dorsal horn of the spinal cord and the brain where impulses from the periphery are modulated. Opiate receptors are also found in peripheral tissues, for example the synovial membrane. Location, classification, and subclassification of opiate receptors are the subject of much ongoing research. The μ-receptors mediate supraspinal analgesia, respiratory depression, bradycardia, physical dependence, and euphoria. The μ-receptors mediate analgesia, hallucinations, sedation, and mydriasis in cats, and δ-receptors modulate μ-receptor activity. Differences in subtype distribution, density, and activity state of opiate receptors cause species-specific effects of opiates. All full μ-receptor agonists are controlled substances (schedule II drugs) because of possible abuse and physical dependence in humans.

The historical reputation of cats for becoming excited after the use of opioids is based on overdose. In contrast to many other species, opioids cause mydriasis in cats. This might impair their vision and cause them to react strangely when treated with an opioid. However, there is enough evidence that opioids at appropriate doses are recommended for the treatment of feline pain (1–6). The choice of opioid depends on the degree of pain expected, the speed of onset and duration of action of the drug, as well as the side-effects that can occur. Full μ-receptor agonists follow a linear dose–response curve, and increasing their dose will increase analgesic effects. Partial agonists and μ-receptor antagonists theoretically follow a bell-shaped dose–response curve, and analgesic effects cannot necessarily be increased by higher doses (Table 18-2).

18.2.1 Morphine

The classic μ-receptor agonist morphine has shown analgesic effects in experimental models and clinical pain in cats without causing signs of excitation at doses of 0.1–0.2 mg/kg. The intramuscular (IM) route is preferred because intravenous (IV) injection can cause histamine release. Onset of action is slow and repeated dosing is required after 2–4 hours. Prolonged use of morphine can cause constipation and urine retention.

18.2.2 Hydromorphone/oxymorphone

Hydromorphone and oxymorphone are both morphine derivatives. They are more potent than morphine and can produce several hours of analgesia in cats. The use of hydromorphone has recently been implicated in postanesthetic hyperthermia in cats.

18.2.3 Pethidine

Pethidine (meperidine) is a μ-receptor agonist and has been widely used in cats. It has a rapid onset of action but also a very short duration of analgesic effect (1–2 hours). IV injection should be avoided, as this might cause excitement and histamine release. Unlike morphine, it relaxes intestinal spasms.

18.2.4 Methadone

Racemic methadone and L-methadone are synthetic μ-receptor agonists with similar properties as morphine. The L-isomer has a higher receptor affinity than the D-isomer, resulting in approximately twice the analgesic effect of the L-methadone compared to the racemic methadone, and doses for racemic and L-methadone should not be confused. Methadone also acts as an N-methyl-D-aspartic acid (NMDA) receptor antagonist and might help to prevent the development of hyperalgesia. In some countries, the veterinary product L-Polamivet contains an anticholinergic to counteract opioid-induced vagal stimulation. Tachycardia can occur when the L-methadone is antagonized with naloxone because of the excess of diphenylpiperidine.

18.2.5 Fentanyl

Fentanyl is a μ-receptor agonist. It is about 50–100 times more potent than morphine and can produce a high level of analgesia. It is effective after IV injection but is also well absorbed through mucous membranes and the transdermal route. A single bolus has a short duration of effect (15–20 minutes). Fentanyl is used as part of neuroleptanalgesic mixtures, balanced anesthetic techniques, and postoperative analgesia. When used in combination with general anesthetics, intermittent positive-pressure ventilation is usually necessary.

Table 18-2. Dosages of opioids for perioperative analgesia in cats

Drug	Dose	Route	Duration/dosing interval
Butorphanol	0.2–0.4 mg/kg	SC/IM/IV	1–2 hours
Buprenorphine	0.007–0.03 mg/kg	SC/IM/IV	4–8 hours
	0.01–0.02 mg/kg	PO	8 hours
Morphine	0.1–0.3 mg/kg	IM	2–4 hours
	0.05–0.1 mg/kg per hour	CRI	12–24 hours
	0.1 mg/kg	Epidural	
Methadone	0.2–0.3 mg/kg	SC/IM/IV	4 hours
	0.05–0.1 mg/kg per hour	CRI	
L-methadone	0.1–0.3 mg/kg	SC/IM/IV	4 hours
Pethidine	2–5–(10) mg/kg	SC/IM	2 hours
	0.5–1 mg/kg per hour	CRI	
Hydromorphone	0.05 mg/kg	SC/IM	2–4 hours
	0.03–0.05 mg/kg	IV	1 hour
	0.005–0.01 mg/kg per hour	CRI	
Oxymorphone	0.03–0.05 mg/kg	SC/IM	4–6 hours
	0.01–0.03 mg/kg	IV	
	0.005–0.01 mg/kg per hour	CRI	
Tramadol	2–4 mg/kg	IV/PO	24 hours
Fentanyl	0.001–0.01 mg/kg	IV/IM	20–30 minutes
	0.01–0.02 mg/kg per hour	CRI intra Sx	
	0.001–0.005 mg/kg per hour	CRI post Sx	
Fentanyl patch Durogesic TTS®	25 μg/hour patch	Transdermal	Onset: 7 hours Approx. 72 hours
Naloxone	0.001–0.01 mg/kg IV to effect	IV	20–40 minutes

SC, subcutaneous; IV, intravenous; IM, intramuscular; PO, peroral; CRI, constant-rate infusion; Sx, surgery.

For continuous controlled administration of fentanyl, transdermal patches (Durogesic TTS) are available. The 25 μg/hour release patches are appropriate for cats. Steady-state plasma concentrations are reached within 6–12 hours in cats and the average duration of analgesia after patch application is approximately 72 hours. However, the fentanyl plasma concentrations after patch placement are very variable, depending on skin permeability and perfusion and body and skin temperature. Therefore, repeated evaluation of the animal for signs of pain or overdose is necessary. The time to onset of effective plasma concentrations of fentanyl has to be bridged with another analgesic. The skin is clipped and cleaned with water before patch placement, without degreasing the skin. After the skin has dried the patch is applied and pressed on to the skin for some seconds. An area where there is not too much movement, for example, the lateral thorax, should be used for patch placement. The time and date of patch placement can be marked on the patch.

18.2.6 Butorphanol

Butorphanol is a μ-receptor antagonist that has a bell-shaped dose–response curve. Recommended doses should not be exceeded. It is not a controlled drug and therefore very popular in veterinary practice. Butorphanol is an effective analgesic for visceral pain but poor for somatic pain. For this reason, it is not the best choice of drug for orthopedic surgical patients. It has a short duration of action and requires frequent redosing (2 hours). Butorphanol has a high affinity for the opioid receptors, and when given for premedication will impair further analgesic therapy with μ-receptor agonists during painful procedures.

18.2.7 Buprenorphine

Buprenorphine is a partial μ-receptor agonist with slow receptor association and dissociation. This results in a slow onset of action even after IV injection (at least 30 minutes)

but also a very long duration of action at the receptor (6–8 hours). Transmucosal absorption through the oral mucous membranes is almost 100% in the cat, and buccal administration with a syringe is effective and well tolerated. Experimental studies on a transdermal delivery patch in cats gave very inconsistent plasma buprenorphine concentrations as well as analgesic effects. Buprenorphine rarely causes dysphoria or vomiting, and it has produced effective analgesia in both experimental cats and in the clinical setting, making it very suitable for perioperative pain treatment in the cat. Buprenorphine is a controlled drug because of possible human abuse and dependence.

18.2.8 Tramadol

Tramadol is an atypical opioid with weak μ-receptor binding activity in combination with serotonin and norepinephrine reuptake inhibition. For cats a dose of 1–2 mg/kg IV and 2–4 mg/kg PO has been recommended but no controlled studies are available.

18.2.9 Opioid antagonists

Naloxone is a pure antagonist at all opioid receptors. It can be used to reverse inadvertent overdose and respiratory depression. Naloxone has a fairly short duration of action, shorter than most agonists, often making redosing necessary. Naltrexone is also a pure antagonist with a longer duration of action than naloxone. Butorphanol and buprenorphine are difficult to antagonize because of their high receptor affinity. Low doses of butorphanol (< 0.1 mg/kg) can be used to reverse respiratory depression induced by pure μ-receptor agonists without fully reversing analgesic effects.

18.3 Non-steroidal anti-inflammatory drugs

NSAIDs exert their main effects by inhibiting cyclooxygenase (COX) isoforms, thereby interfering with the arachidonic acid cascade and preventing the formation of prostaglandins, prostacyclin, and thromboxane. Development of COX2-selective NSAIDs was thought to reduce the potential for toxicity of NSAIDs, but the situation is more complex than initially thought. The deficiency of the glucuronidation pathway in cats results in slow metabolism of several NSAIDs with a prolonged duration of effect, and possible accumulation. Therefore, a dosage and dosing interval transfer from other species must not be made to avoid gastrointestinal and renal toxicity.

The practical advantages of NSAIDs in the perioperative period are their long analgesic action and that they are not controlled substances. Important factors to consider when NSAIDs are used preoperatively are their influence on renal function and coagulation. Renal perfusion will be reduced during general anesthesia, and NSAIDs should be avoided if renal function is already impaired or if the animal is hypovolemic (shock patients). Non-selective or COX1-selective NSAIDs (i.e., acetylasalicylic acid, ketoprofen) can influence coagulation times by inhibiting thromboxane formation, and should not be used when excessive hemorrhage is expected or when coagulopathies are present. Only carprofen and meloxicam are licensed for preoperative use in cats (4–7) (Table 18-3).

Different NSAIDs should not be combined because toxicity is increased. Combinations of NSAIDs and corticosteroids will also increase gastrointestinal toxicity with an increased risk of ulcer formation.

18.3.1 Carprofen

Carprofen has been studied extensively in cats. It has a good safety profile because of limited COX inhibition, and provides effective perioperative analgesia. One dose of carprofen at 4 mg/kg is currently licensed for preoperative use in cats. This will provide analgesia for at least 24 hours. Toxicity with repeated dosing can occur because of a high variability in individual elimination half-life (9–49 hours) in cats. Long-term use is therefore prohibited.

18.3.2 Meloxicam

Meloxicam is a COX2-selective NSAID, licensed in cats to be given as a single subcutaneous injection for preoperative use. In Europe, an oral formula (0.5 mg/ml meloxicam) is now also licensed for long-term use. The oral suspension is provided as a honey-flavored liquid, which is palatable to some cats, and which can be accurately administered by owners. Meloxicam is therefore a good choice of an NSAID drug for perioperative use in orthopedic patients, because therapy can be continued in the postoperative period. Its analgesic efficiency in the perioperative period is comparable to carprofen.

18.3.3 Other NSAIDs

Tolfenamic acid is a COX1-selective NSAID that should not be used preoperatively. When given at the end of anesthesia tolfenamic acid at 4 mg/kg produces analgesia comparable to ketoprofen, carprofen, and meloxicam in the cat.

Ketoprofen is a potent COX inhibitor without any selectivity. It causes thromboxane inhibition and should not be used preoperatively because excessive hemorrhage can occur. When given after anesthesia its analgesic effect is similar to that of tolfenamic acid.

Drug	Dose	Route	Duration/ dosing interval
Carprofen	4 mg/kg single preoperative dose	IV/SC/PO	24 hours (single dose)
Meloxicam	0.2 mg/kg single preoperative dose	IV/SC	24 hours (single dose)
	0.1 mg/kg if to be continued postoperatively	IV/SC	(see Chapter 5 for long-term use)
Vedaprofen	0.5 mg/kg	PO	24 hours (for maximum 5 days)
Acetylsalicylic acid	10–25 mg/kg	PO	48 hours
Piroxicam	0.3 mg/kg	PO	24 hours (for maximum 5 days) Unpredictable enterohepatic circulation possible
Tolfenamic acid	4 mg/kg postoperatively	IV/PO	24 hours
Ketoprofen	2 mg/kg postoperatively	SC/IM/IV PO	24 hours (for maximum 5 days)

Table 18-3. Dosages of non-steroidal anti-inflammatory drugs used for perioperative analgesia in cats

Drug	Dose	Route	Duration/dosing interval
Xylazine	0.2–0.4 mg/kg	SC/IM	2 hours
Medetomidine	0.01–0.020 mg/kg	SC/IM	1–4 hours
	0.005–0.01 mg/kg per hour	CRI	
	0.001–0.005 mg/kg	Epidural	
Romifidine	0.01–0.05 mg/kg	SC/IM	2–4 hours
Ketamine	0.5 mg/kg	IM/IV	1–2 hours
	0.6 mg/kg per hour	CRI	Intra Sx
	0.12 mg/kg per hour	CRI	Post Sx for 24 hours

SC, subcutaneous; IM, intramuscular; IV, intravenous; Sx, surgery; CRI, constant-rate infusion.

Table 18-4. Dosages of analgesic adjuncts used for perioperative analgesia in cats

Piroxicam has been used for its antiangiogenetic effects in canine tumor patients in addition to its analgesic properties. The pharmacokinetics can be unpredictable in cats because of possible enterohepatic circulation.

Vedaprofen is not licensed for use in cats. The gel formula-tion for dogs has been used in cats at 0.5 mg/kg PO q24 hours over 5 days without toxic signs in healthy cats. However, no information exists on its perioperative use and analgesic efficacy.

Phenylbutazone is still licensed in many countries for use in cats. No controlled studies are available on its pharmacokinetic properties or toxicity in the cat. Historical dose recommendations are based on those for chronic pain management. With the availability of the newer NSAIDs with a known safety profile, phenylbutazone should not be used in the cat in the perioperative period.

Paracetamol (acetaminophen), ibuprofen, indomethacin and naproxen are toxic in the cat and must not be used in this species.

18.4 Analgesic adjuncts

In addition to the classic analgesic substances, other classes of drugs have shown advantageous effects in pain management via a variety of different mechanisms. Systemic administration of low-dose ketamine and alpha$_2$ agonists are the most important analgesic adjuncts in the perioperative period (Table 18-4). Systemic lidocaine has also shown prokinetic and anesthetic-sparing effects in various species in combination with other analgesics. However, the cardiovascular depressive effects caused by lidocaine in cats outweigh the anesthetic-sparing effects, so its use in not recommended (8).

18.4.1 Ketamine

Activation of NMDA receptors in the spinal cord plays an important role in the wind-up phenomenon, and ketamine, as a non-competitive NMDA antagonist, might be able to reduce hyperalgesia. Using ketamine as part of the anesthetic protocol can provide pre-emptive analgesia in cats. However, the analgesic effects of ketamine are difficult to prove in experimental cats and it cannot be considered as a stand-alone analgesic, rather as a reinforcing analgesic. Subanesthetic doses of ketamine have been found to reduce opioid requirements.

18.4.2 Alpha$_2$ agonists

Alpha$_2$ agonists are primarily used for their sedative and anesthetic-sparing effects in cats. However, potent analgesia is mediated via alpha$_2$ receptors in the dorsal horn of the spinal cord and can be used to treat severe pain states. Profound sedation and cardiovascular depression are unwanted side-effects, which can be reduced by epidural administration and low-dose constant-rate infusions. The mild sedation in combination with analgesia can be advantageous in the immediate postoperative period in some cats.

References and further reading

1. Taylor PM, et al. Morphine, pethidine and buprenorphine disposition in the cat. J Vet Phamacol Ther 2001;24:391–398.
2. Robertson SA, et al. Changes in thermal threshold response in eight cats after administration of buprenorphine, butorphanol and morphine. Vet Rec 2003;153:462–465.
3. Hofmeister EH, Egger CM. Transdermal fentanyl patches in small animals. J Am Anim Hosp Assoc 2004;40:468–478.
4. Robertson SA, Taylor PM. Pain management in cats – past, present and future. Part 2. Treatment of pain – clinical pharmacology. J Feline Med Surg 2004;6:321–333.
5. Gaynor JS, Muir WW. Handbook of veterinary pain management. St. Louis: Mosby; 2002.
6. Flecknell PA, Waterman-Pearson AE. Pain management in animals. London: WB Saunders; 2000.
7. Slingsby LS, Waterman-Pearson AE. Postoperative analgesia in the cat after ovariohysterectomy by use of carprofen, ketoprofen, meloxicam or tolfenamic acid. J Small Anim Pract 2000; 41:447–450.
8. Pypendop BH, Ilkiw JE. Assessment of the hemodynamic effects of lidocaine administered IV in isoflurane anesthetized cats. Am J Vet Res 2005;66:661–668.

19 Preparation for surgery

K. Voss

Preparation for surgery includes preoperative assessment and stabilization of the patient, an appropriate anesthetic protocol (Chapter 17), and perioperative analgesia (Chapter 18). Aseptic preparation of the surgical site, preparation of the surgical team, and preparation of instruments, implants, facilities, and the environment are essential both to the success of the surgery and to prevent infection of the surgical wound. Antisepsis is defined as the inactivation or destruction of most pathogenic microorganisms on living tissue, and is aimed at limiting bacterial contamination of the surgical site to the lowest possible level. Sterilization is destruction of all microorganisms, usually applied to surgical instruments, implants, and materials.

This chapter focuses on preparation of the patient for surgery and on preparation of the surgical team. Cleaning, sterilization, and maintenance of the surgery theater and surgical materials and implants are described elsewhere.

19.1 Preparation of the patient

As many as 30–60% of feline fracture patients have sustained concurrent and possibly life-threatening injuries (1–3). These injuries have to be treated prior to fracture repair. Management of the polytraumatized cat is described in part 3 of this book.

19.1.1 Preoperative management of the orthopedic patient

Repair of most fractures and joint instabilities can be delayed several days without negatively affecting outcome if the patient is not stable for anesthesia and surgery. However, early treatment and stabilization are preferable for open fractures and joint injuries, joint luxations, fractures with a critical blood supply, and fractures and luxations causing neurological deficits. Fractures in immature cats are at risk for interference with growth potential and joint function if treatment is delayed. Young cats may also be more susceptible to quadriceps contracture after delayed stabilization of femoral fractures.

Fractures and joint injuries distal to the elbow and stifle joint can be stabilized with a splinted bandage until definitive treatment is performed. External immobilization should reduce pain and minimize further vascular damage by limiting motion at the fracture site. Fractures and joint injuries above the elbow and stifle joint are difficult to stabilize securely with external immobilization, and cats should therefore be cage-rested until surgery is performed. If definitive surgery has to be delayed for several days or longer, temporary stabilization with an external skeletal fixator should be considered. Adequate analgesia is provided for every patient with orthopedic injuries (Chapter 18).

Food is withheld for 12 hours prior to surgery in adult patients. Cats less than 4 months of age should only be fasted for 4 hours, because of limited glycogen reserves. The patient must be stable, both cardiovascularly and metabolically, before induction of anesthesia. The packed cell volume should be at least 20% with albumin levels exceeding 20 g/l. Administration of blood products should be considered if the packed cell volume and/or albumin levels fall below these values (Chapter 11). Balanced electrolyte solutions are administered at a rate of 10 ml/kg per hour during preparation of the patient and perioperatively.

19.1.2 Risk factors for surgical infections

Surgical wound infections develop when bacteria enter the wound through the dermal incision, overwhelm the host's defense mechanisms, and start to replicate. Significant factors in the development of surgical wound infection are the number and pathogenesis of the microorganisms, and the effectiveness of the host's defense mechanisms. Local reduction of vascularity, for example due to trauma or implants, is a common factor promoting wound infection. Infections occurring within 30 days of surgery at the surgical site are considered surgical infections. Infections occurring up to 1 year after surgery at the surgical site are considered surgery-related.

Several studies have evaluated the incidence of postoperative wound infection and associated risk factors (Box 19-1). Postoperative wound infection occurs with an overall frequency of 3.0–5.5% (4–6). One prognostic factor for the development of post surgical infection is the degree of wound contamination at the time of incision. Surgical procedures are classified into clean, clean-contaminated, contaminated, and dirty procedures (Table 19-1). Clean and clean-contaminated wounds are less likely to become infected than contaminated or dirty wounds (4–6). The incidence of postoperative wound

Box 19-1. Identified risk factors which increase the risk of surgical infections

Risk factors of surgical infection
Contaminated and dirty surgical wounds
Duration of anesthesia
Duration of surgery
Break in asepsis
Number of persons in the surgery room
Endocrinopathies
Use of propofol
Clipping of hair before anesthetic induction

Surgical procedure	Examples
Clean	Elective procedures Closed fractures No break in asepsis
Clean-contaminated	Minor break in asepsis
Contaminated	Fresh traumatic wounds (<4 hours after trauma) Skin lacerations Grade 1 open fractures
Dirty	Traumatic wounds with devitalized tissue, foreign bodies, delayed treatment (>4 hours after trauma) Grade 2 and 3 open fractures Degloving injuries Bite wounds Abscesses

Table 19-1. Classification of surgical wounds with orthopedic surgery examples

infection for clean and clean-contaminated wounds ranges from 2.5 to 5%, whereas the incidence of postoperative wound infection for contaminated and dirty wounds ranges from 5.8 to 18.1% (4, 5).

Clinical factors associated with an enhanced infection rate are duration of anesthesia (7, 8) and length of surgery (6, 8). Prolongation of anesthesia, especially for preoperative diagnostic procedures, and duration of surgery should therefore be kept as low as possible. A larger number of persons present in the operating room is another factor that increases postoperative wound infection (6). Patients suffering from endocrinopathies also have a higher risk for wound infection (8). The use of propofol for anesthetic induction increases the likelihood of infection by a factor of 3.8 (9). Propofol is a lipid-based emulsion and capable of supporting microbial growth. Opened bottles should be kept in a fridge, and used within 12–24 hours of opening. Clipping of hair before anesthetic induction also renders the surgical site more likely to become infected, compared to clipping shortly after induction just prior to the procedure (5). The use of razors is not recommended, because it causes skin irritation and erosion and thus increases the surgical wound infection rate.

19.1.3 Perioperative antibiotics

Preoperative antibiotic prophylaxis has been shown to decrease postoperative infection rates in elective orthopedic surgical procedures (10). For this reason routine prophylactic perioperative antibiotic treatment is usually recommended, although many orthopedic surgeries are classified as clean procedures. Orthopedic procedures commonly last longer than 90 minutes and local wound factors, such as metallic implants and tissue trauma, may potentiate infection. Additionally, bone and joint infections are difficult to treat in the presence of implants, enhance morbidity, and may negatively influence outcome. Cefazolin is currently considered the antibiotic of choice due to its excellent efficacy against most surgical wound pathogens, its low toxicity, and reasonable cost. The first dose should be administered 30–60 minutes before the surgical incision at a dose of 22 mg/kg. Repeating the dose every 90–120 minutes is commonly recommended, but evidence suggests that a frequency of every 3 hours is sufficient (11).

Antimicrobial therapy is continued postoperatively after contaminated and dirty procedures. A short postoperative course of antibiotics is also indicated in patients with increased susceptibility to infection, such as severely traumatized patients, those with endocrinopathies, malnutrition, and cats with an expected prolonged hospitalization period. Cefazolin is often a good initial choice and can be continued after surgery, but definitive postoperative antimicrobial therapy should be selected according to the results of antimicrobial testing. Anorexia, vomiting, or diarrhea is observed in some cats taking cephalosporins in the postoperative period.

19.1.4 Preparation of the surgical site

Normal bacteria on feline and canine skin include *Staphylococcus* spp., *Micrococcus* spp., *Acinetobacter* spp., *Corynebacterium* spp., *Streptococcus* spp., *Clostridium* spp., *Escherichia coli*, and *Enterobacter* spp. These organisms lodge on hair and skin surfaces, within the superficial cornified layers and in the glands of skin and subcutaneous tissue. The goal of aseptic preparation of the surgical site is reduction of the number of bacteria to levels incapable of producing an infection.

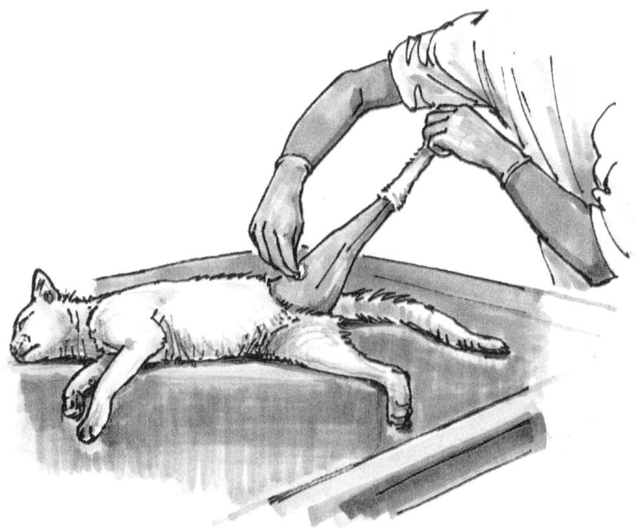

Figure 19-1 The left hindleg of a cat is scrubbed for orthopedic surgery in the preparation room. Note that the whole circumference of the limb is going to be prepared aseptically, allowing free manipulation of the limb during surgery.

Antiseptic agent	Characteristics
Povidone-iodine	Broad-action antiseptic against Gram-negative and Gram-positive bacteria, mycobacteria, and fungi Inactivation of spores only after prolonged application time Reduced action in the presence of blood or necrotic debris May cause skin irritation
Chlorhexidine	Broad-action antiseptic, but better against Gram-negative bacteria than Gram-positive bacteria and fungi Sustained action in the presence of blood and necrotic debris Excellent residual action
Ethyl alcohol	Fast and efficient antibacterial action Enhances action of both iodophors and chlorhexidine Causes tissue necrosis (not to be used in open wounds)

Table 19-2. Type and characteristics of selected antiseptic agents

The hair is clipped after anesthetic induction in a preparation room outside the surgical theater. A minimum of 10–15 cm is clipped around the incision site. For most orthopedic procedures the whole leg is prepared aseptically in order to be able to manipulate and position the leg freely during surgery. Loose clipped hair is immediately removed using a vacuum cleaner. For surgeries not involving the toes and metacarpus or metatarsus, the hair of the feet is not clipped, and the feet are covered with an adhesive or cohesive bandage after the limb was scrubbed. The limb is suspended from the ceiling or an intravenous drip stand to allow access to the whole circumference. Antiseptic scrubs are applied with wet gauze sponges by gentle pressure in a circular motion (Fig. 19-1). Scrubbing starts at the center of the clipped field and then moves towards the edges. The sponge is replaced once it has touched the edges, and a new one is taken to start again at the center. At least 3 minutes of scrubbing is required for all commonly used scrub solutions. After scrubbing is completed, residual debris and loose hairs are removed with antiseptic solutions, and the fur around the edges is flattened away from the incision site. Either 70% ethyl alcohol or tinctures of chlorhexidine or iodine may be used for this purpose.

Both iodophors and chlorhexidine can be used as scrubs and as antiseptic solutions, but they should not be mixed because this reduces efficacy (Table 19-2). Overall, chlorhexidine seems to have some advantages when compared to iodine. It remains effective in the presence of blood, pus, and other organic material, it has a good residual activity for killing bacteria that emerge from sebaceous glands and hair follicles during surgery, and skin irritation is uncommon. Alcohol causes tissue necrosis in open wounds and is therefore avoided in the presence of open wounds. Phenol derivates, another class of antiseptics, should not be used in cats because cats have a defective glucuronide synthesis, and may therefore be more sensitive to phenol toxicity than other species (12).

The patient is positioned on the table inside the surgery room. For orthopedic surgeries, the affected limb is suspended on an intravenous stand or similar, and the surgical site is wiped or sprayed once more with an antiseptic solution to complete the preparation (Fig. 19-2). Orthopedic draping should allow the surgeon to manipulate the leg in different directions without risk of contamination. The body of the patient is covered first with four drapes around the base of the limb. These drapes are applied with approximately 10 cm of double-thickness folds at the edges. They are secured to the skin with Backhaus towel clamps (Fig. 19-3). The clamps should not be repositioned because their tips are contaminated after skin penetration. The foot is then covered with a layer of sterile adhesive draping material (Fig. 19-3). A second layer consisting of a large single sheet with a central opening is then applied over the body with the limb emerging from it. Depending on the draping material used, a third layer should be applied over the second one. Reusable cotton cloth drapes do not prevent bacterial penetration effectively, especially when wet. Their advantage for orthopedic procedures is their good mechanical properties, which give better resis-

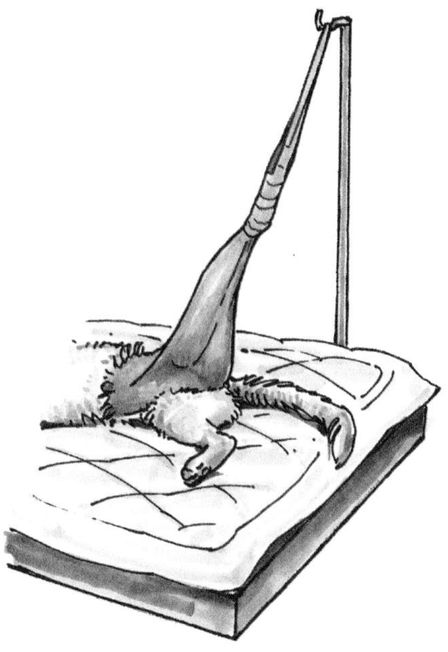

Figure 19-2 The cat is now in the surgical theater. The foot is covered with a clean bandage and the limb is suspended from an intravenous stand.

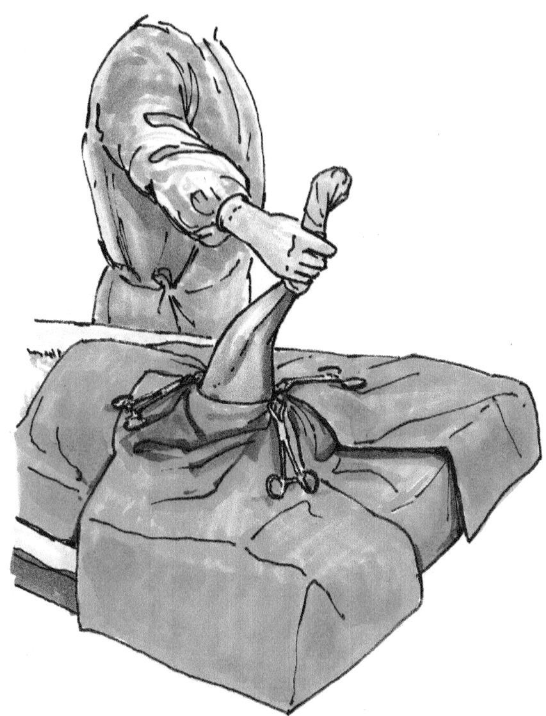

Figure 19-3 Four sterile towels have been placed around the base of the hindlimb, and were fixed with Backhaus towel clamps. The foot is covered with a sterile bandage, meaning that the whole limb protruding from the four towels is now prepared aseptically.

tance to penetration by sharp instruments. If cotton drapes are used, the middle drape should be of water-repellent material to reduce the risk of wetting or strike-through and bacterial penetration.

Special Backhaus forceps with balls at their extremities are employed to the most superficial drapes to stabilize the cables and tubes of the cautery and suction units (Fig. 19-4).

19.2 Preparation of the surgical team

The preparation of the surgical team is aimed at reducing both airborne contamination and contamination from human skin. The number of people, the level of activity in the surgery room, the amount of uncovered skin, and the amount of talking may increase bacterial numbers in the air (6).

Surgical scrub suits are worn to avoid introduction of organisms from the consultation and ward area into the surgery room. The shirt is tucked into the pants. A laboratory coat or overalls are worn on top of the scrub suit if the surgery room is left between surgeries. All people inside the surgery room wear head covers and face masks. It seems reasonable not to wear the same shoes as in the rest of the hospital and on the street, although no difference in floor and air contamination was found between street shoes, dedicated surgery shoes, and shoe covers (13). Face masks protect the wound from saliva drops by redirecting the airflow from the mouth and nose sideways. Masks filter particles for several hours; however, a reduction of air contamination has not yet been shown (14).

Several different options exist for the hand scrub, including iodine, chlorhexidine, and alcohol-based scrubs. Generally

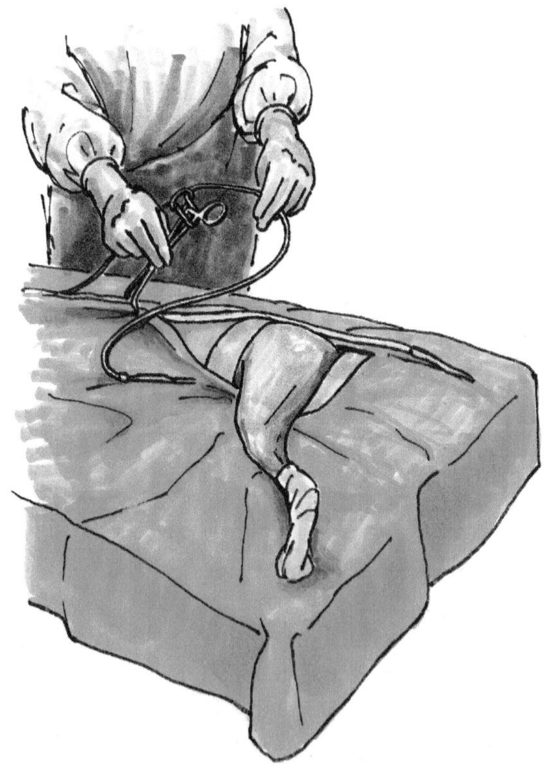

Figure 19-4 Appearance of the completed orthopedic draping. Two large towels with a central opening were added because cotton towels were used (the green ones). The suction tube and the cautery cable are fixed to the superficial towel with a non-penetrating towel clamp.

the first scrub of the day should last 5 minutes and the following scrubs on the same day 2–5 minutes, but the manufacturers' recommendations for the different types of scrub must be followed. The fingernails and nail beds host a high number of bacteria and should be cleaned thoroughly. Gowns should be water-resistant, and made of tough material. Gowns that cover the back of the surgeon are recommended. The gown is put on with the help of an assistant and the hands of the surgeon stay inside the sleeves until the gloves are put on. A closed gloving technique is used. Up to 31% of gloves have perforations at the end of surgery (15), and although perforations have not been associated with increased surgical wound infection rates, probably because surgical hand scrubs have reduced bacterial counts on the skin, the gloves should be exchanged if perforation is noticed intraoperatively. Talc and cornstarch particles may induce inflammatory reactions when entering a wound, and starch causes synovial necrosis in joints (16). Powdered gloves should therefore be cleaned with a sponge soaked in sterile isotonic solution before skin incision.

References and further reading

1. Kolata RJ, et al. Patterns of trauma in urban dogs and cats: a study of 1000 cases. J Am Vet Med Assoc 1974;164: 499–502.
2. Griffon D, et al. Thoracic injuries in cats with traumatic fractures. Vet Comp Orthop Traumatol 1994;7:98–100.
3. Rochlitz I. Clinical study of cats injured and killed in road traffic accidents in Cambridgeshire. J Small Anim Pract 2004;45: 390–394.
4. Vasseur PB, et al. Surgical wound infection rates in dogs and cats. Data from a teaching hospital. Vet Surg 1988;17:60–64.
5. Brown DC, et al. Epidemiologic evaluation of postoperative wound infections in dogs and cats. J Am Vet Med Assoc 1997;210:1302–1306.
6. Eugster S, et al. A prospective study of postoperative surgical site infections in dogs and cats. Vet Surg 2004;33:542–550.
7. Beal MW, et al. The effects of perioperative hypothermia and the duration of anesthesia on postoperative wound infection rate in clean wounds: a retrospective study. Vet Surg 2000;29:123–127.
8. Nicholson M, et al. Epidemiologic evaluation of postoperative wound infection in clean-contaminated wounds: a retrospective study of 239 dogs and cats. Vet Surg 2002;31:577–581.
9. Heldmann E, et al. The association of propofol usage with postoperative wound infection rate in clean wounds: a retrospective study. Vet Surg 1999;28:256–259.
10. Whittem TL, et al. Effect of perioperative prophylactic antimicrobial treatment in dogs undergoing elective orthopedic surgery. J Am Vet Med Assoc 1999;215:212–216.
11. Rosin E, et al. Cefazolin antibacterial activity and concentrations in serum and the surgical wound in dogs. Am J Vet Res 1993;54:1317–1321.
12. Stubbs WP, Bellah JR, et al. Chlorhexidine gluconate versus chloroxylenol for preoperative skin preparation in dogs. Vet Surg 1996;25:487–494.
13. Hambraeus A, Malmborg AS. The influence of different footwear on floor contamination. Scand J Infect Dis 1979;11: 243–246.
14. Shmon C. Assessment and preparation of the surgical patient and the operating team. In: Slatter D (ed.) Textbook of small animal surgery, 3rd edn. Philadelphia: Saunders; 2003: pp. 162–178.
15. Dodds RD, Barker SG, et al. Self protection in surgery: the use of double gloves. Br J Surg 1990;77:219–220.
16. Singh I, Chow WL, et al. Synovial reaction to glove powder. Clin Orthop 1974;99:285–292.

20 Postoperative care

K. Voss, F. Steffen

The aim of postoperative care is to aid a rapid and complete recovery from surgery. Appropriate analgesia, general care, and nutrition must be provided in the early postoperative period. Postoperative analgesia should be a synergistic and a natural extension of pre- and perioperative analgesia and its provision should be considered and planned before surgery according to the severity of pain expected. Nutritional demand is high after injury and major surgery. Cats are peculiar in their eating habits when under stress or in pain, and they may reject food intake. Nutritional support is therefore often required in postoperative management of traumatized cats. Postoperative care also includes instructions for the owners regarding the management of their cat at home. Depending on the type of lesion and the stability achieved at surgery, immobilization of the limb may be necessary for a certain period and this can involve vigilant and intensive postoperative monitoring by the owner. Postoperative care may also require rehabilitation therapy to optimize return to function after orthopedic and neurosurgery.

Postoperative care of patients with fractures or joint injuries, postoperative care of the neurological patient, and nutritional support of critically ill cats are described in the following sections. Analgesia is described in Chapter 18, and physical therapy is covered in Chapter 21.

20.1 Postoperative care of the fracture patient

Most cats recover quickly after fracture repair if they are otherwise healthy. The surgical site should be protected for 2–3 days postoperatively with a sterile dressing to prevent contamination of the skin wound. A light bandage may be applied to help reduce limb swelling and edema in patients with fractures distal to the elbow or stifle joint. Prolonged and unnecessary external immobilization of a limb should be avoided to prevent development of pressure sores, and to allow early weight-bearing, joint motion, and muscle function. Exceptions to this rationale are fractures where stability of the fixation is considered insufficient for immediate weight-bearing, where only small, flexible implants have been used (e.g., metacarpal/metatarsal fracture repair), and in the presence of wounds that are left to heal by second intention. External skeletal fixators are covered with a bandage only for the first few postoperative days to reduce swelling and edema, and until the pin tracts are sealed with granulation tissue. After that only the cut ends of the transosseous pins and the connecting bar are protected to avoid self-trauma.

Cats with uncomplicated fractures can usually be discharged from the hospital the day after surgery, provided the owners are supplied with analgesics to give to the cat (Chapter 18). Cats can be discharged with fentanyl patches, or buprenorphine can be given intrabuccally by the owners after painful procedures; however, there are serious concerns regarding legislation and abuse of these drugs so these only should be dispensed in selected cases. Non-steroidal anti-inflammatory drugs (NSAIDs), especially meloxicam, can be given alone or in combination with opioids. Prolonged use of NSAIDs has a potential to slow down fracture healing (1), but using meloxicam for 3–7 days in the postoperative period will not have a clinically relevant effect.

The owners should be instructed about the normal expected postoperative recovery, possible complications, and their associated signs. Internal fracture fixation should be stable enough to allow the cat to move freely in the house, but running, playing, and jumping on high objects should be prevented. In selected cases with limited fracture fixation stability, the cat might need to be confined to a cage or a single room for 2–4 weeks. Cages should be large enough to include a padded surface for sleeping and resting, room for a litter box or tray, water and food bowls, and some kind of a hiding place, such as a cardboard box. Large dog crates, a rabbit run, or a baby's playpen are suitable.

The time and frequency of clinical and radiographic fracture reassessment depend on the age of the cat, presence of soft-tissue injuries, fracture type, location in the bone, and implants used. As a general rule, radiographs are obtained after 2–3 weeks in immature cats, after 3–4 weeks in young adult cats, and after 4–6 weeks in older cats. Fractures stabilized with external fixators need frequent clinical checks to reduce and manage complications with pin tracts (Chapter 24). Owners of cats treated with external skeletal fixators tend to be more reliable in returning them for follow-up examinations compared to owners of cats treated with internal fixation devices (2).

Rehabilitation therapy is not yet widely used in cats, mainly because of concerns about the cat's dislike for manipulation. Despite this, physical therapy is possible and beneficial in many feline patients, if conducted correctly and with patience

(Chapter 21). Cats with uncomplicated fractures and stable repair usually start to use their limbs the day after surgery, and physical therapy may not be necessary. Owners should be encouraged to observe the degree of lameness and palpate joint range of motion and muscle mass, to be able to evaluate improvement of their cat. Lack of early limb use or failure to improve, reduced range of joint motion, and loss of muscle mass are all indications for rehabilitation therapy if the signs are not associated with complications of the fracture repair. Rehabilitation therapy should be instituted early if indicated.

20.2 Postoperative care of the patient with joint injuries

Severe joint injuries require postoperative immobilization after reconstruction to protect the surgical repair, and allow fibrosis and healing of periarticular tissues. Joint immobilization may involve application of splints, slings, or rigid joint immobilization with a transarticular external fixator, depending on the joint involved and the type of injury sustained. No general rules exist for how long a joint should be immobilized after various injuries and procedures. The need for joint immobilization depends on the injury sustained and the amount of preoperative instability, stability achieved after surgery or reduction, and inherent anatomic stability of a joint.

Immobilization for 10–14 days is usually sufficient, even in the presence of multiple ligamentous injuries, in joints with good stability due to joint congruency and bone conformation, such as the temporomandibular, elbow, and hip joint. In other joints, such as the carpus, tarsus, and stifle, an external splint or transarticular external fixator is often left in place for 3–4 weeks after multiple ligament injuries or luxations. The period of immobilization should be long enough for periarticular scar tissue and fibrosis to develop, providing sufficient stability to withstand weight-bearing and light activity. A soft bandage may be applied for an additional week or two to increase weight-bearing forces slowly. Weight-bearing is important in this phase of healing, as the longitudinal orientation of the collagen fibers depends on the presence of moderate tensile forces across the wound.

Prolonged joint immobilization causes periarticular fibrosis, loss of range of motion, and cartilage softening and degeneration (3). Structural and biochemical cartilage changes can already be apparent after 4 weeks of rigid immobilization (4). Ideally, immobilization should therefore not exceed 4 weeks, although prolonged immobilization may be required in selected cases. For example a transarticular external skeletal fixator applied to a joint with a degloving injury should be left in place until the soft-tissue injuries have healed, which may take longer than 4 weeks. Continuous passive motion has a protective effect on cartilage (5), but this is difficult to perform in cats. A splinted bandage does allow minimal joint motion, and in this respect is preferable over rigid joint immobilization with an external skeletal fixator, but in practice may be more difficult to keep on a fractious cat.

All cats with severe joint injuries should be kept in the house for 3 months to avoid strenuous activity. Analgesia is provided during the early postoperative period as described for fractures. Physical therapy is an important adjunct in the treatment of joint injuries. It is indicated in cats after prolonged joint immobilization to improve range of motion and joint function, and in those that are non-weight-bearing after surgery. Physical therapy is described in Chapter 21.

20.3 Postoperative care of the neurological patient

Postoperative care of neurosurgical patients is labor-intensive and time-consuming, especially in non-ambulatory animals. Pain management (Chapter 18) and adequate nursing care will enhance physical well-being in the recovery period, and encourage food and water intake. Neurosurgical procedures are painful and adequate peri- and postoperative analgesia must be provided. Opioid analgesics are most effective. They are always indicated in the immediate postoperative period, and are usually given for a couple of days in the form of fentanyl patches or subcutaneous or intrabuccal buprenorphine. NSAIDs should be used very cautiously as neurosurgical patients tend to develop gastrointestinal disorders. Hydration and nutrition must be provided until the cat drinks and eats on its own.

Non-ambulatory cats are less prone to decubital ulceration than dogs due to their low body weight, but patients should still be provided with adequate padding in the form of specially manufactured pet bedding (synthetic bedding that is water-repellent) and a carpet or clean towel, and they must be kept clean and dry to avoid urine scald. Grooming care is essential for the well-being of paralyzed cats as they are not able to reach every part of their body. The hair coat should be brushed and cleaned daily to improve mental well-being. A neck brace or buster collar may be necessary to prevent self-mutilation in cats with denervation injury.

The ability to urinate voluntarily is often absent in non-ambulatory cats with spinal cord lesions due to upper motor neuron spasticity of the external urinary sphincter and loss of the detrusor reflex. Manual expression of the urinary bladder or catheterization has to be performed at least two to three times daily in these patients to prevent overdistension of the bladder and urinary infections. Placement of a urinary catheter with a closed urine collection system is indicated when the bladder is difficult to express, and if the patient is difficult to handle. Micturition may be medically supported.

Phenoxybenzamine (0.25–0.5 mg/cat PO BID) is used to relax the internal urinary sphincter. Bethanechol chloride (2 mg/kg PO BID) enhances bladder contractility but should only be given after urethral relaxation.

Cats with fractures and luxations of the spine are kept in a cage for at least 10 days. They are then allowed to move around in the house under supervision if they are ambulatory. Jumping activities must be prevented for about 8 weeks. Physical therapy is of great value, especially in non-ambulatory cats. Physical therapy includes massage and passive movements of paralyzed limbs, and gait exercises to improve neurological recovery. Intensive physical therapy helps in the prevention of joint stiffness and muscle atrophy, and improves circulation and production of collagen. The physical therapy can help decrease tissue adhesions and inflammation. A suggestion for a physical care plan for non-ambulatory animals is given in Box 20-1. Physiotherapists may be able to apply more specific exercises tailored to the problem of the individual patient. Establishing a specific protocol for each patient may be helpful and the owner can be involved in the care after instruction from the veterinarian and physiotherapist. See Chapter 21 for further information about feline physiotherapy.

Box 20-1. Suggestion for physical therapy in a non-ambulatory cat, ideally performed three times daily

Therapeutic hot packing of affected limbs. Place the limb in heated towels or on covered hot-water bottles for approximately 20 minutes

Massage of the paralyzed limbs with simple hand technique, beginning with the distal part of the affected limb. Apply moderate pressure with the fingertips. Knead or twist the skin and larger muscle groups with the palm of the hand

Passive range-of-motion exercises. Hold the foot with one hand and grasp the stifle or elbow with the other. Pull the limb forward and then back in a circling motion. Assess range of motion and repeat the exercise several times.

Flexion/extension exercises. Perform 5–10 flexions and extensions of each joint before flexing the entire limb

Proprioceptive exercises. Support the animal in a standing position and place paws in a correct position. Move the body slightly to and fro under maintenance of a physiological posture

Gait exercises. Support the paretic animal with a sling/towel around the abdomen (and chest if necessary). Follow the movements of the cat slowly and support spontaneous movements. If the cat is reluctant to move with this support, let it move freely in the room

20.4 Nutritional support

Many polytraumatized cats and cats following major surgery are reluctant to eat for several days, and at the same time they have an enhanced nutritional demand. This results in a negative energy balance and patients are at risk for decreased immune competence, decreased tissue synthesis and repair, and altered drug metabolism (6). Overweight cats may also develop hepatic lipidosis during phases of anorexia. Nutritional support should ideally start within 24 hours of injury. The goal is to provide exogenous sources of energy and proteins, thus sparing endogenous sources and preventing a catabolic state and muscle wasting.

An anorexic cat may start eating if the food is prepared according to its preference. The owners can be asked to bring in their cat's favorite diet. The smell of the food plays an important role in dietary preference in cats (7). Most cats like fat, and fat may be used as a flavor enhancer on dried kibble (7). Warming canned food in a microwave enhances the smell of the food and may initiate food intake. Cats reject food if served at temperatures lower than 15°C and higher than 50°C (8). Low-dose intravenous diazepam (0.1–0.2 mg/kg) can be given as an appetite stimulant and is sometimes successful in getting a previously anorexic cat eating again. It should not be used repeatedly to avoid side-effects.

20.4.1 Nutritional needs

Diseased animals have energy requirements near their resting energy requirement (RER) (6). Metabolic rates are enhanced in traumatized patients and patients with sepsis. RER can be easily calculated with the equation shown in Box 20-2. RER of a cat with a body weight of 5 kg is around 200 kcal/day. At least 50% but preferably 100% of RER must be fed daily in the postoperative period (6). Weight loss and muscle wasting indicate insufficient calorie uptake, and in these circumstances energy and protein supplementation should be enhanced. Cats have a higher protein demand than dogs (7), and the protein content of a food should be 6–8 g/100 kcal (6). Nutritional support is required if patients voluntarily consume less than 50% of their RER over the first 24 hours (6).

Other nutritional needs that should be considered in cats are the essential amino acids, especially taurine and arginine, and vitamins. Although most veterinary diets contain arginine, the demand may be higher in cats with traumatic or

Box 20-2. Calculation of resting energy requirements (RER)

Cats larger than 5 lb (2.5 kg) BW: RER kcal/day = 20 × BW lb (= 40 × BW kg)
Cats smaller than 5 lb (2.5 kg) BW: RER kcal/day = 25 × BW lb (= 50 × BW kg)

BW, body weight.

surgical wounds. Arginine supplementation improves nitrogen balance and immune function, and enhances formation of new collagen in traumatized animals (6, 9, 10). The optimal arginine concentration is not known, but 100–400 mg/kg per day has been shown to improve healing of burn wounds in rats (9). Oral supplementation of arginine may therefore be beneficial in polytraumatized cats. Arginine is available as a food supplement for people (Dynamisan).

B-complex vitamins (folic acid, thiamin, and others) are essential for hepatic metabolism of glucose, fat, and protein. All diets contain B-complex vitamins, but they should be supplied when the cat is not eating. Vitamin B can be added to intravenous fluids.

20.4.2 Enteral feeding

Nutritional support may be provided enterally and parenterally. Enteral support is easy to administer and cost-efficient, and is usually adequate for traumatized cats. The most important and practical aspects of enteral nutritional support are summarized in the following section. For a more detailed discussion on nutritional support and parenteral feeding the reader is referred to specialized textbooks.

Enteral feeding can be provided via nasoesophageal tubes, esophagostomy tubes, gastrostomy tubes, and jejunostomy tubes. Advantages, disadvantages, and potential complications of different tubes are summarized in Table 20-1. Nasoesophageal tubes are easy to insert without sedation or anesthesia. They are only indicated in cats requiring short-term nutritional support. In cats with facial trauma, esophagostomy or gastrostomy tubes may be preferred to avoid additional occlusion of the nasal meatus. Gastrostomy tubes can be inserted surgically or percutaneously with or without endoscopic control, and are often used in patients requiring long-term feeding (11–13). Esophagostomy tubes are a viable alternative for long-term feeding (14). They are easier to insert, do not require specialized equipment, and have similar complication rates and owner acceptance as gastrostomy tubes (15). Jejunostomy tubes are rarely necessary or indicated in orthopedic and trauma patients. Insertion of nasoesophageal and esophagostomy tubes is described below.

Only liquid food can be introduced through the small-diameter nasoesophageal tubes. An adequate liquid food for cats is CliniCare Feline (Abbott Laboratories, Chicago, IL). CliniCare has an energy content of 1 kcal/ml and a protein content of 6–8 g/100 kcal. Approximately 200 ml meet the RER of a 5-kg cat. Esophagostomy and gastrostomy tubes allow feeding with blended diets mixed with water. Hills a/d is a high-energy thick liquid diet (Hill's Pet Nutrition, Topeka, KS). It contains 1.3 kcal/100 ml and 8.3 g protein/100 kcal. A cat with a body weight of 5 kg would need about 160 ml/day (Table 20-2). Cats have a stomach capacity of around 5–10 ml/kg body weight during initial food introduction. Maximal stomach capacity is around 50 ml/kg body weight. Enteral feeding should be started by giving small quantities. Most cats tolerate initial quantities of 30–40 ml per meal. If vomiting occurs even smaller amounts should be fed at a higher frequency. In cats that have been anorexic for several days, food has to be introduced slowly, with one-third of RER given on the first day, two-thirds on the second day, and the full dose on the third day.

With both nasoesophageal and esophageal feeding tubes it is extremely important to introduce the food slowly with a syringe to avoid regurgitation and aspiration pneumonia. Sterile saline is injected into the tube before feeding is begun. The position of the tube is checked radiographically if coughing or regurgitation occurs. The tube is cleaned with water after every feeding session to avoid drying of food particles in the tube and tube obstruction. This is especially important in the small-diameter nasoesophageal tubes. Tube position should also be checked if vomiting occurs, as this can result in tube displacement (14).

Insertion of a nasoesophageal feeding tube

Polyurethane or silicon feeding tubes can be used as nasoesophageal tubes. The 5-French size is appropriate for most cats. A drop of lidocaine is placed into the nasal passage before tube insertion. The distance from the nares to the eighth intercostal space is premeasured to estimate the length of tube to be inserted, and a mark is made on the tube at the appropriate point. The tube is then inserted carefully into the ventral meatus and advanced slowly. The head of the cat should be held in flexion during advancement of the tube into the pharyngeal area to reduce the risk of inadvertent tube placement into the trachea (Fig. 20-1A and 20-1B). Most cats will swallow as the tube is passed through the proximal esophageal sphincter. The tube is advanced up to the previously marked point and is then secured to the skin adjacent to the nares with superglue (Fig. 20-1C). Correct positioning of the tube is checked by injection of sterile saline. Coughing

Feeding tube	Advantages	Disadvantages	Potential complications
Nasoesophageal tube	Very easy to place No anesthesia needed No additional trauma/surgery	Only liquid food Only short-term feeding Should not be used in cats with facial trauma	Inadvertent placement into airways Aspiration pneumonia if food is injected too rapidly
Esophagostomy tube	Easy to place Long-term feeding possible Can be removed any time	Anesthesia needed Not for patients with pharyngeal and esophageal trauma	Local infection Inadvertent placement into mediastinum Aspiration pneumonia if food is applied too rapidly
Gastrostomy tube (surgical, percutaneous with/without endoscopic control)	Comfortable for patient Ideal for long-term feeding	Anesthesia needed More difficult to place Special instrumentation needed Must be left in place for at least 10 days	Local infection Inadvertent damage to other organs (percutaneous technique) Septic peritonitis if tube dislodges prematurely (less likely if placed surgically)

Table 20-1. Advantages, disadvantages, and potential complications of different feeding tubes

Product	Energy and proteins contained	Amount to be fed per day
CliniCare Feline (Abbott)	Energy 1 kcal/ml Protein 8.2 g/100 kcal	200 ml
Prescription diet a/d (Hills)	Energy: 1.3 kcal/ml Protein: 8.3 g/100 kcal	160 ml
Two cans prescription diet a/d (Hills) mixed with 50 ml water	Energy: 1 kcal/ml Protein: 8.3 g/100 kcal	200 ml
Reconvalescence support feline (Waltham) 1 sachet (50 g) mixed with 150 ml water	1.2 kcal/ml Protein: 8.7 g/100 kcal	170 ml

Table 20-2. Examples of type and amount of food to be fed. A cat with a body weight of 5 kg needs at least 200 kcal/day to meet the resting energy requirement (RER), with an ideal protein content of 6–8 g/100 kcal

should occur if the tube is inserted in the trachea. An additional test is to attempt air aspiration by attaching a syringe to the tube; air can be aspirated if the tube is in the trachea, but not if it is in the esophagus, because negative pressure created by gentle suction on the syringe will collapse the esophagus. Tubes with radiodense markers are ideal as correct tube placement can be checked radiographically (Fig. 20-2). A nasoesophageal tube can be placed straight after surgery while the cat is still under anesthesia. Direct visualization of the tube with a laryngoscope as it disappears through the upper esophageal sphincter can then be used to verify correct positioning. An Elizabethan collar prevents the cat from removing the tube.

Insertion of an esophagostomy feeding tube

A 10–14 French red rubber tube is commonly used as an esophageal feeding tube. The cat is anesthetized and the left cervical area is aseptically prepared. A curved Kelly forcep is inserted into the cervical esophagus (Fig. 20-3). The tips of the forceps are pressed against the skin, dorsal to the jugular vein. The tube length is premeasured from the tube insertion

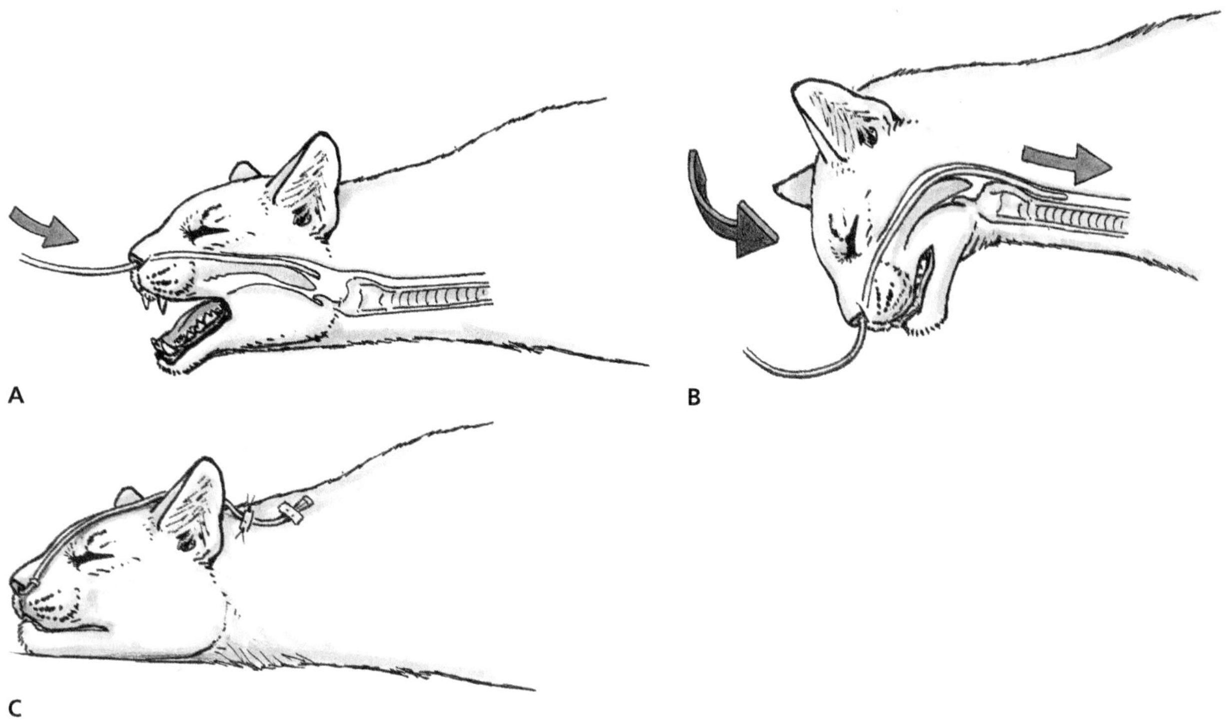

Figure 20-1 Insertion of a nasoesophageal feeding tube.
(**A**) The tube is inserted into the ventral nasal meatus after a drop of lidocaine has been instilled.
(**B**) Flexing the neck of the cat helps direct the tube into the esophagus. Most conscious cats swallow once the tube has entered the esophagus.
(**C**) The tube is inserted the premeasured distance. It can be fixed just laterally to the nasal plane with a drop of superglue. The correct position of the tube is then controlled.

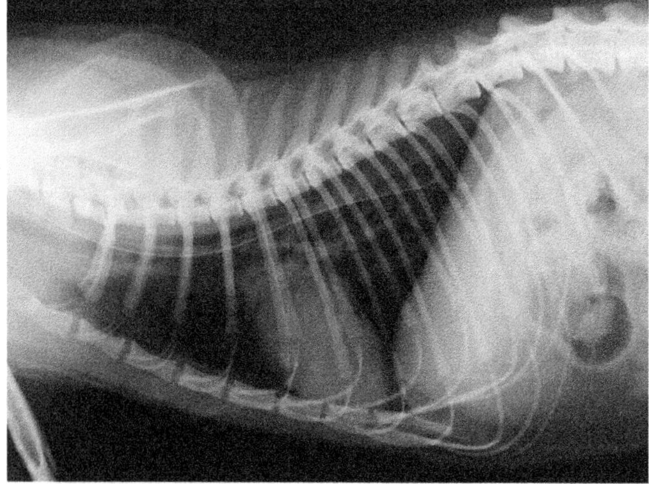

Figure 20-2 Laterolateral radiograph of the thorax of a cat after insertion of a feeding tube. The tip of the tube should be located in the esophagus between the heart base and the cardia, ideally at the eighth intercostal space.

site to the eighth intercostal space. A small longitudinal incision through the overlying skin and esophageal wall is then performed with a scalpel blade. The tip of the tube is securely grasped with the Kelly forceps and retrieved through the oral cavity. The tip of the tube is then redirected and inserted through the proximal esophageal sphincter. The tube end, which is still protruding from the incision site, is carefully retracted to allow advancement of the tip of the tube further down the esophagus without kinking or curling of the tube. Care is taken not to remove the tube inadvertently during this step of the procedure. The tube should be advanced up to the premeasured length and secured to the skin with a Chinese fingertrap suture (Fig. 20-3). The tube insertion site can be protected with a light neck bandage. An Elizabethan collar may have to be applied in cats that scratch at their tube.

Another technique has been described in which the esophagostomy tube is inserted directly into the esophagus, without the need for retrieving it and redirecting it through the oral cavity (16). The tube is inserted with the help of a tube applicator (esophageal feeding tube applicator, Fixomed, Munich, Germany), which allows insertion of the esophageal tube directly in a distal direction after the skin and esophageal wall have been incised with a scalpel blade (Fig. 20-4).

Correct tube positioning is checked radiographically, and by inserting sterile saline before each feeding session, as described above.

Cats can still eat despite the presence of an esophagostomy tube. The tube is removed once the patient has resumed an adequate oral food uptake. The incision is left open for second-intention healing.

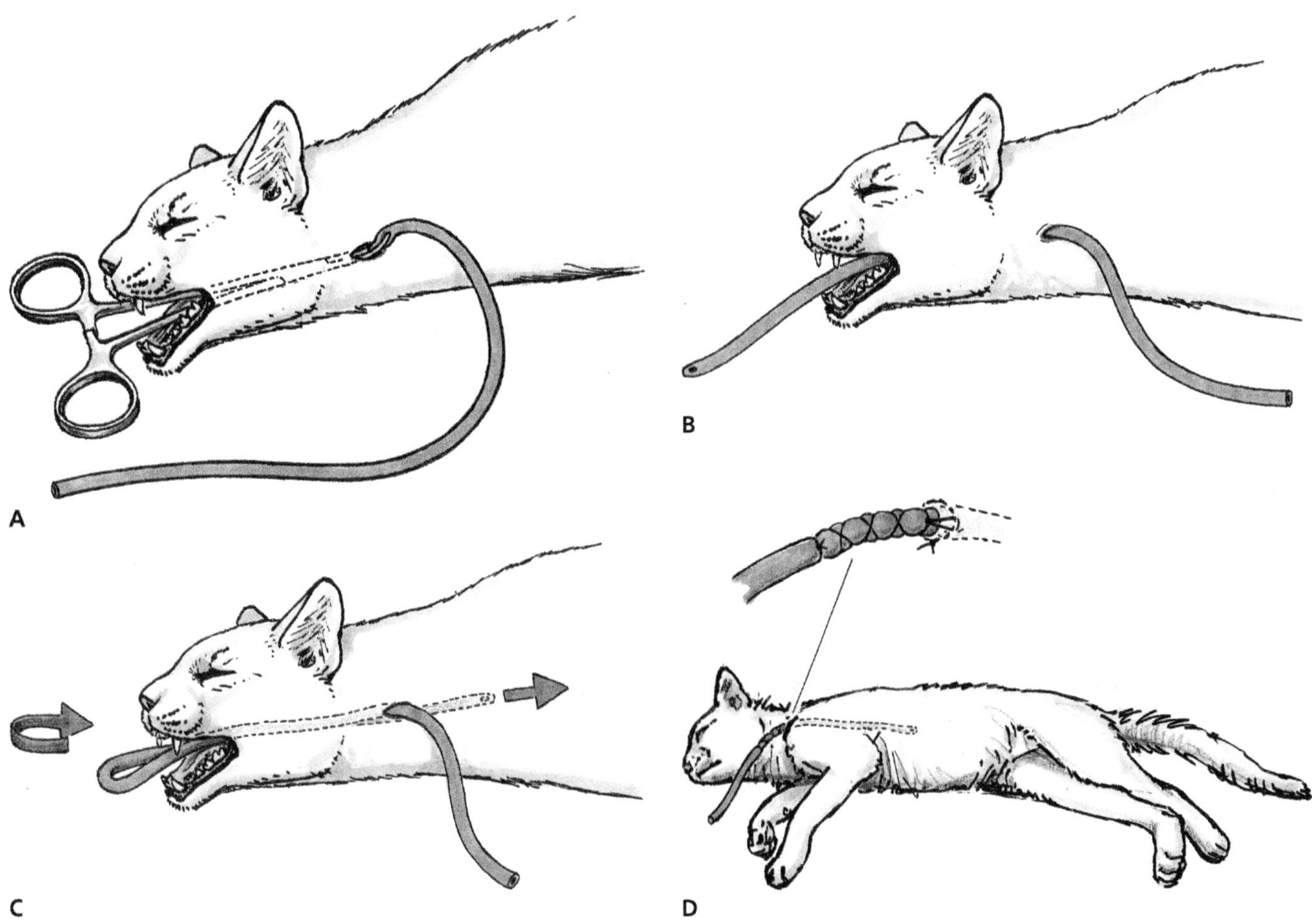

Figure 20-3 Insertion of an esophagostomy feeding tube.
(**A**) A curved Kelly forceps is used to grasp the tip of the esophagostomy feeding tube from the esophageal incision.
(**B**) The tip of the tube is guided through the oral cavity with the help of the Kelly forceps.
(**C**) The tip of the tube is then redirected from the oral cavity into the esophagus. Care must be taken after the tip of the tube passes the incision site to ensure that it is advanced correctly down the esophagus.
(**D**) The tube is inserted the premeasured distance, and is fixed to the skin with a Chinese fingertrap suture.

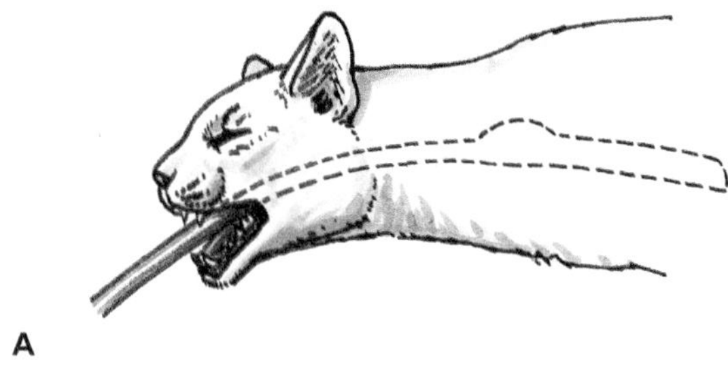

A

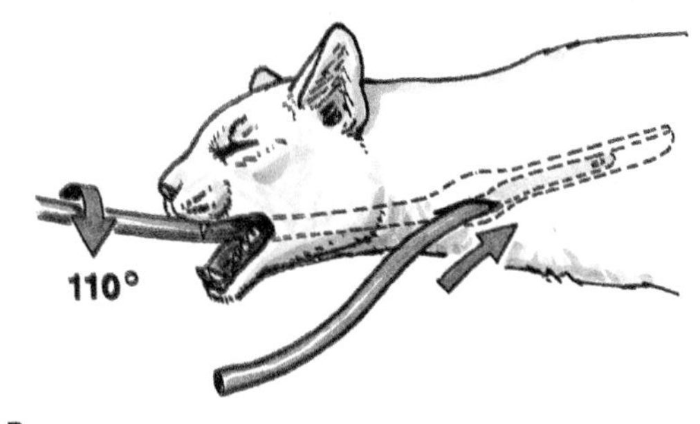

B

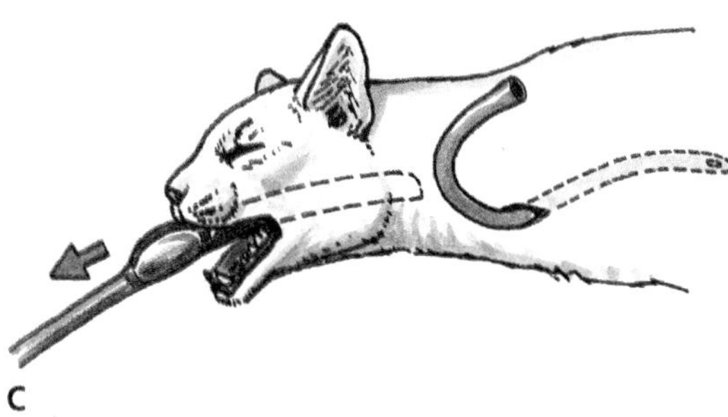

C

Figure 20-4 Insertion of an esophagostomy feeding tube with the help of an applicator.
(**A**) The applicator is inserted into the esophagus.
(**B**) It is then turned until the widened insertion area with its slot can be palpated laterally. The skin and esophageal wall are incised over the slot and a feeding tube is inserted into the esophagus, without the need for redirecting it through the oral cavity.
(**C**) The applicator is turned back and is removed. The tube is fixed to the skin with a Chinese fingertrap suture, as shown in Figure 20-3D. (Reprinted with permission from Von Werthern CJ, Wess G. A new technique for insertion of esophagostomy tubes in cats. J Am Anim Hosp Assoc 2001;37:140–144.)

References and further reading

1. Wheeler P, Batt ME. Do non-steroidal anti-inflammatory drugs adversely affect stress fracture healing? A short review. Br J Sports Med 2005;39:65–69.
2. Emmerson TD, Muir P. Bone plate removal in dogs and cats. Vet Comp Orthop Traumatol 1999;12:74–77.
3. Piermattei DL, Flo GL. Principles of joint surgery. In: Piermattei DL, Flo GL (eds) Small animal orthopedics and fracture repair, 3rd edn. Philadelphia: WB Saunders; 1997: pp. 201–217.
4. Vanwanseele B, et al. The effects of immobilization on the characteristics of articular cartilage: current concepts and future directions. Osteoarthritis Cartilage 2002;10:408–419.
5. Salter RB. The biologic concept of continuous passive motion of synovial joints. The first 18 years of basic research and its clinical application. Clin Orthop Relat Res 1989;242:12–25.
6. Remillard RL. Nutritional support in critical care patients. Vet Clin North Am Small Anim Pract 2002;32:1145–1164.
7. Zaghini G, Biagi G. Nutritional pecularities and diet palatability in the cat. Vet Res Commun 2005;29:39–44.
8. Sohail MA. The ingestive behaviour of the domestic cat: a review. Nutrition Abstracts Rev 1983;53:177–186.
9. Chen X, et al. Dose-effect of dietary L-arginine supplementation on burn wound healing in rats. Chin Med J (Engl) 1999;112: 828–831.
10. Shi HP, et al. Supplemental L-arginine enhances wound healing in diabetic rats. Wound Repair Regen 2003;11:198–203.
11. Mauterer JV, et al. New technique and management guidelines for percutaneous nonendoscopic tube gastrostomy. J Am Vet Med Assoc 1994;205:574–579.
12. Mauterer JV. Endoscopic and nonendoscopic percutaneous gastrostomy tube placement. In: Bonagura JD (ed.) Kirk's veterinary therapy. Philadelphia: WB Saunders; 1995: pp. 669–674.
13. Han E. Esophageal and gastric feeding tubes in ICU patients. Clin Tech Small Anim Pract 2004;19:22–31.
14. Devitt CM, Seim HB. Clinical evaluation of tube esophagostomy in small animals. J Am Anim Hosp Assoc 1997;33: 55–60.
15. Ireland LM, et al. A comparison of owner management and complications in 67 cats with esophagostomy and percutaneous endoscopic gastrostomy feeding tubes. J Am Anim Hosp Assoc 2003;39:241–246.
16. Von Werthern CJ, Wess G. A new technique for insertion of esophagostomy tubes in cats. J Am Anim Hosp Assoc 2001; 37:140–144.

21 Rehabilitation of the cat

S. Hudson

The field of feline rehabilitation has been slow to take hold due to the perceived idea that the cat will not cooperate with the physical therapy modalities or perform therapeutic exercises. However, physical rehabilitation is a very effective modality in cats, provided that feline behavior and personality are taken into account (1). Specific orthopedic conditions that benefit from physical therapy include postoperative fracture repair, postoperative joint repair, and osteoarthritis management.

21.1 Principles of rehabilitation

Physical therapy is the application of techniques that help restore function, improve mobility, relieve pain, and prevent or limit permanent physical disabilities of patients suffering from injuries or disease. Identical modalities and similar exercises used in the human field can be applied to the animal. Studies have shown effectiveness of physical therapy techniques applied to the dog (2, 3). Veterinary physical therapy and rehabilitation is a relatively new field. Certification programs and continuing education programs for canine and equine patients are providing training for veterinarians, veterinary technicians, and physical therapists. There is not currently a program designed specifically for the cat.

Rehabilitation can be used to provide immediate postoperative care, early weight-bearing training, progressive weight-bearing training, advanced conditioning, gait training, management of chronic pain, and conservative management for certain conditions or as an alternative to some surgeries.

The primary focus of rehabilitation immediately following surgery is to reduce pain, swelling, and edema that can result from trauma to tissue. Efforts are made to preserve range of motion and muscle mass to speed return to normal activities. This is usually all passive rehabilitation, and may begin before the cat has fully recovered from anesthesia.

In the early postoperative stage, the goal is to begin to improve strength and endurance of muscles, increase range of joint motion, and improve proprioception. At this stage the cat may be non-weight-bearing or just barely placing a toe of the injured limb on the ground.

As the cat begins to use the injured limb more, the progressive weight-bearing stage begins. The focus in this stage is on increasing muscle strength, endurance, joint range of motion, and proprioception as in the early weight-bearing phase; however, the exercises are longer and more strenuous.

Box 21-1. Important factors for successful rehabilitation therapy in cats

Factors that facilitate productive and safe rehabilitation session

Quiet environment free of other animals
Presence of owner
No rushing
Confident application of modality or introduction of exercise
Sedation
Pain management
Second attempt at an exercise is more difficult than first
Closed area to reduce risk of escaping cat

Gait training is used when the cat moves in a way that is not normal following an injury or procedure. Gait training identifies and addresses the areas that need to improve to produce a normal gait pattern.

Conditioning can be defined as controlled exercise to improve the body composition of an overweight cat. Reduction in body weight and improvement in muscle strength and endurance may be the most important elements to improve the quality of life of the older cat.

Rehabilitation is designed to provide the most complete return to function possible while reducing the risk of additional injury. Factors that facilitate a productive and safe rehabilitation session are summarized in Box 21-1. Not every exercise or modality is well suited for every cat. It is important to have several alternative ways to reach rehabilitation goals.

21.2 Four target areas of rehabilitation

The goal of rehabilitation is restoration of the quality of life and function for the cat through improvement of the bones, joints, and muscles. The four primary target areas of rehabilitation are strength, endurance, range of motion, and proprioception.

21.2.1 Strength

Muscle atrophy can occur due to disease, injury, lack of use, or lack of nerve impulse. Strength activities increase the size of muscle fibers. Increasing strength can help with the stability of the joint.

21.2.2 Endurance

Prolonged contraction of a muscle leads to muscle fatigue due to the inability of the metabolic process of the fibers to supply nutrients at the level required for the workout. Endurance can be defined as the amount of time between the beginning of physical activity and the end because of exhaustion or fatigue. Endurance exercises increase the oxidative capacity of the muscle, making it more resistant to fatigue. Improving endurance helps the cat return to its normal level of activity.

21.2.3 Range of motion

Range of motion is the capability of a joint to go through its complete spectrum of movements. It can be passive or active. Passive range of motion can be defined as what is achieved when an outside force, such as a therapist, causes movement of a joint. It is usually the maximum range of motion. Active range of motion is what can be achieved when opposing muscles contract and relax, resulting in joint movement. Active range of motion is usually less than the passive range of motion.

Range of motion therapy is beneficial in recovery from soft-tissue and joint lesions, maintaining existing joint and soft-tissue mobility, minimizing the effects of contracture formation, assisting neuromuscular re-education, and enhancing synovial movement. Measurement of range of motion can be used to evaluate available motion, determine joint stability, and determine soft-tissue elasticity as well as response to therapy over time. The evaluation of a joint's end feel, which is the quality of the resistance of the joint as the endpoint of a passive movement of the joint, will provide information about the complete range of motion for that joint (Table 21-1).

21.2.4 Proprioception

Proprioception and kinesthesia, the sensation of joint motion and acceleration, are the sensory feedback mechanisms for motor control and posture. These mechanisms along with the vestibular system help the body remain oriented and balanced.

21.3 Passive and active rehabilitation

Rehabilitation can be divided into two specific categories. Passive modalities require no participation from the cat and include cold and heat therapy, passive range of motion, stretching, massage therapy, electrical stimulation, and ultrasound. Active rehabilitation requires active participation from the cat, and includes exercise therapy, gait training, and aquatic therapy.

21.3.1 Passive rehabilitation

Thermal agents

The application of heat or cold is used to increase or decrease the temperature of the tissue around a joint and can be used throughout a rehabilitation program. The use of heat versus cold is determined by the tissue's stage of recovery.

Application of cold therapy. The application of cold is used to reduce bleeding and inflammation, and to decrease pain. Specific indications for the use of cold include musculoskeletal injury following orthopedic surgery, treatment of muscular pain, and postexercise soreness.

Cold can be applied using ice packs, cold packs, or iced towels. In addition, compression can be applied with the cold to help reduce or prevent edema. When applying cold treatments, place a thin layer of material between the cold pack and the cat's skin to increase the comfort level. Placing a towel over the cold pack also avoids loss of cold to the environment. Cold therapy is usually applied for 10 minutes, one to four times a day. Even one application of cold during the first 24 hours of trauma has been shown to be beneficial in the reduction of swelling and pain in the human patient.

Cold should not be applied if the cat has cold hypersensitivity, decreased or absent sensation, and it should not be applied directly over areas with compromised circulation. The skin should be inspected if the cat shows unusual signs of discomfort. Immediately postoperatively, while the cat is still under anesthesia, may be the only time that the cat tolerates the application of cold. Subsequent applications are best performed with the cat resting in the lap of the therapist and a blanket wrapped around the patient.

Application of heat therapy. Superficial heat therapy is used to increase metabolism, increase soft-tissue extensibility, and decrease pain. Heat should only be used after signs of inflammation are gone. Specific uses for heat are for subacute and chronic traumatic and inflammatory conditions, muscle spasm, tissue tightness, adhesions, and pain. In the management of osteoarthritis, heat may be used to help loosen tight muscles around a joint to improve flexibility. Heat is often

End feel	Description	Example (normal)	Example (abnormal)
Bone on bone	Abrupt halt to movement when two hard surfaces meet	Carpal extension Cervical extension	Shoulder flexion
Capsular	Elastic arrest of movement with some give	Hip flexion Shoulder flexion Hip extension Shoulder extension	
Empty	Unable to reach end range due to painful reaction of cat, no tissue tension felt		All joints
Spasm	Muscle spasm actively occurs when attempting range of motion		All joints
Springy block	Rebound of both extreme ends of range of motion due to intra-articular displacement		Common with meniscal injury
Tissue approximation	Range of motion stopped due to secondary engagement against a muscle	Stifle flexion	

Table 21-1. Joint end feels

used within the first days to weeks after surgery, once the initial inflammation has decreased.

Superficial heat can be applied using heat packs (Fig. 21-1). Application time is 10 minutes two to four times per day. Remove the heat source if the cat shows any signs of discomfort.

Heat therapy should not be used if any signs of inflammation are present, such as redness or swelling. Heat should not be used on animals with decreased or absent sensation, over malignancies or over an active infection.

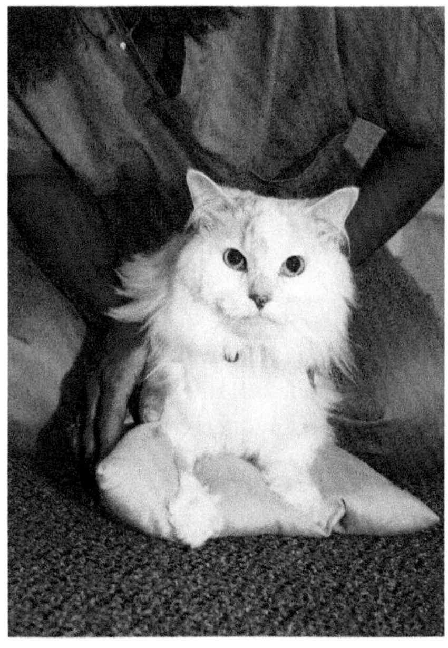

Figure 21-1 Most cats tolerate application of heat well.

Electrical stimulation

Electrical stimulation can be used to increase muscle strength, to attenuate atrophy, for pain control, and to reduce edema. Positive results have been documented with the use of electrical stimulation on the dog (4). It should not be used on cats with pacemakers or seizure disorders. It should also not be used over the trunk of pregnant females, in patients that cannot give feedback, over infected areas, or in areas of thrombosis. Active motion is contraindicated. The animal's reaction to electrical stimulation should be carefully monitored.

Electrical stimulation recruits muscle fibers in reverse of volitional contractions. Electrical stimulation recruits the fast-twitch fibers first. The area to be stimulated must be clipped and cleaned before the electrodes can be properly applied. Two types of current are generally recommended for use on felines: continuous alternating current for pain and edema or pulsed current for strengthening and edema.

Electrical stimulation for pain management. Two waveforms, interferential and premodulated, are generally used for the management of pain due to post-traumatic, postoperative, or chronic pain.

The interferential waveform consists of two channels, each with a sinusoidal waveform, one fixed- and one variable-frequency. The electrodes are positioned so that the two channels cross each other to stimulate large-impulse fibers. These frequencies interfere with the transmission of pain messages at the spinal cord level. Interferential stimulation allows for a deep penetration of the tissue with more comfort and therefore more compliance than a transcutaneus electrical nerve stimulation application.

The premodulated waveform is an amplitude-modulated sine wave that is similar to the beat frequency created by the interferential current. This is often used when the placement of four electrodes cannot be utilized.

The electrode placement should cover the entire area suspected of pain. Specific frequency and phase duration of the stimulation will vary with each patient and condition. There are many electrical stimulation units available with a variety of variables and recommended parameters.

Electrical stimulation for attenuation of muscle atrophy. Two waves that can be used for muscle contraction are high-volt and Russian. Locate the area where the motor nerve enters the muscle. This allows for optimum muscle contraction with as low a current as possible to increase the comfort level of the treatment. Apply the gel to the skin of the cat and place the electrode over the expected area of the motor point. Turn the unit on and move the electrode until the desired contraction is observed. Once identified, the motor points can be marked on the cat with an indelible marker for subsequent treatments.

The optimum time and frequency of treatment are unknown. The generally accepted frequency is 25–50 Hz.

Therapeutic ultrasound

Therapeutic ultrasound is produced by applying an electric current to a crystal. The current causes the crystal to vibrate at a resonant frequency, emitting pressure waves that are absorbed by the tissue (Fig. 21-2).

Therapeutic ultrasound can be used to increase collagen extensibility (stretch), increase blood flow, increase range of motion, decrease pain and muscle spasm, and accelerate wound healing. Ultrasound therapy generates ultrasonic energy in continuous or pulsed form to produce thermal, mechanical, and chemical effects in tissues. Ultrasound is capable of separating collagen fibers and changing the tensile strength of tendons to permit a greater amount of stretching. Use caution when using ultrasound over plastic or metal plate implants because the reflection may cause more intense heating, leading to burns or discomfort.

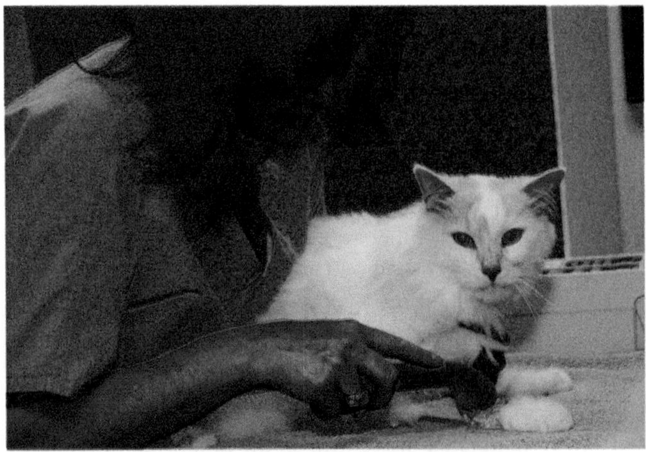

Figure 21-2 Therapeutic ultrasound for a carpal injury.

To begin the treatment, determine the depth of tissue to be treated. Clip hair and clean skin (5). If the depth of tissue to be treated is up is 3 cm, select 3.3 MHz frequency (6, 7). If the tissue to be treated is 2–5 cm in depth, select 1.0 MHz frequency. Then determine the amount of soft tissue in the area. Intensity is the rate at which the energy is delivered into the area. Choose 1–2 W/cm^2 for areas with large amount of soft tissue such as the caudal thigh muscles, choose 1–1.5 W/cm^2 for areas with less soft tissue, and 0.5–1.0 W/cm^2 for areas with little soft tissue such as the carpus.

Choose the mode, pulsed or continuous, depending on the type of thermal effects desired. Both give thermal and non-thermal effects, but the pulsed ultrasound has a lower average energy so the thermal effects are minimal. Pulsed ultrasound is available in 20% pulse and 50% pulse. Pulsed ultrasound is selected when healing effects are desired with minimal heating effects.

Treatment time can be calculated by determining the number of transducer heads that fit into the treatment area and multiplying that number by 2.5. The transducer head is moved at a rate of 4 cm/sec in overlapping circles in the treatment area. Keep the beam at less than 15° to the surface of the skin. Do not select a treatment area that requires more than 20 minutes treatment time. If a large treatment area is desired, select a larger transducer head or divide the area into different treatment session areas. Sessions are usually repeated 2–3 times per week.

The application of therapeutic ultrasound to increase the extension of a joint that has restricted movement can be performed by applying the appropriate frequency and intensity for the proper amount of time to the affected area. After the treatment is complete hold the joint in extension for 2 minutes as the tissue cools in the extended state. Repeat two to three times a week for 6–8 weeks. Heating tissue with ultrasound can provide immediate and residual increase in range of motion if combined with stretching (7).

Massage

Therapeutic massage is the manipulation of soft tissue that includes holding, causing movement, and applying pressure to the body. Massage therapy may improve function of the circulatory, lymphatic, muscular, skeletal, and nervous systems and may improve the rate at which the body recovers from injury or illness. Massage can be used to relax and reduce anxiety of the cat in the postoperative stage of recovery.

Two basic massage techniques are effleurage and pétrissage. Effleurage massage is a gliding stroke using the whole hand. The stroke is applied along the lines of the muscle and affects the superficial tissues. It is mostly used to assist with circulation so the strokes are always performed toward the heart. Pétrissage uses a kneading compression stroke with skin rolling. It is used for muscle tension, knots, and spasms.

Passive range of motion

Passive range of motion is the manipulation of a joint through its maximum flexion and extension angles. It provides controlled movement along the normal lines of stress, which can result in stronger scar and connective tissue. The motion of the joint affects muscles, joint surfaces, capsules, ligaments, fasciae, vessels, and nerves. Reduction in the normal range of motion can be caused by orthopedic or neurological surgery, trauma, immobilization or inactivity.

Range of motion therapy is beneficial in aiding recovery from soft-tissue and joint lesions, maintaining existing joint and soft-tissue mobility, minimizing the effects of contracture formation, assisting neuromuscular re-education, and enhancing synovial movement. It can be used to evaluate available motion, determine joint stability, and determine soft-tissue elasticity. It is possible to identify, and improve a limited range of motion. Passive range of motion can be used to warm up before exercise. It is important to note that passive range of motion will not prevent muscle atrophy or improve strength and endurance, but passive range of motion may be the most important exercise for a cat recovering from restrictive movement caused by splinting or casting.

Phototherapy

Phototherapy is the application of low-power light to areas of the body in order to stimulate healing. It is also known as cold laser, soft laser or low-intensity laser. It can accelerate wound and tissue repair by as much as 30–40%. Cell proliferation and wound healing can be enhanced by 150–200%.

Electromagnetic energy is emitted from the low-power laser and enters the tissue, where it is absorbed by the mitochondria of the cell. The energy is converted to chemical energy within the cell. The permeability of the cell membrane changes, which affects a variety of cell types including macrophages, fibroblasts, endothelial cells, and mast cells.

Phototherapy can be used for soft-tissue injuries such as sprains, strains, and tendonitis, for osteoarthritis, chronic pain, in the wound management of ulcers, pressure sores or burns, for skin infections, and for healing of incision sites (Fig. 21-3).

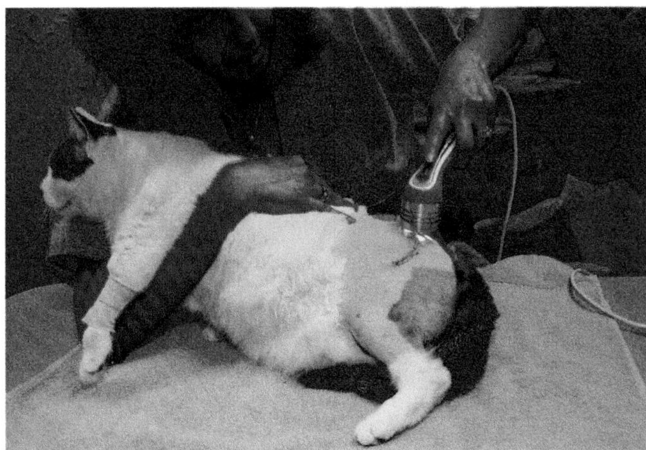

Figure 21-3 Application of cold laser therapy to increase healing following femoral head ostectomy surgery.

To begin phototherapy, remove any dressing and cleanse the wound bed and surrounding tissue. Cover the wound or phototherapy device with clear protective barrier if the skin is broken. Apply the laser with gentle contact for duration of treatment.

21.3.2 Active rehabilitation

Aquatic therapy

Aquatic therapy is the use of the therapeutic properties of water to provide appropriate exercises for strength, range of motion, and endurance, while reducing the risk of injury. It allows for active muscle contraction while limiting weight-bearing. Aquatic therapy is beneficial for soft-tissue injuries, osteoarthritis, postoperative fracture care, muscle weakness, neurological impairment, geriatric care, and postoperative amputee care. It should not be used for cats with cardiac dysfunction, respiratory dysfunction, surface infection, danger of bleeding or hemorrhage, severe peripheral vascular disease, or diarrhea. The therapeutic properties of water include:

- thermal – transfer of heat to the submerged tissue
- buoyancy – the upward thrust of water on a immersed body
- hydrostatic pressure – pressure exerted by water on immersed body
- cohesion – the tendency for water molecules to adhere to each other
- turbulence – the whirlpools in water caused by movement.

The therapeutic thermal effects of water are the same as for superficial heat, but more systemic. The soothing effects of warm water reduce pain and may increase the cat's ability to exert more effort.

The buoyancy property of water is used to increase or decrease the amount of weight-bearing on joints and bones. Reducing the body weight of the cat can reduce the amount of stress on a weak joint to allow the cat to exercise with a more natural gait pattern and move more comfortably.

The effect of hydrostatic pressure increases with water depth. This encourages upward flow of edema. Exercising the cat in deeper water enhances the effect of hydrostatic pressure.

Cohesion and turbulence contribute to the resistance the cat has while moving through the water. The cohesion property of water is used to increase the specific flexion of the joint at water level.

The underwater treadmill provides exceptional therapeutic exercise for the feline (Fig. 21-4). The unique effects of the underwater treadmill include the ability to vary the water depth to increase or decrease the amount of weight-bearing the cat has while exercising, to vary the speed of exercise, and to control the water temperature closely due to the small body of water. Increasing the water temperature can stimulate metabolism, relax tight muscles, help reduce pain, and increase soft-tissue extensibility. Water temperature should be approximately 90–92°F (32–34°C). The normal walking speed for the cat on the treadmill is 0.8–1.3 mph.

Exercise therapy

Feline exercise therapy is an active rehabilitation technique using the cat's natural ability to perform activities. This form of therapy is designed to return the cat to normal function sooner and to lessen the risk of future injuries. The level of each exercise will vary with the condition or postoperative stage of the cat.

An exercise therapy program begins with short-duration, low-impact activities and progresses to longer time periods with more strenuous activities. It is important to modify the program to accommodate the cat's comfort level. The exercise therapy program is divided into three stages: warm-up, the exercise activities, and the postexercise therapy.

The warm-up portion of the program includes assessing the cat's physical and mental condition and preparing the cat for

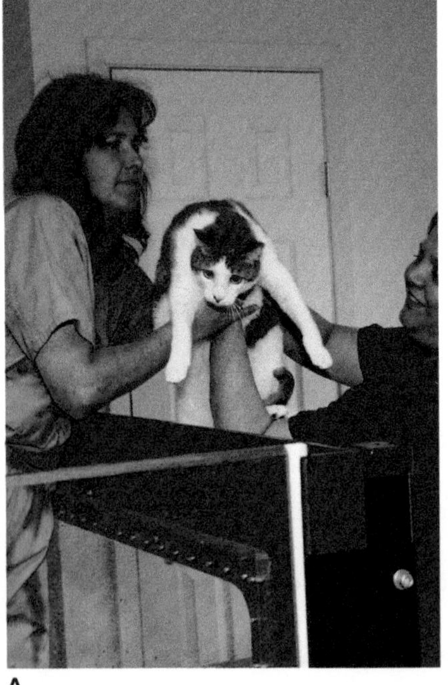

A

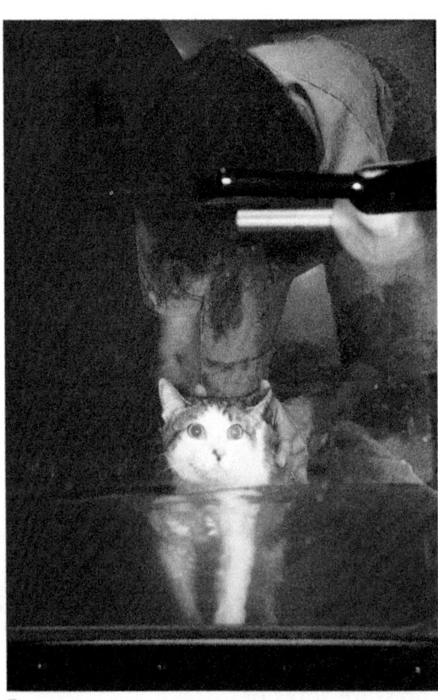

B

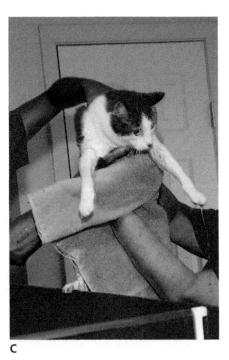

C

Figure 21-4 Aquatic therapy. (**A**) Have the owner hand the cat to the therapist in the chamber with a smooth confident motion, with the cat facing the direction in which it will walk. (**B**) Place the cat in the water. Guide with hands supporting the trunk of the cat if needed. (**C**) When the session is complete, lift the cat from the water and place it on a prepared towel. Have the owner or an assistant gently towel the cat dry. Then turn off and drain the treadmill.

the exercise session. It is important to assess the cat in order to evaluate the impact of previous sessions and to make changes necessary to keep progressing toward therapy goals. The cat is prepared for the exercise session by warming the affected area with a warm pack, passive range of motion, massage, or stretch. A combination of superficial heat and stretch is an excellent way to prepare the cat to get the most from the exercise session.

Gait training

Chronic pain or traumatic injury can cause a cat to alter its movement. This alteration in gait may cause pain or injury to unaffected limbs (8). Gait-training techniques and exercise focus on returning the cat to as near normal movement as possible.

21.4 The rehabilitation program

The rehabilitation program begins with the evaluation of the cat. This evaluation is a combination of subjective and objective information. Subjective information is data provided by the owner, whereas objective information is data collected during the examination. Both are important in determining the current condition of the cat. The owner is the key factor in providing information for the optimal outcome for the cat because the cat will not usually act or behave normally in the clinic environment.

Owner-provided history includes information such as age, breed, the general appearance and disposition of the cat to help determine how cooperative the cat will be, details about the onset of the problem or injury to identify how long the animal has been favoring a leg, and any past pertinent medical history which may indicate that an exercise or modality should or should not be used. The presence of other pets is also a consideration since in the early to middle phase of rehabilitation it is often necessary to restrict unsupervised activity with other animals to reduce the risk of injury. The cat's baseline activity level helps determine the cat's condition and the owner's expectation of what the cat should be able to do after rehabilitation. Identification of medication and supplements the cat is currently receiving and how the owner believes they are or are not working can be helpful in assessing benefits from rehabilitation. Questions should be asked to help determine if the cat's normal activities have changed (9).

Clinical examination should include a lameness evaluation, evaluation of the cat in standing and sitting positions, the cat's ability to rise, appearance of the scar and any discoloration, swelling, edema, or warmth of the affected tissue. These areas are evaluated before and after surgery. Range of motion of the affected and unaffected joints is measured to determine any loss of movement. Both passive and active range of motion can be evaluated.

Determine the cat's body condition (10). Is the cat muscular or weak? Is there a noticeable difference in the muscle mass of the affected limb? Is the cat overweight? If so, how much? After the assessment of the cat's current condition is complete, rehabilitation goals and expectations are determined.

It is important to set reasonable goals at the beginning of the rehabilitation program. Thorough evaluation and assessment of the cat's current condition, the expectations of the cat's owner, and the commitment of the owner to the rehabilitation program provide necessary information to develop the proper program for each cat. Expectations will vary greatly. Owners should be given the information and time to determine their personal rehabilitation goals for their cat.

Goals can be set for each phase of the rehabilitation. For example, phase I: within 1 week, strengthen pelvic limbs so that the cat is able to bear weight for a minimum of 20 seconds without outside support. Phase II: strengthen pelvic limb so the cat is able to walk normally. Examples of rehabilitation programs are listed at the end of this chapter.

21.5 How do you know you have reached a goal?

Outcome measurements ensure that rehabilitation goals are being met. They are vital to providing the information needed to improve or change the rehabilitation protocol to ensure the most benefit for each individual cat. The documentation of the measurements provides progress information to owner, therapist, and veterinarian.

Passive range of motion is measured with a goniometer (Fig. 21-5). A goniometer is a protractor-like instrument with two blades that are attached to a 360° marked hinge that pivots to measure the angle formed by two bones across a joint. The two bones are moved to extreme flexion and extension and a measurement is taken at each extreme. Limited range can be at flexion only, extension only, or both. Range of motion can be limited by pain or a mechanical problem such as contracted muscle. Measurements taken in the conscious cat can indicate pain-free range of motion. Measurements made in the sedated cat can indicate the maximal range of motion, because the cat cannot respond to pain in joint manipulation when sedated. Affected and non-affected joints are measured.

Active range of motion is evaluated by encouraging or allowing the cat to sit, rise, and lie down. The cat can be

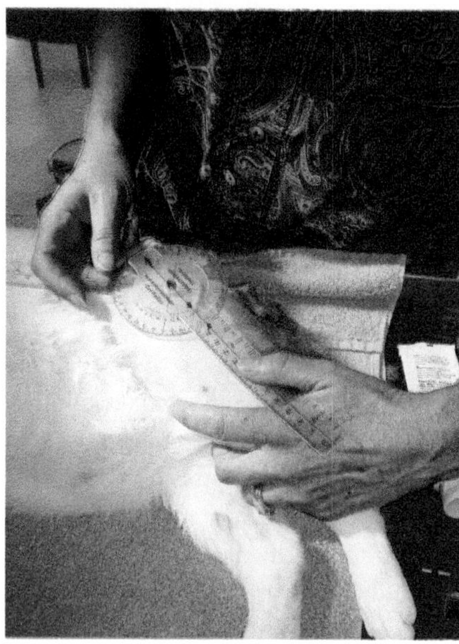

Figure 21-5 Initial goniometry measurements can provide information for planning rehabilitation exercises, and to measure the effectiveness of the interventions.

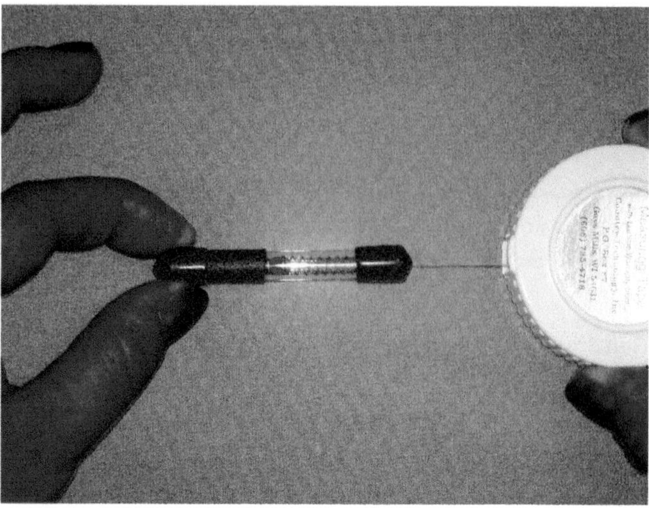

Figure 21-6 The ooliometer has a special gauge at the end of the tape to verify that the same amount of stress is placed on the tape to ensure repeatability of measurement and help give accurate results.

asked to climb stairs or walk over poles for additional data.

Muscle mass. The size of a muscle correlates with the strength of the muscle. Therefore, the circumference of a front or rear leg muscle provides information about how much strength a cat has in one leg compared to the other. Measurement of thigh or arm circumference helps assess changes in muscle mass throughout the rehabilitation program. Sometimes the loss of muscle in a limb can be felt or even seen. The measurement of the circumference is taken with a special measuring tape called an ooliometer (Fig. 21-6). Without this objective tool, expectations can prejudice and alter results (11).

Body composition. Body composition is a term used to describe the percentage ratio of body fat to lean muscle. Measurements can be taken of the circumference of the waist and chest to give objective data of the degree of obesity. Actual weight should also be taken.

Visual analog scale. The visual analog scale (VAS) is a commonly accepted technique for measuring gait, functionality, pain, and performance. For example, in measuring gait, the VAS uses a continuum ranging from walking normally to continuous non-weight-bearing lameness. The evaluator places a mark along a line of a specified length to indicate the cat's performance at a particular gait. Each evaluator must be aware of the criteria used to identify the low and high end of the scale. For example, the definitions shown in Figure 21-7 could be used for this scale. Scores are deter-

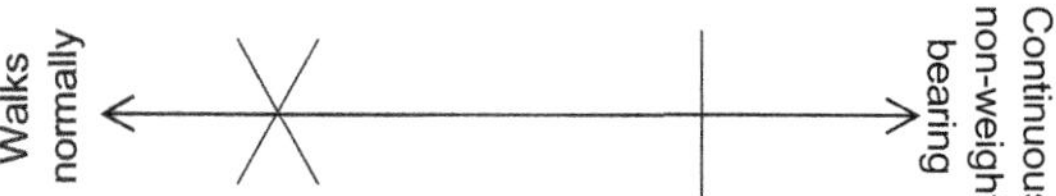

Figure 21-7 Example of visual analog scale. Walks normally: the cat has no lameness; range of motion, swing phase, and stance phase of all four legs are normal. Continuous non-weight-bearing lameness: the cat never places one of the legs down during all phases of movement. Each evaluation on the same gait is performed on the same scale, using a different mark each time.

mined by marking the distance from the left-hand side of the line to the point on the line where the mark is made. The example above uses a 10-cm line to separate the two ends of the continuum. Based on this, the cat would receive a grade of 5 (5 cm distance), indicating that it has a severe weight-bearing lameness. The VAS system is only valid and reliable when the same individual performs the initial and re-evaluations under similar conditions. This is very difficult to perform in a clinical situation with the cat. It may be necessary for the cat to be filmed in its home environment for a more reliable evaluation.

Gait analysis

Motion is a result of a combination of nerves stimulating muscle to move bone. Abnormal motion occurs when this chain of events is disrupted. Gait analysis is performed by most of us on a daily basis. We can recognize if a person walking toward us is graceful or clumsy or if a person running is balanced and fluid or stiff. The same observations are applied to the cat.

Lameness is defined as a difference from normal gait. The walk and trot are the easiest gaits to evaluate for lameness because of the symmetrical movement of the trot and walk. Subjective gait analysis is the most common diagnostic tool to assess lameness in cats. It is best done before touching the cat. It starts by observing the animal while it is still. The analyst looks for conformational abnormalities, such as turned-out toes, or abnormalities in stance, such as the cat holding one leg up or putting most of its body weight on a particular leg. After these observations are noted the animal is analyzed while moving. Gait analysis of the cat should be done in a closed room.

Visual gait analysis is a very difficult outcome measurement to make in a clinic situation. If possible, a videotape of the cat in its home environment will provide a more accurate evaluation of the gait of the cat.

21.6 Examples of exercises

21.6.1 Passive range of motion

General instruction

Lay the cat on its side on a comfortable surface and allow or help the cat to relax. Isolate the affected joint as much as possible so that pain or stiffness elsewhere in the limb does not influence the range of the focus joint.

Carpus

Support the leg with one hand. With the leg in a neutral position begin extension. Continue to extend the carpus to the end feel. Then, to get maximum extension, extend the digits to end feel. Press on the pads of the foot. This will simulate the normal position of the leg during the stance phase of movement, giving the cat proprioception feedback and making it more aware of the leg. Hold for 10 seconds, then release and begin flexion of the carpal joint. Continue flexing the joint until the end feel, then for maximum flexion, flex or fold the digits to the back of the leg. Hold for 10 seconds. Repeat 5–10 times.

Elbow

The carpal joint must be flexed and extended, respectively, to flex and extend the elbow. Begin with the carpal joint supported by one hand and the other behind the elbow. Gently push the elbow into extension end feel. The carpal joint will extend at the same time. Push gently on the carpal joint to get maximum extension of both the carpal joint and elbow. Hold for 10 seconds. Begin the flexion by flexing the carpal joint and then supporting the elbow joint to keep in same location; flex to end feel. Hold for 10 seconds. Repeat 5–10 times.

Shoulder

Begin with one hand supporting the leg in a neutral position. Hold one hand on the top of the shoulder. Begin extending the elbow, which will also extend the carpus (Fig. 21-8). Bring the elbow to end range and continue to push on the elbow gently until the end feel of shoulder is reached. Usually the leg will reach just above the eye if the head is in normal position. Hold for 10 seconds. Begin the flexion. Fold the elbow and gently push up against the supporting hand to end feel. Hold for 10 seconds. Repeat 5–10 times.

Stifle and hock

Combine passive range of motion for these two joints to get maximum extension and flexion. Supporting the tarsus in a neutral position, begin to push the stifle gently into extension until end feel is reached. Gently push on the tarsus to reach maximum extension. Digits can be extended and the pads of the foot pressed as if the cat was standing. Hold for 10 seconds; begin flexion by folding the tarsus to maximum flexion and then folding the knee to maximum flexion. Hold for 10 seconds, and repeat 5–10 times.

Hip

Support the limb and begin to push the stifle gently into extension. Keeping the knee in extension, and one hand on the ischial tuberosity preventing movement, gently bring the leg back until end feel of the hip is reached. Hold for 10 seconds. Begin flexion by folding the stifle and tarsus and bringing the knee up to hip joint end feel. Hold for 10 seconds. Repeat 5–10 times.

21.6.2 Early proprioception exercises

Physioroll

Choose the appropriate-size ball for the cat, and for the type of exercise. The ball should be at the shoulder height of the cat when it is standing. Air can be added or removed to help make the ball the right size. Although many cats may resist being placed on the ball initially, most cats relax after rhythmic movement or bouncing begins (Fig. 21-9).

Standing resistance

Once the cat can stand, gently press on the shoulder, slowly increasing pressure. The cat will push back to remain

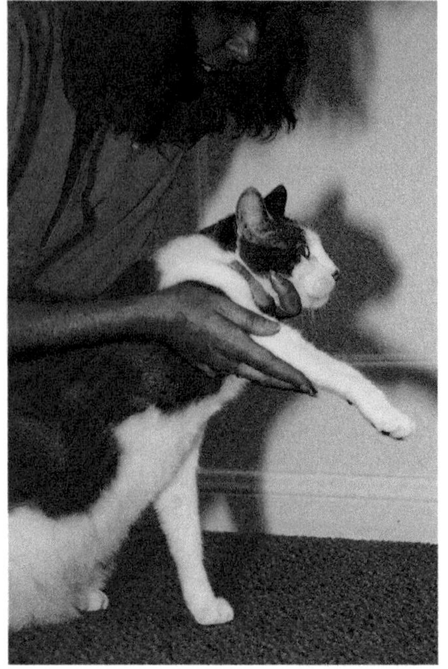

A

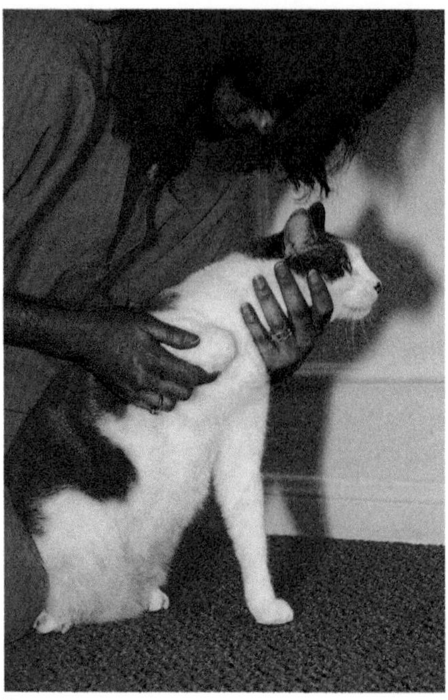

B

Figure 21-8 Cat during passive range of motion exercise. (**A**) Extension and (**B**) flexion of the elbow and shoulder joint.

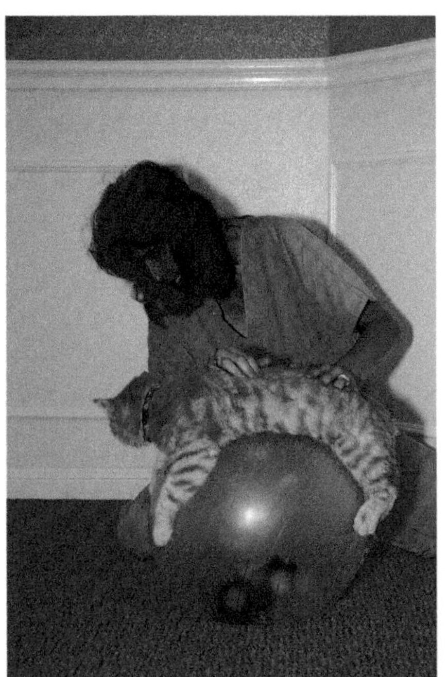

A

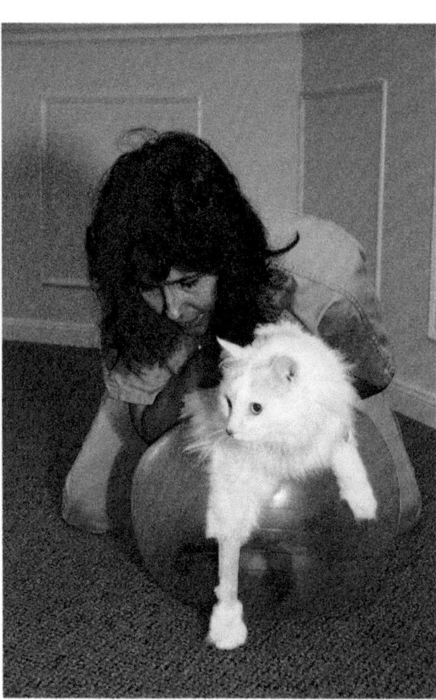

B

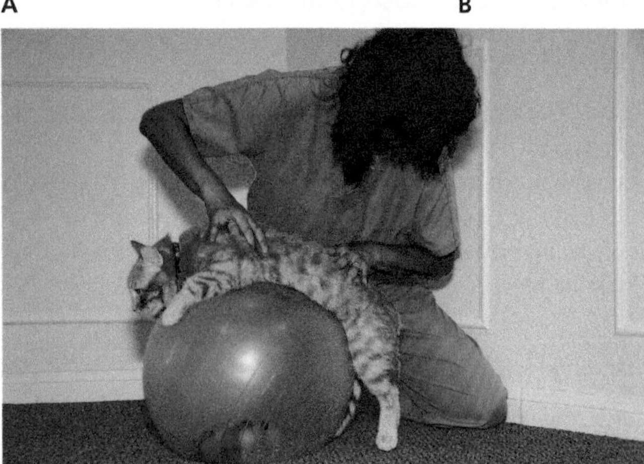

C

Figure 21-9 (**A**) Place the cat on the ball so that the trunk is supported. (**B**) Gently roll the ball until the front legs come in contact with the ground. Hold and bounce gently for 10–20 seconds. (**C**) Then gently roll the ball so the front feet come off the ground and the back feet touch the ground. Gently bounce for 10–20 seconds. The amount of weight can be increased or decreased depending on the amount of roll and pressure on the ball. The cat will use its trunk muscles to stabilize itself.

standing. If the push is too hard, the cat will be knocked off balance. Release the pressure slowly or the cat may fall. Try to keep the cat in the same spot. Shoulder, hip, and trunk on both sides of the cat are good locations for resistance exercises.

Balance board

The balance board is usually 20 inches (approx. 50 cm) with a 14° angle. Homemade versions may vary from these specifications and are still very suitable.

Balance board exercise can assist in the restoration of stability and proprioception of cats following back, rear-limb, or front-limb surgery (Fig. 21-10). It can also be used as an early weight-bearing exercise following knee or hip surgery, elbow or shoulder surgery, or fracture repair. Benefits include improved balance and coordination, better proprioceptive awareness for injury prevention, greater trunk and pelvic girdle stability, and increased leg and ankle range of motion.

21.6.3 Early weight-bearing exercises

One-leg standing

Lift the contralateral leg. Hold for 10–15 seconds. Repeat 2–3 times. Increase time and repetitions as cat's strength is increased.

Cross-leg standing

Lift the contralateral leg. Once the cat is balanced, lift the diagonal rear leg (Fig. 21-11). Hold for 10–15 seconds. Repeat 2–3 times. Increase time and repetitions as cat's strength is increased.

Carts

Carts and slings can be used to support the animal during the early stages of recovery of most neurological conditions. They provide the necessary support for the cat to assist the therapist during range of motion and floor exercises.

21.6.4 Examples of front-limb exercises

Wheelbarrow

Lift both rear legs (Fig. 21-12). Hold for 10–15 seconds. Repeat 2–3 times. Increase time and repetitions as cat's strength is increased.

Down to sit

Start with the cat in the down position. Lure the cat to the sitting position by raising your hand above its head with food in your hand.

Physioroll or physioball

Fold and hold the contralateral limb to the injured limb and roll the cat forward as shown in Figure 12-9. The cat will reach for the ground with the injured limb. Gently bounce with limb on ground.

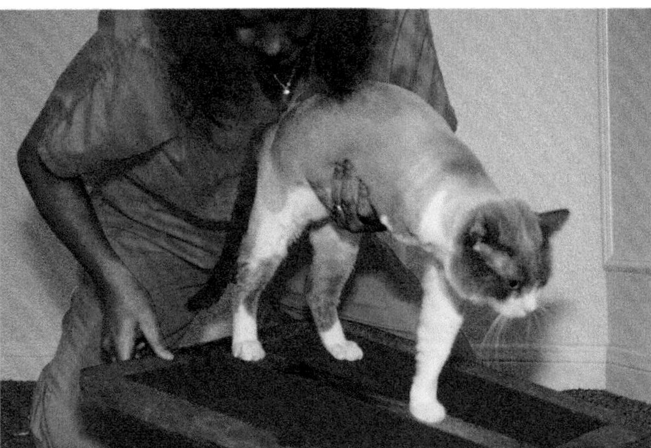

Figure 21-10 Position the cat centrally over the board with feet shoulder-width apart. Begin by slowly moving the board front to back for 20 repetitions. Support the cat as needed. Be sure to keep the rocking motion under control. Then rock from side to side for 20 repetitions. The cat will contract its muscles and shift its weight to stay on the balance board.

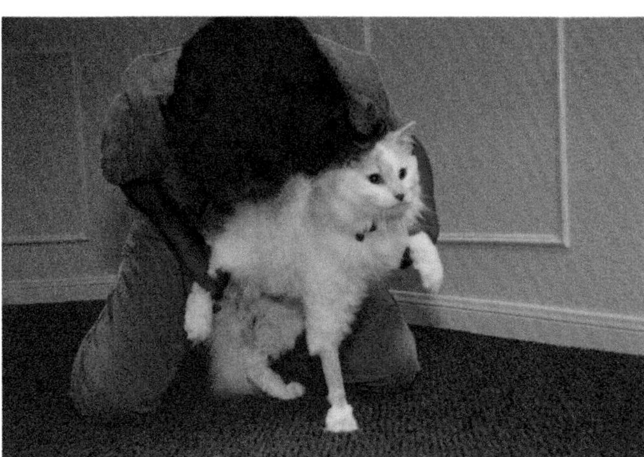

Figure 21-11 Cross-leg standing. The right front limb and the left hindlimb are lifted up.

Trail of treats

Place treats on the floor about 1 foot (30 cm) apart. Allow the cat to walk slowly, sniffing the ground (Fig. 21-13).

Decline and tunnel

Walk the cat down hills or a ramp to encourage front-limb weight-bearing. Similarly, walking through a tunnel will cause the cat to crouch and increase weight-bearing on its front limbs (Fig. 21-14).

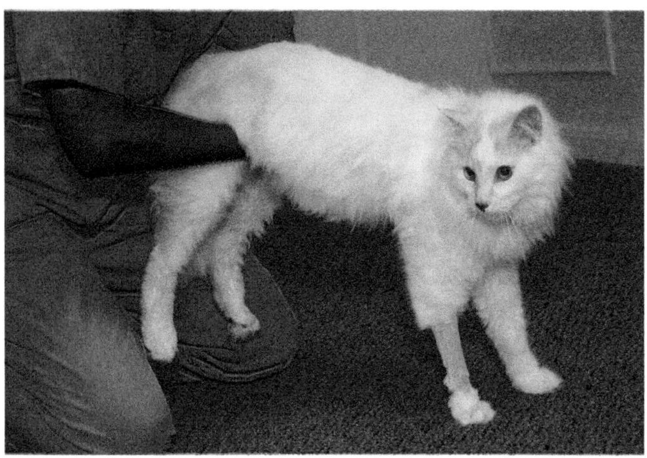

Figure 21-12 Wheelbarrow. When the cat's strength is increased to the point that it is no longer difficult to support its weight in the stationary position, begin to walk slowly forward while holding both rear legs. Begin with 2–3 steps and increase until the cat is able to move forward 10 steps.

21.6.5 Examples of hindlimb exercises

Dancing

Support the cat under its front legs and lift to encourage increased weight-bearing on rear legs (Fig. 21-15). Hold for 10–15 seconds. Repeat 2–3 times. Increase time and repetitions as cat's strength is increased.

Sit to stand

Place the cat in a sit position. Allow or encourage the cat to stand. Repeat several times (Fig. 21-16).

Incline

Inclining improves the strength of the hindlimbs. The cat is led up a ramp or a hill. Gradually increase the inclination grade.

21.6.6 Gait-training exercises

Cavaletti poles can be used to increase range of motion and stride length (Fig. 21-17). Start with poles approximately the same distance apart as the height of the cat's elbow. Encourage the cat to go over the poles. This can be done by luring with food, calling, or allowing the cat to go over the poles into a closet or carrier. Raise, lower, or spread apart the poles to reach desired gait.

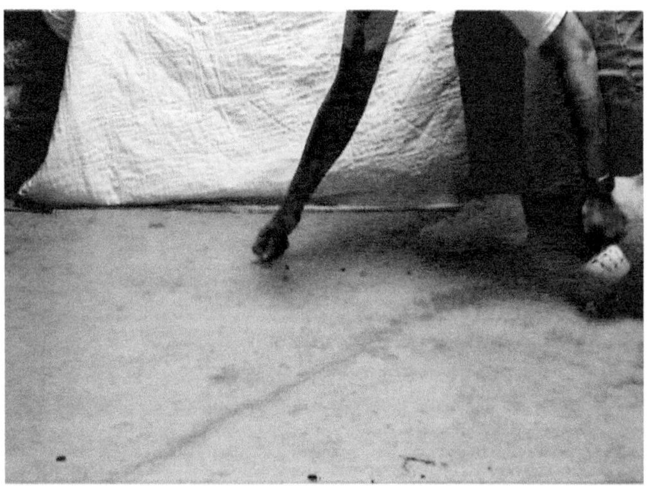

A

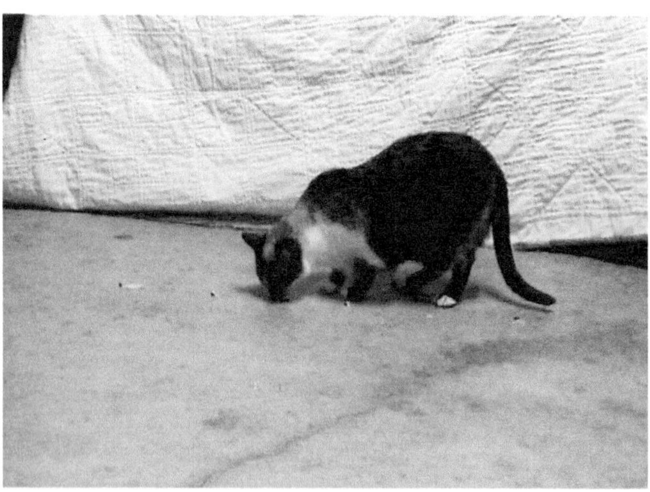

B

Figure 21-13 (**A, B**) Trail of treats. Sniffing or eating from the floor shifts body weight cranially and encourages weight-bearing on both front feet.

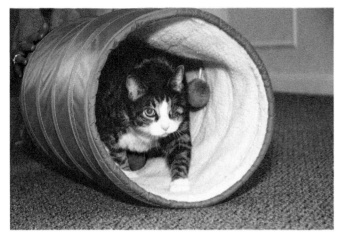

Figure 21-14 Example of walking a cat through a tunnel.

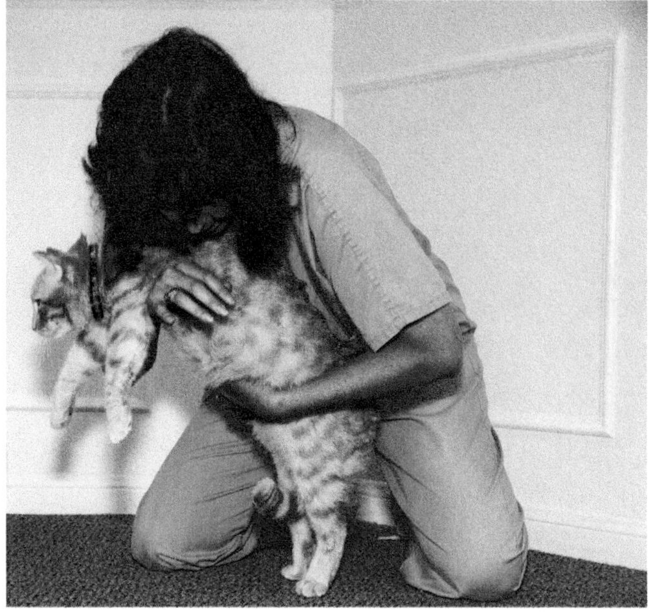

Figure 21-15 Dancing. When the cat's strength is increased to the point that it is no longer difficult to support its weight in the stationary position, begin with 2–3 steps and increase until the cat is able to move forward 10 steps.

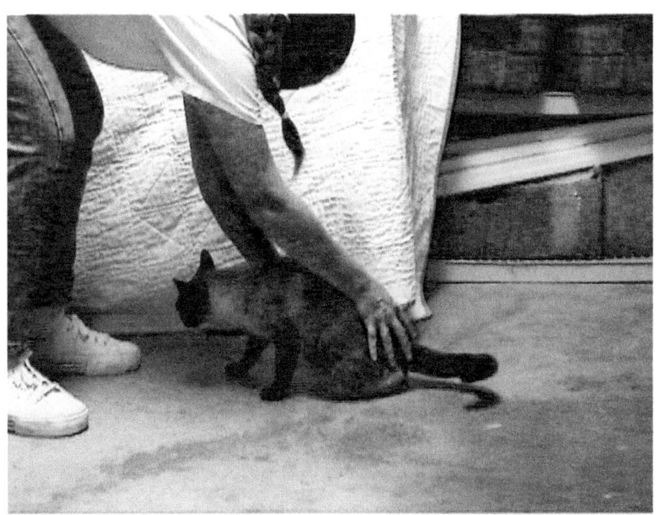

A

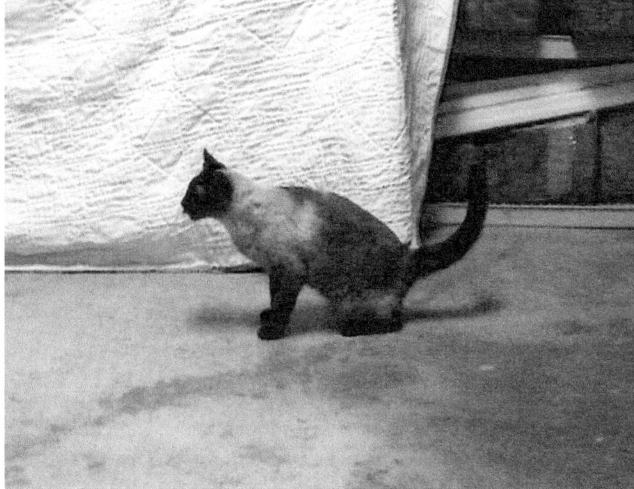

B

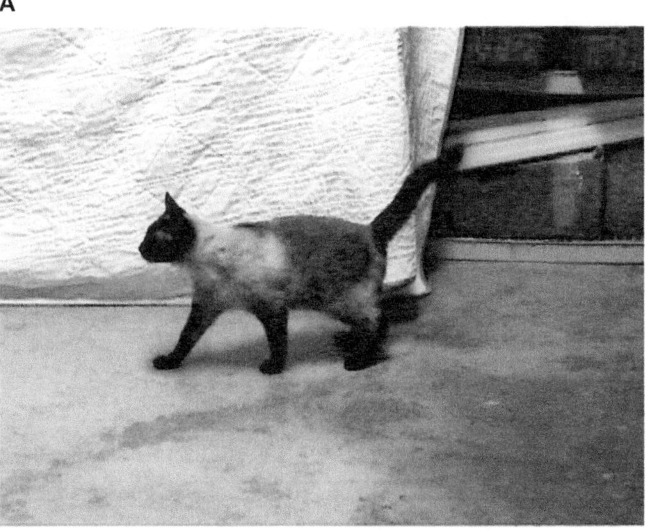

C

Figure 21-16 (**A–C**) Sit-to-stand exercise.

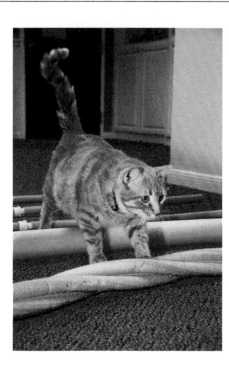

Figure 21-17 Cat walking over Cavaletti pole.

Limb rehabilitation program (Table 21-2)

Back rehabilitation program (Table 21-3)

Obesity program (Table 21-4)

Problem	Exercises	Specific exercises and treatments	Modalities
Loss of range of motion	Passive range of motion		
	Active range of motion	Cavaletti Walking in 6 inches (15 cm) of high grass Walking in 6 inches (15 cm) of water Exercise in underwater treadmill (tarsus)	
Loss of muscle mass	Stationary weight-bearing exercises	One-leg standing Cross-leg standing Sit to stand Down to stand	
	Moving weight-bearing exercises	Slow walking Incline Underwater treadmill Serpentine walking	
Muscle guarding	Physioball	Active stretching Balance board	Massage therapy Therapeutic ultrasound Electrical stimulation for pain control

Table 21-2. Limb rehabilitation program

Table 21-3. Back rehabilitation program

Problem	Specific exercises	Modalities
Rear-limb atrophy	Underwater treadmill Serpentine walking	Massage therapy Electrical stimulation for pain control
Muscle spasm	Physioball Active stretching Balance board	

Table 21-4. Obesity program

Problem	Specific exercises	Modalities
Exercise-intolerant	Underwater treadmill Slow walking	Massage therapy Electrical stimulation for pain control
Joint pain	Physioball Active stretching Balance board Underwater treadmill	Therapeutic ultrasound

References and further reading

1. Overall KL. Clinical behavioral medicine for small animals. St. Louis: Mosby; 1997.
2. Marsolais GS, et al. Effects of postoperative rehabilitation on limb function after cranial cruciate ligament repair in dogs. J Am Vet Med Assoc 2002;220:1325–1330.
3. Millis DL, Levine D. The role of exercise and physical therapy modalities in the treatment of osteoarthritis. Vet Clin North Am Small Anim Pract 1997;27:913–930.
4. Johnson JM, et al. Rehabilitation of dogs with surgically treated cranial cruciate ligament-deficient stifles by use of electrical stimulation of muscles. Am J Vet Res 1997;58:1473–1478.
5. Steiss JE, Adams CC. Rate of temperature increase in canine muscle during 1 MHz ultrasound therapy: deleterious effect of hair coat. Am J Vet Res 1999;60:76–80.
6. Levine D, et al. Effects of 3.3 MHz ultrasound on caudal thigh muscle temperature in dogs. Vet Surg 2001;30:170–174.
7. Draper DO, et al. Immediate and residual changes in dorsiflexion range of motion using an ultrasound heat and stretch routine. J Athletic Train 1998;33:141–144.
8. Rumph PF, et al. Redistribution of vertical ground reaction forces in dogs with experimentally induced chronic hindlimb lameness. Vet Surg 1995;24:384–389.
9. Millis DL, et al. Canine rehabilitation and physical therapy. St. Louis: Saunders; 2004: pp. 416–418.
10. Burkhoder WJ. Precision and practicality of methods assessing body composition of dogs and cats. Compend Continuing Educ Pract Vet 2001;23:1–10.
11. Maylia E, et al. Can thigh girth be measured accurately: a preliminary investigation, J Sport Rehab 1995;8:43–49.

Part 6

Orthopedic materials, instruments, implants, and techniques

Use of the right instruments and implants is critical for success in orthopedic surgery. Although in general the same instruments and implants are used in cats as in dogs, they need to be adapted to the smaller size of the patients. Using instruments or implants that are too large will complicate and lengthen surgery, and cause iatrogenic damage to soft tissues and bone. A large variety of instruments and implants are available on the market, and the information provided in Chapters 23 and 24 is aimed to help in deciding which instruments and implants to use for the treatment of the feline orthopedic patient. Technical guidelines for the correct use of these instruments and implants are also provided.

External coaptation and arthroscopy are techniques of great value in orthopedics if selected for the right indications and performed correctly. External coaptation is often more difficult to apply and maintain in the feline patient, and not all bandaging techniques described for dogs are suitable for cats. Tips for bandages, casts, and slings are described in Chapter 22 and should help the orthopedic surgeon to apply these techniques safely in cats. Arthroscopy is not yet widely used in cats, mainly due to the small size of joints. But, although in its infancy, the use of arthroscopy is already revealing additional information on joint pathology in the feline, as described in Chapter 25.

22 External coaptation

S.J. Langley-Hobbs, M. Keller, K. Voss

External coaptation is an important and versatile therapeutic method for the management of orthopedic cases, but treatment with external coaptation must follow strict indications, and should not be regarded as a cheap substitute for surgical stabilization. External coaptation includes bandages, splints, casts, and slings. Bandages are usually used to protect postoperative wounds, to treat open wounds, and to prevent limb swelling and edema. Incorporation of a splint into the bandage provides additional stability and is often used for temporary immobilization of joint injuries or fractures. Casts are used for the treatment of selected fractures. The main indication for slings is immobilization of joints after closed or open reduction of luxations and to prevent weight-bearing.

Application of bandages, splints, casts, and slings is not without risk. Circulatory stasis and limb swelling, and avascular or pressure necrosis of skin and deeper tissue, may result from improper application or insufficient patient care. Cats may not cope or tolerate the external coaptation. Some cats will refuse to move after immobilization of their leg, whilst others will make determined and sustained efforts to get rid of the external coaptation, sometimes successfully. In most cases, the patients will eventually accept the external coaptation after minutes or hours and adapt to the situation, but in rare cases it may be necessary and safer to sedate the cat or remove the external coaptation to prevent self-trauma. The benefit of the bandage, particularly complex ones such as slings and spica splints, must be weighed against potential problems. There are a number of situations, particularly in emergency situations, where it may be better not to apply an extensive bandage and perhaps cause additional stress to the cat, but to use cage rest, analgesia, and sedation to restrict further damage at the fracture site.

External coaptation is described in several review articles and book chapters (1–5), but the emphasis is on dogs (1–4) rather than cats (5). In the following section, indications, application techniques, and possible complications of external coaptation in the feline patient are described.

22.1 Bandages

The basic functions of a bandage are wound protection, absorption of wound secretions, an aid to hemostasis, compression of soft tissues, stabilization, and to increase patient comfort. True pressure bandages are not necessary and are even dangerous in the cat. A modified Robert Jones bandage or soft padded bandage is usually sufficient; used in the immediate postoperative period they prevent limb swelling and seroma formation, and they are an important part of open-wound treatment. Indications for bandages are summarized in Box 22-1.

A bandage consists of three main layers: the contact layer, the padding layer, and the external layer(s). The technique of application of a soft padded or modified Robert Jones bandage is described in Figure 22-1.

22.1.1 Contact layer

The contact layer protects the wound. Depending on the type of wound treated and the phase of wound healing, either a non-adherent or adherent contact layer is chosen. Non-adherent contact layers are used to protect clean postoperative wounds or healthy granulating and epithelializing traumatic wounds.

In contaminated and dirty wounds, which are left open for secondary wound healing, the contact layer is adapted to the phase of wound healing. Adherent and absorptive contact layers are used in the early inflammatory and exudatory phase of wound healing: dry-to-dry or wet-to-dry bandages are often ideal in this situation (see Chapter 16 on degloving injuries). Non-adherent contact layers are used once the granulation bed has been formed. They will allow wound contraction and epithelialization without damaging the new tissue or healing processes. It is also still possible to alternate the type of contact layer used depending on the appearance of the wound, changing back to an adherent layer if the wound needs further superficial debridement. A variety of non-adher-

Box 22-1 Indications for bandages

- Postoperative bandage after orthopedic procedures on the elbow or stifle joint or distal to them
- Protection of clean and clean-contaminated wounds (dry bandage)
- Treatment of contaminated and dirty wounds (wet-to-dry bandage)
- Minor joint instability

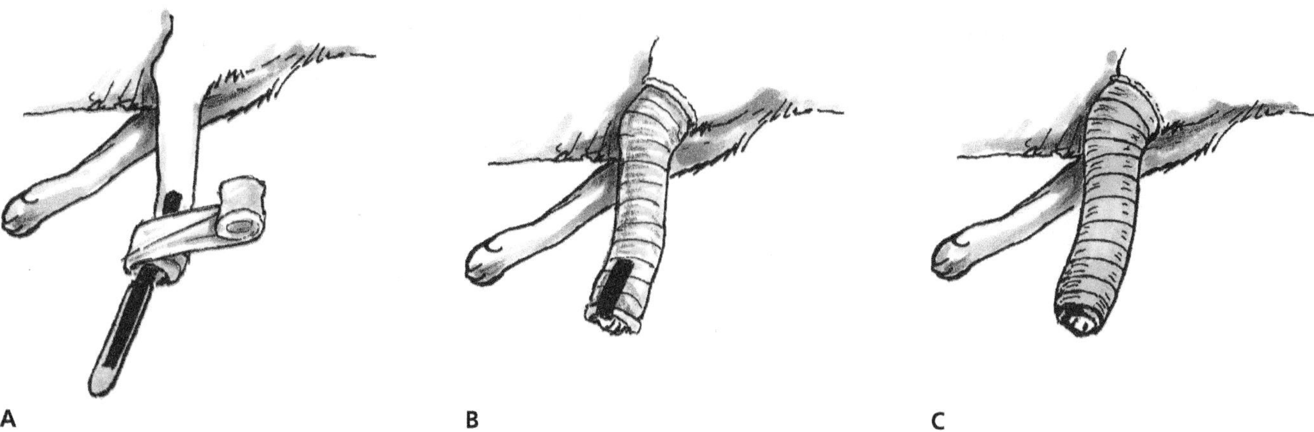

Figure 22-1 Application of a modified Robert Jones bandage (soft padded bandage).
(**A**) One or two strips of adhesive tape (stirrups) with a wooden tongue depressor or spoon adhered to the tape, is/are applied on to the dorsal, medial, or lateral aspect of the metacarpus or metatarsus. Padding is applied from distally to proximally (usually in inward rotation) with about 50% overlap. The bandage is unwound two to three times up and down the limb, giving a total thickness with the 50% overlap of four to six layers.
(**B**) Two or three layers of conforming or elastic gauze are then applied on top of the padding, extending from the distal limb to 1 cm below the proximal edge of the padding. The adhesive tape (stirrup) is reflected up and over the gauze. Moderate tension can help prevent bandage slippage.
(**C**) The outer protective layer is finally applied, extending no further proximally than the conforming gauze.

ent contact layers are available and their properties and uses are summarized in Table 22-1 and examples of the different manufacturers' products are given.

22.1.2 Padding layer

The padding layer creates even compression of soft tissues and protects bony prominences from pressure sores. Non-absorptive padding materials, such as cast padding, are used for soft padded bandages, with or without a splint. Because they do not absorb fluid, they prevent soiling of the bandage from water, urine, or feces. Absorptive cotton padding is used for a modified Robert Jones bandage. The soft cotton allows mild compression of soft tissues without causing vascular compromise. Cotton is also used for wet-to-dry bandages, because it is able to absorb excess fluid (see Chapter 16 on degloving injuries).

22.1.3 External layers

There are often two external layers: an inner layer using some stretchy bandage material (conforming gauze) is used to create compression of the padding layer, and an outer protective layer uses Elastoplast or cohesive bandage (e.g., Vetrap). Care has to be taken not to apply these layers too tightly, as pressure necrosis of the skin occurs easily in cats. Special care must be taken over bony prominences and over implants with minimal soft-tissue covering. Conversely, the bandage must also be tight enough to prevent slippage. Slipping is usually less of a problem in the hindlimbs due to the angulation of the hock joint.

22.2 Splints and casts

Proper immobilization is best achieved with a cast. Splints and bandages (Robert Jones) are best used for temporary immobilization prior to definitive repair. The clinician must be aware of the disadvantages and limitations of casts and splints. Their use is limited to conditions affecting the lower limbs (below the elbow and stifle). To function properly, the joints above and below the affected bone must be immobilized, thus increasing the likelihood of fracture disease. The cast or splint may be bulky and uncomfortable and become self-traumatized, leading to a necessity for replacement. Sores can develop under the cast and some fracture types are poorly immobilized with external coaptation. Despite the disadvantages, external coaptation can be an excellent method of producing rapid uncomplicated fracture healing when used in the correct situations (Fig. 22-2).

Splinted bandages are easier to apply, easier to change, and bear less risk for complications than cylinder casts. They are most often used for temporary immobilization of joints and for the treatment of metacarpal and metatarsal fractures. Casts provide more stability and are mainly used for conservative fracture treatment. They are more difficult to apply and change, and may be more of a risk in terms of vascular compromise of the leg. Indications for splints or casts are listed in Table 22-2.

22.2.1 Splints

For application of a splinted bandage, a soft padded bandage is first used, as described in Figure 22-1. The splint is then

Type of contact layer	Description	Indication	Function	Contraindications, complications, and disadvantages	Advantages
Adherent					
Wet-to-dry	Saline-soaked sterile gauze swabs	Mildly exudative wounds	Superficial debridement	Granulating or epithelializing wounds. Can be painful to remove	Readily available and economic
Dry-to-dry	Dry gauze swabs	Very exudative wounds	Superficial debridement	Granulating or epithelializing wounds. Can be painful to remove	Readily available and economic
Non-adherent					
Film dressings	Absorbent layer between two thin layers of porous film	Post surgical incisions. Granulating epithelializing wound	Pores in film for absorbtion of wound fluid and exchange of gases	Wound can adhere to absorbent layer at pores – causing trauma at removal	Reasonably priced
Film dressings	Single layer of adhesive polyethylene film	Post surgical incision Granulating epithelializing wound	Film allows gas exchange but limits escape of fluid – maintains moist environment	To function properly dressing needs to adhere to skin surrounding wound – do not readily stick to hair	Reasonably priced
Foam dressings	Polyurethane or Silastic foam	Serous exudative wounds	Absorb large amounts of fluid	Moderate in price	Comfortable
Hydroactive	Insoluble polymers or gels	Exudative or granulating and epithelializing wounds	Absorb and retain moisture – moist enviroment promotes autolytic debridement in early stages and fibroplasia and epithelialization in later stages	Expensive	Need less frequent changing than traditional gauze dressings
Hydrocolloid	Layer of carboxmethylated cellulose and gelatin attached to a polyurethane or foam backing	Exudative or granulating and epithelializing wounds	Contact layer adheres to the skin but not to wound – promotes autolytic debridement in early stages and fibroplasia and epithelialization in later stages	Adherence to skin surrounding wound may delay wound contraction. Expensive	Maintains a moist environment at the wound
Alginate	Woven or non-woven pads derived from brown seaweed. Composed of combinations of calcium alginate and sodium alginate	Highly exudative wounds	Gel formed from fibers when calcium exchanged for sodium ions from wound fluid	Expensive	Very hydrophilic. Entraps bacteria as gel removed and antibiotics can be incorporated into dressings
Hydrogel	Insoluble hydrophilic polymers of polyethylene oxide bound to a synthetic sheet or applied as a gel	Gel – irregular wounds. Acute or healing wounds	Absorb large amounts of wound fluid and maintain a moist environment	Needs an overlying layer such as a perforated film or foam dressing to keep gel in apposition with wound. Predispose to excessive granulation tissue	Can be used to deliver antimicrobials

Table 22-1 Different types of contact layers that are available for use under bandages

applied on the outer surface of the conforming gauze (the first external layer), and is secured with an outer external layer of elastic tape or cohesive bandage. Commercially available off-the-shelf splints or spoon splints are particularly useful for temporary and emergency use. Custom-made splints made of cast material can usually be adapted better to the conformation of the leg and are therefore preferable for long-term use. Theoretically, the splint can be applied on any side of the bandage. Placing the splint on the medial or lateral surface of the bandage may help prevent pressure sores at the level of the accessory carpal bone and tuber calcanei. The tarsus should be immobilized in a slightly flexed position to prevent contracture and atrophy of the gastrocnemius muscles. Additionally, some angulation at the hock gives the cat a more normal conformation for weight-bearing, and helps prevent bandage slippage.

Most splints extend to just distal or proximal to the elbow or stifle joint, depending on the indication they are applied for. Only the spica splint extends more proximally, incorporating the affected leg and the torso (Fig. 22-3). It is used to immobilize the elbow joint in extension, for example after closed reduction of elbow luxation.

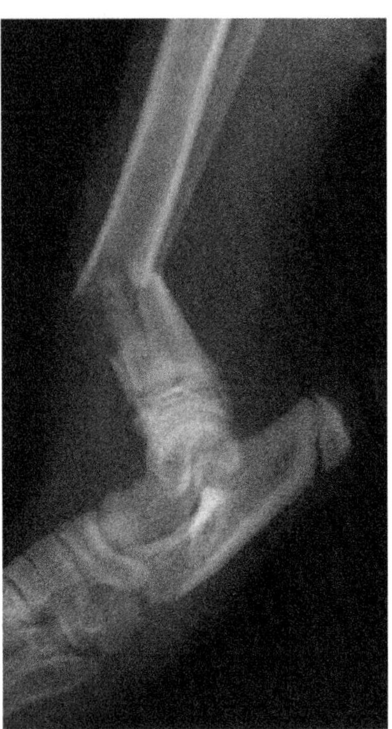
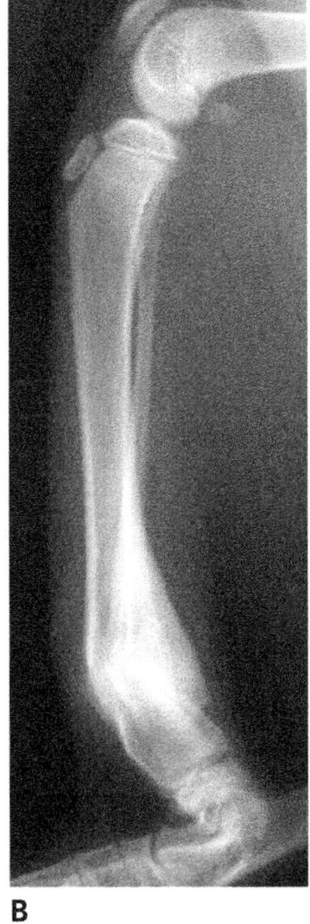

A B

Figure 22-2 Example of a suitable fracture for stabilization with external coaptation.
(**A**) A tibial fracture in a 10-week-old kitten. The fracture was not suitable for internal fixation due to the distal and fissured nature of the fracture and its closeness to the physis.
(**B**) The fracture was stabilized with a cast, and was healed at 6 weeks. There was some craniocaudal angulation, which is remodeling. Note that the growth plate of the distal tibia is still open.

22.2.2 Casts

Cylinder casts encircle the limb to stabilize a fracture temporarily or as definitive fracture treatment. Only non-articular

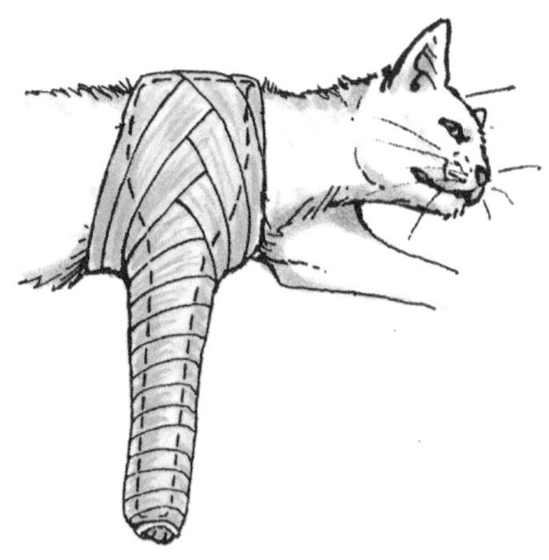

Figure 22-3 Spica splint on the forelimb of the cat. These splints are useful for protection of injuries or surgical repairs of the shoulder or elbow. A bandage is wrapped around the extended leg, and around the thorax, caudal to the opposite leg. The splint is applied along the lateral surface of the limb, extending from the toes to over the dorsal midline.

	Splinted bandage	Cylinder cast
Indications	Immobilization of joints (especially carpus, tarsus, toes; elbow with spica splint) Metacarpal, metatarsal, and phalangeal fractures Protection of tendon sutures (e.g., digital tendon or Achilles tendon) Neurological deficits (e.g., peroneal nerve deficit) Protection of suboptimal surgical fracture repair (radius/ulna, tibia/fibula) Greenstick fractures in very young cats	Fractures of the lower limb: closed, simple, reducible, transverse/interdigitating radius/ulna or tibia/fibula fracture in immature animals At least 50% of the fracture ends should be in contact on orthogonal radiographs Fractures of the radius when the ulna is intact Fracture of the tibia when the fibula is intact

Table 22-2 Indications for splints and casts

fractures distal to the elbow and stifle joint without concurrent soft-tissue injuries are amenable for cast immobilization. Ideal fractures for external coaptation are greenstick or simple transverse fractures in young cats, which can be reduced in a closed manner, and fractures where one bone of a pair (radius and ulna or tibia and fibula) is intact. Following reduction, there should be at least 50% overlap between fracture ends on orthogonal radiographs.

Casts have to be applied with the cat under general anesthesia. Newer synthetic cast materials have largely superseded plaster of Paris. They are less messy to apply, set more quickly, are lighter than plaster of Paris, and they are water-resistant. However, they are not as comformable as plaster of Paris and are more expensive. The synthetic materials include fiberglass impregnated with polyurethane resin, polypropylene with polyurethane resin, and thermoplastics (6). The 5-cm (2-inch) size is appropriate for the cat. The synthetic casting tapes are activated by immersion in water prior to application. To slow down setting of the cast and allow more time to mold it perfectly to the leg of the cat, it can be applied in a dry state (7) or be immersed in cold rather than hot water. This also ensures better lamination of the tapes over joints, such as the tarsus, stifle, and elbow. After application of the tapes in a dry state, a non-elastic bandage soaked with water is used to activate the cast.

Adequate conformity can be achieved by exploiting the elastic properties of the tapes. On the distal part of the limb, the tape is unrolled without applying tension to avoid excessive compression of the sparse soft tissues and potential resulting circulatory compromise. On the proximal part of the limb, some compression of the larger muscle masses is desired to ensure a close fit of the cast to the limb and to compensate for ensuing muscle atrophy. Horizontal rotation of the roll in the area of flexed joints, such as the tarsus, stifle, and elbow, facilitates directional changes and minimizes folds. If folds are created, the tape should be cut through the folds and then smoothed over.

The tapes are unwound with 50% overlap, from distal to proximal and back to distal, resulting in four to six layers (Fig. 22-4). Final small corrections of the setting cast can be done at this stage to optimize the form of the cast for fracture healing and joint conformity. The carpus should be placed in mild internal rotation, 10–15° of flexion, and varus posture. The hock joint should be flexed by approximately 5° from its neutral standing position. Additionally, the cast should be bent slightly to overcorrect the initial angulation of the frac-

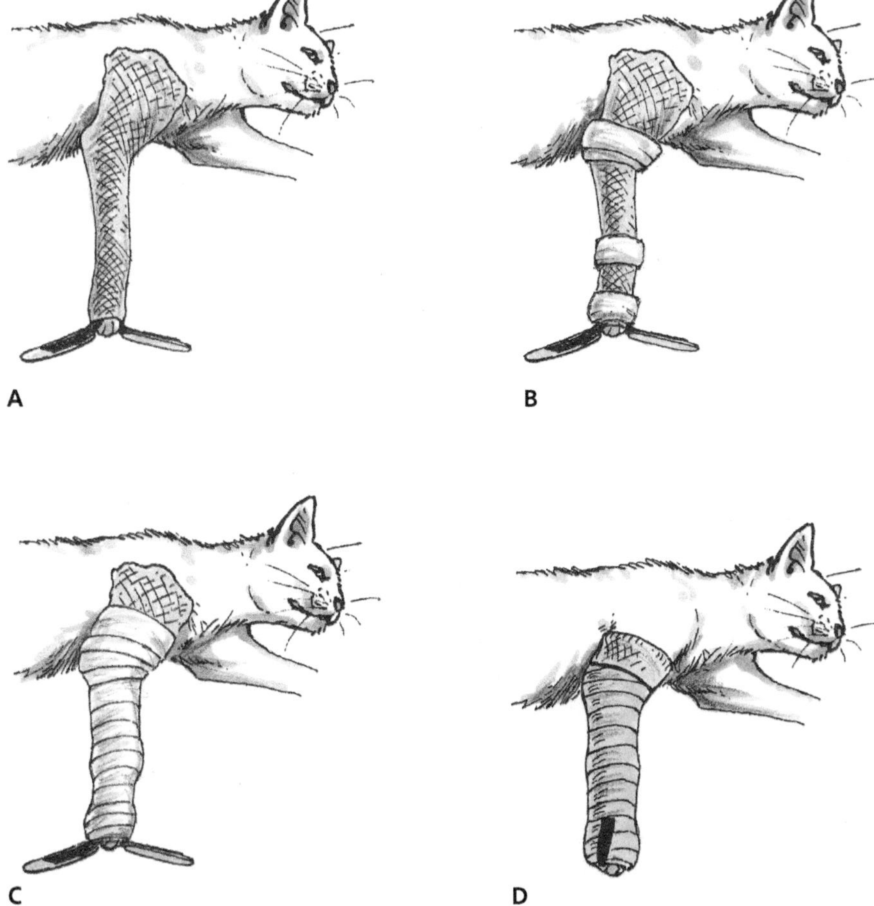

Figure 22-4 Application of a cast.
(**A**) One or two tape stirrups are applied to the distal limb, as described in Figure 22-1. A single layer of thick orthopedic stockinette is applied over the limb.
(**B**) Three or four layers of extra padding are applied over bony prominences at risk for pressure sores (accessory carpal bone and olecranon in the forelimb, tuber calcanei, patella, and the fibular head in the hindlimb). Additionally the distal end of the limb is provided with extra padding.
(**C**) Elasticated gauze or rolled foam underwrap is applied to stabilize and compress the padding.
(**D**) The fracture is reduced, and the cast material applied from distal to proximal and back, in inward rotation. The limb is held with flat hands in slight varus and inward rotation while the casting material hardens. The stockinette and the tape stirrups are reflected back on to the cast.

ture. The stockinette and padding are reflected back using some tension, so that the edges of the cast are bent outward from the limb and fixed with tape (Fig. 22-4). Spending adequate time and care at this stage to ensure the cast fits well, and that the ends are smooth and will not rub or irritate the soft tissue, can be time well spent, as preventing cast-related problems is much easier than trying to deal with cast sores.

The success of fracture reduction is assessed with radiographs. Although perfect anatomic reduction is desirable, satisfactory results can be achieved when at least 50% of the fracture ends are in reduction on both the lateral and craniocaudal view. Slight overcorrection of the initial deformity is optimal.

Hospitalizing the cat for 24 hours is recommended after cast application, so it can be monitored for slippage of the cast or vascular problems of the digits prior to discharge. Written instructions should always be given to owners to help identify potential complications early (Section 22.4).

22.3 Slings, muzzles, and hobbles

Slings are usually applied with the main aim of preventing weight-bearing, although some of the slings have an additional specific function (Table 22-3). Cats may not tolerate slings, and some will attempt amazing contortions in their efforts to remove them. In most cases the patients will eventually accept the sling and adapt to the situation, but in rare cases it may be necessary and safer to sedate the cat or remove the sling to prevent additional injury or damage.

Slings are potentially dangerous if not applied and maintained correctly. To avoid avascular necrosis or venous congestion, the bandage material should never be wrapped circumferentially around a leg. Instead, when bandage material is used in a sling it is folded around the extremity as illustrated in Figure 22-7, below. Adhesive bandage material can be used to reduce slippage of the bandage material on the fur.

22.3.1 Carpal flexion sling or splint

The purpose of a carpal flexion sling or splint is to hold the carpus in sufficient flexion to prevent weight-bearing (Fig. 22-5). The advantage is that the elbow and shoulder are not included, so these joints are able to move freely, which should

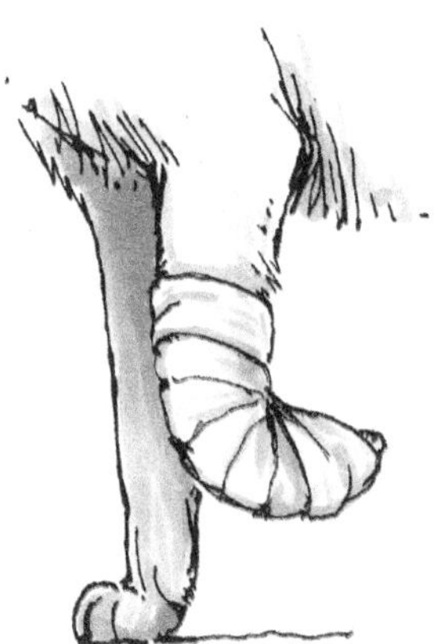

A

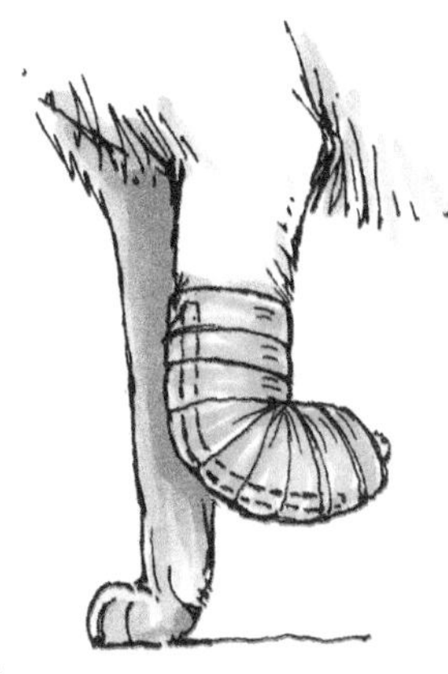

B

Figure 22-5 A carpal flexion splint is designed to prevent weight-bearing while still allowing motion in the elbow and shoulder.
(**A**) The padding layer and gauze are wrapped around the carpal joint in a figure-of-eight pattern. Carpal flexion should not exceed 90°.
(**B**) A splint can additionally be applied on the dorsal aspect of the paw to help maintain carpal flexion.

Sling	Function	Indication	Duration
Tape muzzle	Interarcuate stabilization of mandibular fracture and maxilla	Temporomandibular luxation Selected mandibular fractures	1–2 weeks
Velpeau sling	Flexion of shoulder and elbow joint Prevents weight-bearing	Scapular fractures Scapular dislocation Medial shoulder luxation	7–10 days
Carpal sling	Prevents weight-bearing	Prevention of weight-bearing while maintaining elbow and shoulder mobility	7–10 days
Ehmer sling or Robinson sling	Internal rotation and slight abduction of femur (Ehmer) Prevents weight-bearing	Craniodorsal and caudodorsal hip joint luxations Avoid when possible	7–10 days
Hobble sling	Prevents abduction of hindlimbs	Pelvic floor fractures Ventral hip joint luxation	1–3 weeks

Table 22-3 Function, indication, and suggested duration of application for selected orthopedic slings and miscellaneous bandages

minimize joint stiffness. Its use is indicated after flexor tendon repair, and in some cases after fracture repair of the scapula, humerus, or accessory carpal bone.

A carpal flexion splint may be more comfortable than a sling, and is applied by wrapping the limb from the mid-antebrachium to the toes with a secondary layer of padding material in a figure-of-eight pattern. A layer of stretchy gauze is applied in a similar manner. Cast material is conformed to the cranial or dorsal aspect of the flexed foot; additional strips of padding can be applied beneath the splint if there is insufficient present. The final external layer is applied from the foot to the distal radius. Care must be taken not to overflex the carpus or to apply the bandage too tightly as swelling of the foot can result. The toes should be visible for monitoring purposes, but not protruding.

22.3.2 Velpeau sling

Velpeau slings are designed to prevent weight-bearing in the forelimb. They are indicated for injuries such as a reduced medial shoulder luxation, some fractures of the scapular neck and glenoid, and dorsal dislocation of the scapula. A Velpeau sling keeps the whole thoracic limb flexed (Fig. 22-6). The sling is applied by wrapping a padding layer around the torso and flexed antebrachium. The layers should be wrapped caudal and cranial to the contralateral leg to prevent cranial or caudal bandage slippage. An initial outer layer of less stretchy material is then applied on top. Great care must be taken with Velpeau slings that they are not applied too tightly as constriction can lead to pressure sores, particularly on the flexor aspects of the elbow and carpal joints. The thorax must not be excessively compressed as this can lead to compromised respiration.

Cats can be very adept at removing their legs from Velpeau slings. A Velpeau sling should not be used for too long a period as the elbow and shoulder can become very stiff if immobilized for more than 2 weeks. If immobilization is absolutely needed for more than 2 weeks, the bandage should be removed weekly and physiotherapy applied to the forelimb joints, paying special attention to the elbow joint.

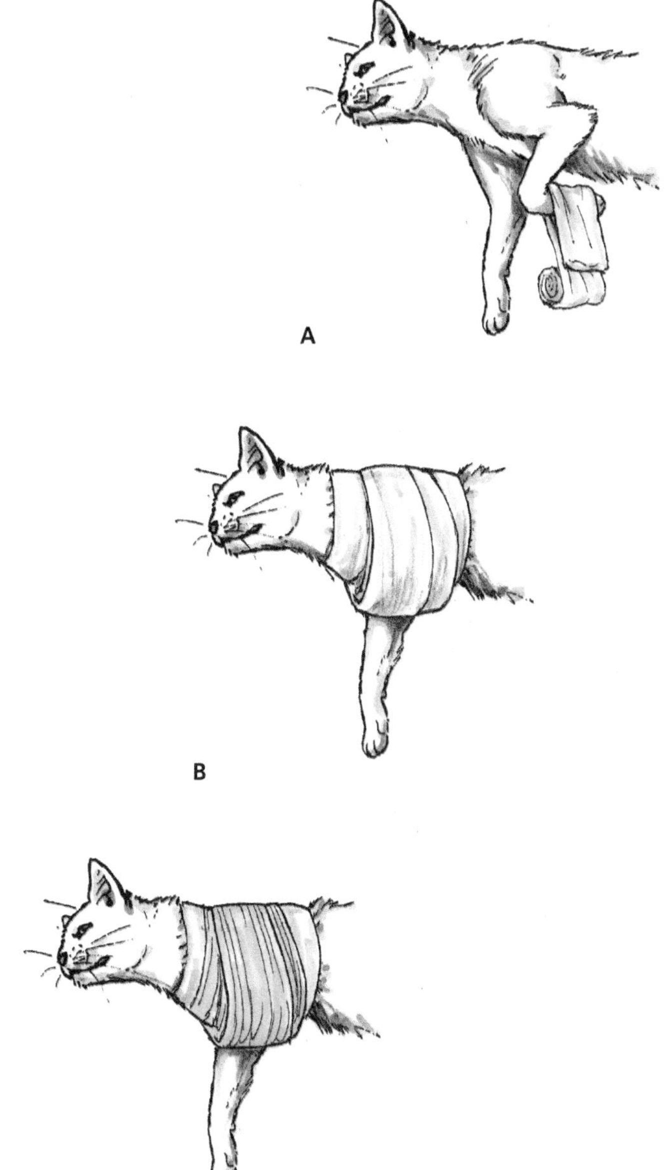

Figure 22-6 A Velpeau sling prevents weight-bearing on the forelimb. (**A**) Padding material is wrapped around the metacarpus. (**B**) While the carpus, elbow, and shoulder are held in moderate flexion, padding material is then wrapped around the thorax of the cat, passing cranial and caudal to the contralateral leg, and incorporating the affected limb. (**C**) Elastic gauze is then applied on top of it. Care should be taken not to apply the bandage too tightly to avoid overflexion of the joints.

22.3.3 Ehmer sling and Robinson sling

Two types of sling are described to prevent weight-bearing of the hindlimbs (4): the Ehmer sling and the Robinson, or pelvic limb, sling.

The main indication of an Ehmer sling is to prevent reluxation after closed reduction of a craniodorsal hip luxation. It is applied across the metatarsus and femur in a fashion that aims to prevent weight-bearing and inwardly rotates and abducts the hip. The stifle and hock are held in marked flexion. The Robinson sling also prevents weight-bearing of the hindlimb by holding the joints in slight flexion, but otherwise allows relatively free movement of joints. The Robinson sling may be indicated for situations where immediate weight-bearing is not desired.

Both of these slings are usually disliked by cats. They are difficult to apply and maintain safely due to the looser skin of cats, which frequently results in slippage of the bandage material down over the stifle joint (Ehmer sling) or down the back (Robinson sling). Applying adhesive elasticated tape directly to the cat's skin or fur may be required to keep these slings in place, but this causes marked patient discomfort,

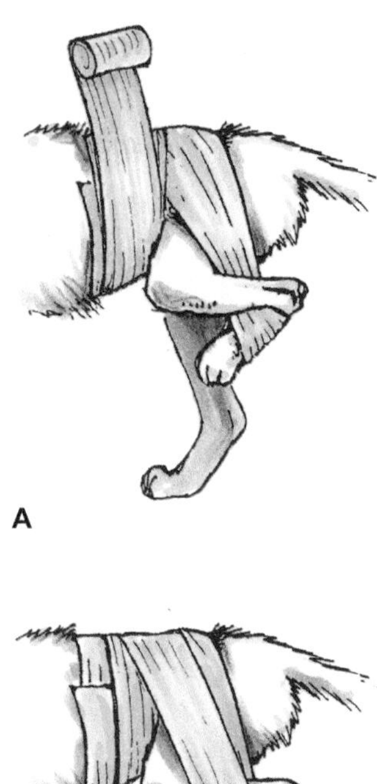

Figure 22-7 Modified Ehmer sling, using self-adhesive bandage material. This sling may be difficult to maintain in position, and removal of the adhesive material from the skin is painful. (**A**) A sling is formed around the metatarsus (never wrap the adhesive bandage material circumferentially around the metatarsus!). The self-adhesive bandage is directed medial to the tibia and lateral to the femur, which results in inward rotation of the femur, and is then wrapped around the caudal abdomen.
(**B**) An additional wrap can be applied from the abdomen around the plantar aspect of the metatarsus for additional stabilization, taking care not to lose internal rotation of the limb.

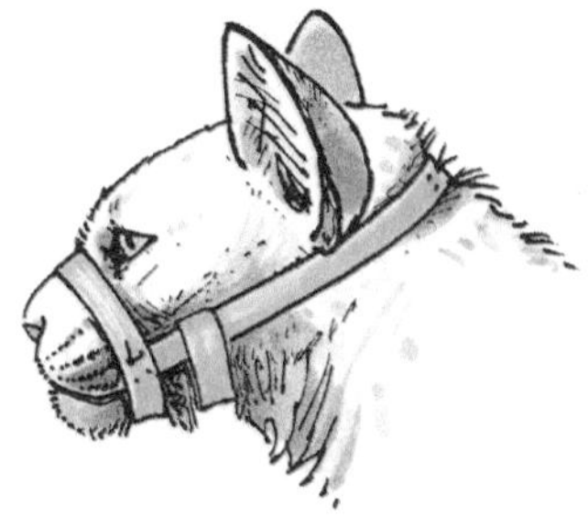

Figure 22-8 A tape muzzle is applied to maintain dental occlusion and limit the ability to open the mouth. An Elizabethan collar is necessary to prevent the cat removing the muzzle.

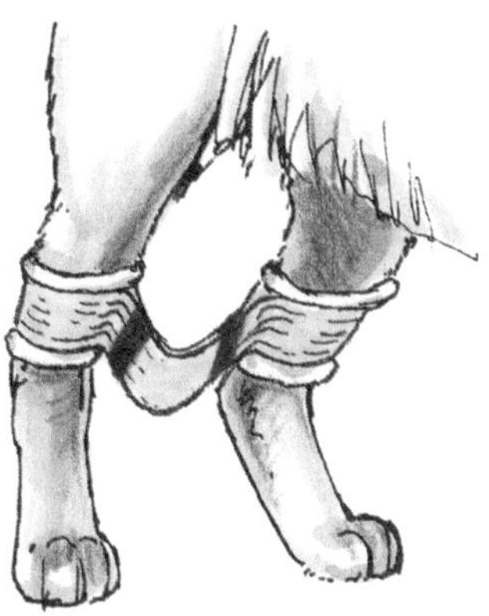

Figure 22-9 Hobble sling. Padding is first applied around each hindlimb, proximal to the tarsus. A self-adhesive bandage is then folded around the padding, and stuck to itself between the legs (never wrap the self-adhesive bandage circumferentially around the limbs!).

damage to the fur and skin, and it is painful to remove the sling. For these reasons, Ehmer and Robinson slings should be avoided in cats wherever possible.

A modified Ehmer sling, incorporated into a body bandage around the caudal abdomen, is shown in Figure 22-7. This sling holds the limb in slight inward rotation by passing the bandage material medial to the tibia and lateral to the femur, but reduces the likelihood of slippage of the bandage material down over the stifle joint. It can be used instead of a traditional Ehmer sling to maintain reduction after hip joint luxation. The sling will only stay in place if adhesive bandage material is applied directly on to the fur and, as stated above, this should be avoided whenever possible.

Complications include slippage of the skin down the back of the cat, foot swelling, and sores at the flexor aspect of the hock if the sling is too tight. Removal of the adhesive bandage material is painful, and usually requires sedation or anesthesia.

22.3.4 Tape muzzles

These are used for stabilization of non-displaced mandibular fractures and after reduction of temporomandibular luxation (see Chapter 26 for indications). They should be applied with the canine teeth slightly overlapped, and tight enough to prevent the cat opening its mouth far enough for malocclusion to occur, but loose enough to allow the cat to open its mouth a few millimeters to lap liquids.

Applying the tape muzzle at this optimal level of pressure is difficult. Strips of zinc oxide tape are used to make the muzzle; two pieces of tape are stuck together (sticky side in), with straps fastened around the head of the cat (Fig. 22-8). A chin strap is a useful addition and an Elizabethan collar is required to prevent the cat attempting to remove the muzzle.

Tape muzzles are of absolutely no use in brachycephalic breeds like the Persian or Chinchilla as the muzzle will not be able to be applied under sufficient tension across the nose or muzzle. In cats with head trauma and mandibular fractures the pharyngeal area and chin may be swollen, bruised, and edematous. These are also contraindications for use of tape muzzles. The muzzle will need regular replacement, and the cat will need meticulous cleaning under and around the muzzle to prevent soreness, as salivation is often excessive.

22.3.5 Tape hobbles

Tape hobbles are used to restrict hindlimb abduction. Their use is indicated for pelvic floor fractures and after treatment of ventral hip dislocation. They can also be used to prevent scratching at a surgical site on the flank, forelimb, or head. Tape hobbles are applied between both hindlimbs with the limbs held at a normal standing width apart, and with enough laxity to allow stepping movements (Fig. 22-9). A layer of

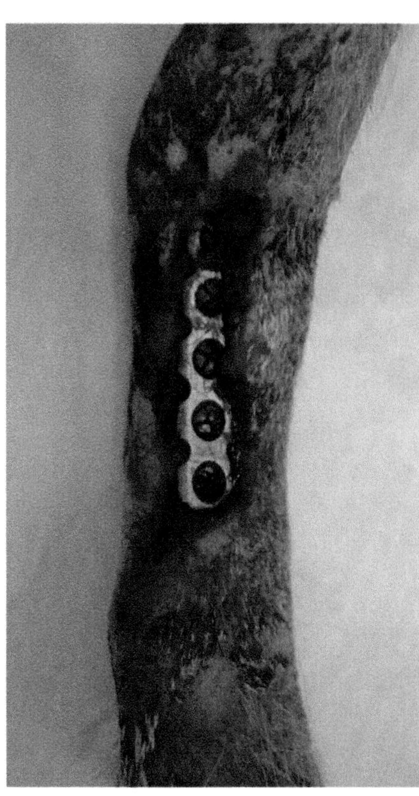

Figure 22-10 Skin slough over a locking plate used for pantarsal arthrodesis, due to pressure necrosis from a bandage that was too tight. Skin is especially subjective to pressure necrosis in areas with minimal soft-tissue cover, and over implants.

padding material is first applied around the hindlimbs just above the hock, and stabilized with conforming gauze. A layer of self-adhesive bandage material is then folded around the padding and is stuck to itself between the limbs. Care must be taken not to apply the hobbles too tightly around the hock as this will impede venous and lymphatic drainage, and may result in an edematous swollen foot.

Hobbles can be applied more proximally on the hindlimb just above the stifles. An additional strip of tape coursing over the back, and connecting the lateral-most aspects of the stifle hobbles, is necessary to prevent ventral slippage. The more proximal hobble may be more effective at preventing hindlimb abduction for ventral hip dislocation; the more distal hobble can be more effective at controlling the distal limb and preventing scratching (2).

22.4 Aftercare for bandages, splints, casts, and slings

Ischemic injury can occur after incorrect application of a bandage, cast, or sling (8) (Fig. 22-10). This can be attributed to direct pressure necrosis related to inadequate or uneven application of padding, or to a tourniquet effect resulting in secondary ischemic edema. All owners of cats discharged with a bandage, splint, or cast should be given written instructions on home care and inspection of all forms of external coaptation (Fig. 22-11).

22.4.1 Bandage, splint, and cast aftercare

If possible, the tips of the third and fourth distal phalanges should be left visible at the bottom of the bandage, splint, or cast for monitoring of toe temperature and swelling, and to check for bandage slippage. Any animal showing signs of pain or licking and chewing, foul odor, swelling of toes, or evidence of slippage should have the external coaptation removed and replaced. All bandages should be reassessed within 24 hours of application to minimize the risks inherent in inadvertent misapplication of the bandage. Bandages placed on limbs with vascular injury or deep lacerations should be rechecked and changed frequently to monitor for increased tissue pressure due to edema (8). Even the simpler bandages have limitations. The Robert Jones bandage, when applied above the elbow or stifle, tends to slip down and form a pendulum of extra weight at or below the joint. If this occurs the bandage should be removed and replaced.

Cats with bandages, splinted bandages, or casts should have regular weekly checks and the external coaptation changed and replaced if there are any concerns. Problems are more likely to develop after a change, so if the cat is comfortable and walking well with the external coaptation at the revisit, and no problems can be identified on external assessment, a change is not always necessary.

A properly applied cast in a mature cat can remain in place for up to 4 weeks. In growing cats, casts should be changed weekly or every second week. Anesthesia or heavy sedation is required for changing of the cast and when fractures are present radiographs should be taken before and after every cast change. Radiographic assessment of fractures should generally be conducted 1 week following cast application and every 2–3 weeks thereafter.

22.4.2 Sling aftercare

Similar to bandage and cast aftercare, cats with a sling should be rechecked on a regular basis for potential problems, especially pressure necrosis. The Ehmer sling in particular bears risks for slippage, and the authors prefer to keep cats with an Ehmer sling in hospital to allow daily checks. Other slings, like the hobble sling or the tape muzzle, are less dangerous.

Slings holding joints in flexion, such as the Velpeau, Ehmer, and carpal sling, should not be left on for longer than 10 days to avoid joint contractures and pain.

The Queen's Veterinary School Hospital
University of Cambridge
Madingley Road Cambridge CB3 0ES

Telephone: Fax:
e-mail:

Sorrel Langley-Hobbs MA, BVetMed, DSAS (Orthopaedics), Dip. ECVS, MRCVS
University Surgeon (Orthopaedics)
European Specialist in Surgery

Homecare of cats with splints, casts, bandages or slings

It is of extreme importance for the well being of your cat that a bandage, splint, cast or sling be well cared for at all times. You, as the pet owner, must assume this responsibility. It should be realised that under certain conditions (i.e. getting wet, slippage from its original position, etc) the bandage, splint, cast or sling may not perform its function properly or may even do severe damage to your cat, such as causing gangrene of the foot.

Your cat should not be allowed outside

Examine the splint bandage or cast at least once daily

Watch for swelling or skin lesions of the leg above the bandage, splint, cast, or sling and feel the toes at least once daily to ensure that your cat has good sensation in them and that the toes have not become swollen or cold. The bandage, splint, cast or sling must be kept dry and clean.

If any of the following events occur, phone your veterinary surgeon

1. Any change in shape of the bandage, splint, cast or sling on the limb.
2. Any excessive chewing of the bandage, splint, cast or sling by the cat.
3. Any sign of excessive discomfort.
4. Any unusual or bad odors coming from the bandage, splint, cast or sling.
5. Any unexplained soiling that was not present before.
6. Any sores that develop at the top or bottom of the splint or cast or around a sling
7. Swelling of the toes, or the leg above the bandage, splint, cast or sling.
8. Inappetance, depression or fever in your cat.

Be sure to make and keep an appointment to have the bandage, splint, cast or sling examined by your veterinary surgeon. No bandage, splint, cast or sling can be worn in complete comfort by a cat and minor licking or chewing is to be expected. **BUT if there is even a suggestion of trouble, it is always better to have your cat examined as soon as possible.**

Figure 22-11 Example of an instruction sheet on bandage, splint, cast, and sling care that can be given to owners. (Adapted from Whittick WG, Egger EL. Principles of fracture management. In: Whittick WG (ed.) Canine othopaedics, 2nd edn. Philadelphia: Lea & Febiger; 1990: p. 232.)

References and further reading

1. Leighton RL. Principles of conservative fracture management: splints and casts. Semin Vet Med Surg (Small Anim) 1991;6: 39–51.
2. Tobias TA. Slings, padded bandages, splinted bandages and casts. In: Olmstead ML (ed.) Small animal orthopaedics. St. Louis: Mosby; 1995: pp. 75–110.
3. Oakley RE. External coaptation. Vet Clin North Am Small Anim Pract 1999;29:1083–1095.
4. DeCamp CE. External coaptation. In: Slatter D (ed.) Textbook of small animal surgery, 2nd edn. Philadelphia: WB Saunders; 2003: pp. 1661–1676.
5. Montavon PM, Vass K. [External coaptation]. In: Horziaek MC, Schmidt V, Lutz H (ed.) Krankherten der Katie, 4th edn. Stultgart: Enke Verlag; 2005: pp. 682–684.
6. Langley-Hobbs SJ, et al. Comparison and assessment of casting materials for use in small animals. Vet Rec 1996;139:258–262.
7. Keller MA, Montavon PM. Conservative fracture treatment using casts. Indications, principles of closed fracture reduction and stabilization, and cast materials. Compend Continuing Educ 2006;28:631–641.
8. Anderson DM, White RAS. Ischemic bandage injuries: a case series and review of the literature. Vet Surg 2000;29:488–498.

23 Orthopedic instrumentation

J.P. Lapish

As the patient size or area of surgery becomes smaller in relation to the surgeon's hand, the tissues must be manipulated increasingly through the medium of surgical instrumentation. Appropriately scaled instruments must be selected to minimize devitalization of the bones and soft tissues. Feline orthopedic surgery will therefore have a greater reliance on instruments than orthopedics on larger patients.

Generally, smaller variants of familiar instruments are selected, but ultimately, within certain parameters, the final choice of instruments will be dictated by surgeon preference. Although the patient is small, the hand of the surgeon remains unchanged; therefore, typically, the working tips of instruments will be scaled down but the handles and often the length will remain unchanged. Surgeons who do not work exclusively with cats will prefer the working distances of the instruments to remain similar across the patient range.

23.1 Instruments used for surgical approaches

23.1.1 Scalpels and blades

For most feline procedures a number 15 blade is appropriate which fits the number 3 or number 7 scalpel handle (Fig. 23-1). Where a sharp pointed blade is required, the number 11 or number 15a are useful choices: both fit the same handles. The smaller Beaver-type handle and blade is preferred if it is necessary to work within joints. The number 65 blade is approximately half the scale of the number 11, and the number 65a blade is even smaller.

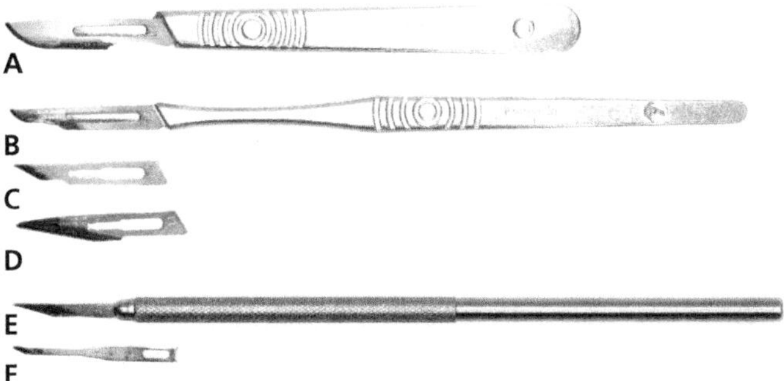

Figure 23-1 Scalpels and blades. (**A**) Number 3 scalpel handle plus number 10 blade; (**B**) number 7 scalpel handle plus number 15 blade; (**C**) number 15a blade; (**D**) number 11 blade; (**E**) Beaver-type handle plus number 65 blade; (**F**) number 65a blade.

23.1.2 Dissecting forceps

Standard dissecting forceps such as Treves are slightly bulky and cumbersome for operating on cats, and the lighter Adson is preferred for soft tissues. The Adson is available in toothed or serrated versions. A microtoothed version, the Adson–Brown, offers a good combination of grip and gentleness, and is mainly used to manipulate tough tissues like fascia. DeBakey pattern forceps, which were developed as an atraumatic forcep for cardiac surgery, have multiple microteeth for an atraumatic grip. The smallest variant is 150 mm (6 inch) with a 1.5-mm jaw width. Dissecting forceps are depicted in Figure 23-2.

23.1.3 Scissors

The preferred dissection scissor for feline orthopedics is the Metzenbaum (Fig. 23-3). Although a similar overall length to the standard surgical Mayo, the Metzenbaum has shorter, finer cutting blades. Appropriate lengths are 180 mm (7 inch) and 145 mm (5.75 inch): the latter are also known as pediatric Metzenbaum or Laheys. The ophthalmic range offers a wide selection if an even smaller scissor is required. The strabismus scissor (Fig. 23-3) is effectively a scaled-down Metzenbaum. The curved Mayo scissor or dedicated suture scissor is used to cut suture material (Fig. 23-3).

23.1.4 Artery forceps

Hemostasis in the cat may be achieved using Halstead mosquito forceps 125 mm (5 inch), either curved or straight (Fig. 23-4). The tip of the instrument is used for clamping small vessels. The Halstead is also ideal for bluntly opening a channel through soft tissues to bone, prior to closed placement of external fixation pins. The closed jaws are placed down a stab incision and gently opened to create a passage.

23.1.5 Retractors

Retraction of the soft tissues around bones and joints is essential to protect them from trauma, to expose the bone or joint under investigation, and to allow in sufficient light for

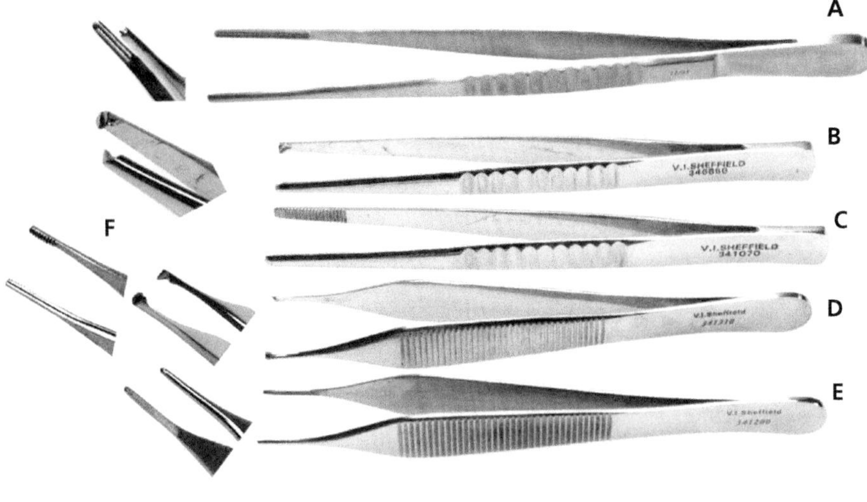

Figure 23-2 Dissecting forceps with close-up views of the tips. (**A**) Debakey: (**B**) Treves; (**C**) dressing; (**D**) Adson; (**E**) Adson serrated; (**F**) Adson Brown tips.

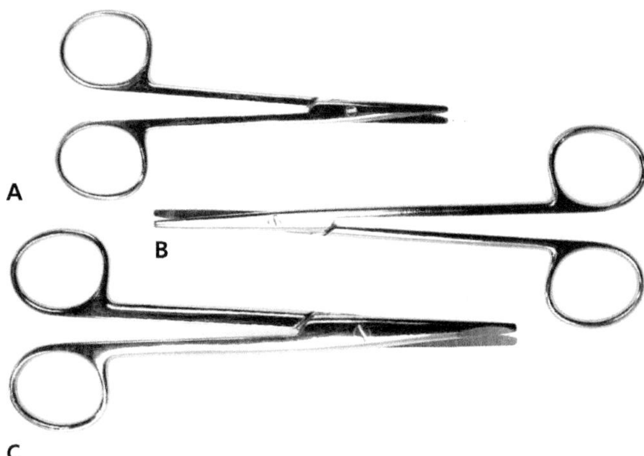

Figure 23-3 Scissors. (**A**) Strabismus; (**B**) Metzenbaum; (**C**) Mayo.

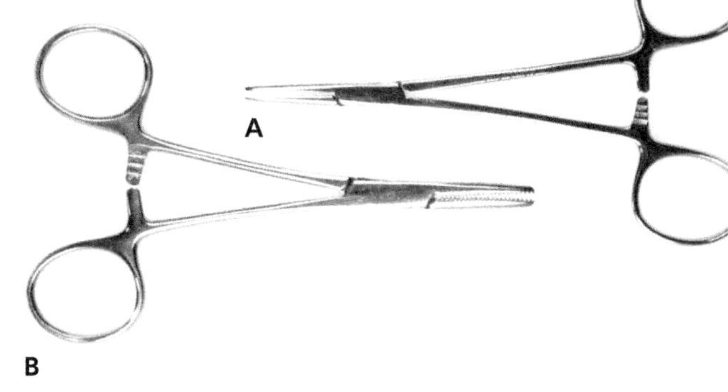

Figure 23-4 Artery forceps. (**A**) Halstead mosquito; (**B**) Spencer Wells.

adequate visualization. Surgeons working without assistance will rely on a wide range of self-retaining retractors to provide exposure (Fig. 23-5). They may be subdivided into two main groups: single-pronged (Gelpi style) and multipronged (Wests or Travers style). Both types are available in smaller variants appropriate for cats. Multipronged retractors are typically used for superficial retraction of skin and muscle, where a relatively wide exposure is necessary. Closer to the bone or joint more focal retraction is obtained by using single-pronged devices. Two single-pronged small Gelpis may be placed at right angles to each other to create a window on to the area of interest.

Hand-held focal retraction offers the most controllable retraction where assistance is available (Fig. 23-6). Single-blade retractors with a blade width of 6 mm or less are preferred. Most of those available to the veterinary surgeon were designed for human finger surgery. Appropriate patterns are the smaller Langenbecks, Meyerdings, and the Senn. The Senn is a double-ended instrument: one end is a single blade 6 mm wide and the other is a sharp multipronged tip with a width of 10 mm.

Hohmann retractors are a specific group of retractors designed both to elevate bone or joint structures while at the same time retracting and flattening soft tissues for improved visual access and manipulation (Fig. 23-6). All have a small tip which is placed behind the bone and a wider proximal blade which, when depressed, pushes the soft tissues away. All require an assistant to maintain retraction. Short-tipped variants with blade widths of 6 or 8 mm are the most useful. Hohmann retractors can also be used as a lever to distract and reduce a fracture.

Although not technically instruments, Penrose drains and woven or umbilical tape have a role to play in soft-tissue retraction, particularly in the protection of nerves and vessels. Passed around the nerve or vessel, these products are used to manipulate its position atraumatically, avoiding contact with metal instruments. A pair of Halstead mosquito forceps clipped on to a Penrose drain offers a degree of self-retaining

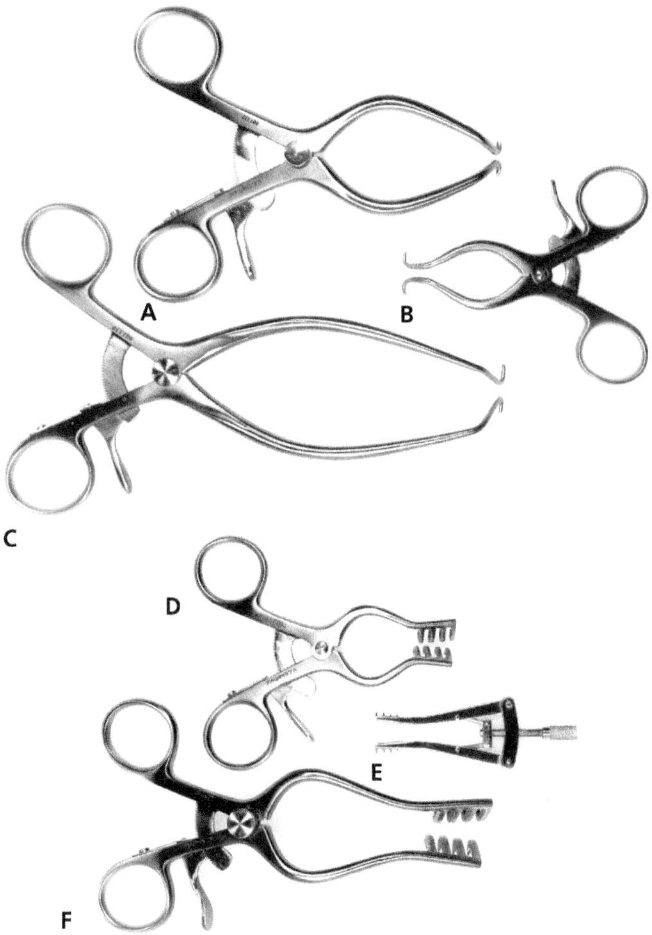

Figure 23-5 Self-retaining retractors. (A) Small Gelpis; (B) mini Gelpis; (C) standard Gelpis with blunt tips; (D) mini Travers; (E) Aln; (F) Weitlaners.

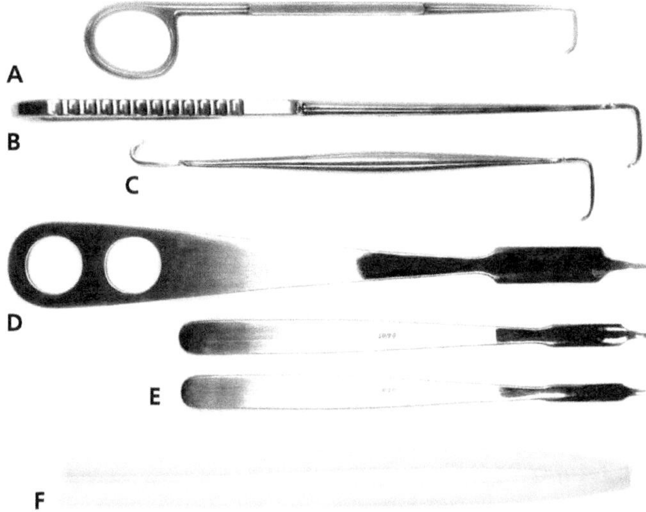

Figure 23-6 Hand-held retractors. (A) Meyerding finger; (B) Langenbeck 6 mm; (C) Senn; (D) Hohmann 12 mm; (E) Hohmann 8 mm; (F) Hohmann 6 mm; (G) Penrose drain.

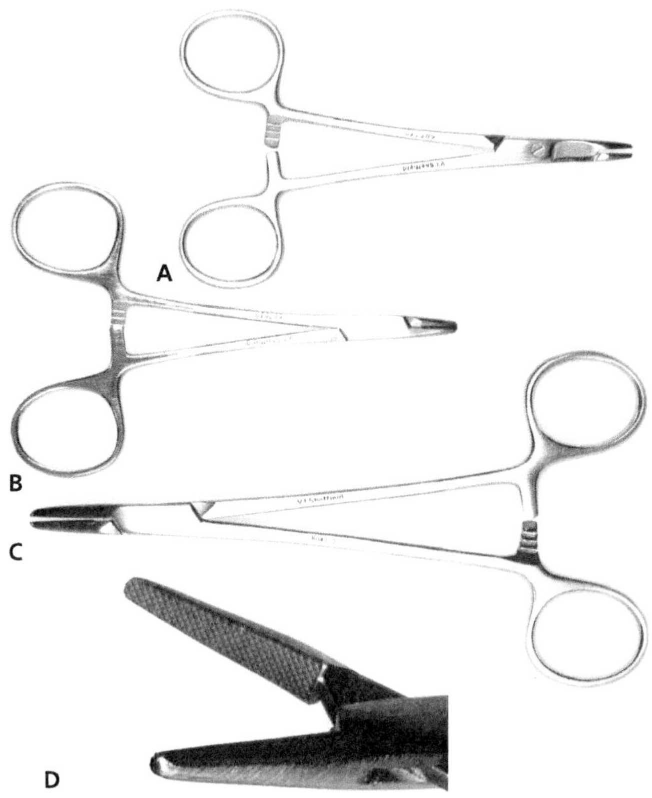

Figure 23-7 Needle-holders. (A) Olsen–Hegar; (B) Mayo–Hegar; (C) DeBakey; (D) microserrated tungsten jaw inserts.

retraction, the weight of the instrument being sufficient to keep the nerve in the desired position. Alternatively, positioning may be controlled by an assistant.

23.1.6 Needle-holders

Needles used in feline surgery are small, and needle-holders with suitable-sized jaws should be selected (Fig. 23-7). It is recommended that a needle-holder with tungsten carbide jaws is used for maximum grip and minimum needle slippage, as the very hard microserrations bite into the relatively soft stainless-steel needle. Many designs are available and typically the needle-holder is the one instrument over which the surgeon likes to express a choice. Recommended are the Mayo–Hegar 125–165 mm (5–6.5 inch). Similar in pattern but lighter are the DeBakey. Non-locking Gillie-type needle-holder/scissors are less reliable, although useful for cutting sutures if an assistant is not available. An alternative to the Gillie as a needle-holder/scissor is the Olsen–Hegar: this has the benefit of a locking action. Tungsten carbide jaw versions are available in 115–165 mm (4.5–6.5 inch). The Derf needle-holder is effectively a scaled-down Mayo–Hegar.

A

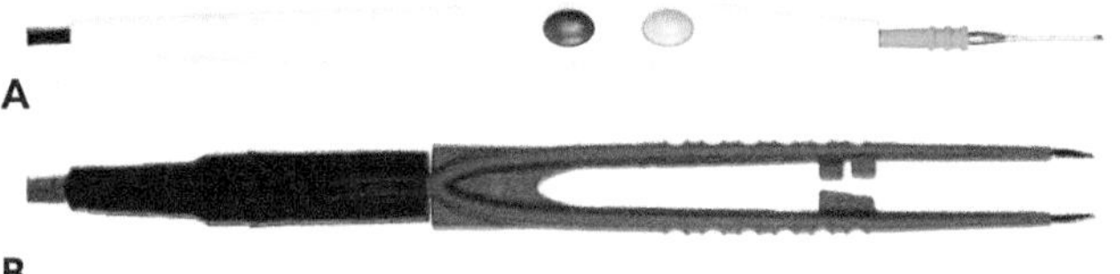

B

Figure 23-8 Electrocautery. (**A**) Monopolar hand piece; (**B**) bipolar hand piece.

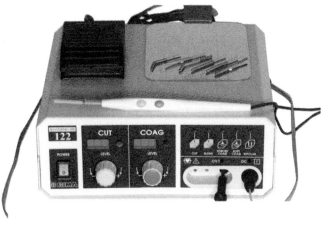

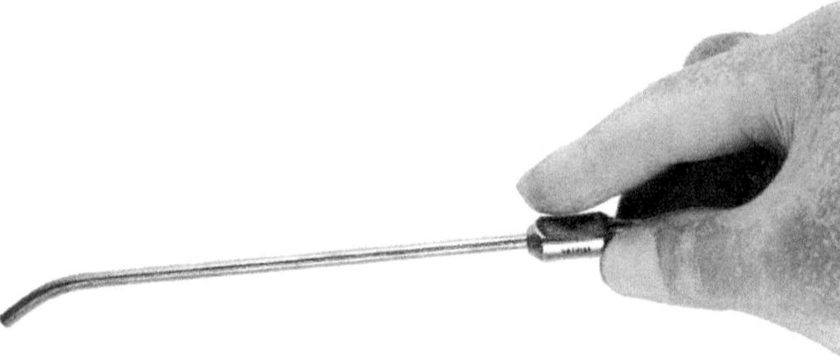

Figure 23-9 Adson suction tip.

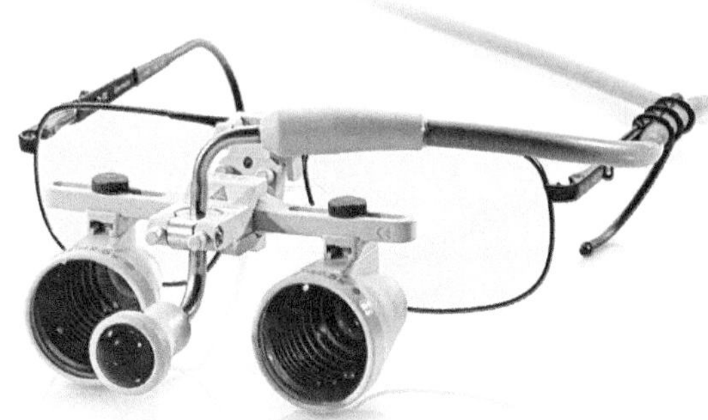

A

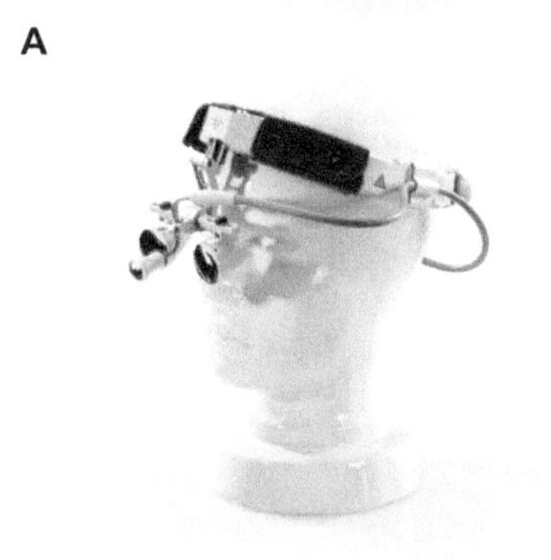

B

Figure 23-10 Binocular loupes and LED light source. (**A**) Loupes and light source on a spectacle frame; (**B**) loupes and light source fitted to a head band.

23.1.7 Ancillary aids

Adequate lighting is a prerequisite for good surgery. A repositionable focal light source is very desirable. Care should be exercised to control the heating and drying effects of good lighting. Ideally an assistant should be delegated the task of keeping tissues moist. Newer LED light sources are able to provide light without heat.

Diathermy facilitates the creation of a blood-free operating site by electrocutting and coagulation (Fig. 23-8). Blood loss is minimized: this may be crucial in severely injured patients. Bipolar diathermy must be used in the proximity of any nerve bundles, and particularly the spine. Dry swabs or sponges are abrasive and will cause damage if used repetitively, particularly if dragged across soft tissues. Conversely, a swab can be an effective means of clearing soft tissue from a bone fragment.

Suction will contribute to a clear operating field. It is particularly desirable in the presence of cooling irrigation. Many tips are available but the most useful are the Adson (4 mm diameter) (Fig. 23-9) or Frazier (2.6 mm diameter) type, which offer fingertip control of suction by an assistant. The suction tips should be exchanged during surgeries exceeding 1.5–2 hours to decrease bacterial contamination.

The bones and joints of cats are small, so the use of binocular loupes, which magnify while maintaining a normal working distance, will significantly improve visualization of the working area (Fig. 23-10). Magnification is especially useful for spinal surgery. A magnification of 2.5 times is sufficient for most procedures. The focal distance should be selected to maintain a normal working distance, usually between 380 and 430 mm. The addition of a loupe light, either fiberoptic or, more economically, LED, will automatically provide surgical light where it is needed.

23.2 Instruments used for osteosynthesis

23.2.1 Powered equipment

Most powered orthopedic equipment is designed for human large-bone surgery. Until recently the industry-standard pneumatic equipment for small canine and feline orthopedics

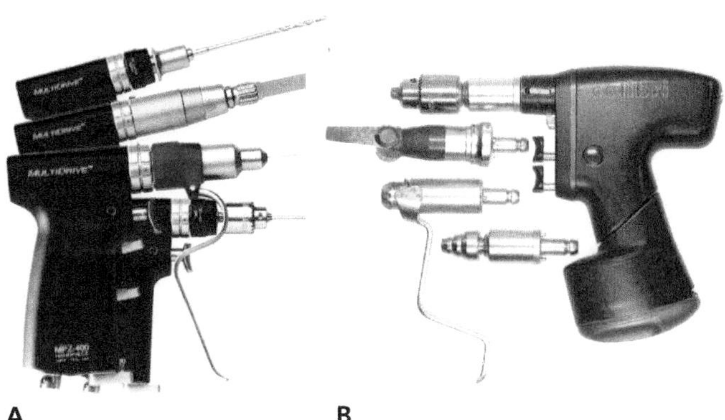

A B

Figure 23-11 Powered orthopedic equipment for feline surgery. (A) DeSoutter MPZ modular system; (B) Synthes Colibri modular system.

was the 3Ms Mini Driver which is no longer available new, although it is still widely used. Alternatives include the pneumatic DeSoutter MPZ system, the cable drive Aesculap Elan or battery-powered Aesculap mini Acculan systems, and the Synthes battery Colibri system. All have their own advantages and pricing. They are modular systems comprising a hand piece with a range of interchangeable attachments, including drill, oscillating saw, and wire driver (Fig. 23-11). Most drills are based on a 4-mm-capacity Jacobs chuck. Some systems have a novel oscillating drill attachment, which generates cleaner and heat-reduced drilling plus minimal soft-tissue wrap-around. All the saws in the systems mentioned will take appropriately sized saw blades for cutting feline bones.

A wire driver is particularly useful in feline orthopedics. Hard wires having a diameter of less than 2 mm are flexible and difficult to drive into bone without bending or at least creating a hole which is less than circular. The interface between pin and bone is reduced if the hole created is not circular, resulting in early implant failure. Wire drivers permit the incremental insertion of wires via a rotating clutch mechanism. Only a short segment of wire is exposed to bending forces at any time. Recreating incremental insertion using a chuck and key is much less convenient and very time-consuming.

All the modular systems described above are powered by low-speed, high-torque motors. They are not suitable for driving high-speed burs, which demand a much higher speed together with low torque. At speeds approaching 100 000 rpm, the burs become self-cleaning to a degree, as bone debris gets spun off. Burs that run at lower speeds very rapidly clog up. The industry standard bur system is the Halls Surgairtome II, driven by an air vane motor (Fig. 23-12). The Surgairtome drives a range of handpiece-fitting burs (shaft diameter 2.34 mm) of a variety of lengths and diameters. Bur construction will be of carbide or a diamond coating. The latter offers a finer cut and better wear characteristics.

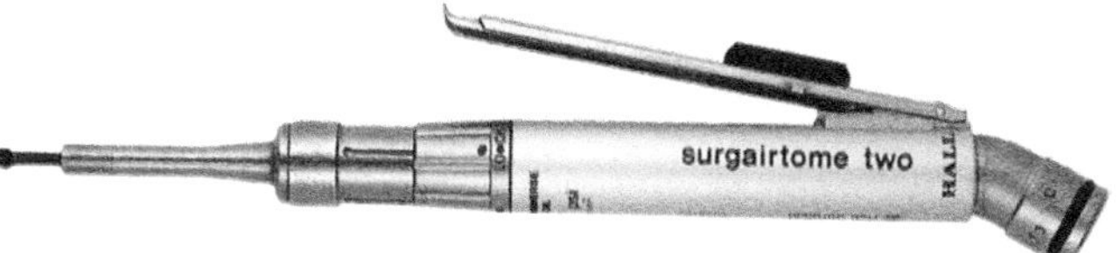

Figure 23-12 The Halls Surgairtome is a high-speed, low-torque air-driven bur system useful for neurosurgery or debridement of articular cartilage prior to arthrodesis.

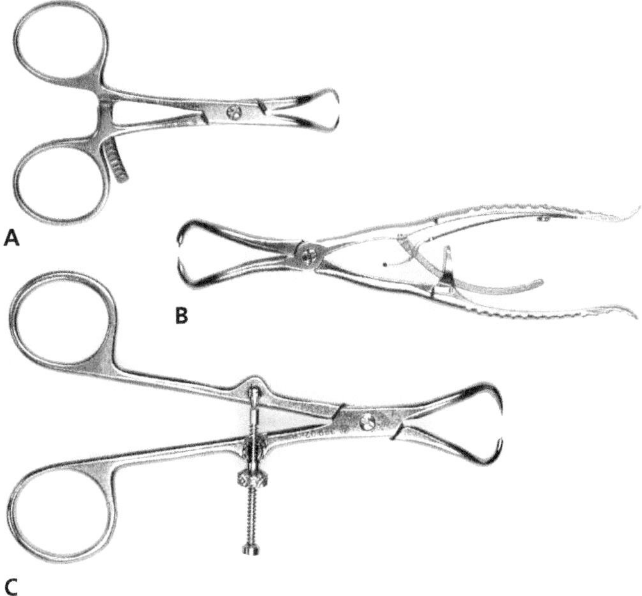

Figure 23-13 Small pointed reduction forceps showing the different closing mechanisms. (A) The ratchet; (B) soft lock; and (C) spin lock mechanism.

23.2.2 Pointed reduction forceps

Pointed reduction forceps are designed to reduce and maintain reduction of bone fragments. Each fragment is compressed at a single point, which is typically critical in its location. The jaws are maintained in position using either a ratchet mechanism or a spin lock mechanism. When dealing with very small fragments, the increments between ratchets can be too large and offer less "feel." The spin lock allows the forceps to be tightened free-hand and the spin lock is spun into position to maintain reduction. A third option available is a "soft lock" mechanism: this utilizes a very fine ratchet and therefore gives much better "feel." All three types are available in a variety of small sizes suitable for cats (Fig. 23-13).

23.2.3 Bone-holding forceps

The distinction between pointed reduction and bone-holding forceps is somewhat arbitrary. Generally, bone-holding

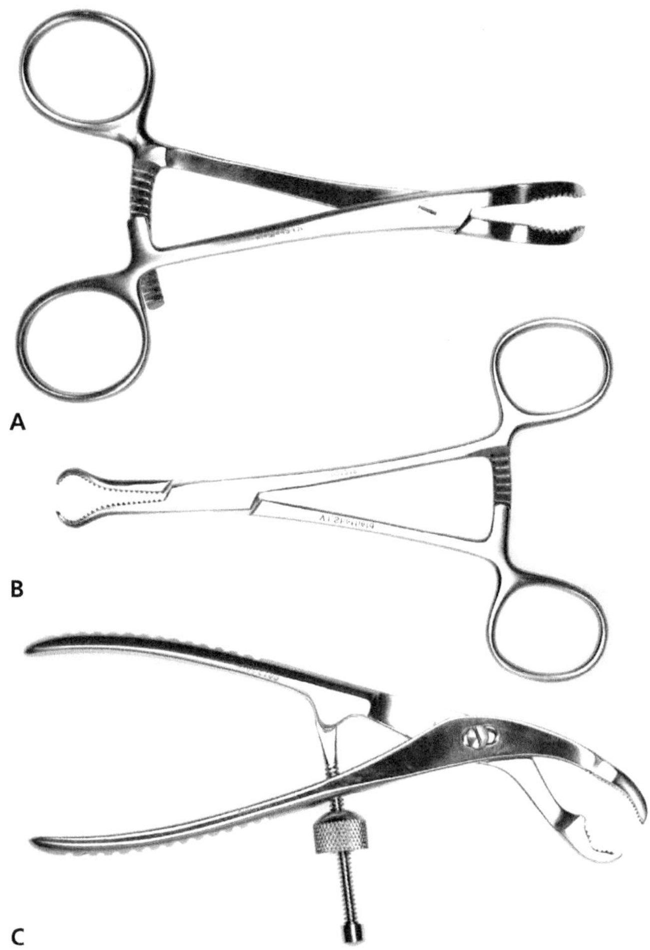

Figure 23-14 Bone-holding forceps. (A) Small curved; (B) small serrated "crab claw"; (C) self-centering, veterinary pattern.

forceps are used to grip and hold bone and move fragments while attempting reduction rather than simply to hold already reduced bone fragments in apposition; the latter is the main task of pointed reduction forceps. The closing mechanisms described for pointed reduction forceps are also available for bone-holding forceps. A wide variety of jaw designs are available to suit different orthopedic situations. There is no such thing as a universal bone-holding forceps. The long bones of cats have a relatively thin cortex and manipulating their fragments requires that the forceps offer support as well as grip. Use of forceps that are too large or have too great a ratchet increment or the wrong-shaped jaw will crush the fragment. A variety of useful designs are illustrated in Figure 23-14.

23.2.4 Bone levers and hooks

Bone fragments in small patients should not be handled with fingers. Fingers obscure the fracture site and devitalize bone and soft tissues. In addition to reduction forceps and bone-holding forceps, it is useful to include a small selection of dental hooks, curettes, and a small Hohmann retractor, together with a very fine periosteal elevator to use as bone levers and probes in any feline orthopedic kit.

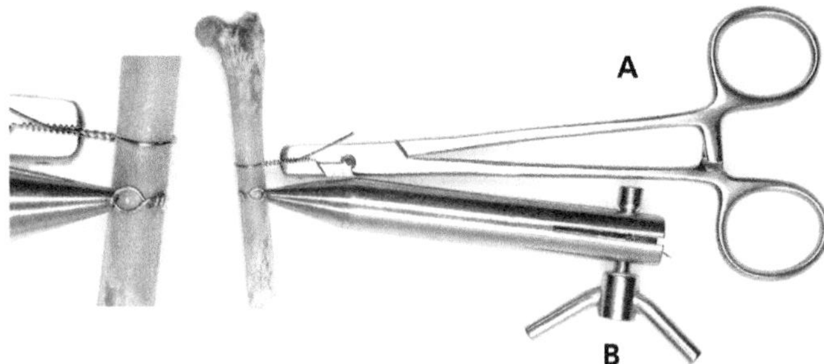

Figure 23-15 (A) The combination wire twister and shear cutter is shown alongside (B) the wire tightener for loop cerclage. Close-ups are on the left.

23.2.5 Instruments for placing orthopedic wire

Cerclage may be applied either as a length of wire twisted around itself or as a wire tensioned against an end loop. The former offers the ability to adjust tension incrementally, but has to be done correctly to avoid weakening the wire at the base of the twist (Chapter 24). The latter is more reliable but does not offer the option of retightening. Both will require dedicated instruments. The use of needle-holders or artery forceps for twisting wire is not recommended. The combination wire twister and shear cutter is appropriate for twisted cerclage. Looped cerclage wire requires its own dedicated tightener (Fig. 23-15). Various designs of wire passer are available for passing wire around bone fragments while minimizing damage to the soft tissues. All consist of a stiff tube curved to match the diameter of the bone. The curved tube is gently pushed around the bone fragment through and past soft tissues. The flexible piece of orthopedic wire is passed into the wire passer, which can then be withdrawn. A wire passer with a diameter of around 20 mm is the most useful in feline orthopedics.

23.2.6 Hard wire and pin insertion

Pins and wires, including external fixation pins, should be driven into bone by pure axial rotation. Anything less will compromise the bone–pin interface which retains the pin in the bone. The ideal instrument is a powered wire driver (Fig. 23-16). Larger, less flexible pins can be driven reasonably well using a hand chuck. A Jacobs chuck consists of a stainless-steel chuck mounted on an anodized aluminum handle. Two capacities are available: the larger 6.35-mm version, and a smaller, lighter 4-mm-capacity version. The latter is recom-

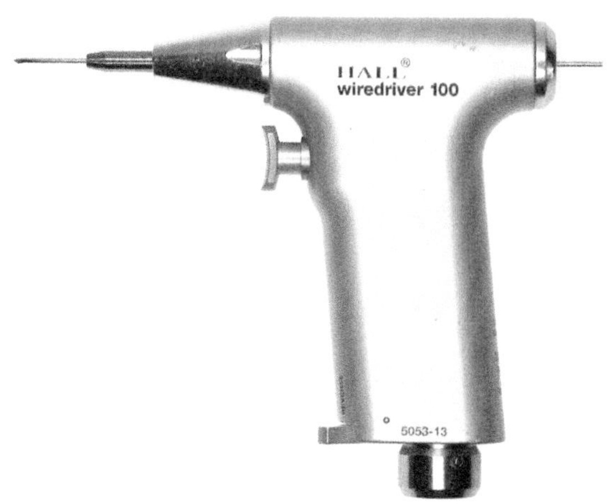

Figure 23-16 An air-powered wire driver.

mended. Pin vices of even smaller capacity are available for wires of 2 mm diameter and less. These vices fit into the palm of the hand, and this allows a purer axial rotation than the larger hand chucks. It should be noted that the chuck key, having approximately 25% of the teeth of the chuck, will wear much faster than the chuck. The key should therefore be replaced more often than the chuck.

Hard wires are typically placed close to joints and their cut end will require management to avoid premature loosening and soft-tissue irritation. The cut ends can be pushed flat to the bone surface using a punch, the end of which is recessed to reduce slippage. Alternatively, the cut end can be bent over and turned to align with inserting ligament or tendons. It is important to maintain the fracture reduction under pressure while bending the wire to avoid destabilization of the fracture. This is achieved using a Kirschner wire bender, an instrument cannulated along its length, and slid down the wire to the bone surface. Applying pressure as well as bending forces means that the repair is not disrupted and that the bend is created sharply at the bone surface.

23.2.7 Cutting bone

If bone is being cut with a view to subsequent reattachment, control and accuracy are very important. A powered oscillating saw with an appropriate blade is then recommended. Bone cutters and osteotomes are less controllable. Cutters can be appropriate in certain circumstances, e.g., tibial crest transplants or femoral head and neck excisions; however, they crush the bone whilst cutting. Osteotomes are difficult to use, because the small size of the cat results in the power from the mallet typically dissipating by movement of the cat or cat limb away from the mallet. Where the bone in question can be supported, a 4- or 6-mm osteotome can be used effectively.

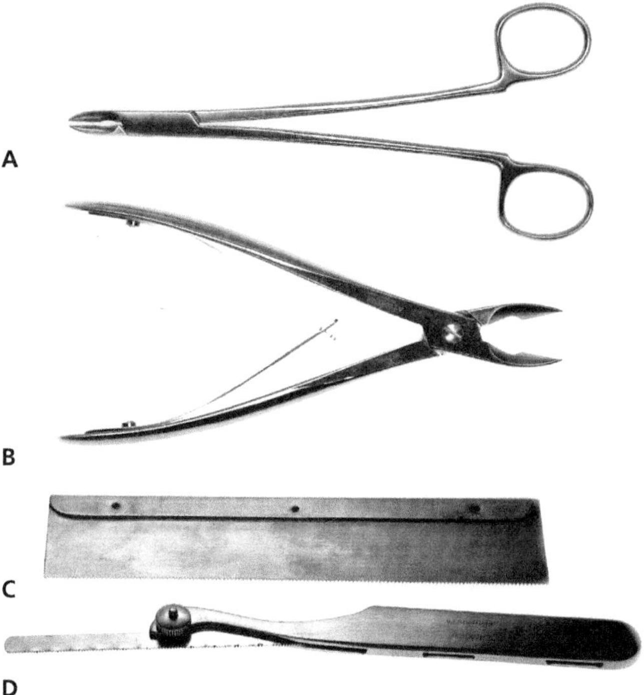

Figure 23-17 Instruments for bone-cutting. (**A**) Fine bone cutters 9 mm jaw; (**B**) bone cutters 11 mm jaw; (**C**) hard back saw; (**D**) adjustable bone saw.

Trochleoplasty is a specific bone-cutting procedure requiring a fine but stiff blade. A stronger piece of metal is run along the back of the blade to stiffen the blade. This type of blade is available as a disposable hobby saw (Xacto), which has the benefit of very fine teeth, or as a surgical hard back saw which can be autoclaved, but whose teeth are a little larger (Fig. 23-17).

23.2.8 Removing bone

Debulking of bone is best achieved using a high-speed bur, so material can be gently incrementally removed. When close to vital structures, particularly the spine, it is desirable that the final overlying layer of bone is removed by hand. It is important that this final layer of bone should only be eggshell thick, as the appropriate-sized rongeurs are not strong enough for thicker bone. When using any rongeur near the spine, it is important to remember that one jaw has to be inserted between the bone and the spinal cord for the opposite jaw to cut against. The jaw inserted must therefore be as small as possible (Fig. 23-18). The jaw width should be between 1.5 and 3.00 mm. However, jaw size is related to strength and these microrongeurs should be reserved for delicate work.

Other useful instruments for removing bone include a selection of dental probes. Sharp probes, such as the Jaquette style, are used for hooking bone fragments away from the

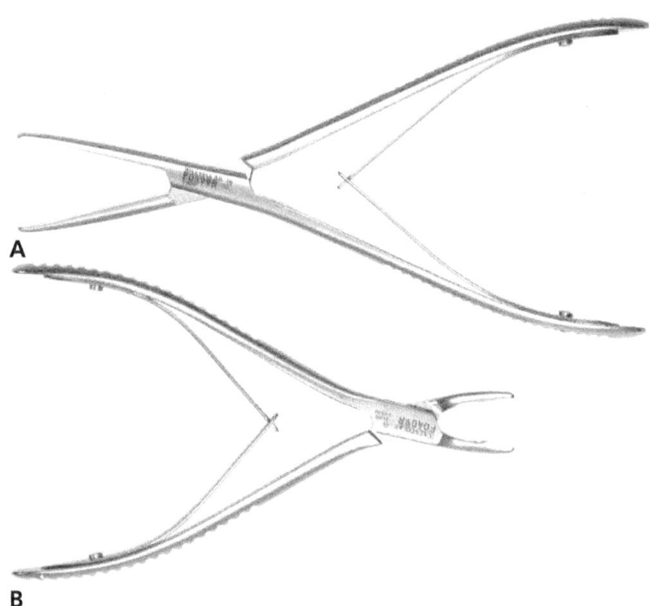

Figure 23-18 Rongeurs. (A) Stellebrink synovectomy rongeurs; (B) micro-Friedman rongeurs.

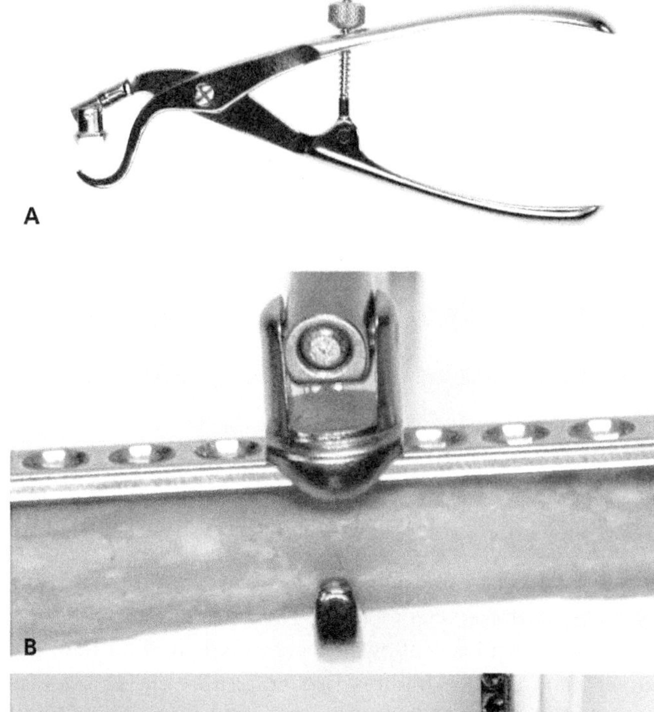

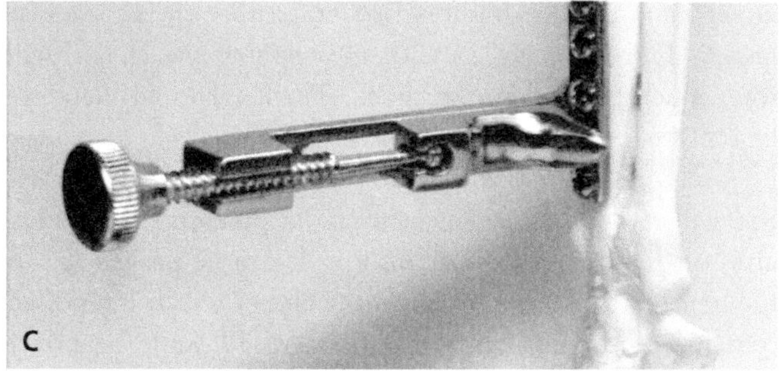

Figure 23-19 Plate bone-holders. (A) Synthes 2.7-mm plate-holding forceps; (B) close-up of (A); (C) cat-sized Lowman clamp.

spine. Dental curettes have a rounded back surface and are therefore more useful when working up against the spine. Most traditional curettes are too large but the House curette, a human ear instrument, is double-ended and appropriately sized.

23.2.9 Plating equipment

Traditionally, plates and screws in the cat have been restricted to 2.7-, 2.0-, and 1.5-mm dynamic compression plate (DCP) systems. Today more options are available, including miniature and 2.4-mm plates and screws, and internal fixators, which involve screws that interlock with the plates (Chapter 24). Each system requires its own dedicated instrumentation.

The Mini AO kit will be described in some detail. For example, for a 2.0-mm position screw the following are required: drill guide, pilot drill (1.5 mm), 1.5/2.0 depth gauge, tap, small countersink, and 1.5 hexagonal or cruciate screwdriver. A lag screw will require in addition a clearance drill of 2.0 mm and a 1.5/2.0 insert sleeve. If applying a DCP, a load/neutral drill guide will also be necessary to position screws appropriately in the plate. If using self-tapping screws the tap is not necessary. The 1.5-, 2.4-, and 2.7-mm screw/plate sets will require a similar array of dedicated equipment.

Locking plates require a threaded drill guide to be placed into the locking hole to ensure that the pilot hole is centered on the plate hole, and is placed at right angles to the plate (Chapter 24). The machine thread on the head of the locking screw is very unforgiving in terms of screw angle.

The inherently unstable construct of bone plate and bone fragment makes the creation of a simple, universal plate-holding forceps difficult. Ratchet-type, jointed instruments work efficiently over a relatively small range of bone diameters. The most efficient bone plate-holding devices are designed to work with a single size of bone plate. In feline fracture orthopedics, useful instruments include the Synthes 2.7 mm plate-holding forceps, and the cat-sized Lowman clamp. The former is a modified Verbrugge forceps, incorporating a sliding self-centering hinge and a hinged jaw. The latter is not hinged and works in a single plane, allowing it to function over a wider range of bone size, and with both 2.0- and 2.7-mm plates (Fig. 23-19).

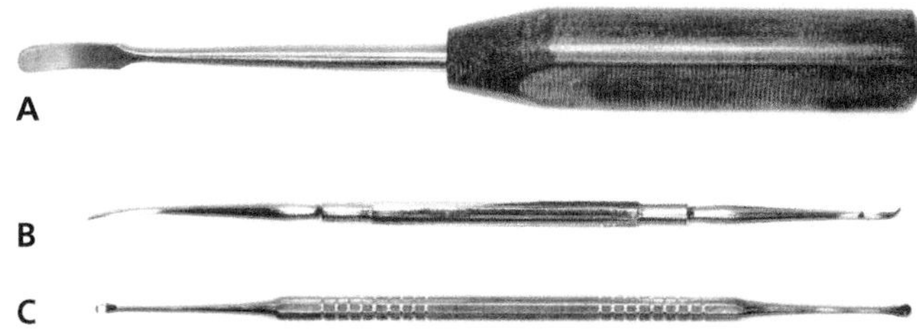

Figure 23-20 Periosteal elevators. (**A**) AO style; (**B**) Freer; (**C**) very fine 2–3-mm periosteal elevator.

23.2.10 Periosteal elevator

A periosteal elevator is used to strip soft tissues from long bones prior to plate fixation (Fig. 23-20). The standard AO-style 6-mm elevator can be slightly large for cats. The Freer elevator is a finer and slightly narrower alternative at 5-mm width. A small double-ended periosteal elevator with 2- and 3-mm tips is an even smaller option. These instruments should be held with the index finger near the working extremity to facilitate control.

References and further reading

Commercial catalogues and websites featuring human hand surgery instruments and veterinary orthopedic specialties illustrate a wide range of small instruments appropriate for feline orthopedics. Catalogues are available from many companies, including:

Aesculap: www.aesculap.de

Synthes: www.synthes.com

Veterinary Instrumentation: www.vetinst.com

24 Orthopedic implants

S.J. Langley-Hobbs, K. Voss, J.P. Lapish, P.M. Montavon

A large variety of orthopedic implants are suitable for use in cats. The commonly applied standard implants include orthopedic wire, Kirschner wires, intramedullary pins, and dynamic compression plates (DCPs). More specialized implants, such as miniaturized and specific plates, internal fixators, and interlocking nails, can be particularly useful for repair of the smaller bones of cats. It is often possible successfully to apply a variety of different implants for stabilization of a fracture, and the choice of which implant to use is based on individual assessment of the cat, including its size, age, and the presence of other injuries, the fracture itself, and the type of fracture healing expected (Chapter 13), the availability of implants, and the experience of the surgeon. An advantage in feline fracture repair is the fairly limited variation of implant sizes that need to be kept in stock because of the similar size range of all domestic cats. Implants suitable for cats and their application techniques are described in the following sections.

24.1 Orthopedic wire

Orthopedic wire is composed of 316 L stainless steel. It is manufactured differently from pins and plates to make it more flexible and malleable. It is available in a variety of diameters, referred to as gauge (G). The 0.8-mm or 22 G wire is usually the most appropriate size to use in cats. The 0.4-mm (26 G), 0.6-mm (24 G), or 1.0-mm (20 G) wire may occasionally be preferred. Orthopedic wire is used for cerclage, hemicerclage, interfragmentary, and tension band wiring. Cerclage refers to a circle of wire that completely encircles the circumference of the bone. Hemicerclage refers to a piece of wire that is placed through holes in the bone, thus partially encircling it. A conversion chart of the metric and imperial wire and pin size system is provided in Table 24-1.

24.1.1 Cerclage and hemicerclage wiring

Cerclage wires must be placed correctly, obeying certain principles (Box 24-1). Wires placed incorrectly will loosen and disrupt blood supply. Subsequent disturbed fracture healing has given cerclage wiring a bad name. However, when used appropriately, they are a useful and economic implant for feline osteosynthesis (see Fig. 37-9, Chapter 37).

Cerclage and hemicerclage are *not* used as the sole method of fixation on any type of long-bone fracture. Most commonly, cerclage wires are combined with an intramedullary pin to repair long oblique fractures. They can also be placed under or over a plate. One study showed that it was preferable to use them under rather than over the plate (1).

There are a variety of methods for tightening and securing the wire with both cerclage and hemicerclage wiring. These include twisting the ends together or using a single- or double-loop knot. Numerous articles discuss the pros and cons and different mechanical characteristics of these different tightening techniques. The twist knot should be appropriate for most feline orthopedic procedures when the correct principles of application are applied. Wire twisters or pliers are used to form the twist. The wire should be pulled tight to the bone before starting the twist. Then, the twist is started by hand before grasping both ends of the wire with the instrument. The instrument is pulled firmly away from the bone while twisting the two ends evenly around each other (Fig. 24-1). The twist is left perpendicular to the bone when there is

Pin size			Wire
Millimeters	Inches	Fractions	gauge
0.4	0.015		24 G
0.6	0.023		
0.8	0.031		22 G
0.9	0.035		
1.0	0.039		20 G
1.1	0.043		
1.2	0.047		18 G
1.6	0.062	1/16	
2.0	0.078	5/64	
2.4	0.094	3/32	
2.5	0.098		
2.8	0.109	7/64	
3.0	0.118		
3.2	0.125	1/8	
3.5	0.140	9/64	
4.0	0.156	5/32	

Table 24-1 Pin and wire size conversion chart

Box 24-1 Principles for use of cerclage wires in feline orthopedic surgery

Use large enough diameter wire – 22 gauge or 0.8 mm is usually appropriate in cats
Apply the wire tightly – movement allows devascularization and demineralization of bone
When applying the wire use a wire passer to disturb surrounding soft tissues minimally and disrupt the blood supply to the bone minimally
Restrict the use of wires to areas where the bone can be reconstructed anatomically – they should not be used to surround unreduced fragments
Only use for oblique fractures; the length of the fracture line should be at least twice the diameter of the bone
A minimum of two wires should be placed for oblique fractures – one alone will act as a fulcrum for bending and if there is only room for one wire, this suggests that the fracture is not oblique enough to be cerclaged
Wires should be placed at least 0.5 cm from the fracture line, and a gap equivalent to between half and the entire bone diameter should be left between the wires
Wires should be placed at the narrowest part of the bone or if the bone is tapered it can be notched or a small K wire placed across the bone (skewer pin) to prevent slippage
When twisting the wire use pliers and pull away from the bone whilst twisting to ensure the wires twist evenly around each other. It should not end up with one piece of straight wire with the other piece wrapped around it, which will loosen
Cut the ends of the wires, leaving three twists or turns – a longer end than this is unnecessary and could lead to soft-tissue irritation
The twist can be left protruding perpendicular to the bone (biomechanically the better option) – unless there is little soft-tissue cover, in which case the twist should be bent over flat on the bone

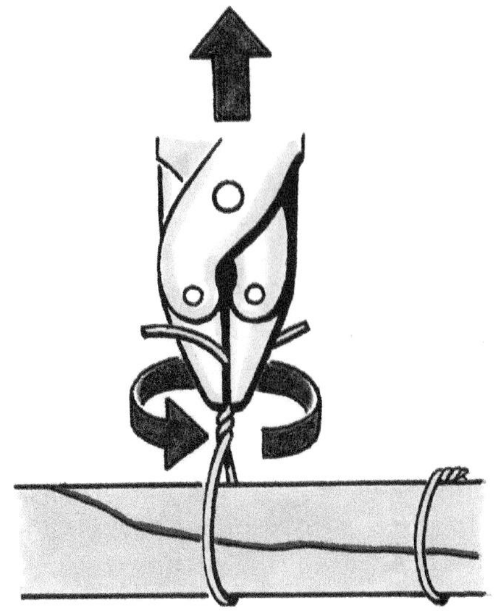

Figure 24-1 Correct application of cerclage wire requires pulling away from the bone as the wire is twisted to ensure an even twist is formed.

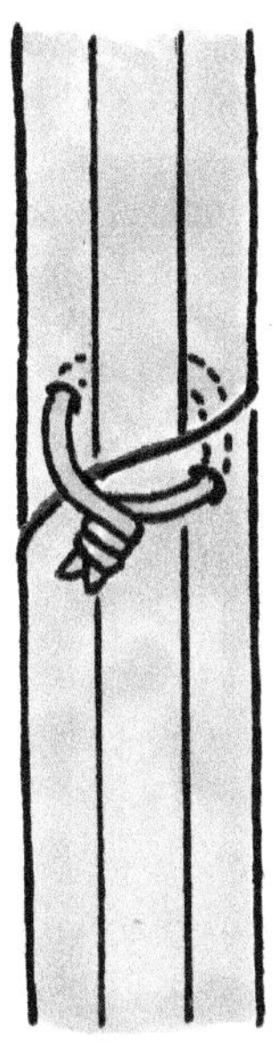

Figure 24-2 A hemicerclage wire in combination with an intramedullary nail. A thick nail is used, filling approximately 70% of the medullary cavity.

enough surrounding soft tissue to prevent irritation, and the ends are cut short, leaving three turns.

Hemicerclage is used less frequently than cerclage. Care must be taken that the wire is tightened sufficiently with this technique, and especial care should be taken when making the holes to thread the wire through so that additional fissures or fractures are not created. The wire inside the medullary canal should wrap around the intramedullary pin so when tightened the pin is pulled against the endosteum (Fig. 24-2). Hemicerclage does not add significantly to fracture stability, and the holes in the bone can weaken the bone further (2).

24.1.2 Interfragmentary wiring

Interfragmentary wires are placed through holes in bone in a manner similar to a suture. Interfragmentary wiring is used as the primary fixation device for simple fractures of the flat bones of the skull or scapular body (Fig. 24-3). They are not appropriate for full weight-bearing bones. Small-diameter wire (0.4–0.6 mm) should be selected as larger-diameter wire will be more difficult to tighten, and may cut through the thin bone.

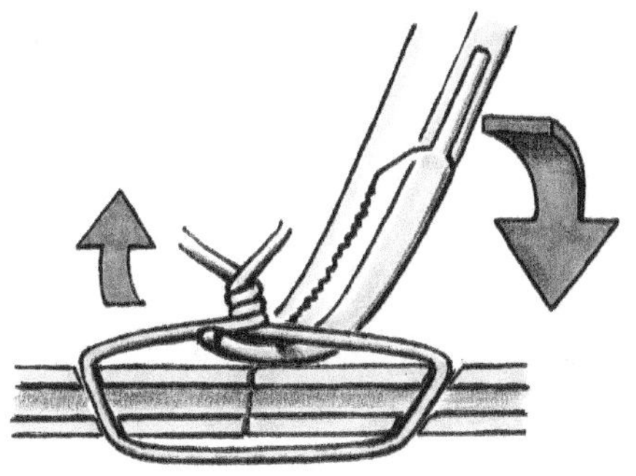

Figure 24-3 Application of an interfragmentary wire. The holes for the wires to pass through are drilled in a slightly oblique direction towards the fracture to facilitate wire insertion. The tip of a mosquito forceps helps tension the wire.

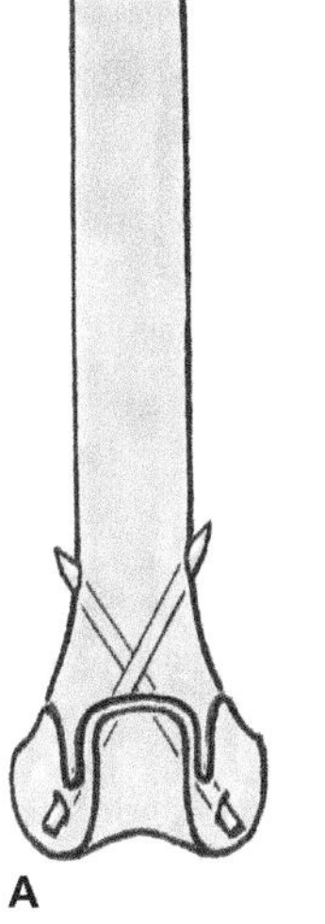

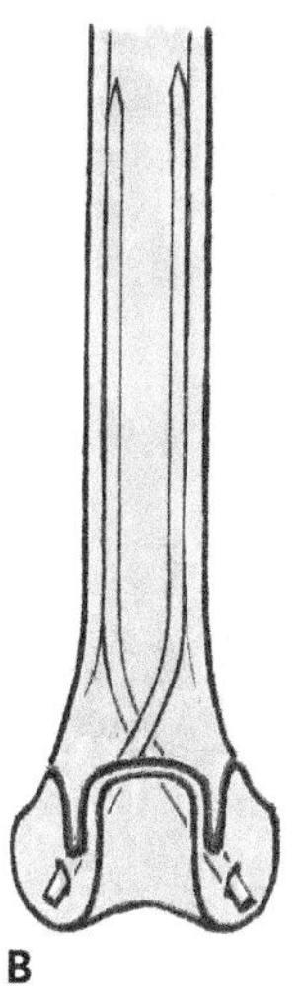

Figure 24-4 Example for (**A**) cross pinning and (**B**) dynamic intramedullary pinning of a Salter and Harris type I fracture of the distal femur.

24.2 Kirschner wires

Kirschner wires (or K wires) are semirigid pins made of 316 L stainless steel. They are available from 0.6- to 3.0-mm diameter, and their length ranges from 150 to 300 mm. Kirschner wires exist with pointed tips on one or both ends. These are usually trocar-type tips. Small Kirschner-type pins with trocar tips are also available with a threaded section, either on the end of the pin or in the center. Further details on threaded pins are described in the section on external skeletal fixation (ESF) implants, below. A conversion chart of the metric and imperial wire and pin size system is provided in Table 24-1.

Kirschner wires can be applied for many indications and purposes in feline orthopedics. Smooth pins are used for intramedullary nailing, for cross and parallel pinning, for tension band fixation, and for skewer pins. Kirschner wires can also be used as transosseus pins for ESF. Most commonly, threaded pins are used for this indication.

24.2.1 Cross and parallel pinning

The main indication for cross pinning and parallel pinning is for repair of physeal fractures. Rotational stability is provided because two pins are inserted across the fracture. Cross pinning is used for Salter Harris type I and II fractures of the distal humerus, radius, femur, and tibia. Parallel pinning is indicated to repair Salter I and II fractures of the proximal humerus, distal femur, and proximal tibia, and to stabilize fractures of the femoral capital physis and femoral neck.

Appropriately sized small-diameter smooth K wires are selected according to the size of the fragment. Their size may range from 0.6 to 1.6 mm, depending on the size of the cat and fragments, and location of the fracture. The K wires are best inserted by low-speed battery drilling. Insertion with an oscillating mode is useful if this facility is available and has the advantage of preventing soft tissue from twisting around the pin during insertion. Anatomic fracture reduction is necessary to achieve sufficient stability with cross and parallel pinning. With cross pinning, care has to be taken that the pins cross above the fracture line (Fig. 24-4). Insufficient rotational stability is achieved if they cross at the level of the fracture. In oblique fractures, the pin oriented more parallel to the fracture line is inserted first to prevent distraction of the fracture.

In certain locations, such as the distal humerus or femur, the K wires are sometimes inserted too parallel to the long axis of the bone, causing the pins to glance off the inner surface of the transcortex without penetrating it. If this occurs, the pins can be advanced further proximally into the medullary cavity, similar to Rush pinning. A spring-like effect is created by enhanced contact with the inner surface of the cortex to compensate for the lack of cortex penetration. This technique has been termed dynamic intramedullary pinning (3) (Fig. 24-4).

With the right indications, few complications are encountered with cross or parallel pinning. Intraoperative complications include pin placement into a joint and subperiosteal pin placement resulting in reduced holding power. Thorough knowledge of regional anatomy helps avoid poor placement of pins. Late complications are mainly attributed to pin migration. Fracture instability should be suspected if pins migrate, and the affected pin may have to be replaced or a different implant system applied if healing is not advanced sufficiently. Because cross pins penetrate the cortex in highly functional areas near joints, it may be beneficial to remove them after the fracture has healed.

24.2.2 Skewer pin

When cerclage wires are applied on hourglass-shaped bones or around oblique fractures the use of an adjunctive K wire

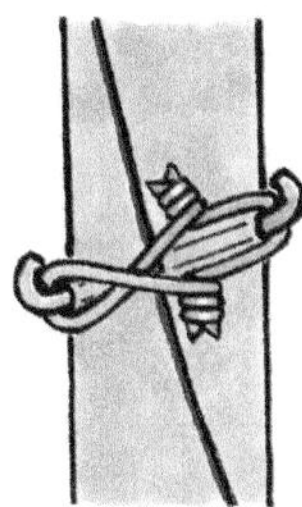

Figure 24-5 Close-up of a skewer pin. The figure-of-eight wire is anchored around the pin ends and compresses the fracture fragments.

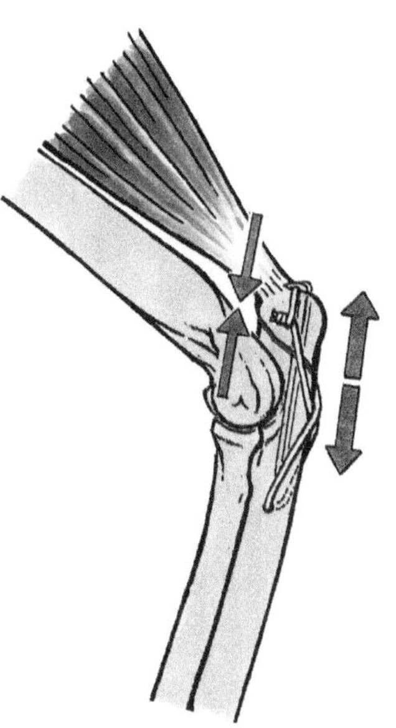

Figure 24-6 Tension band fixation of a simple proximal olecranon fracture. The wire does not cross over the fracture site.

across the bone can prevent wire slippage towards the narrower part of the bone and improve the function of the cerclage. This technique has been termed the skewer pin technique. After reduction of the fracture, a 0.9- or 1.1-mm K wire is directed across the bone, between fragments, just off perpendicular to the fracture plane. If the fracture is more transverse, the K wire must be directed at an angle between perpendicular to the long axis of the bone and the angle of the fracture. Once the K wire is inserted, either a full cerclage or a piece of orthopedic wire in a figure-of-eight fashion is positioned around it. Tightening of the wire provides some interfragmentary compression, prevents slippage of the K wire, and improves stability of the construct (Fig. 24-5). The most common clinical applications for a skewer pin are long oblique fractures of the ilium (Chapter 35).

24.2.3 Tension band fixation

A tension band wire is used to secure avulsion fractures. The tension band works on the principle that active distracting forces are counteracted and converted into compressive forces.

Tensile forces are exerted by the pull of ligaments or contraction of muscles on small fracture fragments. These fractures are termed avulsion fractures. Avulsion fractures in the cat include those of the olecranon, greater trochanter, medial malleolus, acromion of the scapula, os calcaneus, and tibial tuberosity. These tension forces can be overcome and converted into compressive forces by inserting two parallel K wires across the fragment, and a figure-of-eight tension band wire on the tension or distraction side (Fig. 24-6).

The K wires act as an anchor point for the tension band, and if two are placed, they will counteract rotational forces. The figure-of-eight wire can also be placed through a predrilled hole instead of being anchored around the pin ends. This can be advantageous as it avoids tendon compression compared to placing the wire around the pin ends, for example during the repair of olecranon fractures, and it also places the wire closer to the fracture, which makes it stronger. The principles for applying pins and tension band wires are listed in Box 24-2.

Complications include placement of the hole for the tension band wire too superficially, risking wire pull-out, placement of the K wires too close to the fracture, resulting in loss of fixation, using orthopedic wire of too small a diameter so it breaks, and compression of soft-tissue structures below the implants. Close attention to insertion technique and knowledge of regional anatomy should avoid most complications.

24.3 Intramedullary pins

Intramedullary pins are often termed Steinmann pins. Steinmann pins are larger than K wires. Similar to K wires, they are round pins composed of 316 L stainless steel. They usually have a point at both ends but are available with only one pointed end. The point is usually a trocar tip, but bayonet, diamond points, and threaded ends are also available. They are usually 250- or 300-mm long. Kirschner wires are often appropriately sized for intramedullary pinning in cats, especially in smaller bones and younger animals.

Intramedullary pinning is used for diaphyseal and metaphyseal fractures of long bones including the femur, humerus, ulna, tibia, and metatarsal and metacarpal bones. Its application, insertion, and final position cause minimal damage to the periosteal blood supply, which can be an advantage in young animals. The radius is the only long bone not suited for intramedullary pinning, as insertion of a pin would cause damage to the carpal or elbow joint. Metacarpal and metatarsal bones also do not have sites for easy insertion of intramedullary pins, but by burring a small slot in the distal end of the bone, the pins can be inserted into the medullary canal without trauma to the articular surfaces.

Intramedullary pins are well suited for resisting bending forces, but lack rotational and axial stability. They should not be used as a sole method of fixation except in the rare interdigitating transverse fracture or in very young kittens less than 3 months of age. Otherwise they should be combined with cerclage or hemicerclage wires, plates, or ESF.

Box 24-2 Principles for application of pin and tension band to an avulsion fracture

1. Reduce the fracture indirectly by extension of the joint and the use of Allis tissue forceps on the tendon or a pointed dental hook. Do not grasp the fragment itself as it is mainly composed of cancellous bone and may be crushed or fragment further
2. Place two small K wires perpendicular to the fracture and parallel to each other
3. Pins are placed through the fragment and into the parent bone until the ends just penetrate the far bone cortex
4. A transverse hole is drilled through the diaphysis distal to the fracture site at a distance approximately equal to the distance of the pins above the fragment. The hole is drilled superficially but deep enough to engage sufficient bone to prevent pull-out*
5. Large-gauge orthopedic wire is inserted in a figure-of-eight pattern through the hole and around the protruding K wires (or through a second hole in the fragment). Using two pieces of wire allows making a twist on both sides for better distibution of tension.
6. The wire is twisted using two twists until the twist is taken up. The wire should not cross directly over the tracture line.
7. The K wires are bent over, initially in a direction that will ensure they lie flat against the bone; they are then rotated over the figure-of-eight tension band wire, opposite to the pull of the wire, and the ends of the K wires are cut short
8. Tightening of the figure-of-eight tension band wire is completed and the ends are twisted and flattened prior to cutting so three or four twists remain

*The hole can be drilled and the orthopedic wire placed prior to K wire placement to prevent interference with intramedullary implants.

Although a general recommendation is to use a pin size which fills at least 70% of the medullary cavity, this applies to situations where intramedullary pins are used as the main method of fixation, for example in combination with cerclage wires. Thinner pins occupying only 30–40% of the intramedullary canal are chosen if the pin is combined with a plate or an external fixator to leave room for placement of screws or transosseous pins (4). Intramedullary pins are always inserted prior to antirotational implants. This helps in fracture reduction and alignment.

A Jacob's chuck or slow-speed battery drill is used for insertion of intramedullary pins. Pins can be inserted in a retrograde or normograde manner (Fig. 24-7). Retrograde insertion means that the insertion of the pin begins at the fracture site. The pin is retrieved from the proximal end of the bone until it is flush with the fracture. The fracture is then reduced and the pin is advanced into the distal fragment. Normograde insertion begins at one end of the bone (usually proximal). The pin is advanced to the level of the fracture, the fracture is reduced, and the pin is further advanced. Regardless of which method is used, the pin is driven distally until resistance is felt when the pin starts to touch the distal cortex or subchondral bone. Comparison with a pin of the same length helps to assess depth of insertion of the pin into the bone and thus avoid inadvertent joint penetration. It is also important to avoid overdistraction, which will create a gap at the fracture, and may predispose to delayed union or non-union, particularly in the tibia.

Normograde pinning is generally preferred, because with retrograde pinning the exit point of the pin is poorly controlled. This is especially true in the femur and tibia. Retrograde pinning of the femur carries the risk of sciatic nerve injury (5) (Chapter 37), and retrograde pinning of the tibia causes the pin to impinge on the patellar tendon (6) (Chapter 39).

Complications associated with intramedullary pins include loosening and migration, bending, and breakage. A massive embolic shower of fat occluding the pulmonary capillaries has been reported in one young cat that died during intramedullary pin advancement for a humeral fracture (7).

24.4 Interlocking nails

An interlocking nail is a stainless-steel intramedullary pin with holes in it. It is connected to the bone by implants placed through the holes, usually through the use of a temporary jig that is removed after implant placement. The advantage of this implant system is that rotation, compression, and nail migration are prevented, and the location of the nail inside the bone, close to the neutral axis, is a biomechanically advantageous position with excellent resistance to bending. Interlocking nails are the implants of choice in humans for the fixation of femoral, tibial, and humeral fractures. They have been used in cats for the stabilization of femoral, humeral, and tibial fractures (8–12). Their application in cats is limited by the size of the bone affected and the nature of the fracture. Suitable fractures are mid-diaphyseal, simple or comminuted fractures in straight bones. Distal fractures in either the humerus or tibia may not be suitable for interlocking nails because of the narrowness of the intramedullary canal, precluding placement of the pin distal enough in the bone. Interlocking nails have been used mainly for femoral fractures in cats.

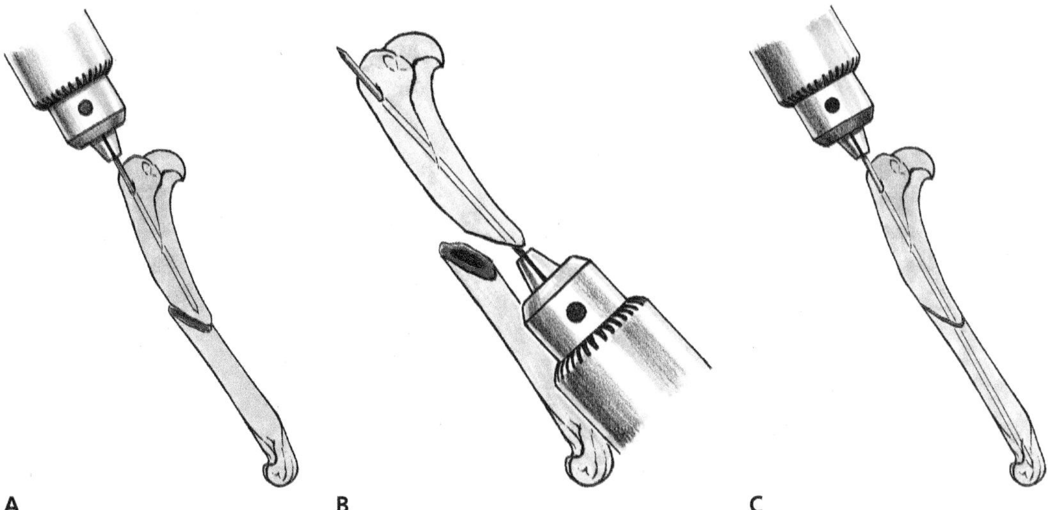

Figure 24-7 Intramedullary pinning of the humerus.
(**A**) For normograde insertion, the pin is started from the craniolateral aspect of the humerus and aimed distally and medially.
(**B**) For retrograde insertion, the pin is started from the fracture site and aimed proximally and laterally.
(**C**) For both insertion techniques the fracture is then reduced and the pin is passed from the proximal fragment into the distal fracture fragment.

24.4.1 Interlocking nail systems

Specialized equipment is necessary for placing interlocking nails in cats. Several interlocking nail systems have been reported in the literature; however, not all the systems are commercially available. The use of the veterinary interlocking nail (VIN: Numédic Company, Cholet, France) was reported in 43 cats with femoral, tibial, or humeral fractures (10). The third-generation nails for use in cats are 4 mm in diameter with a trocar tip on one end and a slot on the other to accept the removable sliding jig. They are used with specific interlocking screws with a 2-mm core. The nail has one proximal and two distal holes and is available in six lengths (92, 100, 109, 119, 130, and 142 mm). Another interlocking intramedullary nail system (INN; Mizuho Ikakogyo, Tokyo) was successfully used in femoral fractures in cats (8). These nails are 4 mm in diameter, 60, 70, 80, 90, or 100 mm in length, with holes at 10-mm intervals, and are used with 2.0-mm screws.

Another interlocking nail system (ILN) is marketed by Innovative Animal Products (Fig. 24-8). Nails suitable for cats are available in 4.0- and 4.7-mm diameter; both are used with 2.0-mm self-tapping screws or bolts. They have three to four pre-placed holes per nail, 11 mm apart. The solid cross-locking bolt has self-tapping threads below the head of the bolt that engage in the near cortex. The bolts are provided in one length and then cut to the measured bone length, which eliminates having to keep a large bolt inventory.

Additionally, a smaller 3.5-mm titanium nail (Fixomed, Munich, Germany) has recently been introduced for the repair of femoral fractures in cats (12).

Two additional devices can be used to stabilize further ILN repair of inadequately stabilized diaphyseal fractures in cats and dogs (11). The first is an axial extension for the ILN that connects to a conventional type I ESF via a short connecting bar for femoral and humeral fractures. The second is hybrid ILN bolt/ESF pins that were used to lock the ILN and serve as the transosseous pins for a type I ESF for femoral, humeral, and tibial fractures.

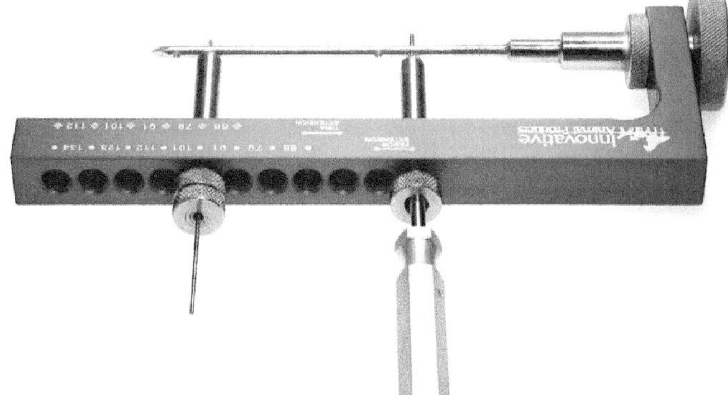

Figure 24-8 The interlocking nail system and jig (Innovative Animal Products).

24.4.2 Application principles

Specific guidelines for application are dependent on the nail system. The following description applies to the ILN system (Innovative Animal Products), which is the system with which the authors are most familiar (Fig. 24-9).

The size and length of nail are selected prior to surgery by comparing the ILN nail templates with the radiographs. A limited open approach for nail placement in the distal medullary canal is generally necessary for the upper limb bones. Closed application may be possible in the tibia, as the thin surrounding soft tissue makes palpation and fracture reduction easier. The nail is usually placed in a normograde fashion after a hole has been predrilled with a K wire. Care is taken to advance the K wire in the correct direction down the intramedullary canal. The hole is gradually enlarged using sequentially larger K wires and Steinmann pins, and finally using a reamer from the interlocking nail instrument kit. The appropriate-length and diameter nail is then placed into the bone using the insertion tool. When the nail has been inserted far enough into the bone the insertion handle is detached and replaced with the jig. Insertion sleeves are placed into the relevant hole in the jig, corresponding to the distal hole in the nail. A trocar is used to make a small notch or impression on the bone, aimed to prevent the drill bit slipping on the curved bone surface. A hole is then drilled across both cortices of the bone, using the appropriate additional drill sleeves. The direction of the drill has to be correctly oriented in the anticipated direction of the nail hole. The depth of the hole is measured and the correct-length screw or bolt (cut to length) inserted. The fracture is checked for correct rotational alignment prior to placing screws in the proximal nail. Further screws or bolts are added in a similar manner until all nail holes are filled. The jig is then detached from the bone. Additional fixation devices such as cerclage wires can be considered in simple fractures if fracture configuration is appropriate. Fewer complications are seen if additional implants are not used in comminuted fractures (10).

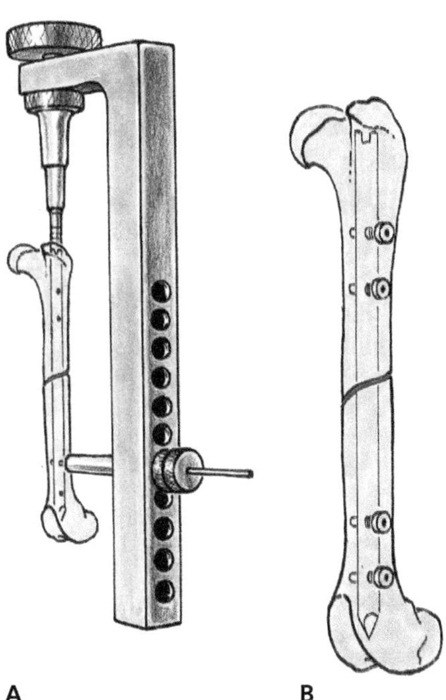

Figure 24-9 Interlocking nail insertion technique. (**A**) The nail is inserted in a normograde fashion and, with the jig in place, drill holes are made through the holes in the nail and 2.0-mm bolts are placed. (**B**) The final result after jig removal. The bolts lock the nail to the bone, preventing rotation and axial compression of the fracture and migration of the nail.

Complications with interlocking nails include delayed or non-union, missed nail holes, implant failure (nail and pin), and the windshield wiper effect where the distal piece of bone rotates on a single screw.

24.5 External skeletal fixation (ESF)

ESF is a versatile method for both fracture repair and treatment of other orthopedic conditions. The main advantages of ESF for fracture repair are preservation of blood supply in the fracture region and the possibility of closed reduction of a fracture. Opportunity for postoperative revision of fracture reduction also exists. Comminuted and open fractures are the main indications for fracture stabilization with ESF. Temporary fracture and joint immobilization, stabilization after soft-tissue repairs, correction of limb deformities, and distraction osteogenesis are other indications.

A disadvantage of ESF is morbidity due to pin tract inflammation, especially if the transosseous pins are inserted in areas with a large muscle mass or in highly mobile areas, such as near the larger joints, especially the stifle and elbow. Postoperative management is more cumbersome compared to plate osteosynthesis, and minor complications occur more frequently. Despite this, fracture fixation with ESF is a versatile method in orthopedic surgery of the cat. Different ESF systems, application principles, postoperative management, and possible complications are described in the following section.

24.5.1 Transosseus pins

Several pin types can be used as transosseus pins, including smooth K wires, negative-profile threaded pins, or positive-profile threaded pins (Fig. 24-10). Positive-threaded pins provide the best resistance to pull-out. Pins used for ESF are classified as half pins if they penetrate only one skin surface, and as full pins if they transfix the limb and penetrate two

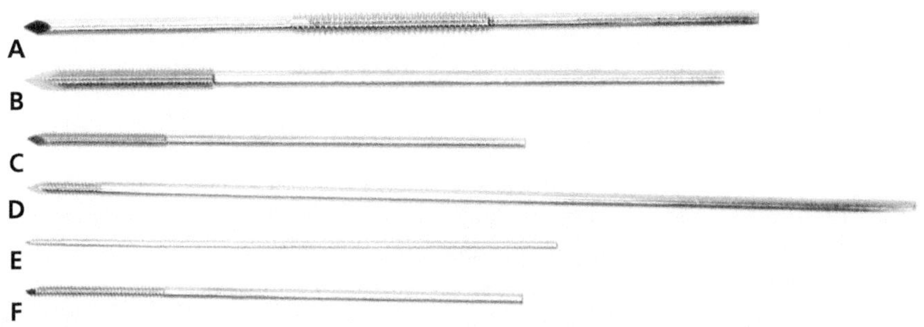

Figure 24-10 Transosseus pins. (**A**) Positive-profile centrally threaded 2.0-mm pin. (**B**) Positive-profile end-threaded 2.0-mm pin. (**C**) Positive-profile end-threaded 1.6-mm pin. (**D**) Negative-profile threaded 1.6-mm pin. (**E**, **F**) Negative-profile 1.2-mm pins with different-length threaded portions.

skin surfaces. Positive-threaded half pins only have a thread at the end of the pin, whereas positive-threaded full pins have their thread in the center.

Negative-profile threaded pins are available with 1.2–2.0-mm outer diameters. Although the thread provides improved bone-holding power compared to smooth pins, the thread–pin interface is a weak point of these pins, making them prone to bending or breakage if placed incorrectly. To avoid this complication, the short threaded tip of the pin should only engage the transcortex so the thread–pin interface is located inside the medullary cavity, where it is protected from bending or breaking.

Pins where the threaded section is larger than the core size of the pin are known as positive-profile pins. Pins with a core diameter of 1.6–2.4 mm can be used in cats. These pins do not have the stress riser or weak point at the pin–thread junction but they are slightly more expensive than the negative-profile pins. The size of the overall pin, including the thread, must be considered when used in a cat. Using too large a pin of more than 25% of the width of the bone can result in iatrogenic fracture.

24.5.2 External skeletal fixation systems

Several different ESF systems are available for feline orthopedics. They differ with regard to implant sizes, costs, ease of application, overall stability, and indications (Table 24-2).

Kirschner Ehmer external skeletal fixation system

The original small Kirschner Ehmer (KE) system is still widely used in cats (Fig. 24-11). Single clamps are designed to accommodate transosseous pins up to 2-mm diameter and a 3-mm bar (Table 24-3). Double clamps designed to connect two bars are also available. The KE ESF has been used successfully for both fracture repair and transarticular ESF in cats. The system is relatively simple but has some disadvantages compared to some of the newer ESF systems, including the necessity to pre-place all clamps on the bars prior to ESF assembly, and the inability to place large positive-profile threaded pins through the pre-placed clamps. These disadvantages have been largely overcome by the introduction of split clamps and KE plus clamps, respectively.

SK external skeletal fixation system

A widely used system in the USA is the IMEX miniature SK ESF system (13) (Fig. 24-11). The single pin-gripping clamps and double clamps for rod-to-rod articulations are made of aluminum. They accommodate a 3.2-mm stainless-steel connecting rod and 0.9–2.5-mm diameter transfixation pins (Table 24-3). The stainless-steel rods can be cut to the desired length and can be contoured. To tighten the clamps, 7-mm wrenches are needed. The miniature SK ESF is a stable system usable for both fracture repair and transarticular ESF. One of its main advantages is the relatively large size of connecting rod. Larger connecting rods have been shown to have a positive effect on overall frame stiffness, if fewer than two full pins are used (14). This means that simpler frames can be applied with the SK ESF system compared to other systems with sustained stability. Simpler frames have the advantage of causing less morbidity from the interaction of the pins with the musculature.

Meynard external skeletal fixation system

An ESF system widely used in Europe is the Meynard system (15) (Fig. 24-11). The Meynard clamps are inexpensive and are available in three sizes. They each accommodate variable pin and external bar sizes (Table 24-3), which makes the system quite versatile for different indications, including transarticular ESF. The holding power of the clamps has been shown to be inferior to others, and the large size of the clamps limits the closeness of adjacent pins, but the system has been applied with good clinical results in cats (15).

Tubular external skeletal fixation system (FESSA)

The tubular ESF (FESSA: Medical Solution) is widely used in cats in some countries in Europe (16, 17). It consists of a stainless-steel tube, designed for use as a type 1 ESF. The tubes are available in 6-, 8-, and 12-mm diameters in various lengths, but the 6- and 8-mm tubes are mainly used in cats (Table 24-3). The external tube has four rows of holes along its longitudinal axis. The non-threaded holes accommodate the transosseous pins, and the opposing threaded holes accommodate set screws for securing the pins (Fig. 24-12). An Allen key is supplied to tighten the screws. The main advantages of the system are the stable but light-weight tube, and the possibility of inserting a large number of transosseous pins of different diameters over a small distance. Six pins can be inserted over a distance of 15 mm with the 6-mm tube, whereas only three screws can be inserted in the same area with a 2.0-mm DCP (17). There are also no clamps, which are usually the weak link in an external fixator. Fractures with small metaphyseal or epiphyseal fragments are ideal indications for the tubular ESF.

The maximum outer pin diameter that can be inserted through the tubes is 2 mm for the 6-mm tube, and 2.5 mm for the 8-mm bar (Table 24-3). With the exception of the first pin, which can be inserted before the tube is placed on to it, only smooth or negative-threaded pins can be used with the 6-mm tube, because even the smallest positive-threaded pins do not fit through the holes. It is advantageous to use at least a few negative-profile threaded pins (Ellis pins) to enhance pull-out strength as the pins are usually placed perpendicular

System	Advantages	Disadvantages	Indications
Kirschner Ehmer system	Readily available Simple to use Lighter and less bulky than SK clamps	Cannot add positive-profile threaded pin through preplaced clamps unless use KE plus clamps Cannot add or remove clamps from middle of bar	Fractures Transarticular fixation
SK external skeletal fixator	Versatile Stable clamps Large connecting bar allows use of simple constructs Threaded bar for distraction osteogenesis and circular rings for hybrid frames available	Heavy weight Too large for immature cats	Fractures Transarticular fixation Distraction osteogenesis
Meynard system	Inexpensive Versatile Usable with all types of transfixation pins All types of constructs possible	Clamp stability Clamps bulky, limiting closeness of pins	Fractures Transarticular fixation
Tubular external skeletal fixator (FESSA)	Light weight No large clamps More transosseous pins can be inserted over a small distance compared to other systems	Pins have to be inserted perpendicular to external tube Only non-threaded or negative-threaded pins fit through holes (with the 6-mm tube)	Fractures of straight bones Ideal for distal metaphyseal fractures of tibia and radius and ulna
Acrylic pin external fixator (APEF)	Economic Light weight Radiolucent Pins can be inserted from different angles and no limit to closeness	More difficult to remove frame or adjust it	Transarticular frames Mandibular fractures Radius and ulnar fractures
Ring fixator	Small pins cause minimal morbidity Useful for small epiphyseal fragments Combine with linear fixator to make hybrid frames	Technically more difficult to apply Requires specialized equipment	Lower-limb fractures or joint injuries Small epiphyseal/ metaphyseal stabilization

Table 24-2 Disadvantages and advantages of the external skeletal fixation systems used in cats

to the bar and parallel to each other. Smaller pins, however, can be inserted obliquely through adjacent holes (Fig. 24-12). An additional adaptation is that the 6-mm tubes can be inserted and connected to the 8-mm tube, and connectors are available to assemble two tubes at an angle (Fig. 24-13).

Acrylic external fixator systems

An alternative to clamps and bars is to replace them with acrylic (Fig. 24-14). The small APEF system (Innovative Animal Products) has a 15-mm diameter column designed for cats and toy breed dogs. This system has the advantage that pins can be placed from any direction, there is no maximum pin size that can be used (Table 24-3), positive-profile threaded pins can easily be placed, and the frame is light and relatively radiolucent. Disadvantages include increased difficulty in adjusting the fixator postoperatively, and implant removal involves cutting the pins or the acrylic bar.

IMEX miniature circular external skeletal fixation system

The IMEX miniature circular ESF system is specifically designed for small patients, including toy breed dogs and cats. A ring ESF system is especially useful for fractures with

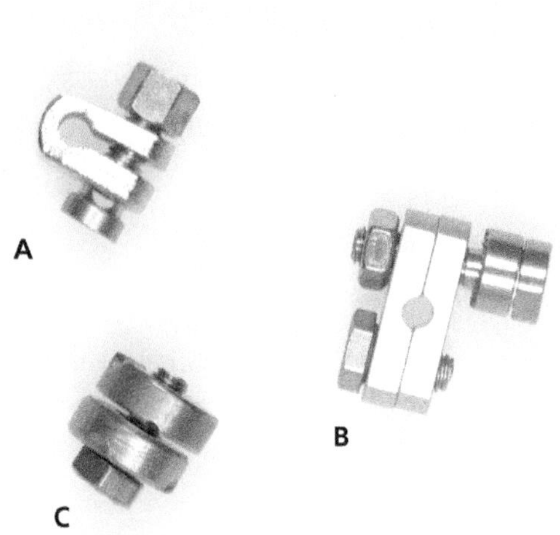

Figure 24-11 Clamps from different external fixation systems.
(A) Kirschner Ehmer (KE) clamp.
(B) SK external skeletal fixation clamps.
(C) Meynard external skeletal fixation clamp.

a small fragment close to a joint. Using a ring fixator enables two small pins to be placed into a small fragment close together in a similar plane, but from different angles. The two pins are then secured to the ring using SK clamps. The full aluminum rings are slotted for freedom in wire position and they can be cut at holes to convert into arches or half-rings. Most often 1-mm stopper wires with trocar point are used for cats and small dogs. A wire tensioner is not necessary with miniature frames.

The completed ring can be connected to further rings, which may be indicated for correction of limb deformities. A ring can also be connected to a linear frame, using mini hybrid rods. The combination of a ring with the linear system is called a hybrid frame.

24.5.3 Application principles

ESFs may be applied after closed or open reduction of the fracture. The ESF should be designed to have appropriate

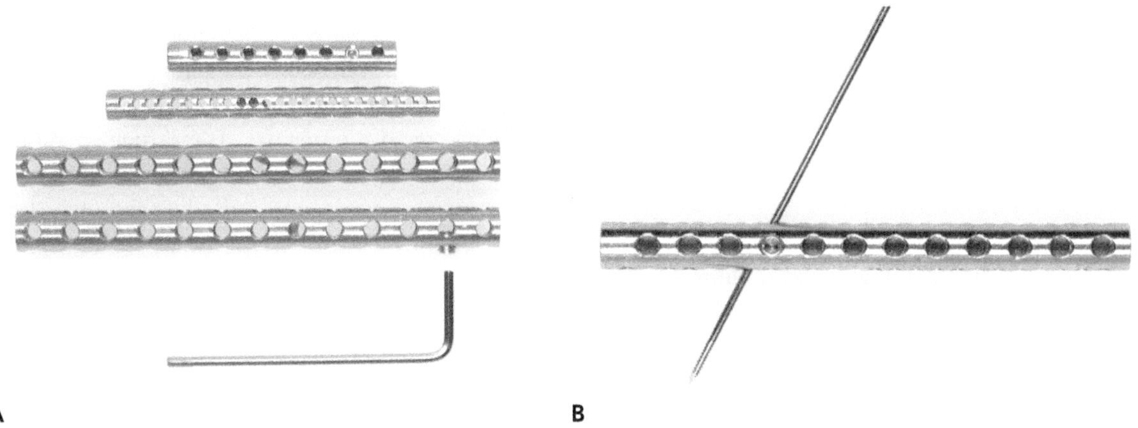

Figure 24-12 The FESSA tubular external skeletal fixation system.
(A) Two different lengths of the 6-mm tube and the 8-mm tube are shown. The screws are tightened to hold the pins secure using an Allen key.
(B) It is possible to angle small pins through two adjacent holes in the tubular bar, but normally the pins are inserted perpendicular to the bar.

System	Clamps	External bar	Pin sizes
Kirschner Ehmer (KE) clamps	Small KE clamps	3 mm	Up to 2.0 mm (the smallest size varies)
SK external skeletal fixator	Mini SK clamps	3.2-mm	0.9–2.5 mm
Ring fixator	Mini SK clamps	4-mm threaded rod	1 mm
Meynard system	Meynard clamps	K wire or Steinmann pin	All sizes
Tubular external skeletal fixator (FESSA)	Screws	6-mm external tube 8-mm external tube	Maximum pin size 2.0 mm Maximum pin size 2.5 mm
Acrylic systems	Acrylic or epoxy putty clamps	Acrylic bar or stainless-steel bar	All sizes

Table 24-3 Size guide for the different external fixation systems used in cats

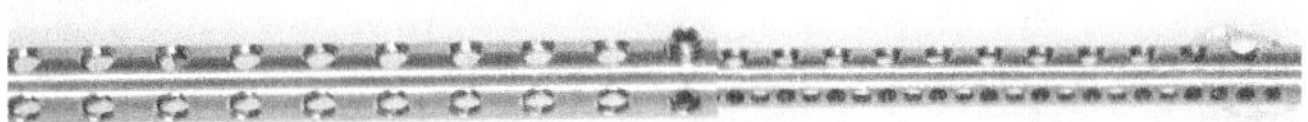

A

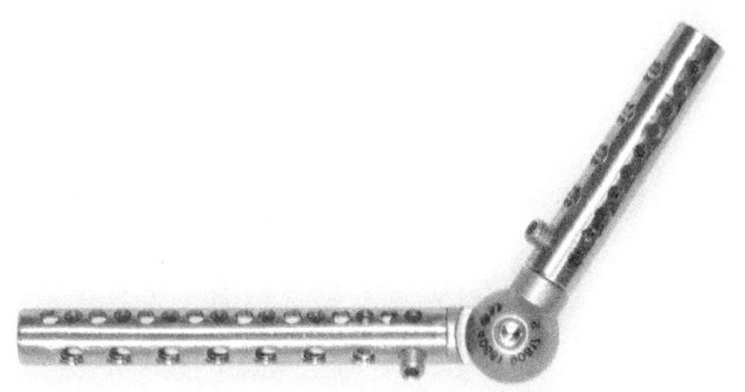

B

Figure 24-13 Options for connecting the FESSA tubes. (**A**) The 6-mm tube can be inserted into the 8-mm tube, allowing insertion of a larger number of pins even in very small fragments. (**B**) Tube connectors allow angulation of the tubes for use in a transarticular fashion.

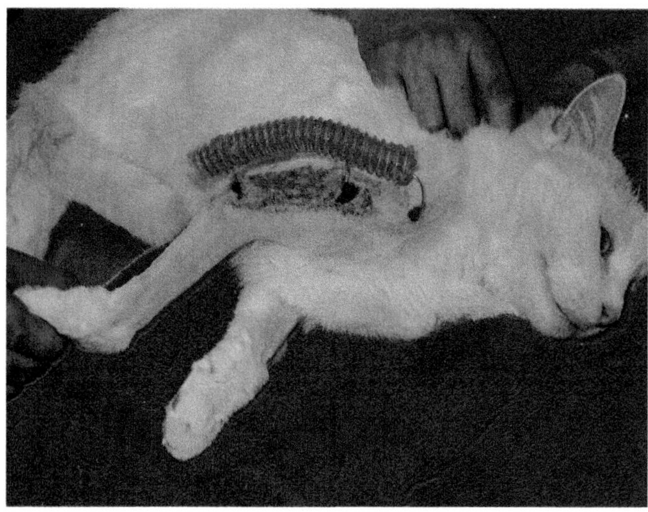

Figure 24-14 Polymethyl methacrylate (PMMA) in plastic tubing, forming the external skeletal fixation bar, on a cat with a humeral fracture. (Courtesy of Erick Egger.)

stability for the severity of the fracture and the anticipated healing time. Frame stability depends on several variables, such as frame configuration, number of pins inserted per fragment, pin size and length, and location and size of the connecting bar. Unilateral (type Ia), unilateral biplanar (type Ib), bilateral (type IIb), and bilateral biplanar (type III) frames are increasingly stiffer (Fig. 24-15). A type I construct provides sufficient stability in many feline fractures, especially if a large connecting bar is used. Low-stiffness frames were used in radial and tibial fractures (1a, 1b, 2b) in cats with no fixation failure (18). Bilateral frames have the disadvantage that the transosseous pins have to be inserted through areas with large muscle mass, which may cause morbidity. They should therefore only be used in heavy cats and in fractures which are expected to heal slowly. Insertion of an intramedullary pin and connecting its end to the external bar is another option to enhance frame stability (19) (Fig. 24-16). This tie-in configuration is especially useful in fractures of the humerus and femur (20, 21).

Techniques for increasing stiffness of the ESF construct are listed in Box 24-3. The number of pins influences ESF stability, which increases when up to four pins are used per fragment (22). A minimum of two pins per main fracture fragment should always be used. Pins are placed according to the far–near, near–far principle. The stiffness of a pin is inversely proportional to the third power of pin length; the external bar is therefore placed as near as possible to the skin to reduce pin length.

Using transosseous pins with a diameter of 20–25% of bone diameter is generally recommended. Pins are inserted in the areas with the least muscle mass and should not interfere with joint and muscle function. The pin–bone interface is the weakest point in most ESF constructs. Holding power of the pins is influenced by pin type and insertion technique. The use of threaded pins enhances the pin–bone interface and therefore pin-holding strength (23). Smooth pins should be inserted with an angle of around 70° to the long axis of the bone to reduce the risk for pulling out of the bone. Thermal and structural damage to the cortex during pin insertion is reduced by predrilling a hole with a drill bit and by inserting the pin using low-speed power drilling (24). Predrilling is recommended for positive-threaded pins, and is performed with a drill bit 10% smaller than or the same size as the core diameter of the pin.

The first pins to be inserted are the most distal and proximal ones. The ESF bar is then connected to the first two pins. Clamps have to be pre-placed with the KE system. With other systems additional clamps can be added to the frame as more transosseous pins are placed. The clamps are tightened around the first two pins and bone alignment and fracture reduction are checked. Additional pins are added to the bone, alternating between the distal and proximal fracture fragments. Limb alignment is constantly reassessed. Skin tension around pins should be checked at the end of surgery by flexing and extending the leg. Any tension or skin puckering around the pin insertion site should be eliminated by enlarging the skin incision.

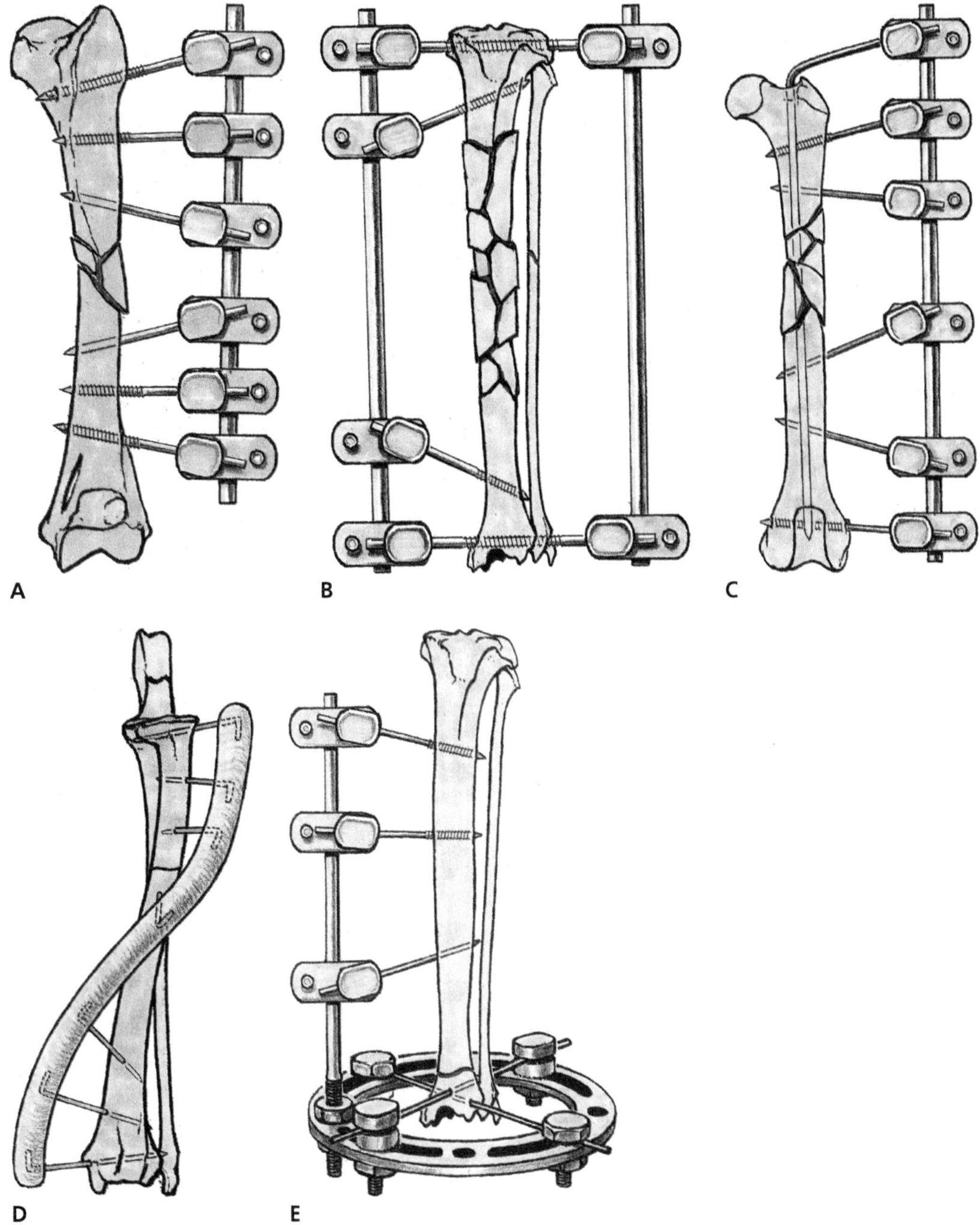

Figure 24-15 External skeletal fixation frame types useful in cats.
(**A**) Type Ia – unilateral.
(**B**) Type IIb – bilateral.
(**C**) Tie-in configuration.
(**D**) Freeform.
(**E**) Hybrid ring fixator.

Knowledge of local anatomy and a drill sleeve must be used to protect surrounding soft tissues and avoid damage to nerves and vessels.

24.5.4 Postoperative treatment and complications

Gauze sponges are placed around the pins, between the skin and the external bar to prevent infection of the pin tracts and to stabilize the soft tissues around the pins. A bandage is applied to cover all metal. The bandage is changed 2–3 days after surgery and then removed. The pin insertion sites are cleaned from debris with a diluted povidone-iodine or chlorhexidine solution. After several days, granulation tissue forms within the pin tracts, resulting in an enhanced resistance to infection. Bandages are then left off and the sharp pin ends and clamps are covered with strips of self-adhesive bandage.

Complications after ESF occur in up to 100% of cases according to the literature (25). The majority of complications are minor and do not interfere with fracture healing and outcome. Pin tract drainage is the most common complication. Minor pin tract drainage consists of serous secretion around the pin entrance site, only minimal inflammatory signs, and no patient discomfort. Major pin tract drainage includes excessive and/or purulent discharge, significant inflammatory signs, and patient discomfort. Secondary infection is present and affected pins might be loose. In rare cases the infection progresses to a focal osteomyelitis, visible as excessive periosteal reaction, cortical lysis, and increased intramedullary density on radiographs. The main cause of pin tract drainage is a loose pin or motion of soft tissues around the pin. Excessive motion causes tissue necrosis and an environment for potential infection. Pins should therefore be inserted without tension on soft tissues. Threaded pins give improved purchase in bone and are less likely to loosen and pull out. Treatment of minor pin tract drainage consists of cleaning of the pin entrance site, application of topical antiseptic or antibiotic solutions, and stabilizing bandages. If major pin tract drainage is present it is likely that the pin is loose and affected pins need removal; antibiotics alone will not usually solve the problem.

Pin loosening causes pin tract discharge and patient discomfort. Pins are considered loose if they can be turned by hand. Premature pin loosening can be secondary to inadequate pin insertion techniques, or to an unstable fracture repair causing excessive stress at the pin–bone interface. Also, continuous motion due to delayed fracture healing can cause pin loosening over time. Loose pins are removed and additional ones placed if fracture healing has not advanced sufficiently.

Pin breakage during insertion or at a later date has mainly been associated with the use of negative-threaded pins and occurred in more than 10% of pins in one study (17). Another study looked at Ellis pins in 70 dogs and cats and found no problems with any of the pins when used appropriately, with the thread–pin intersection located inside the medullary cavity (26). Adequate-sized smooth or positive-threaded pins rarely break. Affected pins have to be replaced if fracture stability is not sufficiently advanced.

Iatrogenic fractures through pin holes are rare, but can occur if oversized pins are used, if pins are placed too close together, too close to the fracture, or if they are inserted through pre-existing fissure lines. Antebrachial fractures, transarticular fixators, and animals having had previous revision surgery or more than one injured limb were at increased risk of fracture after ESF in one study (Langley-Hobbs, unpublished data). Unrestricted activity of the patient can also predispose to fracture.

Box 24-3 Methods of increasing stiffness of external skeletal fixators

Use four pins maximum per fracture fragment
Use biggest pin possible but not more than 25% of bone diameter
Place pins in a near–far fashion
Angle pins to reduce pin pull-out
Use positive-profile pins
If using negative-profile pins, place thread pin interface inside bone
Place bar close to bone
Bilateral/biplanar > bilateral > unilateral (type III > type II > type I)
Clamp should be oriented with nut/bolt closest to leg
Predrill holes to minimize loosening
Consider fracture biomechanics and design frame appropriately

24.6 Bone screws

The small size of feline bones limits the sizes of screws that can be used. Appropriate screw sizes usually are 1.5, 2.0, 2.4, and 2.7 mm. Even smaller screws, such as 1.0 or 1.3 mm, are indicated for small or thin bones, for example the metacarpi, toes, or maxilla. In general, the screw size selected should not be greater than 20–25% of the bone diameter to avoid a risk of iatrogenic fracture. Only cortical screws are used, as cancellous screws are not available in small-enough sizes. Screws are available as self-tapping or non-self-tapping screws. Table 24-4 details the different screw sizes and drills to be used for placing the screws.

Self-tapping screws are designed so that once a pilot hole is drilled into bone, they can be inserted by simply screwing them in. A thread does not need to be cut. The pilot hole is

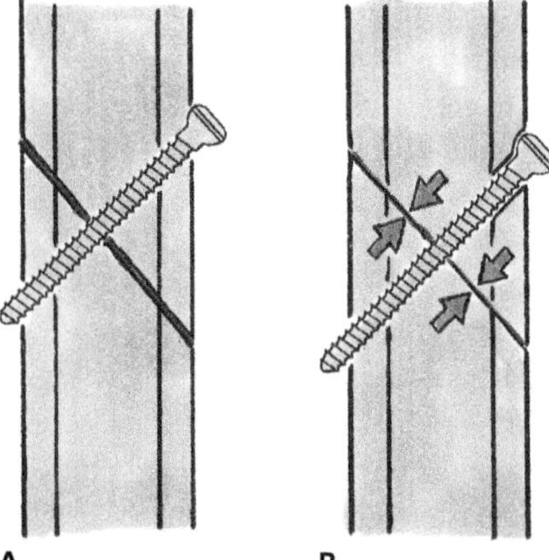

Figure 24-16 (**A**) A position screw engages both bone cortices and is usually used through a plate hole. With a lag screw (**B**), the thread only engages the far cortex. This results in interfragmentary compression as the screw is tightened.

Screw type	Cortex self-tapping and non-self-tapping			
Screw diameter (mm)	1.5	2.0	2.4	2.7
Drill bit (mm) for glide hole	1.5	2.0	2.4	2.7
Drill bit (mm) for thread hole	1.1	1.5	1.8	2.0
Tap (mm) for non-self-tapping screws	1.5	2.0	2.4	2.7

Table 24-4 Summary of commonly used screw sizes in cats and their appropriate drill bits and taps

somewhat larger than the core of the screw. Because the screw has to cut its own thread as it is inserted, it encounters resistance, particularly in thick cortical bone. Theoretically, the resistance during screw insertion may be such that the torque required to drive the screw is greater than the tolerance of the screw and the screw may break, especially with very small screws. The bone that compacts around the screw during insertion can improve pull-out resistance, an advantage in both osteopenic patients and cancellous bone. If removed carefully the screw can be reinserted, but care has to be taken not to place the screw in a different angle or it will cut a new thread.

Non-self-tapping screws require a predrilled pilot hole, followed by careful cutting of a thread in cortical bone with a tap that corresponds exactly to the profile of the screw thread. As the thread is cut with the same-size tap as the screw thread, the thread has a deeper bite into bone, but it is still important that the screw is carefully inserted into the tapped hole. The low resistance to insertion generates less heat. It is easy to remove and replace screws as necessary.

24.6.1 Plate screws

Bone screws are most commonly applied in conjunction with plates. Bicortical screws are usually used for securing bone plates to the bone. The technique for insertion involves drilling an appropriate-sized hole through both bone cortices. Then, with the plate in position, the depth of the hole is measured using a depth gauge. A screw is selected that is either at least as long as the measured depth or 2 mm longer than the measured length to ensure that the threads on the screw adequately engage the far or trans cortex. The screw is inserted until it is finger-tight. It is recommended to retighten each screw three times after application of all screws into the plate.

24.6.2 Positional screws

Positional screws engage both cortices and do not result in interfragmentary compression (Fig. 24-16). Positional screws can be used to secure fracture fragments together, although lag screws are usually used for this purpose. Insertion of a positional screw can be safer in very small fragments, where drilling of the larger gliding hole would carry a risk of creating fragmentation of the smaller piece of bone. In this situation the fracture line should be compressed with bone-holding forceps prior to screw insertion.

24.6.3 Lag screws

The thread of a lag screw only engages the far or trans cortex, but not the near or cis cortex. The bone fragments are therefore compressed together as the screw is tightened (Fig. 24-16). The main clinical indication for lag screws is interfragmentary compression of intra-articular fractures. Oblique diaphyseal fractures or fractures with large bone fragments can also be reduced and stabilized with lag screws. Lag screws are preferable to cerclage wires because they provide better interfragmentary compression. A lag screw can also be placed through a plate hole. Lag screws can also be used as an alternative to a tension band (see section above), but most feline avulsion fractures are small, and the presence of a gliding drill hole and pressure from the screw head can cause further fragmentation of the small piece of bone. Screws are never used in isolation for repair of diaphyseal fractures.

To insert a fully threaded screw as a lag screw, the near cortex must first be drilled with a hole equal in size to the diameter of the screw threads, meaning that the screw threads do not engage the near cortex. This is called the glide hole. An insert guide is then placed in the glide hole to ensure that the hole in the far cortex is drilled at the correct angle. A drill bit equal in diameter to the screw core is then drilled in the far cortex with the fragments in anatomic reduction. This is the thread hole. The corresponding thread is cut into the far cortex, and the screw is inserted.

The lag screw must be inserted in the middle of the fragment equidistant from the fracture edges, and directed at a right angle to the fracture plane to achieve maximal interfragmentary compression. Shearing forces are introduced during tightening of the screw if the screw is not inserted perpendicular to the fracture plane, and the fragments will shift. Screws inserted at right angles to the fracture plane

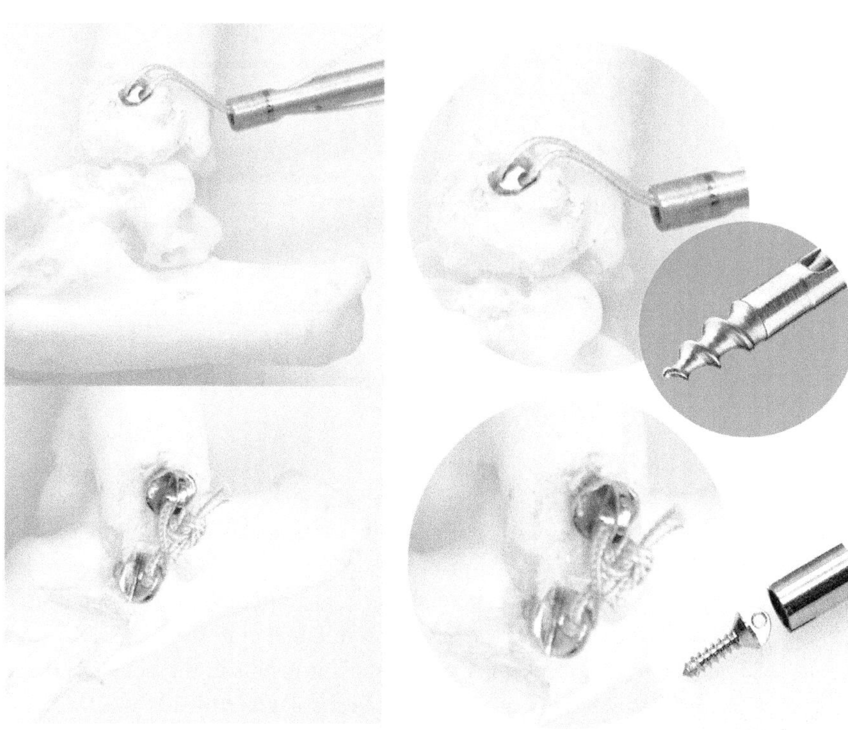

Figure 24-17 Suture anchors shown separately and in situ in plastic bone models.

Suture anchor	Size (mm) × length	Drill bit size (mm)	Size of hole for suture or suture size	Additional equipment
Screw and washer	1.5, 2.0, 2.7	1.1, 1.5, 2.0	Any	Tap and screwdriver
Bonebiter	2.0	1.5	5 braided or 50 lb	Combination driver set
	5.0	2.5	80 lb	
IMEX suture anchor	4.0 × 6 mm	2.7	1.1 mm	Suture anchor driver Suture anchor tap
Arthrex – bioabsorbable PLLA screw	3.0 × 8 mm	–	2-0	Insertion tool
Suture screw – Veterinary Instrumentation	2.0 × 6 or 10 mm	1.5	1.0 mm	Insertion tool – 2.0 mm
	2.7 × 8 or 14 mm	2.0	1.5 mm	Insertion tool – 2.7 mm

Table 24-5 Summary of suitable suture anchors for use in cats

provide maximum interfragmentary compression but minimal axial stability. A screw inserted at 90° to long axis of bone provides maximum axial stability but can cause shift of fragments. Therefore, when using more than one screw it is best to have the first screw perpendicular to the fracture line, and the second one perpendicular to the long axis of the bone.

24.6.4 Suture anchors

Suture anchors are used for securing ligament prostheses to bone, for reattachment of joint capsule, or anchoring avulsed tendons. They are usually small metal implants that are placed in drill holes in the bone. They are either designed to lie completely under the bone, therefore causing no interference to joint range of motion, or they protrude slightly from the bone and the suture is threaded through the protruding eye (Fig. 24-17). Suture anchors have been used in cats for cruciate surgery, collateral ligament ruptures, elbow and coxofemoral luxation, and tendon avulsions. There are several different designs available and some of the smaller sizes of these designs are suitable for use in cats (Table 24-5). Alternatively, a small conventional screw, with or without washer, can be used with the suture anchored around the screw head.

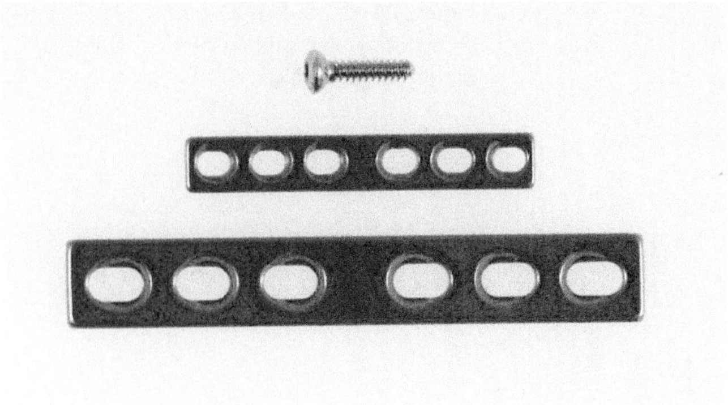

Figure 24-18 Dynamic compression plates. 2.0-mm DCP, 2.7-mm DCP, and 2.0-mm screw shown as a size guide.

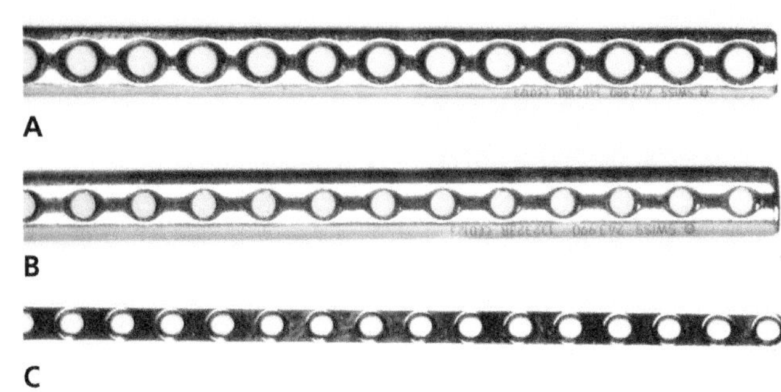

Figure 24-19 Veterinary cuttable plates. (A) 2.0/2.7 mm; (B) 1.5/2.0 mm; and (C) 1.5 mm.

24.7 Bone plates

One of the primary aims and objectives in the treatment of fractures is early return to full function of the injured limb. Bone plates are ideal for accomplishing this goal because they are applied internally and have the potential to restore rigid stability to the reconstructed fractured bone.

24.7.1 Types of plate

Several types of plate are available. They differ regarding strength and shape, design of the plate holes, and indications. Most of the plates described below are used for fracture repair, and some of them have been designed for specific locations and fracture types. Specific plates are also available for arthrodesis and stifle joint surgery.

Dynamic compression plates

The 2.0- and 2.7-mm DCPs (Fig. 24-18) are both used in feline fracture repair, but have their limitations. The 2.7-mm plate used with 2.7-mm screws is often too big for all but the largest cats and the largest cat bones, like the femur. The distance between screw holes in the 2.7-mm plate also limits the number of screws that can be inserted into a fragment. The 2.0-mm is usually too small, short, and weak for diaphyseal fractures in cats. The 2.0-mm plate is available in two thicknesses. Plates with six holes or fewer are only 1.0 mm thick and very weak. Plates of 7–12 holes in length are available in 1.5-mm thicknesses. The thicker plates are significantly stiffer.

There is a new plate, the 2.4-mm limited contact-dynamic compression plate (LC-DCP). This is available in both titanium and stainless steel and is used with 2.4-mm screws. Titanium is slightly weaker than stainless steel and can bend if used as a buttress plate for diaphyseal cat fractures. The stainless-steel 2.4-mm plate is a very useful implant for feline diaphyseal fracture repairs.

The design of the screw holes in DCPs is based on the spherical gliding principle developed by AO and patented by Synthes. The spherical screw head glides towards the center of the plate as the screw is tightened, until the deepest portion of the plate hole is reached. This results in the bone fragment attached to the screw being displaced towards the fracture, which results in compression of the fracture line. The DCP drill guide accommodates two guides at each end of the instrument – the neutral (green) or load (gold). A maximum of four screws can be inserted in the load mode for each plate, so when the 2.7-mm plate and the load guide are used, the fracture is compressed approximately 0.8 mm for each screw inserted, giving a maximum amount of compression of 3.2 mm. With the 2.0-mm plate the fracture is compressed 0.6 mm for each screw, inserted in a load fashion, giving a maximum of 2.4 mm of compression.

Veterinary cuttable plates

The veterinary cuttable plate (VCP) (Fig. 24-19) has rapidly become popular, filling a gap in the market for long-bone fracture repair in cats. It comes in two main sizes, 2.0/2.7 mm and 1.5/2.0 mm, and each plate is designed to take two different cortical screw sizes. There is also a 1.5-mm plate that only takes 1.5-mm screws. The standard uncut length of either size plate is 300 mm. The 1.5/2.0-mm plate is 1.0 mm thick and the 2.0/2.7-mm plate is 1.5 mm thick. Both plates are 7 mm wide. The holes are round and equally spaced in all plates and all sizes. A small amount of compression can be achieved by drilling the screw hole slightly eccentrically and away from the fracture line.

The plates were developed because the 2.0-mm DCP plates were often too short or too weak and the 2.7-mm too thick, too wide, or the 2.7-mm screws too large for small bone fragments (exceeding 25% of bone diameter and thus weakening the bone). The distance between screw holes in the 2.7-mm plate also limits the number of screws that can be inserted into a fragment.

The stiffness of cuttable plates can be enhanced by stacking two plates of the same size or two plates of different sizes. This gives five different thicknesses and stiffnesses (Table 24-6). The thicker and longer plate is placed adjacent to the bone. Screw size is determined by the largest screw that will fit the smaller plate. Stacking can be full-length (both plates same length) down to half-length, where the upper plate is half the length of the lower plate. However, when using plates of different lengths it can be difficult to place screws in the holes in the lower plate adjacent to the cut end of the plate. Stacked plates should be contoured simultaneously by placing a screw through both plates, at each end, to prevent sliding of plates relative to each other during contouring. The cuttable plate has been compared to the stiffness of other small bone plates (27) (Table 24-7). Single and stacked VCPs were stiffer than miniplates accepting 1.5 and 2.0 mm screws, but less stiff than the 2.7-mm DCP.

Veterinary cuttable plates (mm)	Thickness (mm)	Width (mm)	Length (mm)
1.5/2.0	1.0	7	300
2.0/2.7	1.5	7	300
1.5/2.0 and 1.5/2.0	2.0	7	300
1.5/2.0 and 2.0/2.7	2.5	7	300
2.0/2.7 and 2.0/2.7	3.0	7	300

Table 24-6 The veterinary cuttable plates, sizes and lengths when used alone or stacked

The cuttable plate can be easily cut through a plate hole to the desired length using standard pin cutters. It can also be customized into a hook plate (28). These can be very useful for very distal or proximal epiphyseal or avulsion fractures with small fragments to reduce.

The cuttable plate has been used successfully in many fractures, including long-bone repair in cats and for pelvic fracture repair. The ability to place many screws within a short distance is very useful in multifragmented fractures and often makes the bone plate construct stronger than a larger plate with fewer screws.

Reconstruction and adaptation plates

Reconstruction plates (Fig. 24-20) are characterized by notches between the holes which allow the plates to be contoured in three planes so they can be bent, twisted, and curved to allow accurate contouring and reconstruction to awkwardly shaped bones like the pelvis or mandible, and in the vicinity of joints. The notches make them weaker than a similar-size DCP so care should be taken when using them in areas with high load. They should not be used as buttress plates. They are available as 2.7-mm plates and a thinner version, called an adaptation plate, is available in the 2.0-mm size.

Acetabular plates

The 2.0-mm acetabular plate may be of use in acetabular fractures in cats. Sizes 0 and 1 take 1.5- and 2.0-mm screws (Fig. 24-21). However the feline pelvis has quite a straight,

Plate(s)	Screw (mm)	Stiffness (N/mm) (SD)
1.5-mm straight miniplate	*1.5*	*67 (10.8)*
2.0-mm DCP	*2.0*	*134 (12.7)*
2.0-mm straight miniplate	*2.0*	*190 (23.2)*
1.5/2.0 VCP	1.5	340 (10.4)
1.5/2.0 VCP	2.0	356 (13.3)
2.0/2.7 VCP	2.0	542 (31.5)
2.0/2.7 VCP	2.7	578 (30.6)
1.5/2.0 VCP + 1.5/2.0 VCP	**1.5**	**600 (9.0)**
1.5/2.0 VCP + 1.5/2.0 VCP	**2.0**	**638 (21.2)**
1.5/2.0 VCP + 2.0/2.7 VCP	**2.0**	**828 (32.0)**
2.0/2.7 VCP + 2.0/2.7 VCP	**2.0**	**938 (50.6)**
2.0/2.7 VCP + 2.0/2.7 VCP	**2.7**	**1066 (46.6)**
2.7-mm DCP	*2.7*	*1507 (30.5)*

DCP, dynamic compression plate; VCP, veterinary cuttable plate.
Normal font, VCPs; *italics,* other plates; **bold,** stacked VCPs.
Reproduced with permission from Fruchter AM, Holmberg DL. Mechanical analysis of veterinary cuttable plate. Compend Continuing Educ 1991;4:116–119.

Table 24-7 Calculated slopes (stiffness) from the force versus displacement curves of 13 bone plate and screw combinations

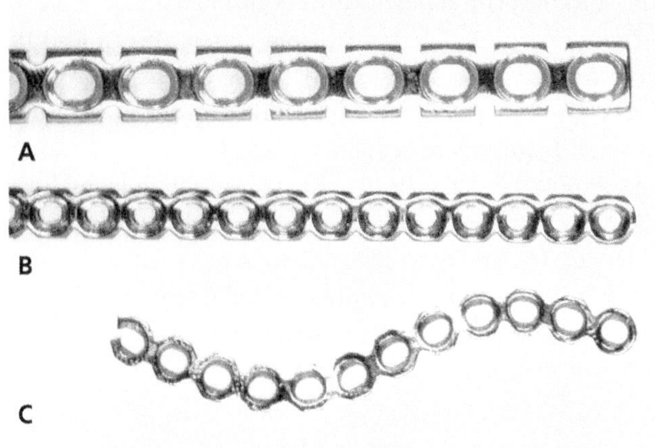

Figure 24-20 Reconstruction and adaptation plates. (**A**) 2.7 mm; (**B**) 2.0 mm; (**C**) 1.5 mm.

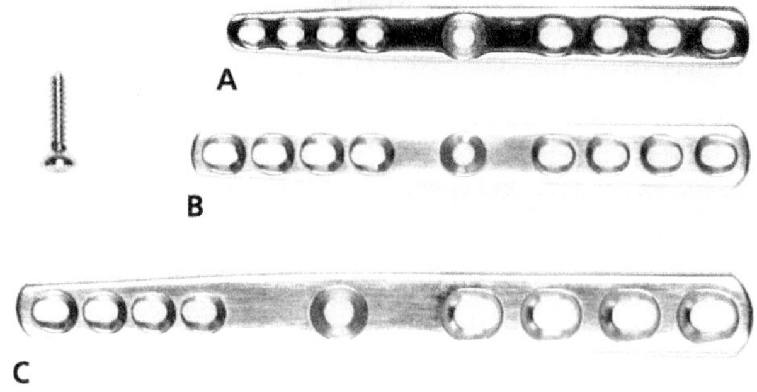

Figure 24-22 Pancarpal arthrodesis plates. (**A**) 1.5/2.0 mm; (**B**) 2.0/2.0 mm; and (**C**) 2.0/2.7 mm. A 2.0-mm screw is shown for size comparison.

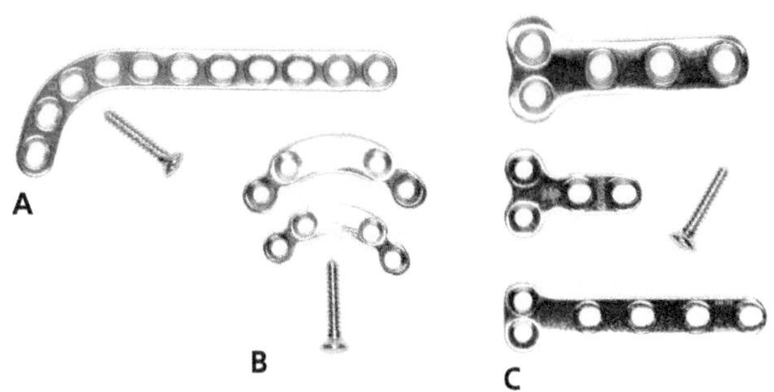

Figure 24-21 Miniplates with specialized shapes. (**A**) The 2.0-mm supracondylar distal femoral plate; (**B**) size 0 and 1 acetabular plates; (**C**) finger T plates and a 1.5-mm/2.0-mm AO T-plate. 2.0-mm screws are shown as a size guide.

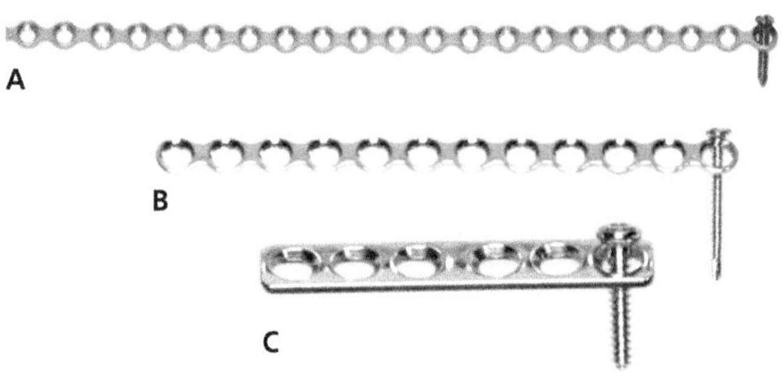

Figure 24-23 Miniaturized plates. These plates are cuttable, and the screws are self-tapping. (**A**) A 1.0-mm maxillofacial miniplate; (**B**) a reconstruction plate of the 1.3-mm Compact Hand system; (**C**) a 2.0-mm dynamic compression plate for comparison.

flat dorsal surface and straight plates also work well in this area.

Distal femoral plate

Distal femoral plates have been designed to match the caudal curvature of the lateral aspect of the femoral condyle (Fig. 24-21). The plate is indicated for repair of supracondylar femoral fractures, and facilitates insertion of screws into the small distal fragment.

Pancarpal arthrodesis plate

Dependent on patient and bone size, the 2.0/2.7, 2.0/2.0 or the 1.5/2.0 mm pancarpal arthrodesis plate (Fig. 24-22) can be used in cats for both pancarpal arthrodesis and pantarsal arthrodesis.

Miniaturized plates

A minifragment plate is a general description for plates designed for use with 2.0- and 1.5-mm cortex screws. They are available as straight mini-DCP, round and oval hole miniplates, mini L-plates, mini T-plates (Fig. 24-21), or cuttable plates. Indications include repair of long-bone fractures in small cats, repair of articular fractures, and stabilization of pelvic, metacarpal, metatarsal, and digital fractures (29). Veterinary T-plates are available in 2.0-mm sizes that take 2.0- or 1.5-mm screws, useful for fractures with a small epiphyseal fragment such as distal radial, tibial fractures, and scapular neck fractures.

The application of even smaller plates and screws is desirable for some indications in feline orthopedics. Specialized miniplates are available from human hand and maxillofacial implant systems. The cuttable 1.3-mm reconstruction plates from the Compact hand system (Synthes) are an appropriate size for repair of fractures of the maxilla, carpal, and tarsal bones, metacarpi, metatarsi, and digits (Fig. 24-23). A 1.0-mm drill bit and a cruciform screwdriver are used to insert the 1.3-mm self-tapping screws.

Another system that can be used for stabilization of very small and thin bones is the 1.0-mm Compact maxillofacial miniplate system. This consists of a variety of preshaped

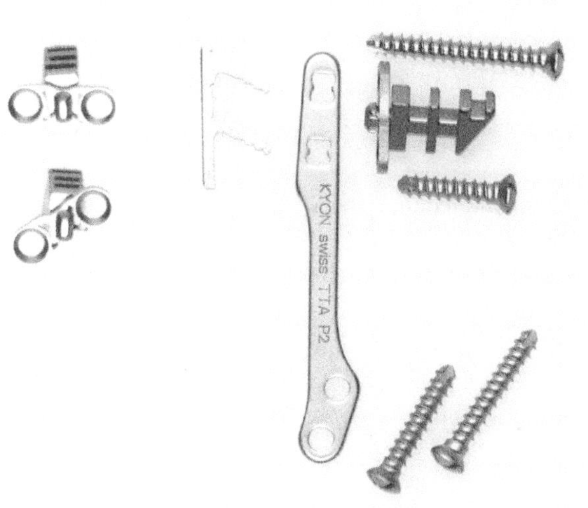

Figure 24-24 Implants designed for management of cats with cranial cruciate ligament deficiency. Tibial tuberosity advancement plate with corresponding prongs and screws.

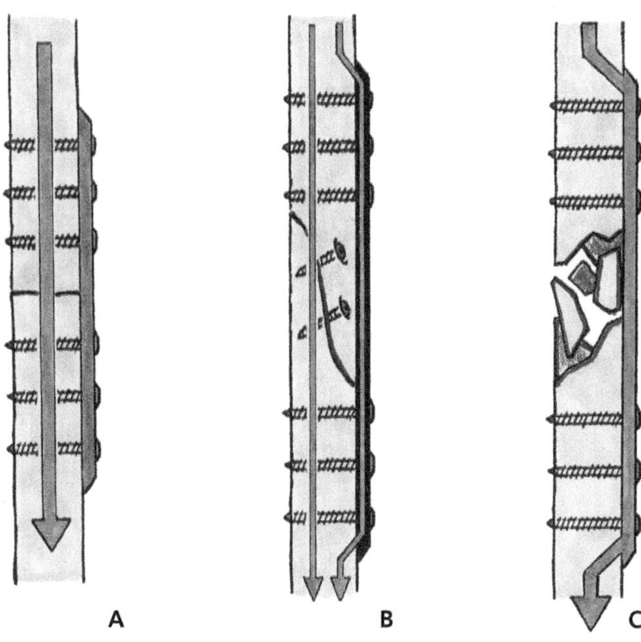

Figure 24-25 The three basic functions of plates. (**A**) Compression function; (**B**) neutralization function; (**C**) buttress function.

titanium reconstruction plates, including cuttable plates (30). The corresponding screws are self-tapping and require a 0.7-mm drill bit for the core hole and a cruciform screwdriver to insert them. Emergency screws with a thread diameter of 1.2 mm are also available for use when the smaller screw threads strip in the bone. These plates are too weak to withstand bending forces, so they are strictly used on the tension side of a fracture. Indications for their application are the same as for the 1.3-mm Compact Hand plates, but the 1.3-mm plate is stronger and offers more bending stability.

Tibial tuberosity advancement (TTA) plates

Plates have been specially developed to stabilize the tibial tuberosity after its osteotomy and are known as TTA plates (Fig. 24-24). The technique is indicated to treat cranial cruciate ligament ruptures or patellar luxation. These plates act as a tension band and can also be employed to stabilize osteotomies and avulsion fractures of other apophyses, such as the greater tubercle of the humerus, the olecranon, and the greater trochanter.

The plates are made of pure titanium. A fork with prongs is adapted to be inserted into holes at the proximal part of the plate. A branch connects the proximal part of the plate with the distal part, where two holes for screw fixation are present. The smallest plate with only two prongs and two holes for 2.4-mm screws is indicated for cats. The holes for the prongs are first drilled with a 2.0-mm drill bit angled distally into the piece of bone to be stabilized. The branch part of the plate can be contoured to fit the surface and shape of the bone. The plate is secured to the main fragment with 2.4-mm self-tapping titanium screws after drilling the screw holes.

A bone spacer of 3.5 mm is used to advance the tibial tuberosity to treat cranial cruciate ligament deficiency in cats (Chapter 38).

Tibial plateau leveling osteotomy (TPLO) plates

A specific plate (Fig. 24-25) designed for TPLO, a procedure for the treatment of cranial cruciate ligament rupture, has been used successfully in cats with cranial cruciate rupture. The 2.0-mm plate is suitable for cats. It has six holes, three in the nose or proximal end, which are oval-shaped to allow compression, and three round holes on the straight aspect. It is designed to fit the shape of the proximal tibia after contouring. It can be used after cranial closing wedge osteotomy or after creation of a circular tibial plateau osteotomy. The plate is made of stainless steel. Locking titanium TPLO plates are also available.

24.7.2 Principles of plate application

Plates for fracture repair should be applied using the tension band principle, with the plate being applied on the tension side of the bone. This gives the benefit of dynamic compression, especially after full reconstruction of the bone. The plate should span the length of the bone for optimal load sharing between the plate and implants, and it should be contoured to the shape of the bone to maintain anatomic reduction.

Table 24-8 Bone plates for feline orthopedic surgery, their indications and sizes

Size of plate	Plate type	Indications
2.7	Dynamic compression plate	Diaphyseal fractures of the femur, humerus, and tibia
	Reconstruction plate	Distal femoral fractures
2.4	Limited-contact dynamic compression plate	Diaphyseal fractures of the femur, humerus, and tibia
2.0	Dynamic compression plate, miniplate with oval holes	Diaphyseal fractures of the radius, femur, humerus and tibia, arthrodeses, pelvic fractures
	Veterinary cuttable plates (2.0/2.7 and 1.5/2.0 mm)	Fractures of the long bones (femur, humerus, tibia, and radius)
		Pelvic fractures
	Reconstruction plate	Acetabular fractures, flat-bone fractures
	Acetabular plate	Acetabular fractures
	T- and L-miniplates	Flat-bone fractures
		Fractures with small epiphyseal fragments
1.5	Miniplate with round holes	Skull fractures, metacarpal and metatarsal fractures
1.3	Compact Hand plates	Skull fractures, metacarpal and metatarsal fractures
1.0	Titanium micro maxillofacial plate	Facial fractures – mandibular and maxillary

Bending and twisting are usually necessary. Pre-stressing the plate is advisable for simple transverse fractures as it aids in minimizing the gap on the far or trans cortex and aids in compressing the fracture site. This is achieved by leaving a very small gap of less than 1 mm between the plate and bone at the fracture site. Selection of proper plate size and screws is important: too weak an implant will bend or break, whereas too large tends to destroy blood supply and result in bone necrosis and soft-tissue damage. Table 24-8 gives appropriate plate and screw sizes to use in feline bones.

An absolute minimum of two screws or four cortices is applied either side of a fracture, but where possible a minimum of three screws or six cortices should be aimed for. It is usually preferable to use the longest plate possible to distribute the load better and avoid stress risers at the ends of the plate. It is not necessary to fill every plate hole but screws should be inserted in a near–far manner with screws placed close to the fracture and at the proximal and distal aspects of the bone. The minimum distance a screw is placed from the fracture line should be at least the diameter of the screw.

The fracture may lend itself to lag screws being inserted through plate holes. The size of screw to use is dictated to a certain extent by the plate; for example, the 2.0-mm screws are used with 2.0-mm plates. The holding power of a screw diminishes, and the risk for iatrogenic fracture increases, as the diameter of the screw approaches 40% of the diameter of the bone, so use of too large a screw is not recommended. The 2.0- and 2.4-mm screws are generally recommended in all except the largest cats and bones (e.g., the femur), where 2.7-mm screws may be used. Avoid leaving a single empty screw hole over the fracture. This will act as a stress riser and the plate may fatigue and break at this point.

Plates may be applied to achieve one of the following three functions (Fig. 24-25).

Compression plate

Static compression is achieved by the application of a self-compressing technique with a DCP (Fig. 24-25). This aids in improved load sharing of the fracture fragments, and improves fixation stability. Fractures suitable for applying axial compression include simple transverse fractures or short oblique fractures with an angle of less than 45°.

During weight-bearing every bone has a tension and compression side (Table 24-9). Dynamic compression results from the muscular tension across the bone during weight-

Bone	Tension side
Femur	Lateral
Tibia	Cranial or medial
Humerus	Cranial or lateral – proximal humerus
	Caudal or medial – distal humerus
Radius	Craniomedial or cranial
	Medial – distal radius
Ulna	Caudal – proximal ulna (olecranon)

Table 24-9 The tension sides of the long bones

bearing, when the plate is applied to the tension side of the bone. This is known as the tension band principle. Therefore, plates are preferably applied to the tension side of the bone.

Neutralization plate

A neutralization plate is applied to the tension side of the bone, after the fracture is reduced and stabilized by other means to neutralize or overcome the torsional, bending, compressive, or distraction forces to which the fractured bone may be subjected during healing (Fig. 24-25). Interfragmentary compression is applied prior to plate application by lag screws or cerclage wires that are used to reconstruct the cylinder of bone. Fractures suitable for neutralization plates include oblique or multifragmentary fractures that can be anatomically reconstructed.

Buttress plate

A buttress plate is used to shore up fragments of bone, whilst maintaining bone length and orientation of the main fragments (Fig. 24-25). Fractures suitable for plates applied in buttress function are unreconstructable or severely comminuted fractures. A relatively larger and longer plate is selected when the plate is being used in buttress function. The implants should be applied in a manner that minimally disturbs the blood supply to the bone. The plate is precontoured with the help of radiographs of the normal bone and a cat skeleton. It can be inserted through small stab incisions in the skin, and is then slid under muscle bellies and secured to the proximal and distal ends of the bones, taking care to achieve correct rotational alignment. This technique is also known as minimally invasive plate osteosynthesis (MIPO) or biological plating.

24.7.3 Postoperative treatment and complications

Complications are rare after adequate plate osteosynthesis. Implant failure, iatrogenic fracture, delayed union and non-union, and osteomyelitis are possible complications (Chapter 13). Plate breakage is rare in cats. Screw pull-out or plate bending are more likely complications.

Indications for plate removal are listed in Box 24-4. It is important not to remove plates too early, or refracture may occur. This is when a fracture of bone occurs in a region of a previous fracture that appears to have undergone sound union both clinically and radiographically. It commonly results from premature implant removal.

Box 24-4 Indications for bone plate removal

- Plate is loose or broken
- Plate causes irritation when it ends close to a joint
- Plate acts as a thermal conductor causing lameness in cold weather
- Plate causes stress protection or interferes with the vascular supply to the bone, resulting in osteoporosis under the plate
- Plate crosses a growth plate in an immature cat
- Plate causes irritation – lick granuloma occasionally seen with superficial plates
- Infection – if the fracture is stable then the plate should be left in place until healing has occurred prior to plate removal
- Plate causes a stress riser and there is concern that the bone will fracture at the plate–bone junction
- Routine removal – some surgeons will routinely remove the plate once the bone has healed – this should generally not be done sooner than 5 months after fracture repair in an adult animal

24.8 Internal fixators

Internal fixators, or locking plates, have gained popularity in both human and veterinary surgery (31, 32) during the last few years. Internal fixators have a locking mechanism between the plate hole and the screw heads, resulting in a stable fixation and fixed angle of the screw heads in the plate. This has several advantages over conventional plates. The inherent stability between the screws and the plate renders screw loosening less likely, and allows insertion of fewer screws and monocortical screws with sustained stability. Additionally, the plate is not pressed on to the underlying bone during screw insertion, thus preserving periosteal blood supply, and reducing or eliminating pressure necrosis of the cortex. Because the plates can be applied with a small gap between the bone and plate, precise plate contouring is less critical for maintaining fracture reduction, and less tissue dissection is required to apply the plate. Overall, this technique is more rapid than conventional plating, partly because self-tapping screws are used.

Indications for application of internal fixators for long-bone fractures include fractures in young cats with softer bones, older cats with osteopenia, comminuted fractures, fractures in the vicinity of joints, and for treatment of complications, especially if vascularity is poor. Stabilization of complex fractures with two plates placed orthogonally on the diaphysis or metaphysis is rendered possible by inserting monocortical screws. Other applications are pelvic fractures, and certain spinal fractures and/or luxations (32, 33). Internal fixators can also be used for temporary splinting of intertarsal fractures and instabilities (34), and for carpal and tarsal arthrodeses.

24.8.1 Internal fixator systems

Despite the numerous advantages of internal fixators, the high implant costs have prevented widespread use of these implants so far. A system from human surgery, which has been used by the authors in over 100 feline cases, is described in detail below. Other locking plates have recently become available at reduced costs for veterinary use (Königsee Implantate, Kyon). Application principles for these implants may vary slightly depending on the design of the plate holes and screw heads, the use of self-tapping or non-self-tapping screws, and plate strength.

Unilock mandible locking plates

The 2.0/2.4 Unilock mandible locking plate system (Synthes) was originally designed for mandibular surgery in humans. The locking mechanism consists of a thread in the plate hole and a corresponding thread on the screw head (Fig. 24-26). Both locking and non-locking screws (screws with and without a threaded head) can be used through the same plate holes. All screws are self-tapping. The plates are reconstruction plates and are available in different forms and lengths. They can also be cut and bent in three dimensions. The implants are made of titanium, reducing the risk of infection.

The 2.0-mm plate comes in three different thicknesses, 1.0, 1.3, and 1.5 mm, which all accept the same 2.0-mm locking and non-locking screws (Fig. 24-27). Non-locking emergency screws with a diameter of 2.4 mm can also be inserted if a smaller screw thread strips in the bone. The 2.0-mm plates are mainly used for the repair of metaphyseal long-bone fractures, pelvic fractures, intertarsal instabilities, carpal and tarsal arthrodeses, and spinal fractures.

The 2.4-mm plates are 2.5-mm thick (Fig. 24-28). Two different sizes of locking screws can be inserted, 2.4- and 3.0-mm screws, but the 2.4-mm screws are mainly used in cats. Non-locking 2.4-mm screws and non-locking emergency

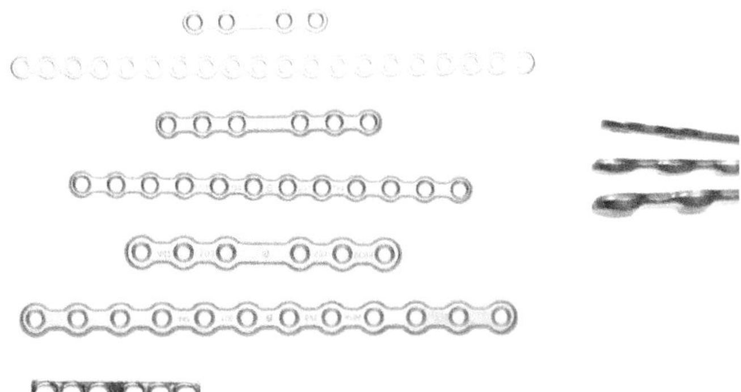

Figure 24-27 A selection of 2.0-mm Unilock plates. They are available in three different thicknesses that are all used with 2.0-mm screws. The 1.3- and 1.5-mm thick plates are used most commonly. A 2.0-mm dynamic compression plate is shown for comparison.

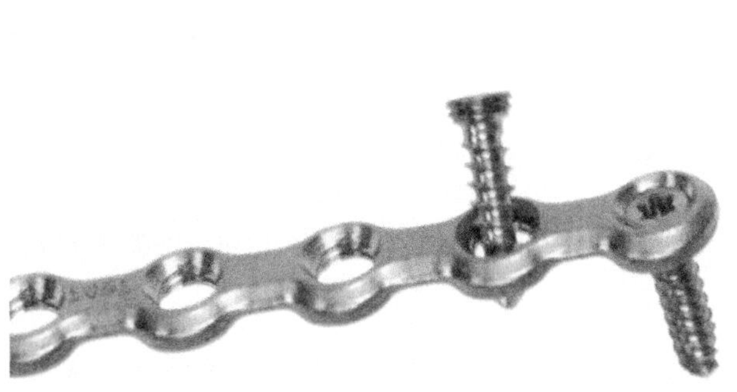

Figure 24-26 A 2.0-mm Unilock plate and the locking threaded head screw. The threaded screw heads engage into the threaded plate hole once the screw is fully inserted.

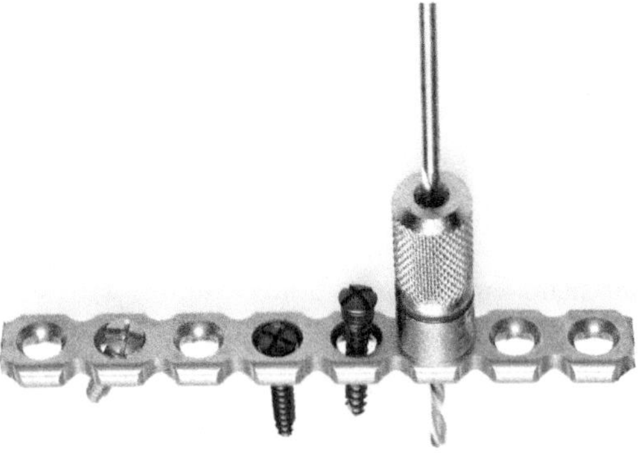

Figure 24-28 A 2.4-mm Unilock plate. The purple screws have a threaded head, allowing engagement into the threaded plate hole. The special drill guide shown is needed to ensure screw insertion perpendicular to the plate. The golden screws do not have a threaded head, and can be angled like conventional screws.

screws with a diameter of 2.7 mm are also available. The 2.4-mm plates are suitable for osteosynthesis of diaphyseal long-bone fractures.

A 1.5-mm drill bit is required for the 2.0-mm screws, and a 1.8-mm drill bit for the 2.4-mm screws. Because the screw heads have a cruciform recess, a corresponding cruciform screwdriver is used. The locking screws must be inserted perpendicular to the plate to achieve maximal locking stability. This is performed with the help of a special threaded drill guide, which centers the drill precisely over the plate hole (Fig. 24-28).

24.8.2 Application principles

The application principles described here are based on recommendations from human medicine and on a retrospective evaluation of consecutive clinical cases with long-bone fractures, stabilized with the Unilock system (Voss, unpublished data).

The plates are only roughly contoured to the shape of the bone. Repeated bending back and forth should be avoided, because it weakens the titanium plates. The plates can be applied with a small gap between the implant and the bone to avoid compression of bone and periosteum and allow for ingrowth of vessels. Gaps larger than 1 or 2 mm should be avoided. The reduced contact between plate and bone allows preservation of the periosteum and soft-tissue attachments in the fracture area. Internal fixators are most commonly used in buttress function for the repair of comminuted fractures. Screws are then only inserted into the main proximal and distal fragments. Internal fixators can also be applied in neutralization function in the presence of simple transverse fractures, or after interfragmentary compression of long oblique fractures with a lag screw.

Positioning of the plate over the bone has to be carefully maintained while inserting the first locked screw, because the locking screws cannot be angled as in conventional plates. The first screw is only fully tightened after partial insertion of a second screw to avoid rotation of the plate during screw tightening. Based on clinical experience with the 2.4-mm Unilock system, two screws per main fragment result in sufficient stability for the treatment of long-bone fractures. A third screw may be added if there is enough room.

The holes for the locking screws are drilled perpendicular to the plate using the special drill guide shown in Figure 24-28. The self-tapping locking screws can be inserted both monocortically and bicortically. As a rule of thumb, monocortical screws are used in the diaphysis of long bones, where a thick cortex is present. Bicortical screws are inserted in soft bone, such as the cancellous bone of the epiphysis and metaphysis of long bones, and also in the diaphysis of immature cats, where screw pull-out is more likely. Bicortical screws are avoided in the diaphysis of older cats, as iatrogenic fissures or fractures may occur. The advantage of monocortical screw placement is particularly beneficial for avoiding screw insertion into joints or the spinal canal. In areas where angling of the screws is necessary, for example to avoid penetration of a joint, a non-locking screw can still be inserted through the plate hole. Monocortical screws also allow placement of two plates perpendicular to each other, or on the medial and lateral aspect of the bone.

24.8.3 Postoperative treatment and complications

Complications are rare after application of the Unilock system. Implant failure was not observed in a series of consecutive clinical cases of cats with long-bone fractures (Voss, unpublished study). Screw pull-out may occur if the screws have not been fully seated in the bone, for example if they only engage the cranial or caudal edge of a cortex. This problem may occur unnoticed during surgery, because the surgeon's feel for the screw-holding power in the bone during tightening of the screw is not as good as when conventional screws are used. A locked screw has a stable appearance after tightening, even if not inserted into bone at all.

Iatrogenic fractures/fissures may occur in the diaphysis of older cats if bicortical screws are inserted. A possible reason for this complication is that shear forces may be created in the transcortex during screw tightening and locking of the screw heads in the plate holes. Therefore only monocortical screws should be used in the diaphysis of older cats with brittle bones. For the same reason, care is also taken if the internal fixator is used together with an intramedullary pin. The screws are forced to lock perpendicular to the plate during tightening, which creates shear forces when the screw tips touch the intramedullary pin. In cats even the shortest 6-mm long screws are often too long to be inserted without coming into contact with the pin.

References and further reading

1. Willer RL, et al. Comparison of cerclage wire placement in relation to a neutralisation plate. A mechanical and histological study. Vet Comp Orthop Traumatol 1990;3:90–94.
2. Roe SC. External fixators, pins, nails, and wires. In: Johnson AL, Houlton JEF, Vannini R (eds) AO principles of fracture management in the dog and cat. Switzerland: AO Publishing; 2005.
3. Whitney WO, Schrader SC. Dynamic intramedullary cross pinning technique for repair of distal femoral fractures in dogs and cats: 71 cases. J Am Vet Med Assoc 1993;191: 1133–1138.
4. Hulse D, et al. Effect of intramedullary pin size on reducing bone plate strain. Vet Comp Orthop Traumatol 2000;13: 185–190.
5. Withrow SJ. Sciatic nerve injuries associated with intramedullary fixation of femoral fractures. J Am Vet Med Assoc 1977;13: 562–568.

6. Payne J, et al. Comparison of normograde and retrograde intramedullary pinning of feline tibias. J Am Anim Hosp Assoc 2005;41:56–60.
7. Schwarz T, et al. Fatal pulmonary fat embolism during humeral fracture repair in a cat. J Small Anim Pract 2001;42:195–198.
8. Endo K, et al. Interlocking intramedullary nail method for the treatment of femoral and tibial fractures in cats and small dogs. J Vet Med Sci 1998;60:119–122.
9. Larin A, et al. Repair of diaphyseal femoral fractures in cats using interlocking intramedullary nails: 12 cases (1996–2000). J Am Vet Med Assoc 2001;219:1098–1104.
10. Duhautois B. Use of veterinary interlocking nails for diaphyseal fractures in dogs and cats: 121 cases. Vet Surg 2003;32:8–20.
11. Basinger RR, Suber JT. Two techniques for supplementing interlocking nail repair of fractures of the humerus, femur, and tibia: results in 12 dogs and cats. Vet Surg 2004;33:673–680.
12. Scotti SA, et al. Retrograde placement of a novel 3.5 mm titanium interlocking nail for supracondylar and diaphyseal femoral fractures in cats. Vet Comp Orthop Traumatol 2007;20: 211–218.
13. Toombs JP, et al. The SKTM external fixation system: description of components, instrumentation, and application techniques. Vet Comp Orthop Traumatol 2003;16:76–81.
14. Bronson DG, et al. Influence of the connecting rod on the biomechanical properties of five external skeletal fixation configurations. Vet Comp Orthop Traumatol 2003;16:82–87.
15. Font J, et al. A review of 116 clinical cases treated with external fixators. Vet Comp Orthop Traumatol 1997;4:173–182.
16. Reichler IM, et al. Der Tubuläre Fixateur Externe (F.E.S.S.A.): Klinische Anwendung zur Frakturversorgung bei 6 Zwerghunden und 20 Katzen. Kleintierpraxis 1997;42:407–419.
17. Haas B, et al. Use of the tubular external fixator in the treatment of distal radial and ulnar fractures in small dogs and cats. Vet Comp Orthop Traumatol 2003;16:132–137.
18. Gemmill TJ, et al. Treatment of canine and feline diaphyseal radial and tibial fractures with low-stiffness external skeletal fixation. J Small Anim Pract 2004;45:85–91.
19. Aron DN, et al. Experimental and clinical experience with an IM pin external skeletal fixator tie-in configuration. Vet Comp Orthop Traumatol 1991;4:86–94.
20. Langley-Hobbs SJ, et al. Use of external skeletal fixators in the repair of femoral fractures in cats. Vet Comp Orthop Traumatol 1996;37:95–101.
21. Langley-Hobbs SJ, et al. External skeletal fixation for stabilisation of comminuted humeral fractures in cats. J Small Anim Pract 1997;38:280–285.
22. Briggs BT, Chao EYS. The mechanical performance of the standard Hoffman–Vidal external fixation apparatus. J Bone Joint Surg Am 1982;64A:566–573.
23. Bennett RA, et al. Comparison of the strength and holding power of 4 pin designs for use with half pin (type I) external skeletal fixation. Vet Surg 1987;16:207–211.
24. Egger EL, et al. Effect of fixation pin insertion on the bone–pin interface. Vet Surg 1986;15:246–252.
25. Marcellin-Little DJ. External skeletal fixation. In: Slatter D (ed.) Textbook of small animal surgery. Philadelphia: WB Saunders; 2002: pp. 1818–1834.
26. Beck AL, Pead MJ. The use of Ellis pins (negative profile tip-threaded pins) in external skeletal fixation in dogs and cats. Vet Comp Orthop Traumatol 2003;16:223–231.
27. Fruchter AM, Holmberg DL. Mechanical analysis of veterinary cuttable plate. Compend Continuing Educ 1991;4:116–119.
28. Robins GM, et al. Customized hook plate for metaphyseal fractures, nonunions and osteotomies in the dog and cat. Vet Comp Orthop Traumatol 1993;6:56–61.
29. Montavon PM, et al. The mini instrument and implant set and its clinical application. Vet Comp Orthop Traumatol 1988;1: 44–51.
30. Von Werthern CJ, Bernasconi CE. Application of the maxillofacial mini-plate Compact 1.0 in the fracture repair of 12 cats/2 dogs. Vet Comp Orthop Traumatol 2000;13:92–96.
31. Savoldelli D, Montavon PM. Clinical handling: small animals. Injury 1995;26:47–50.
32. Keller M, et al. The ComPact UniLock 2.0/2.4 system and its clinical application in small animal orthopedics. Vet Comp Orthop Traumatol 2005;18:83–93.
33. Voss K, et al. Use of the ComPact UniLock System for ventral stabilization procedures of the cervical spine: a retrospective study. Vet Comp Orthop Traumatol 2006;19:21–28.
34. Voss K, et al. Internal splinting of dorsal intertarsal and tarsometatarsal instabilities in dogs and cats with the ComPact UniLock 2.0/2.4 System. Vet Comp Orthop Traumatol 2004; 17:125–130.

A selection of websites for further information on the implants described above:

Animal Care: www.animalcare.co.uk/orthopaedics.html.
Eickemeyer: www.eickemeyer.de.
IMEX Veterinary: www.imexvet.com.
Innovative Animal Products: www.innovativeanimalproducts.com.
Königsee Implantate: www-koenigsee-implantate.de.
Kyon: www.kyon.ch.
Medical Solution: www.medical-solution.ch.
Synthes Veterinary: www.synthesvet.com.
Synthes: www.synthes.com.
Veterinary Instrumentation: www.vetinst.com.

25 Feline arthroscopy

B. Beale

Feline arthroscopy – is it possible? Is it useful? Is it practical? Arthroscopy is a valuable tool for the diagnosis and treatment of conditions affecting the joints of cats. The arthroscope can be inserted into the shoulder, elbow, hip, and stifle of the cat to allow a direct view of the joint in a minimally invasive manner. The arthroscope is also used to evaluate joints approached by routine arthrotomy. The arthroscope provides magnification and an ability to reach poorly accessible areas of the joint, improving the view of structures within the joint. Even if you never actually performed a procedure completely arthroscopically, the arthroscope can be used to improve the effectiveness and accuracy of the general veterinary surgeon performing joint surgery in the cat.

This chapter is organized to avoid repetition. Instrumentation, patient preparation, and postoperative care are similar for all joints. The chapter will also focus on the most common indications for feline arthroscopy. The shoulder, elbow, hip, and stifle of the cat can be examined arthroscopically, but the stifle is much more frequently examined. Arthroscopy is used for evaluation of joint conditions (e.g., cranial cruciate disease, shoulder ligamentous damage), removal of loose joint bodies (e.g., elbow dysplasia), and treatment of meniscal damage. For information on arthroscopy the reader is reminded to review other sources, listed at the end of this chapter (1–4). The purpose of this contribution is to introduce the reader to basic arthroscopy of the cat and is not intended to be a complete review of the topic.

25.1 Arthroscopic instrumentation

The instrumentation used for arthroscopy in cats is similar to that used in small dogs. An arthroscope, cannula, camera, monitor, light source, fluid delivery and collection system, and assorted hand instruments are required (Fig. 25-1). Instrument cannulas, radiofrequency or cautery units, and motorized shavers may also be useful.

25.1.1 Arthroscope and cannula

The arthroscope is a rigid telescope that transmits an image to the camera and monitor. The arthroscope contains a series of lens or fiberoptics that produce the image. The arthroscope is inserted into a cannula which acts to protect the scope and provides a continuous portal into the joint. The arthroscope attaches to the cannula with a coupling mechanism. A light cable attaches to the cannula to provide the illumination needed to produce a quality image. Fluid tubing also attaches to the cannula, allowing fluids to be continuously delivered into the joint to improve the quality of the image (Fig. 25-2).

Arthroscope diameters commonly used in feline arthroscopy include 1.9–2.7 mm. The cannula is first introduced into the joint through a stab incision in the skin and fascia. A conical or sharp obturator is locked in the cannula and the cannula is carefully pushed into the saline-distended joint. The cannula may be available in a smaller and a larger diameter, depending on the manufacturer. The smaller-diameter cannula can be inserted more easily, but allows less fluid flow into the joint due to the reduced space between the cannula wall and the arthroscope. Another advantage of the smaller scope and cannula is greater mobility in small joints such as the elbow or hock. The advantage of larger arthroscopes is

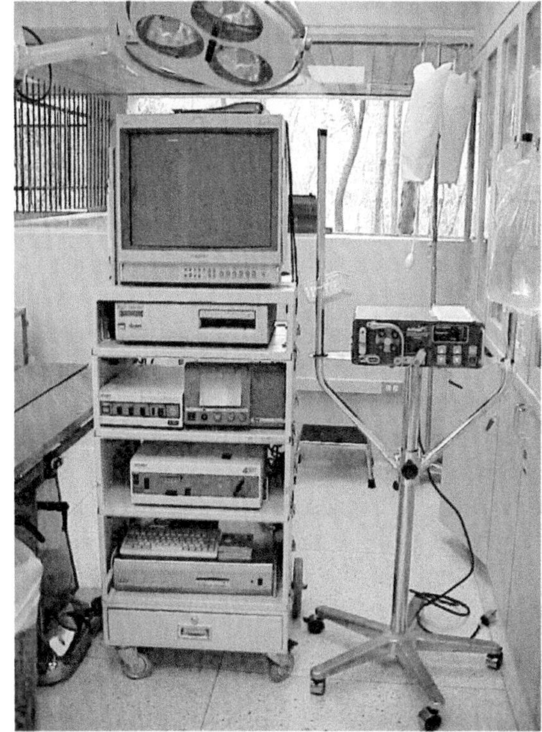

Figure 25-1 The arthroscopic tower includes a cabinet, monitor, camera control box, light source, cautery or radiofrequency unit, digital image capture device, and printer.

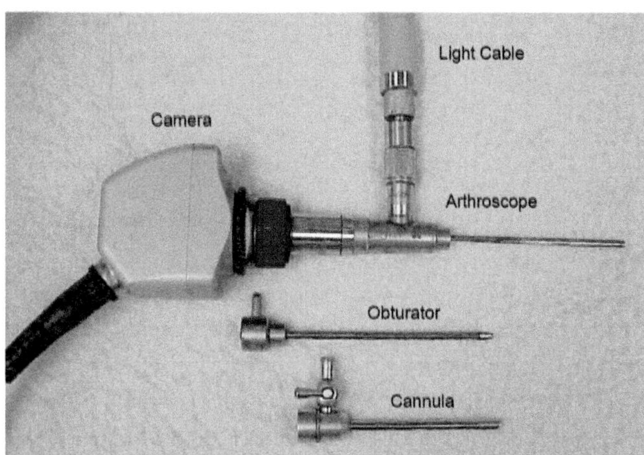

Figure 25-2 A cannula is inserted into the joint using an obturator. The arthroscope is attached to a camera head and light cable. The arthroscope is inserted into the cannula to view inside the joint. Fluid tubing is attached to the cannula.

a larger field of view and greater resistance to bending and therefore greater durability. Smaller cannulas are most often used in the cat.

Arthroscopy of the feline shoulder, elbow, and hip is usually performed with a 1.9-mm arthroscope. Arthroscopy of the feline stifle is usually performed with a 2.3-, 2.4-, or 2.7-mm arthroscope. The 30° arthroscope is the most common employed in feline arthroscopy. Working length refers to the overall length of the shaft of the telescope and is usually designated as short or long. Short arthroscopes (8.5 cm) are recommended for feline arthroscopy due to the ease of handling in smaller joints and less susceptibility to damage from bending.

The light post on the arthroscope is the site of attachment of the fiberoptic cable that will provide lighting within the joint. The light post can be rotated around the arthroscope, changing the arthroscopic field of view. This maneuver is an important concept of arthroscopy. Use of the light post to change the field of view reduces the need to move the tip of the arthroscope to achieve the same result. Reduced manipulation of the arthroscope decreases the chance of iatrogenic trauma to the joint surface and unintentional withdrawal of the scope from the joint.

Arthroscopes are fragile and can be easily damaged during surgery, cleaning, or storage. Not only are arthroscopes expensive to buy initially, they are also expensive to repair or replace. Thus, they should be handled with extreme care. Many manufacturers offer repair or replacement warranties that often provide a replacement or loan within 24 hours. Proper methods of cleaning and storage have been described (1). In my experience most damage to arthroscopes is caused by the surgeon or technician and not as a result of manufacturing problems. Damage during surgery can occur if too much bending pressure is applied to the scope or if the glass at the end of the scope is scratched or broken due to a direct blow with a hand instrument, shaver blade, or cautery tip.

25.1.2 Arthroscopic cameras

The arthroscopic image is projected on to a monitor screen by means of a video camera system. The camera system comprises a control unit and a camera head. Most cameras contain either one or three semiconducting chips. Three-chip cameras give greater resolution than one-chip cameras; however, three-chip cameras can be significantly more expensive than single-chip cameras. Newer single-chip cameras provide an excellent image and are appropriate for most applications. Most camera heads should fit most arthroscope eye pieces regardless of manufacturer, but it is advisable to ensure compatibility before purchasing components from different manufacturers. Some camera heads will have buttons that permit white balance, image printing, or zoom. The control box converts the electronic image information into a standard video signal and relays the image to the monitor. The control box is usually specific to the camera head and therefore the camera head and control box must be from the same manufacturer. Camera heads may be sterilized by autoclave, ethylene oxide gas or cold sterilization, according to manufacturer's recommendations.

25.1.3 Monitors

The arthroscopic image is visualized on a color monitor. Monitors for arthroscopy should have a high horizontal resolution of at least 450 lines and a large screen (20 inches (50 cm) or greater). Medical-grade monitors are available and provide the best image, but household monitors may provide adequate image quality at a lower cost. Most monitors will have S-video or red, green, blue (RGB) inputs which enable higher-quality video imaging.

25.1.4 Light source

Light sources provide illumination within the joint for visualization. Light source bulbs may be tungsten-halogen, or xenon. Xenon lamps provide increased light intensity and higher color temperature as compared to halogen and therefore provide higher visual clarity and color rendition. Xenon light sources are more expensive than halogen but are generally recommended for superior image quality. The light from the light source is transferred to the arthroscope through a fiberoptic cable that attaches to the light post on the arthroscope. The connection for the fiberoptic cable must be compatible with the light source and the camera. The light cable may be sterilized by ethylene oxide gas, Cidex soaking, or autoclave, depending on manufacturer's recommendations. The light cable is composed of numerous glass fibers that may be broken if the cable is bent or wound too tightly; therefore it should be handled carefully. The fiberoptic cable will also heat up significantly and should never be placed directly against the patient or draping materials as it may cause burning.

25.1.5 Storage of arthroscopic images

Documentation of arthroscopic procedures provides a permanent visual resource that is invaluable for historical archiving of arthroscopic findings and therapy, and for client and professional communication. Arthroscopic images can be stored as digital images or as printed photos. Methods used to collect and store the images include video tape recording, digital still image capture, and color printing. A household video camera provides an excellent and convenient means of documenting patient data. The video camera typically attaches to the arthroscopic camera using an S-video cable.

25.1.6 Arthroscopic irrigation

A constant and reliable flow of fluid across the tip of the arthroscope and through the joint is vital to give adequate visualization. Fluid expands the joint, provides clear fluid for visualization, and clears the joint of debris and contamination. Irrigation also increases pressure within the joint and this suppresses bleeding during the procedure. Irrigation systems must provide a minimum pressure necessary to distend the joint and maintain flow without exceeding safe pressures, which could result in extravasation of fluid into the adjacent soft tissues. Recommended pressures in most feline arthroscopy are between 25 and 50 mmHg. As previously described, fluid is directed into a Luer-Lok connector on the arthroscope cannula and enters the joint via the space between the telescope and the cannula. Fluid may be pressurized either by gravity flow or by an electric fluid pump (Fig. 25-3). Both systems have advantages and selection often depends upon the joint being operated and surgeon preference. Gravity remains an effective method of fluid delivery for most procedures that do not involve fluid suction or long-term use of shaving devices.

25.1.7 Egress systems

Maintenance of appropriate fluid flow through the joint during arthroscopy also necessitates establishment of adequate outflow or egress. Maintenance of fluid outflow can be particularly challenging in small-animal arthroscopy due to the small size of the joints. Use of standard outflow cannulas in smaller joints, particularly the elbow, may result in significant iatrogenic cartilage trauma. The use of needles may

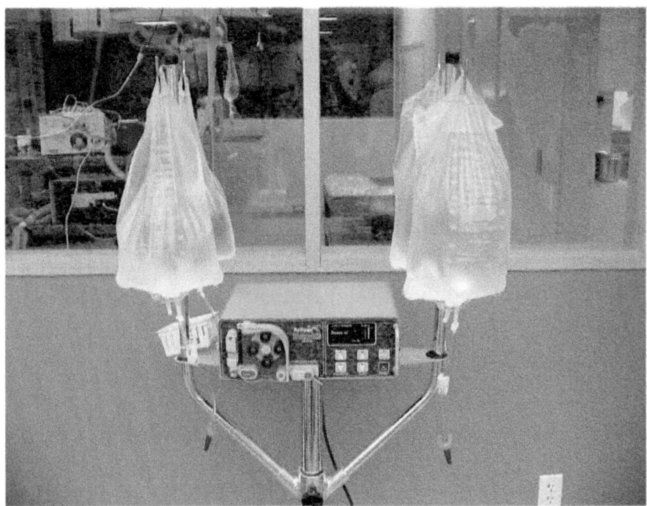

Figure 25-3 Sterile fluids are administered continuously through the cannula into the joint using a fluid infusion pump (shown) or by hanging a bag of fluids attached to a pressure bag.

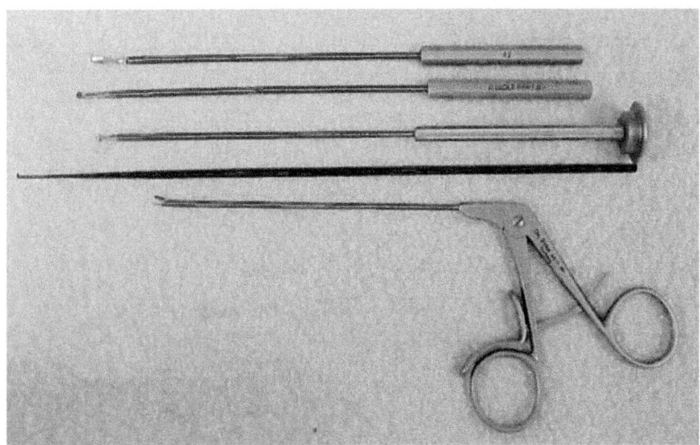

Figure 25-4 Hand instruments are used to treat various conditions when used with arthroscopy. Commonly used instruments (from top to bottom) include a banana knife, curette, hand bur, probe, and a grasper.

minimize trauma due to their size, although the sharp tips may damage the cartilage and the narrow tube may frequently become clogged. Selection of the appropriate outflow instrument will be based primarily on the size of the joint being operated. If the outflow cannula is not providing adequate fluid evacuation, the instrument portal can be increased in diameter to permit fluid to egress alongside operative instruments.

25.1.8 Hand instruments

Hand instruments for small-joint arthroscopy must combine small diameter with excellent mechanics to provide high accuracy and reliability while minimizing iatrogenic trauma and instrument failure. Basic recommended arthroscopic hand tools include a probe, grasping forceps, biting forceps, arthroscopic knife, curette, and a hand bur (Fig. 25-4).

Probes are usually right-angle in design with a tip of approximately 1–3 mm in length. Probes are used to palpate surfaces and manipulate tissues within the joint. In small-animal arthroscopy right-angle probes are used to palpate articular cartilage for pathology and to manipulate flaps, meniscal injuries, and bone fragments. Many bucket-handle tears are missed because non-displaced meniscal tears cannot be seen. The probe can be used to pull the torn portion of the meniscus cranially, allowing identification and treatment using partial meniscectomy.

Grasping forceps are available as locking and non-locking types. Grasping forceps designed specifically for arthroscopic use are usually more sturdy and have a locking mechanism that aids in tissue removal. The grasping surface may be smooth or serrated. It is recommended to have a large grasping forceps with serrated teeth for removal of large bone chips and cartilage flaps. A small grasping forceps is also useful for delicate tissue manipulation in narrow joint spaces.

Biting or punch forceps are used to debride soft tissues and may also be referred to as basket forceps. Punch forceps have a sharp hollow lower anvil and an upper punch that can be used to remove small pieces of soft tissue, including synovium or meniscus. Variations in design include straight or side-biting and differences in diameter and length. A small- or medium-diameter straight punch forceps is most useful in small-animal arthroscopy for debriding synovium that is obscuring the view, obtaining a synovial biopsy, or debriding a meniscal injury.

Arthroscopic knives are useful in small-animal arthroscopy for treating meniscal injuries, tenodesis, and cutting soft-tissue attachments to bony fragments. Knives may be straight, curved, or hooked, and the choice depends upon the procedure being performed. A knife set is not mandatory for basic small-animal arthroscopy; however, purchase of straight and hook knives is recommended for advanced techniques.

Small-diameter curettes are very useful in small-joint arthroscopy for elevation of bone fragments and debridement of cartilage and bone. Generally, a straight curette will be easier to insert into the joint and will be adequate for most applications. Loop or ring curettes are also available specifically for arthroscopic use.

Curettage and abrasion of bone or cartilage can be performed with a hand bur. The instrument is a round bur on the end of an arthroscopic handle. Alternatively a bur from a power shaver may be used in a similar manner.

25.1.9 Instrument cannulas

Arthroscopic instruments may be inserted into the joint through a portal with or without a cannula (Fig. 25-5). The major advantage of working through a cannula is the ease of instrument insertion. Without a cannula it may be difficult to switch instruments and identify the portal, particularly if the portal was poorly made. Repeated attempts to insert an instrument through a poorly defined portal can lead to soft-tissue trauma and fluid extravasation. The major disadvantage of using a cannula is the limited diameter of the instruments that will fit into the cannula.

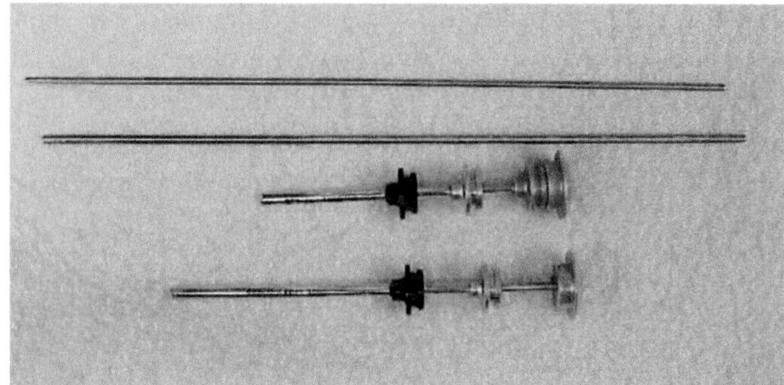

Figure 25-5 An instrument cannula can be used to maintain an instrument portal. Hand instruments can be moved in and out of the joint easily through the portal. The cannula size can be progressively increased over a series of "switching sticks" to allow removal of larger fragments.

Instrument cannulas are available in numerous diameters and lengths. For small-joint arthroscopy, cannulas of inner diameter of 2.3–3.5 mm are most appropriate. Lengths of 4–5 cm are appropriate. Most cannulas come with both sharp and blunt obturator, although the blunt obturator should be used whenever possible. Small-joint cannula systems should also include a set of switching sticks and/or switching tubes. This technique permits the progressive dilation of the portal and subsequent insertion of larger cannulas. To work with this system, a relatively small cannula and obturator is inserted first into the joint. A switching stick is then placed through the cannula and the cannula withdrawn. A larger cannula or dilation tube is then placed over the stick and the process is repeated until the desired cannula is in place. The use of cannulas depends upon the joint being operated, the instruments being used, and the surgeon's preference. Although a cannula system is not necessary for small-joint arthroscopy, it is useful to have a system for particular situations and it may be easier for the inexperienced arthroscopist to work through cannulas.

25.1.10 Motorized shavers

Motorized shavers are designed to debride soft and hard tissues rapidly. The small-joint shavers can be used in the elbow, shoulder, and stifle of cats. Power shavers comprise a control box, a hand piece, and a shaver tip (Fig. 25-6). The

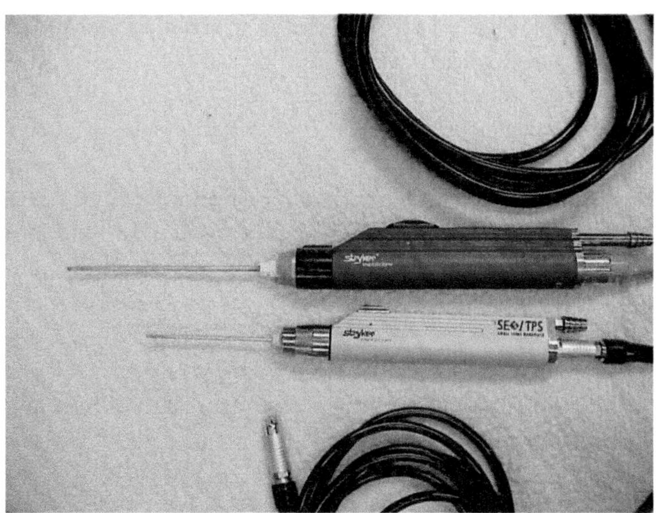

Figure 25-6 A power shaver is a useful instrument to remove synovium, torn ligament fibers, meniscal tears, cartilage flaps, or eburnated subchondral bone.

control box includes the power supply and basic operational controls. Most shavers permit variation of speed and direction, including forward, reverse, and oscillation. Speed control is important as debridement of different tissues with different shaver blades requires different speeds. The shaver is generally controlled with a foot pedal. The hand piece has a switch that controls the amount of suction pressure.

Shaver blades come in numerous styles and diameters that are designed for either soft-tissue or hard-tissue debridement. The diameter of shaver blades used in cats typically ranges from 2.0 to 3.5 mm. Soft-tissue shaver blades include guarded sharp cutters and aggressive cutters. Sharp cutter blades have a simple sharp-edged cup whereas aggressive cutters have a toothed cup. Both can be used for debridement of fat or synovium in small joints. Aggressive cutters are more effective if a large amount of tissue must be removed or if the target tissue is expected to be denser due to chronic synovitis. When using an aggressive cutter to debride the fat pad of the stifle, it is helpful to apply limited suction to the unit and use the shaver at a relatively slow speed. Operation of the shaver at higher speeds limits the amount of tissue that can be drawn into the shaver blade. Shaver blades for debridement of bone are round or oval-shaped guarded burs. Full-radius shaver blades are useful to debride necrotic cartilage, soft bone, or small amounts of synovium or fat pad.

25.1.11 Electrocautery and radiofrequency

Electrocautery and radiofrequency are used to generate heat for cauterization of vessels, debridement of tissues, or shrinking of collagen. Electrosurgical tips specifically designed for underwater arthroscopic application are available for use with standard electrocautery generators. These instruments may be used for cautery of small vessels and special tips are designed for cutting soft tissues. Special tips are also available to ablate or shrink soft-tissue structures. Small probe sizes (1.0–2.5 mm) should be used in most feline arthroscopic procedures.

25.2 Patient preparation and positioning

Patients should be positioned in a routine fashion for exploratory surgery of the joint. Clip and prepare the patient as if an open arthrotomy were to take place. The reason for this strategy is that the arthroscopy procedure may need to be aborted for technical reasons and an open arthrotomy performed. This will occur more frequently when the surgeon is beginning to learn arthroscopy. The arthroscope can still be used to improve the surgeon's view even if an arthrotomy is performed. The surgeon and assistant generally stand on the same side of the table when performing arthroscopy.

25.3 Postoperative care

Lavage of the joint should be performed at the conclusion of arthroscopy to remove debris. If an instrument cannula is being used, the joint can be lavaged with inflow through the arthroscope cannula and outflow through the instrument cannula. If an instrument cannula was not used, lavage can be achieved by connecting the fluid line to the egress needle and removing the arthroscope from its cannula, leaving the cannula in the joint to allow fluid egress. Once the joint has been thoroughly lavaged, remove the arthroscope cannula and suture the arthroscope and instrument portals with nylon in a cruciate pattern through the skin. Bupivacaine may then be injected into the joint to provide topical anesthesia. Postoperatively, a bandage may be placed on the limb for 24 hours if there is significant swelling around the joint from fluid extravasation. Cold therapy applied 2–3 times a day for several days will help provide analgesia and decrease swelling. The duration of activity restriction depends on the procedure. Activity should generally be restricted for 2 weeks following arthroscopy. Further restriction may be needed depending on the orthopedic procedure performed at the time of arthroscopy (e.g., cruciate ligament repair requires 2 months of minimal activity).

25.4 Arthroscopy of the shoulder

25.4.1 Patient position

The patient should be in lateral recumbency with the target shoulder up. The lateral aspect of the shoulder will be approached. Slight traction should be placed on the leg while holding the leg parallel to the floor.

25.4.2 Recommended arthroscope size

This is 1.9, 2.3, or 2.4 mm.

25.4.3 Portal sites for shoulder arthroscopy (3)

The portal sites used for feline shoulder arthroscopy are similar to the canine (Fig. 25-7). Arthroscope, egress, and instrument portals are typically used. The egress portal is established first. Insert a 20-gauge needle from the craniolateral aspect of the shoulder over the greater tubercle towards the craniomedial aspect of the joint near the origin of the biceps tendon. In most cases, when the egress portal is properly placed, synovial fluid is easily aspirated. If synovial fluid is not aspirated and the surgeon believes the joint has been entered, saline can be instilled into the joint. If the needle is located in the joint, fluid is easily instilled and reverse pressure is felt on the syringe plunger as the joint capsule fully distends. Approximately 3–6 ml of fluid is needed to distend most feline shoulder joints. The arthroscope portal is established second. The arthroscope cannula with the attached conical obturator is inserted. Standard scope insertion site is based on localization of the acromion of the scapula and approximation of the location of the joint surface. Place a finger on the acromion and then move distally until the approximate level of the joint is reached. Estimation of this level is assisted by evaluation of the lateral radiographic view. A 22-gauge needle may be inserted at the location of the proposed scope port to ensure proper port location. The needle should pass easily into the joint perpendicular to the long axis of the limb.

To insert the scope use a number 11 blade to make a 2–3-mm stab incision through the skin and superficial soft tissues. The incision should not be continued full-thickness through the joint capsule or the joint distension will be eliminated and it will allow excessive extravasation of fluid into the surrounding soft tissues. The instrument portal is established if a biopsy of intra-articular tissue is desired or if treatment of joint pathology is required. The craniocaudal and proximodistal position of the instrument portal relative to the acromion can be estimated from the lateral radiograph. This site is approximately 1 cm caudal and slightly distal to the caudal edge of the acromion. It is best to learn to triangulate the instrument portal site relative to the position of the arthroscope tip within the joint. A 20-gauge 1-inch (2.5-cm) needle is used as a guide needle to locate the appropriate site for the instrument portal. The guide needle must penetrate the skin surface at a 75–90° angle and maintain this orientation through the soft tissues. As the needle enters the joint and is seen on the monitor (be sure the scope and light post are directed toward the point of entry), the surgeon can assess correct placement of the portal relative to the lesion to be treated. One has the impression that the needle is entering at a very oblique angle. This is the illusion created by the 30 fore-oblique arthroscope and not the real penetration angle.

The most common reason for failing to locate the appropriate instrument portal site is entering the skin and soft tissue at too oblique an angle. When one enters at too oblique an angle, the triangulation needle (to locate the instrument port) crosses the arthroscope and cannot be visualized on the

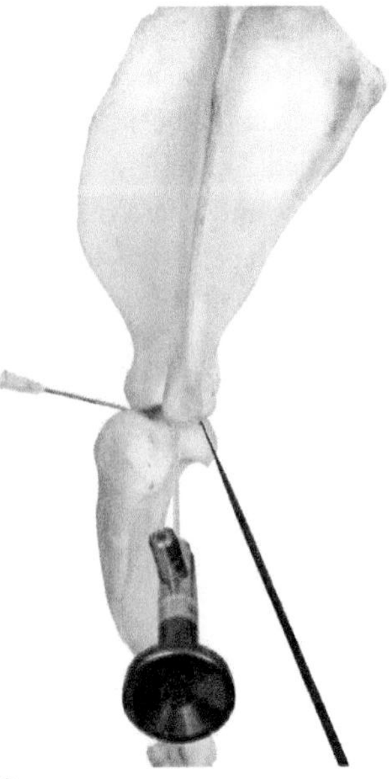

A

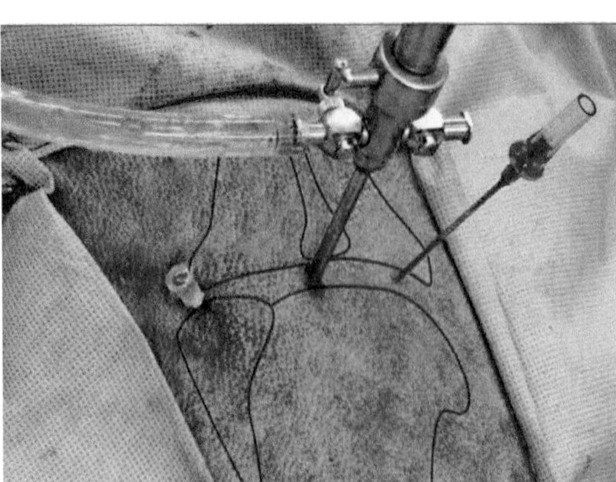

B

Figure 25-7 The portals for the shoulder are lateral, as shown in (**A**) and (**B**). The arthroscope portal is distal to the acromion process of the scapula. The instrument portal is typically caudal and the egress portal is cranial to the arthroscope portal. The instrument and egress portals are occasionally exchanged depending on the site of the lesion to be treated.

monitor. Once the appropriate site for the instrument portal has been confirmed by observation of the needle on the monitor, the portal site is prepared for instrumentation. A number 11 scalpel blade can be inserted adjacent to the needle into the joint. The opening can then be enlarged with Metzenbaum scissors or a series of increasing-diameter instrument cannulas. If different-sized cannulas are needed, a switching stick is used to change out cannulas.

25.4.4 Surgical anatomy

The initial step in shoulder arthroscopy should be a thorough systematic exploration of the joint. Developing a standardized pattern for examination of the joint will help the development of arthroscopic skills and ensure that all accessible areas of the joint are examined. An example of standard shoulder joint examination would be to visualize the:

- Biceps tendon (Fig. 25-8)
- Medial glenohumeral ligament (Fig. 25-9)
- Subscapularis tendon
- Humeral head (Figs 25-10 and 25-11)
- Glenoid cavity (Fig. 25-10)
- Caudal joint pouch

The joint is explored by changing the field of view of the arthroscope using a combination of techniques. Actual movement of the scope should be minimized to avoid inadvertent withdrawal of the scope from the joint. The field of view can be changed in three ways:

1. by advancing or withdrawing the tip of the arthroscope slightly
2. by leaning the arthroscope proximally, distally, cranially, and caudally
3. by rotating the light cable to change the orientation of the beveled lens.

Pathological lesions are evaluated and treated using hand instruments or the motorized shaver through the instrument portal.

25.4.5 Indications for shoulder arthroscopy

Shoulder arthroscopy is occasionally performed in cats. Indications for shoulder arthroscopy may include diagnosis

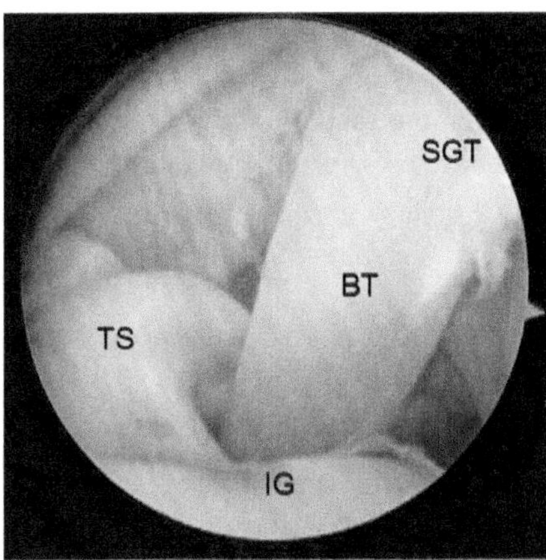

Figure 25-8 The normal biceps tendon (BT) of the cat appears similar to that of the dog. The tendon originates from the supraglenoid tuberosity (SGT) of the scapula. The tendon crosses the joint space and enters the tendon sheath (TS) at the intertubercular groove (IG) of the humerus. A portion of the tendon within the sheath can be assessed by flexing the shoulder.

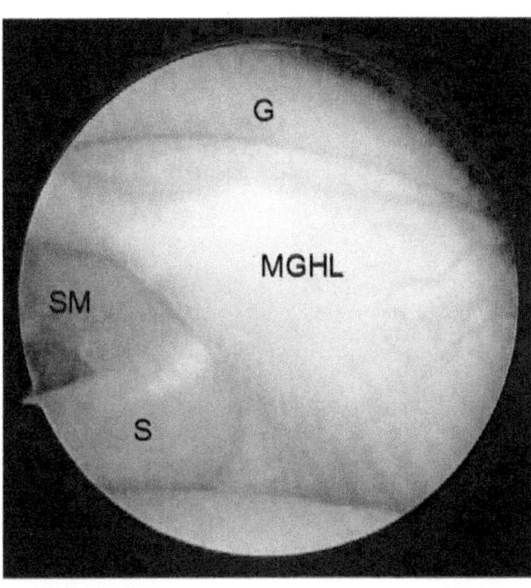

Figure 25-9 Structures that should be assessed on the medial aspect of the shoulder include the medial glenohumeral ligament (MGHL), subscapularis tendon (S), glenoid rim (G), and synovial membrane (SM).

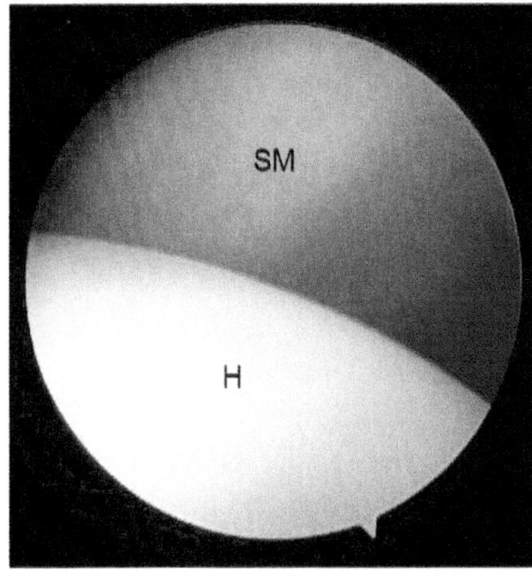

Figure 25-10 The humeral head (H), glenoid cavity, and synovial membrane (SM) can be evaluated in the caudal joint space.

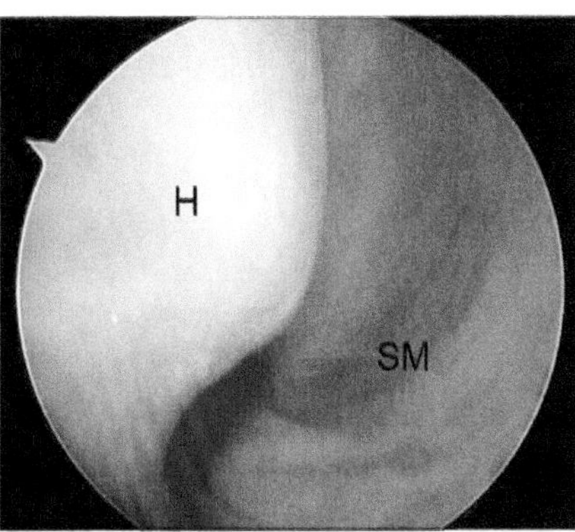

Figure 25-11 The humeral head (H) and synovial membrane (SM) are visible in the caudomedial joint pouch.

and therapy of infectious, neoplastic, traumatic, developmental, and degenerative diseases. Minimally invasive synovial biopsy may be performed. Biopsies of the synovium are usually obtained with a small biter forceps. The sharp biting action of these instruments permits rapid biopsies in a single step. Biopsies of cartilage or soft bone may be performed with very small trephines or a meniscal vascular punch. The most common application of shoulder arthroscopy in cats has been for the diagnosis and therapy of traumatic and degenerative diseases, specifically ligamentous injury, osteoarthritis, and synovitis. The list of indications for shoulder arthroscopy in cats will likely expand in the future as new pathological conditions are discovered during exploratory arthroscopic examinations of cats having painful conditions of the shoulder.

Ligamentous injury

Feline patients may have ligamentous damage of the shoulder similar to that found in canine patients. Injury to the medial supporting structures of the joint appears to be most common. The medial glenohumeral ligament, subscapularis tendon, and joint capsule may be torn or stretched. In a study by Ridge (3) the medial glenohumeral ligament in the cat appeared as a single band and was not Y-shaped as in dogs. Arthroscopy can be used to assess the integrity of these structures. The structures can be probed to assess for tightness. Thermal shrinkage of these tissues can be attempted using a radiofrequency probe in an attempt to tighten the medial tissues and restore stability. A minimally invasive surgical approach can be performed to reconstruct the ligamentous structures if needed.

Osteoarthritis and synovitis (Figs 25-12–25-14)

Arthroscopy of the shoulder has limited use in the management of osteoarthritis and synovitis in cats. The underlying cause of osteoarthritis should be identified and eliminated if possible. Arthroscopic exploration of the joint can be used to obtain synovial biopsies for histopathology and culture and sensitivity. Loose osteochondral fragments can be removed using grasping forceps. Areas of full-thickness cartilage wear can be treated. A description for treatment of damaged regions of the articular cartilage is described below in elbow osteoarthritis.

25.5 Arthroscopy of the elbow

25.5.1 Patient position

The patient should be in lateral recumbency with the target elbow down. The medial aspect of the elbow will be approached.

25.5.2 Recommended arthroscope size

This is 1.9 mm.

25.5.3 Portal sites for elbow arthroscopy

The portal sites used for feline elbow arthroscopy are similar to the canine (Fig. 25-15). Arthroscope, egress, and instrument portals are typically used. The egress portal is established first. Insert a 20-gauge needle from the medial aspect of the elbow over the medial epicondyle crest, towards the tip of the anconeal process. In most cases, when the egress portal is properly placed, synovial fluid is easily aspirated. If synovial fluid is not aspirated and the surgeon believes the

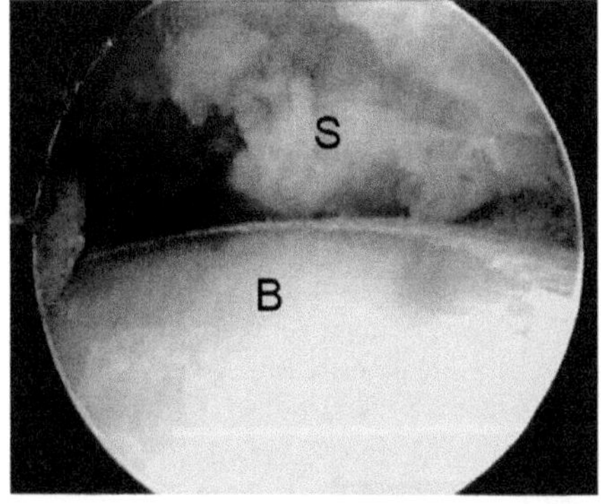

Figure 25-13 The bone of the humeral head (B) is eburnated following grade 4 cartilage erosion. Chronic inflammation of the synovial membrane is seen (S).

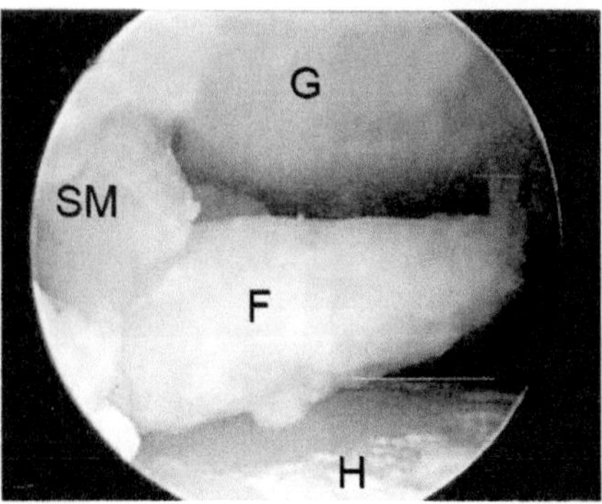

Figure 25-12 A bone fragment (F), proliferative synovial membrane (SM), glenoid (G), and eburnated bone of the humeral head (H) can be seen in this feline patient with chronic shoulder osteoarthritis of unknown cause.

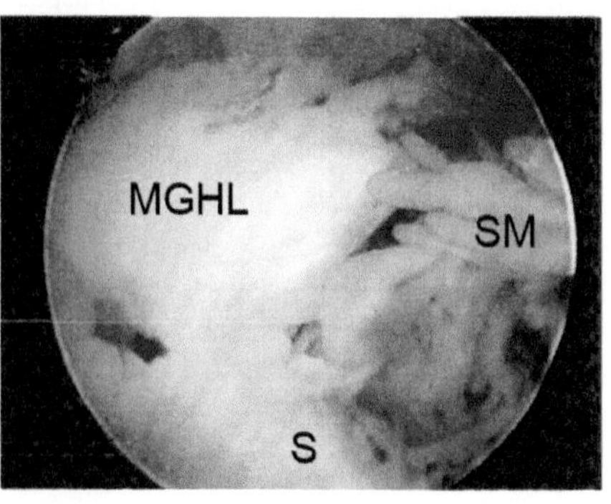

Figure 25-14 The medial glenohumeral ligament (MGHL) and subscapularis tendon (S) are intact in this feline patient with chronic inflammation of the synovial membrane (SM).

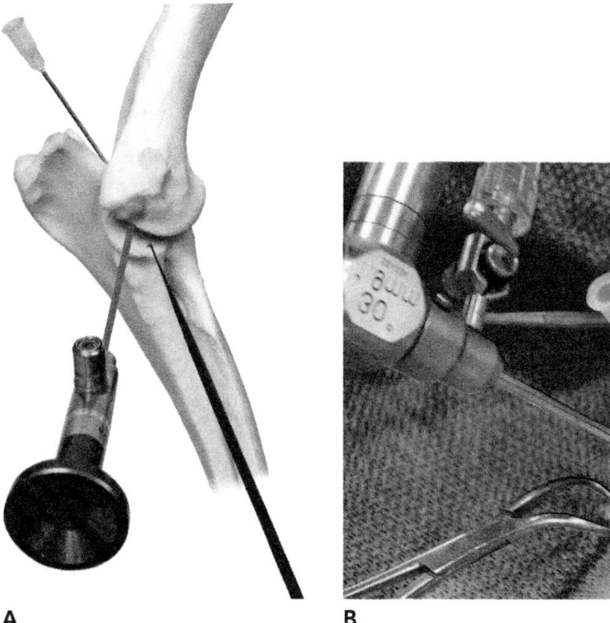

Figure 25-15 The portals for the elbow are medial, as shown in (**A**) and (**B**). The arthroscope portal is usually 5–7 mm distal and caudal to the medial humeral epicondyle of the humerus in the cat. The instrument portal (probe) is cranial and the egress portal (needle) is caudal and proximal to the arthroscope portal.

joint has been entered, saline can be instilled into the joint. If the needle is located in the joint, fluid is easily instilled and reverse pressure is felt on the syringe plunger as the joint capsule fully distends. Approximately 1–4 ml of fluid is needed to distend most feline elbow joints. The arthroscope portal is established second. The arthroscope cannula with the attached conical obturator is inserted. Standard scope insertion site is based on localization of the medial epicondyle and approximation of the location of the joint surface. Place a finger on the medial epicondyle and then move distally until the approximate level of the joint is reached. Estimation of this level is assisted by evaluation of the lateral radiographic view. Next move the finger approximately 4–5 mm caudal to this point for arthroscope insertion. A 22-gauge needle may be inserted at the location of the proposed scope port to ensure proper port location. The needle should pass easily into the joint perpendicular to the long axis of the limb.

To insert the scope use a number 11 blade to make a 2–3-mm stab incision through the skin and superficial soft tissues. The incision should not be continued full-thickness through the joint capsule or the joint distension will be eliminated and it will allow excessive extravasation of fluid into the surrounding soft tissues. The elbow should be positioned at the edge of the table or a bolster placed under the elbow to use as a fulcrum. Have the assistant maintain a slight valgus force (mild downward pressure) to the foot to open the medial compartment of the joint.

Once in the joint, remove the obturator from the cannula. Fluid will flow freely from the cannula, confirming correct placement. Attach the fluid ingress line to the cannula and insert the arthroscope. The instrument portal is established last and is used for insertion of a variety of instruments, including small-joint graspers, right-angled probes, small-joint shavers, and curettes.

Once the joint has been thoroughly explored, position the arthroscope to visualize the craniomedial portion of the joint. Insert a 22-gauge needle into the joint caudal to the medial collateral ligament while observing arthroscopically. Once the needle has been visualized and the internal and external positioning are judged to be satisfactory, use a number 11 blade to make a 3–5-mm longitudinal incision directly adjacent to the needle. Insert a small blunt trochar into the joint at a similar angle to the needle. If an instrument cannula is going to be used it should be inserted at this time.

The obturator is removed and the portal enlarged as needed using Metzenbaum scissors or a hemostat to spread the opening. A cleanly created, large portal will allow easy insertion of all necessary instruments without the need for a cannula. A larger portal also allows egress fluid to drain more effectively with fewer tendencies to extravasate into the subcutaneous tissues.

25.5.4 Surgical anatomy

The initial step in elbow joint arthroscopy should be a thorough systematic exploration of the joint. Developing a standardized pattern for examination of the joint will help the development of arthroscopic skills and ensure that all accessible areas of the joint are examined. An example of standard medial elbow joint examination would be to visualize and image each area of the medial joint as follows:

- Anconeal process (Fig. 25-16)
- Trochlear notch
- Lateral coronoid process (Fig. 25-17)
- Medial coronoid process
- Radial head (Figs 25-17 and 25-18)
- Medial collateral ligament
- Medial humeral condyle (Fig. 25-19)

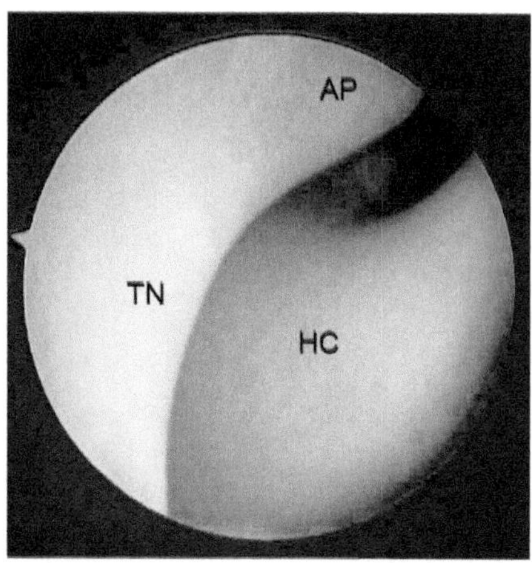

Figure 25-16 The anconeal process (AP) of the cat is slightly smaller than the dog. The trochlear notch of the ulna (TN) and humeral condyle (HC) are similar to the dog.

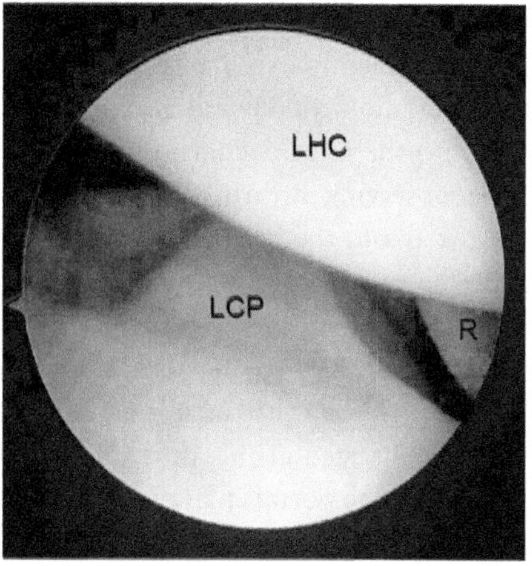

Figure 25-17 Structures that should be assessed on the lateral aspect of the elbow include the lateral coronoid process (LCP) and the lateral aspect of the humeral condyle (LHC) and radial head (R).

The joint is explored by changing the field of view of the arthroscope using a combination of techniques. Actual movement of the scope should be minimized to avoid inadvertent withdrawal of the scope from the joint. The field of view can be changed in three ways:

1. by advancing or withdrawing the tip of the arthroscope slightly
2. by leaning the arthroscope proximally, distally, cranially, and caudally
3. by rotating the light cable to change the orientation of the beveled lens.

Pathological lesions are evaluated and treated using hand instruments or the motorized shaver through the instrument portal.

25.5.5 Indications for elbow arthroscopy

Indications for elbow arthroscopy in cats may include diagnosis and therapy of infectious, neoplastic, traumatic, developmental, and degenerative diseases. Arthroscopy provides a means of minimally invasive synovial biopsy in cases of immune-mediated arthritis or neoplasia. Biopsies of the synovium are usually obtained with a small biter. The sharp biting action of these instruments permits rapid biopsies in a single step. Biopsies of cartilage or soft bone may be performed with very small trephines or a meniscal vascular punch. The most common application of elbow arthroscopy in cats has been for the diagnosis and therapy of developmental and degenerative diseases, specifically fragmentation of the medial coronoid process (FCP) and osteoarthritis.

Fragmentation of the medial coronoid process

Feline patients may have degenerative changes of the elbow similar to that found in canine patients with elbow dysplasia (Figs 25-20 and 25-21). Periarticular osteophytes, joint

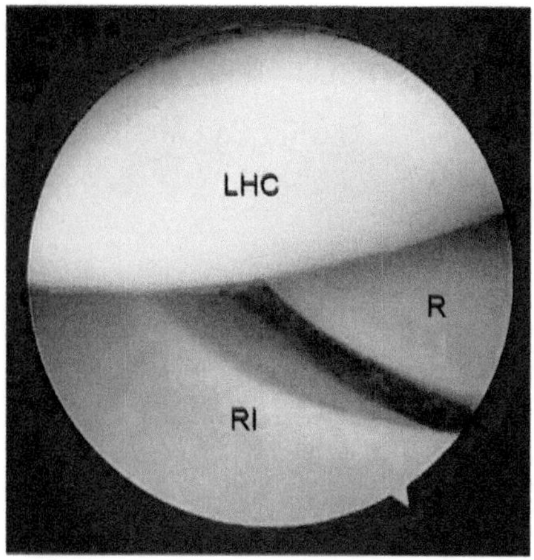

Figure 25-18 Structures that should be assessed centrally in the elbow include the radial incisure of the ulna (RI), lateral aspect of the humeral condyle (LHC), and radial head (R).

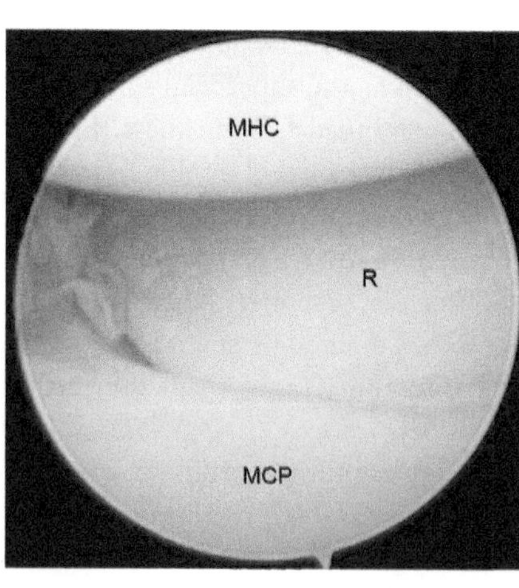

Figure 25-19 Structures that should be assessed on the medial aspect of the elbow include the medial coronoid process (MCP), medial aspect of the humeral condyle (MHC) and radial head (R).

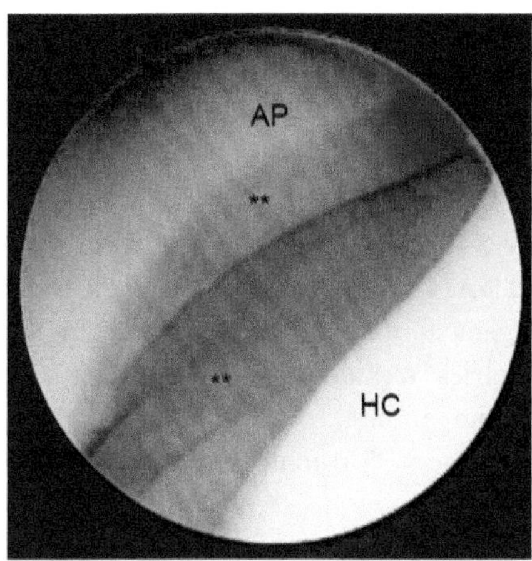

Figure 25-20 Fragmented medial coronoid process of the elbow is a form of elbow dysplasia. This condition may affect dogs or cats. Typical pathological changes include erosion of cartilage from the medial humeral condyle (**) from the anconeal process (AP) and caudal aspect of the trochlea of the humeral condyle (HC). Fragmentation of the medial coronoid process leads to loose osteochondral fragments within the joint.

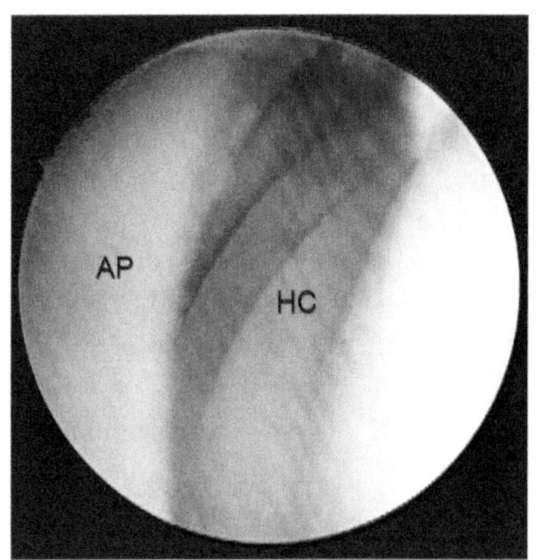

Figure 25-21 This feline patient with elbow dysplasia has changes that are identical to those seen in canine patients. Note the full-thickness cartilage erosion of the humeral condyle (HC) and anconeal process (AP) and grooves in the subchondral bone of the humeral condyle.

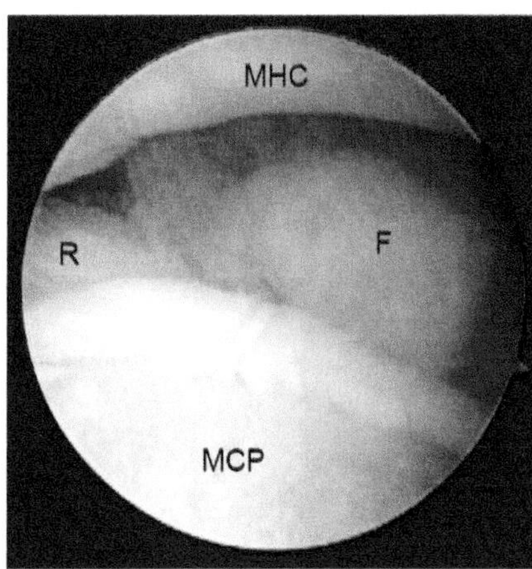

Figure 25-22 A fragment (F) from the medial coronoid process (MCP) of this cat has shifted cranial to the radial head (R) Medial humeral condyle (MHC).

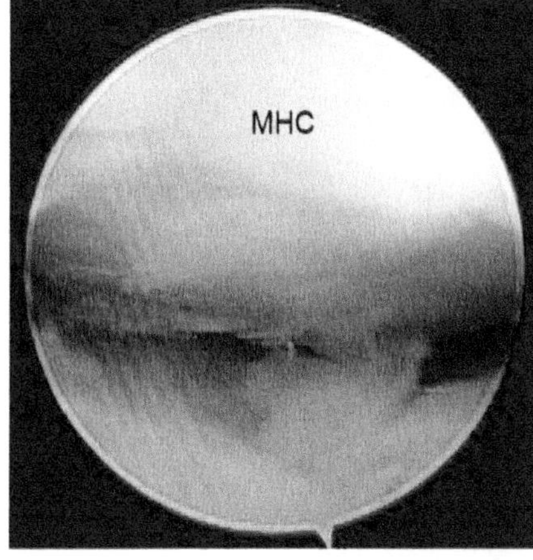

Figure 25-23 Full-thickness cartilage erosion of the Medial humeral condyle (MHC) occurs in cats with elbow dysplasia.

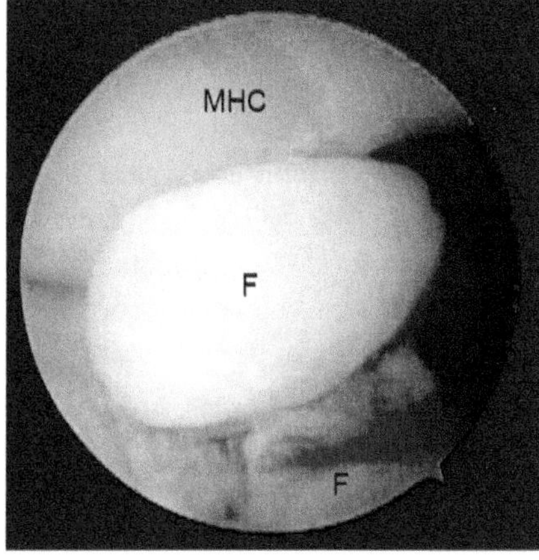

Figure 25-24 Multiple fragments (F) are often found in patients with fragmented medial coronoid process. The fragments are typically located near the medial coronoid process and the medial aspect of the humeral condyle (MHC) or cranial to the radial head.

capsule thickening, and mineralized free bodies are seen radiographically in affected cats. The mineralized free bodies may be found both inside the joint and within the soft tissues around the joint (Fig. 25-22). FCP has been identified arthroscopically in cats (4). The cause of this condition is unknown, but developmental, degenerative, and traumatic causes are considered most likely. The lesion is characterized by fragmentation of the cartilage and subchondral bone in the cranial and lateral aspect of the medial coronoid, and grade II to grade IV cartilage erosion over the medial coronoid process (Fig. 25-23).

When an FCP fragment initially separates, it may remain in its original location. Insert a small curette or probe into the joint to dislodge the fragment. A small grasper or small shaver blade is used to remove the fragment. Multiple fragments are often seen (Fig. 25-24). Avoid iatrogenic cartilage damage by carefully manipulating the working instruments. The assistant must be cautioned not to move abruptly or iatrogenic cartilage damage may occur. Remove multiple fragments individually (Fig. 25-25).

Larger and more chronically migrated fragments become more difficult to remove because of their size, location, and soft-tissue attachments. Fragments may continue to grow

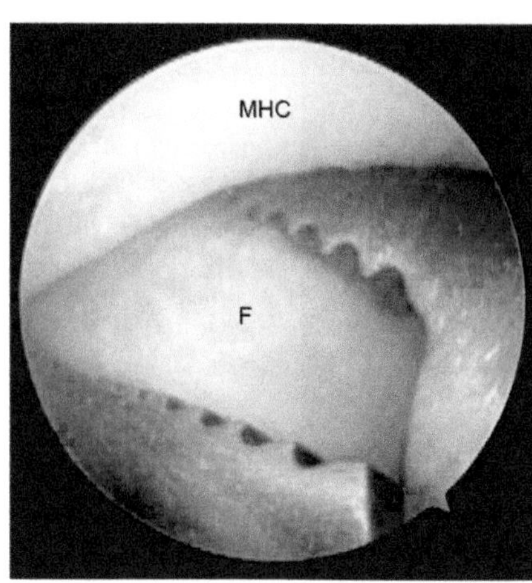

Figure 25-25 A grasper is used to remove a fragment (F) arising from the medial coronoid process. Medial humeral condyle.

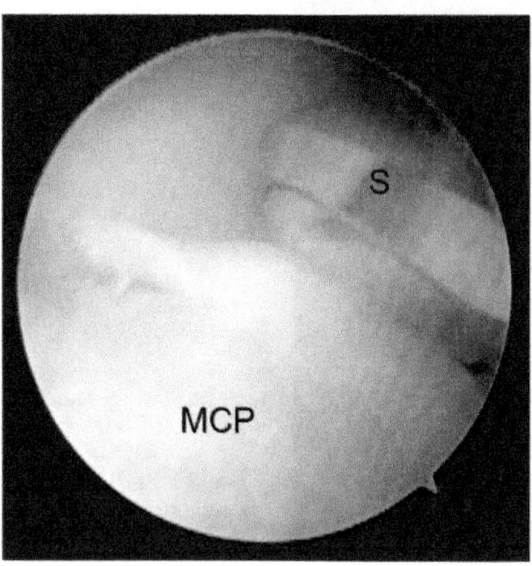

Figure 25-26 A motorized shaver (S) is used to remove osteochondral fragments, necrotic cartilage, and sclerotic bone of the medial coronoid process (MCP).

once migrated and become very large. To remove these fragments with a grasper alone, insert a locking grasper and remove the fragment in one piece or use the grasper to break it into smaller parts, always being careful to avoid damage to adjacent cartilage. Alternatively, insert a small-joint shaver with a shielded bur and suction (Fig. 25-26). Using the shield to protect the radial head, humerus and remaining coronoid, bur the fragment down to a size that can be removed or bur away the entire fragment.

Fragments may migrate cranially to a point where they cannot be reached with a bur or grasper. In this case, insert a 5-0 curette and pass the tip of the curette medial and cranial to the fragment. Then use the tip of the curette to push parts or the entire fragment back into the working space. This technique is difficult at first but with practice will permit retrieval of most cranially migrated fragments. Once the fragments have been completely removed, lavage the joint to remove any remaining bone debris. If osteochondritis dissecans or additional cartilage damage is identified, treat as described in the following sections. At the conclusion of the procedure inject bupivacaine if desired, and close the skin wounds.

Postoperatively, pain can be managed with cold therapy and appropriate doses of non-steroidal anti-inflammatory drugs (NSAIDs), chondroprotectants, or narcotics. Pain is usually minimal. Adequan is a good consideration for feline patients with FCP and can be given at a dose of 2 mg/kg, IM or SQ, every 5–7 days for eight treatments. Activity should be restricted for 4 weeks. The prognosis following arthroscopic management of FCP in the cat has yet to be determined and likely varies tremendously with severity of disease, function of the animal, postoperative management, and patient temperament. Fortunately, complications are rare and minor.

Osteoarthritis of the elbow

Arthroscopy has limited use in the management of elbow osteoarthritis in cats. The underlying cause of osteoarthritis should be identified and eliminated if possible. Arthroscopic exploration of the joint can be used to obtain synovial biopsies for histopathology and culture and sensitivity. Loose osteochondral fragments can be removed using grasping forceps. Areas of full-thickness cartilage wear can be treated. Management of articular cartilage lesions is based on the concept that providing blood, with mesenchymal stem cell precursors, access to the lesion encourages healing by the formation of fibrocartilage. Several methods have been described to achieve this. Abrasion arthroplasty involves uniform removal of subchondral bone until bleeding is achieved. This can be accomplished in the feline elbow by use of either a curette or bur attachment on a small-joint shaver. The shaver is usually more rapid and efficient and generally just as accurate. Another method of treatment for grade IV lesions is microfracture. In this technique, numerous microcracks are created in the subchondral bone plate to allow bleeding at the lesion surface. Microfracture awls are available for small-joint arthroscopic use. Alternatively, a small microfracture pick may be created by bending the end of a 0.035- or 0.045-inch K wire to about a 45° angle. The wire is then secured into a Jacobs chuck.

25.6 Arthroscopy of the hip

25.6.1 Patient position

The patient is positioned in lateral recumbency with the target hip-up. The lateral aspect of the hip will be approached. Slight traction should be placed on the leg while holding the leg parallel to the floor.

25.6.2 Recommended arthroscope size

This is 1.9, 2.3 or 2.4 mm.

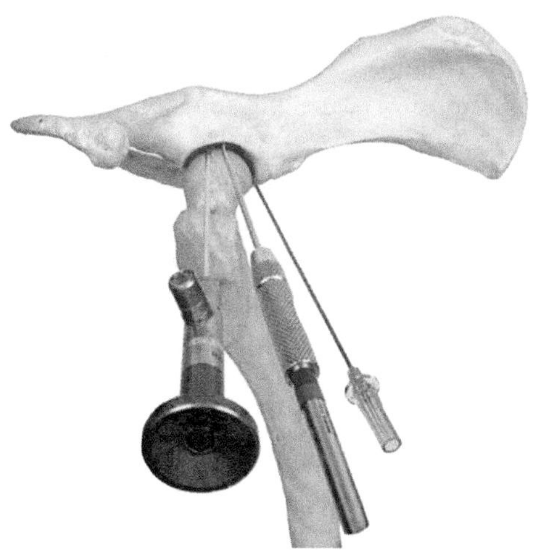

A

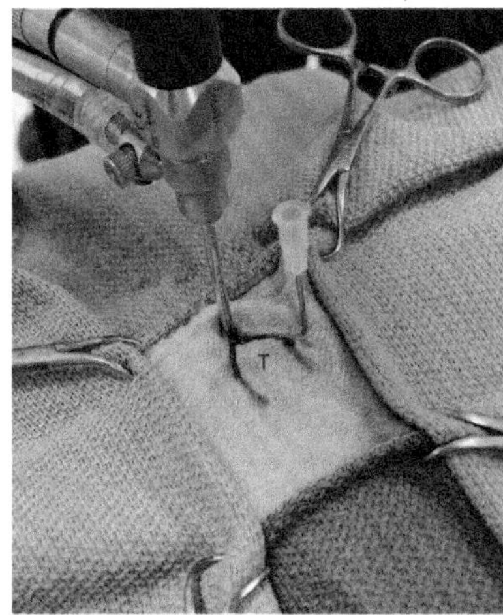

B

Figure 25-27 The portals for the hip are lateral, as shown in (**A**) and (**B**). The arthroscope portal is proximal to the greater trochanter. The instrument portal is slightly cranial and the egress portal is more cranial to the arthroscope portal.

25.6.3 Portal sites for hip arthroscopy

The portal sites used for feline hip arthroscopy are similar to the canine (Fig. 25-27). Arthroscope, egress, and instrument portals are typically used. An instrument portal may not be needed in all cases. The arthroscope portal is established first. The joint capsule must initially be distended. Insert a 20-gauge needle from the lateral aspect of the hip just proximal to the greater trochanter. The needle should be directed perpendicular to the long axis of the limb. In most cases, when the needle is properly placed, synovial fluid is easily aspirated. If synovial fluid is not aspirated and the surgeon believes the joint has been entered, saline can be instilled into the joint. If the needle is located in the joint, fluid is easily instilled and reverse pressure is felt on the syringe plunger as the joint capsule fully distends. Approximately 3–6 ml of fluid is needed to distend most feline hip joints. The needle is quickly removed.

The arthroscope cannula with the attached conical obturator is inserted. Standard scope insertion site is based on localization of the greater trochanter of the femur and approximation of the location of the joint surface. Place a finger on the greater trochanter and then move proximally just over its proximal edge. To insert the scope use a number 11 blade to make a 2–3-mm stab incision through the skin and superficial soft tissues. The incision should not be continued full-thickness through the joint capsule or the joint distension will be eliminated and it will allow excessive extravasation of fluid into the surrounding soft tissues. The egress portal is established second. A 20-gauge needle is placed in the craniolateral joint space just cranial and distal to the arthroscope portal. The lateral radiograph should be used to estimate the location of the craniolateral joint space. If the needle is properly placed, fluid should flow freely from the egress needle. The instrument portal is established if probing, biopsy, or treatment of joint pathology is required. The instrument portal can be placed at the site of the egress portal. An instrument cannula can be used, allowing the portal to have dual actions – acting as an instrument and an egress portal. Alternatively the instrument portal may be established halfway between the arthroscope and egress portals.

25.6.4 Surgical anatomy

The initial step in hip arthroscopy should be a thorough systematic exploration of the joint. Developing a standardized pattern for examination of the joint will help development of arthroscopic skills and ensure that all accessible areas of the joint are examined. An example of standard hip joint examination would be to visualize the:

- Femoral head (Figs 25-28 and 25-29)
- Acetabulum (Figs 25-28 and 25-29)
- Labrum (Fig. 25-29)
- Synovial membrane
- Round ligament (Fig. 25-30)

The joint is explored by changing the field of view of the arthroscope using a combination of techniques. Actual movement of the scope should be minimized to avoid inadvertent withdrawal of the scope from the joint. The field of view can be changed in three ways:

1. by advancing or withdrawing the tip of the arthroscope slightly
2. by leaning the arthroscope proximally, distally, cranially, and caudally
3. by rotating the light cable to change the orientation of the beveled lens.

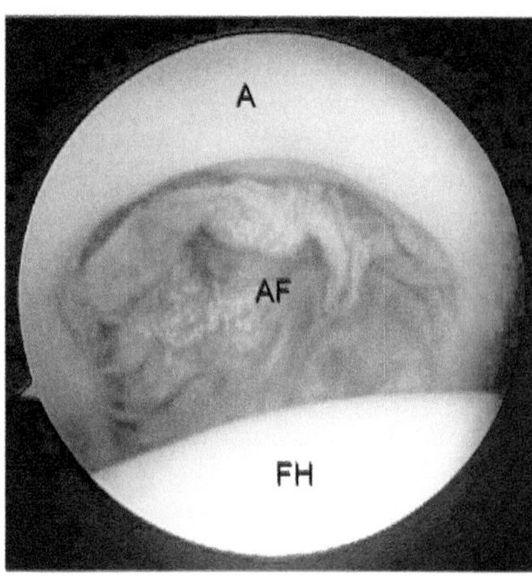

Figure 25-28 The acetabulum (A), acetabular fossa (AF), and femoral head (FH) are easily accessed during hip arthroscopy in cats.

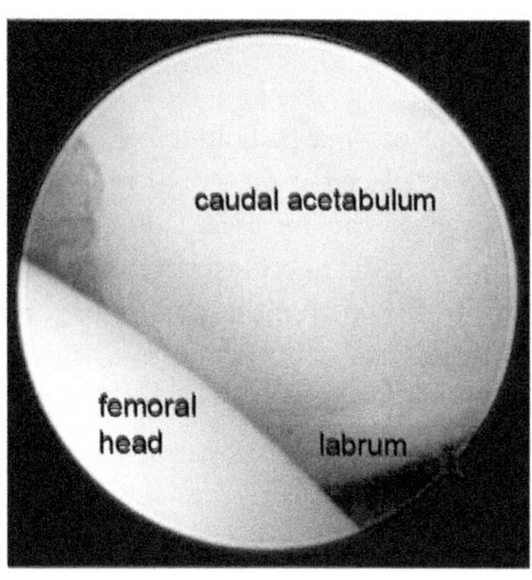

Figure 25-29 The acetabulum, femoral head, and labrum of the hip joint can be seen arthroscopically.

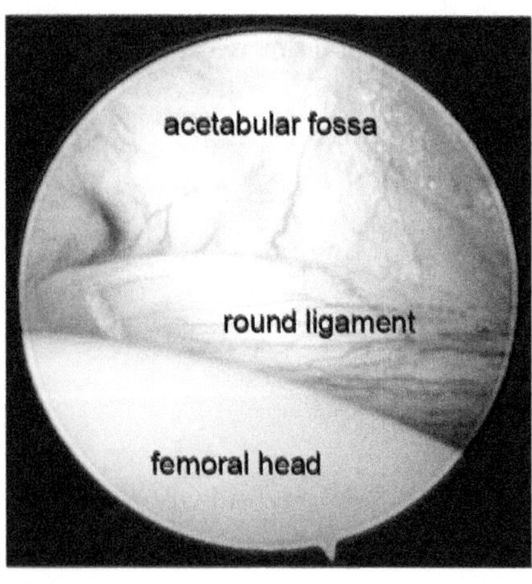

Figure 25-30 The round ligament can be evaluated as it courses from the acetabular fossa to the femoral head by applying traction to the leg and advancing the tip of the scope towards the medial aspect of the hip joint.

Pathological lesions are evaluated and treated using hand instruments or the motorized shaver through the instrument portal.

25.6.5 Indications for hip arthroscopy

Hip arthroscopy is occasionally performed in cats. Indications for hip arthroscopy may include diagnosis and therapy of infectious, neoplastic, traumatic, developmental, and degenerative diseases. Minimally invasive synovial biopsy may be performed. The most common application of hip arthroscopy in cats has been for the diagnosis and therapy of traumatic and degenerative diseases, specifically hip dislocation, and osteoarthritis. The list of indications for hip arthroscopy in cats will likely expand in the future as new pathological conditions are discovered during exploratory arthroscopic examinations of cats having painful conditions of the hip.

Hip dislocation

Feline patients may incur cartilage damage of the hip as a sequela to traumatic dislocation. The arthroscope can be used to assess damage to the acetabulum, articular cartilage, and joint capsule prior to determining a definitive surgical plan. If closed reduction is to be performed, the arthroscope can be used to guide removal of debris and hematoma from the acetabulum. The swollen round ligament and avulsed fracture fragments can be debrided to facilitate reduction. The arthroscope can also be used to confirm reduction of the hip following closed reduction. If substantial damage to the joint capsule or articular cartilage is seen, the surgeon may opt to perform a total hip replacement or a femoral head and neck ostectomy using traditional techniques.

Osteoarthrtitis and synovitis

Arthroscopy of the hip has limited use in the management of osteoarthritis and synovitis in cats. The underlying cause of osteoarthritis should be identified and eliminated if possible. Arthroscopic exploration of the joint can be used to obtain synovial biopsies for histopathology and culture and sensitivity. Loose osteochondral fragments can be removed using grasping forceps. Areas of full-thickness cartilage wear can be treated. A description for treatment of damaged regions of the articular cartilage is described above, in the section on elbow osteoarthritis.

25.7 Arthroscopy of the stifle

25.7.1 Patient position

The patient is positioned in dorsal recumbency with the stifle hanging off the end of the table. It is helpful to tilt the table slightly with the head up and the stifle down. The cranial aspect of the stifle will be approached. The stifle should be unconstrained so that flexion and extension can be achieved.

25.7.2 Recommended arthroscope size

This is 1.9, 2.3, 2.4 or 2.7 mm.

25.7.3 Portal sites for stifle arthroscopy

The portal sites used for feline stifle arthroscopy are similar to those for the canine (Figs 25-31 and 25-32). Arthroscope, egress, and instrument portals are typically used. The egress portal is placed first (Fig. 25-33). A stab incision is made lateral to the insertion of the patellar tendon just proximal to the tibial plateau. The obturator for the matched-egress cannula is inserted into the joint in a distal to proximal and lateral to medial direction. The obturator is directed into the trochlear groove, under the patella, exiting the suprapatellar joint pouch medial to the insertion of the quadriceps. The cannula is inserted over the obturator and pushed carefully into the joint while the stifle is held in extension (Fig. 25-34). The obturator is removed. The cannula can then be carefully maneuvered into the medial joint pouch (Fig. 25-35). The scope portal is created next. The arthroscope is inserted through the previous craniolateral stab incision in the same direction as was used for the egress obturator (Fig. 25-36). The instrument portal is made at the same level as the scope portal but is medial to the insertion of the patellar tendon. A small portion of the patellar fat pad may need to be removed

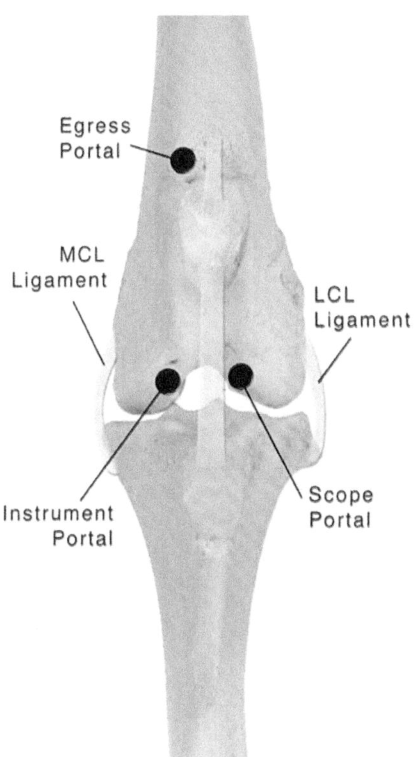

Figure 25-31 The portals for the stifle are shown in Figures 25-31 and 25-32. The arthroscope portal is lateral to the patellar tendon and just proximal to the tibial plateau. The instrument portal is medial to the patellar tendon. The egress portal is located in the medial aspect of the suprapatellar pouch.

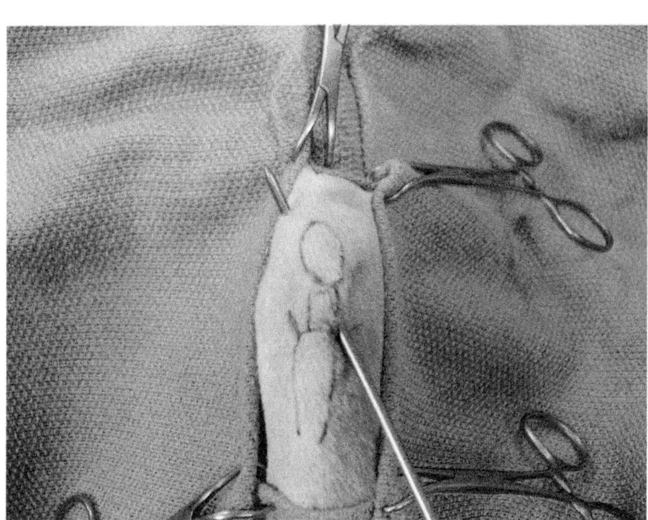

Figure 25-33 The egress portal is placed in retrograde fashion. An obturator is first passed from the arthroscope portal, under the patella, exiting at the medial aspect of the suprapatellar pouch.

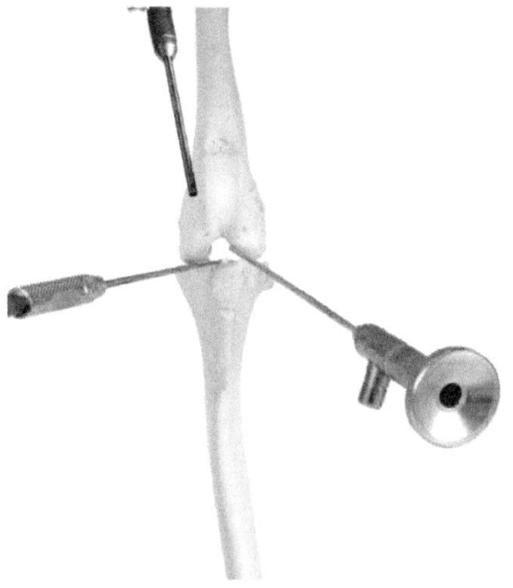

Figure 25-32 Portal positions for stifle arthroscopy in the cat.

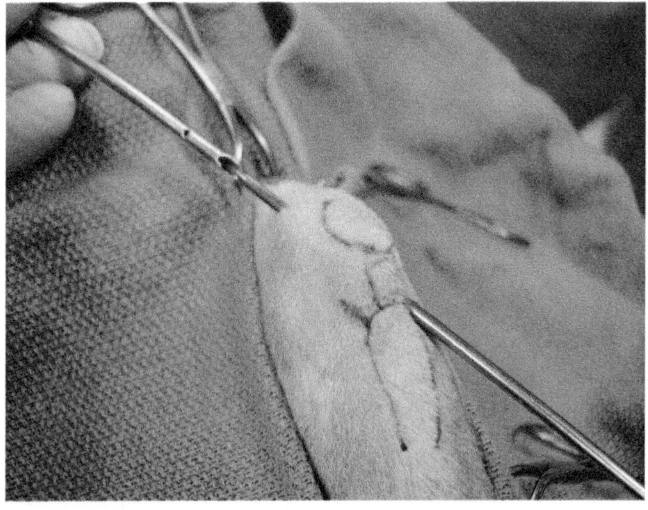

Figure 25-34 The egress cannula is inserted into the joint by sliding the cannula over the obturator.

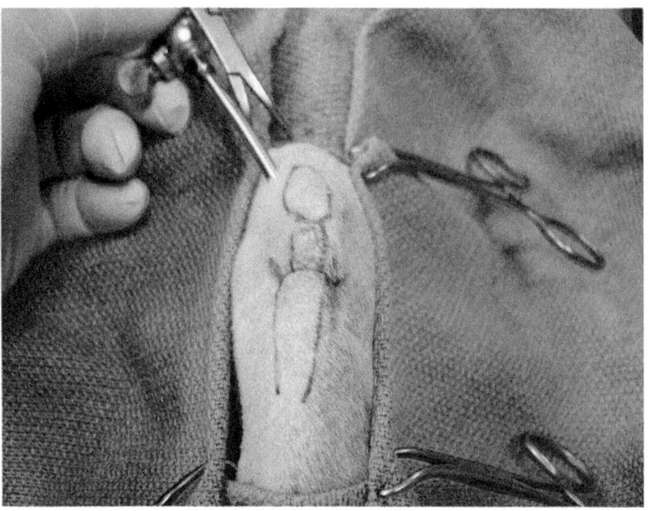

Figure 25-35 The obturator is removed and the cannula is positioned in the medial gutter of the joint.

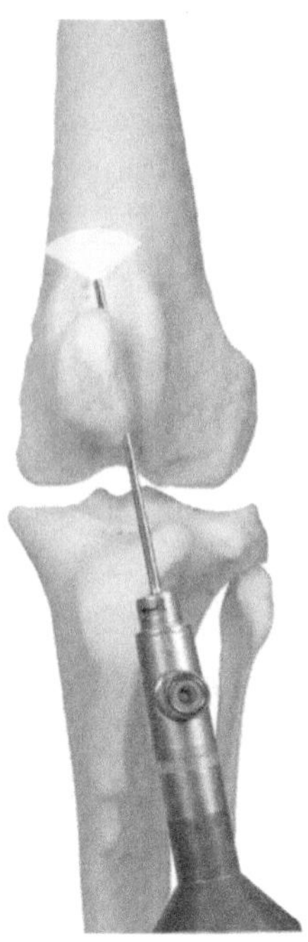

Figure 25-37 Examination of the stifle joint begins in the trochlear groove with the arthroscope positioned as shown.

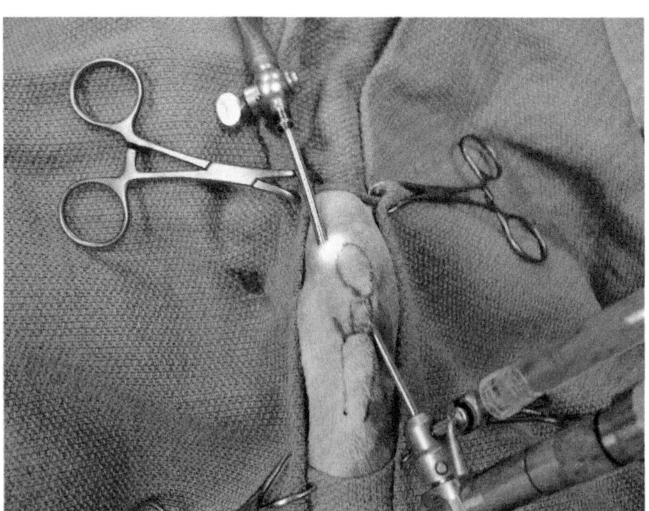

Figure 25-36 The arthroscope is placed into the joint through the arthroscope portal.

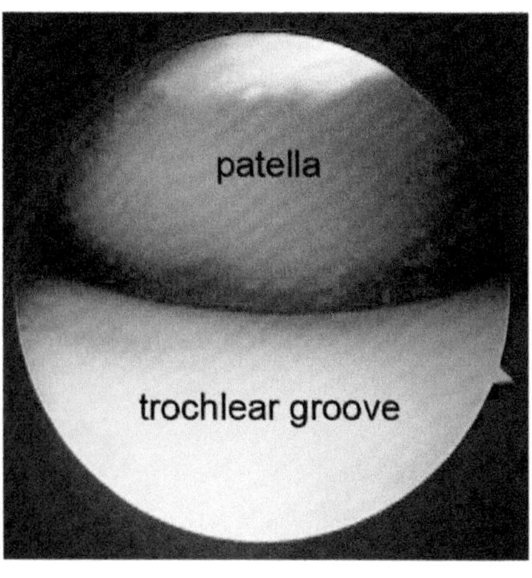

Figure 25-38 The trochlear groove is examined for cartilage wear below the patella.

using hand instruments or a motorized shaver to allow an adequate view of the intercondylar notch, cruciate ligaments, articular cartilage, and menisci. An attempt can be made to retract the fat pad distally using a probe or small retractor placed into the joint through the instrument portal rather than removed with the shaver.

25.7.4 Surgical anatomy

The initial step in stifle arthroscopy should be a thorough systematic exploration of the joint. The proximal aspect of the stifle is evaluated first (Fig. 25-37), followed by the distal compartment. Developing a standardized pattern for examination of the joint will help development of arthroscopic skills and ensure that all accessible areas of the joint are examined. An example of a standard stifle joint examination would be to visualize the:

- Supratrochlear joint pouch
- Trochlear groove (Fig. 25-38)
- Patella (Figs 25-39 and 25-40)
- Lateral joint compartment (Fig. 25-41)
- Articular surface of the femoral condyles (Fig. 25-42)
- Medial joint compartment (Fig. 25-43)
- Cranial cruciate ligament (Figs 25-44 and 25-45)

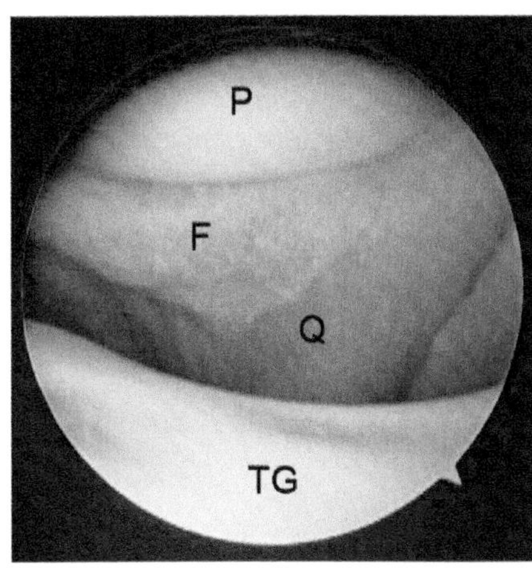

Figure 25-39 The arthroscope is advanced and the light cable is turned to view the underside of the proximal pole of the patella (P), trochlear groove (TG), fat within the joint (F), and the insertion of the quadriceps tendon (Q).

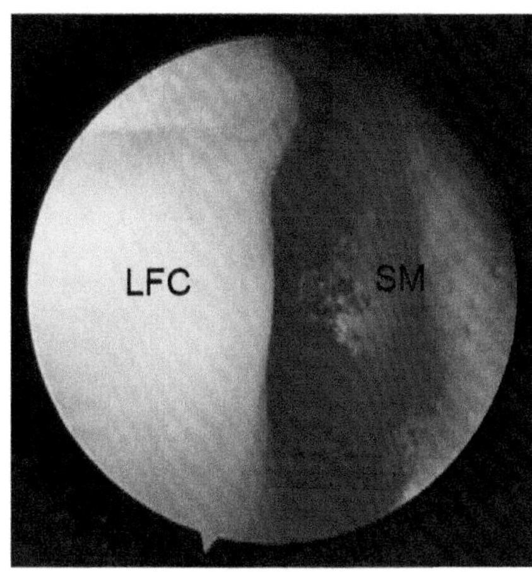

Figure 25-42 The lateral femoral condyle (LFC) is evaluated for cartilage wear and osteophyte formation near the synovial membrane (SM) attachment.

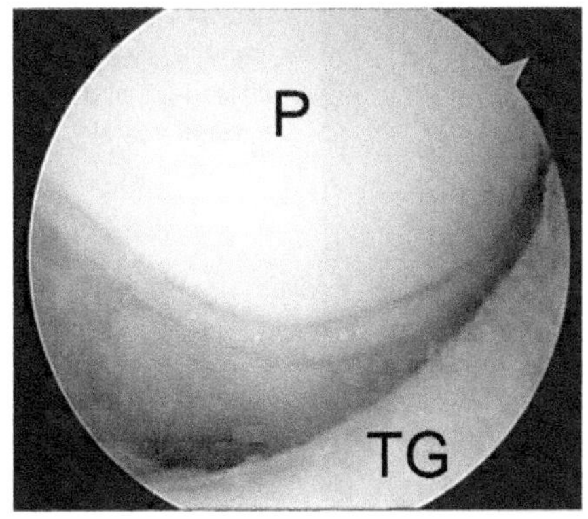

Figure 25-40 The arthroscope is withdrawn slightly, maintaining the position of the light cable to view the remaining portion of the patella (P) and trochlear groove (TG).

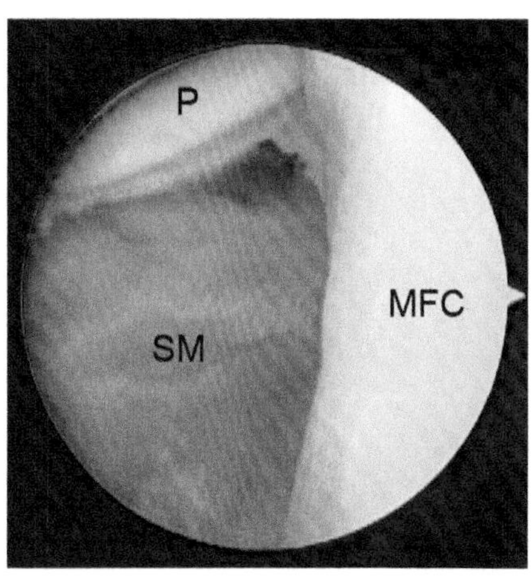

Figure 25-43 The tip of the arthroscope is carefully moved into the medial gutter to evaluate the medial femoral condyle (MFC) and synovial membrane (SM). The patella (P) will occasionally be seen if it shifts medially due to tension placed on the soft tissues during placement of the egress cannula.

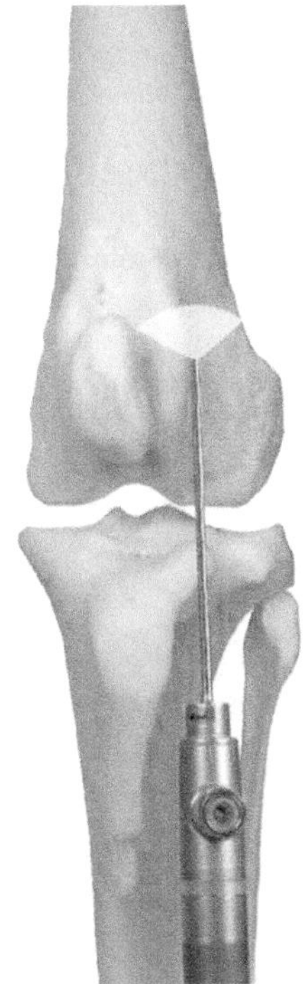

Figure 25-41 The tip of the arthroscope is carefully moved into the lateral gutter to evaluate the lateral joint pouch.

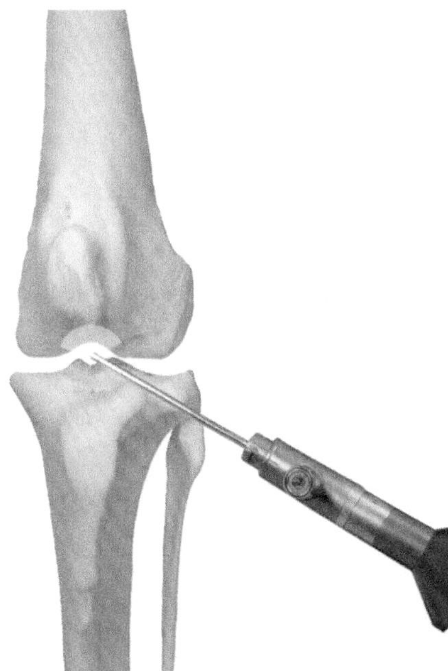

Figure 25-44 The tip of the arthroscope is carefully moved into the intercondylar notch and the stifle is slowly flexed to view the cruciate ligaments and menisci.

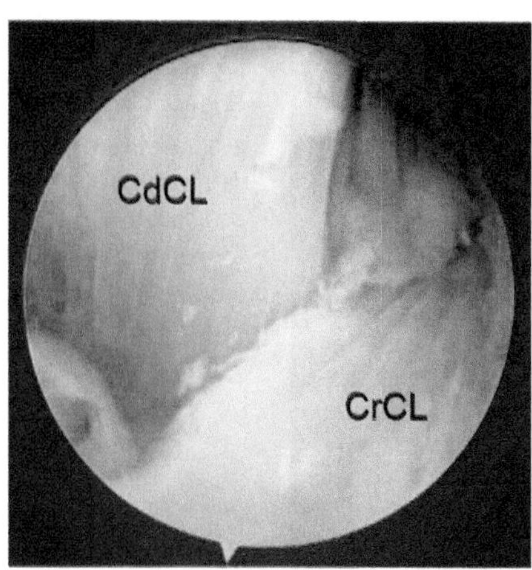

Figure 25-45 The normal cranial cruciate ligament (CrCL) and caudal cruciate ligament (CdCL) are seen within the intercondylar notch. A portion of the fat pad may have to be retracted or removed to evaluate the ligaments adequately.

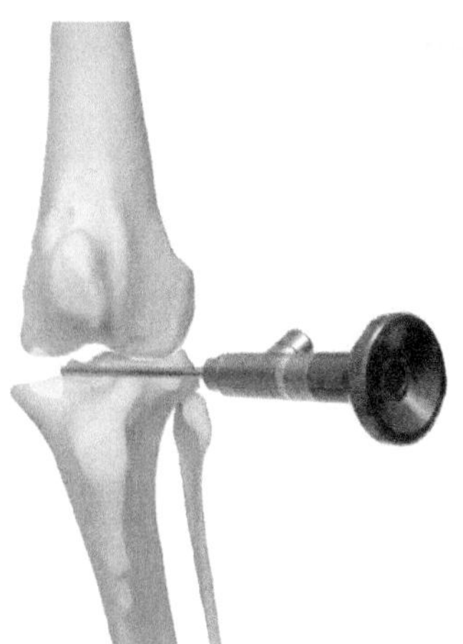
Figure 25-48 The arthroscope is positioned to view the medial meniscus. Complete evaluation of the medial meniscus requires rotation of the light cable to change the position of the beveled lens of the arthroscope.

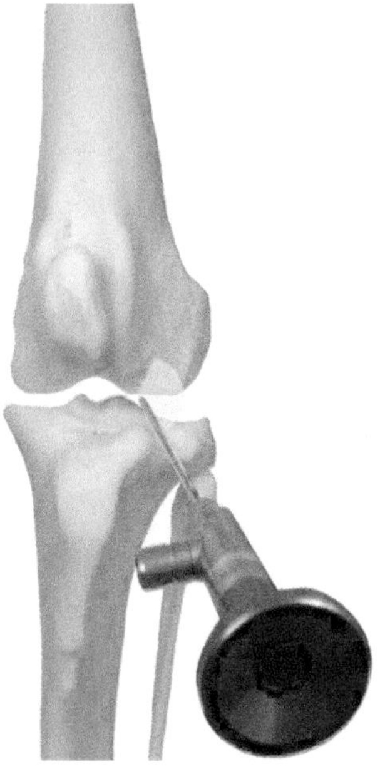
Figure 25-46 The arthroscope is positioned to view the lateral meniscus. Note the position of the light cable.

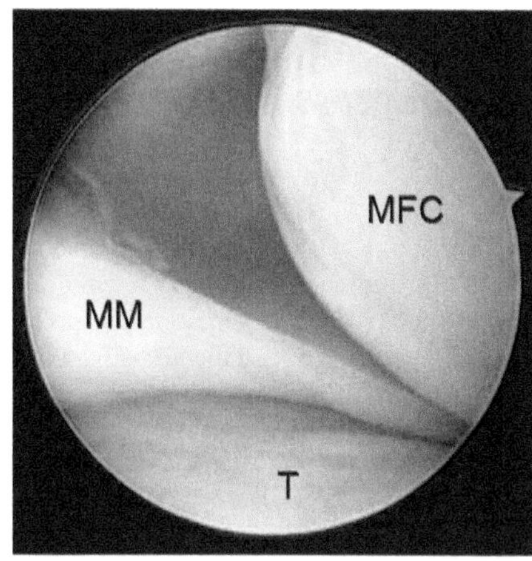

Figure 25-49 Appearance of the normal medial meniscus (MM), tibial plateau (T), and medial femoral condyle (MFC).

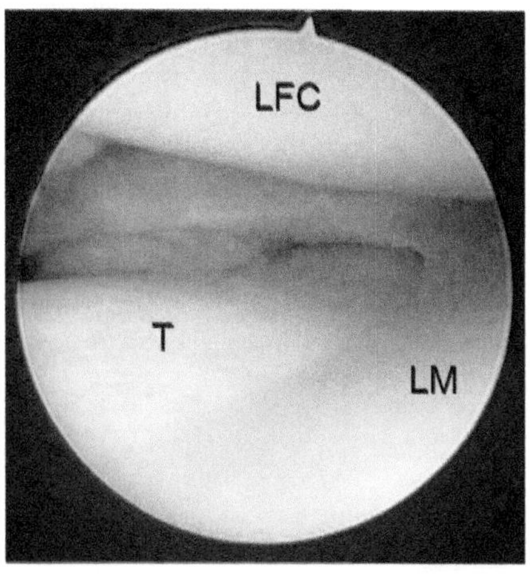

Figure 25-47 Appearance of the normal lateral meniscus (LM), tibial plateau (T), and lateral femoral condyle (LFC).

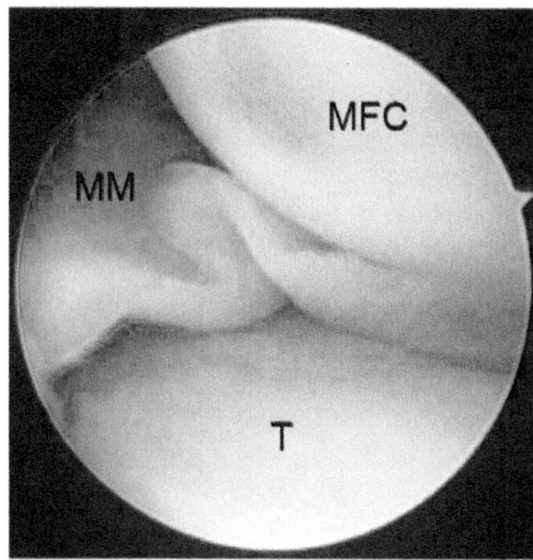

Figure 25-50 The medial meniscus (MM) seen in this view has a small fold due to compression between the medial femoral condyle (MFC) and tibial plateau (T) as the stifle is flexed. This is a normal meniscus and should not be mistaken for a tear.

- Caudal cruciate ligament
- Lateral meniscus (Figs 25-46 and 25-47)
- Medial meniscus (Figs 25-48–25-50)
- Articular surface of the tibial plateau

The joint is explored by changing the field of view of the arthroscope using a combination of techniques. Actual movement of the scope should be minimized to avoid inadvertent withdrawal of the scope from the joint. The field of view can be changed in three ways:

1. by advancing or withdrawing the tip of the arthroscope slightly

2. by leaning the arthroscope proximally, distally, cranially, and caudally
3. by rotating the light cable to change the orientation of the beveled lens.

Pathological lesions are evaluated and treated using hand instruments or the motorized shaver through the instrument portal. The cruciate ligament debris is removed to allow a better view of the menisci. The lateral meniscus is evaluated by applying a mild varus pressure to the joint while simultaneously rotating the stifle internally. The medial meniscus is evaluated by applying a mild valgus pressure to the joint while simultaneously rotating the stifle externally.

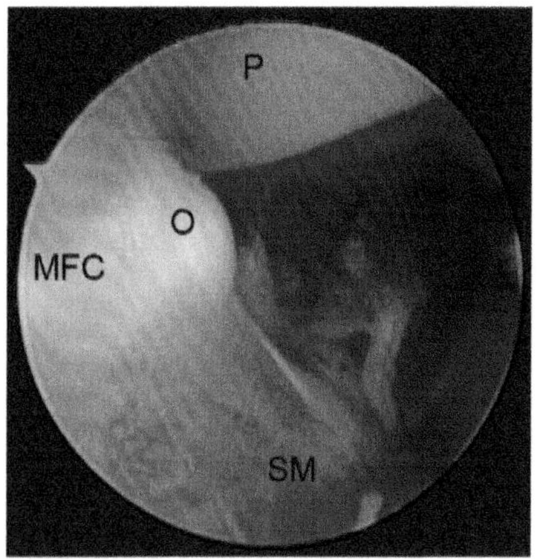

Figure 25-51 A small osteophyte (O) can be seen at the junction of the medial femoral condyle (MFC) and synovial membrane (SM) in this cat with a torn cranial cruciate ligament. Patella (P).

25.7.5 Indications for stifle arthroscopy

The stifle is the most common joint in the cat evaluated arthroscopically. Conditions that may benefit from arthroscopy include cruciate ligament disease, multiligamentous instability, osteochondrosis, meniscal tears, and meniscal mineralization. Minimally invasive synovial biopsy may also be performed.

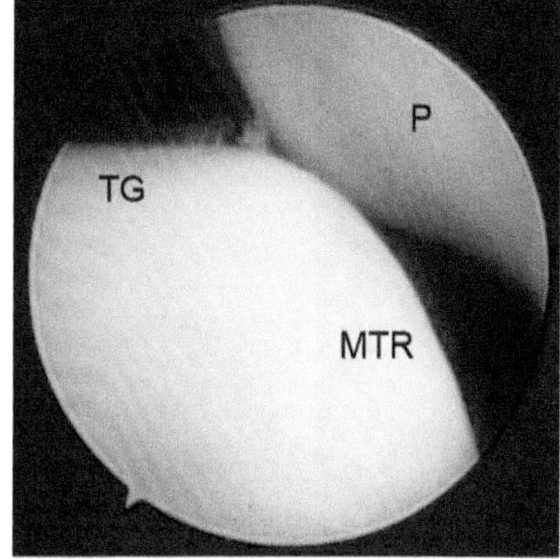

Figure 25-52 The patella (P) is positioned medial to the medial trochlear ridge (MTR) in this feline patient with medial patellar luxation. Note the shallow trochlear groove (TG) and the focal area of cartilage wear at the proximal extent of the MTR.

Cranial cruciate ligament disease

Injury to the cranial cruciate ligament in cats occurs commonly. Treatment options include conservative management and surgical management. Most orthopedic surgeons recommend surgical management as the best and most predictable option. Arthrotomy and extracapsular stabilization of the stifle have traditionally been used in surgical management. Arthroscopic evaluation of the stifle offers advantages compared to arthrotomy. Arthroscopic evaluation of the stifle offers a minimally invasive method of evaluating all regions of the stifle under magnification and in a fluid medium. This allows more critical evaluation of the condition of the articular cartilage, synovial membrane, cranial and caudal cruciate ligaments, and medial and lateral menisci. Documentation of the condition of the joint is important and easily performed at the time of arthroscopy. Examination of the cranial cruciate ligament and menisci can be accomplished and a diagnosis made prior to making a more invasive arthrotomy. This becomes particularly important for confirmation of partial tears of the cranial cruciate ligament and meniscal tears. The degree of cartilage damage associated with osteoarthritis can also be assessed and this may help the surgeon plan a long-term therapeutic regime following surgery (Fig. 25-51).

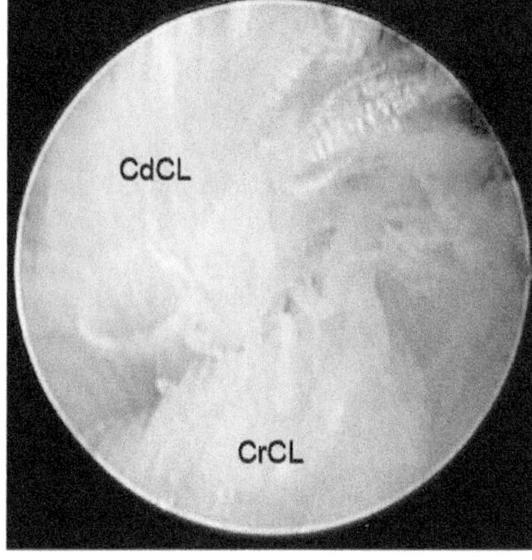

Figure 25-53 This cat has a tear of the cranial cruciate ligament (CrCL). The caudal cruciate ligament (CdCL) is visible behind the torn fibers of the CrCL.

The proximal aspect of the joint is evaluated first. The degree of synovitis and presence of osteophytes are assessed by positioning the arthroscope in the medial and lateral gutters of the joint. The condition of the articular cartilage in the trochlear groove and trochlear ridges can be assessed with the tip of the arthroscope positioned within the trochlear groove. Patellar position and integrity of the subpatellar articular cartilage are evaluated (Fig. 25-52). The distal aspect of the joint is assessed after retraction or removal of a small portion of the infrapatellar fat pad. The intercondylar notch is best examined with the stifle positioned in flexion.

The cranial cruciate ligament should be assessed for changes in vascularity, tautness, and fiber damage (Fig. 25-53). Complete tears of the ligament may be characterized by the typical

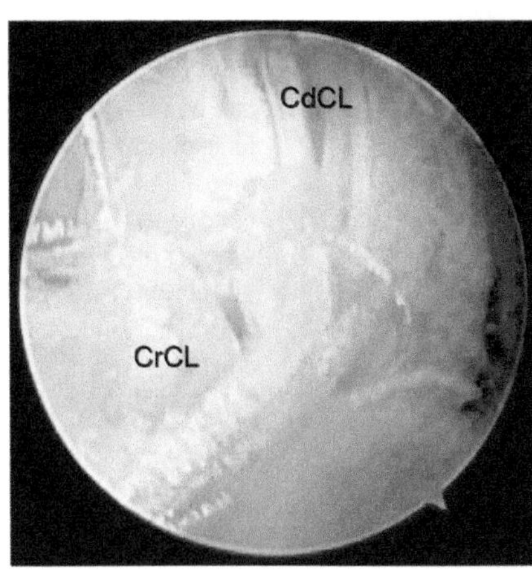

Figure 25-54 The arthroscope is advanced towards the cranial cruciate ligament (CrCL) to evaluate the torn fibers. Caudal cruciate ligament (CdCL).

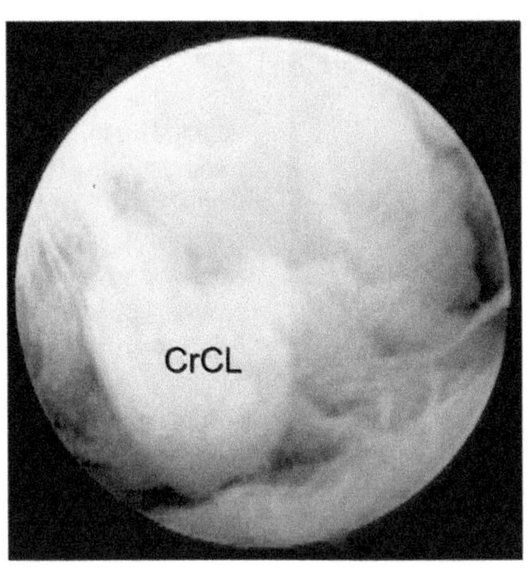

Figure 25-55 A complete tear of the cranial cruciate ligament (CrCL) is seen in this feline patient.

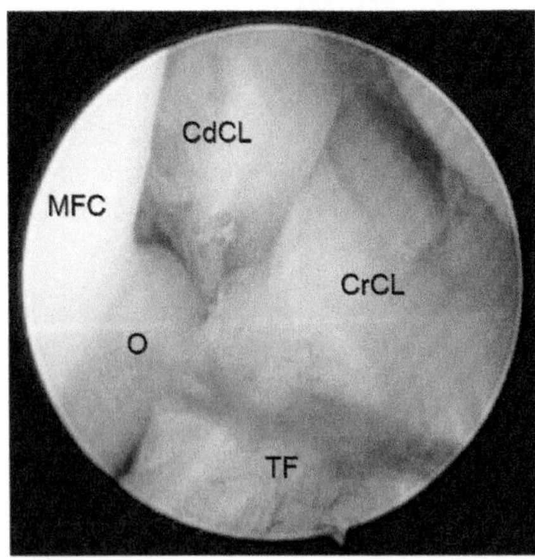

Figure 25-56 A partial tear of the cranial cruciate ligament (CrCL) is seen in this feline patient. The torn fibers (TF) are seen in the craniomedial band of the CrCL adjacent to an osteophyte (O) off the medial femoral condyle (MFC) in the intercondylar notch. Caudal cruciate ligament (CdCL).

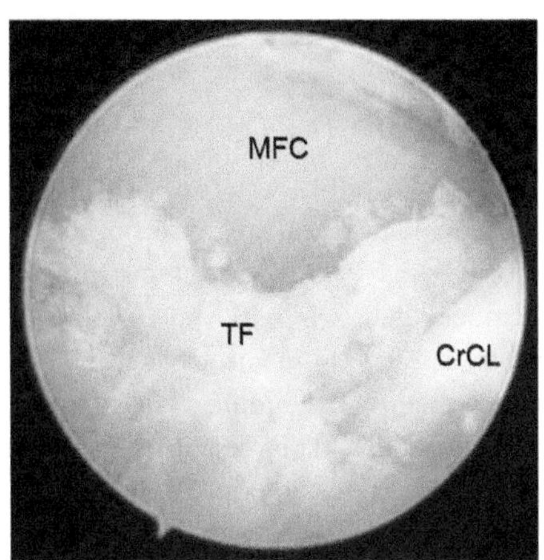

Figure 25-57 A partial tear of the cranial cruciate ligament (CrCL) is seen in this feline patient. The torn fibers (TF) are at the insertion of the craniomedial band of the CrCL on the tibia near the medial femoral condyle (MFC).

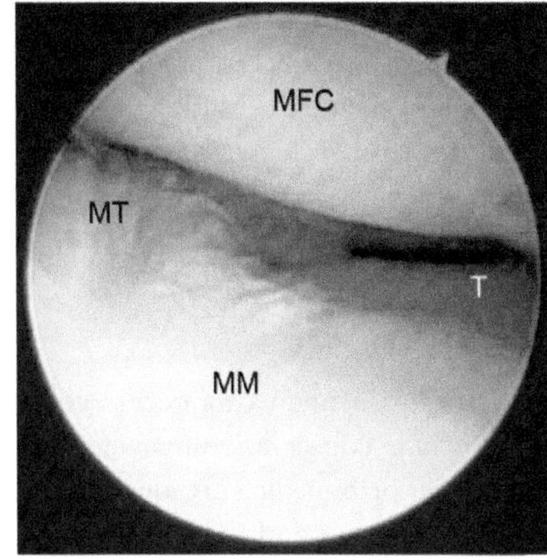

Figure 25-58 Radial tears (MT) of the medial meniscus (MM) are present in this feline patient with a partial tear of the cranial cruciate ligament. Medial femoral condyle (MFC), tibial platean (T)

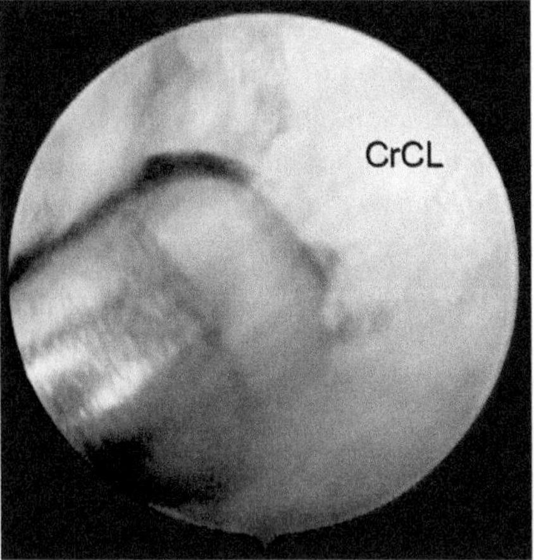

Figure 25-59 A motorized shaver is used to remove torn fibers of the cranial cruciate ligament (CrCL).

appearance of torn collagen fibers and hematoma formation if the tear is acute (Figs 25-54–25-56). Partial tears of the ligament may be easily observed or may be apparent only after careful probing of the ligament (Figs 25-57–25-59). Occasionally partial tears are characterized by fiber stretching and not total fiber disruption. The ligament should be carefully probed to assess tension within the ligament. Although the fibers are not completely disrupted, the ligament is non-functional and stabilization is indicated. Damaged fibers of the cranial cruciate ligament are excised using hand instruments or a motorized shaver (Figs 25-60 and 25-61). The radiofrequency probe can be used to remove small por-

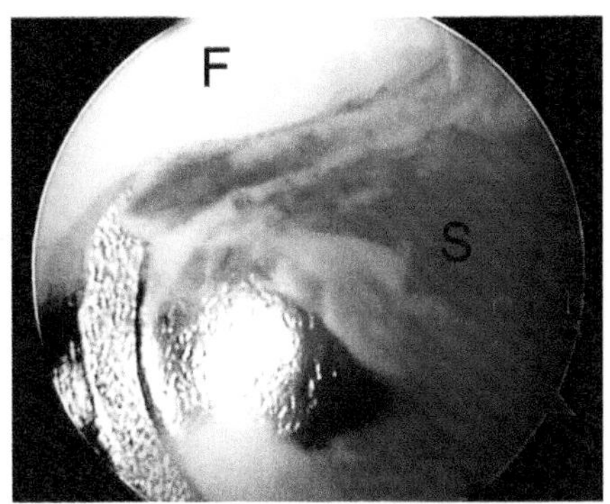

Figure 25-60 A motorized shaver is used to remove hyperplastic synovial tissue (S) adjacent to the femoral condyle (F).

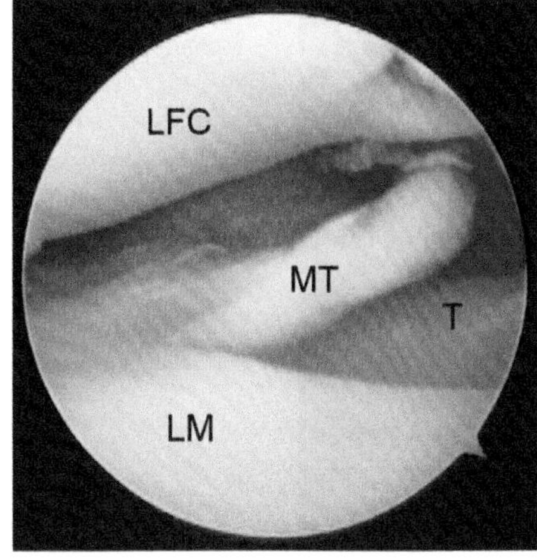

Figure 25-62 A radial tear (MT) of the lateral meniscus (LM) is seen in this feline patient. Lateral femoral condyle (LFC), tibial plateau (T).

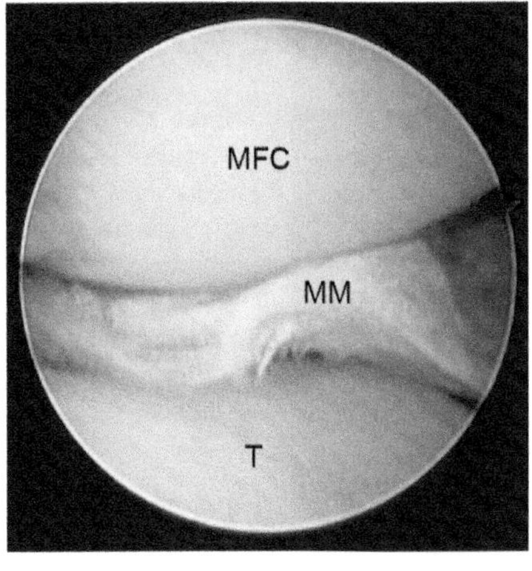

Figure 25-61 A bucket-handle tear of the medial meniscus (MM) is seen between the medial femoral condyle (MFL) and the tibial plateau (T).

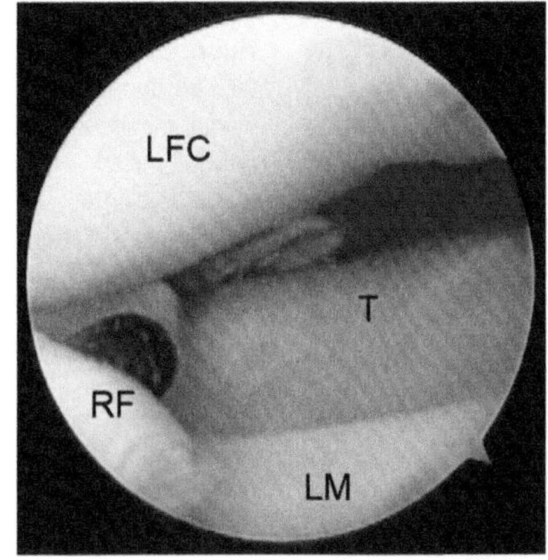

Figure 25-63 Small radial meniscal tears can be removed by partial meniscectomy using a radiofrequency probe (RF). Lateral femoral condyle (LFC), tibial plateau (T), meniscus (LM).

tions of torn fibers in areas that cannot be accessed with the shaver or hand instruments.

The caudal cruciate ligament should be assessed in a similar manner to the cranial ligament. Perhaps the greatest advantage of arthroscopic evaluation of the stifle is assessment of the menisci. The magnification provided by the arthroscope allows a better view of tears that might otherwise be missed during arthrotomy. The menisci should be carefully probed for tears. Bucket-handle tears of the posterior horn of the medial meniscus are the most common tears found. Radial tears are also commonly seen and may affect the medial or lateral menisci (Fig. 25-62–25-65).

Partial meniscectomy is performed, removing only the damaged portion of the meniscus. Partial meniscectomy can be performed arthroscopically using hand instruments, a motorized shaver, or a radiofrequency probe. This procedure can be challenging and a miniarthrotomy can be used if needed to complete the procedure. Release of the meniscal tibial ligament (meniscal release) can be performed arthroscopically in the cat if desired as a means of preventing meniscal tears in the future. Stabilization of the stifle is generally achieved using an extracapsular technique through a minimally invasive approach to the lateral aspect of the stifle.

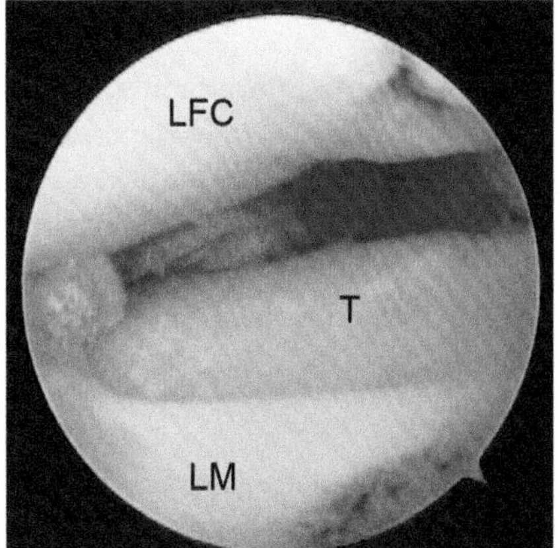

Figure 25-64 Appearance of the lateral meniscus (LM) following partial meniscectomy. Lateral femoral condyle (LFC), tibial plateau (T).

Multiple ligamentous instability

Multiple injuries are common stifle injuries in the cat. Arthroscopic evaluation of these patients commonly reveals injuries to the cranial cruciate ligament, caudal cruciate ligament, collateral ligaments, and medial and lateral menisci. The arthroscope is useful in assessing the extent of damage

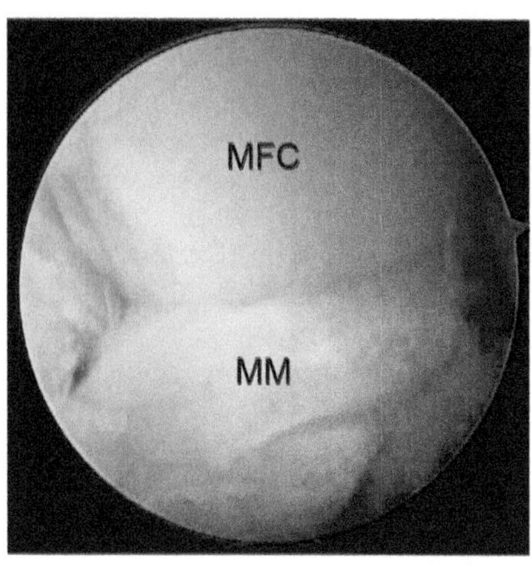

Figure 25-65 Appearance of a large bucket-handle tear of the medial meniscus (MM). Medial femoral condyle (MFC).

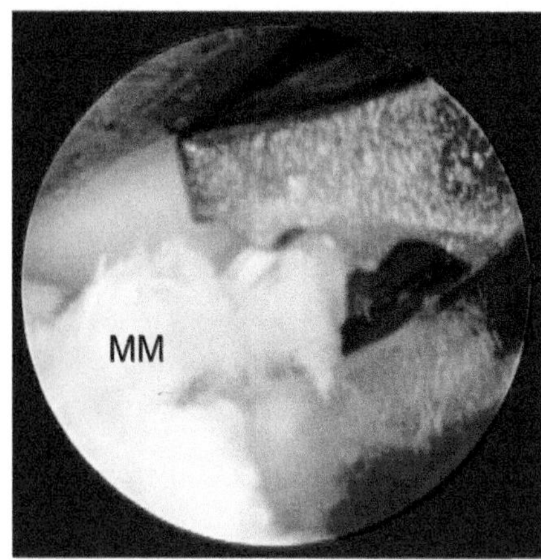

Figure 25-67 A punch forcep is used to cut the attached portion of the torn medial meniscus (MM), allowing removal of the damaged meniscal tissue.

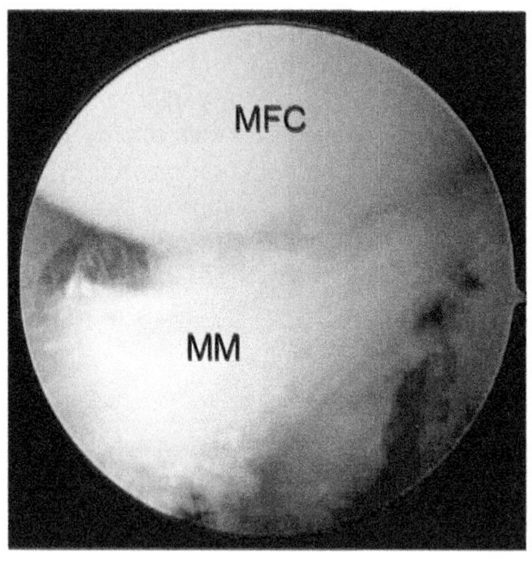

Figure 25-66 The torn portion of the medial meniscus (MM) is pulled forward using a probe in preparation of partial meniscectomy. Medial femoral condyle (MFC).

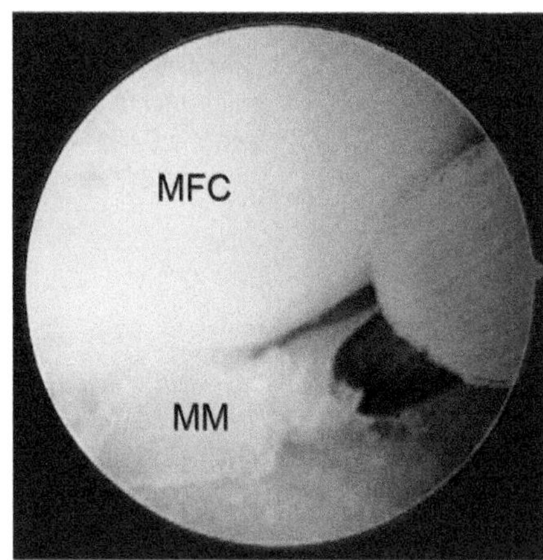

Figure 25-68 Small remnants of the torn medial meniscus (MM) can be removed with a radiofrequency probe. Medial femoral condyle (MFC).

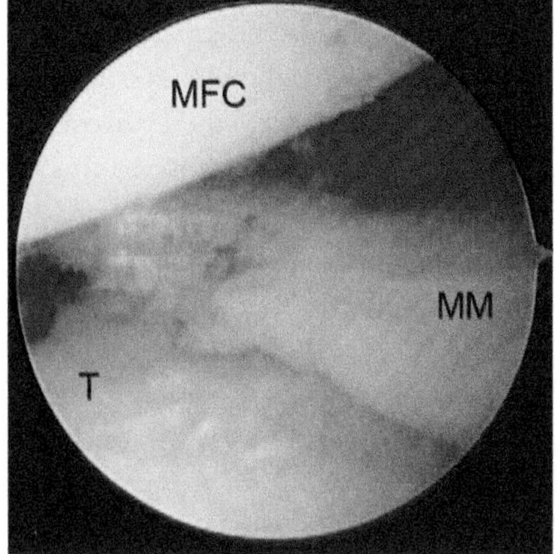

Figure 25-69 Appearance of the cranial aspect of the medial meniscus (MM) following partial meniscectomy. Medial femoral condyle (MFC), tibial plateau (T).

and assisting in surgical treatment. An arthrotomy is usually needed, but the scope can be used to magnify the areas of interest and confirm adequate treatment. The stifle can be stabilized using a transarticular pin, transarticular external fixator, or reconstruction of the torn ligaments. The arthroscope can be used to help guide the surgeon in proper placement of a transarticular pin.

Medial meniscal tear

Tears of the medial meniscus are most commonly seen in cats with tears of the cranial cruciate ligament or multiple ligament instability. Isolated medial meniscal tears are very rare. Occasionally, meniscal tears occur a period of time after conservative or surgical treatment of a torn cranial cruciate ligament. The posterior horn of the medial meniscus is the portion of the meniscus that is at greatest risk of tearing. Bucket-handle tears are commonly seen in this region (Fig. 25-66). Arthroscopic partial meniscectomy is achieved by placing tension on the damaged portion of the meniscus using a grasper or probe (Fig. 25-67). The cranial and caudal attachments of the torn portion of the meniscus ("the bucket-handle") are transected using a biting punch forcep (Fig. 25-68), a meniscal knife, or a radiofrequency probe (Fig. 25-69). The grasper and cutting device can be placed though

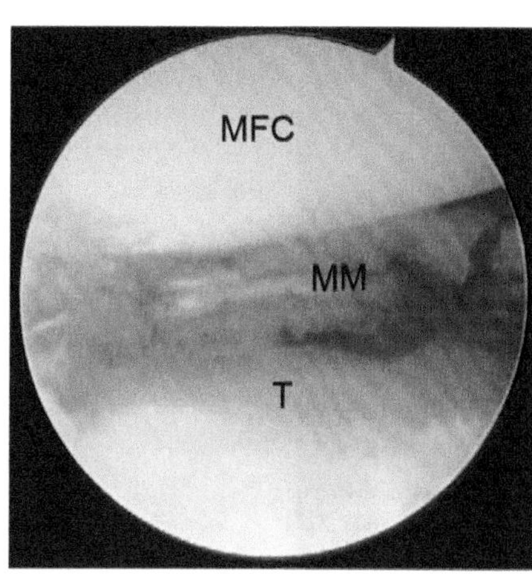

Figure 25-70 Appearance of the caudal aspect of the medial meniscus (MM) following partial meniscectomy. Medial femoral condyle (MFC), tibial plateau (T).

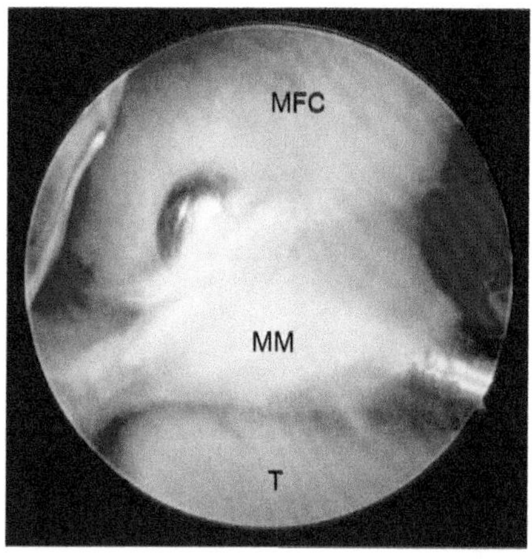

Figure 25-71 The medial meniscus (MM) should be probed to avoid missing a tear that might not be seen upon initial inspection. Medial femoral condyle (MFC), tibial plateau (T).

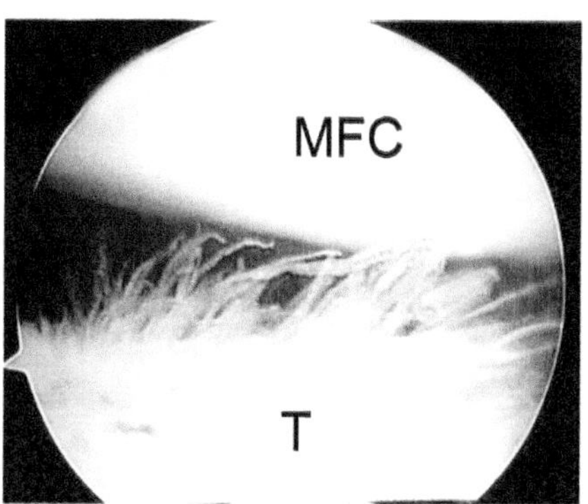

Figure 25-72 Fibrillation of the cartilage on the tibial plateau (T) is seen in this feline patient with a cranial cruciate ligament tear. Medial femoral condyle (MFC).

the same instrument portal; the portal may need to be enlarged to accommodate both instruments. Alternatively, a second instrument portal can be made adjacent to the first instrument portal. The damaged portion of the meniscus is removed (Figs 25-70 and 25-71). The surgeon should always probe the remaining portion of the meniscus to be sure that a second or third tear is not present (Fig. 25-72).

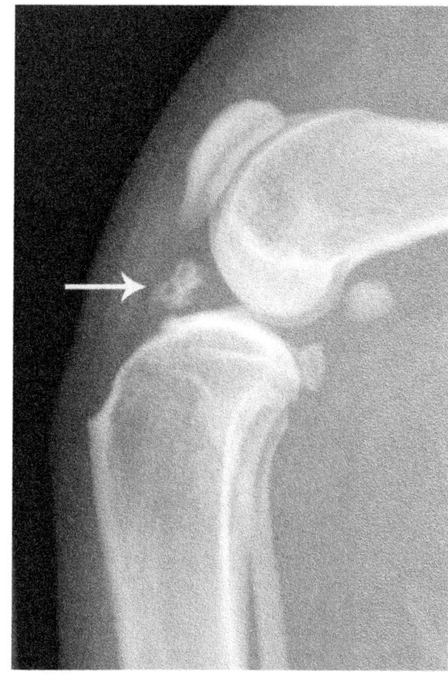

Figure 25-73 Mineralization (arrow) of the meniscus, torn cruciate ligament fibers, and synovial membrane commonly occur caudal to the patellar tendon in feline patients. Many patients with this condition have a chronic tear of the cranial cruciate ligament.

Meniscal mineralization

Meniscal mineralization is seen more commonly in cats than dogs. Mineralization may be seen in the cranial and caudal aspect of the stifle. Mineralization is most commonly found in the region of the medial meniscus near the insertion of the cranial cruciate ligament (Fig. 25-73). It appears that most cats having meniscal mineralization have some degree of cranial cruciate ligament disease. It is unclear whether lameness in affected feline patients is due primarily to the mineralized tissue, a tear of the cranial cruciate ligament, or both. The cranial cruciate ligament commonly has a complete or partial tear. Mineralization is found not only in the meniscus, but it may also be found in the synovium, infrapatellar fat pad, and insertion of the cranial cruciate ligament. The mineralized tissue can be quite large, leading to abrasion of the adjacent articular cartilage of the femoral condyle. The mineralized tissue may also include variable amounts of the intermeniscal ligament and lateral meniscus. Arthroscopic examination of the intercondylar notch is usually difficult until the mineralized tissue is removed (Figs 25-74–25-78). The tissue can be removed using a motorized shaver or hand instruments. A miniarthrotomy may be needed to view the mineralized tissue better and facilitate excision. Ligament reconstruction and treatment of meniscal injury may also be needed following removal of the mineralized tissue. Relief of clinical signs is generally seen following treatment. Free-floating osteochondral fragments are occasionally seen in the stifle of the cat. The source of the fragments may be associated with osteochondrosis, osteophytosis, or dystrophic mineralization (Figs 25-79 and 25-80).

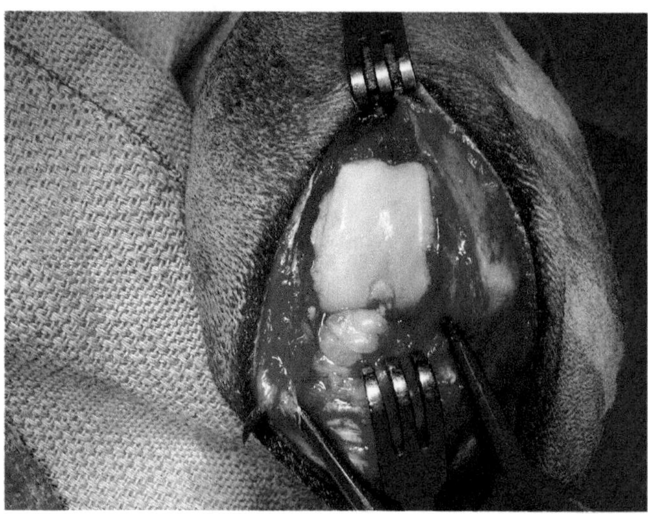

Figure 25-74 Gross appearance of a mineralized body in the stifle joint of a cat.

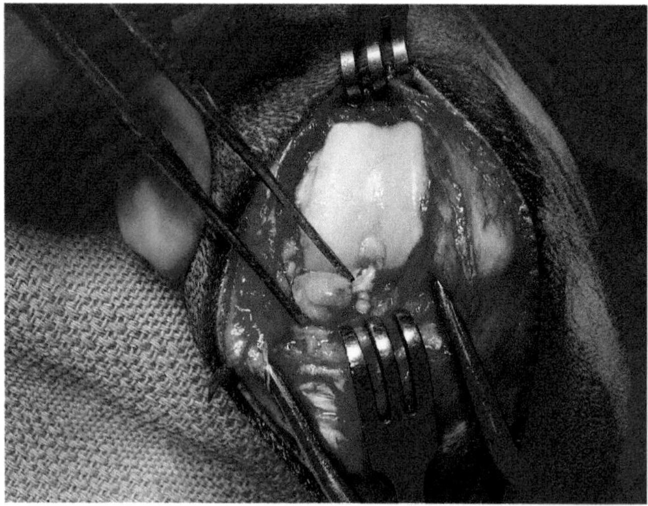

Figure 25-75 The mineralized body is grasped and resected.

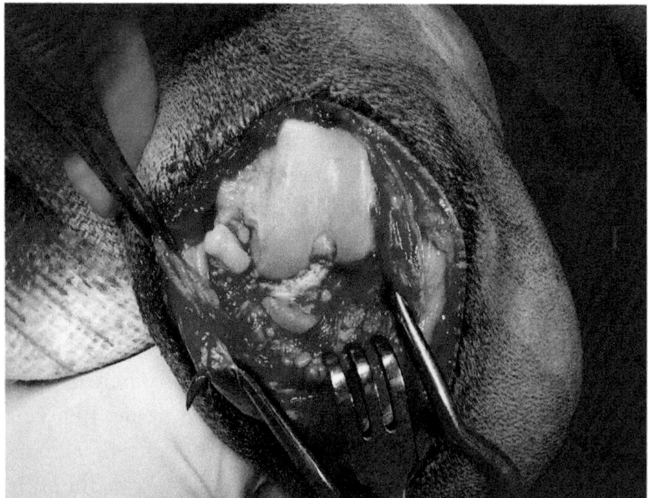

Figure 25-76 Appearance following removal of a mineralized body. Note the intimate association with the cranial horn of the medial meniscus and insertion of the cranial cruciate ligament.

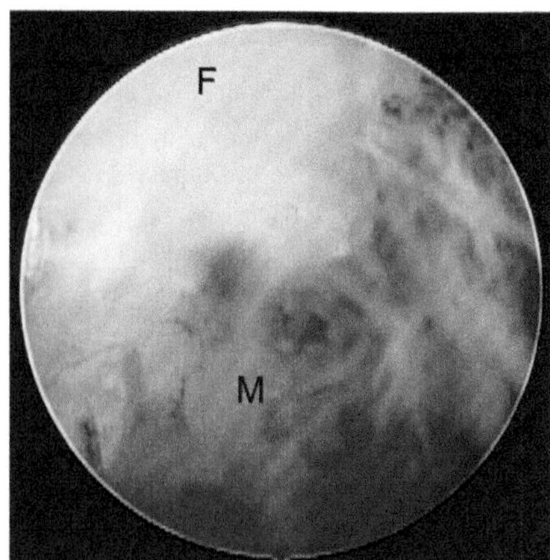

Figure 25-77 Meniscal mineralization (M) is difficult to evaluate arthroscopically due to hyperplastic synovium and the cranial location of the lesion. Femur (F).

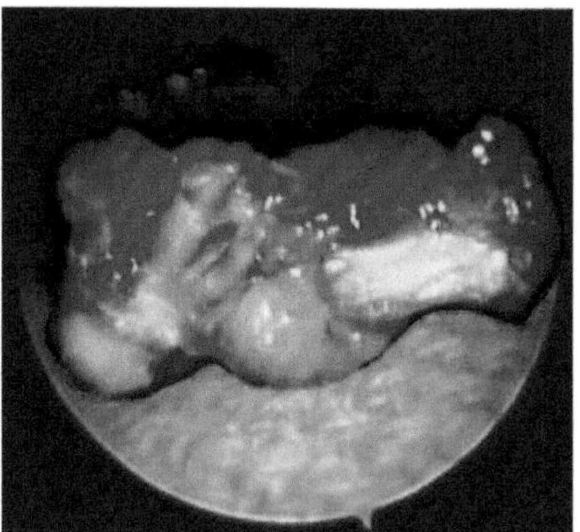

Figure 25-78 Appearance of excised mineralized tissue as viewed through the arthroscope.

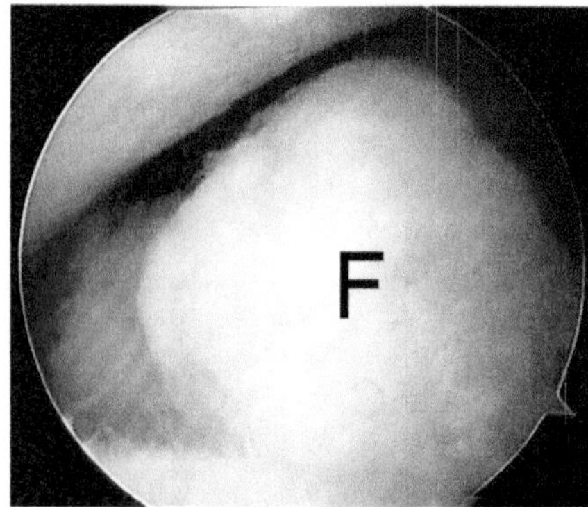

Figure 25-79 Free-floating osteochondral fragments (F) are occasionally seen in the stifle of the cat. The source of the fragments may be associated with osteochondrosis, osteophytosis, or dystrophic mineralization.

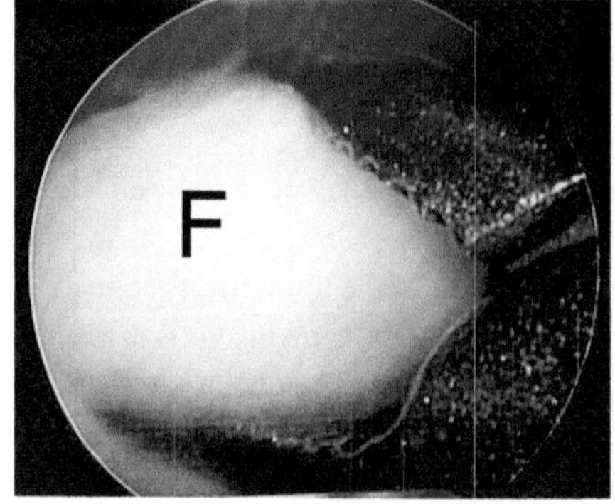

Figure 25-80 Free-floating osteochondral fragments (F) are usually easily removed with a grasper.

References and further reading

1. Beale BS, Hulse DA, Schutz KS, Whitney WO. Small animal arthroscopy. Philadelphia: Saunders; 2003.
2. Chamness CJ. Endoscopic instrumentation. In: Tams TR (ed.) Small animal endoscopy, 2nd edn. St. Louis: Mosby; 2001; pp. 1–16.
3. Ridge PA. Feline shoulder arthroscopy: a cadaveric study. In: Scientific proceedings of the British Small Animal Veterinary Association 49th annual congress 2006, Birmingham, UK, p. 17.
4. Staiger BA, Beale BS. Use of arthroscopy for debridement of the elbow joint in cats. J Am Vet Med Assoc 2005;226:401–403.

Part 7

Treatment of selected surgical diseases and injuries

This part of the book is designed to deliver easily accessible information for the operating room or during consultations. It is organized according to the anatomic location of the orthopedic condition and injury. Surgical techniques, that have worked well on feline patients in our hands, and that are based on referenced literature and the knowledge and philosophy described in the previous parts of the book, have been chosen. Surgically relevant anatomy, diagnostic aids, an overview of treatment options, specific surgical techniques, and postoperative treatment and prognosis are covered for each anatomic area and problem. Surgical approaches are only described in detail when anatomic differences exist between dogs and cats. For all standard approaches we refer to *An Atlas of Surgical Approaches to the Bones and Joints of the Dog and the Cat* (1).

26 Mandible and maxilla

K. Voss, S.J. Langley-Hobbs, S. Grundmann, P.M. Montavon

Traumatic mandibular and maxillary fractures are common in the feline patient. The incidence of mandibular fractures has been described as 16% of all fractures (2). Motor vehicle accidents tend to cause severe and multiple head injuries, whereas falls from a height are more likely to result in simple fractures, such as symphyseal separations or a traumatic split palate. Traumatic luxation of the temporomandibular joint is also common in cats. The main goal of treatment for mandibular and maxillary trauma is restoration of dental occlusion and function of the temporomandibular joint, essential for feeding and grooming. Cats with mandibular and maxillary fractures often have suffered concurrent critical injuries, such as brain trauma, shock, and injuries to the upper or lower airways. These conditions must be diagnosed and treated prior to addressing the bony lesions. Initial stabilization, general care, anesthesia, postoperative care, and nutritional support are as important, or more so, than the actual fracture repair in these patients (Chapters 11, 12, 17, and 20).

26.1 Surgical anatomy

The mandible consists of the mandibular body and the mandibular ramus. The fibrocartilaginous symphysis joins the right and left halves of the mandible. The mandibular body hosts the roots of the teeth of the lower arcade, and the mandibular canal, containing the mandibular alveolar artery and the inferior mandibular nerve. Knowledge of the topographical anatomy helps avoid iatrogenic damage from incorrect implant placement. The mandibular ramus has three bony prominences: the angular process, the condylar process of the temporomandibular joint, and the large coronoid process dorsally. The masseteric fossa of the mandibular ramus is the insertion site of the thick masseter muscle. The bone is very thin in this region, and implants for repair of fractures of the mandibular ramus must be placed near the thicker coronoid crest rostrally, and along the caudoventral border to achieve sufficient bone purchase.

The facial and palatine regions are shorter in cats than in other species. This is even more pronounced in brachycephalic breeds with disturbed endochondral ossification. The incisive, nasal, maxillar, palatine, and zygomatic bones are connected as suture-type articulations, and form the upper part of the face, containing the nasal cavity, the cranial part of the frontal sinus, and the tooth roots of the upper arcade. For simplicity, these bones are summarized as maxillary bones in the following text. The infraorbital artery and the maxillary nerve exit the infraorbital foramen of the maxillary bone, ventral to the orbit.

The feline temporomandibular joint is a very stable hinge joint due to close congruity between the mandibular fossa of the temporal bone and the condylar process of the mandible (3). Cats have a large retroarticular process caudally, and also a large bony process rostral to the temporomandibular joint, contributing to joint stability (3). The temporomandibular joint contains a fibrocartilaginous meniscus.

26.2 Diagnosis and general considerations

Nearly 70% of cats with fractures of the mandible and maxilla have associated injuries of the head, including nasal trauma resulting in epistaxis, brain trauma, and ocular injuries (4). Brain trauma occurred in 15% of the cats in this survey (4). Repeated neurological examinations should therefore be conducted to detect for evidence of brain trauma, and instigate appropriate treatment if necessary. Epistaxis associated with head trauma can be severe enough to cause anemia (4), and changes in packed cell volume should be monitored prior to anesthesia. Cats with head trauma should be placed in an oxygen cage because breathing may be impaired due to occlusion of the nasal passages and sublingual and pharyngeal swelling. Additionally, oxygen supplementation is helpful in preventing cerebral hypoxemia in patients with brain trauma. Antibiotic prophylaxis is indicated because many of the fractures are open and oral surgery cannot be performed under aseptic conditions.

Mandibular and maxillary fractures are diagnosed by clinical examination of the oral cavity. A thorough palpation is often only possible once the cat is sedated or under general anesthesia. Separation of the mandibular symphysis (Fig. 26-1) and fractures of the mandibular body are easily detected and palpable. Lesions of the caudal part of the mandibular body, the ramus of the mandibular body, and the temporomandibular joint are not as obvious due to the overlying muscle mass, but these should be suspected if dental malocclusion is present and no other injuries are readily visible. An open wound or hematoma is often present intraorally with

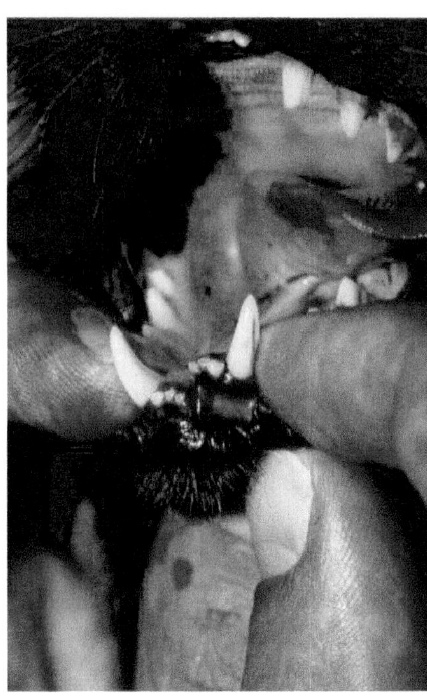

Figure 26-1 Cat with a symphyseal separation.

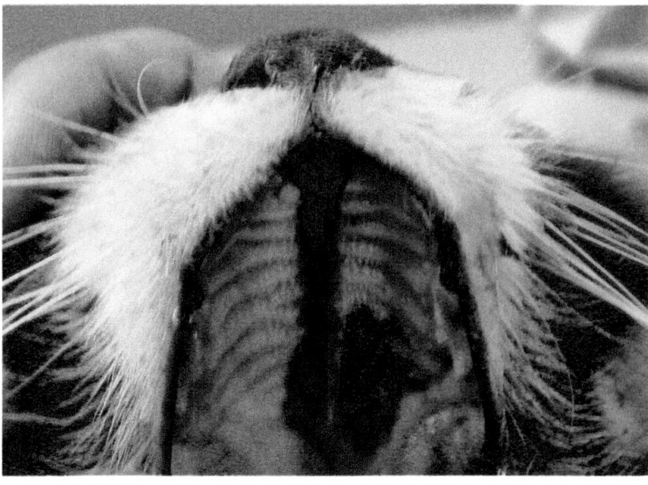

Figure 26-2 Cat with a traumatic split palate after a fall from a height. The wide gap between the oral and nasal cavities is unlikely to heal without surgical intervention in this case.

fractures of the mandibular ramus that extend through the coronoid crest.

The hard palate should be inspected for the presence of a split and, if present, stability and width of the fracture assessed (Fig. 26-2). Significant instability of the two halves indicates concurrent fractures of the facial bones. Facial fractures cause local swelling, exophthalmos, and scleral bleeding, epistaxis, and facial asymmetry. They are often compression fractures with inherent stability.

Ankylosis of the temporomandibular joint is a rare complication of trauma or neoplasia, and results in inability to open the mouth. Another disease interfering with mastication is the locking-jaw syndrome, which has been reported in the Persian cat (5). Oral neoplasia is relatively common in cats and is summarized in Chapter 8. The reader is referred to oncological textbooks for in-depth information on oral neoplasia.

Radiographs are obtained under general anesthesia once the patient has been adequately stabilized. Intubation is usually necessary because of upper-airway obstruction secondary to retropharyngeal and laryngeal swelling. Dorsoventral and laterolateral radiographs of the head, oblique radiographs of the mandibular body and temporomandibular joints, and intraoral radiographs of the rostral mandible or maxilla need to be obtained depending on the clinical fracture localization. The temporomandibular joints are best assessed on dorsoventral radiographs and on 20° lateral oblique views (6). Superimposition of bony structures makes radiographic diagnosis of caudal mandibular and maxillary fractures difficult. A computed tomography scan displays fractures more accurately in these cases.

It is common that the fracture line runs through the alveolus of a tooth. However, the affected tooth should only be removed if luxated or loose. Stable teeth are left in place because they contribute to fracture stability.

Restoration of dental occlusion is the most important goal with osteosynthesis of mandibular and maxillary fractures. The presence of an endotracheal tube does not allow complete closure of the mouth, which is necessary to evaluate dental occlusion adequately during surgery. Other intubation methods must therefore be used in some cases to be able to close the mouth completely during surgery, especially for the repair of multiple or comminuted fractures. Intubation through a pharyngotomy incision is a good solution, and is described in Figure 26-3. Alternatively, tracheal intubation can be used.

It is also essential when planning the surgery that consideration is made as to how the cat will eat postoperatively. Placement of a feeding tube can be done prior to fracture fixation (Chapter 20).

26.3 Stabilization techniques

Mandibular fractures can be classified into separations of the mandibular symphysis, fractures of the mandibular body, and fractures of the mandibular ramus. Fractures of the maxilla include fractures of the hard palate and the facial bones, or a combination of the two. Dental occlusion and fracture stability are the two most important factors to consider when deciding on the best choice of treatment. Conservative treatment can be appropriate for stable fractures with correct occlusion. Mandibular and maxillary fractures causing malocclusion and unstable fractures must be reduced

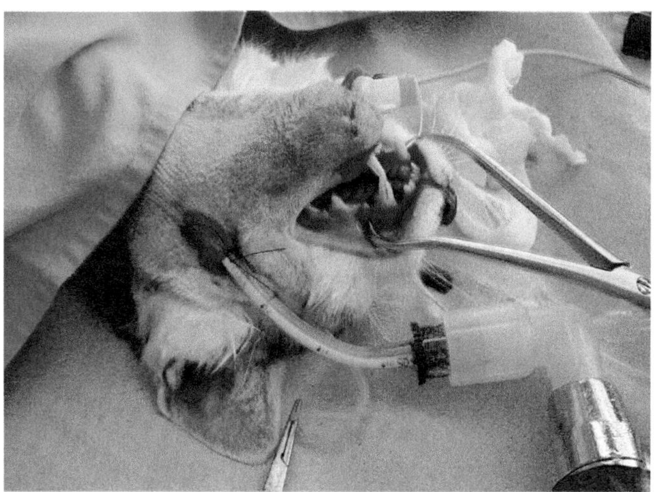

Figure 26-3 Cat with pharyngotomy intubation. The tube was first inserted orally. A pharyngeal incision was then performed in the piriform fossa, caudal to the mandibular ramus. The oral tube end was redirected through the pharyngeal incision with the help of mosquito forceps. The connecting device of the tube was temporarily removed during redirection. The endotracheal tube was secured to the skin with sutures.

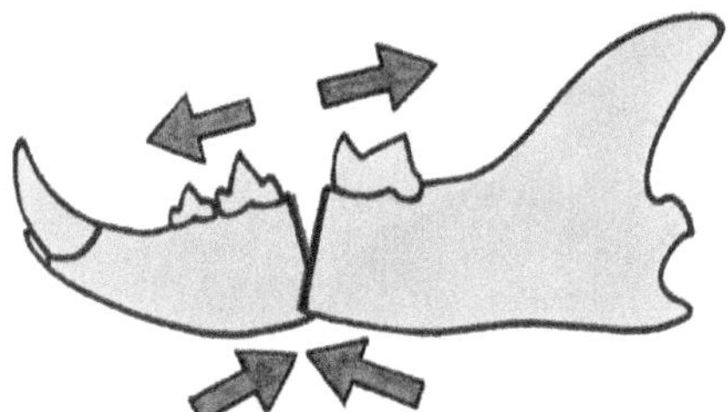

Figure 26-4 The tension side of the mandibular body is located at its alveolar border, the compression side at the ventral border.

and surgically stabilized. Unstable fractures cause pain due to motion of fracture fragments, which precludes food uptake and carries the risk of non-union, or malunion development.

In general, internal fracture repair is preferable to indirect fracture stabilization with interarcuate immobilization techniques because it allows a faster return to normal food uptake and grooming. Interarcuate immobilization can be the treatment of choice for more complicated fractures, and fractures involving the caudal aspects of the jaw that are not amenable to primary repair. Internal fixation of mandibular and maxillary fractures requires small implants and a precise surgical technique to achieve perfect reduction and sufficient implant stability in the small and flat bones. Orthopedic wire, miniplates, internal fixators, and external skeletal fixators can be used. The tension side of the mandibular body is located orally at the alveolar border of the mandibular body (Fig. 26-4), so implants should be positioned orally from a biomechanical point of view (4, 7). This can be difficult to achieve because damage of the tooth roots and the mandibular canal must be avoided.

A selection of treatment options for the different types of fracture is summarized in Table 26-1.

26.3.1 Interdental wiring

True interdental wiring is not possible in the cat, because the small size and shape of the teeth prevent stable anchorage of the wire around the base of the teeth. A modification of interdental wiring, with the wires passing through predrilled holes in between the tooth roots, is sometimes used for bilateral fractures of the rostral mandible or maxilla.

26.3.2 Interfragmentary wiring

Interfragmentary wires can be applied to stabilize simple fractures of the mandibular body and ramus. Interfragmentary wires have to be positioned perpendicular to the fracture line to prevent shearing of the fragments while tightening the wire. The holes to pass the wire through are located about 5 mm away from the fracture line, and they are drilled in a oblique direction towards the fracture to facilitate insertion of the wire medially (Fig. 26-5). A piece of 0.5–0.6-mm orthopedic wire is usually used. Interfragmentary wires are most stable if positioned at the tension side of a fracture, which is the alveolar border of the mandible. The tooth roots should be avoided.

26.3.3 Plating

Reconstruction plates are useful for the mandible and maxilla because they are easy to contour in all directions. The flat bones of the mandible and maxilla offer little bone purchase for screws, especially in areas with thin cortices. Miniaturized screws with a small-thread pitch provide better screw-holding power in the thin bone compared to standard screws. The smallest plates and screws are the 1.0- and 1.3-mm reconstruction plates from human maxillofacial and hand implant systems (Chapter 24). These are especially useful for areas with very thin bone, such as the mandibular ramus, and the facial bones of the maxilla. These small plates are too weak to withstand bending and compression forces, and should always be applied to the tension side of a fracture. The small screws can be placed in between the teeth or the tooth roots, allowing the plate to be positioned at the alveolar border of the mandible.

Stronger plates, such as the 1.5/2.0-mm veterinary cuttable plate, the 2.0-mm dynamic compression plate, or a 2.0-mm locking plate (Chapter 24) are required to repair comminuted fractures. These larger plates have to be applied on the biomechanically less ideal ventral border of the mandibular

Localization of lesion	Type of lesion	Treatment options
Mandibular symphysis	Separation	Cerclage wire Hemicerclage wire Screw
Mandibular body	Bilateral rostral fracture	Interdental wiring External skeletal fixation
	Simple fracture	Interfragmentary wiring Plates Internal fixator
	Comminuted fracture	Plates Internal fixator External skeletal fixation Interarcuate immobilization
Mandibular ramus	Simple fracture	Plates Interfragmentary wiring Conservative treatment
	Comminuted fracture	Plates Interarcuate immobilization Conservative treatment
Temporomandibular joint	Luxation	Closed reduction and tape muzzle
	Fracture/luxation	Closed reduction and rigid interarcuate immobilization Excisional arthroplasty (for chronic cases)
Maxilla	Split palate	Conservative treatment for small and stable fractures Skewer pin for large and unstable fractures
	Combination of intraoral and facial fracture	Skewer pin Plates
	Facial compression fracture	Conservative treatment Plates Mandibular–maxillary realignment

Table 26-1. Mandibular and maxillary fractures and conditions of the temporomandibular joint with possible treatment options. Several techniques may have to be combined in the presence of more than one injury

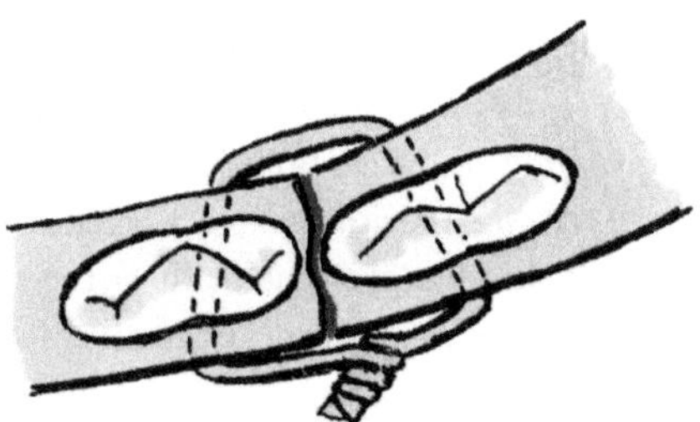

Figure 26-5 Interfragmentary wiring for stabilization of a simple mandibular body fracture. The wire is inserted in a slight oblique direction. Tooth roots are avoided by drilling the holes in between them.

body, because 2.0-mm screws are too large to be inserted at the alveolar border without causing damage to the tooth roots.

26.3.4 External skeletal fixation

External skeletal fixation can also be used to stabilize mandibular body fractures. Main indications are comminuted unilateral or bilateral mid-body fractures, and grade 3 open fractures. Smooth or negative-threaded 1.0–1.4-mm transosseous pins are used. The pin ends are best connected with an external bar made of dental acrylic or polymethyl methacrylate, because it can be molded to the shape of the mandible and avoids using heavy clamps and bars which limit the choices for pin placement. Pharyngeal intubation is always

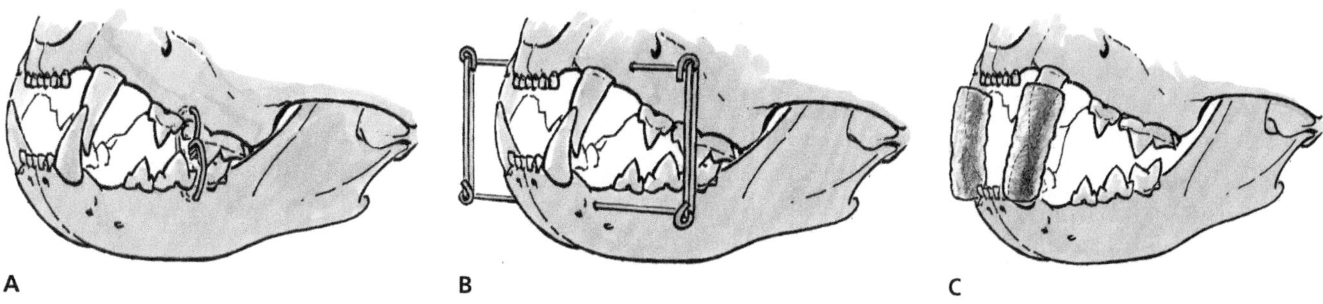

Figure 26-6 Different techniques for interarcuate immobilization.
(**A**) Interarcuate wiring is usually performed bilaterally. Tension can be exerted on the mandible in a caudal or cranial direction by inserting the wire obliquely.
(**B**) Transarticular external skeletal fixation with elastic bands allows restricted jaw motion. Care is taken to prevent the elastic bands rubbing on the skin. A rigid bar and clamps could be used instead of the rubber band.
(**C**) Dental composite fixation of both the left and right canine teeth. This technique is least invasive, but requires specialized equipment.

performed to allow intraoperative closure of the mouth for control of reduction and dental occlusion.

26.3.5 Interarcuate immobilization

Interarcuate immobilization is a practical option for mandibular fractures that are difficult to repair by internal fixation, and to prevent reluxation after closed reduction of a temporomandibular luxation. Cats with interarcuate immobilization are only able to lick liquid food, are unable to groom themselves, and can develop local dermatitis due to dribbling of saliva. Frequent cleaning of the lips, cheeks, and chin is necessary. Interarcuate immobilization is contraindicated in cats with intraoral and pharyngeal swelling and significant occlusion of the nasal passages, and in the presence of vomiting. Several methods of interarcuate immobilization can be applied, including tape muzzle, interarcuate wiring, external skeletal fixation, and composite fixation techniques. Where possible, the mouth is left slightly open to allow uptake of liquid food, but many cats with interarcuate immobilization require insertion of a feeding tube to assure adequate nutrition. Depending on the indication, the interarcuate immobilization devices are removed after 10 days to 4 weeks. An Elizabethan collar is usually necessary as cats resent this form of fixation and will make attempts to remove the implants.

Tape muzzles

A tape muzzle can only be applied in cats with a long nose. It should allow the cat to open the mouth slightly, but the tips of the canine teeth must overlap to prevent lateral deviation of the hemimandible. The muzzle is not stable if the canine teeth are broken or absent. The main indication for tape muzzles is temporary immobilization after closed reduction of temporomandibular luxation to prevent reluxation. The technique for application of a muzzle is described in Chapter 22.

Interarcuate wiring

Interarcuate wiring provides more stability than a tape muzzle, but less than other techniques. A 0.6- or 0.8-mm wire is inserted through predrilled holes in the oral border of the maxilla and mandible, and is tightened just enough for the cat to open the mouth a few millimeters (Fig. 26-6). The holes are usually drilled between the premolar and molar tooth roots. Interarcuate wiring is performed bilaterally in most cases to enhance shearing stability, but the wire is sometimes applied to one side only for correction of lateral deviation of the lower jaw. Instructions to the owners and wire cutters must be provided to be able to release the fixation immediately in case of vomiting.

Transarticular external skeletal fixator

A bilateral transarticular external skeletal fixator with elastic bands, or with clamps and short connecting bars, is another method of interarcuate stabilization (8). Kirschner wires are placed horizontally across the mandible, just caudal to canine teeth, and across the maxilla just dorsal to the hard palate. The ends of the Kirschner wires are twisted and connected to each other with small elastic bands (Fig. 26-6). The twists prevent the elastic bands rubbing against the skin, or slipping off the ends of the pins. As an alternative, external skeletal fixation clamps and bars can be used instead of elastic bands to create rigid immobilization. With this technique, the cat benefits from having intact canine teeth as the correct occlusion of the teeth helps maintain both the teeth and fracture fragments in correct alignment.

Dental composite fixation

Composite splints can be used to bond maxillary to mandibular canine teeth in functional occlusion. The technique is less invasive than others, because the fixation connects directly to the teeth without the need for bone exposure and placement of internal implants (9, 10). Fixation of both the left and right side is more stable than unilateral fixation. The canine teeth are first cleaned with an ultrasonic scaler. Then the enamel is acid-etched with 37% phosphoric acid, rinsed, and dried. A bonding agent is applied and light-cured. The mouth is fixed in a semiopened position with composite resin, placed around the canine teeth in 2-mm thick layers. The layers are each light-cured for approximately 30 seconds.

26.4 Fractures of the mandible

Mandibular symphyseal separation is the most frequent injury, followed by fractures of the mandibular body (4, 11). As many as 68% of mandibular fractures are open (11). Fractures of the mandibular ramus are less frequent, possibly because the vertical ramus is protected by the zygomatic arch and overlying masseter muscle.

26.4.1 Approaches to the mandible

A ventral approach is preferable for fractures of the mandibular body since it reduces the risk of contamination from the oral cavity and allows wound drainage. The skin incision for the approach to the rostral part of mandibular body is performed directly over the bone (12). A midline skin incision followed by retraction of the skin edges can be used for bilateral fracture repair.

The caudal mandibular body and the mandibular ramus are also approached via a ventral skin incision centered on the bone (12). Elevation of the digastric muscle is necessary to reach the caudal mandibular body. The masseter muscle is elevated from its insertion on the masseteric fossa and is retracted dorsolaterally to expose the mandibular ramus.

26.4.2 Symphyseal separation

Mandibular symphyseal separations are caused by falls from a height in most cases (4, 11) (Fig. 26-1). They are treated surgically to restore stability between the two hemimandibles. Application of a cerclage wire is an easy and reliable technique, and is most commonly used (Box 26-1). Other possibilities include insertion of a hemicerclage wire or an interfragmentary screw (Box 26-1). These techniques provide better stability against shear forces and are sometimes indicated, for example to repair oblique or comminuted fractures or to perform revision surgeries (Fig. 26-9). Cerclage wires are removed after 4–6 weeks.

26.4.3 Fractures of the mandibular body

Fractures of the mandibular body are usually located just caudal to the canine teeth, or they involve the mid-body of the mandible.

Rostral fractures usually run through the caudal alveolar canal of the canine teeth, and can be bilateral, resulting in an unstable rostral fragment (Fig. 26-10). These fractures are difficult to stabilize with hemicerclage wires and plates, because the large roots of the canine teeth occupy most of the rostral aspect of the mandible. A modified interdental wiring technique or an intraoral splint is best used to treat these fractures (Box 26-2).

Mandibular mid-body fractures are usually bilateral or are accompanied by a symphyseal separation (4). Both situations result in instability of the lower jaw and require surgical treatment (Fig. 26-12). The mandibular body is easy to approach, and internal fixation allows early function and immediate oral food uptake postoperatively. Several implants, such as orthopedic wire, miniplates, internal fixators, and external skeletal fixators, can be chosen to stabilize mandibular body fractures.

Simple and reducible multifragmentary fractures are treated with interfragmentary wiring or plate fixation (Box 26-3). Implants are best positioned at the tension side on the alveolar border of the mandible. The 1.3-mm reconstruction plates from the human hand surgery set (Chapter 24) are a good size for this application. They are strong enough for application on the tension side, and the screws are small enough to fit in between the tooth roots (Fig. 26-12). Alternatively, a 1.5- or 2.0-mm dynamic compression plate or a 2.0-mm locking plate can be used. Larger plates are positioned on the ventral side of the mandibular body to avoid damage of the tooth roots by the larger-diameter screws.

Comminuted fractures are stabilized with plates and internal or external fixators (Box 26-4). Relatively strong implants, such as a 2.0-mm dynamic compression plate or a 2.0-mm locking plate, are recommended for comminuted fractures. Accurate plate contouring is essential to ensure perfect fracture reduction, thereby preventing postoperative dental malocclusion. Locking plates have the advantage of improved stability in soft bone and in cases where fewer than three screws can be inserted per fragment. External skeletal fixation is often reserved for severely comminuted and open fractures, but it is also useful for simple and mildly comminuted fractures, particularly if small plating equipment is not readily available. It has the advantage of not requiring an open approach to the fracture. Instead, fracture reduction is

Box 26-1. Stabilization of a mandibular symphyseal separation

A small longitudinal skin incision is made on the chin ventral to the symphysis.

Cerclage wire: A 0.6–0.8-mm piece of orthopedic wire is threaded through a prebent 18-gauge hypodermic needle that has been placed from the skin incision along the lateral aspect of the bone to penetrate the oral mucosa just caudal to the canine tooth (Fig. 26-7). The needle is then withdrawn and placed in the same fashion to exit just caudal to the other mandibular canine tooth. The orthopedic wire is directed through the tip of the needle back to the ventral chin skin incision (Fig. 26-7). The wire ends of the cerclage are twisted ventrally while reduction is controlled manually. The wire must be tightened sufficiently until no motion can be elicited between the two mandibles. The wire twist is left protruding from the ventral aspect of the chin for ease of removal after healing.

Hemicerclage wire: This technique prevents shearing and can be used for revision surgeries. A ventral approach to the mandibular symphysis is performed, and the fracture is reduced. A hole is drilled just caudal to the tooth roots of the canine teeth, perpendicular to the symphysis. A hemicerclage wire is inserted through the hole and is tightened ventrally as described above (Fig. 26-8A).

Positional screw: A positional screw can be used if fracture comminution is present, which would prevent stable fixation with wiring techniques. A 1.5- or 2.0-mm positional screw is inserted across the rostral mandible, caudodorsal to the tooth roots of the canine teeth (Fig. 26-8B).

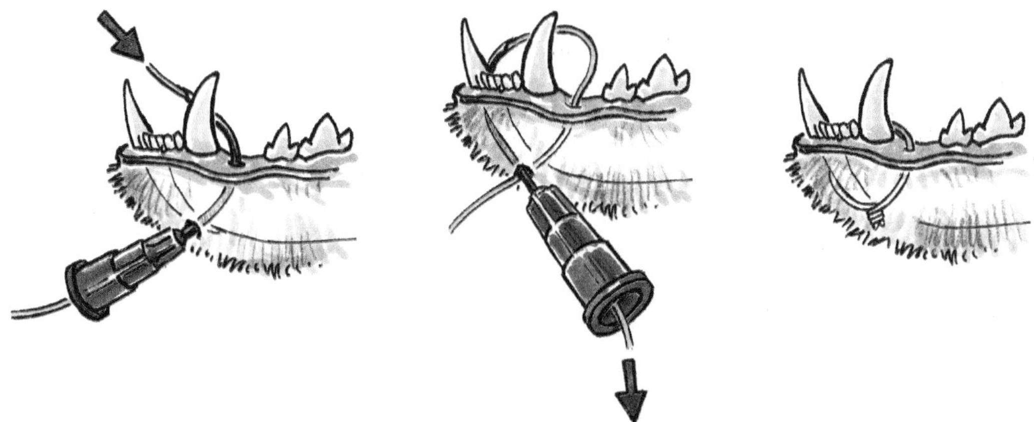

Figure 26-7 Cerclage wiring for stabilization of mandibular symphyseal separation. A piece of orthopedic wire is inserted from ventrally through a prebent hypodermic needle, exiting just caudal to the canine tooth. The wire is redirected through a hypodermic needle, inserted on the contralateral side. The wire ends are twisted and cut short.

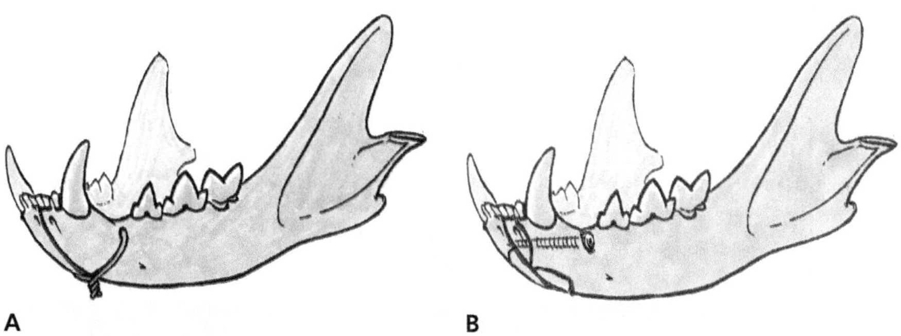

Figure 26-8 Other options for stabilization of mandibular symphyseal separations.
(**A**) Stabilization of symphyseal separation with a hemicerclage wire. Note that the wire is located further caudal to avoid the roots of the canine teeth.
(**B**) Insertion of an interfragmentary positional screw for fixation of a symphyseal separation with comminution of the fracture ends.

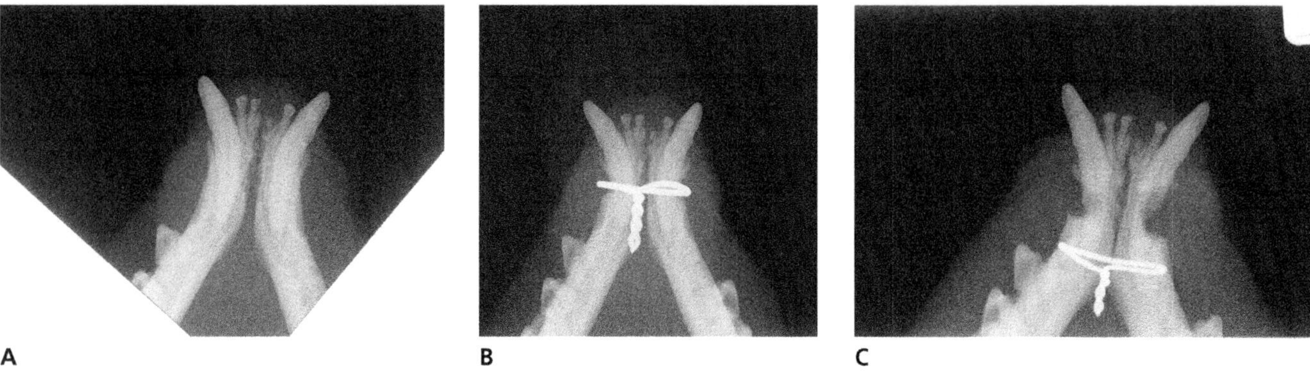

Figure 26-9 A rare case of failure of a cerclage wire after symphyseal separation.
(**A**) Preoperative radiographs of a cat with symphyseal separation.
(**B**) Instability of the initial cerclage wire resulted in non-union and bone resorption below the wire 6 weeks postoperatively.
(**C**) Revision surgery was performed using a hemicerclage wire placed further caudally.

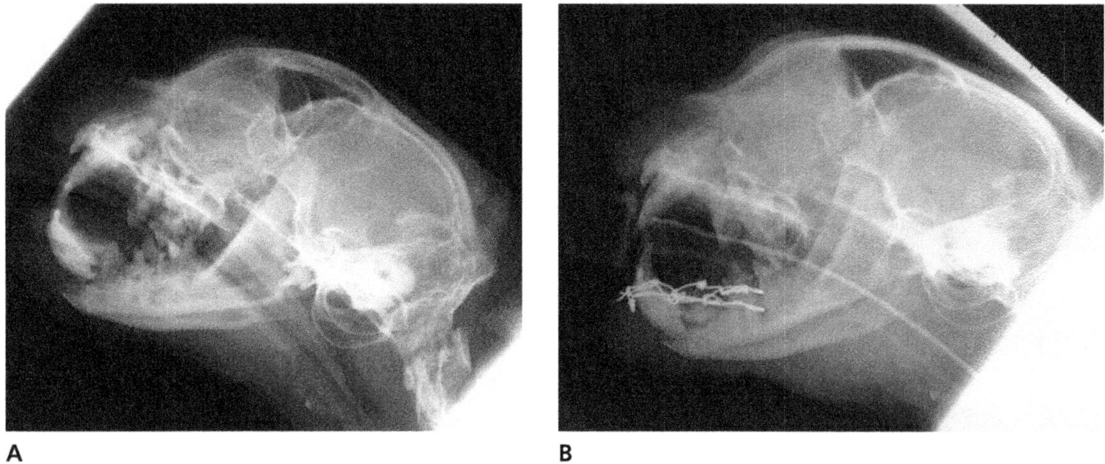

Figure 26-10 (**A**) Preoperative and (**B**) postoperative laterolateral radiographs of a cat with a bilateral rostral mandibular fracture. The rostral mandible is fractured bilaterally along the caudal alveolar canal of the canine teeth. Modified interdental wiring was used to stabilize the fracture. There is slight overreduction, but the wire will adjust to the tensile forces present on the alveolar border.

Box 26-2. Modified interdental wiring for bilateral rostral mandibular body fractures

Holes are predrilled in the alveolar border of the mandible between the teeth with a small Kirschner wire. A piece of 0.4–0.5-mm orthopedic wire is inserted into these holes in loops. The wire is passed through the loops intraorally. The loops are tightened individually over the intraoral wire (Fig. 26-11). Alternatively, a 0.6-mm Kirschner wire can be used as an intraoral splint, around which the wire loops are anchored. The oral part of the splint can be reinforced with dental composite if deemed necessary.

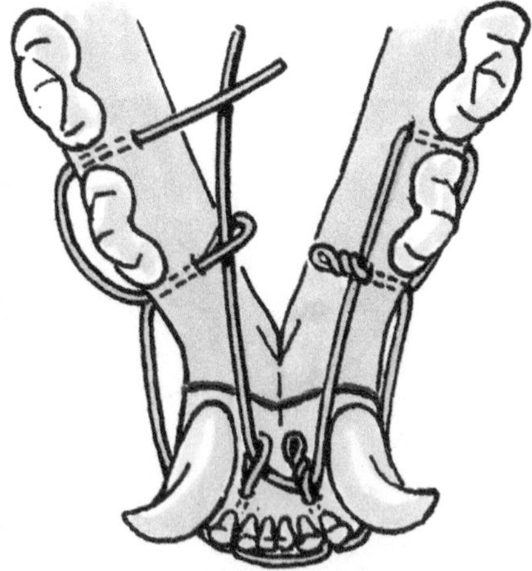

Figure 26-11 Modified interdental wiring of a bilateral rostral mandibular body fracture. The wire loops are twisted intraorally.

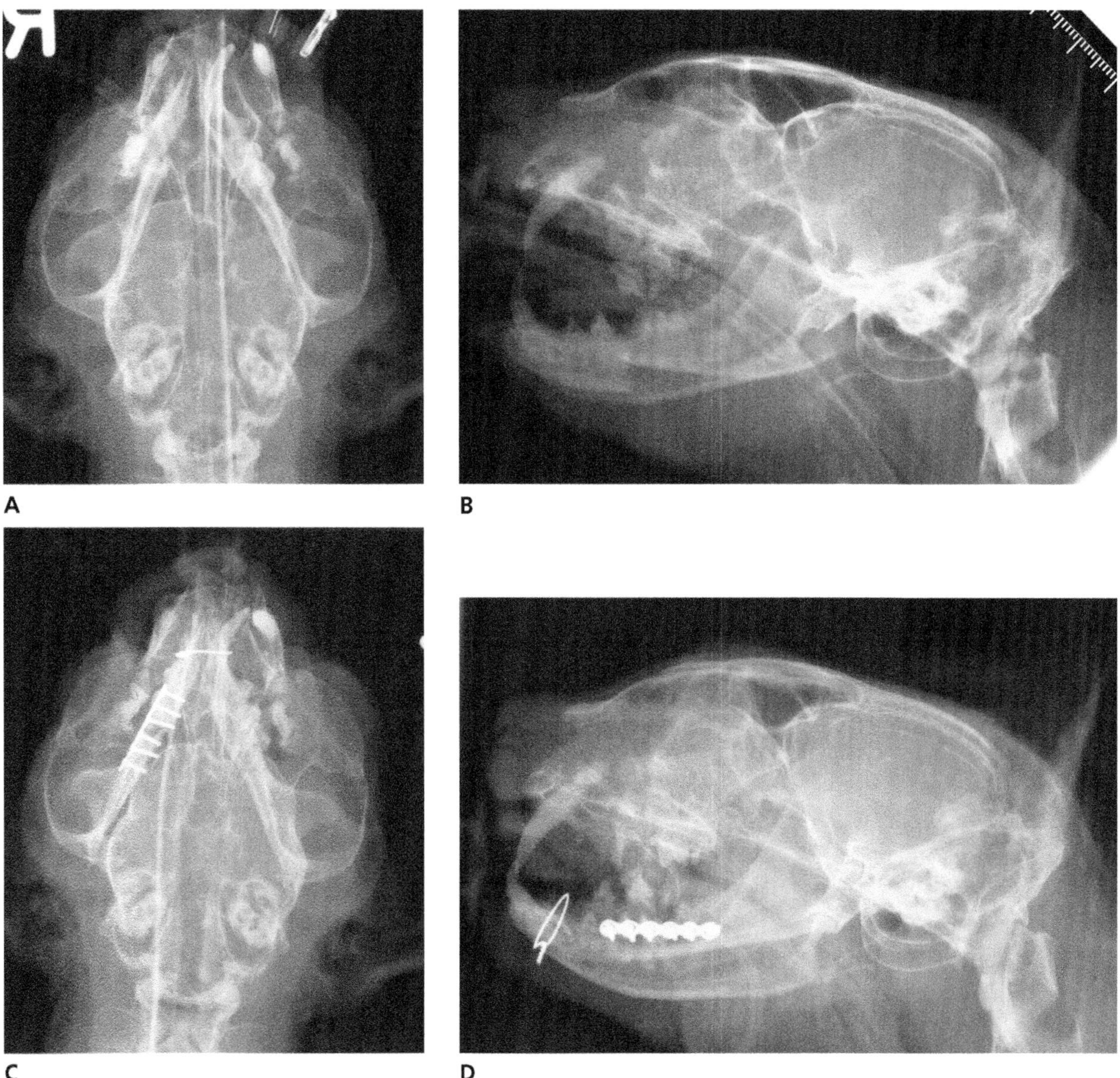

Figure 26-12 (**A**, **B**) Preoperative and (**C**, **D**) postoperative radiographs of a cat with a displaced simple fracture of the right mandibular body and symphyseal separation. The mandibular body fracture was anatomically reduced to restore dental occlusion and stabilized with a six-hole 1.3-mm reconstruction plate along the alveolar border. The symphysis was stabilized with a cerclage wire.

indirectly assessed from maintaining normal dental occlusion.

26.4.4 Fractures of the mandibular ramus

Many fractures of the mandibular ramus are minimally displaced because of the large muscle masses covering the region. These fractures can be treated with interarcuate immobilization or may require no stabilization at all if normal dental occlusion is maintained.

Displaced fractures causing malocclusion have to be reduced and stabilized with plates or hemicerclage wires (Box 26-5). The bone of the masseteric fossa is very thin and does not provide much holding power for implants. Therefore, implants are positioned along the thicker rostral coronoid crest of the mandible, which has the additional advantage of being the tension side of the bone.

Simple fractures are usually stabilized with one or two interfragmentary wires using a ventral approach. They can also be treated with miniplates applied along the rostral coronoid crest. The 1.0-mm compact maxillofacial plates or the 1.3-mm compact hand plates (Chapter 24) are a suitable size for the thin bone (Fig. 26-16). An additional plate can be applied along the ventral mandibular rim if deemed necessary for stability.

As an alternative, slowly absorbable suture material can be used instead of orthopedic wire. This may be used if the fracture is open to the oral cavity, avoiding the risk of infection around the implants. The suture can then be applied

Box 26-3. Stabilization of simple and reducible multifragmentary fractures of the mandibular body

A ventral approach is performed to the lateral side of the mandibular body. Anatomic fracture reduction is essential to restore dental occlusion.

Interfragmentary wiring: A 0.6–0.8-mm orthopedic wire is inserted on the oral side of the mandible through two predrilled holes, around 5 mm away from the fracture line (Fig. 26-13A). The location of the drill holes is also dictated by the location of the tooth roots, which should be avoided. An additional wire can be placed at the aboral side of the mandible to enhance neutralization of shear and rotational forces. In case of a butterfly fracture, the ventral wire is inserted in a figure-of-eight fashion incorporating the butterfly fragment (Fig. 26-13B). The wires are not overtightened to avoid tearing through the thin bone.

Plating: A 1.3- or 1.5-mm plate is used for tension band application along the alveolar border of the mandible. The screws are inserted between the teeth or in between the tooth roots. At least two and preferably three screws are inserted per fragment (Fig. 26-13C). If larger plates are used, they should be positioned along the ventral border of the mandible (Box 26-4).

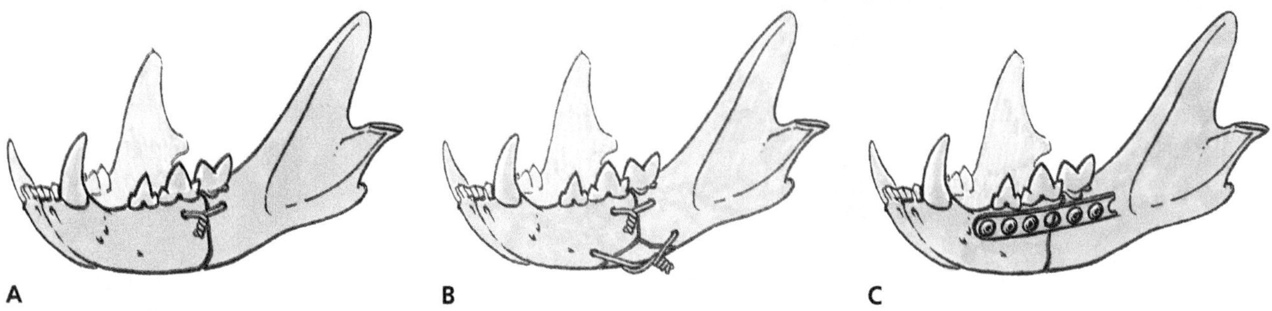

Figure 26-13 Options for stabilization of reducible mandibular body fractures.
(**A**) Stabilization of a simple fracture with an interfragmentary wire, positioned at the oral tension side. An additional wire inserted at the aboral border would improve stability.
(**B**) Interfragmentary wiring technique for butterfly fractures. The ventral figure-of-eight wire incorporates and stabilizes the butterfly fragment.
(**C**) Stabilization of a simple mandibular body fracture with a 1.5-mm miniplate. The plate is positioned on the tension side and the screws are inserted in between teeth and tooth roots.

directly from the oral cavity, provided that fracture stability is judged to be sufficient for only one suture to be placed at the rostral mandibular angle.

Interarcuate stabilization is a valid alternative to primary fracture repair, especially in multifragmentary fractures. Interarcuate stabilization maintains accurate dental occlusion during the early stages of fracture healing. Techniques for interarcuate stabilization are described above and are shown in Figure 26-6. Both dental bonding and bilateral external skeletal fixator technique provide sufficient stability of adequate duration. An endotracheal tube is placed via a pharyngostomy incision to enable control of correct dental occlusion if the external skeletal fixator technique is chosen. Interarcuate immobilization is usually required for a time period of 2–3 weeks if used for fracture stabilization. Mobility can be gradually enhanced with the external skeletal fixator technique, by exchanging the rigid rod and clamp fixation with elastic bands (Fig. 26-6).

26.5 Disorders of the temporomandibular joint

Disorders of the temporomandibular joint include fractures and luxations, which are seen most frequently, and ankylosis of the joint, most commonly occurring as a sequel to trauma. Another condition affecting mandibular–maxillary function is the locking-jaw syndrome.

26.5.1 Fractures and luxations

The temporomandibular joint usually luxates in a rostrodorsal direction, but caudal luxations are also observed. Temporomandibular joint luxations can occur uni- or bilaterally. Unilateral luxations result in deviation of the mandible towards one side. Bilateral luxations cause rostral or caudal translation of the mandible in relation to the maxilla. Rarely,

Box 26-4. Stabilization of comminuted fractures of the mandibular body

Intubation through a pharyngeal incision is required for the repair of multiple or comminuted fractures to allow intraoperative closure of the mouth and control of dental occlusion. The mandibular body is approached from ventral for plate osteosynthesis. Closed reduction is performed when an external skeletal fixator is used.

Plating: A 1.5/2.0 veterinary cuttable plate or a 2.0-mm dynamic compression plate is contoured and applied laterally along the ventral border of the mandibular body. The mouth is kept closed during insertion of the screws. At least two, but ideally three, screws are inserted per main fragment. Interposed free fragments containing teeth are correctly aligned and incorporated in the fixation to restore dental occlusion (Fig. 26-14A).

Internal fixator: A 2.0-mm locking plate is preferred over a conventional plate in cases with soft bone and limited room for screw insertion. Insertion of two locking screws per main fragment provides superior stability compared to standard screws. Plate contouring is less critical for fracture reduction than with conventional plating, but maintenance of correct dental occlusion is still essential.

External skeletal fixation: External skeletal fixation is a good treatment option for bilateral comminuted and/or open fractures. Two to three 1.0–1.4-mm smooth or negative-threaded pins are inserted into the main fragments. Avoid passing the pins across both hemimandibles unless correct occlusion is maintained. Additional pins can be placed into larger interposed fragments. The ends of the transosseous pins are bent perpendicular to the skin. Dental acrylic or polymethyl methacrylate is prepared and molded around the pin ends when it has a doughy consistency (Fig. 26-14B). The mouth is kept closed during application of the acrylic to control occlusion. Soft tissues are protected with wet sponges to avoid heat damage while the acrylic is applied.

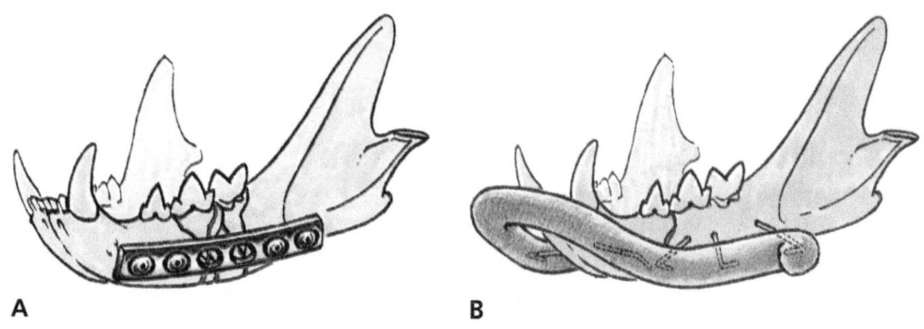

Figure 26-14 Options for repair of comminuted fractures of the mandibular body.
(**A**) Stabilization of a unilateral comminuted fracture with a 2.0-mm dynamic compression plate applied along the ventral border of the mandible. A locking plate could have been used instead.
(**B**) Stabilization of a bilateral comminuted fracture with an acrylic external skeletal fixator.

the mouth is kept open in a locked position because of impingement between the coronoid process and the zygomatic arch (Fig. 26-17). Luxation of the temporomandibular joint can be associated with fractures of the bony prominences of the temporal bone, or fractures of the mandibular condyle. These fractures may be difficult to detect on radiographs.

Temporomandibular joint luxations are treated by closed reduction (Box 26-6). Interarcuate immobilization for 1–2 weeks helps to prevent reluxation and allows fibrous healing of the periarticular structures. Techniques for interarcuate immobilization are described in Figure 26-6. A tape muzzle provides sufficient stability in the absence of fractures, but more stable techniques may be required in the presence of articular fractures (Fig. 26-19).

The mandibular condyles can also fracture in the absence of luxation of the temporomandibular joint. These fractures are usually only minimally displaced and difficult to stabilize with internal implants due to their small size and location (13, 14). Interarcuate immobilization is not required in cases with normal dental occlusion, but liquid or soft food is given for approximately 2–3 weeks. Interarcuate immobilization for approximately 14 days should be provided in cases with deviation of the mandible and poor dental occlusion (Fig.

Box 26-5. Stabilization of fractures of the mandibular ramus

A ventral approach with partial elevation of the masseter muscle from its fossa is used for interfragmentary wiring and plate osteosynthesis.

Interfragmentary wiring: Interfragmentary wiring is only indicated for treatment of simple fractures. One 0.5–0.6-mm wire is placed through predrilled holes at the rostral coronoid crest, and one at the ventral margin of the ramus. The fracture is reduced and the wires are tightened carefully to prevent pull-out (Fig. 26-15A).

Plating: Plating can be used for simple and multifragmentary fractures. A 1.0-mm compact maxillofacial plate or a 1.3-mm compact hand plate is positioned along the rostral coronoid crest of the vertical ramus using at least two or three screws per fragment (Fig. 26-15B). This may be sufficient in simple fractures, but an additional plate placed along the ventral margin of the ramus does enhance fixation stability. A second plate is always indicated in other than simple fractures.

Interarcuate stabilization: Interarcuate stabilization can be used to treat simple and comminuted fractures, but is mainly indicated for stabilization of fractures not amenable for primary fixation, considering the postoperative morbidity associated with it. See description above and Figure 26-6.

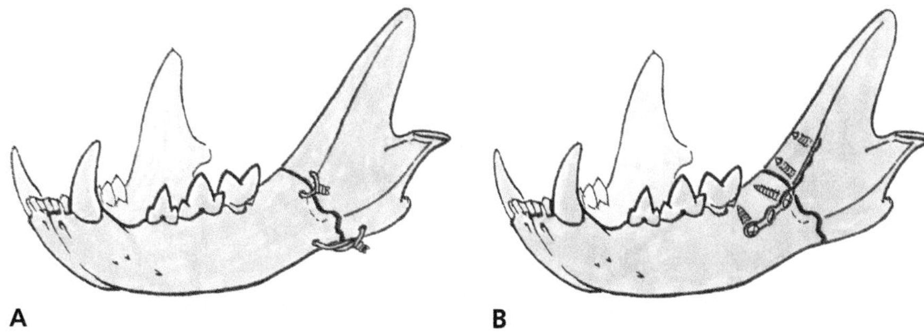

Figure 26-15 Options for stabilization of fractures of the mandibular ramus.
(**A**) Stabilization of a simple fracture with two interfragmentary wires.
(**B**) Stabilization of a butterfly fracture with a miniplate positioned along the rostral coronoid crest as tension band. A second plate, or an interfragmentary wire, could be placed along the ventral border for additional stability.

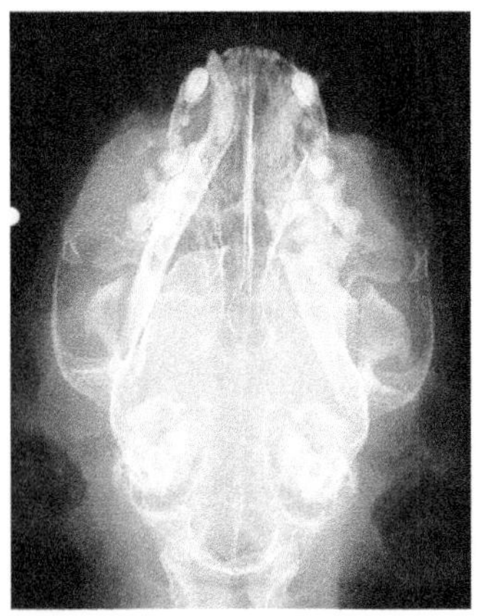

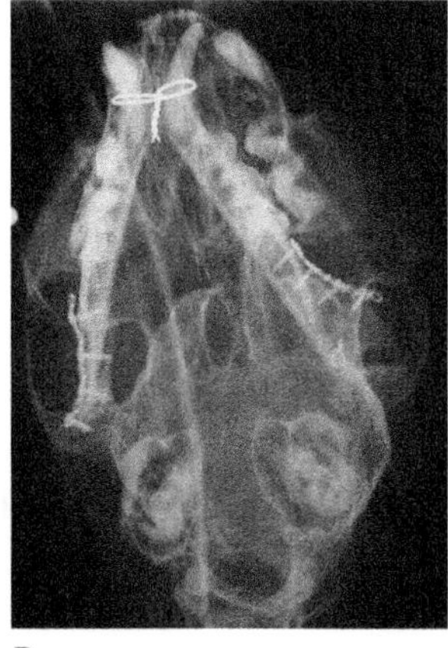

Figure 26-16 (**A**) Preoperative and (**B**) postoperative radiographs of the skull of a cat with bilateral mandibular ramus fractures, and a symphyseal separation. The mandibular fractures were each stabilized with a 1.0 mini maxillofacial plate positioned along the rostral coronoid crest. A small interfragmentary wire was placed additionally across the ventral aspect of the fracture on the right side. The mandibular symphysis was repaired with a cerclage wire.

26-6). Traction may have to be used while applying the devices to restore dental occlusion.

Most cats regain satisfactory function of the temporomandibular joint, although in some patients non-union, persistent instability, and periarticular fibrosis or mineralization may result in temporomandibular joint ankylosis (see below).

26.5.2 Ankylosis of the temporomandibular joint

Ankylosis of the temporomandibular joint is a rare chronic condition causing significant patient morbidity due to difficulty or inability to feed and lack of grooming behavior.

True ankylosis involves the temporomandibular joint itself, whereas false ankylosis is caused by periarticular structures. True ankylosis is more common in cats (15). Temporomandibular joint ankylosis is usually a sequel of trauma, such as temporomandibular joint luxations and fractures, or fractures of the zygomatic arch (15–17). It may also occur sec-

Box 26-6. Closed reduction of the temporomandibular joint

Closed reduction of the temporomandibular joint luxation can be performed with the help of a pencil. The pencil is interposed between the involved upper and lower molars. Firm digital compression rostrally causes distraction of the temporomandibular joint (Fig. 26-18). The pencil is then rotated to shift the mandible in a caudal direction for rostral luxations (Fig. 26-18), or in a rostral direction for caudal luxations. Additional traction with pointed reduction forceps applied to the caudoventral border of the mandible may be necessary to achieve reduction. A snapping sensation is usually felt while reducing the joint. Occlusion, mobility, and stability are tested after reduction. Failure to achieve stable reduction often indicates the presence of concurrent fractures.

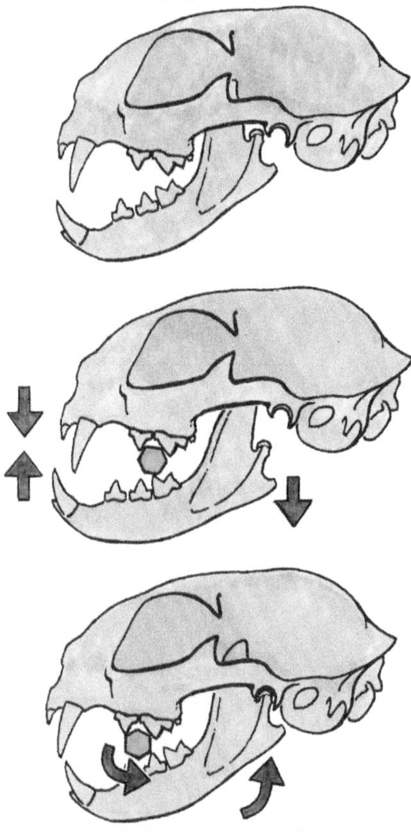

Figure 26-18 Diagram showing reduction of a rostral temporomandibular joint luxation with the help of a pencil. The pencil is used to create distraction of the temporomandibular joint (arrows). The mandible is then shifted caudally by rotating the pencil around its axis (arrows), while the jaws are still compressed rostrally.

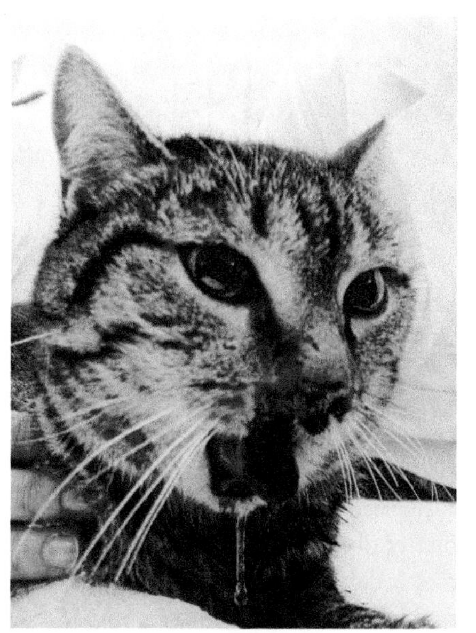

Figure 26-17 Cat with bilateral temporomandibular joint luxation. The mouth is locked in an open position because of impingement of the coronoid process and the zygomatic arch. Additional injuries included a cleft palate and a symphyseal separation.

ondary to infection, tumors, and temporomandibular dysplasia (18).

Clinical signs include progressive difficulty with eating, limited mobility of the lower jaw, and inability to open the mouth. Residual opening of the mouth can be as little as 4–8 mm (15). Ankylosis can occur uni- or bilaterally. Radiographs or computed tomography scans of the head and the temporomandibular joints are obtained to detect fractures and luxations, or callus formation (Fig. 26-20). Oblique 20° lateral views of the mandible have been recommended as the best view for looking at the temporomandibular joints in cats (6).

Conservative treatment is usually unsuccessful (15), and is therefore only tried in less severe or early cases. It involves stretching of the jaws under general anesthesia. Recurrence is prevented by manually forcing the jaws open several times

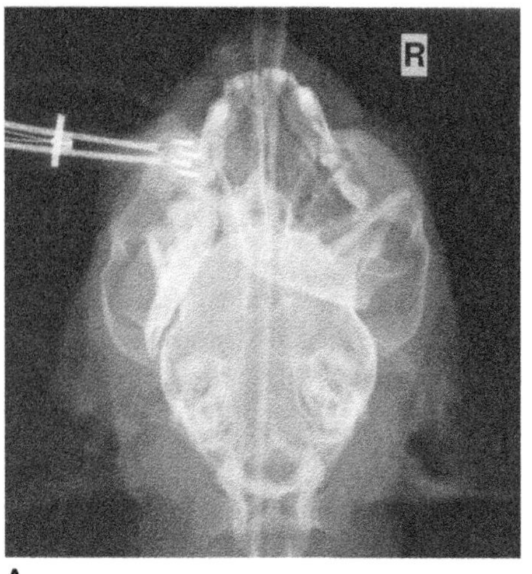

A

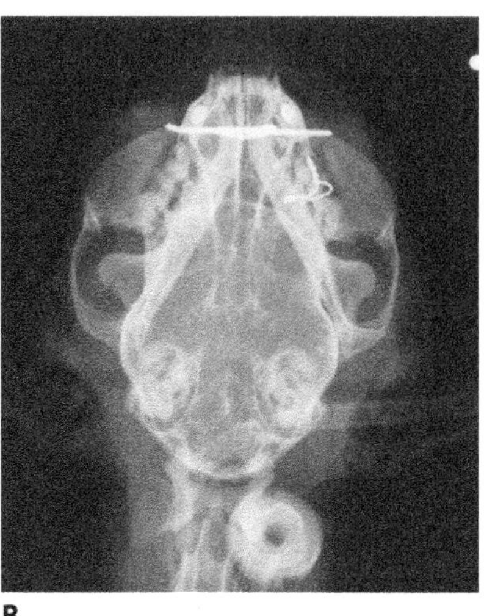

B

Figure 26-19 (**A**) Preoperative and (**B**) postoperative radiographs of the cat shown in Figure 26-17. Bilateral rostral luxation of the temporomandibular joints is seen on preoperative radiographs. Also note the displacement of the right coronoid process over the zygomatic arch, which prevented closure of the mouth (**A**). Closed reduction and interarcuate stabilization with a wire was performed. The cleft palate and symphyseal separation were also stabilized.

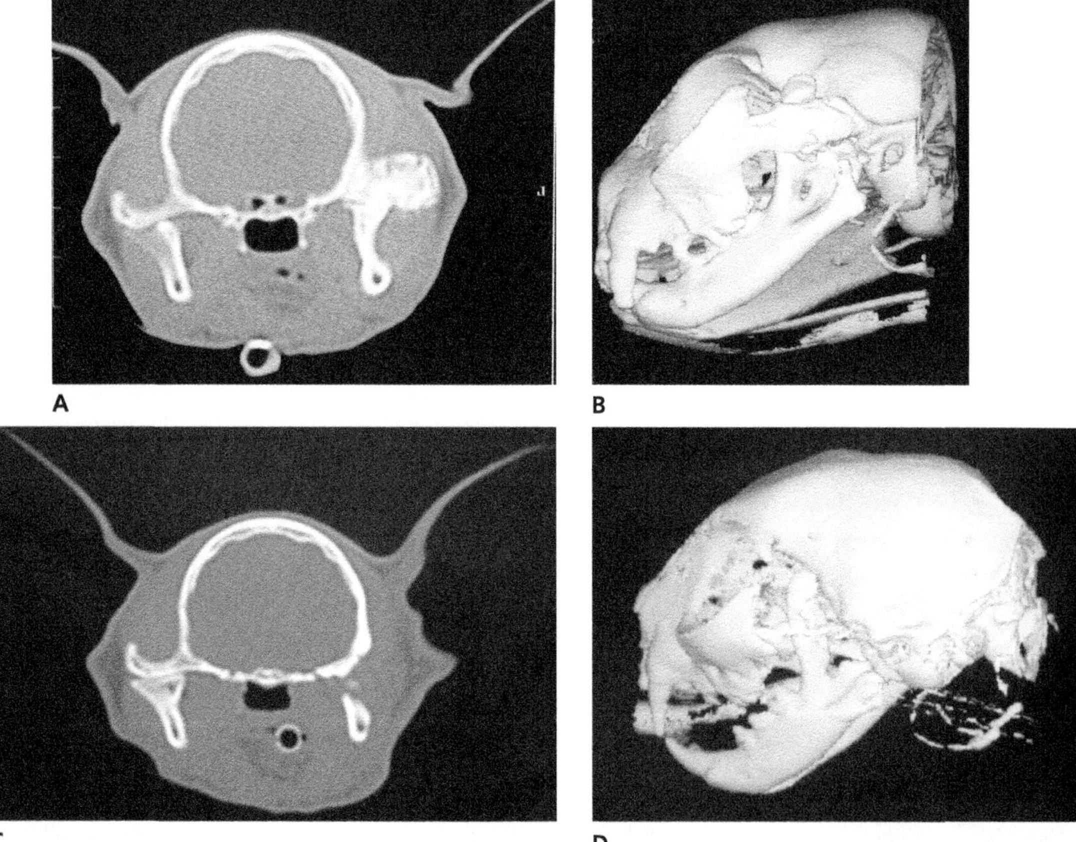

Figure 26-20 (**A**, **B**) Preoperative and (**C**, **D**) postoperative computed tomography scans of a cat with left temporomandibular joint ankylosis. New bone formation is seen in the area of the temporomandibular joint on both transverse section (**A**) and three-dimensional reconstruction (**B**). Surgery involved removal of the condylar process of the mandible, the mandibular fossa of the temporal bone, and most of the zygomatic arch (**C**, **D**).

a day, and by administration of corticosteroids. However, most cats have to undergo excisional arthroplasty of the temporomandibular joint to treat true ankylosis, or excision of parts of the zygomatic arch for false ankylosis (Fig. 26-20 and Box 26-7) (15, 19). Surgical excision of the affected tissue immediately and markedly improves range of motion, and long-term prognosis is good in most cases (15–17). Surgery is performed bilaterally if necessary. Manual opening of the jaws several times a day should be instituted postoperatively to prevent recurrence.

Box 26-7. Excisional arthroplasty of the temporomandibular joint

Normal tracheal intubation is difficult or even impossible, depending on the residual opening of the mouth. Intravenous anesthesia, blind intubation, or intubation through a tracheotomy incision can be used instead. Performing a mandibular symphysiotomy allows opening of the unaffected hemimandible and normal tracheal intubation in unilateral cases. A symphysiotomy can also help in bilateral cases, because it is easier to evaluate intraoperatively if all adhesions have been removed when each hemimandible can be moved independently.

The skin is incised along the ventral border of the zygomatic arch, followed by subperiosteal elevation of the masseter muscle (Fig. 26-21). Branches of the facial nerve and the maxillary artery and vein course through that region and must be preserved. The joint capsule is incised, and the condylar process and all reactive tissue and new bone around are excised with scissors and rongeurs or burs (Fig. 26-21). Parts of the mandibular ramus, condylar process of the mandible, and zygomatic arch may have to be removed additionally.

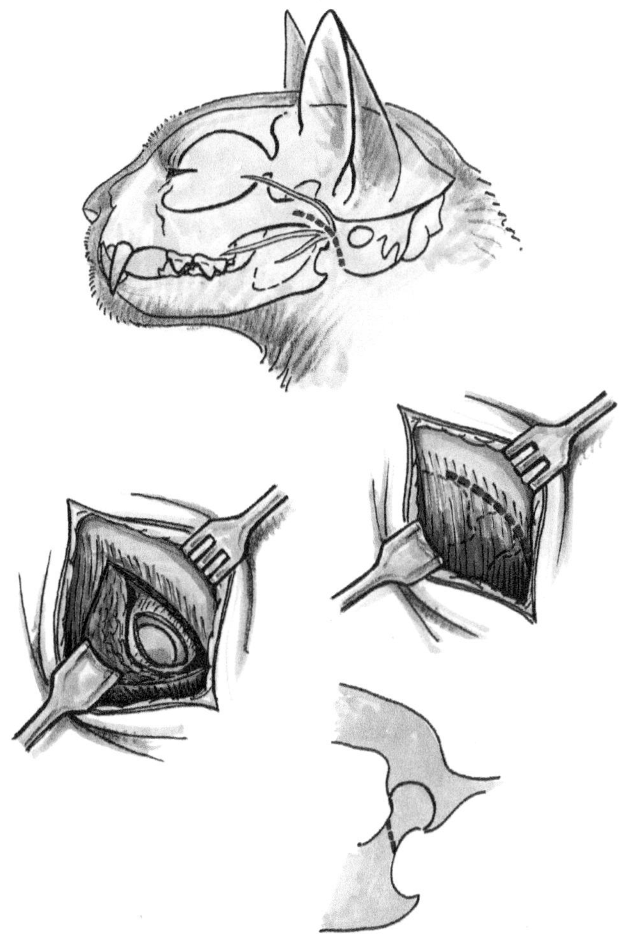

Figure 26-21 Excisional arthroplasty of the temporomandibular joint. The skin is incised along the ventral border of the zygomatic arch. Note that branches of the facial nerve course nearby. They must be preserved. Subperiosteal elevation of the masseter muscle from the ventral border of the zygomatic arch allows access to the temporomandibular joint. The condylar process is removed with rongeurs (dotted line). Additional removal of periarticular fibrosis or calcification may be necessary to achieve good mobility.

26.5.3 Locking-jaw syndrome

The open-mouth locking-jaw syndrome is caused by impingement of the mandibular coronoid process on the zygomatic arch. Locking occurs after opening of the mouth during yawning, grooming, or vocalization, and prevents closure of the mouth. Locking of the jaw causes distress, and affected cats often paw at their faces or vocalize. The duration of the locking period may last from a couple of seconds to several days. The malpositioned mandibular coronoid process can often be palpated as a protrusion lateral to the zygomatic arch. Manual correction can be achieved under sedation by further opening of the mouth followed by medial pressure on the coronoid process and closure of the mouth.

Persian cats are overrepresented in the literature (5, 20, 21), indicating that the brachycephalic formation of the skull is involved in the pathogenesis of locking-jaw syndrome, but other breeds can also be affected (22). Temporomandibular joint dysplasia or laxity and traumatically induced conformational changes of the mandible or zygomatic arch are other described inciting causes (5). Radiographs or computed tomography scans can be performed to investigate for an underlying cause.

Surgery usually involves partial resection of the portion of the zygomatic arch. The mouth is manually locked when the cat is anesthetized to facilitate identification of the site of impingement during surgery. The skin is incised along the ventral border of zygomatic arch, and the masseter muscle is elevated. The portion of the zygomatic arch that the coronoid process is interfering with is then resected with rongeurs. Alternatively, the tip of the coronoid process coming in contact with the zygomatic arch can be ostectomized (22). Prognosis is good with both techniques if sufficient bone was removed.

Symphyseal laxity and overriding of the molar teeth were considered causative factors in one cat (21). This cat was successfully treated with mandibular symphysectomy and symphyseal arthrodesis, which prevented independent movement of the hemimandibles and interference of the lower molars with the upper molars.

26.6 Fractures of the maxillary bones

Fractures of the maxilla can involve the hard palate, the facial bones, or a combination of the two. Traumatic split palate is the most common fracture type. A computed tomography scan is superior to standard radiographs to outline maxillary fractures. Many fractures of the maxillary bones can be treated conservatively. Surgery is indicated to close any communication between the oral and nasal cavities, and to restore occlusion if the maxillary teeth are maloccluded.

26.6.1 Approaches to the maxillary bones

The facial bones are approached by incision of the buccal mucosa lateral to the teeth, and elevating it from the underlying bone. A surgical approach is not necessary to repair a traumatic split palate.

26.6.2 Traumatic split palate

Mid-sagittal fractures through the hard palate usually occur after falls from a height (Fig. 26-2). The resulting connection between mouth and nose allows water and food to lodge in the nasal cavity, causing septic rhinitis and potentially aspiration pneumonia. Choice of treatment largely depends on the size of the defect. Rapid spontaneous healing often occurs if the fracture is stable and minimally displaced. Cats with small defects are treated conservatively, but are re-examined after approximately 5 days to evaluate healing of the defect. Surgery is indicated if the defect is not closing. Larger defects and split palate with instability require surgical correction (Box 26-8). Wound dehiscence is a common complication after repair of only the soft tissues, due to tension, impaired blood supply, and mobility. Significantly displaced split palates are therefore best stabilized surgically with a pin or a skewer pin. The wound edges can be additionally apposed

Box 26-8. Stabilization of a traumatic split palate

The fracture can be reduced by gently applying pointed bone reduction forceps across the maxilla. Care is taken not to cause folding of the hard palate, because this would result in inward deviation of the upper molars and malocclusion. The torn mucosa can be apposed with simple interrupted sutures after the fracture is stabilized, although this is not necessary if the fracture is adequately reduced.

Skewer pin: A 0.6–0.8-mm Kirschner wire is inserted at the level of the premolars, from the lateral alveolar border ventrally across the nasal floor to exit on the contralateral side. This may cause temporary nasal bleeding. Both pin ends are bent and cut short to avoid mucosal trauma, migration of the pin, and distraction of the fracture. A 0.6-mm orthopedic wire is then anchored around the pin ends in a figure-of-eight pattern and is tightened on the buccal mucosal surface (Fig. 26-22). Overtightening of the wire is avoided. This type of fixation compresses the split palate.

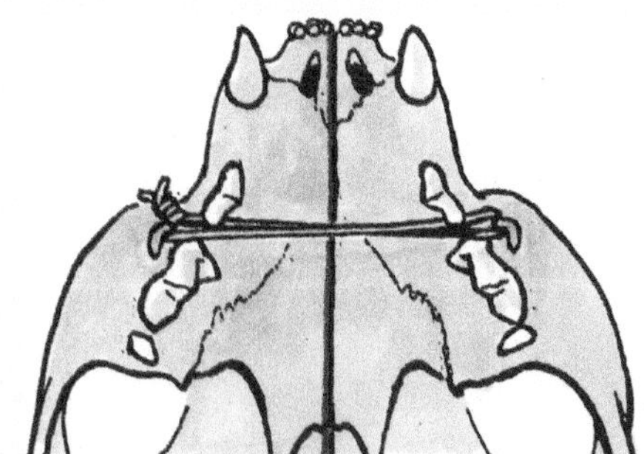

Figure 26-22 Stabilization of a traumatic split palate with a skewer pin and placement of a transoral figure-of-eight wire across the pin ends. This type of fixation provides intertragmentary compression.

with fine absorbable suture material. Implants are removed after approximately 6 weeks.

26.6.3 Fractures of the incisive, nasal, maxillary, and zygomatic bones

Fractures of the facial bones are often minimally displaced compression fractures that cause no malocclusion or instability. More commonly, they cause occlusion of the nasal passages. Instability and malocclusion occur if both the hard palate and the facial bones are fractured, resulting in a free bone fragment. These unstable fractures are usually treated surgically with the goal of restoring dental occlusion. Another indication for surgery is to relieve severe nasal compression caused by impacted facial fractures. Impression fractures of the zygomatic arch can cause injuries and compression of the eye globe, which would also be an indication for open reduction and surgical stabilization.

The facial bones of cats are very thin and miniaturized implants, such as maxillofacial miniplates, are required for surgical stabilization (Chapter 24). Interfragmentary wiring is another possibility in simple fractures, but thin wire and meticulous technique must be used to prevent tearing out of the bone. The facial bones are reached through a buccal approach.

A useful alternative option in some cases to restore dental occlusion is to realign the mandible to match the maxillary malalignment. This can be done by malaligning a concurrent mandibular symphyseal separation or by performing an osteotomy of the mandibular symphysis to realign the mandible with the maxillary malalignment (23).

26.7 Postoperative treatment and prognosis

Nutritional support is of particular concern in the postoperative treatment of cats with mandibular and maxillary fractures and luxations. Cats tend to start eating surprisingly early and well after stable internal fixation of simple mandibular fractures, often requiring no special nutrition besides avoidance of dry food.

Cats with multiple mandibular and maxillary fractures, concurrent brain trauma, occlusion of the nasal passages, and cats with interarcuate immobilization frequently need assistance in postoperative feeding. Although interarcuate stabilization should allow uptake of liquid foods, it usually takes several days until the patients have adapted to the situation and start feeding on their own. Many cats with facial trauma have occluded nasal passages. These patients may not eat because the ability to smell is an important factor for food uptake in cats (24).

Nutritional support can be provided through nasoesophageal, esophageal, and gastric feeding tubes (Chapter 20). Nasoesophageal feeding tubes are used if short-term nutritional support is necessary, and if nasal passages are not occluded. Esophageal tubes are the best choice for most cats with severe facial trauma and need for prolonged artificial feeding (Chapter 20).

Dental occlusion, food uptake, and general health are parameters used for assessment of clinical outcome. Radiographic evaluation of fracture healing is not usually necessary. Intraoral implants, such as cerclage wires for fixation of symphyseal separation, and skewer pin fixation of traumatic split palate are removed after approximately 4–6 weeks.

Overall, the prognosis is good for mandibular fractures (4, 11). Cats with multiple mandibular fractures have a higher risk for complications such as malocclusion (11). Dental surgery, such as shortening of the canine teeth, may be needed for chronic cases. Although many mandibular fractures are open fractures, the incidence of soft-tissue infection or osteomyelitis has been reported to be low in cats (11).

References and further reading

1. Piermattei DL, Johnson KA. An atlas of surgical approaches to the bones and joints of the dog and the cat, 4th edn. Philadelphia: WB Saunders; 2004.
2. Hill FWG. A survey of bone fractures in the cat. J Small Anim Pract 1977;18:457–463.
3. Caporn TM. Traumatic temporomandibular joint luxation. Comparative anatomy of the temporomandibular joint. Vet Comp Orthop Traumatol 1995;8:58–60.
4. Battier B, Montavon PM. A retrospective clinical study of the fractures and luxations of the mandible in the cat. Schweiz Arch Tierheilkunde 1989;131:77–80.
5. Lantz GC. Intermittent open-mouth locking of the temporomandibular joint in a cat. J Am Vet Med Assoc 1987;190: 1574.
6. Ticer JW, Spencer CP. Injury of the feline temporomandibular joint: radiographic signs. Vet Radiol Ultrasound 1978;19: 146–156.
7. Piermattei DL, Flo GL. Fractures and luxations of the mandible and maxilla. In: Piermattei DL, Flo GL (eds) Small animal orthopedics and fracture repair. Philadelphia: WB Saunders; 1997: pp. 659–675.
8. Baines SJ, Langley-Hobbs S. Horner's syndrome associated with a mandibular symphyseal fracture and bilateral temporomandibular luxation. J Small Anim Pract 2001;42:607–610.
9. Bennett JW, et al. Dental composite for the fixation of mandibular fractures and luxations in 11 cats and 6 dogs. Vet Surg 1994; 23:190–194.
10. Legendre L. Maxillofacial fracture repair. Vet Clin North Am Small Anim Pract 2005;35:985–1008.
11. Umphlet RC, Johnson AL. Mandibular fractures in the cat. A retrospective study. Vet Surg 1988;17:333–337.
12. Piermattei DL, Johnson KA. The head. In: Piermattei DL, Johnson KA (eds) Surgical approaches to the bones and joints of the dog and cat, 4th edn. Philadelphia: WB Saunders; 2004: pp. 33–45.

13. Salisbury SK, Cantwell HD. Conservative management of fractures of the mandibular condyloid process in three cats and one dog. J Am Vet Med Assoc 1989;194:85–87.
14. Lantz GC. Surgical correction of unusual temporomandibular joint conditions. Compend Continuing Educ 1991;13: 1570–1583.
15. Meomartino L, et al. Temporomandibular ankylosis in the cat: a review of seven cases. J Small Anim Pract 1999;40:7–10.
16. Sullivan M. Temporomandibular ankylosis in the cat. J Small Anim Pract 1989;30:401–405.
17. Okumura M, et al. Surgical correction of temporomandibular joint ankylosis in two cats. Aust Vet J 1999;77:24–27.
18. Eisner ER. Bilateral mandibular condylectomy in a cat. J Vet Dent 1995;12:23–26.
19. Bennett D, Campbell JR. Mechanical interference with lower jaw movement as a complication of skull fractures. J Small Anim Pract 1976;17:747–751.
20. Oakes MG, et al. Intermittent open mouth locking in a Persian cat. Vet Comp Orthop Traumatol 1990;3:97–99.
21. Reiter AM. Symphysiotomy, symphysiectomy, and intermandibular arthrodesis in a cat with open-mouth jaw locking – case report and literature review. J Vet Dent 2004;21:147–158.
22. Hazewinkel HAW, et al. Mandibular coronoid process displacement: signs, causes, treatment. Vet Comp Orthop Traumatol 1993;6:29–35.
23. Buchet M, Boudrieau RJ. Correction of malocclusion secondary to maxillary impaction fractures using a mandibular symphyseal realignment in eight cats. J Am Anim Hosp Assoc 1999;35:68–76.
24. Zaghini G, Biagi G. Nutritional pecularities and diet palatability in the cat. Vet Res Commun 2005;29:39–44.

27 Scapula

K. Voss, S.J. Langley-Hobbs, P.M. Montavon

The scapula is a mobile bone, protected by an extensive muscle mass. Fractures of the scapula are therefore rarely encountered. When they do occur, they may be after motor vehicle accidents, falls from a height, or dog bites. Animals with scapular fractures will have suffered concurrent thoracic trauma due to the proximity of the scapula to the thoracic wall (1). Cats with spinal fractures and luxations had a relatively high incidence of scapular fractures in one study (2). Cats with scapular fractures may also have sustained injuries of the brachial plexus or the subscapular nerve. Avulsion of the scapula, where the medial muscular attachment to the body wall is disrupted, is another injury occasionally seen. The disconnection between the scapula and the body wall then causes the scapula to dislocate dorsally during weight-bearing.

27.1 Surgical anatomy

The scapula consists of the scapular body, the scapular spine with the acromial process, the scapular neck, and the glenoid cavity for articulation with the humeral head. The scapular body is flat and very thin; the thickest bone is found at the base of the scapular spine. The scapular spine ends distally in the acromion process. The acromion of cats has two bony prominences: the hamatus and the suprahamatus processes. The suprahamatus process curves off in a caudodistal direction, and is also called the metacromium (Fig. 27-1). The acromion serves as origin for the acromial part of the deltoid muscle.

The short scapular neck has an oval shape and is thicker than the scapular body. It ends in the glenoid cavity, which articulates with the head of the humerus. The supraglenoid tuberosity is located at the craniodorsal edge of the glenoid cavity, and is the origin of the tendon of the biceps muscle. Another prominent process in the cat protrudes from the craniomedial aspect of the glenoid, the coracoid process (Fig. 27-1). The suprascapular nerve courses from cranial to caudal along the lateral border of the scapular neck, just under the acromion process. It innervates the supra- and infraspinatus muscles and must be protected during surgery.

The scapula is connected to the body wall by several muscles. The deep muscle group includes the serratus ventralis and rhomboid muscles, which originate from the ribs and spine and insert on the dorsal border of the scapular body. Their main function is to support the trunk against gravity when the cat is weight-bearing. The superficial muscle group includes the trapezius, latissimus, and superficial pectoral muscles. These are more important for mobility.

27.2 Stabilization techniques

Scapular fractures can involve the thin scapular body, the scapular spine and its distal processes, the scapular neck, and the glenoid cavity of the shoulder joint. Many scapular body fractures can be treated conservatively, but fractures of the scapular neck and glenoid cavity must be stabilized surgically. This is difficult to achieve due to the extensive surgical approaches necessary for adequate exposure, and the small fragment sizes. Small T- or L-plates are most commonly used. A summary of scapular fractures and their treatment options is provided in Table 27-1.

27.3 Fractures of the body and spine

The clinical signs associated with fractures of the scapular body and spine are often less severe than those seen with fractures of other bones. Some affected cats are still weight-bearing, and pain can be difficult to localize clinically. Neurological signs associated with brachial plexus injury (Chapter

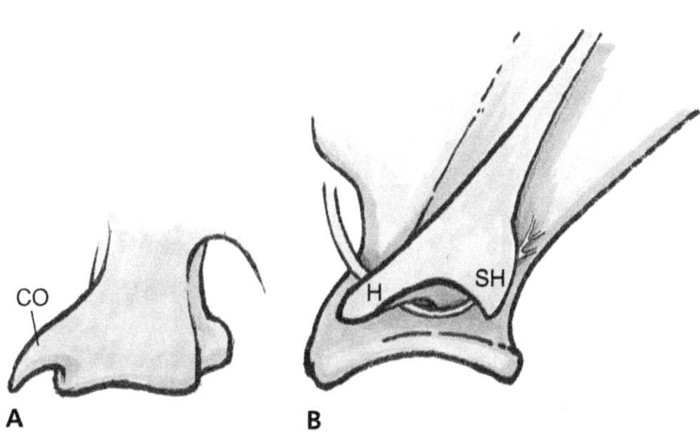

Figure 27-1 Anatomy of the left distal scapula. The acromion has two bony prominences: the hamatus (H), and the suprahamatus (SH) processes. The suprascapular nerve courses along the lateral side of the scapular neck (**B**: lateral view). Another process, the coracoid process (CO), is present on the craniomedial aspect of the glenoid cavity (**A**: cranial view).

Table 27-1. Fractures of the scapula and their treatment options

Fracture localization	Fracture type	Treatment options
Scapular body and spine	Mild to moderate displacement	Conservative
	Severe displacement, simple	Interfragmentary wiring Internal splint
	Severe displacement, comminuted	Internal splint Plate
Acromion process	Avulsion	Tension band repair
Scapular neck	Extra-articular	Cross pins Plate Internal fixator
	Intra-articular	Interfragmentary lag screw and: – cross pins – plate – internal fixator
Supraglenoid tubercle	Avulsion	Tension band repair Lag screw

15) can occur simultaneously and may be the main reason for presentation (Fig. 27-2).

27.3.1 Approaches to the scapular body, spine, and acromion process

The scapular body, spine, and acromion are approached through a lateral incision performed directly along the spine of the scapula (3). Cranial elevation and retraction of the supraspinatus muscle and/or caudal elevation and retraction of the infraspinatus muscle from the spine and body are necessary to access the scapular body.

27.3.2 Fractures of the scapular body

Many fractures of the scapular body show little displacement due to the protection and splinting by the surrounding muscles, and can be treated conservatively (Fig. 27-2). The scapular body is a flat bone with an abundant blood supply and fractures usually heal well with cage rest alone.

Indications for open reduction and internal stabilization are grossly displaced or folded fractures, and fractures resulting in spatial displacement of the scapular neck and glenoid cavity, altering the biomechanics of the shoulder joint, and impeding joint function. Simple fractures can be stabilized with interfragmentary wiring (Box 27-1). It is advantageous to place the wires near the scapular spine, and/or the cranial or caudal scapular rim, where the bone is slightly thicker. Repair of transverse fractures of the scapular body can also be achieved by anchoring an additional figure-of-eight wire in the scapular spine in a tension band fashion. Application of interfragmentary wires bears the risk of the implants tearing out of the thin and fragile bone.

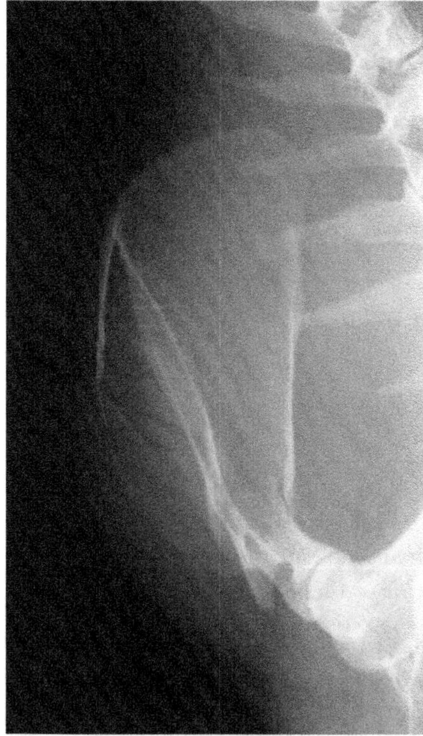

Figure 27-2 Radiograph of the scapula of a cat, presented with neurological deficits associated to a brachial plexus avulsion. A comminuted fracture of the scapular body with minimal displacement of the fragments is visible. This fracture can be treated conservatively.

An internal splint or a bone plate is more appropriate for stabilization of comminuted fractures (Box 27-1). The internal splint is easy to apply, no specialized implants are needed, and it provides good stability in cats. Small-diameter wires, a careful insertion technique, and the application of moderate tension while tightening of wires are necessary to prevent

Box 27-1. Stabilization of scapular body fractures

A lateral approach with partial elevation of the supra- and infraspinatus muscles from the scapular spine is performed.

Interfragmentary wiring: Small-diameter wires (0.5–0.6 mm) are used in the thin bone of the scapular body for the repair of simple fractures. Interfragmentary wires can be placed at the cranial and/or caudal border of the scapular body. As an alternative to an additional interfragmentary wire at the base of the scapular spine, a figure-of-eight tension band wire can be positioned over the spine of the scapula (Fig. 27-3A).

Internal splinting: This technique can be used for simple and comminuted fractures. A 0.9- or 1.0-mm Kirschner wire is inserted in the proximal main fragment through the thicker bone of the base of the spine. It is inserted midway and then bent to form a U-shaped splint. The fracture is reduced and the splint is adapted along the base of the spine to the main distal fragment. The U-shaped Kirschner wire is stabilized to the scapular spine with 0.5- or 0.6-mm hemicerclage wires (Fig. 27-3B). Additional wires can be inserted into the proximal or intermediate fragments if deemed necessary.

Plating: Plates can also be applied to stabilize simple and comminuted fractures. A 1.5/2.0-mm veterinary cuttable plate is positioned with its convex surface lying along the base of the scapular spine in order to achieve better bone contact (Fig. 27-3C). At least three 1.5-mm screws are inserted at an angle into the junction between body and spine to achieve as much bone purchase as possible. Do not overtighten the screws or the threads will strip.

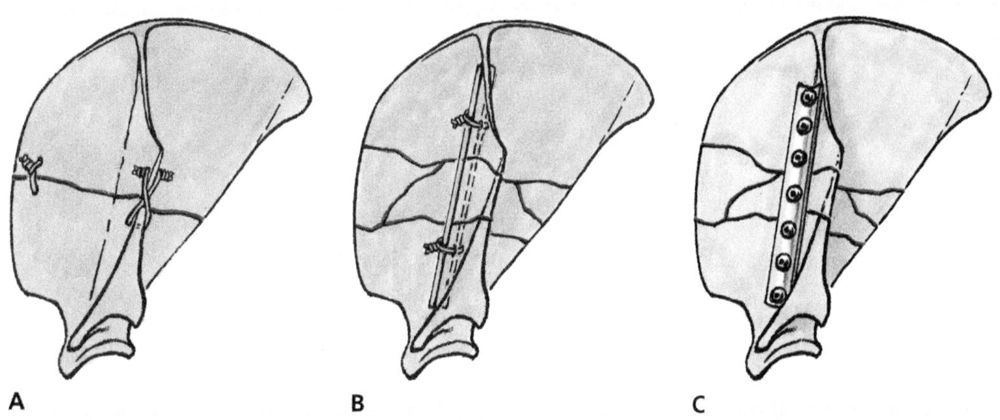

Figure 27-3 Options for stabilization of fractures of the scapular body.
(**A**) Reduction of a simple transverse scapular body fracture with interfragmentary wire and a tension band wire applied lateral to the scapular spine.
(**B**) Splinting of a comminuted scapular body fracture with a U-shaped Kirschner wire anchored to the scapular spine with hemicerclage wires.
(**C**) Stabilization of a comminuted scapular body fracture with a reversed 1.5/2.0-mm veterinary cuttable plate positioned cranial to the scapular spine.

additional damage to the bone. Plates are positioned along the base of the scapular spine, where most bone can be purchased. The use of veterinary cuttable plates is most often recommended (4). The 1.5/2.0-mm veterinary cuttable plate can be reversed to match the groove between scapular body and spine, and it allows the insertion of more screws over the same distance when compared to other plates.

27.3.3 Fractures of the scapular spine and acromion process

Fractures of the scapular spine and acromion process are rare (Fig. 27-4). The spine can be avulsed from the scapular body. Reattachment of the spine to the body with cerclage wires may be necessary if displacement is severe or if lameness persists with conservative treatment.

The acromion process is the origin of the acromial head of the deltoid muscle, which courses distally and covers the scapular neck. Fractures of the acromion process or, more commonly, osteotomy of the acromion needed to expose the scapular neck and shoulder joint, require surgical repair. The distal pull of the deltoid muscle results in distal displacement of the acromion after fracture, and impingement of the suprascapular nerve may occur. The distally directed muscle forces can be adequately counteracted with a tension band fixation. The size of the acromion and the spine of the scapula can make it difficult to insert a Kirschner wire for the tension

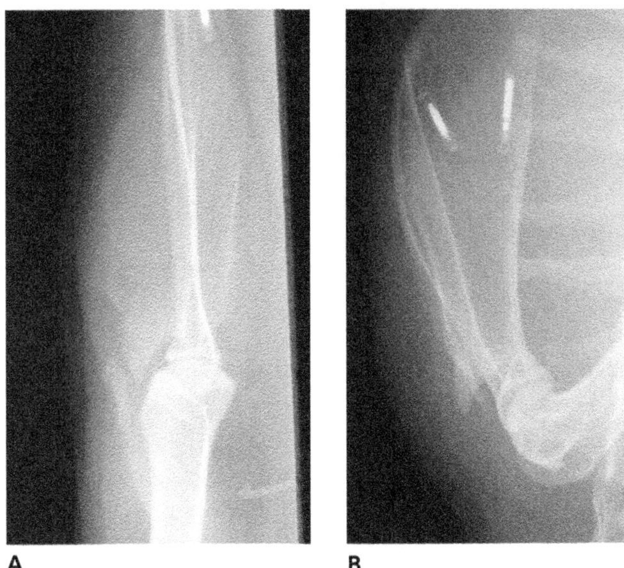

Figure 27-4 (**A**) Craniocaudal and (**B**) oblique views of the scapula of a cat with a fracture of the suprahamate process. The cat presented with a mild sudden-onset forelimb lameness. Conservative treatment was successful in this case.

band fixation. A figure-of-eight wire can be used in a tension band fashion instead (Box 27-2).

27.4 Fractures of the scapular neck and glenoid cavity

Fractures of the distal scapula are classified into non-articular fractures of the scapular neck and articular fractures involving the glenoid cavity. The latter include avulsion fractures of the supraglenoid tuberosity and articular T- or Y-fractures. All fractures of the distal scapula result in shoulder joint dysfunction and chronic pain if left untreated (5).

27.4.1 Approaches to the distal scapula

The scapular neck and glenoid cavity are best approached via a craniolateral approach to the shoulder joint (3). The acromial head of the deltoid muscle originates from the acromion process and overlies the scapular neck. Dissection between the deltoid muscle and the supraspinatus muscle, followed by cranial retraction of the distal supraspinatus muscle, allows access to the craniolateral part of the scapular neck and the supraglenoid tuberosity.

Osteotomy of the acromion with its origin of the deltoid muscle is necessary to visualize the entire scapular neck and glenoid cavity. Both the hamatus and suprahamatus processes should be osteotomized in one piece because reattachment of this relatively large piece of bone is easier than when only the hamatus process is cut. The osteotomy is performed by making two cuts (Box 27-2). Care is taken not to injure the suprascapular nerve on the craniolateral surface of the scapular neck. The acromion is reattached with a tension band before closure (Box 27-2).

A craniomedial approach to the shoulder joint allows access to the supraglenoid tuberosity and the insertion site of the biceps tendon (3).

27.4.2 Extra-articular fractures of the scapular neck

Extra-articular fractures of the scapular neck interfere with shoulder joint function by creating malalignment of the glenoid cavity. The distal fragment is usually displaced caudomedial to the scapular body, and in the absence of internal fixation, delayed union, non-union, or malunion is likely to result. The suprascapular nerve can be trapped between the fracture fragments or can become enclosed in the fracture callus during healing. Fractures of the scapular neck are therefore treated surgically (Box 27-3).

Most fractures of the scapular neck are simple transverse fractures. Cross pinning can result in sufficient fracture stability if anatomic fracture reduction is achieved. Plates offer more stability and are always indicated to repair comminuted or unstable fractures. A 2.0-mm T- or L-plate can be positioned just cranial to the spine and around its distal base, allowing insertion of at least two screws in the distal fragment (Fig. 27-7). Alternatively, a 1.5/2.0-mm veterinary cuttable plate or a 2.0-mm locking plate can be used if the distal fragment is large enough to place two screws.

27.4.3 Intra-articular fractures of the scapular neck and glenoid cavity

Intra-articular fractures of the scapular neck and glenoid cavity are rare in cats. They are classified into T- or Y-fractures of the scapular neck, and avulsion fractures of the supraglenoid tuberosity or the glenoid rim.

T- or Y-fractures of the scapular neck and glenoid are difficult to stabilize because of the small fragment sizes. Lateral exposure requires osteotomy of the acromion process (Box 27-2) and additional exposure can be achieved by osteotomy of the greater tubercle to reflect the supraspinatus muscle from the craniolateral aspect of the joint. The intra-articular part of the fracture is addressed first. The fragments are reduced anatomically and stabilized in compression with a 2.0-mm lag screw, or with a threaded Kirschner wire if the fragments are too small to insert a screw. The neck of the scapula is then repaired with a plate or internal fixator, as shown in Box 27-3. The 2.0-mm T- or L-plates or the 1.5/2.0-mm veterinary cuttable plates are good implant

Box 27-2. Osteotomy of the acromion process and tension band repair of fractures or osteotomies of the acromion

A lateral approach to the distal spine of the scapula and the acromion process is used.

Osteotomy of the acromion process: One hole is predrilled proximal and one distal to the osteotomy site for later stabilization, as described below. Two osteotomy cuts are then made to be able to remove both the hamatus and suprahamatus processes in one piece and facilitate later reduction and stabilization (Fig. 27-5A).

Tension band repair: One hole is drilled through the base of the spine where the bone is thickest, and one hole is drilled through the acromial process, proximal to the hamatus and suprahamatus processes. A small-diameter wire (0.6-mm) is inserted in a figure-of-eight fashion through the predrilled holes and is carefully tightened on both sides. The wire should not cross exactly over the fracture or osteotomy line (Fig. 27-5B).

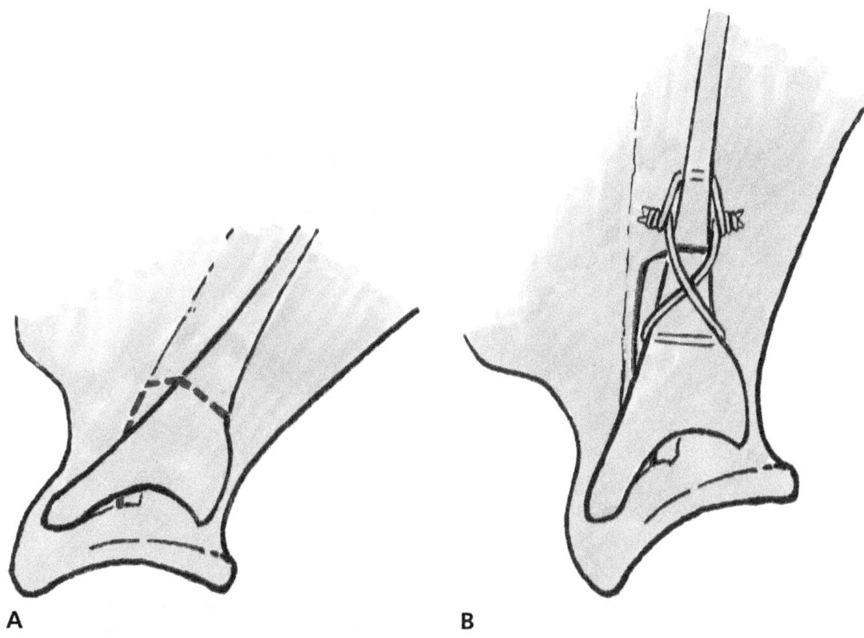

Figure 27-5 Osteotomy of the acromion and its fixation. (**A**) Two cuts are performed perpendicular to each other. The resulting step shape of the osteotomy facilitates later repair. (**B**) Tension band wire for repair of fractures or osteotomies of the acromion.

choices. Internal fixators offer better stability when fragment size only allows insertion of one or two screws into the distal fragment.

Avulsion fractures of the supraglenoid tuberosity are rare. The avulsed fragment is usually pulled distally through the biceps muscle. Anatomic reduction and stable fixation are necessary to restore the biceps tendon mechanism, and shoulder joint stability and congruity. A craniomedial approach is best used to repair fractures of the supraglenoid tuberosity. The avulsed fragment is anatomically reduced and reattached with a lag screw and antirotational pin if the fragment is large enough, or a tension band repair (Fig. 27-1).

In addition to supraglenoid fractures, fractures of the glenoid rim could theoretically occur at any other location. Large fragments should be stabilized in anatomic reduction with a small lag screw or threaded pin. Fragments too small to be reattached are resected.

27.5 Scapular avulsion

The scapula is connected to the body wall by both deep and superficial muscles. The deep muscle group holds the body up towards the scapula when the cat is standing, and is composed of the serratus ventralis, trapezius, and rhomboideus muscles. These insert at the cranial angle and dorsal border of the scapula. Rupture of the deep muscle group causes the scapula to shift dorsally, and prevents the cat maintaining normal posture during weight-bearing. Jumps, falls, and bite wounds are common traumatic causes (6). There is one case report of feline scapular avulsion in the literature (7). Fracture of the body of the scapula may coexist.

The characteristic dorsal displacement of the scapula is easily observed and palpable (Fig. 27-8). The proximal part of the scapula displaces laterally if the distal limb is adducted. The function of the limb is initially impeded but with time

Box 27-3. Stabilization of extra-articular scapular neck fractures

A craniolateral approach to the shoulder joint is performed. This may give sufficient exposure for cross pinning, but osteotomy of the acromion process helps to visualize and reduce the fracture and is advised for plating procedures. The fracture is reduced carefully without damaging the suprascapular nerve.

Cross pinning: Cross pinning is only used for simple transverse fractures. One 0.9–1.2-mm Kirschner wire is driven from the supraglenoid tuberosity into the caudoproximal portion of the scapular neck/body, and one pin is driven from proximal to the fracture line into the caudodistal aspect of the scapular neck (Fig. 27-6A).

Plating: Plating can be used for both simple and comminuted fractures of the scapular neck. A 2.0-mm L- or T-plate is contoured to the scapular neck and distal scapular body, cranial to the spine of the scapula. The plate is positioned as far distally as possible to allow insertion of three screws into the scapular neck (Fig. 27-6B) but care must be taken not to insert screws into the concavity of the glenoid and thus penetrate the shoulder joint. Three screws are positioned into the scapular body proximal to the fracture. They are angled in a caudal direction to achieve better bone purchase at the base of the spine.

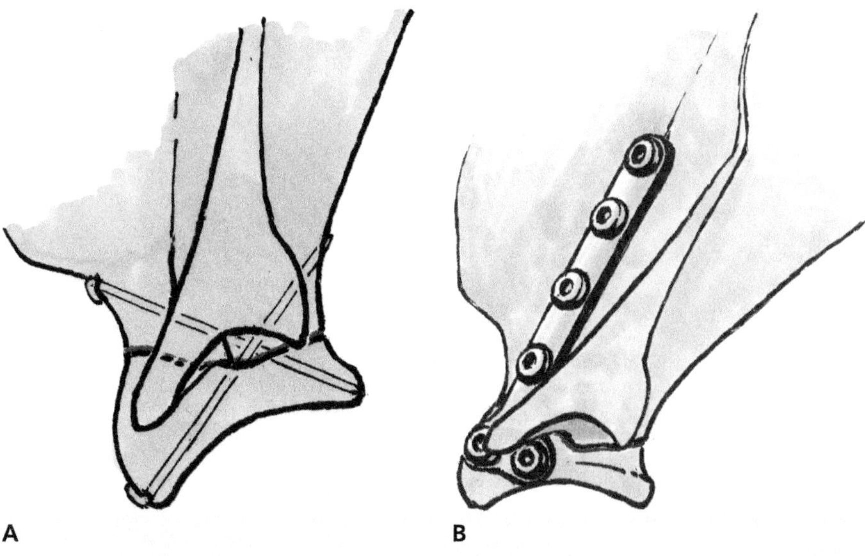

Figure 27-6 Options for stabilization of an extra-articular fracture of the scapular neck. (**A**) Cross pinning of a simple transverse scapular neck fracture. (**B**) Stabilization of a scapular neck fracture with a 2.0-mm L-plate.

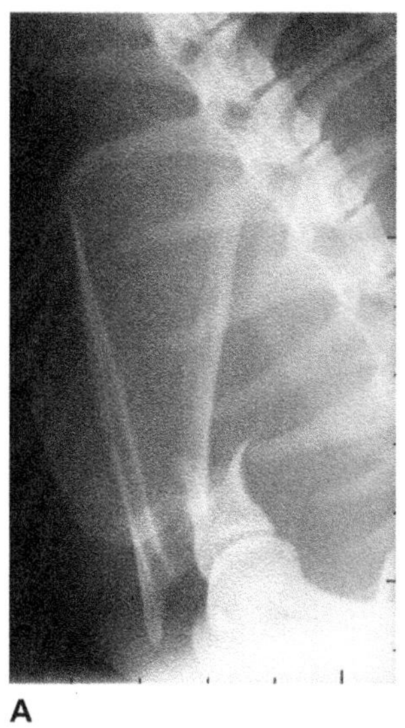

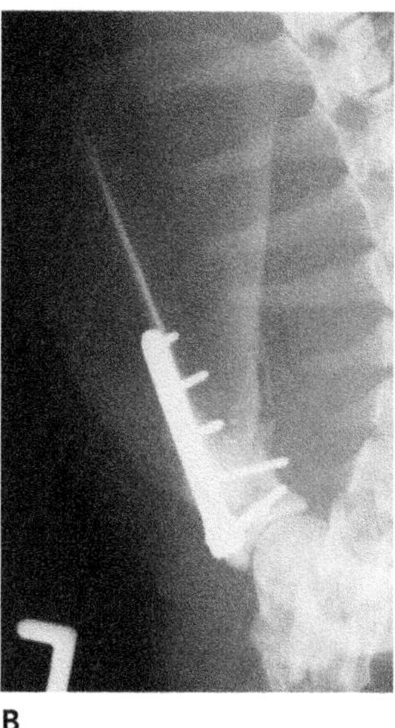

A B

Figure 27-7 (**A**) Preoperative and (**B**) postoperative radiographs of a cat with an extra-articular fracture of the scapular neck. The distal fracture fragment is displaced in a caudomedial direction (**A**). The fracture was stabilized with a 2.0-mm T-plate, which allowed insertion of three screws into the distal fragment.

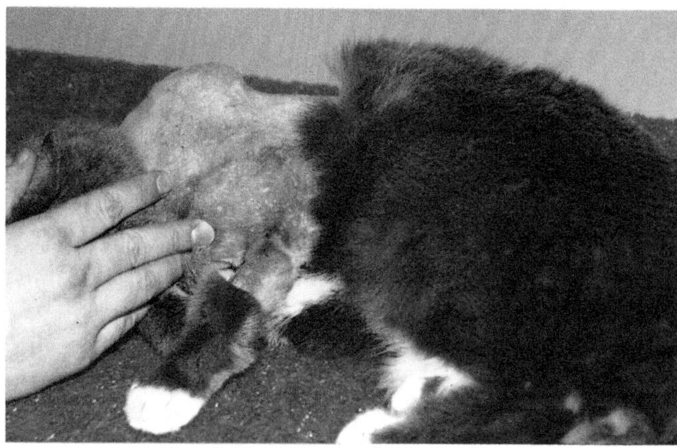

Figure 27-8 A cat with disruption of the scapula from the thoracic wall. Note the marked dorsal dislocation of the scapular body, exaggerated by pressing the bone dorsally. (Courtesy of James L. Cook.)

the cats start to use their leg again, although the scapula usually remains dorsally dislocated without surgical treatment. A Velpeau sling may be a successful treatment option for acute dislocation (8).

The goal of surgery is temporarily to stabilize the scapular body to the body wall in its anatomic position until fibrous healing has occurred. Repair can be achieved by reattaching the bone to the serratus ventralis muscle with non-absorbable sutures secured through small holes in the scapula. If the soft-tissue repair is tenuous, a wire can be placed carefully around an adjacent rib (Box 27-4).

27.6 Postoperative treatment and prognosis

Postoperative immobilization of the scapula and shoulder joint is difficult. Cage rest is sufficient in most cases, but fixation stability may not be sufficient to allow weight-bearing after repair of scapular neck fractures in some cats. Weight-bearing should also be prevented after dorsal dislocation of the scapula. A Velpeau sling stabilizes the shoulder joint in flexion and prevents weight-bearing of the limb. It is applied for 1 week after repair of fractures of the scapular neck and glenoid cavity where fixation stability is deemed insufficient, and after repair of dorsal dislocation of the scapula. It should not be used after avulsion fractures of the supraglenoid tuberosity, because flexion of the shoulder creates additional tensile stress on the fracture. Cats that will not tolerate a Velpeau sling can be prevented from weight-bearing by application of a carpal flexion splint, which is also left in place for 7–10 days. Application of Velpeau slings and carpal flexion splints is described in Chapter 22.

Prognosis for return to full function after fracture of the scapular body is excellent with both conservative and surgical treatment in the absence of neurological deficits. If nerves have been injured, the prognosis is dependent on recovery from the neurological deficits. The most devastating neurological injury is trauma to the brachial plexus, which almost always includes the nerve roots of the radial nerve (Chapter 15).

Prognosis after fracture of the scapular neck and glenoid depends on fracture reduction and fixation stability. A long-term follow-up study of 20 dogs with articular fractures of

Box 27-4. Stabilization of a scapular avulsion

The surgical approach is along the dorsal border of the scapula. The torn muscles are sutured where possible. Sutures can be anchored through holes drilled into the cranial angle and dorsal border of the scapula to reattach an avulsed serratus muscle. One or two holes are then drilled near the caudal scapular angle. A piece of 0.4–0.6-mm orthopedic wire is passed though the holes and carefully around the dorsal aspect of the fourth or fifth rib (Fig. 27-9). The wire is tightened enough to prevent dorsal displacement.

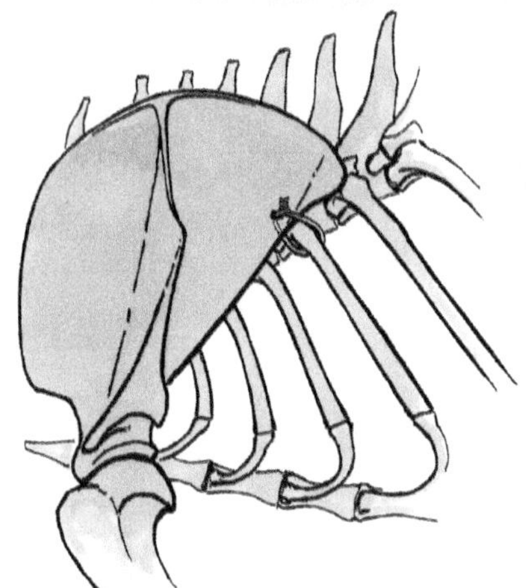

Figure 27-9
Position of an orthopedic wire around the dorsal aspect of the fourth or fifth rib and through a hole in the caudal rim of the scapula to help stabilize the scapula to the thoracic wall after luxation.

the scapula showed that only 15% of animals were free from clinical signs (5). Anatomic alignment and reduction of the glenoid cavity and stable fracture fixation are crucial for success, but may be difficult to achieve.

References and further reading

1. Tomes PM, et al. Thoracic trauma in dogs and cats presented for limb fractures. J Am Vet Med Assoc 1985;21:161–166.
2. Voss K, Montavon PM. Tension band stabilization of fractures and luxations of the thoracolumbar spine in dogs and cats: 38 cases (1993–2002). J Am Vet Med Assoc 2004;225:78–83.
3. Piermattei DL, Johnson KA. An atlas of surgical approaches to the bones and joints of the dog and the cat, 4th edn. Philadelphia: WB Saunders; 2004.
4. Piermattei DL, Flo GL. Fractures of the scapula. In: Piermattei DL, Flo GL (eds) Small animal orthopedics and fracture repair. Philadelphia: WB Saunders; 1997: pp. 221–227.
5. Johnston SA. Articular fractures of the scapula in the dog: a retrospective study of 26 cases. J Am Anim Hosp Assoc 1993;29: 157–164.
6. Piermattei DL, Flo GL. The shoulder joint. In: Piermattei DL, Flo GL (eds) Small animal orthopedics and fracture repair. Philadelphia: WB Saunders; 1997: pp. 228–260.
7. Leighton RL. Feline scapular luxation repair. Feline Pract 1977;7:59.
8. Parker RB. Scapula. In: Slatter D (ed.) Textbook of small animal surgery, 2nd edn. Philadelphia: WB Saunders; 2003: pp. 1703–1710.

28 Shoulder joint

K. Voss, S.J. Langley-Hobbs

Both traumatic and orthopedic diseases of the shoulder joint are rarely diagnosed in cats. Treatment options therefore have to be largely extrapolated from what is known in dogs, although shoulder joint instability and luxation, rupture or tenosynovitis of the biceps tendon, glenoid dysplasia, and osteochondrosis have been described in case reports (1–9). Shoulder joint instability and luxation, shoulder joint dysplasia, and conditions of the biceps tendon are described in the following sections, and osteoarthritis and osteochondrosis are covered in Chapter 5.

28.1 Surgical anatomy

The feline shoulder joint has some anatomic differences compared to the canine shoulder, especially at the distal aspect of the scapula and the acromion (Chapter 27). An ossified clavicle is present, which is visible on radiographs cranial to the shoulder joint.

The shoulder joint has a wide range of motion, not only in extension and flexion but also in abduction and adduction and in external and internal rotation (10). The glenoid provides little coverage of the humeral head, and the joint is mainly stabilized by the joint capsule, the glenohumeral ligaments, and the tendons and muscles spanning the joint. The lateral and medial glenohumeral ligaments are confluent with the joint capsule and can be difficult to visualize in cats. The medial glenohumeral ligament courses from the rim of the glenoid to insert caudal to the lesser tubercle. An additional ligament strand is present in the cat between the coracoid process and the lesser tubercle (10). Clinically important tendons that cross the joint include the biceps tendon, originating on the supraglenoid tubercle, and the tendons of the supra- and infraspinatus muscles, inserting craniomedial and lateral to the greater tubercle, respectively.

28.2 Diagnosis and treatment options

Clinical features of shoulder joint conditions include lameness, pain on manipulation of the shoulder joint, and possibly instability. Instability and luxation of the shoulder joint are caused by rupture of the joint capsule and associated ligaments, or they can rarely be associated with shoulder joint dysplasia.

Animals with luxation of the shoulder joint are usually non-weight-bearing and carry the limb in a flexed position. With medial shoulder luxation the foot is rotated externally; with lateral luxation it is rotated internally. The greater tubercle is displaced and palpable when the luxation is lateral. Medial and lateral shoulder stability is evaluated by abducting and adducting the shoulder while it is held in extension, and by performing a mediolateral drawer test. Normal range of motion has been described as ranging from 95° to 100° from maximal abduction to adduction. Range of motion in internal and external rotation is around 60–70° (10). Craniocaudal and mediolateral drawer tests are additionally performed to evaluate craniocaudal and mediolateral stability. Clinical findings are best compared to the contralateral side. Anesthesia may be necessary to reduce the stabilizing effects of the cuff muscles during palpation.

Radiographs are taken to rule out fractures of the scapular neck, glenoid, or proximal humerus. Shoulder joint luxation is readily seen on radiographs. Both mediolateral and craniocaudal radiographs should be obtained and the films carefully screened for the presence of degenerative joint disease and/or dysplasia. Ultrasonography of the biceps tendon is a noninvasive tool that is useful if lesions of the biceps tendon are suspected clinically or on radiographs (Chapter 2). Arthrography may also help to obtain additional information (Chapter 2). Diagnostic arthroscopy can be performed to inspect the joint for signs of osteochondrosis, collateral ligament ruptures, or biceps tendon disease or rupture (Chapter 25). Table 28-1 provides a summary of diseases and trauma of the shoulder joint.

28.3 Approaches to the shoulder joint

The shoulder joint can be approached from craniomedial, cranial, craniolateral, and caudal directions. The craniomedial approach to the shoulder joint (11) is performed to access the biceps tendon, the supraglenoid tubercle, and the medial glenohumeral ligament, and is used for medial transposition of the biceps tendon. The cranial approach (11) involves osteotomy of the greater tubercle and is used for lateral transposition of the biceps tendon. A craniolateral approach with osteotomy of the acromion process may be used to access the lateral part of the joint capsule and the lateral glenohumeral ligament (11). A caudal approach is chosen if osteochondrosis of the humeral head is suspected (11).

Type of lesion	Further classification	Treatment options
Shoulder dysplasia		Conservative Arthrodesis in severe cases
Biceps tenosynovitis or biceps tendon rupture		Conservative Tenodesis, tenotomy
Shoulder joint luxation	Rupture of collateral ligaments and joint capsule	Closed reduction and conservative treatment Surgical stabilization
Shoulder joint instability	Collateral ligament sprain	Conservative treatment Surgical stabilization if no improvement
Fractures (for further information on humeral and scapula fractures, see Chapters 27 and 29)	Avulsion of the supraglenoid tubercle	Tension band fixation
	Unreconstructable fractures	Arthrodesis Amputation

Table 28-1. Injuries of the shoulder joint and treatment options

28.4 Dysplasia of the shoulder joint

Dysplasia of the glenohumeral joint has been described in two case reports (8, 9). The altered conformation of the joint results in secondary degenerative joint changes, and was considered the cause for concurrent tenosynovitis of the biceps tendon in one cat (8). In the other cat, dysplasia of the shoulder joint was associated with osteochondrosis (9). Clinical symptoms include lameness and/or reluctance to move, and pain during manipulation. Radiologically, glenohumeral incongruity and degenerative joint changes are seen. Treatment options include conservative treatment with chondroprotective agents and pain medication in cats with mild lameness (see treatment of osteoarthritis in Chapter 5). Arthrodesis of the shoulder joint can be considered in cats with severe lameness, if they do not respond to conservative treatment (9).

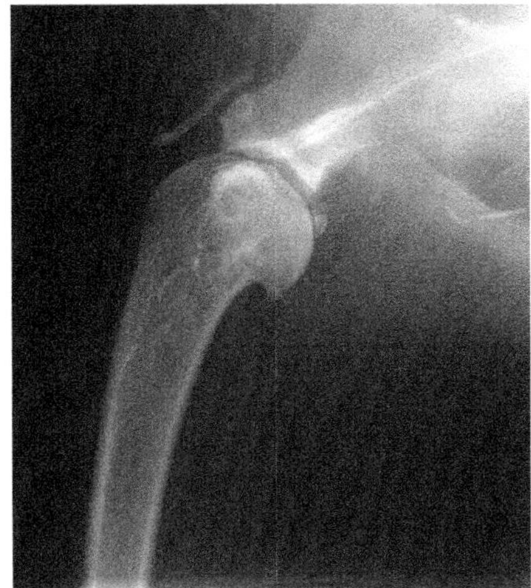

Figure 28-1 Mediolateral radiograph of the shoulder joint of a cat with two ossified bodies at the caudal aspect of the glenoid. These most likely represent accessory centers of ossification. Osteoarthritis of the shoulder is also present.

28.5 Biceps tenosynovitis or rupture

Bicipital tenosynovitis is a common clinical complaint in large-breed dogs. In cats, it is only described in detail in one case report (8), and was thought to be secondary to increased joint laxity associated with glenohumeral dysplasia and incongruity. Another report mentions a cat with arthroscopically diagnosed acute biceps tendon laceration, but the case was not described in greater detail (6). One of the authors has seen a biceps tendon rupture in association with a shoulder luxation in a cat.

The $3\frac{1}{2}$-year old cat in the case report mentioned above (8) presented with weight-bearing forelimb lameness. Pain could be elicited by flexion of the glenohumeral joint and pressure on the biceps tendon. Radiographs revealed glenohumeral incongruity and degenerative joint changes. Bicipital tenosynovitis was diagnosed by ultrasound and arthrography, and was confirmed during surgery. Constriction of the biceps tendon by the transverse ligament was relieved and osteophytes in the bicipital groove were removed. Lameness resolved initially, but recurred 6 months after surgery. The degenerative joint changes had markedly progressed at that time.

Other possible treatment options for bicipital tenosynovitis include intra-articular injection of long-acting corticosteroids, and tenodesis or tenotomy (also see Chapter 25).

28.6 Accessory centers of ossification

Accessory centers of ossification can sometimes be seen on the caudal and medial aspect of the glenoid cavity in some cats (Fig. 28-1). These are presumed to be incidental findings and not fracture fragments or joint mice because they are generally seen in cats being radiographed for reasons other than lameness. However, in cats with clinical signs attributed to the shoulder joint they may be considered a cause of lameness. Arthroscopy or arthrotomy for fragment debridement can be curative (J. Cook, personal communication).

28.7 Shoulder joint instability and luxation

Instability of the shoulder joint and traumatic scapulohumeral luxation is rare in cats. Lateral luxation of the shoulder joint was described in two case reports (2, 3). The authors have seen two cats with a medial shoulder luxation (Fig. 28-2). Shoulder instability is difficult to evaluate clinically and confirm radiographically. Cases with suspected instability of the shoulder joint are therefore often treated conservatively with restricted activity and pain medication (Chapter 5). Diagnostic arthroscopy would be the treatment of choice in unclear cases in which lameness does not resolve after 4–6 weeks of conservative treatment. Surgical stabilization can be performed as described below in cats with confirmed rupture of the medial and/or lateral glenohumeral ligaments.

For shoulder joint luxation, closed reduction followed by external immobilization and limited activity for another 4–6 weeks is usually attempted first. Closed reduction is performed with the cat under general anesthesia. Medial or lateral pressure is applied to the greater tubercle and humeral head while the leg is held in extension, depending on the direction of luxation. A Velpeau sling (Chapter 22) is advised for medial luxations, and a spica splint (Chapter 22) in slight abduction is advised for lateral luxations to prevent reluxation. External immobilization is needed for at least 7 days. Surgical stabilization is indicated if reluxation occurs.

Scapulohumeral luxation may be accompanied by avulsion fractures of the humeral head (3) or of the glenoid cavity (Fig. 28-2). Internal stabilization is always performed if fractures are involved with the luxation. Avulsion fractures are repaired with small lag screws or a tension band repair.

Surgical techniques described for stabilization of the glenohumeral joint are capsulorrhaphy (Box 28-1), prosthetic collateral ligament replacement (Box 28-1), and medial or lateral transposition of the biceps tendon. Extrapolated from the literature in dogs (12–14), capsulorrhaphy and prosthetic collateral ligament replacement are likely to result in sufficient stability in cats, and do not alter regional anatomy. Lateral or medial transposition of the biceps tendon as described for dogs may be performed in cats if imbrication of the joint capsule and collateral ligament prosthesis is insufficient to maintain shoulder stability. Medial transposition of the biceps tendon is used for medial luxation and lateral transposition for lateral luxation of the shoulder joint. The authors have no experience with transposition of the biceps tendon in cats.

Another option for treating cases where soft-tissue techniques do not result in sufficient stability is temporary stabilization of the joint with an internal fixator (15) (Box 28-1). An internal fixator is used because the shoulder joint is not amenable for transarticular stabilization with an external

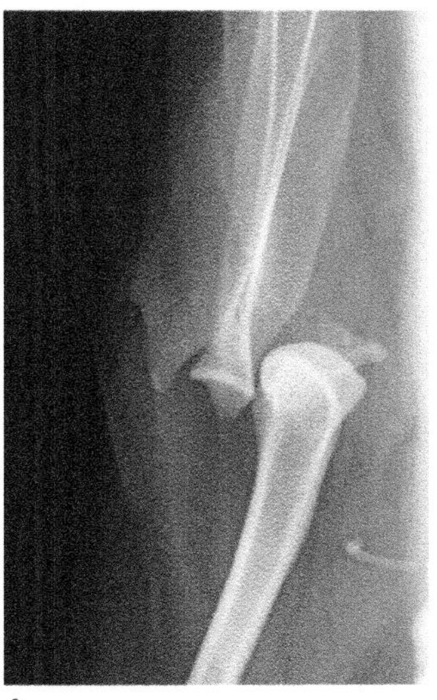
A

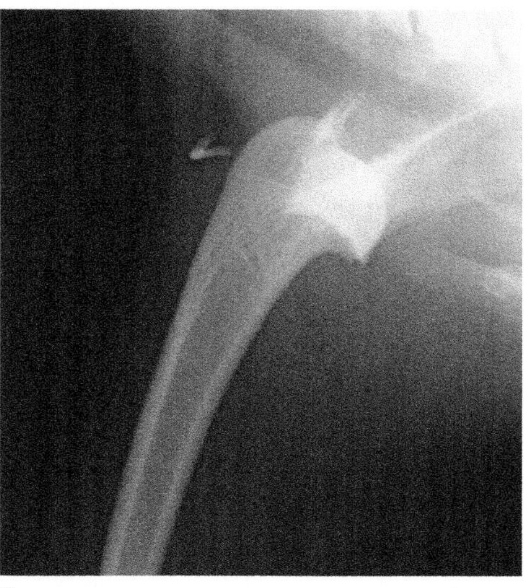
B

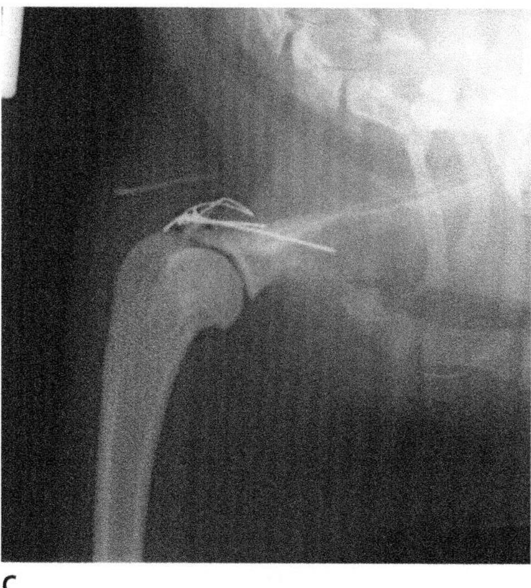
C

Figure 28-2 Pre- and postoperative radiographs of a cat with medial shoulder luxation and an avulsion fracture of the supraglenoid tuberosity.
(A) Preoperative craniocaudal radiograph demonstrating medial shoulder luxation and an avulsion fracture of the glenoid cavity. Also note the abnormal position of the clavicle.
(B) Mediolateral radiograph of the luxated joint. The avulsed supraglenoid tuberosity is seen proximal to the greater tubercle.
(C) A craniomedial approach to the shoulder joint was performed, the torn medial joint capsule and glenohumeral ligament were repaired with sutures, and the supraglenoid tuberosity was reattached with a tension band fixation.

Box 28-1. Options for stabilization of the shoulder joint

Medial instability or luxation: A craniomedial approach to the shoulder joint is performed. If the joint capsule is not torn, it is incised together with the overlying tendon of the subscapular muscle. The joint is inspected for the presence of other injuries. The joint capsule and the tendon of the subscapular muscle are imbricated with horizontal mattress sutures, using non-absorbable monofilament suture material. Any other ruptured tendons are also sutured. A prosthetic ligament is applied additionally if residual instability is present after imbrication:

Technique 1 – using screws or suture anchors: One screw or suture anchor is placed at each of the insertion sites of the medial glenohumeral ligaments and a non-absorbable figure-of-eight suture is anchored and tightened around the screws or suture anchors (Fig. 28-3A).

Technique 2 – using bone tunnels: A hole is drilled from lateral to medial through the center of the humeral neck and a similar hole is created in the neck of the scapula. Care must be taken to avoid injury to the suprascapular nerve. One or two strands of 0 or 1 polybutester are passed from lateral to medial through the scapular tunnel and from medial to lateral through the humeral tunnel and tied in moderate tension (Fig. 28-3B).

Lateral instability or luxation: A cranial approach with osteotomy of the greater tubercle or a craniolateral approach with osteotomy of the acromion process is performed. The joint capsule is incised, if not torn, to inspect and flush the joint. The capsule is then carefully imbricated with non-absorbable monofilament suture material. An additional prosthetic ligament could be used to enhance stability similar to the techniques described above.

Transarticular stabilization with an internal fixator: A 2.0-mm internal fixator is contoured to the cranial aspect of the shoulder joint. There should be a small gap between the shoulder joint and the plate to avoid damaging periarticular structures. The supraspinatus muscle is partially elevated. The locking plate is fixed proximally to the cranial angle of the scapular body and spine with three screws, and distally to the proximal humerus with three or four screws (Fig. 28-3C). The internal fixator is removed after 3–4 weeks.

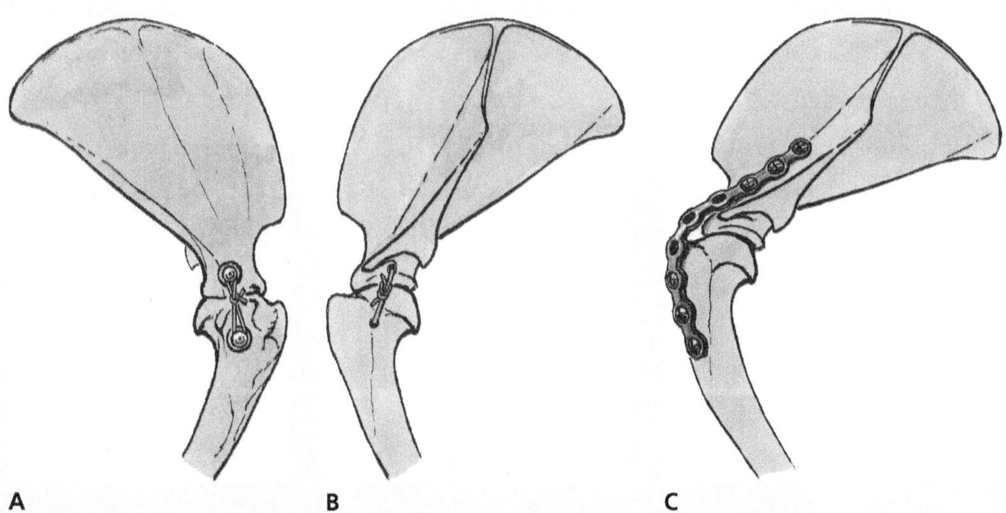

Figure 28-3 Stabilization of medial or lateral shoulder joint instabilities.

(A) A medial glenohumeral ligament prosthesis is attached using suture screws with washers. The screws are placed at the insertion sites of the medial glenohumeral ligament.

(B) A prosthetic collateral ligament is anchored through bone tunnels in the scapula and humerus.

(C) Temporary transarticular stabilization with an internal fixator maintains reduction and allows healing of periarticular structures in severely unstable shoulders.

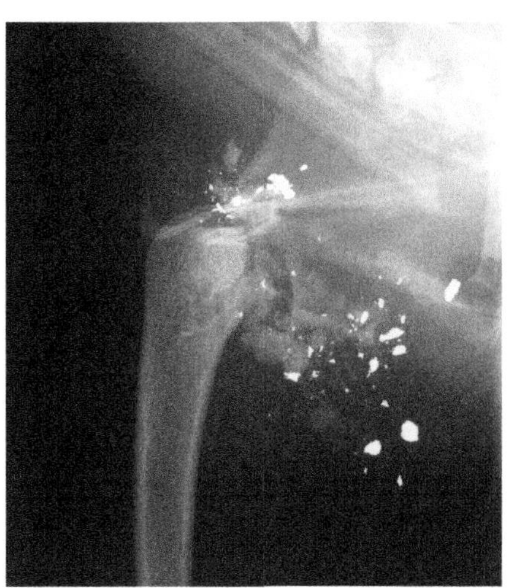

Figure 28-4
A cat of unknown age with a severely comminuted fracture of the shoulder joint caused by a gunshot. Both articular surfaces are destroyed and arthrodesis is the only treatment option.

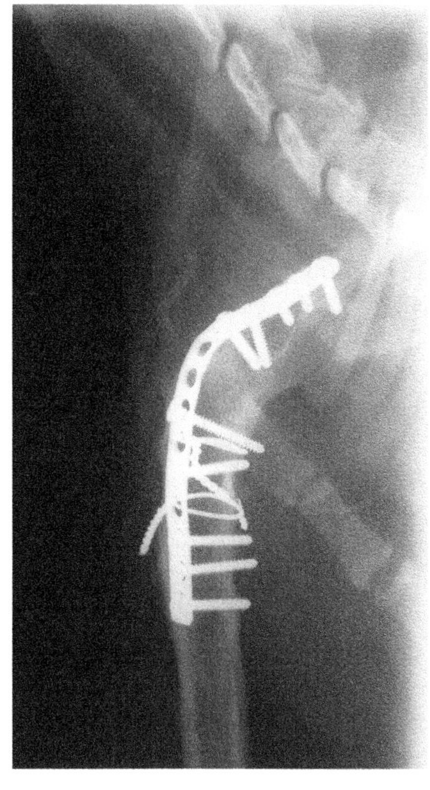

Figure 28-5
A cat with a healed arthrodesis of the shoulder joint performed 5 years earlier following a gunshot injury. Limb function was good.

skeletal fixator. The implants are removed after approximately 3 weeks.

28.8 Fractures of the shoulder joint

Fractures involving the shoulder joint are exceedingly rare, but fractures of the glenoid cavity, avulsion of the supraglenoid tubercle, and fractures of the humeral head can occur. Gunshot injuries commonly involve the proximal forelimbs and can cause devastating shoulder joint injuries (Fig. 28-4). Repair of fractures of the scapular neck are described in Chapter 27 and fractures of the proximal humerus in Chapter 29. Avulsion fractures of the glenoid rim or supraglenoid tuberosity are reattached with a tension band fixation or a lag screw (Fig. 28-2). Arthrodesis should be performed in cases where the articular surfaces cannot be reconstructed. Limb amputation may be another salvage procedure in selected cases (Chapter 41).

28.9 Arthrodesis of the shoulder joint

Arthrodesis of the shoulder joint is a salvage procedure rarely performed in cats. Indications are non-reconstructable joint fractures or luxations (Fig. 28-5), and shoulder joint disease causing significant clinical signs which do not resolve with other treatment. A literature review revealed only one case report on shoulder arthrodesis in a cat as a treatment of glenoid dysplasia (9). Functional outcome was not reported in detail.

Arthrodesis of the shoulder joint is performed with a cranially applied plate (Box 28-2). The standing angle of the shoulder joint in cats is 105–115° (10), so the shoulder should be fused with an angle of approximately 105–110°. At least four screws should be placed in the proximal humerus, and four screws in the scapular neck and base of the scapular spine. Ideally an additional lag screw is inserted through the plate across the shoulder joint (16). Osteotomy of the greater tubercle may have to be performed to be able to position the plate and preserve the tendon of insertion of the supraspinatus muscle (17). Suitable plates for cats include a long 2.0-mm dynamic compression plate, a 2.0/2.7- or 1.5/2.0-mm veterinary cuttable plate, or a 2.0-mm internal fixator. The use of pins and wires in a tension band technique could also be considered, but the authors have not tried this method in cats.

28.10 Postoperative treatment and prognosis

External immobilization for 10 days is recommended after surgical repair of a shoulder joint luxation to provide additional stability to the joint until fibrous healing of the joint capsule and ligaments has begun. A Velpeau sling is applied for medial luxations, and a spica splint for lateral luxations (Chapter 22). Some cats may resent the sling or splint, and it may be safer and easier just to provide cage rest for these patients. External immobilization should not be necessary after fracture repair. Activity is restricted for 4–6 weeks after surgery of the shoulder joint by keeping the cats indoors or in a cage.

Prognosis for return to full function is likely to be good if adequate joint stability and congruity is achieved. A chronic luxation, instability, or incongruity will result in varying degrees of osteoarthritis, pain, and lameness.

Box 28-2. Arthrodesis of the shoulder joint

A combined craniolateral and cranial approach to the shoulder joint with tenotomy of both the acromial head of the deltoid and either a tenotomy of the supraspinatus muscle or osteotomy of the greater tubercle, to reflect the supraspinatus muscle, is performed. The biceps tendon is severed. The cartilage from the glenoid cavity and the humeral head is burred away with a high-speed bur. Take care not to remove too much bone from the glenoid. The suprascapular nerve and caudal circumflex humeral artery are preserved.

A 2.0/2.7- or 2.0/1.5-mm veterinary cuttable plate, a 2.0-mm dynamic compression plate, or a 2.0-mm locking plate is contoured to the cranial part of the base of the spine of the scapula, and to the cranial humerus. The 2.0/2.7-mm veterinary cuttable plate has the advantage of enabling the use of 2.0-mm screws in the thin bone of the base of the scapula, and 2.7-mm screws in the proximal metaphysis of the humerus. The plate must be long enough for placement of at least four screws proximal and distal to the osteotomy.

The shoulder joint can be temporarily stabilized with pins while the plate is applied. It is fused with a flexion angle of approximately 105–110° (Fig. 28-6). At least four screws should be inserted into the base of the spine of the scapula and the scapular neck, and four screws into the humerus. One lag screw is placed through the plate and across the scapulohumeral joint (Fig. 28-6).

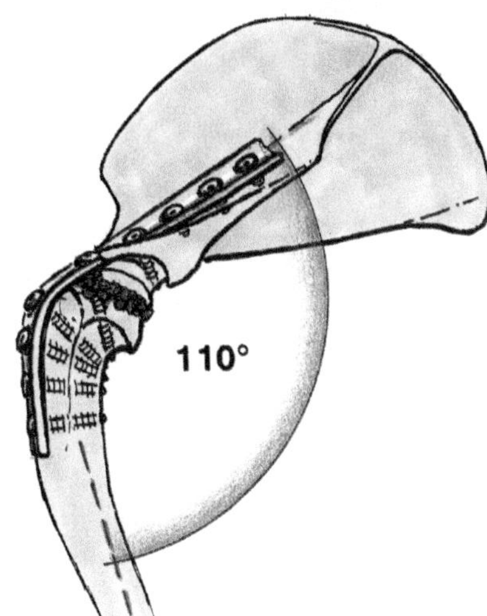

Figure 28-6 Arthrodesis of the shoulder joint. A 10-hole plate is applied to the cranial surface of the humerus and scapular neck along the base of the spine of the scapula. Four screws are inserted into the scapula and four screws into the humerus. One lag screw crosses the osteotomy.

References and further reading

1. Petersen CJ. Osteochondritis dissecans of the humeral head of a cat. NZ Vet J 1984;32:115–116.
2. Vaughan LC. Dislocation of the shoulder joint in the dog and cat. J Small Anim Pract 1967;8:45–48.
3. Bedford PG. Dislocation of the shoulder joint with fracture of the caput humeri in a cat. J Small Anim Pract 1969;10: 519–522.
4. Schrader SC. Orthopedic surgery. In: Sherding RG (ed.) The cat: diseases and clinical management. New York: Churchill Livingstone; 1994: pp. 1649–1709.
5. Bardet JF. Diagnosis of shoulder instability in dogs and cats: a retrospective study. J Am Anim Hosp Assoc 1998;34:42–54.
6. Bardet JF. Lesions of the biceps tendon. Diagnosis and classification. Vet Comp Orthop Traumatol 1999;12:188–195.
7. Butcher R, Beasley K. Osteochondritis dissecans in a cat? Vet Rec 1986;118:646.
8. Scharf G, et al. Glenoid dysplasia and bicipital tenosynovitis in a Maine coon cat. J Small Anim Pract 2004;45:515–520.
9. Christiansen E, Schneider-Heiss M. Schultergelenkdysplasie bei einer Katze. Kleintierpraxis 1999;44:117–119.
10. Roos H, Brugger S. Functional and applied anatomy of the shoulder joint of the domestic cat. Tierarztl Prax 1993;21:265–270.
11. Piermattei DL, Johnson KA. An atlas of surgical approaches to the bones and joints of the dog and the cat, 4th edn. Philadelphia: Saunders; 2004.
12. Prostredny JM, et al. Use of a polybutester suture to repair medial scapulohumeral luxation in the dog: three cases. J Am Anim Hosp Assoc 1993;29:180–183.
13. Ringwood B, et al. Medial glenohumeral ligament reconstruction for ex-vivo medial glenohumeral luxation in the dog. Vet Comp Orthop Traumatol 2001;14:196–200.
14. Fitch R, et al. Clinical evaluation of prosthetic medial glenohumeral ligament repair in the dog (ten cases). Vet Comp Orthop Traumatol 2001;14:222–228.
15. Post C, et al. Temporary transarticular stabilization with a locking plate for medial shoulder luxation in a dog. Vet Comp Orthop Traumatol 2008;21:166–170.
16. Johnson AL, Houlton JEF. Arthrodesis of the shoulder. In: Johnson AL, Houlton JEF, Vannini R (eds) AO principles of fracture management in the dog and cat. Stuttgart: Thieme; 2005: pp. 435–439.
17. Fowler JD, et al. Scapulohumeral arthrodesis: results in seven dogs. J Am Anim Hosp Assoc 1988;24:667–672.

29 Humerus

K. Voss, S.J. Langley-Hobbs, P.M. Montavon

The incidence of humeral fractures in cats is reported to be between 5% and 13% of all fractures (1, 2), with the humeral shaft and the supracondylar area fractured most often (2, 3). Falls from a height, motor vehicle accidents, and gunshot wounds often result in comminuted fractures (3, 4). These can be challenging to stabilize, especially if they involve the supracondylar area. Concurrent thoracic injuries, such as lung contusions and pneumothorax, can be encountered due to the proximity of the thorax.

29.1 Surgical anatomy

The humerus in cats is straighter and more slender than in dogs. Important anatomic differences between the humerus in dogs and cats exist, mainly affecting the distal part of the bone. Cats lack the supratrochlear foramen, but they have a supracondylar foramen proximal to the medial epicondyle. The bony bridge of the medial aspect of the supracondylar foramen is confluent with the medial epicondyle. The median nerve and the brachial artery course through the supracondylar foramen, and iatrogenic damage to these structures should be avoided (Fig. 29-1).

Important nerves are encountered during surgical approaches to the humerus. The radial nerve courses laterally across the middle third of the humerus, in a slightly oblique caudal to cranial direction, before it divides into its sensory and motor branches. It is located superficial to the brachialis muscle. Medially, a neurovascular bundle, containing the median, musculocutaneous, and ulnar nerves, and the brachial artery and vein, is located at the caudal edge of the biceps brachii muscle. The bundle divides distally, with the median nerve and brachial artery coursing through the supracondylar foramen in a cranial direction, and the ulnar nerve continuing in a caudal direction.

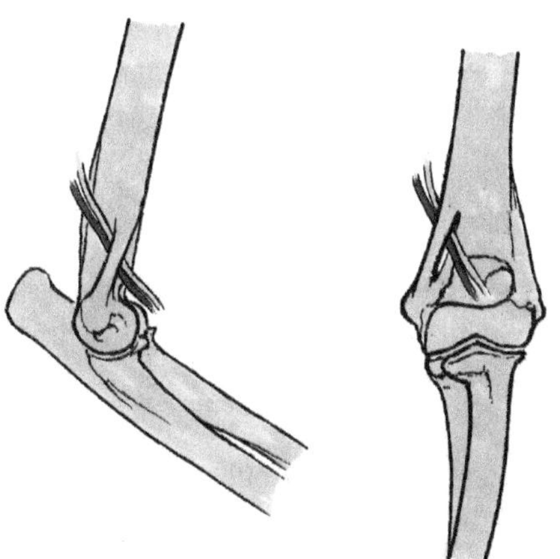

Figure 29-1 Anatomy of the medial aspect of the left distal humerus. The median nerve and brachial artery course through the supracondylar foramen in a caudal to cranial direction.

29.2 Stabilization techniques

Internal stabilization is required for nearly all fractures of the humerus, because the bone is not amenable to stable external coaptation. Only rare greenstick fractures in kittens and some pathological fractures can be treated with cage rest alone. General considerations on intramedullary pinning and nailing, external skeletal fixation, and plating of humeral fractures are described in the following sections. A summary of feline humeral fracture types and their preferential stabilization methods is provided in Table 29-1.

29.2.1 Intramedullary pinning

Intramedullary pins have to be combined with antirotational implants in all cases, except the occasional simple transverse interdigitating fracture in the immature cat. Insertion of an intramedullary pin improves construct stability of plates and external fixators by adding to the resistance to bending forces, and it also aids the spatial alignment of the main bone fragments in comminuted fractures.

Placement of an intramedullary pin into the humerus can be performed in a normograde or retrograde fashion. The area for insertion of a normograde intramedullary pin is the craniolateral aspect of the greater tubercle (Fig. 29-2). After penetration of the cortex, the pin is advanced in a distomedial direction. For retrograde pinning, a double-pointed Kirschner wire is inserted from the fracture site, and is retrograded along the lateral cortex to exit through the proximolateral aspect of the greater trochanter. The fracture is then reduced and the pin is advanced into the distal fracture fragment with the help of a Jacobs chuck, until resistance to its passage is felt and/or the fracture line starts to distract. The pin can often only be inserted into the distal central humerus proximal to the condyle, and not right into the medial aspect of the condyle, as is usually recommended in dogs. The elbow joint is manipulated through its range of motion to exclude inadvertent placement of the pin into the elbow joint. The

Fracture localization	Fracture type	Stabilization methods
Proximal humerus	Salter and Harris type I	Parallel pinning Tension band fixation
Diaphysis	Simple transverse or short oblique	IM pin and ESF Compression plate Internal fixator
	Simple long oblique and reducible multifragmentary	IM pin and cerclage/hemicerclage wires Lag screw(s) and neutralization plate Lag screw(s) and internal fixator
	Comminuted	Interlocking nail ESF ± IM pin Buttress plate ± IM pin Internal fixator
Distal humerus	Supracondylar, simple	IM pin and Kirschner wire Cross pins/dynamic pins Compression or neutralization plate Internal fixator
	Supracondylar, comminuted	ESF ± IM pin Buttress plate ± IM pin Double plating Internal fixator (single or double)
	Lateral portion of the condyle and Salter and Harris type IV	Transcondylar lag screw and Kirschner wire
	Intracondylar T- or Y-fracture	Transcondylar lag screw and: – IM pin with Kirscher wire – neutralization plate – internal fixator
	Intracondylar fracture with supracondylar comminution	Transcondylar lag screw and: – ESF – buttress plate – double plating – internal fixator (single or double)

Table 29-1. A summary of feline humeral fractures and selected treatment options
IM pin, intramedullary pin; ESF, external skeletal fixator.

proximal end of the intramedullary pin is then either cut short or bent laterally if it is to be connected to the bar of an external skeletal fixator in tie-in configuration.

The size of pin used is affected by the size and anatomy of the cat, fracture type and location, and type of ancillary implants used. A pin is selected to fit the smallest diameter of the distal intramedullary canal in the supracondylar region, or to fit the medullary canal of the medial epicondyle. Advancing the pin distally into the medial epicondyle results in firm anchorage of the distal pin end, which is especially important in the treatment of distal fractures. However, an intramedullary canal distal to the supracondylar foramen is only present in less than half of cats, and its diameter only allows insertion of a maximum pin size of 1.6 mm (5) (Fig. 29-2). The distal end of the intramedullary pin is seated at the end of the distal humeral canal, just above the supratrochlear fossa in all other cats (Fig. 29-2). A maximum pin size of 2.4 mm can be used in these cases (5). The presence or absence of an intramedullary canal distal to the supracondylar foramen can be evaluated on appropriately positioned preoperative radiographs or

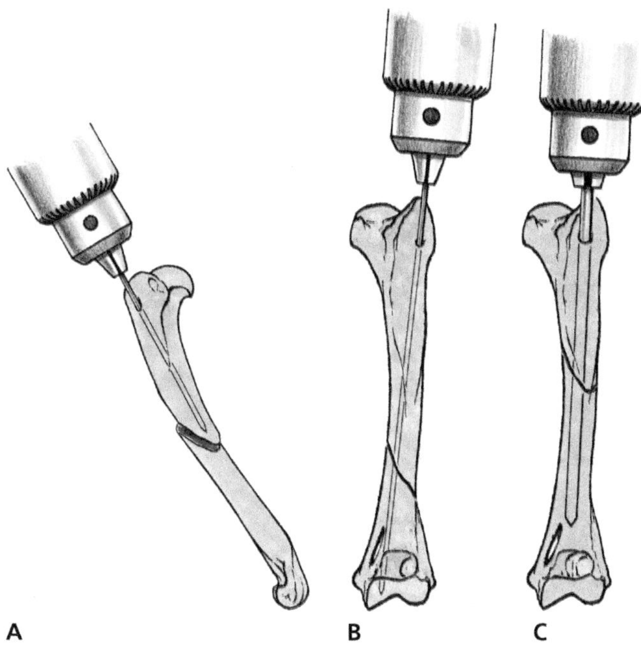

Figure 29-2 Diagram showing normograde intramedullary pinning of the humerus. (**A**) The entry site of the pin is on the craniolateral aspect of the greater tubercle. (**B**) In around 50% of cats, a small-diameter intramedullary pin can be inserted right into the medial epicondyle. (**C**) In cats without a medullary cavity extending into the medial epicondyle, a larger-diameter pin can be inserted instead into the distal aspect of the humeral medullary cavity.

during surgery with the help of a small-diameter Kirschner wire as a probe.

29.2.2 Interlocking nailing

The application of an interlocking nail for stabilization of feline humeral fractures has been described (6, 7). This implant is only useful for proximal to mid-diaphyseal fractures due to the narrow size of the intramedullary canal in the distal humerus of the cat. There should be room to place two screws distal and proximal to the fracture, with the middle screws placed a minimum distance, equivalent to at least one screw diameter, from the fracture line.

The 4.0-mm nail with 2.0-mm screws or bolts is the most useful size for all but the largest cat, where the 4.7-mm nail may work. An open surgical approach is generally recommended, and the nail should be tested for fit in the distal humeral medullary canal where the bone is narrowest. Placement of a too large an interlocking nail will result in fissuring and further fracturing of the bone. Alternative implant systems should be applied if the nail is considered too large. Normograde or retrograde placement of the nail is possible. Normograde placement may require a slightly more proximal nail entry point. The nail is aimed down the middle of the medullary canal with the tip ending in the supracondylar area. The proximal humeral bone has a thin cortical shell and a high proportion of cancellous bone. In dogs it was found that two screws must be placed distal to the tricipital line to prevent screw loosening and collapse of the repair (6).

29.2.3 External skeletal fixation

External skeletal fixation is a versatile method for stabilization of humeral fractures, especially useful for the common comminuted fractures of the distal diaphysis and supracondylar area, which have little distal bone stock to insert other implants (4). However, the transosseous pins can create irritation of the mobile soft-tissue structures, particularly near the elbow joint. A stable construct and appropriate postoperative care help to minimize pin tract complications (Chapter 24).

Only type I or modified type II constructs can be used in the feline humerus due to the proximity of the thoracic wall on the medial side. Placement of an intramedullary pin adds to stability, especially if used as a tie-in configuration (8). The tie-in configuration also prevents migration of the intramedullary pin. Two to three transosseous pins are needed per fragment in combination with an intramedullary pin, depending on fracture type, location, and severity (Chapter 24). Three pins should be inserted per fragment if the fixator is used as the sole method of fixation. Closed fracture reduction is rarely possible, and a limited open approach is usually helpful. An open approach also allows visualization and protection of the radial nerve during fracture reduction and pin insertion.

Transosseus pin size should not exceed 25% of the bone diameter, usually allowing the use of 2.0-mm positive-threaded pins in the proximal half of the humerus, and 1.6-mm positive- or negative-threaded or smooth pins in the distal half of the humerus. Transosseous pins can be placed safely in the proximal third of the humerus where there are no important neurovascular structures. In the distal humerus, pins should be inserted at least 2 cm proximal to the medial epicondyle to avoid penetration of the supracondylar foramen and associated nerves and vessels (5). Transosseous pins distal to that are angled in a laterodistal to proximomedial direction to avoid the foramen. A transcondylar pin is indicated if fracture configuration or the presence of a large intramedullary pin precludes insertion of two pins between the distal fracture end and the supracondylar foramen. A transcondylar pin is inserted from just cranial to the lateral epicondyle, and exits the bone craniodistal to the medial epicondyle. A pin size between 1.5 and 2.0 mm is recommended (5).

29.2.4 Plating

Plate osteosynthesis is generally a good choice of treatment for fractures of the humeral diaphysis, with the exception of open fractures, or comminuted distal fractures, which do not permit insertion of a sufficient number of screws in the distal fragment.

The humeral diaphysis is unique in that plates can be positioned laterally, cranially, and medially. The convex dorsolateral surface is the tension side of the proximal humerus, and the mediocaudal surface is the tension side of the distal humerus. Accordingly, plates are positioned cranially or laterally for fractures of the proximal half of the diaphysis. The lateral approach is easier and less invasive than the medial approach in the proximal half of the humerus, but care has to be taken to preserve the radial nerve. Medial plating is better for distally located fractures, because the medial approach to the distal humeral requires less tissue dissection (9). Additionally, the straighter shape of the medial side of the distal humerus eases plate contouring. The medial approach also allows visualization and proximal or distal retraction of the median nerve and the brachial artery within the limits of the supracondylar foramen. This facilitates screw placement in distally located fractures, while minimizing the risk for iatrogenic damage of these vital structures.

Suitable plates for fractures of the shaft of the humerus are the 2.7-mm dynamic compression plate (DCP), the 2.4-mm limited contact-dynamic compression plate (LC-DCP), and the 2.0/2.7-mm veterinary cuttable plate. Veterinary cuttable plates are preferred in the distal, narrow region, as they allow insertion of 2.0-mm screws. A 2.0-mm DCP may be used for simple diaphyseal fractures in small cats, and for supracondylar fractures. The plate is applied in compression, neutralization, or buttress function, depending on fracture configuration, and type of plate used. Principles of plate function and application are described in Chapters 13 and 24. Pre-contouring the plate prior to surgery is advantageous in the presence of comminuted fractures. The plate and rod configuration can be used for stabilization of comminuted fractures.

29.2.5 Internal fixators

Internal fixators, for example the Unilock mandible locking plates, are valuable for buttress fixation of comminuted fractures of the humeral diaphysis. They preserve the local vascularity, and their application requires less tissue dissection compared to conventional plating (Chapter 24). They are also indicated for diaphyseal fracture repair in immature cats, as the periosteal blood supply is left undisturbed. The 2.4-mm Unilock plate is used for most diaphyseal fractures, and the 2.0-mm plate may be applied in smaller and immature cats.

Internal fixators have advantages over conventional plating, especially when used for the repair of supracondylar fractures of the humerus. The small distal fragment and the close vicinity of the elbow joint make screw placement difficult in this location. The small distal fragment often only allows insertion of two screws, and the stability of internal fixators is superior to conventional plating in situations where few screws are inserted per bone fragment. Internal fixators can also be applied with monocortical screws, therefore reducing the risk of screw insertion into the elbow joint. Bilateral plating is also easier when monocortical screws are used, and is a very helpful technique for the repair of comminuted fractures of the supracondylar region. Additionally, accurate plate contouring is not as critical as compared to conventional plates. The 2.0-mm Unilock plates are a suitable size for fractures of the distal humerus.

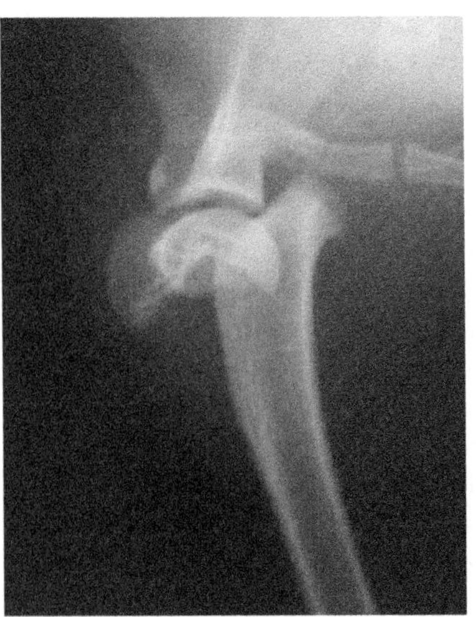

A

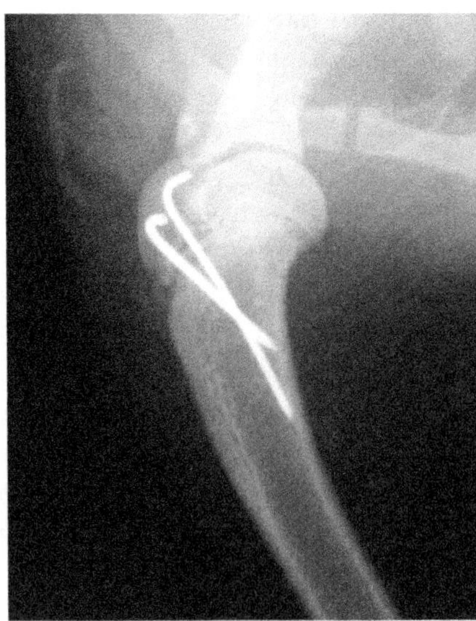

B

Figure 29-3 (**A**) Preoperative and (**B**) postoperative radiographs of a Salter and Harris type I fracture of the proximal humerus in an 11-month-old cat, stabilized with two pins.

Box 29-1. Stabilization of Salter and Harris type I fractures of the proximal humerus

A craniolateral approach is made to the proximal humerus. The shoulder joint is held in extension to reduce the fracture. Distal traction is applied on the humeral shaft with the help of pointed reduction forceps, followed by levering the proximal epiphysis into place. The proximal epiphyses are slightly V-shaped, which allows control of reduction, and gives some inherent stability after fracture reduction. Reduction is maintained manually or with the help of pointed reduction forceps during pin insertion.

Parallel pinning: A 0.8–1.2-mm Kirschner wire is inserted at the proximal ridge of the greater tubercle, and is advanced perpendicular across the fracture surface into the caudal cortex of the proximal humeral metaphysis. A second pin is inserted parallel to the first one (Fig. 29-4A).

Tension band repair: The two parallel pins are inserted first. A hole is then drilled through the cranial cortex of the proximal metaphysis, at a distance from the fracture line approximating the distance between the proximal pin ends and the fracture. A piece of 0.6–0.8-mm orthopedic wire is placed in a figure-of-eight fashion through the hole and around the pin ends (Fig. 29-4B). Overtightening of the tension band wire is avoided, as this could cause the fracture gap to open on the caudal aspect.

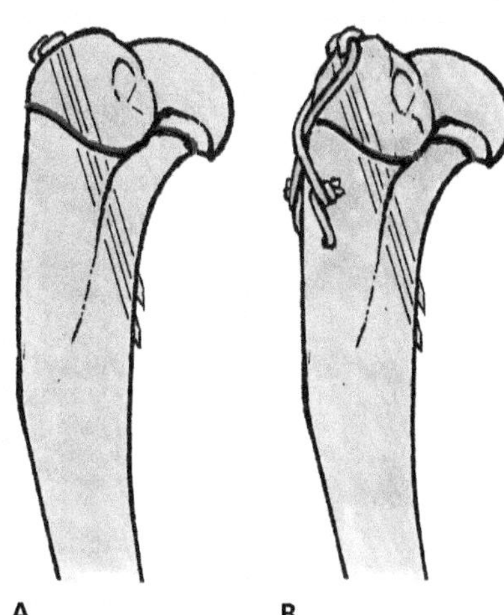

Figure 29-4 Stabilization methods for Salter and Harris type I fractures of the proximal humerus. (**A**) Parallel pinning is preferable for immature cats. (**B**) Tension band repair. This technique can be used in mature cats without further growth potential.

29.3 Fractures of the proximal humerus

Fractures of the proximal humerus are uncommon. They include physeal fractures in young cats, and proximal metaphyseal fractures.

29.3.1 Approaches to the proximal humerus

The proximal humeral metaphysis and shaft are exposed via a craniolateral approach, extending from the proximal end of the greater tubercle distally (10). Extension of the approach proximally allows access to repair Salter and Harris type I fractures of the proximal humerus. Articular fractures of the humeral head requiring anatomic reconstruction of the fragments necessitate a more extensive approach for adequate exposure of the articular surface. An approach to the craniolateral region of the shoulder joint with either tenotomy of the deltoid and infraspinatus muscles or osteotomy of the acromion process or greater tubercle (10) may be necessary.

29.3.2 Salter and Harris fractures

Fractures of the proximal humeral physis are rare (2). The proximal humerus has two epiphyses, one for the greater tubercle and one for the humeral head. Both epiphyses break off the humeral metaphysis like a cap in Salter and Harris type I fractures (Fig. 29-3). The distal fragment is usually displaced caudally and laterally (11). Parallel pinning is the treatment of choice for these fractures in growing cats, because further physeal growth is possible, and parallel pinning can allow this (Fig. 29-3). A tension band repair offers more stability but may result in physeal closure if applied in cats with further growth potential (Box 29-1). The tension band repair is also indicated to repair osteotomies of the greater tubercle, which are sometimes performed as part of the surgical approach to the shoulder joint (Chapter 28).

29.3.3 Proximal metaphyseal fractures

Proximal metaphyseal fractures are most often caused by gunshot injuries. They are otherwise uncommon because the cross-sectional area is larger in the proximal humerus compared to distal, and the bone is cancellous in nature and therefore less brittle (12). Simple fractures can be stabilized with a cranial plate or with an intramedullary pin with an antirotational device, such as an external skeletal fixator. Comminuted fractures caused by gunshot wounds require external skeletal fixation, with or without an intramedullary pin.

Pathological fractures secondary to nutritional or inherited bone diseases have a tendency to involve the proximal metaphysis of the humerus (Chapter 4). Undisplaced pathological compression fractures can be treated conservatively with cage rest. Intramedullary pinning in combination with an external skeletal fixator is used to stabilize displaced pathological fractures. Smaller and more flexible implants than normal should be used in the osteoporotic bone (Chapter 13).

29.4 Diaphyseal fractures of the humerus

Diaphyseal fractures of the humerus usually occur between the middle and distal third of the bone. The radial nerve crosses the diaphysis on the lateral aspect of the bone, and is therefore vulnerable to traumatic or iatrogenic injury. Function of the radial nerve should be assessed preoperatively. Response to spinal reflex testing may be difficult to interpret in the presence of a humeral fracture, but sensitivity of the dermatome of the radial nerve on the dorsum of the paw can be used for assessment of sensory function of the radial nerve (Chapter 1).

Cats younger than 1 year tend to have simple fractures, whereas older cats are more likely to have comminuted fractures (2). Stabilization of diaphyseal fractures is possible with virtually any of the implants available for treatment of long-bone fractures (Table 29-1). The final choice of implant is therefore based on general fracture assessment, as discussed in Chapter 13. The surgeon must be familiar with the specific anatomy of the feline distal humerus. Preoperative radiographs of the opposite humerus help to evaluate the anatomic shape of the bone.

29.4.1 Approaches to the humeral diaphysis

The shaft of the humerus can be approached from both laterally and medially. The lateral approach to the shaft of the humerus (10) is better suited for the proximal and middle humeral diaphysis. The most important structure encountered is the radial nerve, which courses along the brachialis muscle in a caudoproximal to craniodistal direction. For exposure of the humeral diaphysis, the brachialis muscle and the radial nerve are retracted caudally or cranially with Hohmann retractors or with a Penrose drain around the structures.

During the medial approach to the shaft of the humerus (10), the medial neurovascular bundle, consisting of the median, musculocutaneous, ulnar nerve, and brachial artery and vein, has to be identified below the deep brachial fascia. The distal humeral shaft is exposed by cranial retraction of the brachiocephalic muscle, and caudal retraction of the triceps muscle. Extending the medial approach proximally requires incision and elevation of the pectoral muscles, and cranial retraction of the biceps muscle.

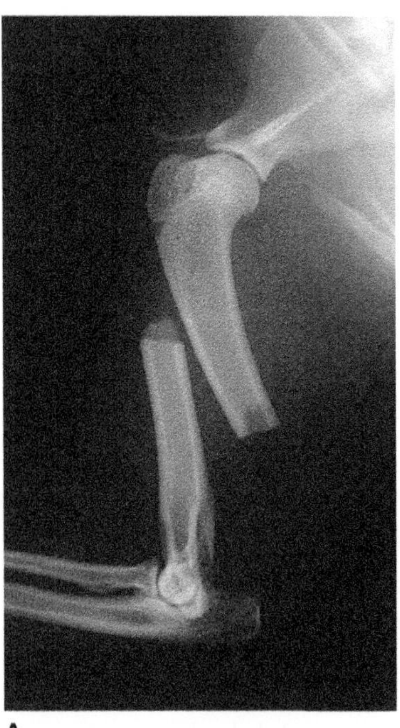
A

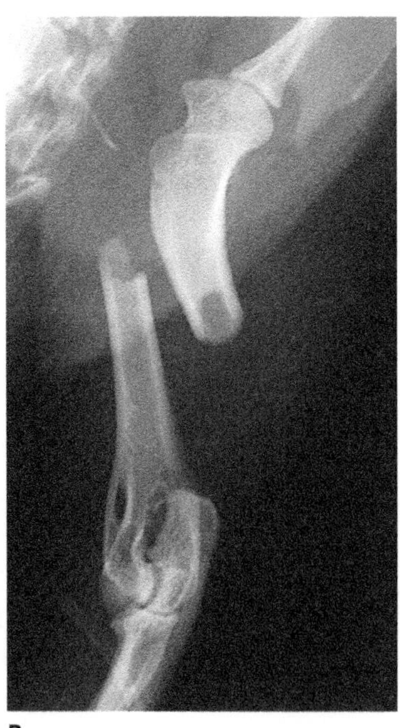
B

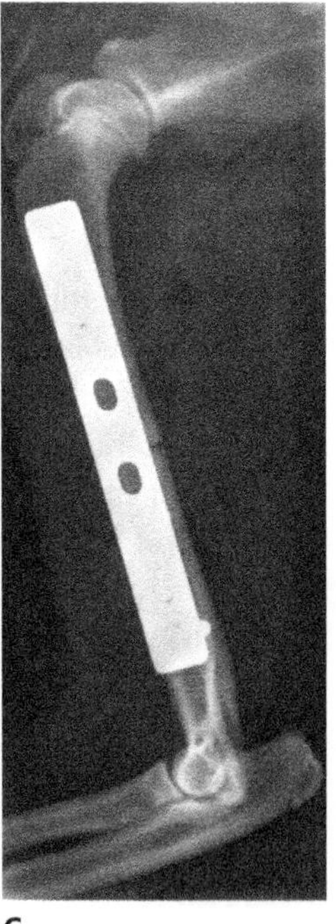
C

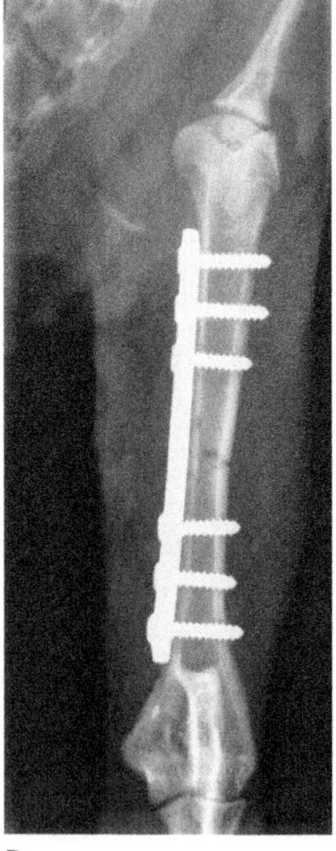
D

Figure 29-5 (**A, B**) Preoperative radiographs of a cat with a simple mid-diaphyseal fracture, (**C, D**) stabilized with a medially applied 2.7-mm DCP. Lateral plating could also have been used in this case.

Box 29-2. Stabilization of simple and short oblique fractures of the humeral diaphysis

A lateral approach to the humeral diaphysis is used for external skeletal fixation and lateral plating, whereas a medial approach is used for medial plating.

Intramedullary pin and external skeletal fixator: An intramedullary pin of a pre-selected size is inserted until its distal end is seated just proximal to the supratrochlear fossa. One 1.6–2.0-mm positive-threaded or two 1.4–2.0-mm smooth transosseous pins are inserted in the main fragments to prevent rotational stability. Smooth pins are angled about 70° to the long axis of the bone to prevent pull-out (Fig. 29-6A).

Plating: Plates are usually applied cranially for proximally located fractures (Fig. 29-6B), laterally for fractures in the mid-diaphyseal area (Fig. 29-6C), and medially for fractures of the distal third of the shaft (Fig. 29-6D). A minimum of three to four screws should be used per fracture fragment. Interfragmentary compression can be applied when a dynamic compression plate is used. It is usually sufficient to insert one screw per fragment eccentrically to achieve compression.

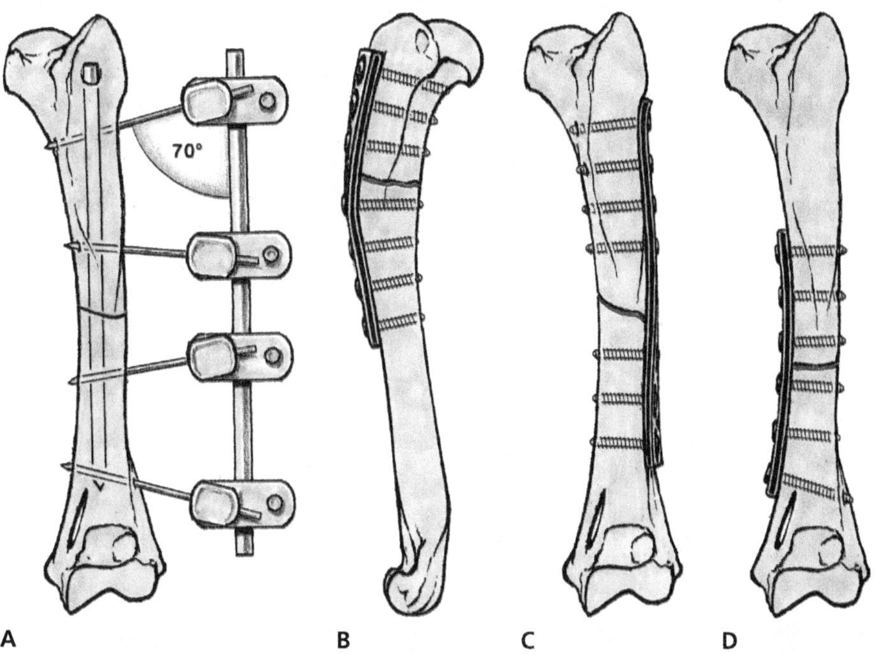

Figure 29-6 Stabilization options for simple transverse fractures of the humeral shaft.
(**A**) Simple transverse fracture stabilized with an intramedullary pin and a type I external skeletal fixator with two smooth pins per fragment. Note the 70° angle between pins and bone.
(**B**) Simple transverse fracture of the proximal humerus stabilized with a cranial plate.
(**C**) Simple transverse fracture of the humeral mid-shaft repaired with a lateral plate.
(**D**) Distally located simple transverse fracture fixed with a medial plate.

29.4.2 Simple transverse and short oblique fractures

Simple transverse and short oblique fractures usually occur in the middle and distal third of the humeral shaft. These fractures are best treated with a plate or with an intramedullary pin and external skeletal fixator (Box 29-2).

External skeletal fixation is mainly used in young cats. Although minimally displaced fractures could be reduced in a closed manner, an open approach is usually preferred to aid accurate implant placement and visualize and preserve the nerves. A relatively large intramedullary pin is selected to provide bending stability. The external skeletal fixator is then only needed to provide rotational stability, and insertion of two transosseus pins per fragment is sufficient.

Plate osteosynthesis is advantageous in cats which are difficult to handle, in avoiding the morbidity associated with transosseus pins, and is preferred in older cats with the longer healing times expected (Fig. 29-5).

29.4.3 Long oblique and multifragmentary reducible fractures

Anatomic reduction of long oblique fractures and multifragmentary reducible fractures enhances bone contact and stability. Long oblique fractures can be stabilized with an intramedullary pin in combination with antirotational implants, or with an interfragmentary lag screw and a plate in neutralization function (Box 29-3).

Box 29-3. Stabilization of long oblique and multifragmentary reducible fractures of the humeral diaphysis

Fractures in the middle to proximal region of the humerus are best approached from lateral, whereas fractures of the distal portion of the humeral shaft are best approached from medial.

Intramedullary pin and cerclage wire: This technique is indicated for long oblique fractures. A pin diameter approximately 70% of the medullary canal is inserted normograde or retrograde, as described in Figure 29-2. Two or more 0.8-mm cerclage wires are then positioned approximately 5 mm away from the proximal and distal ends of the fracture line (Fig. 29-7A). Care is taken not to engage soft tissues between the bone and wires.

Lag screws and neutralization plate: This technique can be used for both long oblique and multifragmentary reducible fractures (Fig. 29-7B and C). The fracture fragments are anatomically reduced and temporarily stabilized with pointed reduction forceps, and a 2.0-mm lag screw is inserted perpendicular to the fracture line(s) for interfragmentary compression. The plate is then applied across the primary repair in neutralization function, with at least three screws in the proximal and the distal fragment. Alternatively, the lag screws can be inserted through the plate if fracture configuration allows (Fig. 29-7C).

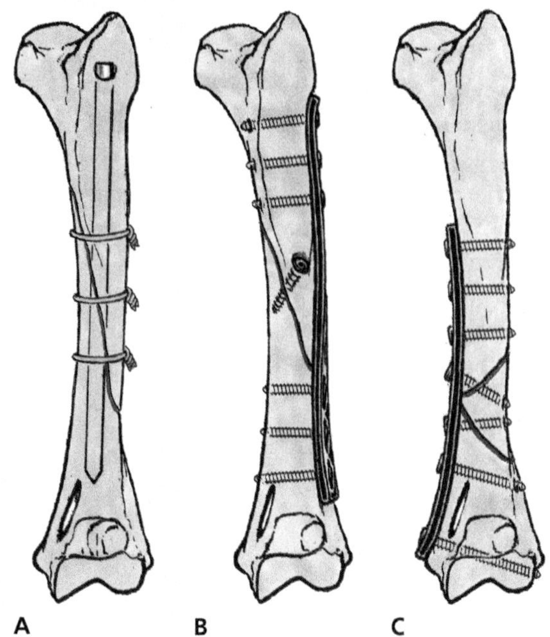

Figure 29-7 Anatomic reduction and stable fixation of simple oblique and multifragmentary reducible fractures.
(**A**) Stabilization of a long oblique fracture with an intramedullary pin and three cerclage wires.
(**B**) Stabilization of a long oblique fracture with a lag screw and a lateral neutralization plate.
(**C**) Reducible butterfly fracture in the distal shaft of the humerus, stabilized with a medial plate. Two lag screws are inserted through the plate holes.

Fractures with one or even two large intermediate fragments can also be repaired with lag screws or cerclage wires, and a neutralization plate (Box 29-3). Anatomic repair of fractures requires extensive dissection of soft tissues, and should only be attempted if anatomic reduction seems possible from the preoperative radiographs, and it is felt that this will enhance fixation stability. Alternatively, multifragmentary fractures can be treated like comminuted fractures with a minimally invasive approach and stabilization of only the main fragments in functional reduction. Plates are usually positioned cranially in the proximal third, laterally in the mid-diaphysis, and medially in the distal diaphysis.

29.4.4 Comminuted fractures

External skeletal fixators are most commonly used to repair comminuted fractures of the humeral shaft, especially for fractures extending into the distal diaphysis. The configuration of the external skeletal fixator is selected according to the expected healing time, the degree of fracture comminution, soft-tissue damage, and age of the cat (Box 29-4). An intramedullary pin facilitates spatial alignment and fracture reduction, and enhances bending stability of the construct. A double bar can be used to provide better bending stability in the absence of an intramedullary pin (Fig. 29-8). Modified type II or even transarticular constructs may be needed for severely comminuted fractures and very distally located fractures (Box 29-5).

Interlocking nailing, plate osteosynthesis, with or without an intramedullary pin, and internal fixators are other options for stabilization of comminuted fractures of the humerus (Box 29-4). Internal stabilization should be considered, especially in cats that are difficult to handle or to keep indoors. Plates are applied laterally if the fracture extends into the proximal diaphysis, and medially if the fracture is located distally. As many comminuted fractures are located

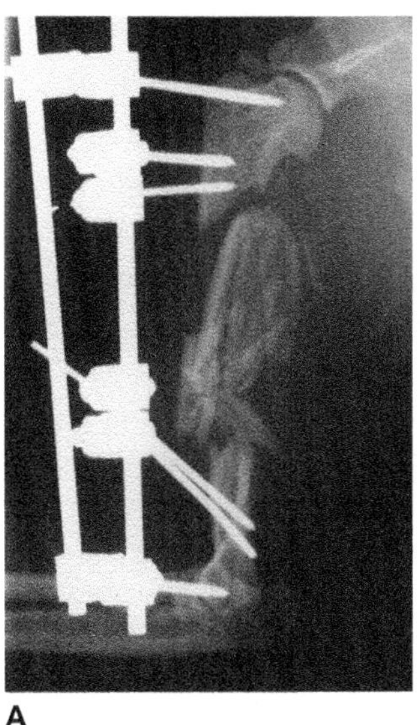
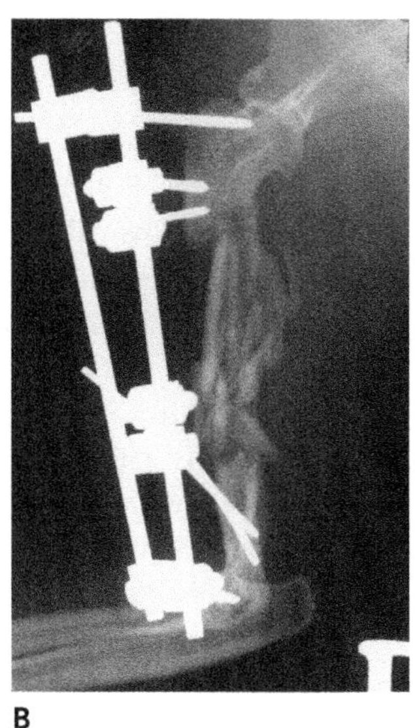
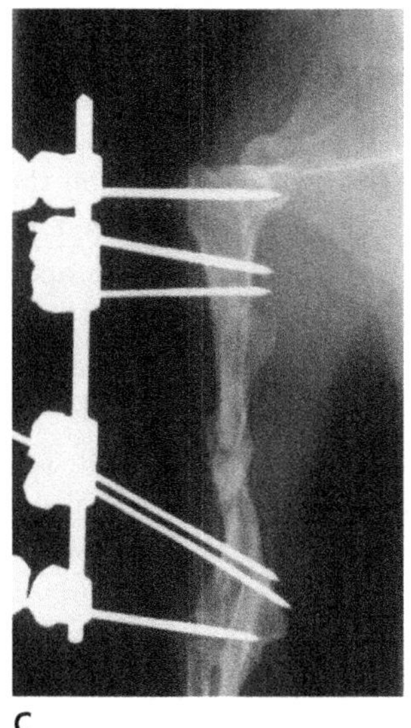
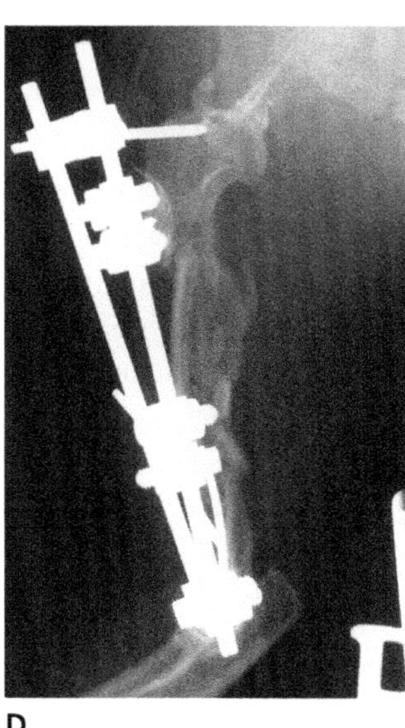

A B C D

Figure 29-8 External skeletal fixation of a highly comminuted fracture of the humeral shaft. (Reproduced with permission from: J Small Anim Pract 1997;37:280–285.)
(**A**, **B**) Immediate postoperative radiographs showing a type I external skeletal fixator. A double connecting bar was used to enhance bending stability.
(**C**, **D**) Progression of healing at 6 and 12 weeks postoperatively.

in the distal third of the humerus, it can be difficult to insert a sufficient number of screws in the distal fragment. Internal fixators have advantages over conventional plates in this situation.

29.5 Fractures of the distal humerus

Fractures of the distal humerus include supracondylar fractures, fractures of the lateral portion of the humeral condyle, intracondylar T- or Y-fractures, intracondylar fractures with supracondylar comminution, and Salter and Harris fractures of the distal growth plate. Supracondylar and intracondylar fractures are most common (3, 13).

29.5.1 Approaches to the distal humerus

The supracondylar area of the humerus can be approached from medially, laterally, and caudally (10). The medial approach is indicated for stabilization of supracondylar humeral fractures, because less dissection is necessary and placement of implants is facilitated when compared to a lateral approach. The median nerve and brachial artery coursing through the supracondylar foramen are protected. The neurovascular bundle can carefully be moved proximally and distally within the foramen to create room for insertion of pins or screws. If necessary, the foramen can be opened with rongeurs to prevent damage or compression of the neurovascular bundle.

A lateral and medial approach to the distal humerus may have to be performed simultaneously to allow reduction and stabilization of intracondylar or supracondylar fractures, especially if comminuted. Osteotomy of the olecranon improves visualization of the caudal aspect of the humeral condyle and can be used for intracondylar fractures if required.

29.5.2 Supracondylar fractures

Simple supracondylar fractures in young cats can be repaired with pins (Box 29-5). Anatomic fracture reduction is necessary for fixation stability if using pinning techniques. Dynamic intramedullary pinning and stabilization with an intramedullary pin and a Kirschner wire have been described (14). It can be difficult to insert the pins into the medial epicondyle in cats in the absence of a medullary canal distal to the supracondylar foramen. Medial plating is an option for both simple and multifragmentary supracondylar fractures (Box 29-5). Plating offers more stability, and in dogs it has been shown to be associated with lower complication rates when compared to stabilization with screws or pins and wires, particularly in adult animals (15).

Supracondylar fractures in cats are often comminuted, and their surgical repair can be a challenge. Comminuted supracondylar fractures may be stabilized with an external fixator, especially if the distal fragment does not offer enough room for plating (Fig. 29-11 and Box 29-5). Type I constructs are

Box 29-4. Stabilization of comminuted fractures of the humeral diaphysis

A medial or lateral approach is made, depending on the technique selected. Cancellous bone grafting should be considered if large fracture gaps are present, and an open approach has been used. Otherwise it is preferable to disturb the fracture site minimally. Fracture alignment is facilitated by insertion of an intramedullary pin prior to application of an external skeletal fixator or a plate. The pin should occupy a maximum of one-third of the distal medullary canal to allow transosseous pins or screws to be placed.

Interlocking nail: The use of interlocking nails is limited to diaphyseal fractures of the humerus, where there is sufficient bone for insertion of two bolts or screws distally and proximally (Fig. 29-9A). Nails with a diameter of 4.0 mm and with 2.0-mm screws are most commonly used.

External skeletal fixation: Configuration of the external skeletal fixator depends on fracture severity and location, but type I constructs are usually adequate for diaphyseal fractures. At least three pins must be inserted per fragment if no intramedullary pin is used (Fig. 29-9B). Two pins per fragment can be sufficient in the presence of an intramedullary pin (Fig. 29-9C). Pin size is usually 2.0 mm to 1.6 mm in the proximal humerus, and 1.6 mm or smaller in the distal humerus. Insertion of pins into the supracondylar foramen is avoided, either by angling the pins in a proximomedial direction, or by insertion of a transcondylar pin (Fig. 29-9D).

Buttress plate: The plates are applied in buttress function, with or without an intramedullary pin. Stacked 2.0/2.7-mm veterinary cuttable plates or a 2.7-mm dynamic compression plate can be used. At least six cortices must be engaged with the screws in both the proximal and distal main fragment in the absence of an intramedullary pin. Four cortices should be sufficient with the plate and rod configuration (Fig. 29-9E).

Internal fixator: A 2.4-mm Unilock plate is applied in a similar fashion as a buttress plate. The screws can be inserted bicortical or monocortical, and should engage at least four cortices in each main fragment. If possible, bicortical screws are used at the proximal and distal end of the plate, and monocortical screws in the middle of the diaphysis.

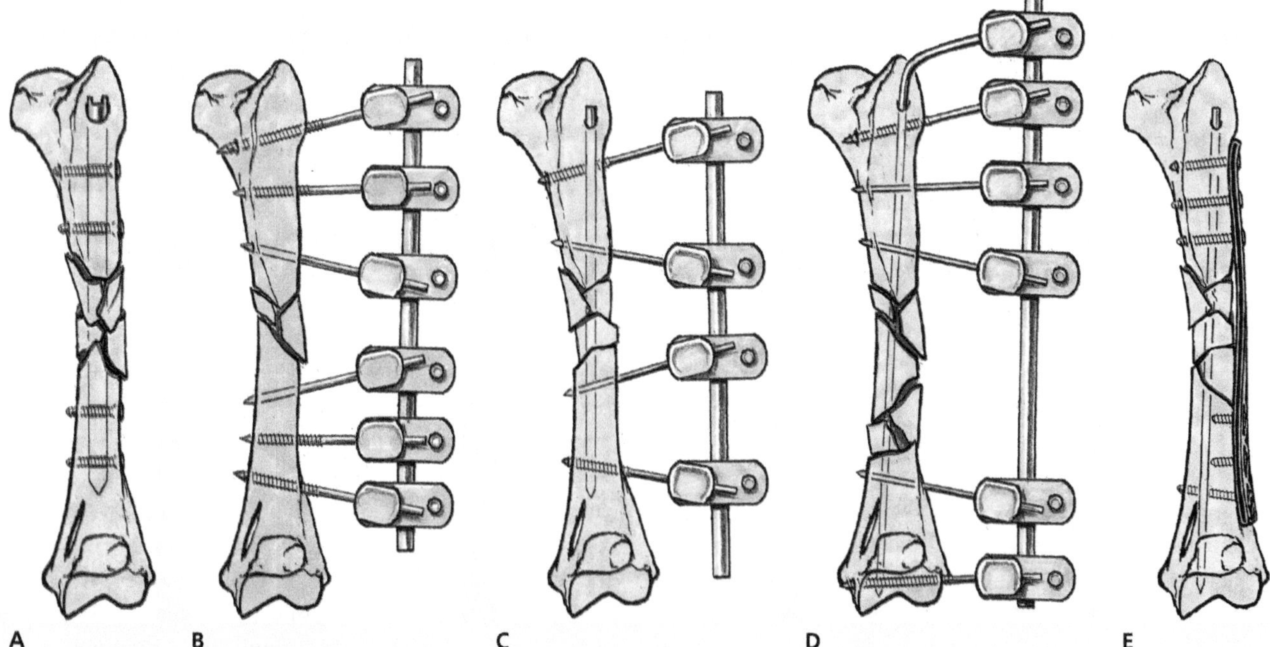

Figure 29-9 Stabilization methods for comminuted fractures of the humeral shaft.
(**A**) Comminuted mid-third humeral shaft fracture treated with an interlocking nail.
(**B**) Mildly comminuted fracture stabilized with a type I external skeletal fixator, using three pins per fragment.
(**C**) Mildly comminuted fracture stabilized with an intramedullary pin and a type I external skeletal fixator. The pins are angled at 70° to the long axis of the bone.
(**D**) Stabilization of a more distally located fracture with an external skeletal fixator in tie-in configuration, using a positive-threaded 1.6-mm transcondylar pin.
(**E**) Mid-diaphyseal comminuted fracture stabilized with a plate and rod technique.

Box 29-5. Stabilization of supracondylar humeral fractures

A lateral approach is performed for pinning and for external skeletal fixation. A medial approach is used for medial plating. Cancellous bone graft should be applied in severely comminuted fractures. The supracondylar foramen may be opened with rongeurs if nerve compression is present.

Pinning techniques: In cats with a medullary canal in the medial epicondyle, a 1.2–1.6-mm intramedullary pin is inserted from the greater tubercle into the medial epicondyle. A Kirschner wire is then drilled from just caudal to the lateral epicondyle through the distal lateral metaphyseal ramus to exit the craniomedial cortex of the humeral diaphysis (Fig. 29-10A). Alternatively, two 1.2–1.4-mm Kirschner wires are inserted as cross pins or dynamic intramedullary pin in cats without an intramedullary canal in the medial epicondyle (Fig. 29-10B).

Plating: Medial plating is indicated for simple and mildly comminuted fractures. A 2.0-mm dynamic compression plate or 1.5/2.0-mm veterinary cuttable plate is positioned caudomedially along the medial epicondylar crest (Fig. 29-10C). The most distal screw is directed cranially into the humeral condyle. The median nerve and brachial artery are visualized, and can be moved within the supracondylar foramen to allow insertion of an additional screw in this area. Double plating is also possible and should be considered in comminuted fractures (see Box 29-7, below).

Internal fixator: A 2.0-mm Unilock plate is applied in a similar fashion as described for conventional plating, but the locking screws can be inserted monocortically. The most distal screw often has to be angled to be inserted into the condyle. A standard screw must then be used for this purpose. Bilateral application is useful in comminuted fractures.

External skeletal fixation: An intramedullary pin is inserted into the medial epicondyle, if possible. It is later connected to the external bar in a tie-in configuration to avoid pin migration. A 1.6-mm transcondylar end-threaded or centrally threaded transfixation pin is inserted first, depending whether a type I or a modified type II (Fig. 29-10D) external skeletal fixator is to be used. It is started from just cranial to the lateral epicondyle and exits the bone craniodistal to the medial epicondyle to avoid joint penetration. The most proximal pin is then inserted, and the connecting bars applied. Two more half pins are inserted proximally and one distally.

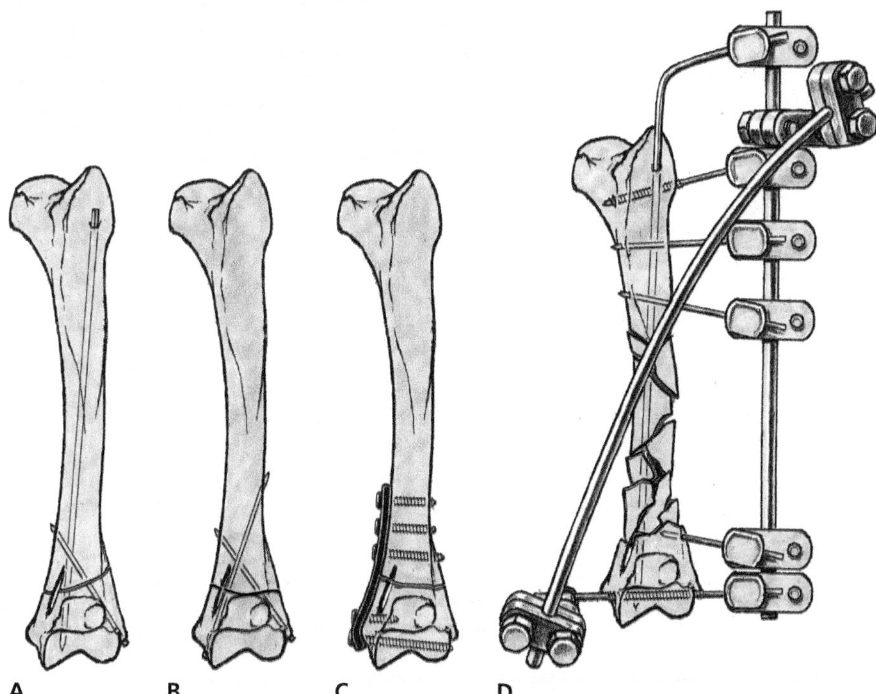

Figure 29-10 Stabilization methods for supracondylar humeral fractures. (**A**) A simple oblique supracondylar fracture, stabilized with an intramedullary pin and lateral Kirschner wire. This technique only applies in cats with a distal intramedullary canal. (**B**) Repair of a simple supracondylar fracture with cross pins. Instead of penetrating the transcortex, the pins could also be inserted far proximally along the inner cortical surface as dynamic intramedullary pins. (**C**) Stabilization of a simple supracondylar fracture with a medial plate. (**D**) A severely comminuted fracture treated with a modified type II external skeletal fixator in tie-in configuration.

adequate if the distal fragment allows insertion of two pins, and if an intramedullary pin is also placed. A modified type II external skeletal fixator provides more stability than a type I external fixator, and may be used in severely comminuted fractures, and fractures with a very small distal fragment (16). Medial or bilateral plating are other options for treating comminuted supracondylar fractures. Double plating is easier with internal fixators than with conventional plates, because of the possibility of monocortical screw insertion. Bilateral plating is further described under stabilization of intracondylar fractures of the humerus.

29.5.3 Fractures through the humeral condyle

Fractures through the humeral condyle are classified into simple fractures of the lateral portion of the humeral condyle, where the medial portion remains attached to the humeral shaft (Fig. 29-12), and T- or Y-intracondylar fractures, where

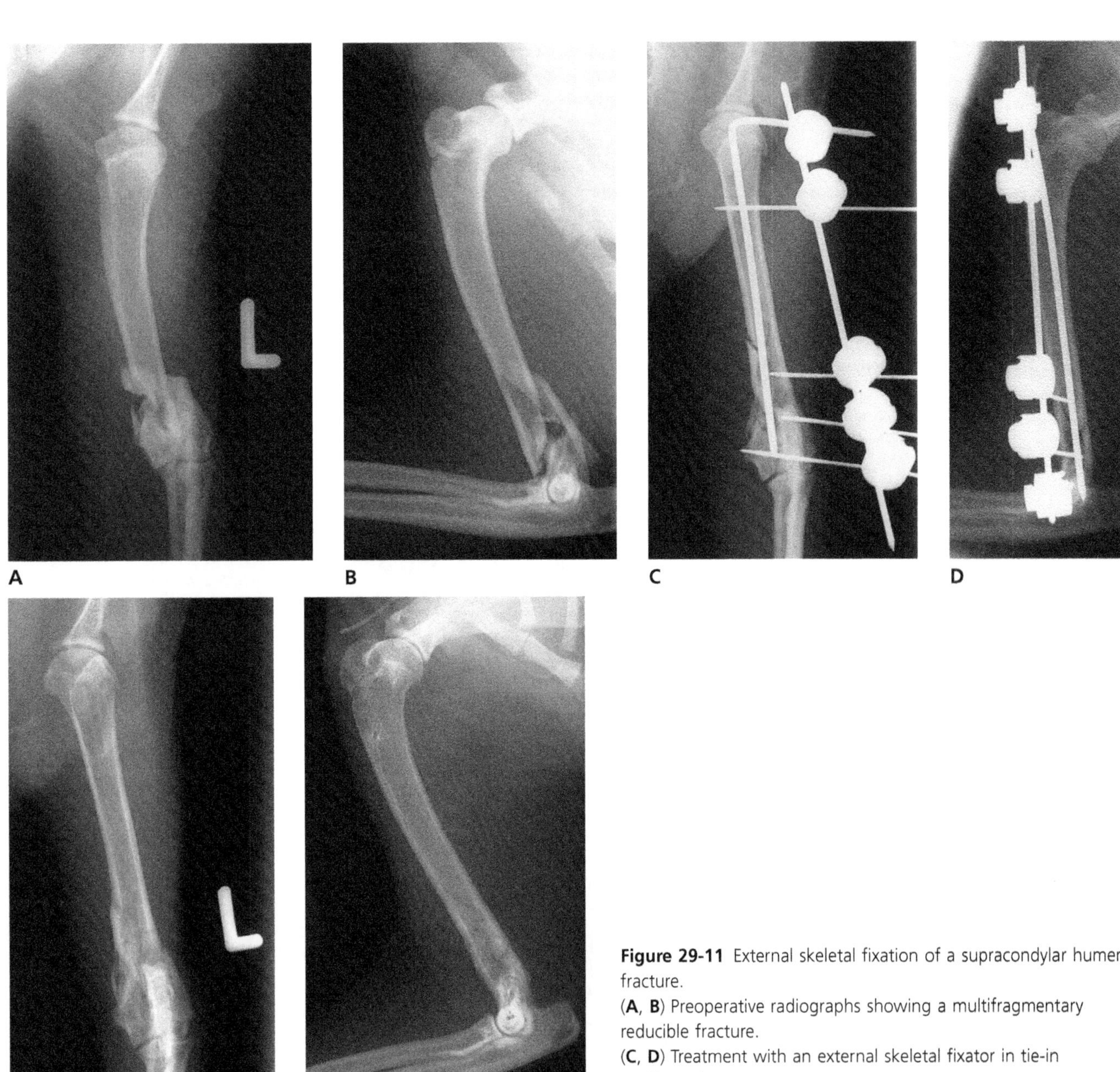

Figure 29-11 External skeletal fixation of a supracondylar humeral fracture.
(**A, B**) Preoperative radiographs showing a multifragmentary reducible fracture.
(**C, D**) Treatment with an external skeletal fixator in tie-in configuration.
(**E, F**) Three-month follow-up radiographs showing healing of the fracture.

both the lateral and medial portions of the condyle are broken off the shaft (Fig. 29-13). The supracondylar part of the fracture may be simple or comminuted.

Fractures of the lateral portion of the humeral condyle occur only infrequently in adult cats (Fig. 29-12). Cats with fractures of the lateral portion of the condyle are usually immature, and the fracture is then classified as a Salter and Harris type IV fracture. These fractures should be anatomically reduced to restore elbow joint congruity, and stabilized with a 1.5- or 2.0-mm transcondylar lag screw (Fig. 29-12 and Box 29-6). Either an antirotational pin or another screw angled along the lateral epicondylar crest is added to provide rotational stability.

Most fractures through the humeral condyle in cats are intracondylar fractures combined with a supracondylar fracture, resulting in detachment of both the medial and lateral portion of the condyle from the shaft. Simple T- or Y-fractures can occur, but comminution of the metaphyseal part of the fracture is present in most cases (13). Comminuted articular fractures of the distal humerus are among some of the most difficult to repair in cats. The humeral condyle and articular surface have to be anatomically reduced and stabilized with a lag screw. Then, depending on the fracture configuration and degree of comminution, plates, internal fixators, or external fixators are added to address the supracondylar part of the fracture (Box 29-7). The small condylar fragments and the presence of a transcortical lag screw often render insertion of a sufficient number of screws difficult, and bilateral plating is usually necessary to achieve adequate stability (Fig. 29-13). Internal fixators are ideal for this purpose because monocortical screws can be used, and fixation stability is better than with conventional plates if only two screws

A

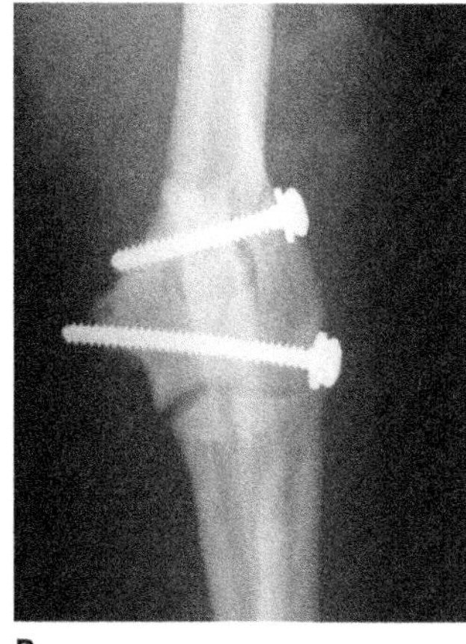

B

Figure 29-12 (**A**) Preoperative and (**B**) postoperative radiographs of an adult cat with a fracture of the lateral portion of the humeral condyle. The articular surface is reconstructed and stabilized anatomically with a transcondylar lag screw. A second screw is used as an antirotational implant.

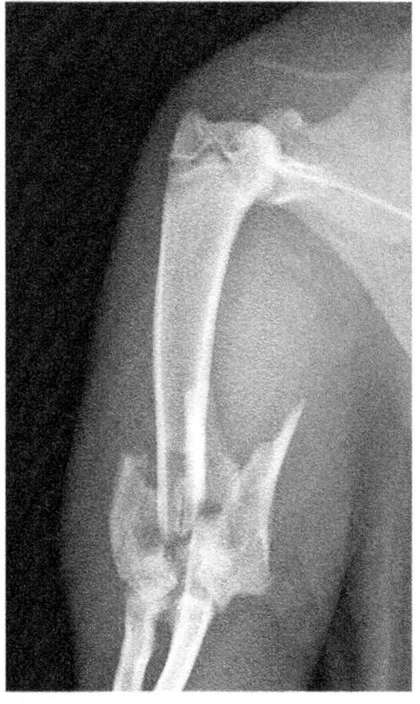

A

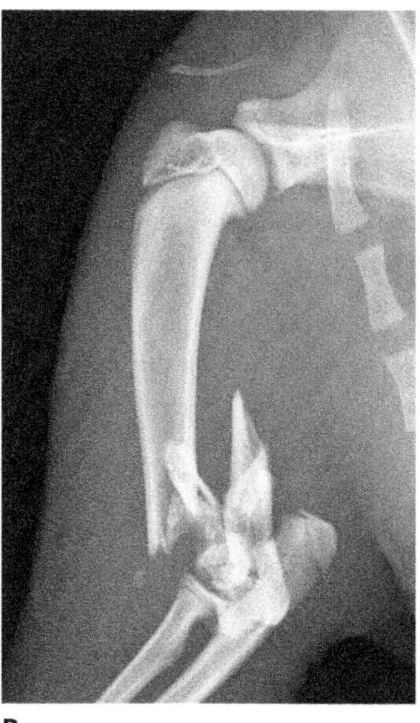

B

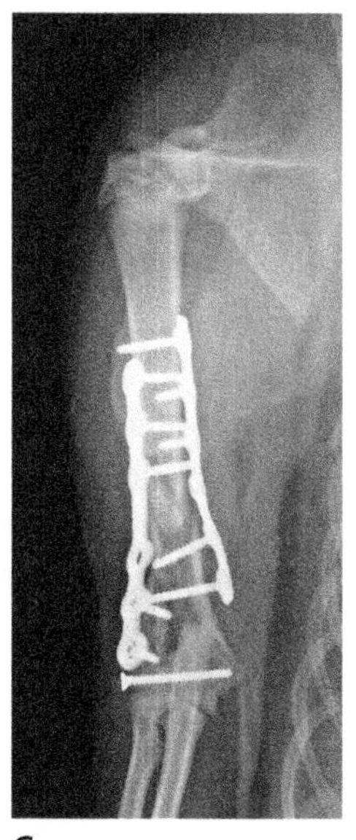

C

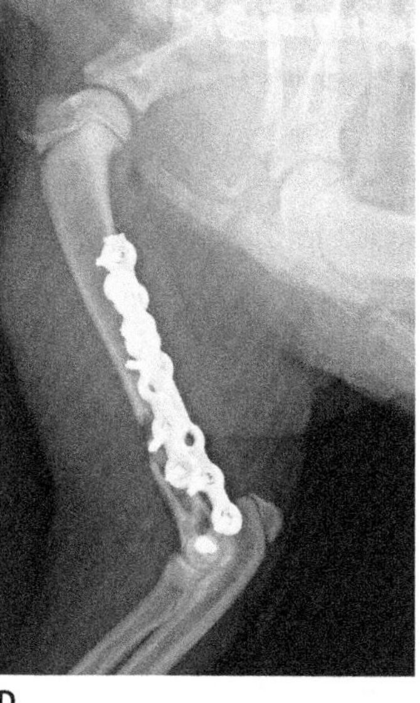

D

Figure 29-13 (**A**, **B**) Preoperative and (**C**, **D**) postoperative radiographs of an intracondylar fracture with supracondylar comminution. The condyle was first anatomically reduced and stabilized with a transcondylar lag screw. The supracondylar part of the fracture was then bridged with two 2.0-mm locking plates. Note that monocortical screws can be used with locking plates. The medially applied plate could have been positioned further distally, taking care not to injure the structures in the supracondylar foramen.

Box 29-6. Stabilization of a fracture of the lateral portion of the humeral condyle

A craniolateral approach to the elbow joint is performed. A 1.5–2.0-mm lag screw is inserted from just cranial to the lateral epicondyle to slightly caudodistal to the medial epicondyle (Fig. 29-14). The gliding hole into the lateral epicondyle can be drilled from the lateral aspect of the bone after the fracture has been reduced and stabilized with pointed bone reduction forceps. A C-shaped drill guide is useful for this method. An alternative is to drill the gliding hole from the fracture surface towards the lateral aspect of the bone before the fracture is reduced. This may facilitate correct screw placement, but involves more dissection and manipulation of the fragments. After the gliding hole has been drilled and the fracture reduced, a drill guide is inserted into the gliding hole to assist in directing the drill bit for the thread hole. The lag screw is inserted. A small Kirschner wire is inserted into the lateral epicondylar crest to provide rotational stability before the screw is tightened.

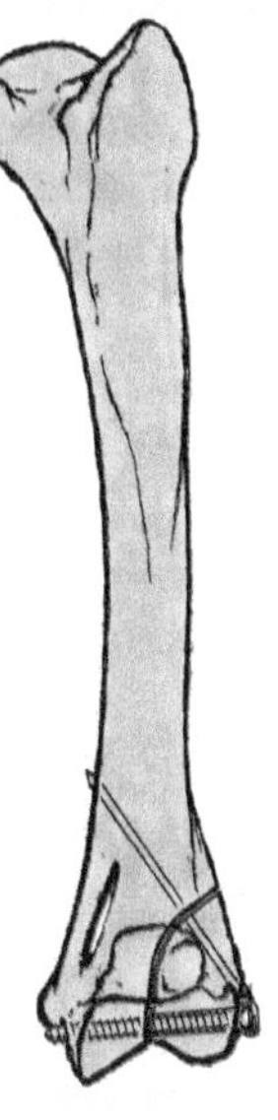

Figure 29-14 Stabilization of a fracture of the lateral portion of the humeral condyle with a transcondylar lag screw and an antirotational pin.

can be inserted distally. Cancellous bone graft should be used in fractures with supracondylar comminution to enhance fracture healing.

29.5.4 Salter and Harris fractures

Salter and Harris fractures of the distal humeral physis are rare, and only occur in very young cats before physeal closure at 16–18 weeks of age (17). Salter and Harris type IV fractures are seen most often (3). Anatomic alignment and stabilization of the joint surface are classically achieved with an intercondylar screw and an antirotational pin, as described above (Fig. 29-16). The small size and soft bone quality of the condyle in a young cat often preclude the use of lag screws. As an alternative, a 1.5-mm positional screw or a small threaded Kirschner wire may be used as transcondylar implants after reduction and careful compression of the fracture with pointed bone reduction forceps (18).

29.6 Postoperative treatment and prognosis

Postoperative treatment depends on the implants used. Cats with stable internal fixation of humeral fractures are confined to the house for around 6 weeks. Radiographs are taken between 4 and 6 weeks postoperatively in adult cats, and after 2 weeks in growing cats with physeal fractures. Postoperative treatment of cats after external skeletal fixation is more time-consuming compared to postoperative treatment after plate osteosynthesis. Gentle physiotherapy after all forms of fracture fixation is likely to improve functional outcome, especially in cats with restricted elbow function.

Healing of fractures of the humeral shaft is usually good, even after severely comminuted fractures. Ten comminuted fractures of the humeral shaft healed without major complications in a study evaluating 13 cats (4). Complications encountered in three cats included non-union, refracture after implant removal, and a stiff elbow joint. Healing times were 5–6 weeks for mildly comminuted fractures, and 10–11 weeks for severely comminuted fractures (4).

Outcome after distal humeral fractures depends on the ability to restore elbow congruity and achieve stable fixation. Approximately 90% of dogs and cats were described as having a good to excellent functional outcome after fractures of the distal shaft and supracondylar region, and after simple fractures of the lateral portion of the condyle (15). Intracondylar T- or Y-fractures had a less favorable outcome, with only around 50% of patients regaining satisfactory or good function (15). In a report on five cats with T- or Y-fractures and supracondylar comminution, three cats regained good

Box 29-7. Stabilization of intracondylar humeral fractures with supracondylar comminution

Both a lateral and medial approach have to be performed. An olecranon osteotomy could be made to reflect the triceps muscle, and improve visualization. The articular part of the fracture is always treated first. It is anatomically reduced and stabilized with a lag screw, as described in Box 29-6.

Medial (Fig. 29-15A) or bilateral plates or internal fixators (Fig. 29-15B) or an external skeletal fixator (Fig. 29-15C) are then used to stabilize the supracondylar part of the fracture. Bilateral plating is advised for severely comminuted fractures, and is facilitated if an internal fixator is used.

The presence of the intracondylar lag screw does not allow for easy insertion of a transcondylar transosseus pin if external skeletal fixation is used, but it may be possible to insert small Kirschner wires. These are inserted proximal to the screw, either monocortically or bicortically. Bicortical pins are positioned under visual control and retraction of the median nerve and brachial artery. At least three transosseus pins are used in the proximal fragment.

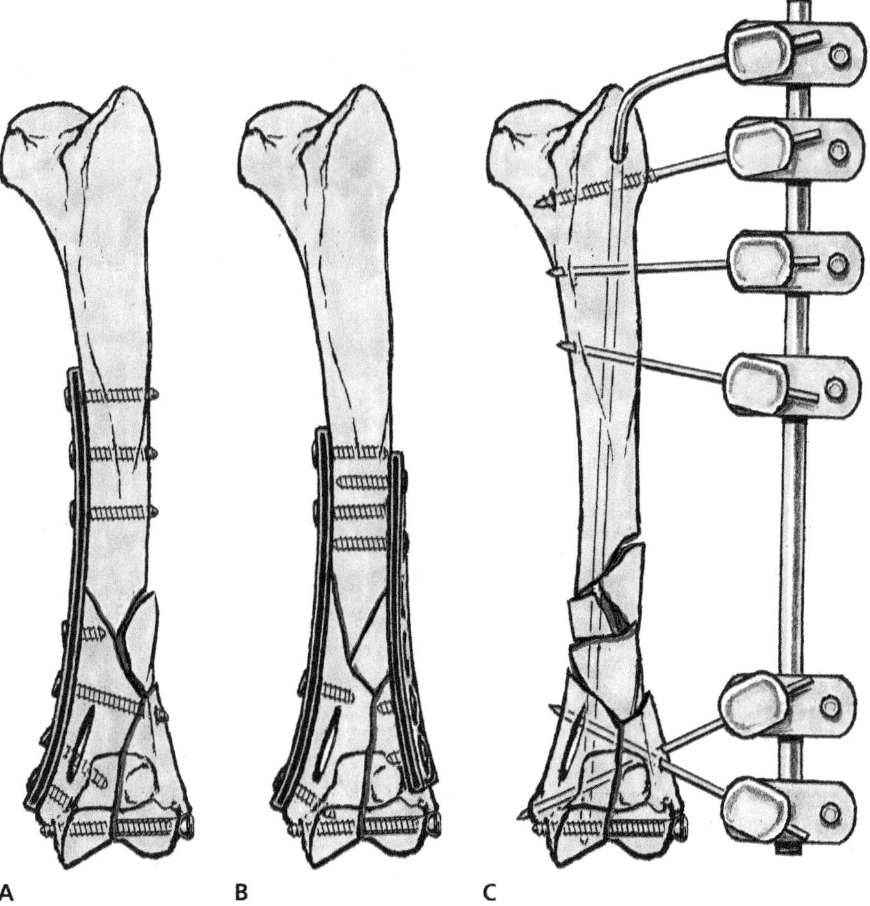

Figure 29-15 Stabilization methods for intracondylar humeral fractures with supracondylar comminution.
(**A**) Repair with a lag screw, and a medial plate.
(**B**) Stabilization with a lag screw, and both a medial and lateral plate. Bilateral plating offers more stability than medial plating alone.
(**C**) Fixation using a lag screw, and an external skeletal fixator in tie-in configuration.

function, one cat was persistently lame, and the limb of one cat had to be amputated following fixation failure (13). The authors have seen the development of periarticular ossification in a few cats with severe elbow fractures, resulting in decreased range of motion in the joint.

Plates are not routinely removed after healing of humeral fractures, because the approach is relatively invasive and bears the risk for iatrogenic nerve damage. An indication for implant removal is irritation of the elbow joint by periarticular implants.

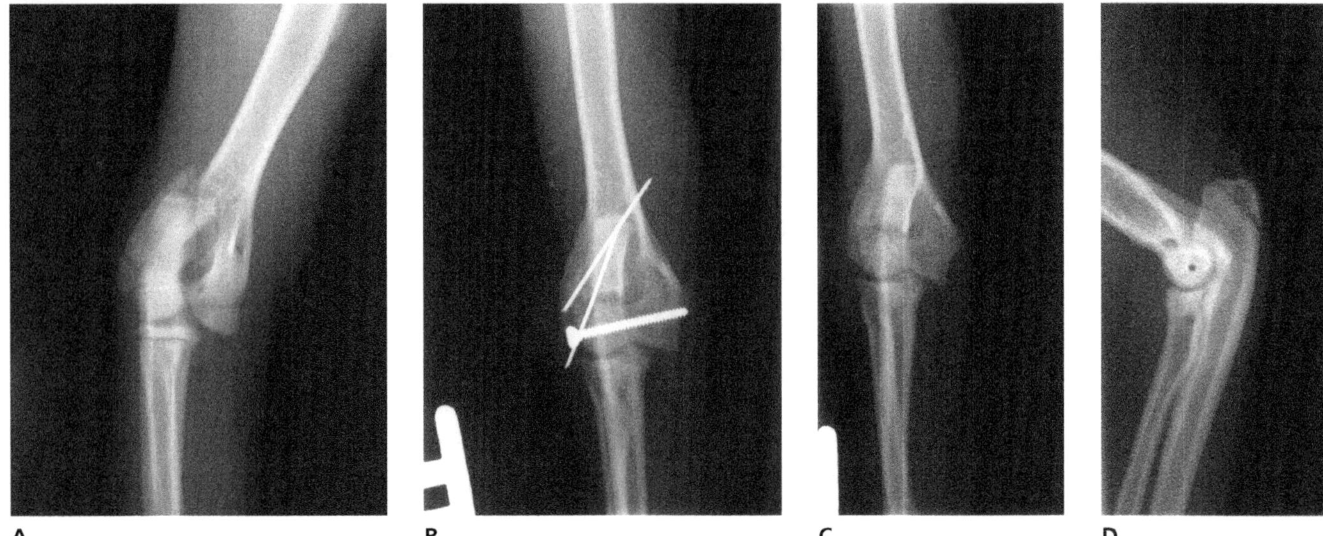

Figure 29-16 A Salter and Harris type IV fracture in a 4-month-old cat.
(**A**, **B**) Pre- and postoperative radiographs. Anatomic reduction and stabilization was achieved with a 1.5-mm lag screw and two small Kirschner wires.
(**C**, **D**) Radiographs 8 weeks postoperatively after implant removal, showing the healed fracture.

References and further reading

1. Hill FWG. A survey of bone fractures in the cat. J Small Anim Pract 1977;18:457–463.
2. Staimer MS. Humerusfrakturen bei der Katze. Dissertationschrift. München: Ludwig-Maximilians-Universität; 1980.
3. Vannini R, et al. An epidemiologic study of 151 distal humeral fractures in dogs and cats. J Am Anim Hosp Assoc 1988;24: 531–536.
4. Langley-Hobbs SJ, et al. External skeletal fixation for stabilisation of comminuted humeral fractures in cats. J Small Anim Pract 1997;38:280–285.
5. Langley-Hobbs SJ, Straw M. The feline humerus. An anatomical study with relevance to external skeletal fixator and intramedullary pin placement. Vet Comp Orthop Traumatol 2005;18: 1–6.
6. Moses PA, et al. Intramedullary interlocking pin stabilisation of 21 humeral fractures in 19 dogs and one cat. Aust Vet J 2002;32: 336–343.
7. Duhautois B. Use of veterinary interlocking nails for diaphyseal fractures in dogs and cats: 121 cases. Vet Surg 2003;32:8–20.
8. Aron DN, et al. Experimental and clinical experience with an IM pin external skeletal fixator tie-in configuration. Vet Comp Orthop Traumatol 1991;4:86–94.
9. Harari J, et al. Medial plating for repair of middle and distal diaphyseal fractures of the humerus in dogs. Vet Surg 1986; 15:45–48.
10. Piermattei DL, Johnson, KA. An atlas of surgical approaches to the bones and joints of the dog and the cat, 4th edn. Philadelphia: WB Saunders; 2004.
11. Tomlinson JL. Fractures of the humerus. In: Slatter D (ed.) Textbook of small animal surgery, 3rd edn. Philadelphia: WB Saunders; 2003: pp. 1905–1918.
12. Turner TM. Fractures of the proximal humerus. In: Johnson AL, Houlton JEF, Vannini R (eds) AO principles of fracture management in the dog and cat. Stuttgart: Thieme; 2005: pp. 203–208.
13. Macias C, et al. Y-T humeral fractures with supracondylar comminution in five cats. J Small Anim Pract 2006;47:89–93.
14. Piermattei DL, Flo GL. Fractures of the humerus. In: Piermattei DL, Flo GL (eds) Small animal orthopedics and fracture repair. Philadelphia: WB Saunders; 1997: pp. 261–287.
15. Vannini RS, et al. Evaluation of surgical repair of 135 distal humeral fractures in dogs and cats. J Am Anim Hosp Assoc 1988;24:537–542.
16. Klause SE, et al. A modification of the unilateral type 1 ESF configuration for primary or secondary support of supracondylar humeral or femoral fractures. Vet Comp Orthop Traumatol 1990;3:130–134.
17. Smith RN. Fusion of ossification centres in the cat. J Small Anim Pract 1969;10:523–530.
18. Morshead D, Stambaugh JE. Kirschner wire fixation of lateral humeral condylar fractures in small dogs. Vet Surg 1984;13: 1–5.

30 Elbow joint

K. Voss, S.J. Langley-Hobbs, P.M. Montavon

Elbow luxations and articular fractures of the distal humerus are the most common injuries of the elbow joint. Humeral fractures are described in Chapter 29, and ulnar and radial fractures in Chapter 31. A variety of different types of elbow luxation are observed in cats, in contrast to dogs where lateral elbow luxations make up the vast majority of cases. Anatomic differences may be responsible for this. Other injuries, like avulsion fractures or collateral ligament sprains, are also diagnosed.

The elbow joint of older cats is more commonly affected by osteoarthritis when compared to other joints of the appendicular skeleton (1–3), but underlying disease processes have not yet been described. A variety of other elbow diseases such as synovial cysts, elbow epicondylitis, synovial osteochondromatosis, elbow dysplasia, or congenital elbow luxation, may also be encountered, but information on these conditions is scarce. Diseases and traumatic injuries to the elbow joint are summarized in the following sections. Please also see Chapters 5 and 25.

30.1 Surgical anatomy

The elbow joint consists of three combined articulations: the humeroradial, humeroulnar, and radioulnar articulation. The shape and orientation of the feline trochlea humeri is different to that of the dog, and lead to medial movement of the radius and ulna during flexion of the elbow joint (4). The radioulnar joint allows rotation of the ulna around the radial head, which is necessary for the high degree of pronation and supination seen in felines.

Differences exist between cats and dogs regarding anatomy of the ligaments and the types of luxations seen. Similar to the dog, the collateral ligaments of the elbow in cats consist of two parts each, but their course and relative strength differ (Fig. 30-1). The ulnar part of the lateral collateral ligament is broader than the radial part, and it courses caudally to insert on the lateral coronoid process (4, 5). The ulnar part of the medial collateral ligament is also broader than the radial part of the medial collateral ligament (4, 5). The ulnar parts of the collateral ligaments are taut throughout the range of motion, whereas the radial parts are lax in flexion, allowing an increased range of rotation of the radial head (4). The annular ligament surrounds the radial head. It originates from the lateral collateral ligament, and inserts on the medial coronoid processes of the ulna (4). Cats lack the strong interosseous ligament between radius and ulna that is seen in dogs (5).

30.2 Diagnosis and treatment options

A summary of diseases and injuries of the elbow joint is provided in Table 30-1. Lameness varies from acute non-weight-bearing to chronic low-grade lameness, depending on the cause of the elbow disorder. The elbow is palpated to detect periarticular enlargement or fibrosis or alteration in normal anatomy and palpable bony landmarks. Pain and range of motion are evaluated by manipulating the joint through flexion and extension, and pronation and supination. Osteoarthritis and other chronic conditions often cause subtle clinical signs. Large fluid-filled structures adjacent to the joint may be consistent with synovial cysts. The insertion site of the flexor tendons on the medial humeral epicondyle may be painful on palpation in the presence of medial epicondylitis.

Pain, abnormal joint configuration, reduced range of motion, and crepitation are usually easily palpable in acute injuries, such as elbow luxations or fractures. In cases with lateral elbow luxation, the radial head and proximal ulna can be palpated lateral to the humeral condyle. The integrity of the collateral ligaments can be tested with the Campbell test, as shown in Figure 30-2.

Radiographs of the elbow joint are taken to detect signs of degenerative joint disease, luxations, and fractures. A sesa-

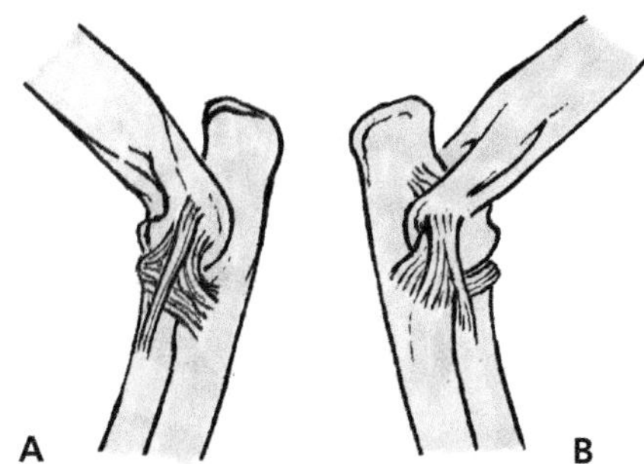

Figure 30-1 Anatomy of the collateral ligaments of the elbow in cats. The ulnar parts of both the lateral (**A**) and medial (**B**) collateral ligaments are broader than the corresponding radial parts. The annular ligament has an additional attachment to the humeral epicondyle on the lateral side.

Type of lesion	Further classification	Treatment options
Elbow dysplasia and congenital luxation	Dysplasia Congenital luxation of the radial head	Depends on individual case
Synovial cysts		Conservative, aspiration of the cyst
Disorder of tendons	Epicondylitis, avulsion of flexor tendons	Conservative Surgical
	Triceps tendon rupture	Tendon suture
Elbow instability	Collateral ligament sprain	Conservative Collateral ligament prostheses
Elbow luxation	Elbow luxation with intact radioulnar joint	Closed reduction followed by conservative treatment Open reduction and collateral ligament prostheses
	Luxation of the radial head	Open reduction and temporary positional screw between ulna and radius
	Complex elbow luxation with disruption of the radioulnar joint	Open reduction and temporary positional screw between radius and ulna, and collateral ligament prostheses
Fractures	Medial epicondylar crest	Conservative Excision of fragment and suture anchorage of flexor muscles
	Anconeal process	Excision of fragment

Table 30-1. Injuries of the elbow joint and possible treatment options

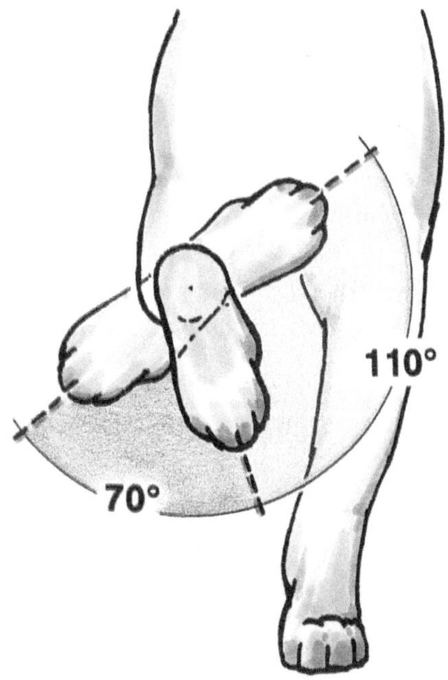

Figure 30-2 Campbell test. Elbow and carpal joint are held in 90° of flexion and supination and pronation movements are performed. Approximately 110° of supination, and up to 70° of pronation, is normal. Supination is exaggerated in the presence of lateral collateral ligament rupture. Subluxation of the radial head may also be felt laterally. Pronation is exaggerated in the presence of medial collateral ligament rupture.

moid bone in the tendon of origin of the supinator muscle is present in around 40% of cats (6). It is located at the cranio-lateral aspect of the head of the radius, and should not be mistaken for a pathological condition. Stress radiographs can help to confirm medial or lateral collateral ligament strain if elbow instability is suspected from clinical findings. Arthrography can confirm the presence of synovial cysts.

30.3 Approaches to the elbow joint

Surgery of the elbow joint in cats is most often performed to reduce and stabilize elbow luxations. Lateral and medial approaches may have to be combined.

A lateral approach allows access to the lateral epicondyle of the humerus, the head of the radius, the lateral coronoid process of the ulna, and the lateral collateral ligament (7). The head of the radius and the lateral coronoid process of the ulna can be reached by blunt separation of the extensor muscles. The superficial branch of the radial nerve lies between the lateral head of the triceps and the brachialis muscle, and runs cranial and distal to the elbow joint. Care must be taken not to injure the thin deep motor branch of the radial nerve, which courses between the extensor carpi radialis muscle and the supinator muscle, innervating the extensor muscle group.

The caudal humeroulnar part of the elbow joint is also approached from lateral (7), but the incision is located more caudally between the humeral epicondylar crest and the olecranon. Incision and elevation of the anconeus muscle allow visualization of the caudal humeroulnar joint, including the anconeal process.

The medial humeral epicondyle, the medial coronoid process of the ulna, and the medial collateral ligament are approached through a medial intermuscular approach (7). The medial coronoid process is relatively large in cats and almost completely covers the radial head. The ulnar nerve lies just caudal to the medial epicondylar crest. The median nerve and brachial artery pass through the supracondylar foramen and run further cranially below the pronator muscle.

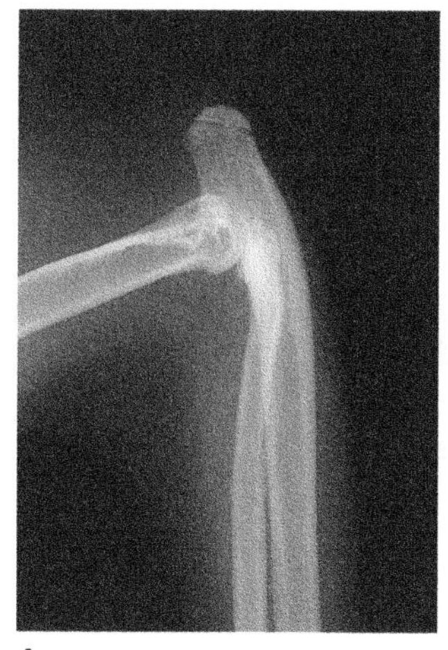

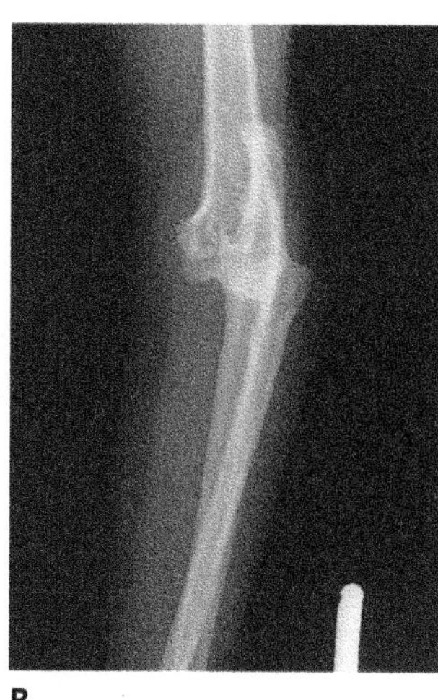

A B

Figure 30-3 (**A**) Mediolateral and (**B**) craniocaudal radiographs of the left elbow of a 1-year-old cat with congenital caudolateral luxation of the radial head. The condition was present bilaterally without causing marked clinical signs.

30.4 Elbow dysplasia and congenital elbow luxation

The high incidence of degenerative changes of the elbow joint in cats raises the question of whether underlying causes, such as elbow dysplasia, could play a role in the disease process. Fragmentation of the medial coronoid process of the ulna was considered a possible cause for osteoarthritis in the elbow joints of one cat, explored arthroscopically (8) (Chapter 25), and the authors have seen bilateral radioulnar incongruency in one cat with elbow osteoarthritis. However, as information in feline literature on elbow dysplasia is nearly non-existent, treatment options in affected cats have to be extrapolated from dogs (Chapter 25).

Congenital elbow luxation has been described in two case reports. The radial head was displaced laterally in one case (9), and caudolaterally in the other case (10). Affected cats can have a surprisingly good limb function (9), and the condition may go unnoticed by the owners (Fig. 30-3). Synostosis between the proximal radius and ulna can be present, and was considered a possible cause for elbow luxation in one report (10). A similar condition is described in children, where a developmental arrest of longitudinal segmentation during fetal life causes congenital synostosis between the radius and ulna, leading to asynchronous growth of the proximal radius and ulna, resulting in congenital elbow luxation (11). Treatment mainly depends on the severity of clinical signs. Most cats can probably be managed conservatively, and arthrodesis of the elbow should be reserved as a salvage procedure in cases with marked clinical disability.

30.5 Synovial cysts

Synovial cysts are periarticular swellings lined with synovial membrane-like cells and containing synovial fluid. Although synovial cysts can theoretically originate from any synovial joint, reports only describe cysts of the elbow joints in cats (12–14). A proposed mechanism for the development of synovial cysts in humans is herniation of the synovial membrane through the joint capsule, possibly secondary to trauma or osteoarthritis. Synovial cysts of the elbow are usually associated with degenerative joint disease in elderly cats (13, 14).

Affected cats usually present with a mild lameness. The cysts can be palpated as large fluid-filled structures adjacent to the elbow joint, protruding between muscle bellies, and extending towards proximally and/or distally. Radiographs demonstrate soft-tissue swelling and degenerative changes of the elbow joint (Fig. 30-4). Retrieval of synovial fluid out of the cyst supports the diagnosis. Contrast arthrography confirms the diagnosis by demonstrating the articular origin of the mass, and it can be used to outline the extent of the cyst.

Surgical resection of synovial cysts at the level of their origin at the joint capsule appears to be the treatment of choice in dogs. However, neither needle drainage nor surgical resection of the synovial cysts was successful in preventing recurrence of the cyst in most of the reported cats (13). It is therefore suggested to treat the underlying elbow osteoarthritis (Chapter 5), and to aspirate the cysts periodically to control their size (13).

30.6 Elbow epicondylitis

Avulsion and calcification of the antebrachial flexor tendons at their insertion site on the medial epicondyle of the humerus is a rare condition in dogs (15, 16). The inciting cause is unknown, but trauma or overuse may cause partial or complete avulsion of the flexor muscles from the medial epicon-

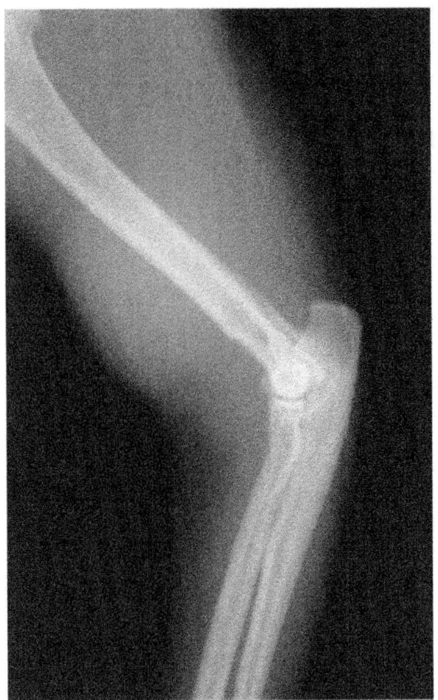

Figure 30-4 Mediolateral radiograph of the elbow joint of a 15-year-old cat with a synovial cyst. The cyst is visible as a large soft-tissue swelling proximal to the elbow. Note also the presence of elbow osteoarthritis.

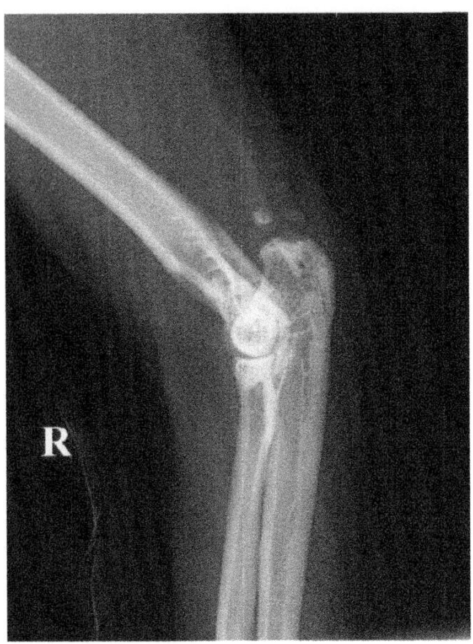

Figure 30-6 Radiographs of a cat with triceps tendinopathy. Similar changes were present in the contralateral leg. Treatment consisted of reinforcement by imbrication of the triceps tendon.

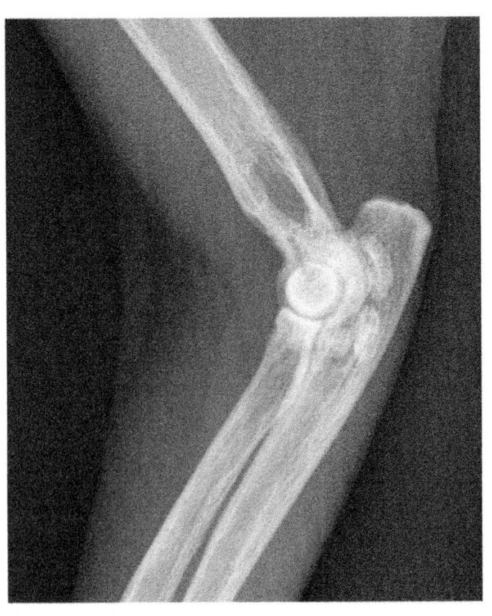

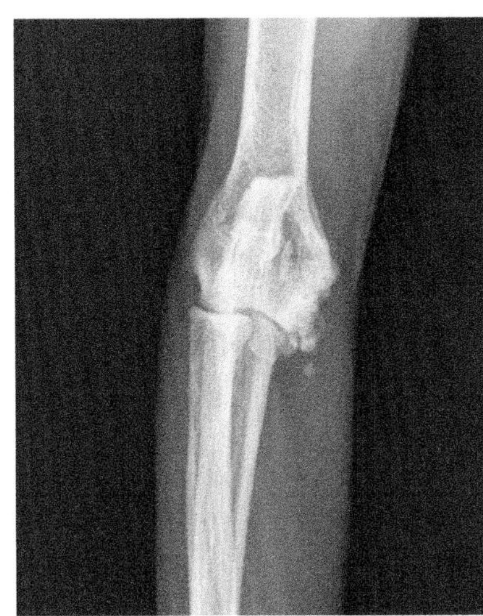

Figure 30-5 Radiographs of a 16-year-old cat with medial epicondylitis of the elbow. Several mineralized bodies are present in the area of the flexor tendons caudal and distal to the medial epicondyle, on both (**A**) the mediolateral and (**B**) craniocaudal radiograph. The medial epicondyle has a rounded and irregular appearance (**A**).

dyle, resulting in epicondylitis, insertion tendinopathy, and dystrophic calcification of the flexor muscles.

A similar condition also occurs in cats. Affected cats can be asymptomatic, or are presented with mild lameness. Pain can often be elicited by digital pressure on the flexor muscles and medial epicondyle. Radiological signs in chronic cases include foci of mineralization in the area of the attachment of the flexor muscles on the medial epicondyle or distal to it, and a rounded and irregular medial epicondyle on mediolateral radiographs (Fig. 30-5). The condition could be a sequel to traumatic avulsion, or it could be caused by repetitive strenuous activity, such as jumping down from a height. Osteoarthritis of the elbow joint can be present concurrently.

Treatment consists of surgical removal of calcified tendon and muscle tissue if the cat is lame at presentation. The humeral head of the flexor carpi ulnaris muscle seems to be affected most commonly. The tendons of the flexor muscle are in close association with the joint capsule, and care is taken during removal of the calcified tissue not to damage the joint capsule. The debrided flexor tendons are then reattached to the surrounding tendons and muscle fascia with mattress sutures. Postoperatively, a modified Robert Jones bandage is applied for 10 days. The carpal joint is immobilized in slight flexion to reduce the tension on the flexor muscles. Activity should be restricted for another 4 weeks.

30.7 Avulsion of the triceps tendon

Avulsion of the triceps tendon was recently described in two cats with a history of falls or jumps from a height (17, 18). One of the cats had histopathological evidence of a pre-existing tendinopathy prior to complete rupture (18). Chronic tendinopathy may result in radiographic changes, as shown in Figure 30-6. The authors have also seen a cat with an avulsed triceps tendon after pin and tension band wire repair of an olecranon fracture.

Diagnosis of triceps tendon avulsion is obtained by clinical signs of a dropped elbow and inability to keep the elbow extended during weight-bearing, palpation of the integrity of the tendon, radiographs to detect avulsion fractures or fragments, and possibly ultrasononography.

The triceps tendon must be reattached to the tuber olecrani to restore resistance to weight-bearing forces. One or several modified locking-loop or three-loop pulley sutures (Chapter 16) are anchored through holes drilled into the tuber olecrani. Non-absorbable monofilament or braided composite suture material is used. Postoperatively, the elbow is kept in an extended position with the help of a splinted bandage, spica splint, or transarticular external skeletal fixator (18) for around 3 weeks. Activity is restricted for another 2–3 months.

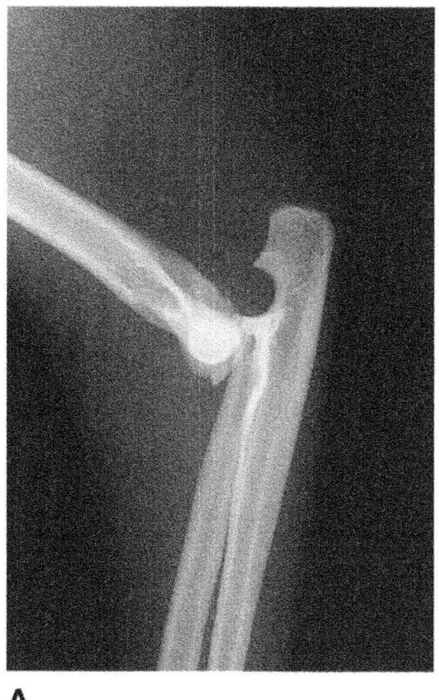
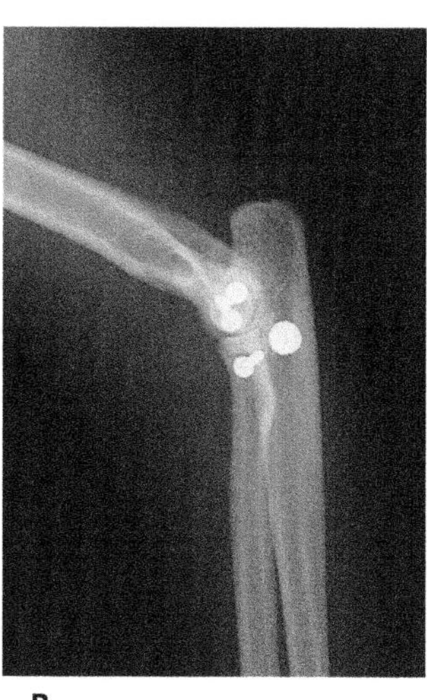

A B

Figure 30-8 (**A**) Preoperative and (**B**) postoperative mediolateral radiographs of a cat with caudal elbow luxation. Instability persisted after closed reduction. Both collateral ligaments were sutured and medial and lateral ligament prosthesis applied, using 1.5- and 2.0-mm screws and polypropylene sutures.

30.8 Elbow luxations

Traumatic luxation of the feline elbow joint can be classified into one of three types: elbow luxation with an intact radioulnar joint; luxation of the radial head, often accompanied by an ulnar fracture and then called a Monteggia lesion; and elbow luxation with concurrent disruption of the radioulnar joint, thus a combination of the first two types.

30.8.1 Elbow luxation with intact radioulnar joint

These injuries are the classical form of elbow luxation, and are characterized by an intact connection between the proximal radius and ulna. Lateral elbow luxation is most common, due to bony restriction of the prominent medial epicondyle (Fig. 30-7), but caudal luxations also occur in the feline patient (Fig. 30-8). Medial elbow luxation is exceedingly rare. The elbow is a very stable joint due to its bony anatomy. Considering the force necessary for elbow luxation to occur, the collateral ligaments are likely to be damaged in most cases. Instability of the collateral ligament support was clinically diagnosed after closed reduction of elbow luxations in 60% of cases in a study including dogs and cats (19).

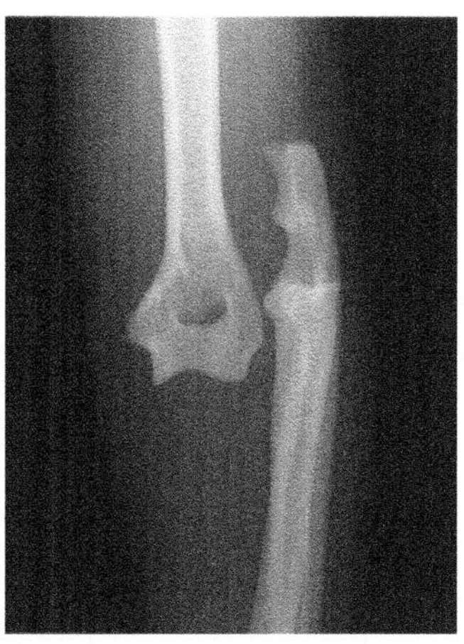
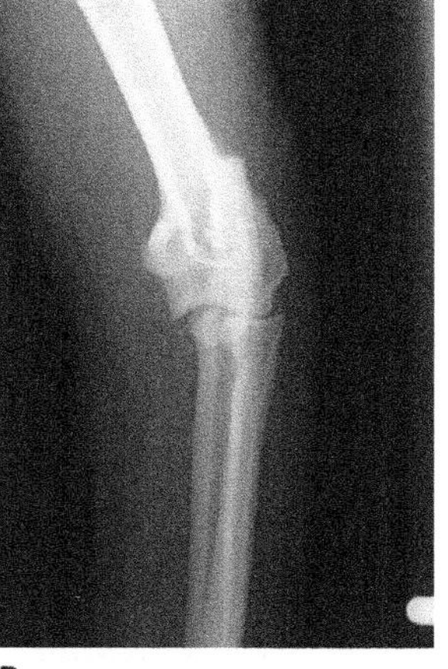

A B

Figure 30-7 Craniocaudal radiographs of a cat with lateral elbow luxation, (**A**) before and (**B**) 10 days after closed reduction. The elbow was considered stable enough for conservative treatment with a spica splint after closed reduction.

The reduction of acute elbow luxations is attempted in a closed manner (Box 30-1). A decision between conservative treatment and surgical stabilization has to be made once the joint is reduced. The decision is based on clinical elbow stability, which is evaluated by the Campbell test, as described above (Fig. 30-2). If stability is considered adequate, a spica splint is applied for 10 days (Chapter 22). The spica splint immobilizes the elbow in extension, thus reducing the risk of reluxation. Some cats do not tolerate the spica splint well. Cage rest alone, or application of a transarticular external skeletal fixator, can be used in these cats, depending on elbow stability.

Indications for surgery are elbow luxations that cannot be reduced in a closed manner, for example chronic elbow luxations, and elbow joints with marked instability after closed reduction. Surgical stabilization of the collateral ligaments reduces the risk of reluxation, and is likely to reduce instability-related degenerative joint changes. According to the anatomic course of the ligaments, the medial collateral ligament should be reconstructed from the humerus to the ulna, and the lateral collateral ligament from the humerus to the radius (Box 30-2).

Box 30-1. Closed reduction of a lateral elbow joint

Closed reduction of the elbow joint is performed under general anesthesia. The aim of the first manipulation is to bring the anconeal process back into the caudal humeral fossa while the elbow joint is held in flexion and pronation (Fig. 30-9). The anconeal process is then used as a fulcrum to reduce the radial head, while the elbow joint is gradually extended (Fig. 30-9). Considerable force may be necessary to reduce an elbow joint and care should be taken not to injure the cartilage by performing unnecessary manipulations. If closed reduction is not possible without risking damage, then open reduction should be attempted.

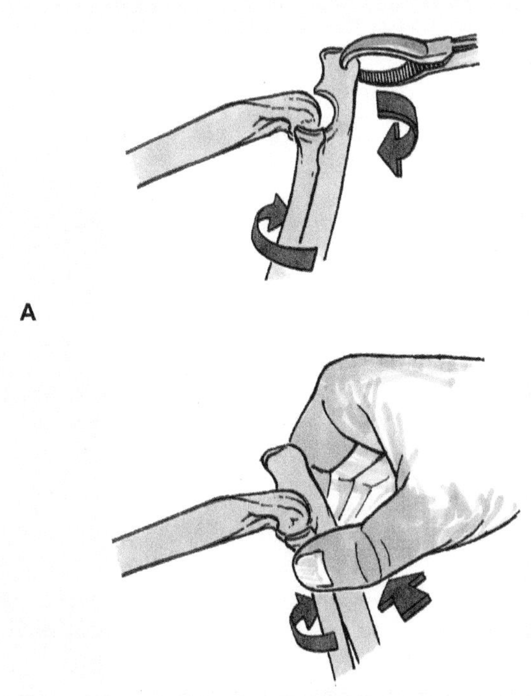

Figure 30-9 Closed reduction of a lateral elbow luxation. (**A**) The anconeal process is levered into the fossa olecrani of the humerus by digital manipulation or with the help of bone-holding forceps positioned on the olecranon, with the elbow joint held in flexion and the antebrachium in pronation. (**B**) The elbow is then slowly extended while exerting digital pressure on the radial head in a medial direction.

30.8.2 Luxation of the radial head and Monteggia lesions

Traumatic luxations of the radial head usually take place in conjunction with an ulnar fracture, but isolated luxations of the radial head also occur. The combination of luxation of the radial head and an ulnar fracture is called a Monteggia lesion. The ulna is usually fractured through its proximal diaphysis, causing separation of the radioulnar joint by disruption of the annular ligament. The injury is due to a fall in most cases and concurrent injuries are frequent (20). Monteggia lesions have been classified into four types, according to the direction of luxation of the radial head (20, 21). The radial head can luxate cranially (type I), caudally (type II), or laterally (type III). An additional fracture of the proximal radial diaphysis is present in type IV lesions. Type I injuries are most common (Fig. 30-11).

Luxations of the radial head and Monteggia lesions are always treated surgically in order to restore the weight-bearing humeroradial axis. Suturing the annular ligament as the only means of stabilization often results in reluxation of the radial head (20). A temporary positional screw is preferably placed between the proximal ulna and radius to add stability until the ligament and periarticular tissues have healed (Box 30-3). The radial neck in cats is narrow, so screw placement bears the risk for iatrogenic fracture of the bone. This risk is minimized by insertion of a 1.5-mm screw into the slightly larger radial head, close to the elbow joint. The screw is removed after approximately 4–6 weeks.

The ulnar fracture is stabilized surgically, because instability of the ulna increases load-sharing of the radius, and enhances the risk for reluxation of the radial head (Box 30-3). Simple reducible ulnar fractures can be stabilized with a caudally positioned figure-of-eight wire and/or an intramedullary pin. Application of a lateral plate provides more stability and is always indicated for comminuted fractures.

30.8.3 Elbow luxation with disruption of the radioulnar joint

Cats can sustain elbow luxation with concurrent disruption of the radioulnar joint. An ulnar fracture is present in most cases (Fig. 30-13). These injuries are similar to Monteggia lesions, but the humeroulnar joint is also luxated. Two of the anatomic differences in the ligamentous support of the elbow and proximal radius and ulna may predispose cats to this type of injury. First, the annular ligament has an attachment to the lateral humeral condyle together with the lateral collateral ligament, which may result in simultaneous damage to both the annular and the lateral collateral ligaments. Secondly, cats lack the strong interosseus ligament between the radius and ulna (5), resulting in a weaker connection between the radial and ulnar diaphyses.

Meticulous reconstruction of all ruptured ligaments is necessary to achieve correct reduction and adequate stability of these highly unstable joints (Fig. 30-13). The elbow is first approached by a lateral intermuscular approach. The humeroulnar joint is reduced, followed by reduction of the radial head. The injury is then treated like a Monteggia lesion as described above, including suturing of the annular ligament,

Box 30-2. Open reduction of lateral elbow luxation with ligament reconstruction

A lateral approach is performed for open joint reduction and for application of a lateral ligament prosthesis. A medial approach is used for a medial ligament prosthesis. A bilateral approach is needed to reconstruct both the medial and lateral collateral ligaments.

Open reduction: Open reduction is performed on the flexed joint with the help of Metzenbaum scissors or mosquito forceps inserted from laterally. The instrument is placed in the intracondylar area to open the joint. It is then twisted round and used as a fulcrum to reduce the joint. The manipulations are performed carefully to prevent additional damage to the cartilage.

Lateral collateral ligament prosthesis: The ligaments are sutured if possible. A 1.5-mm screw is inserted into the lateral humeral epicondyle, and another one into the radial head (Fig. 30-10A). A figure-of-eight non-absorbable suture is anchored around the screw heads. An additional suture prosthesis can be applied between the screw in the humeral epicondyle and another screw in the proximal ulna in cases with a tendency to luxate caudally.

Medial collateral ligament prosthesis: The medial collateral ligament is nearly always damaged with lateral elbow luxations, and is usually explored and treated first. Torn ligaments are sutured if possible. Because the larger part of the medial collateral ligament inserts on the medial coronoid process of the ulna, one 1.5-mm screw is inserted into the medial humeral epicondyle, and one into the proximal ulna (Fig. 30-10B). Non-absorbable suture material is anchored around the screws in a figure-of-eight fashion.

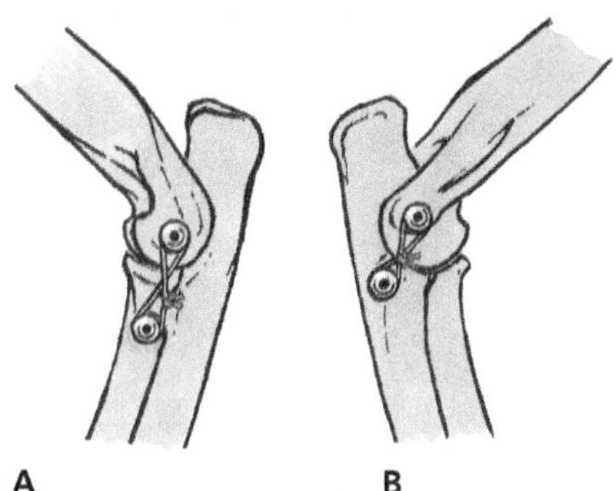

Figure 30-10 Positioning of the screws for collateral ligament prostheses.
(**A**) Ligament prosthesis of the lateral collateral ligament: the figure-of-eight suture anchored around the screws mimics the radial part of the lateral collateral ligament.
(**B**) Ligament prosthesis of the medial collateral ligament: the figure-of-eight suture anchored around the screws mimics the ulnar part of the medial collateral ligament.

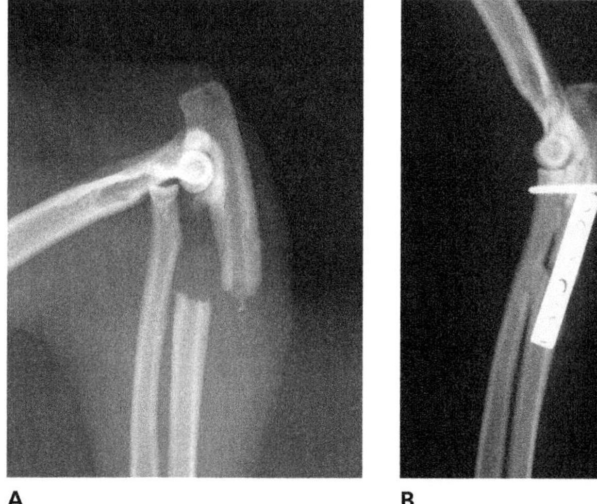
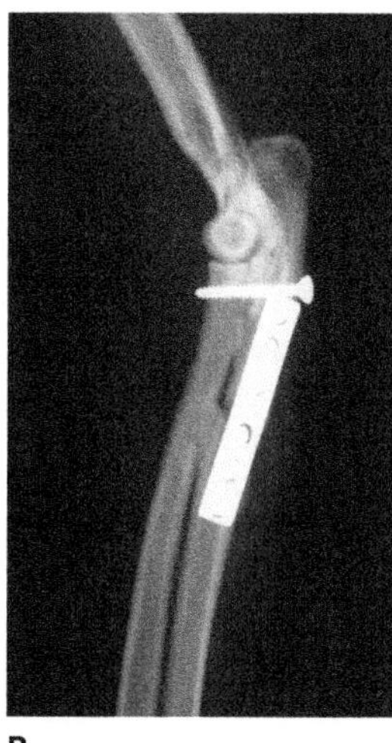
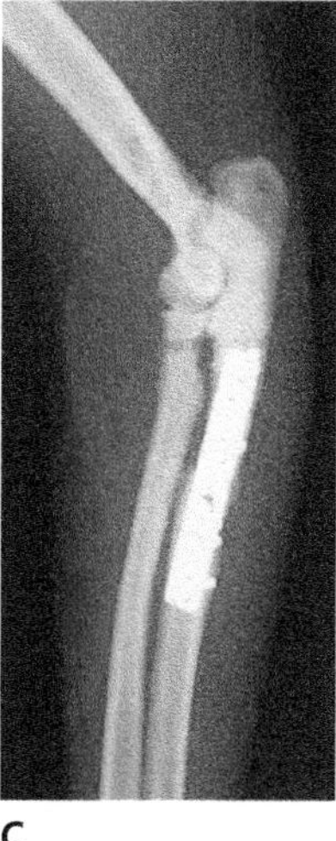

Figure 30-11 (**A**) Preoperative, (**B**) postoperative, and (**C**) follow-up radiographs of a cat with a type I Monteggia lesion.
(**A**) The radial head is luxated cranially, the proximal ulnar diaphysis is fractured, and the radioulnar joint is separated.
(**B**) A 1.5-mm positional screw was placed from the ulna into the radial head, and the ulnar fracture was stabilized with a laterally applied 1.5-mm miniplate.
(**C**) Radiographs after removal of the positional screw 1 month postoperatively. The elbow joint is congruent and the ulnar fracture has nearly healed.

Box 30-3. Internal fixation of Monteggia lesions

The skin incision is performed caudolaterally over the proximal ulna. An intermuscular lateral approach to the elbow joint is used to reach the radial head. The ulnar fracture and the radial head are reduced. A pair of pointed bone reduction forceps can be placed very carefully across the radial head and the proximal ulna to help maintain reduction. Care is taken to achieve a functional pronation and supination position for the antebrachium. A 1.5-mm positional screw is then inserted from the caudal aspect of the ulna into the center of the radial head, as close to the elbow joint as possible (Fig. 30-12). The repair of the ulnar fracture should provide axial stability. Simple ulnar fractures may be repaired with a caudally placed figure-of-eight tension band wire (Fig. 30-12) and/or an intramedullary pin. Comminuted fractures are stabilized with a laterally applied 1.5- or 2.0-mm plate. The annular ligament is identified and sutured if possible.

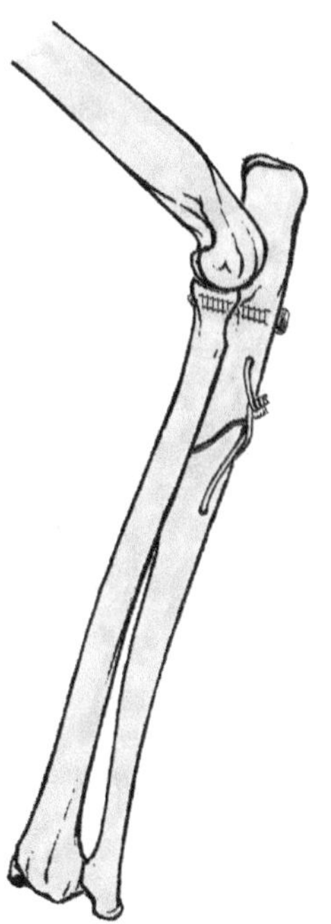

Figure 30-12 Stabilization of a Monteggia lesion. A 1.5-mm positional screw is inserted from the ulna across the radioulnar joint into the radial head. A simple ulnar fracture can be repaired with a caudally applied figure-of-eight wire.

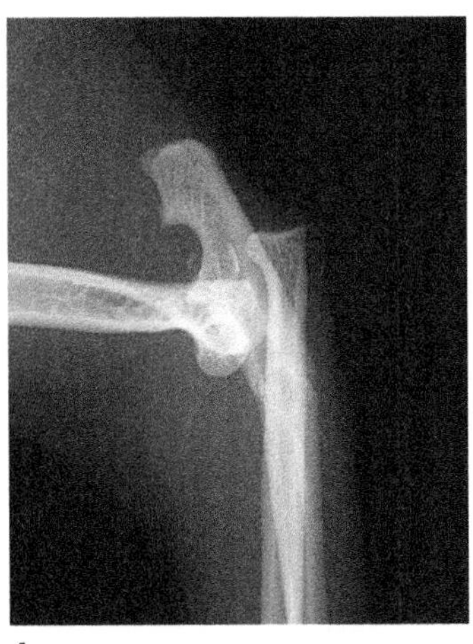

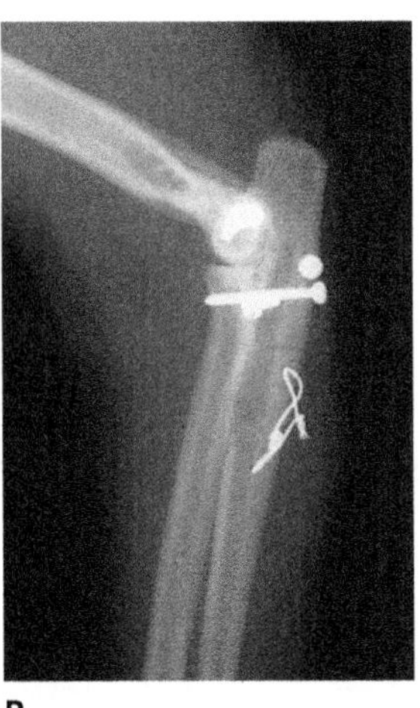

A B

Figure 30-13 (**A**) Preoperative and (**B**) postoperative mediolateral radiographs of a cat with elbow luxation and concurrent Monteggia lesion. Both the humerulnar joint and the radioulnar joint are disrupted and the proximal ulna is fractured. Surgery consisted of reduction of the joints, stabilization of the radioulnar joint with a positional screw, and repair of the ulna with a caudally applied figure-of-eight wire. Lateral and medial collateral ligament prostheses were additionally applied.

insertion of a positional screw between the ulna and radial head, and repair of the ulna fracture. The lateral collateral ligament is sutured and a lateral ligament prosthesis is applied. Finally, a medial intermuscular approach to the elbow joint is conducted to repair the medial collateral ligament.

30.9 Fractures of the elbow joint

The most common fractures involving the elbow joint are distal humeral fractures, followed by fractures of the olecranon. These are described in Chapters 29 and 31.

Fractures of the medial epicondylar crest are sometimes observed as a cause of lameness. They are likely to be avulsion fractures of the origin of the antebrachial flexor tendons (Fig. 30-14). Chronic medial epicondylitis and lameness can develop if these lesions are left untreated (see above). Because the avulsed fragment is too small to be reattached, the condition is treated conservatively if not associated with severe or ongoing clinical symptoms, or the fragment is removed using a medial approach and the avulsed flexor tendons are sutured to the surrounding tissue.

The authors have seen one cat with a traumatic fracture of the anconeal process, resulting in lameness (Fig. 30-15). As the anconeal fragment was too small to be reattached, it was excised using a caudolateral approach to the elbow joint. Lameness resolved after excision of the fragment.

30.10 Arthrodesis of the elbow joint

Arthrodesis of the elbow joint is a salvage procedure for the treatment of disabling elbow joint conditions, such as severely comminuted joint fractures, articular gunshot wounds, mal-

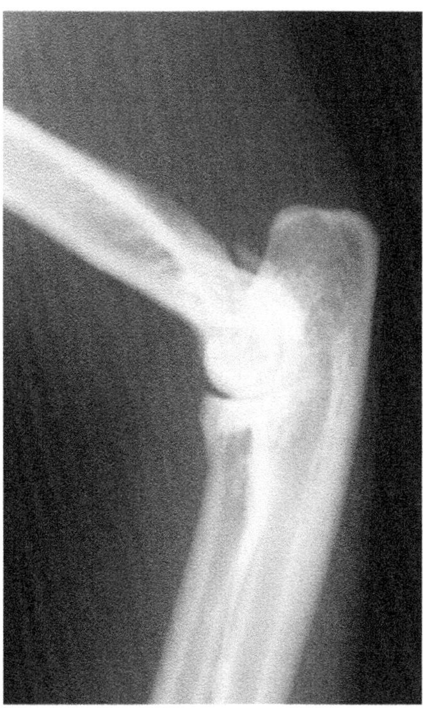

Figure 30-14 Mediolateral radiograph of a cat with an acute lameness of unknown origin. A fracture fragment is visible at the origin of the flexor tendons at the caudal aspect of the medial epicondyle. Untreated, it may lead to medial epicondylitis.

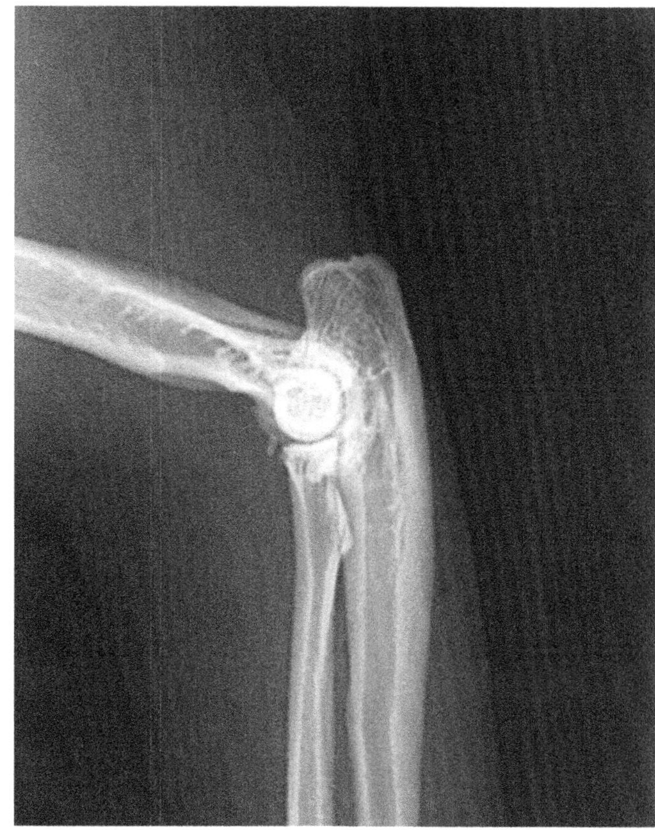

Figure 30-15 Mediolateral radiograph showing traumatic fracture of the anconeal process. The cat was presented with a moderate-grade lameness and pain could be elicited on extension of the elbow joint. Removal of the fragment resulted in resolution of clinical signs.

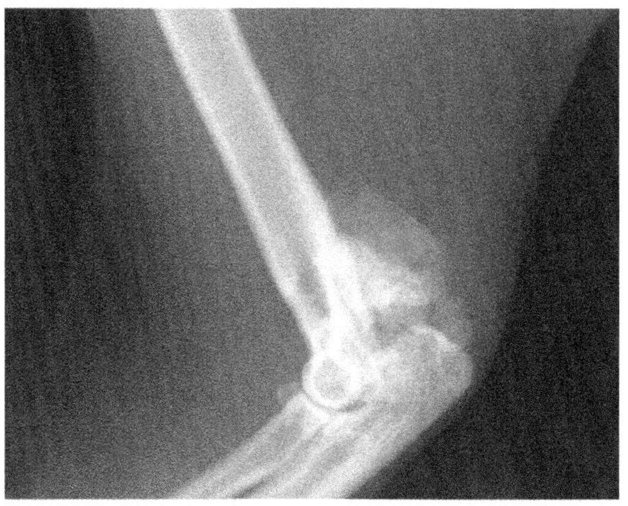

A

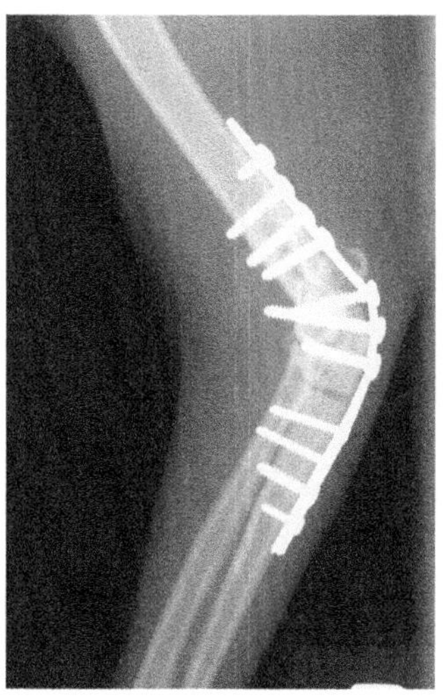

B

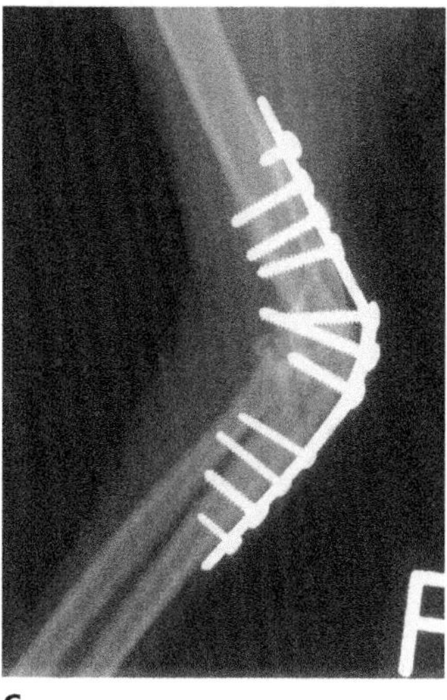

C

Figure 30-16 Example of an elbow arthrodesis.
(**A**) The 5-year-old cat was presented with forelimb lameness and elbow pain. Periarticular soft-tissue calcification is seen in the area of insertion of the triceps muscle. Histologically, the lesion was classified as localized ossifying myositis, Resection was attempted but the lesion recurred 11 months later with accompanying pain and lameness.
(**B**) An arthrodesis of the elbow joint was performed, using a 1.5/2.0-mm veterinary cuttable plate. 1.5-mm screws were used in the ulna, one of which stripped so the hole was left empty.
(**C**) Three-week postoperative radiographs taken when the spica splint was removed; progress is satisfactory.

Box 30-4. Arthrodesis of the elbow joint

A lateral approach to the elbow joint is performed and the olecranon process is osteotomized. The proximal ulna must be prepared on the caudal aspect to create a smooth surface for the plate to lie on (Fig. 30-17A). It can be contoured with rongeurs, an osteotome, an oscillating saw, or bur. The articular cartilage of the humeroradial and humeroulnar contact surfaces is completely removed with a bur. The joint is temporarily stabilized in 135° with a transarticular pin, and limb alignment in valgus and varus and internal and outward rotation is checked. A long 2.0-mm dynamic compression plate or a 2.0/2.7-mm veterinary cuttable plate is contoured to the caudal surface of the humerus and ulna. The first screw is inserted through the distal humerus into the radial head. The second screw is inserted from the proximal ulna into the humeral condyle. The third screw is placed through the ulna and the radial head (Fig. 30-17B). The screw holes proximally and distally are filled. Monocortical screws in the most proximal and distal plate holes can help decrease the stress riser effect. Copious bone graft is applied into and around the joint surfaces. The osteotomized olecranon process is reattached to the medial epicondyle with a lag screw or a tension band repair (Fig. 30-17C).

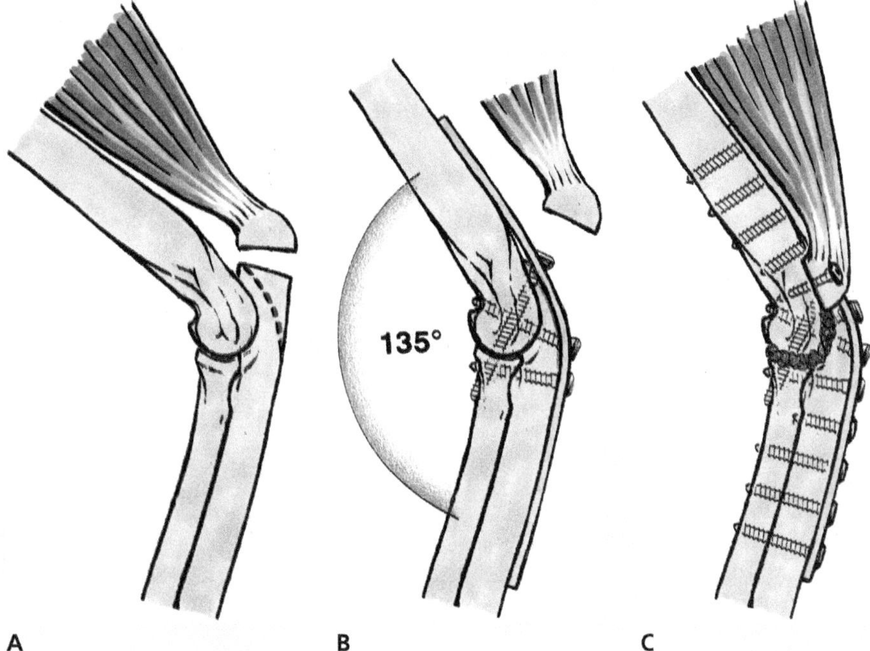

Figure 30-17 Diagrams showing the different steps of an elbow arthrodesis. (**A**) The olecranon process is osteotomized, and the proximal ulnar surface has been contoured to allow plate application.
(**B**) The joint is stabilized in an 135° angle with a Kirschner wire, and the plate is secured to the caudal surface with one screw through the humerus and radial head, one screw through the ulna and humeral condyle, and one screw through the ulna and radial head.
(**C**) All plate holes are filled with screws, and the olecranon process is attached to the medial humeral epicondyle with a lag screw.

unions of articular elbow fractures, chronic traumatic luxations, congenital elbow luxation, and also periarticular diseases resulting in loss of elbow function (Fig. 30-16, Box 30-4). Arthrodesis is only performed if pain does not resolve and joint function cannot be restored by other means.

Arthrodesis of the elbow has been described in three cats (22). It was performed with plate fixation in two cats, and with external skeletal fixation in the third cat. One of the cats with plate arthrodesis sustained a fracture of the radius and ulna just distal to the end of the plate. Functional outcome in the other two was good to moderate. The less than ideal function in one cat was attributed to a too-extended joint angle (22). The best functional outcome was achieved with a joint angle of 135° (22).

30.11 Postoperative treatment and prognosis

30.11.1 Elbow luxations

Postoperative radiographs are performed to evaluate joint congruity and position of the screws. A spica splint can be applied for 10 days after lateral elbow luxation to reduce the risk of reluxation. The spica splint holds the elbow in extension, which causes the anconeal process to remain in the humeral fossa, and helps to prevent reluxation. Some cats do not tolerate the spica splint well, and cage rest alone may be more appropriate for these cats after stable surgical repair. Cats with Monteggia lesions should have their elbows stabilized in moderate flexion with a splinted bandage for 10 days, because overextension of the elbow would facilitate cranial luxation of the radial head. Positional screws between the radius and ulna are removed after 4–6 weeks to allow a return of supination and pronation, which are important for normal gait and limb function in cats.

Prognosis for return to function after luxation of the elbow is good with appropriate treatment, although reduction in range of motion and osteoarthritis are likely to occur (20). Complications are reluxation after inadequate stabilization, iatrogenic fractures through the radial neck caused by positional screws between the radius and ulna, or screw breakage, and osteoarthritis.

30.11.2 Elbow arthrodesis

Cats with arthrodesis of the elbow joint need external support for around 4 weeks. A splinted spica bandage should be applied, reaching as proximally as possible. The carpal joint can be immobilized in slight flexion, which will prevent weight-bearing. Initial follow-up radiographs are performed after 6 weeks.

Elbow arthrodesis is considered to result in less than ideal function in dogs by some authors (23). Clinical experience with elbow arthrodesis in cats is scarce, but it appears to be a technique with a high potential for complications and failures. Described complications include fracture of the radius and ulna, and suboptimal limb function (22). Amputation of the limb is a viable alternative after failed arthrodesis of the elbow joint.

References and further reading

1. Hardie EM, et al. Radiographic evidence of degenerative joint disease in geriatric cats: 100 cases (1994–1997). J Am Vet Med Assoc 2002;220:628–632.
2. Godfrey DR. Osteoarthritis in cats: a prospective series of 40 cases. Proceedings of the BSAVA Meeting 2003; Birmingham, UK. J Small Anim Pract 2003:418.
3. Clarke SP, Bennet D. Feline osteoarthritis: a prospective study of 28 cases. J Small Anim Pract 2006;47:439–445.
4. Vollmerhaus B, et al. Anatomic fundamentals and species-specific movements of the elbow joint and proximal radioulnar joint of domestic cats. Tierarztl Prax 1993;21:163–171.
5. Frewein J, Vollmerhaus B. Anatomie von Hund und Katze. Berlin: Blackwell; 1994.
6. Wood A, et al. Anatomic and radiographic appearance of a sesamoid bone in the tendon of origin of the supinator muscle of the cat. Am J Vet Res 1995;56:736–739.
7. Piermattei DL, Johnson KA. Surgical approaches to the bones and joints of the dog and cat, 4th edn. Philadelphia: WB Saunders; 2004.
8. Staiger BA, Beale BS. Use of arthroscopy for debridement of the elbow joint in cats. J Am Vet Med Assoc 2005;226:401–403.
9. Valastro C, et al. Congenital elbow subluxation in a cat. Vet Radiol Ultrasound 2005;46:63–64.
10. Rossi F, et al. Bilateral elbow malformation in a cat caused by radio-ulnar synostosis. Vet Radiol Ultrasound 2003;44:283–286.
11. Cleary JE, Omer GE Jr. Congenital proximal radio-ulnar synostosis. Natural history and functional assessment. J Bone Joint Surg 1985;67:539–545.
12. Prymak C, Goldschmidt MH. Synovial cysts in five dogs and one cat. J Am Anim Hosp Assoc 1991;27:151–154.
13. Stead AC, et al. Synovial cysts in cats. J Small Anim Pract 1995;36:450–454.
14. White JD, et al. What is your diagnosis? J Feline Med Surg 2004;6:339–344.
15. Zontine WJ, et al. Redefined type of elbow dysplasia involving calcified flexor tendons attached to the medial humeral epicondyle in three dogs. J Am Vet Med Assoc 1989;194:1082–1085.
16. Meyer-Lindenberg A, et al. Vorkommen und Behandlung von knöchernen Metaplasien in den am medialen Epikondylus des Humerus entspringenden Beugesehnen beim Hund. Tierarztl Prax 2004;32:276–285.
17. Liehmann L, Lorinson D. Traumatic triceps tendon avulsion in a cat. J Small Anim Pract 2005;47:94–97.
18. Clarke SP, et al. Avulsion of the triceps tendon insertion in a cat. Vet Comp Orthop Traumatol 2007;20:245–270.
19. Savoldelli DM, et al. Traumatic elbow luxation in the dog and the cat: perioperative findings. Schweiz Arch Tierheilkd 1996;138:387–391.
20. Schwarz PD, Schrader SC. Ulnar fracture and dislocation of the proximal radial epiphysis (Monteggia lesion) in the dog and cat: a review of 28 cases. J Am Vet Med Assoc 1984;185:190–194.
21. Bado J. The Monteggia lesion. Springfield, IL: Charles C Thomas; 1962.
22. Moak PC, et al. Arthrodesis of the elbow in three cats. Vet Comp Orthop Traumatol 2000;13:149–153.
23. Piermattei DL, Flo GL. The elbow joint. In: Piermattei DL, Flo GL (eds) Small animal orthopedics and fracture repair. Philadelphia: WB Saunders; 1997: pp. 288–320.

31 Radius and ulna

K. Voss, S.J. Langley-Hobbs, P.M. Montavon

Fractures of the radius and ulna often occur after a fall from a height, and are therefore more commonly encountered in urban areas (1, 2). The paired bones are usually fractured simultaneously. Stabilization of the radius alone is sufficient in many cases, but fixation stability can be enhanced by additional stabilization of the ulna, especially in proximal fractures. Range of motion in pronation and supination is greater in cats than in dogs and is essential for normal gait and grooming activities. Care should be taken to maintain pronation and supination, and to avoid formation of a synostosis between the radius and ulna, by correct implant positioning and adequate fracture reduction.

31.1 Surgical anatomy

The radius is a slender bone, with the radial neck being the narrowest area. Its small diameter can make it difficult to insert implants. Although the radius carries most of the weight through its articulation with the lateral portion of the humeral condyle proximally and the radial carpal bone distally, the ulna is thicker than the radius in cats (3). The radius and ulna twist around each other, the radius being located craniolateral to the ulna proximally, and medial to the ulna distally.

The radius and ulna are connected to each other by an interosseus membrane, but the strong interosseus ligament present in dogs is lacking (4). This could possibly contribute to the pronounced supination and pronation in cats. Pronation and supination motion also derives from the proximal and distal radioulnar joints. These small synovial joints allow the radius and ulna to rotate around each other.

The olecranon process of cats is relatively smaller than in the dog, and its caudal surface curves cranially, whereas in the dog it curves caudally. The caudal ulna surface in the cat also differs from the dog (5) in that its surface is convex from proximal to the midshaft, and then concave distally. These differences should be taken into account when repairing fractures in this area.

Another anatomic difference between dogs and cats is the shape of the distal ulnar growth plate. Whereas the distal ulnar physis is cone-shaped in dogs, it is straight in cats (4), This anatomic difference might account for the low incidence of antebrachial growth deformities in this species.

31.2 Stabilization techniques

Radius and ulnar fractures can be treated with external coaptation, external skeletal fixation, and plating. Casts can be used to stabilize greenstick and simple transverse diaphyseal fractures of both the radius and ulna, or fractures of either radius or ulna, when the other bone is intact. The radius is not amenable to intramedullary pinning, because the pin would have to be inserted through the articular cartilage of the radiocarpal joint. Intramedullary pins can be used to stabilize fractures of the ulna.

In diaphyseal fractures of the radius and ulna only the radius is stabilized in many cases, but additional stabilization of the ulna can enhance fixation stability in many instances, especially when the fracture affects the proximal antebrachium, where the cross-section of the ulna is greater than the radius, and pronation and supination movement is high. Radius and ulnar fracture types and their possible stabilization methods are summarized in Table 31-1.

31.2.1 Intramedullary pinning of the ulna

Intramedullary pinning of the ulna can be used in conjunction with external skeletal fixation or plating of the radius. It enhances bending stability, and also provides axial compression stability in cases with a simple fracture of the ulna. Intramedullary pinning of the ulna is therefore most useful in simple ulnar fractures, accompanying comminuted fractures of the radius. The intramedullary pin is either inserted normograde, starting at the proximocaudal aspect of the olecranon, just caudal to the insertion site of the triceps tendon (Fig. 31-1), or retrograde from the fracture site. Pin size is selected according to the diameter of the intramedullary cavity of the distal ulna, and on how far distally it is intended to insert the pin. A 1.0–1.4-mm pin is usually used.

31.2.2 External skeletal fixation of the radius

External skeletal fixation is indicated for comminuted or open fractures of the radial diaphysis and metaphyses. A type I or modified type I external skeletal fixator usually results in sufficient stability. Transosseous pins are inserted from medial

Table 31-1. Radius and ulnar fractures and possible treatment options

Fracture localization	Fracture type	Stabilization methods
Proximal ulna	Salter and Harris type I	Tension band repair
	Extra-articular	Tension band repair
	Intra-articular simple	Plate ± figure-of-eight wire Tension band repair
	Intra-articular comminuted	Plate ± figure-of-eight wire
Proximal radius	Salter and Harris type I	Cross pins
	Proximal metaphyseal	Plate Internal fixator ESF
Diaphysis radius and ulna	Simple transverse or short oblique	External coaptation Compression plate radius ± IM pin ulna ESF radius ± IM pin ulna Internal fixator ± IM pin ulna
	Long oblique or reducible multifragmentary	Neutralization plate radius ± IM pin ulna ESF radius ± IM pin ulna Internal fixator ± IM pin ulna
	Comminuted	ESF radius ± IM pin ulna Buttress plate radius ± IM pin ulna Buttress plates radius and ulna Internal fixator(s)
Distal radius	Simple metaphyseal fracture	ESF Plate Internal fixator
	Comminuted metaphyseal fracture	ESF Internal fixator
	Salter and Harris type I and II fractures	Cross pins
Distal ulna	Styloid process fracture	Conservative (carpal joint stable) Tension band repair (carpal joint instability)

IM, intramedullary; ESF, external skeletal fixator.

in the mid-diaphyseal and distal area of the radius to avoid irritation of the extensor muscles and tendons. In the most proximal aspect of the bone, pins impinge less soft tissue if inserted from lateral, and a curved bar can be used to connect the distal pins medially to the proximal pins laterally. A more stable type II or modified type II external skeletal fixator can be considered if prolonged fracture healing is expected, for example in older cats with severely comminuted or open fractures.

For fractures located in the distal third of the radius, the tubular external fixator is a useful implant because it allows insertion of a larger number of transosseous pins over a small distance (Chapter 24).

External skeletal fixators can be applied to the radius in a closed or open fashion. However, insertion of the transosseous pins in a mediolateral direction is difficult due to the flat shape of the radius, especially in the proximal third of the bone. A minimally invasive approach is therefore often used to visualize the bone. Pin size is restricted by the small craniocaudal diameter of the radius. Transosseous pin sizes of 1.2–1.4 mm are usually adequate in the distal third of the radius, and even smaller pins may have to be inserted into the proximal third of the radius. As positive-threaded pins are only available in sizes 1.6 mm and larger, smooth or negative-threaded pins are commonly used. Care is taken not to engage the ulna with the pins.

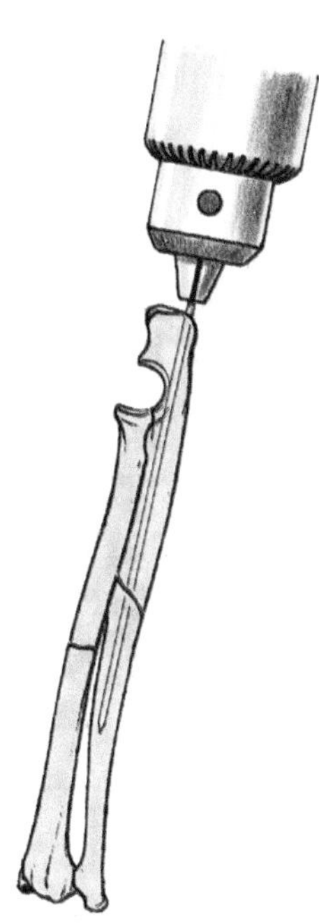

Figure 31-1 The entry site for intramedullary pinning of the ulna is located on the olecranon, just caudal to the insertion of the triceps tendon. Note the rounded form of the proximal ulna. The pin is then advanced distally. As the diameter of the medullary canal is narrowest distally, pin size dictates how far the pin can be inserted.

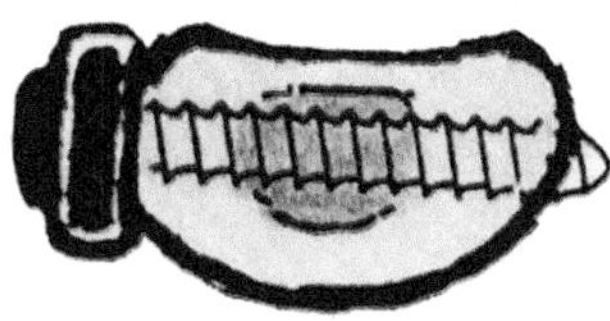

Figure 31-2 Cross-sectional area of the distal two-thirds of the radial diaphysis. Insertion of a screw in the mediolateral plane provides more bone purchase than if inserted in the craniocaudal plane.

31.2.3 Plating of radius and ulna

Plates can be positioned on the lateral, dorsal, or medial aspect of the radius, depending on fracture location. Lateral plating is rarely performed, but is an option for fractures located in the proximal radial metaphysis. Dorsal plating can be used for fractures involving the whole diaphysis of the radius. Medial plating is used for fractures located in the distal third of the radius, and has several advantages over dorsal plating in this area (6). The mediolateral plane offers more bone purchase for the screws than the dorsocaudal plane (Fig. 31-2). Smaller screws can be used in the mediolateral plane with sustained pull-out strength compared to screws placed in the craniocaudal plane (7). A medial plate is also positioned closer to the tension side of the radius, which is located caudomedially in the distal radius, and the plate has a better resistance to bending than a dorsal plate. Additionally, there is no need for lateral retraction of the extensor tendons if the plate is applied medially, thus reducing the risk of valgus malpositioning and external rotation. Complications with tendons crossing the plate are also avoided.

The 1.5/2.0-mm veterinary cuttable plate (VCP) and the 2.0-mm dynamic compression plate (DCP) are most commonly used. Screw size should not exceed the diameter of the intramedullary cavity to avoid cortical damage or iatrogenic fractures. Dorsally applied plates are generally used with 2.0-mm screws. The mediolateral plane may be too narrow to insert 2.0-mm screws in small cats, but both the 1.5/2.0-mm VCP and the 2.0-mm DCP can also be used with 1.5-mm screws for medial plating. The 1.5- and 2.0-mm screws have been shown to have a similar holding power (8).

Plate osteosynthesis is also possible to stabilize ulnar fractures located in the middle and proximal ulna. Indications for plate osteosynthesis of the ulna include intra-articular olecranon fractures, and comminuted fractures of the radius and ulna, where additional stabilization of the ulna contributes to fixation stability. Plates are best applied to the flat lateral surface of the ulnar shaft. A 1.5/2.0-mm VCP or a 2.0-mm DCP with 1.5- or 2.0-mm screws is used. Plates can be applied laterally or caudally for the repair of olecranon fractures. Lateral plating is easier and preferable in many cases because the caudal proximal ulna is thin and curved, making caudal plate contouring and screw insertion technically difficult.

31.2.4 Internal fixators

Internal fixators can be used instead of conventional plates. The main indications to use these more expensive implants are fractures close to the carpal and elbow joint, where the small fragment does not allow insertion of three screws, as needed for conventional plating. Insertion of two screws in a small fragment near a joint gives better stability when locked screws are used with an internal fixator. Plates from the 2.0-mm Unilock system (Chapter 24) are a suitable size for radial and ulnar fractures.

31.3 Fractures of the proximal radius and ulna

Fractures of the proximal radius and ulna accounted for 24% of the fractures in one survey (9). Treatment goals are anatomic reduction and rigid stabilization to restore elbow joint congruity and stability. Fractures of the proximal radius usually involve the metaphyseal area. The ulna is usually fractured concurrently when the radius is fractured, but fractures of the proximal ulna also occur in isolation. They can be classified into fractures through the olecranon physis, articular and non-articular fractures of the olecranon, and fractures of the proximal metaphysis of the ulna.

31.3.1 Approaches to the proximal radius and ulna

A lateral intermuscular approach is best performed to access the radial head and proximal metaphysis of the radius (10). The radial head is palpable under the extensor muscle group. The thinner motor branch of the radial nerve courses below the extensor carpi radialis muscle, and must be identified and spared.

For fractures involving both the proximal radial metaphysis and diaphysis, a medial approach to the shaft of the radius is extended proximally (10) to be able to apply a plate on to the dorsal aspect of the proximal radius. The medial attachment of the pronator muscle to the radius can be severed and the muscle is retracted medially. The median nerve courses below the pronator muscle and must be left intact. The supinator muscle may also have to be elevated and retracted laterally to gain exposure of the most proximal parts of the radius.

The olecranon and proximal metaphysis of the ulna are exposed by a lateral skin incision (10). Periosteal elevation of the anconeus muscle, the ulnaris lateralis muscle, and the flexor muscles on the medial side may be necessary for complete fracture exposure. Elevation of the anconeus muscle allows access to the caudolateral part of the humeroulnar joint, and is necessary for visual control of reduction of intra-articular olecranon fractures (10).

31.3.2 Fractures of the proximal radius

Fractures of the proximal third of the radius were more common in cats than fractures of the distal bone in one survey (9). True metaphyseal fractures of the proximal radius are rare; they are more commonly located in the proximal diaphysis. The proximal radial physis closes between 20–28 weeks of age (11). Salter and Harris fractures could therefore theoretically occur in cats younger than 5–6 months of age, but have not been encountered by the authors in this species.

Fractures of the proximal radius are often accompanied by ulnar fractures and/or luxations of the radial head (Chapter 30). Laterally or dorsally applied plates or internal fixators can be applied for stabilization if the proximal fragment allows insertion of a sufficient number of screws. Only 1.5–2.0-mm screws can be used due to the small diameter of the proximal radius, especially in the lateromedial direction, and meticulous technique is used to prevent iatrogenic fractures or invasion of the joint. Both the 2.0-mm DCP and the 1.5/2.0-mm VCP allow insertion of 1.5- and 2.0-mm screws. Transarticular external skeletal fixation is also possible.

Complications and revision surgeries are common with combined fractures of the proximal radius and ulna (9). Plating is associated with a higher success rate than external skeletal fixation, and the authors also recommend concurrent stabilization of the ulna in these cases (see below).

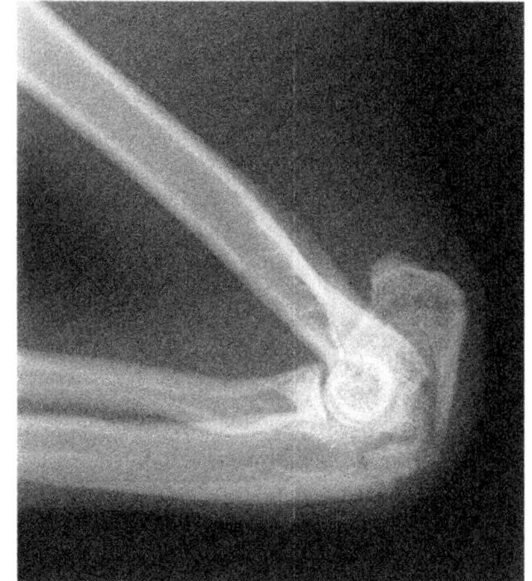

A

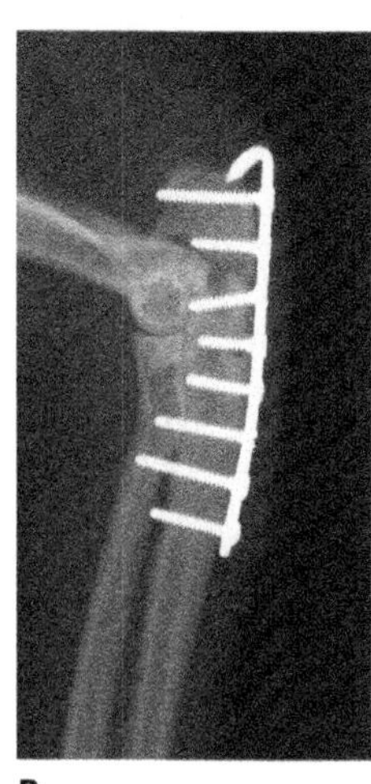

B

Figure 31-3 (**A**) Preoperative and (**B**) postoperative radiographs of a cat with an intra-articular comminuted fracture of the olecranon. The fracture was anatomically reduced and stabilized with a caudally applied 1.5/2.0-mm veterinary cuttable plate. A hook was created at the proximal plate end by cutting through a plate hole to provide additional fixation of the proximal fragment.

31.3.3 Fractures of the proximal ulna

Fractures of the proximal ulna may involve the anconeal process (Chapter 30), the olecranon, or the proximal ulnar metaphysis.

Olecranon fractures are classified into physeal, intra-articular, and extra-articular fractures. The proximal fragment is always displaced in a proximocranial direction due to the pull of the triceps muscle (Fig. 31-3). A tension band repair is required to counteract the action of the triceps muscle and to provide interfragmentary compression. Two parallel inserted Kirschner wires and a caudally applied figure-of-eight wire are usually used to stabilize physeal fractures and simple extra-articular fractures of the olecranon (Box 31-1). In dogs, the pins are directed towards the cranial cortex of the ulna distal to the trochlear notch, because pin anchorage in the cranial cortex of the ulna improves stability compared to leaving them free in the medullary canal. The shape of the proximal ulna in cats makes angling the pins in this direction difficult, and most pins are inserted as intramedullary pins. Tension band wiring of olecranon fractures has been associated with a high complication rate in one survey (9). Careful care in selection and obeying the correct principles for application can improve success (Chapter 24).

Plate osteosynthesis is preferred for intra-articular fractures of the olecranon. The 1.5/2.0-mm VCP or a 2.0-mm DCP

Box 31-1. Stabilization of fractures of the olecranon

A caudolateral approach to the olecranon is performed. Accurate reduction of the joint surface of the ulnar notch can be checked by elevating the anconeus muscle to gain access to the caudolateral aspect of the elbow joint.

Tension band repair: The tension band fixation is used for physeal fractures and simple extra-articular fractures. Two parallel 0.8–1.2-mm Kirschner wires are inserted from caudolateral and caudomedial to the insertion site of the triceps tendon into a distal direction down the intramedullary canal. One hole is drilled through the ulnar metaphysis distal to the fracture, and one through the olecranon, passing cranial to the Kirschner wires. A piece of 0.6–0.8-mm orthopedic wire is placed through these holes in a figure-of-eight fashion (Fig. 31-4A). Alternatively, the figure-of-eight wire can be anchored around the pin ends proximally, but care is taken not to strangulate the insertion of the triceps tendon.

Plating: Plate osteosynthesis is the method of choice for intra-articular and comminuted fractures. The plate is applied to the lateral (Fig. 31-4B) or caudal (Fig. 31-4C) surface of the olecranon and proximal ulna. At least two 1.5- or 2.0-mm screws must be inserted into the proximal fragment. Slight overbending of the plate across the fracture site is necessary to avoid opening of the fracture at the articular surface for caudal plating. Lateral plating is preferred for comminuted fractures. A caudal figure-of-eight wire can be placed additionally to enhance resistance to tension.

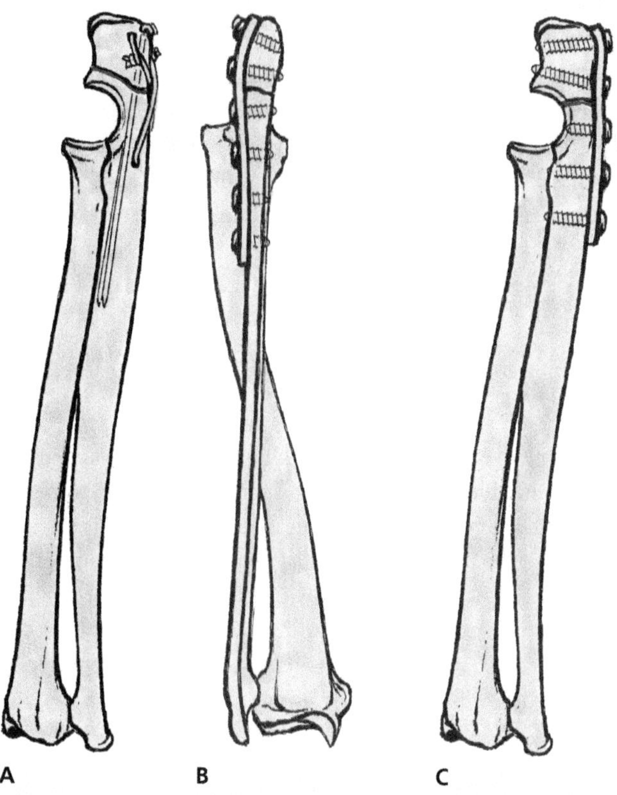

Figure 31-4 Tension band fixation of fractures of the olecranon. (**A**) A simple extra-articular fracture of the olecranon, stabilized with a tension band using two parallel Kirschner wires and a caudal figure-of-eight wire. (**B**) An intra-articular fracture of the olecranon repaired with a lateral plate. (**C**) A simple intra-articular fracture of the olecranon, repaired with a caudal plate in tension band function.

can be applied to the lateral or caudal surface of the olecranon (Box 31-1). Plates applied to the caudal surface have the better tension band effect. A hook plate can be created to achieve additional holding power (Fig. 31-3) (12). Plates applied to the lateral surface have a larger moment of inertia and provide better resistance to bending forces. Lateral plating is therefore preferred for comminuted fractures of the olecranon.

Proximal metaphyseal fractures of the ulna are located distal to the annular ligament, and are often associated with fractures of the proximal radius, or with luxation of the radial head. The latter is called a Monteggia lesion and is described in Chapter 30. Isolated fractures of the proximal ulna distal to the elbow joint are rare. These fractures should be stabilized because the pull of the triceps muscle results in twisting of the proximal fragment and opening of the fracture site caudally. This carries the risk of a delayed or non-union if the fracture is left untreated. Intramedullary pins, figure-of-eight wires, or a lateral plate can be used to stabilize these fractures.

31.4 Diaphyseal fractures of the radius and ulna

Many of the diaphyseal fractures of the radius and ulna are simple transverse fractures, but small fracture fragments or fissure lines are often present. The fractures usually involve the middle third of the diaphyses (9). Treatment options in general include conservative treatment with a cast, plate osteosynthesis, and external skeletal fixation. Intramedullary pinning is not performed in the radius, but can be used in the ulna.

It is often sufficient to stabilize the radius alone, but additional fixation of the ulna should be considered in some cases, especially in mid-diaphyseal and proximal physeal fractures. Additional stabilization of the ulna is advantageous in fractures where healing is expected to be long. For example, in comminuted fractures in older cats, and where fixation stability of the radius alone is critical, it also aids reduction of the radial fracture when the ulnar fracture is simple. Stabilization of both radius and ulna is also considered in heavy cats or if immediate weight-bearing is expected due to concurrent injuries to other limbs. It is easiest to stabilize the bone with less fracture comminution first to achieve fracture alignment.

Pronation and supination movement is crucial for a normal feline gait and activity, and must be preserved by avoiding inadvertent insertion of screws or pins from the radius into the ulna, by inserting short screws or pins, and by correct fracture alignment. Pronation and supination are checked both with the elbow in extension and in flexion. The paw is normally held in supination, which is more pronounced when the elbow is flexed, compared to when it is extended.

31.4.1 Approaches to the radial and ulnar diaphyses

A medial approach to the radial shaft is performed to repair fractures of the radial diaphysis (10). Application of the plate to the proximal bone when using a dorsal plate requires elevation and medial retraction of the pronator muscle. The median nerve courses below the pronator muscle and must be spared. The ulna is approached via a caudolateral incision directly over the bone.

31.4.2 Simple transverse and short oblique fractures

Simple transverse or short oblique fractures of the radius can generally be treated conservatively or surgically. Good indications for conservative treatment with a cast are greenstick fractures in immature cats, reducible fractures in young cats (Fig. 31-5), and those rare cases where only the radial or the ulnar shaft is broken. The technique for cast application is described in Chapter 22.

Surgical stabilization is indicated if closed reduction is not possible, if the fracture fragments are grossly unstable after reduction, and if fracture healing is expected to take longer

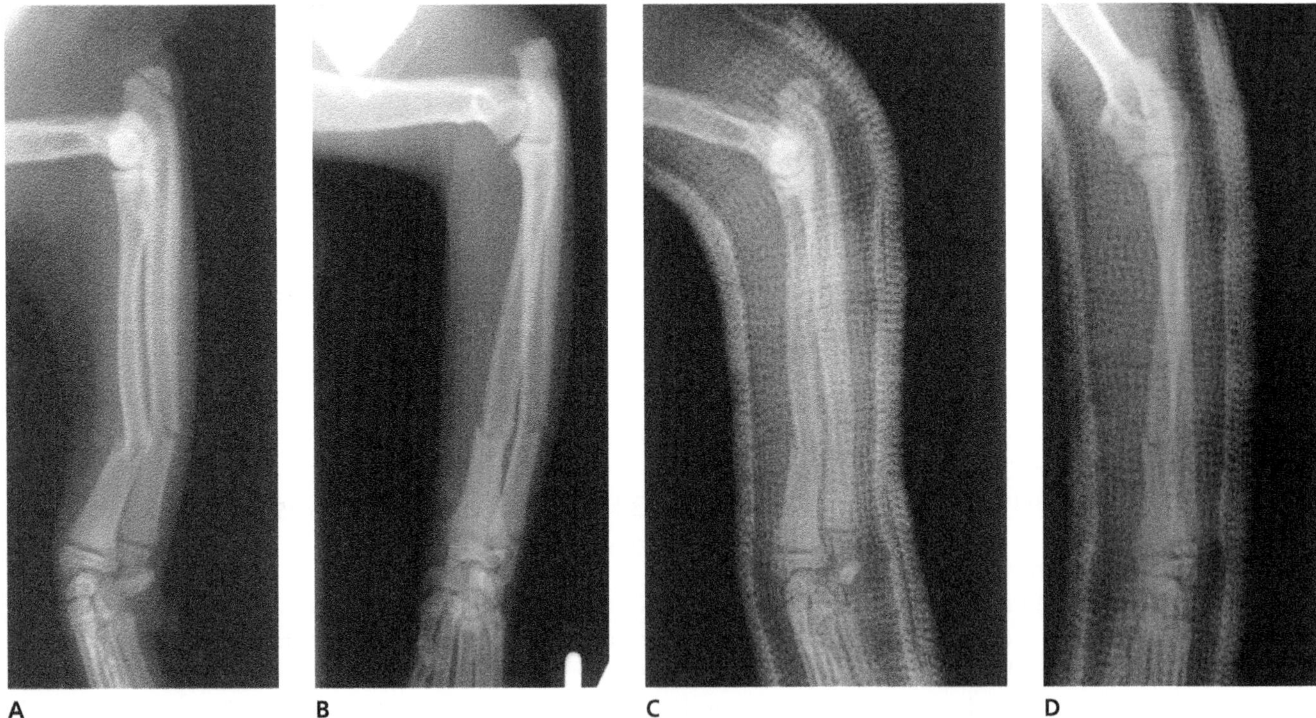

Figure 31-5 (**A**, **B**) A minimally displaced simple transverse fracture of the distal third of the radial and ulnar diaphysis in a 4-month-old cat, (**C**, **D**) treated with a cast.

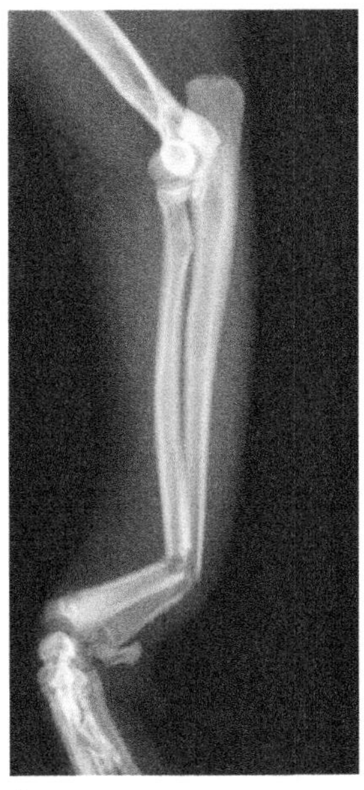

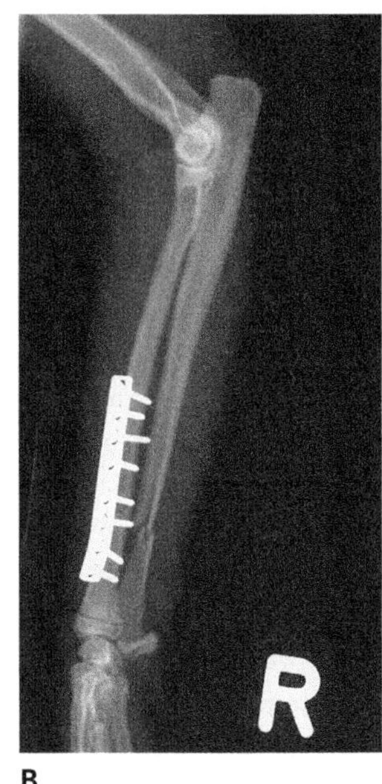

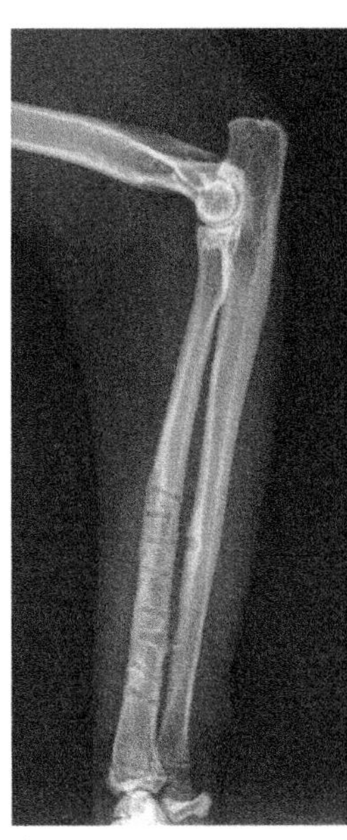

Figure 31-6 (**A**) Preoperative, (**B**) postoperative, and (**C**) follow-up radiographs at 4 months of a 1-year-old cat with a distal diaphyseal radius and ulnar fracture. A 2.0-mm dynamic compression plate with 1.5-mm screws was applied to the medial aspect of the radius, and uncomplicated fracture healing resulted.

than 4–6 weeks in mature cats. Internal stabilization can also be justified in fractures theoretically amenable to closed reduction and external coaptation, because it allows a faster return to function, requires less frequent follow-up examinations, and reduces the potential risks of cast-associated complications, such as pressure sores, loss of reduction, and joint fibrosis.

Both plates and external skeletal fixation can be used to treat simple or short oblique fractures of the radius. Plates are usually applied medially (Fig. 31-6) or dorsally, depending on fracture localization (Box 31-2). Lateral plating can also be used for fractures located very proximal in the radial diaphysis, because the lateral approach is least invasive here. A medially applied type I external skeletal fixator is usually used for simple fractures. Pin insertion is easier distally compared to proximally, because of the lack of soft tissues overlying the distal radius. The tubular external skeletal fixator is ideal due to its low weight, absence of bulky clamps, and the possibility of inserting a large number of transosseous pins over a small distance (Fig. 31-8).

Additional stabilization of the ulna enhances fixation stability, and may be performed in selected cases (Fig. 31-9). Simple fractures of the ulnar diaphysis can be easily stabilized with an intramedullary pin, or a laterally applied plate.

31.4.3 Long oblique and multifragmentary reducible fractures

Long oblique and multifragmentary reducible fractures are rarely encountered in the radius. Application of a lag screw and a neutralization plate, application of a buttress plate, or external skeletal fixation could theoretically be used.

Long oblique fractures are occasionally seen in the ulna. Anatomic reduction and stable fixation of the ulna fracture can enhance overall fixation stability, especially in the presence of a comminuted fracture of the radius. Possible fixation choices for long oblique ulna fractures include intramedullary pinning, lag screw fixation, and lateral plating.

31.4.4 Comminuted fractures

Comminuted fractures of the radial and ulnar diaphyses are always stabilized surgically with a plate or an external skeletal fixator (Box 31-3). Internal stabilization of both the radius and the ulna is advisable (Fig. 31-8), because the 2.0-mm DCP and the 1.5/2.0-mm VCP may be too short, or too weak, respectively, to provide sufficient stability if applied in buttress function.

Dorsal plating is chosen for radial fractures extending into the proximal to middle third of the diaphysis, whereas medial plating is preferred for fractures located in the middle to distal radial diaphysis. Dorsal plating carries the risk of stabilizing the fracture in external rotation and/or valgus, because the extensor tendons have to be retracted laterally to be able to apply the plate. Closed fracture reduction followed by external skeletal fixation is technically difficult in cats. Interdigitation of ulnar fragments may render closed reduction difficult, and insertion of transosseous pins into the narrow radial shaft is problematic without visual control,

Box 31-2. Stabilization of simple transverse or short oblique fractures of the radial and ulnar diaphysis

A medial approach is performed to reach the radial diaphysis for open fracture reduction and plate application. If the fracture is located in the proximal radial diaphysis, a lateral approach is used.

External skeletal fixation: A type I external skeletal fixator is applied medially after closed or open fracture reduction for fractures located in the distal half of the radial diaphysis (Fig. 31-7A). At least three transosseous pins with a diameter of 1.2–1.6 mm are inserted per fragment. Alternatively, a modified type I external fixator with an acrylic bar can be used for fractures located in the proximal half of the diaphysis, because proximally it is easier to insert the transosseus pins from laterally (Fig. 31-7B).

Dorsal plating: Dorsal plating is used for fractures located in the proximal half of the radius. The pronator muscle has to be elevated and retracted medially. The plate is contoured to the dorsal radial surface and is secured using at least three 2.0-mm screws proximally and distally. A 1.0–1.4-mm intramedullary pin can be inserted into the ulna to enhance fixation stability (Fig. 31-7C).

Medial plating: The plate is applied to the medial surface of the radius for fractures located in the distal half of the radius (Fig. 31-7D). The plates have to be contoured along the medial epiphysis distally, and care is taken not to insert the most distal screw into the radiocarpal joint: 2.0-mm screws can be used in the distal metaphysis, but 1.5-mm screws are preferred in the narrow diaphysis. This is possible with both the 1.5/2.0-mm veterinary cuttable plate and the 2.0-mm dynamic compression plate. An intramedullary pin can be inserted into the ulna if deemed necessary for fixation stability.

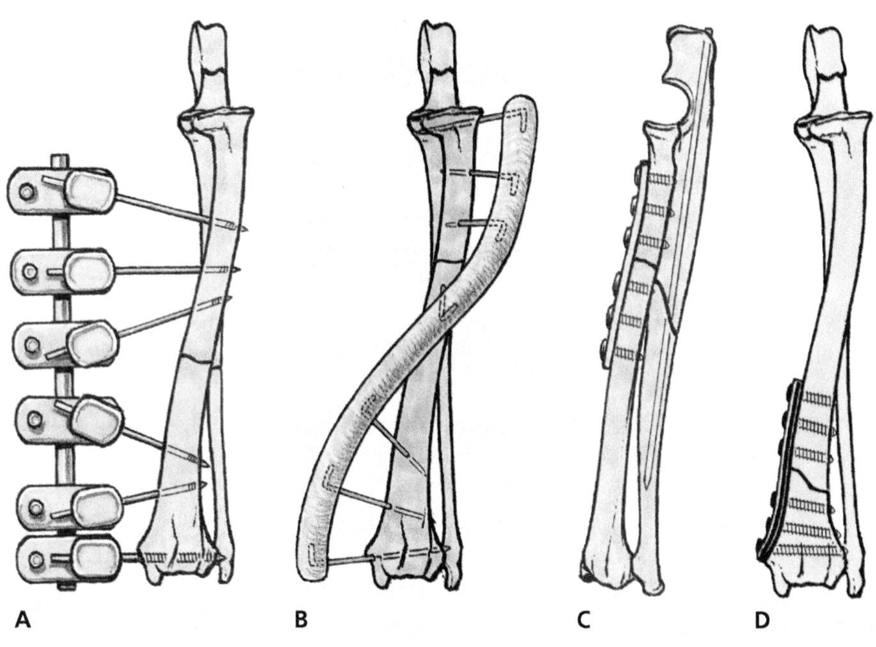

Figure 31-7 Stabilization options for simple transverse or short oblique fractures of the radial and ulnar diaphysis.
(**A**) Application of a type I external skeletal fixator for a simple transverse fracture of the mid-diaphysis of the radius.
(**B**) A modified type I external skeletal fixator with an acrylic bar for the repair of a fracture located in the proximal half of the radius.
(**C**) Stabilization of a simple radial fracture located in the proximal aspect of the diaphysis with a dorsally applied plate. The ulnar fracture is additionally stabilized with an intramedullary pin.
(**D**) Medial plating for stabilization of a short oblique fracture of the distal radial shaft.

especially in the proximal radial diaphysis. A minimally invasive approach to the radius is therefore commonly used for application of a type I, modified type II, or type II external skeletal fixator.

Concurrent simple transverse or oblique fractures of the ulna are best stabilized with an intramedullary pin. Comminuted fractures can be repaired with a laterally applied 2.0-mm DCP or 1.5/2.0-mm VCP if they are located in the proximal, thicker portion of the ulna.

31.5 Fractures of the distal radius and ulna

Fractures of the distal radius and ulna are less common in cats, as compared to dogs (9). They include fractures of the distal radial growth plate, metaphyseal and epiphyseal fractures, and fractures of the radial or ulnar styloid processes. Most of these fractures interfere with congruity and/or stability of the carpal joint, and must be treated surgically to restore anatomy and function of the carpal joint.

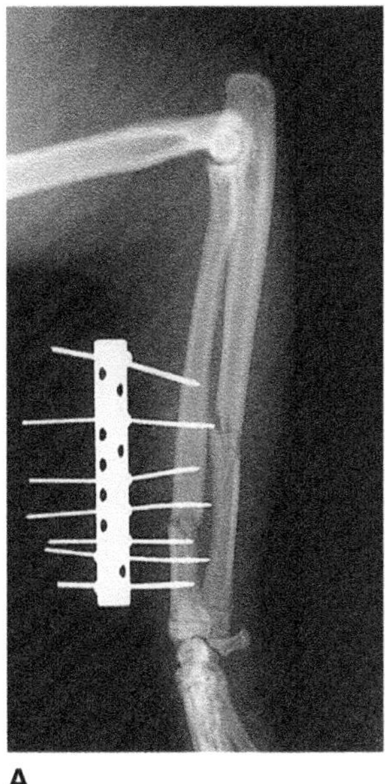
A

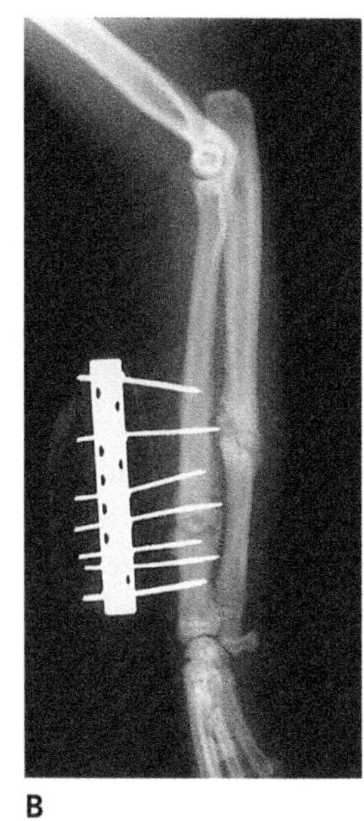
B

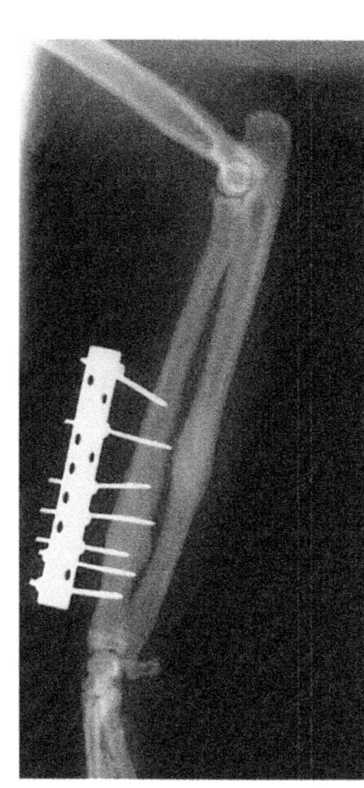
C

Figure 31-8 (**A**) Postoperative, and (**B**) follow-up radiographs at 1 month and (**C**) 2 months of distal diaphyseal radial fracture in a 10-month-old cat, stabilized with a medially applied tubular external skeletal fixator, using three small pins distally and four proximally. This semirigid fixation and the young age of the cat resulted in a large callus formation.

Premature closure of the radial physis is a potential complication in immature cats after physeal fractures (Chapter 13). Control radiographs should be obtained 2 weeks after the injury in all immature cats having sustained trauma to the distal antebrachium to be able to detect early signs of premature closure of the radial physis. The distal growth plate of the ulna seems less vulnerable to premature closure compared to dogs, probably because it is oriented perpendicular to the long axis of the radius, and does not have a conical shape as in dogs.

31.5.1 Approaches to the distal radius and ulna

The distal radius is approached via a medial or craniomedial incision. A medial approach is chosen for repair of fractures of the distal metaphysis of the radius. A craniomedial approach is performed for open reduction and internal fixation of Salter and Harris fractures of the distal radial physis. The styloid process of the ulna is approached from laterally.

31.5.2 Distal metaphyseal fractures of the radius

Distal metaphyseal fractures of the radius in cats are best treated with external skeletal fixation, because the small distal fragment precludes insertion of a sufficient number of screws for plate osteosynthesis (Box 31-4). The tubular external fixator (Chapter 24) is most useful, as more pins can be inserted over a small distance than with other systems, making it an ideal system for metaphyseal fractures of the radius (13). The 6-mm tube of the system allows insertion of six transosseous pins over a distance of 1.5 cm (13).

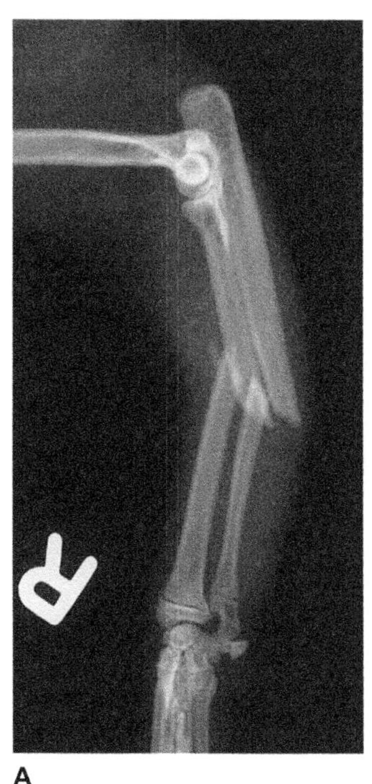

A

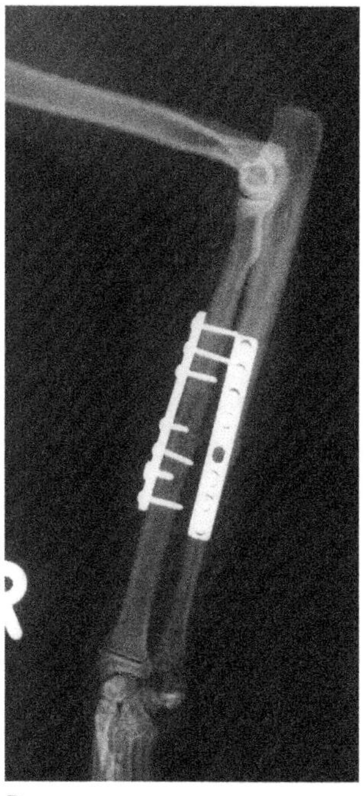

B

Figure 31-9 (**A**) Preoperative and (**B**) postoperative radiographs of a cat with a mid-diaphyseal fracture of the radius and ulna. Both bones were plated with a 2.0-mm dynamic compression plate and 1.5-mm screws. The cat had two other legs injured concurrently, so it required stable fracture fixation.

Alternatively, a modified type II external skeletal fixator (Box 31-4), a hybrid circular external skeletal fixator, Kirschner wires in a cross-pinning fashion, or a 2.0-mm internal fixator can be used to stabilize the small distal fragment. At least two screws must be inserted per fragment with an internal fixator.

Box 31-3. Stabilization of comminuted fractures of the radial and ulnar diaphysis

The radius is approached from medially and the ulna from laterally. Application of cancellous bone graft should be considered in severely comminuted radial fractures, and in the presence of fracture gaps. The ulna is reduced and stabilized first if it is a reducible fracture, because this facilitates fracture reduction.

External skeletal fixation: A medial type I external skeletal fixator is applied for mildly comminuted fractures as described in Box 31-2 (Fig. 31-10A). A modified type II or a type II external skeletal fixator provides more stability in severely comminuted radial fractures (Fig. 31-10B). Full pins must be angled in a dorsolateral direction to avoid inadvertent engagement of the ulna. At least one full pin and one half pin should be inserted into the distal fragment, and at least one full pin and one half pin or three half pins into the proximal fragment. Transosseous pins with a diameter of 1.2–1.6 mm are used. Positive-threaded 1.6-mm pins can only be inserted into the distal radial metaphysis.

Plating of the radius: A medial plate is used for fractures located in the distal half of the radius (Fig. 31-10C), and a dorsally applied plate for fractures extending into the proximal radius. At least three screws must be inserted into the proximal and distal fragment. The 1.5/2.0-mm veterinary cuttable plate should be used in sandwich or stacking function to enhance bending stability. Care is taken to avoid malpositioning of the distal fragment in valgus and external rotation.

Plating of the proximal ulna: The plate is applied to the lateral surface of the ulna with three screws distal and proximal to the fracture (Fig. 31-10C).

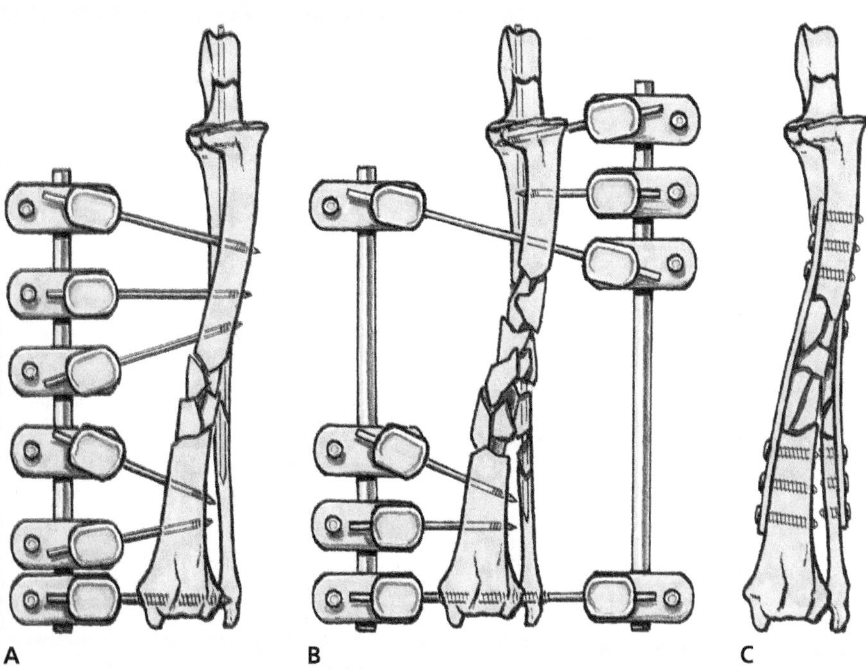

Figure 31-10 Stabilization options for comminuted fractures of the radial and ulnar diaphyses.
(**A**) Type I external skeletal fixation of a mildly comminuted fracture of the radial diaphysis. An intramedullary pin is used to stabilize a concurrent simple ulnar fracture.
(**B**) Stabilization of a severely comminuted fracture of the radius with a type II external skeletal fixator. An intramedullary pin in the ulna is used additionally.
(**C**) Stabilization of a comminuted fracture of both radius and ulna with buttress plates.

Fractures extending into the radiocarpal joint are rare. Most of these are comminuted and render joint reconstruction impossible, thus necessitating pancarpal arthrodesis (Chapter 32). If fragment numbers and sizes allow anatomic reconstruction of the radial joint surface, lag screws can be used for stabilization.

31.5.3 Salter and Harris fractures of the distal radius and ulna

The distal radial physis closes between 14 and 20 months of age in intact cats (11), and even later in neutered cats (14–16). Fractures of the distal radial physis carry the risk of

Box 31-4. External skeletal fixation of distal metaphyseal fractures of the radius

A medial approach to the distal radius is performed.

Tubular external skeletal fixator: A 6-mm tube is used. The first transfixation pin is inserted parallel to the distal radial joint surface, close to the joint. The direction of this first pin is most important, as the tube will be positioned perpendicular to that pin, and dictates the direction of all future pins. A positive-threaded 1.6-mm pin can usually be used. The connecting tube is then assembled over the pin. The fracture is reduced and the most proximal pin is inserted next. At least two, preferably three, 1.2–1.4-mm pins are required proximal and distal to the fracture. Ellis pins can be used to enhance pull-out strength because the transosseous pins are all inserted parallel to each other (Fig. 31-11A).

Modified type II external skeletal fixator: A centrally threaded 1.6-mm transfixation pin is inserted from medial across the radial epiphysis, parallel to the radial carpal joint and in a craniolateral direction to avoid the ulna. A 1.2–1.4-mm Ellis pin is inserted as the most proximal pin. The fracture is reduced and the pins are connected with the external bar medially. One more pin is drilled into the distal fragment, and at least two more pins are inserted into the proximal fragment. The lateral aspect of the distal full pin is connected to the external bar with a second connecting bar, curved cranially around the radius (Fig. 31-11B).

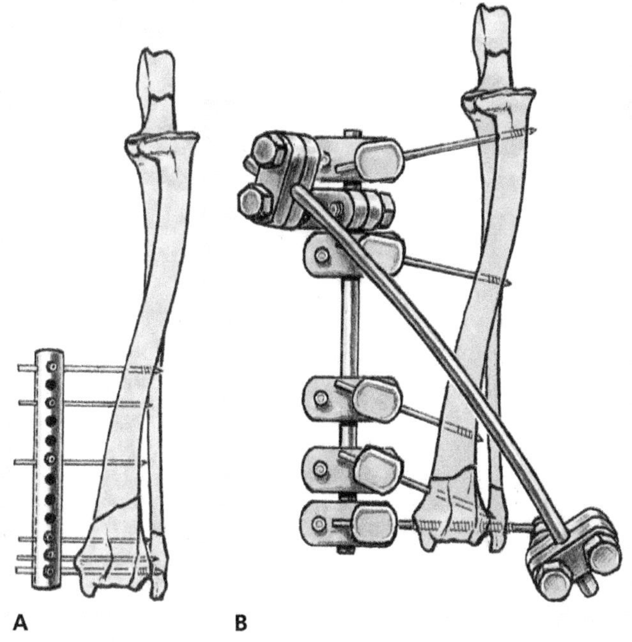

Figure 31-11 External skeletal fixation of distal metaphyseal fractures of the radius.
(**A**) Application of a 6.0-mm tubular external skeletal fixator, using one positive-threaded pin distally, and one Ellis pin proximally.
(**B**) Stabilization with a modified type II external skeletal fixator.

premature physeal closure, depending on the age of the cat at the time of trauma. Radial shortening and limb deformity may result (Chapter 13). The mean length of the feline radius was approximately 70 mm in 5-month-old cats, and around 85–100 mm in 20-month-old cats, with neutered cats having the longest radial length (16). These numbers indicate that if premature physeal closure occurs at an age of 5 months, loss of radial length can be expected to be 15–30%. Carpal incongruity is likely to occur in addition to the loss of radial length (17).

Salter and Harris type I and II fractures of the distal radial physis can be treated conservatively with a cast if they are not displaced or if they can be reduced in a closed manner. Reduction and surgical stabilization are necessary if the fracture is displaced and/or considered unstable after reduction (Fig. 31-12). Cross pinning is commonly used (Box 31-5). Salter and Harris fractures of the distal ulna may occur together with distal radial fractures. They are not usually primarily stabilized, but a small intramedullary pin can be inserted from the distal aspect of the ulnar styloid if deemed necessary.

Control radiographs should be performed in every case of distal radial or ulnar physeal fracture after 2–3 weeks to detect radiographic signs of premature physeal closure.

31.5.4 Fractures of the styloid processes of the radius and ulna

Fractures of the ulnar styloid process are occasionally encountered. Because the styloid process of the ulna is the attachment site for the lateral collateral ligament of the carpus, carpal instability may occur. However, many fractures of the ulnar styloid process in cats do not result in carpal instability. Stress radiographs have to be performed for evaluation of lateral stability of the antebrachiocarpal joint. Ulnar styloid fractures are treated conservatively with a splinted bandage

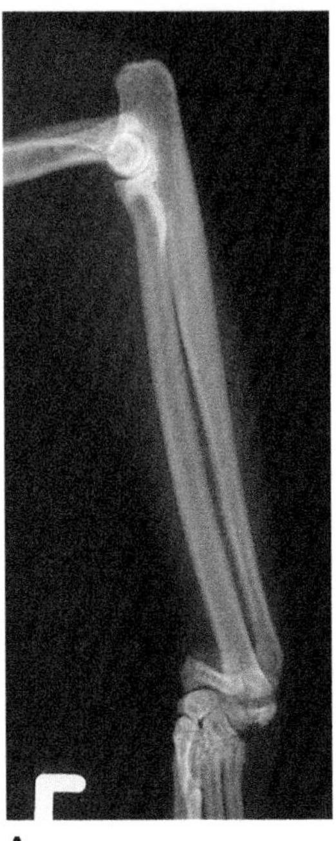
A

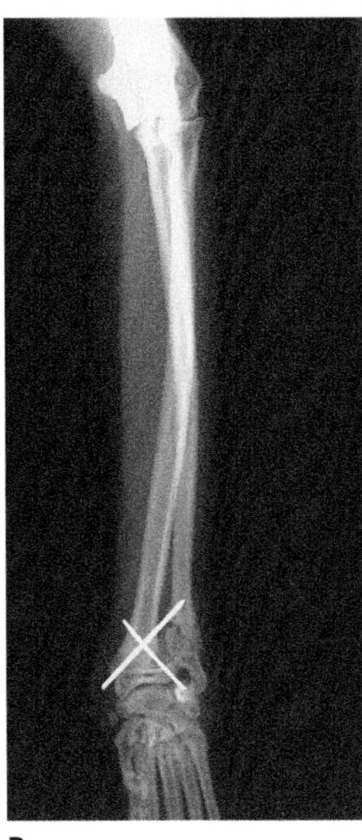
B

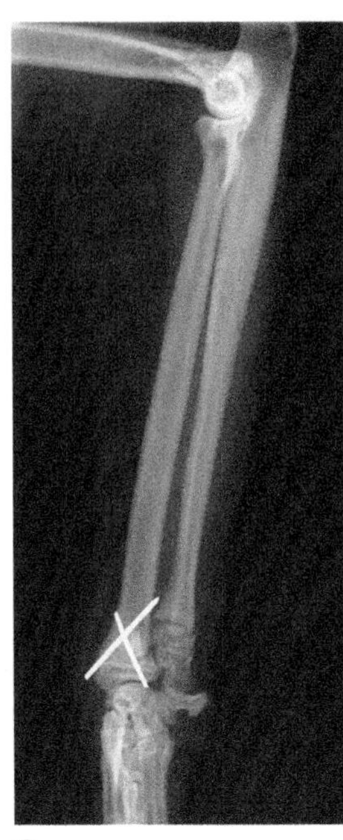
C

Figure 31-12 (**A**) Preoperative, (**B**) postoperative, and (**C**) follow-up radiographs of a cat with a distal radial physeal fracture, stabilized with cross pins. Follow-up radiographs at 3 weeks showing good progression of healing.

Box 31-5. Stabilization of Salter and Harris type I and II fractures of the radius

A craniomedial approach to the distal radius is performed. The distal fragment is usually displaced in a caudal direction. The fracture is reduced manually with the carpal joint in flexion and avoiding iatrogenic injury of the fracture surface of the distal fragment, where the proliferating cells of the growth plate are located. Two 0.8–1.0-mm Kirschner wires are inserted in a cross-pin fashion. One Kirschner wire is inserted from the radial styloid process across the fracture line into the lateral cortex of the radius. The second Kirschner wire is inserted from the laterodistal edge of the radius into the caudomedial cortex of the radius, or from the ulnar styloid process into the radius (Fig. 31-13). A separate small skin incision may be necessary for the lateral pin to be placed. In young cats with soft bones the pins are not bent to avoid the risk of tearing them out of the bone; instead, they are cut short.

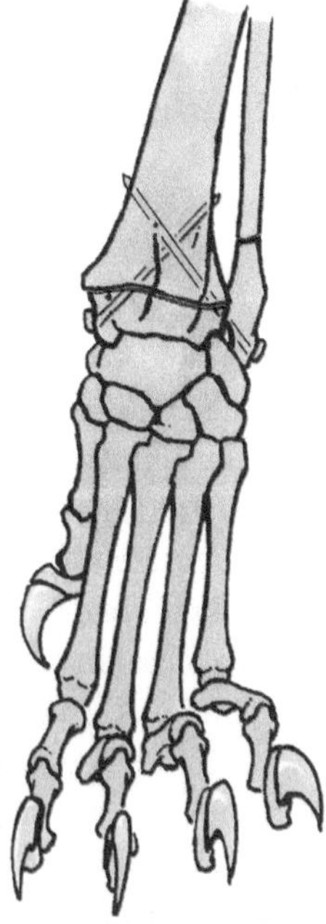

Figure 31-13 Cross pinning of a Salter and Harris type I fracture of the distal radius. The lateral pin is inserted through the ulnar styloid process. This is especially important if the ulnar styloid process is displaced from the radius preoperatively.

Box 31-6. Stabilization of fractures of the ulnar styloid process

A lateral approach to the ulnar styloid process is performed. Adequate reduction of the fracture is necessary to achieve stability and congruity of the carpal joint. The distal part of the fractured ulna is stabilized to the radius with two parallel pins or a tension band repair. One or two 0.6-mm Kirschner wires are inserted from the ulnar styloid process, and are driven into the distal radius. A 0.5-mm wire is inserted in a figure-of-eight fashion around the distal pin ends and through a hole drilled into the radius (Fig. 31-14).

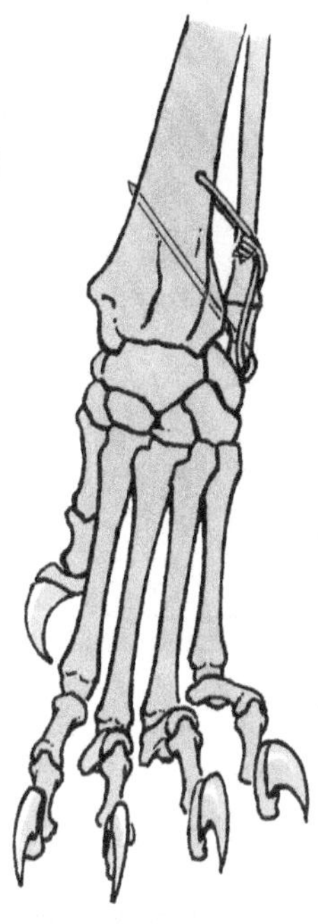

Figure 31-14 Diagram showing tension band repair of a fracture of the ulnar styloid process.

for 2–3 weeks if the carpal joint is considered stable. If ulnar styloid fractures are associated with antebrachiocarpal instability, the distal fragment is reattached with a tension band fixation (Box 31-6).

Ulnar styloid fractures in young cats have been associated with the development of premature closure of the distal radial growth plate (Chapter 13) (17). Control radiographs are therefore taken 2–3 weeks after the trauma in growing animals to rule out radial physeal damage.

31.6 Postoperative treatment and prognosis

Activity is restricted to cage rest or confinement to the house after all fractures of the radius and ulna. External coaptation is usually unnecessary for diaphyseal fractures. In fractures, where the stability achieved with surgery is suboptimal for immediate weight-bearing, external coaptation with a splinted bandage should be considered for 2–3 weeks. A modified Robert Jones bandage is used to limit elbow flexion after comminuted fractures of the proximal ulna. A splinted bandage is also normally applied after repair of Salter and Harris fractures of the distal radius for 10 days.

Control radiographs are performed after 4–6 weeks in adult cats, and after 2–3 weeks in immature cats. They are absolutely mandatory in immature cats with trauma to the distal antebrachium to be able to evaluate further radial growth. Initial radiological signs of premature closure of the distal radial physis include narrowing of the growth plate, and changes in shape of the growth plate (Fig. 31-15). Treatment of premature physeal closure of the radius is described in Chapter 13.

Repair of radial and ulnar fractures in cats was associated with a high failure rate with the initial intervention, and 17 out of 36 cases required revision surgery (9). Fractures of the proximal radius and ulna seem to be especially prone to complications and failures, and fractures of the proximal ulna were described to have a higher risk for non-unions (18). A meticulous technique and attention to performing accurate fracture reduction and stabilization of both the ulna and radius should lead to an increased success rate.

Functional outcome after proximal radial and ulnar fractures is good if anatomic reconstruction of the elbow joint was achieved. Osteoarthritis will develop in most cases with fractures involving the elbow joint.

Prognosis for return to function is usually excellent after diaphyseal fractures of the radius and ulna, provided that correct limb alignment was achieved during surgery. Possible complications are the development of synostoses between the radius and ulna. Synostosis is rare in cats and more likely to occur after comminuted fractures, or if radial implants are placed inadvertently into or close to the ulna. Degenerative

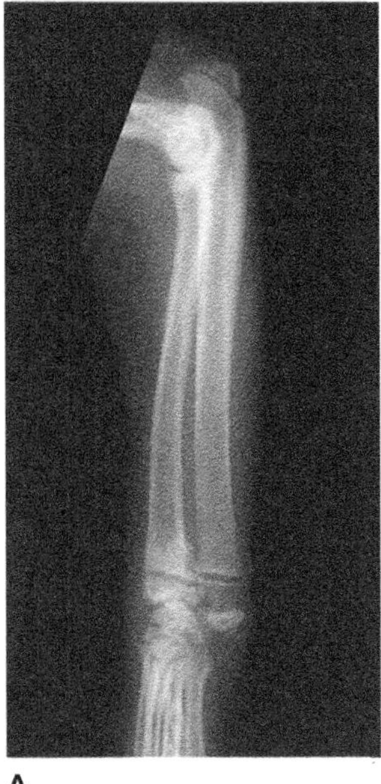
A

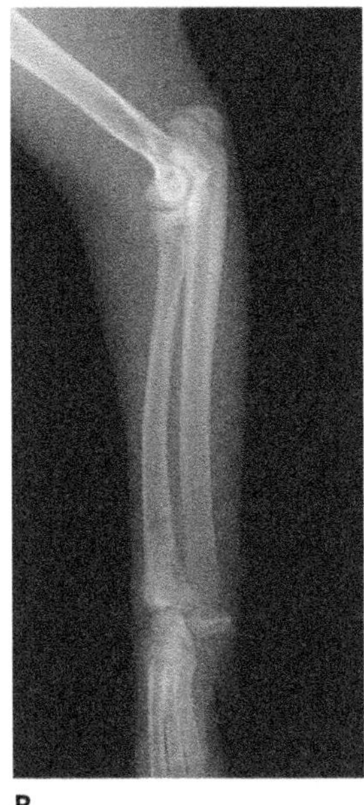
B

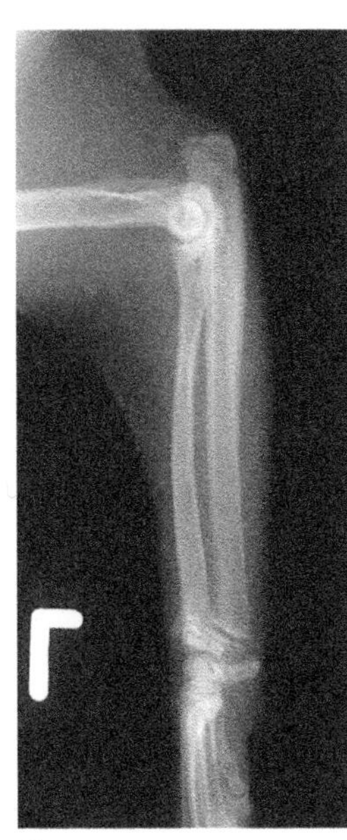
C

Figure 31-15 Cat with premature closure of the distal radial physis. Serial radiographs of a 6-month-old cat with a minimally displaced Salter and Harris type I fracture of the distal radial physis, which was treated conservatively with a splinted bandage. Note the irregular physis 2 weeks after the injury (**A**), and the subsequent narrowing and dorsal tilting 4 weeks (**B**) and 7 weeks (**C**) postinjury. Also note that the ulnar physis was narrowed 4 weeks after injury (**B**), but had widened again after 7 weeks (**C**).

joint disease may develop in the elbow or carpal joint, if the fixation resulted in length discrepancy between the radius and ulna.

The prognosis for distal radial and ulnar fractures is good after stable fixation if congruity of the antebrachiocarpal joint was preserved. Healing of Salter and Harris fractures of the distal radius is usually rapid due to the young age of cats and the good metaphyseal blood supply. Premature closure of the distal radial physis can occur after both Salter and Harris fractures of the distal radius and fractures of the ulnar styloid process (Fig. 31-15).

References and further reading

1. Whitney WO, Mehlhaff CJ. High-rise syndrome in cats. J Am Vet Med Assoc 1987;191:1399–1403.
2. Kapatkin AS, Matthiesen DT. Feline high-rise syndrome. Compend Continuing Educ 1991;13:1389–1394.
3. Harari J. Treatments for feline long bone fractures. Vet Clin North Am Small Anim Pract 2002;32:927–947.
4. Frewein J, Vollmerhaus B. Anatomie von Hund und Katze. Berlin: Blackwell; 1994.
5. Nunamaker DM. Fractures of the radius and ulna. In: Newton CD, Nunamaker DM (eds) Textbook of small animal orthopaedics. Philadelphia: Lippincott; 1985: pp. 365–373.
6. Sardinas JC, Montavon PM. Use of a medial bone plate for repair of radius and ulna fractures in dogs and cats: a report of 22 cases. Vet Surg 1997;26:108–113.
7. Linn LL, et al. Extraction resistance of 2.7 mm medio-lateral-placed cortical screws compared with 2.7 mm and 3.5 mm cranio-caudal-placed cortical screws in canine cadaver radii. Vet Comp Orthop Traumatol 2001;14:1–6.
8. Kudnik ST, et al. In vitro comparison of the holding power of 1.2 mm, 1.5 mm, and 2.0 mm orthopaedic screws in canine radii. Vet Comp Orthop Traumatol 2002;15:78–84.
9. Wallace AM, et al. Radius and ulna fractures in cats: a retrospective study of 38 cases. BSAVA Meeting 2007; Birmingham, UK.
10. Piermattei DL, Johnson KA. An atlas of surgical approaches to the bones and joints of the dog and the cat, 4th edn. Philadelphia: WB Saunders; 2004.
11. Smith RN. Fusion of ossification centres in the cat. J Small Anim Pract 1969;10:523–530.
12. Robins GM, et al. Customized hook plate for metaphyseal fractures, nonunions and osteotomies in the dog and cat. Vet Comp Orthop Traumatol 1993;6:56–61.
13. Haas B, et al. Use of the tubular external fixator in the treatment of distal radial and ulnar fractures in small dogs and cats. Vet Comp Orthop Traumatol 2003;16:132–137.
14. May C, et al. Delayed physeal closure associated with castration in cats. J Small Anim Pract 1991;32:326–328.
15. Houlton JE, McGlennon NJ. Castration and physeal closure in the cat. Vet Rec 1992;131:466–467.
16. Root MV, et al. The effect of prepuberal and postpuberal gonadectomy on radial physeal closure in male and female domestic cats. Vet Radiol Ultrasound 1997;38:42–47.
17. Voss K, Lieskovsky J. Trauma-induced growth abnormalities of the distal radius in three cats. J Feline Med Surg 2007;9:117–123.
18. Nolte DM, et al. Incidence of and predisposing factors for nonunion of fractures involving the appendicular skeleton in cats: 18 cases (1998–2002). J Am Vet Med Assoc 2005;226:77–82.

32 Carpal joint

K. Voss, S.J. Langley-Hobbs, P.M. Montavon

Carpal injuries occur after both falls from a height and motor vehicle accidents. Hyperextension injury at the level of the carpometacarpal joint was the most frequent, and medial collateral ligament strain the second most common injury in a personal survey of feline carpal injuries. Intercarpal ligamentous injury and luxation of the radial carpal bone were diagnosed only infrequently. Fractures of the carpal bones are exceedingly rare, with the exception of fractures of the accessory carpal bone. Knowledge of carpal anatomy and a thorough clinical and radiological examination are required to diagnose correctly the exact type and site of carpal injury. Anatomy of the carpal joint and the diagnosis and treatment options of the most common carpal injuries in cats are described in the following sections.

Osteoarthritis of the carpal joint is rare, but the carpi are commonly affected in cats with polyarthritis. The carpal joint is also prone to open injuries, such as degloving injuries and cat bite wounds. These conditions are described in Chapters 5 and 14.

32.1 Surgical anatomy

The carpal joint consists of two rows of bones and three joint levels, the antebrachiocarpal, the middle carpal, and the carpometacarpal joints. The individual bones are connected to the joint capsule and there are numerous short ligaments, most of them only spanning one joint level. The ligaments are stronger on the palmar side of the joint, and these resist the tensile forces during weight-bearing together with the palmar fibrocartilage. These ligaments are damaged in hyperextension injuries.

Recent publications have addressed anatomy of feline carpal ligaments (1, 2). The medial collateral ligament of the antebrachiocarpal joint in cats has anatomic and functional differences to the ligament in the dog (1). It consists of only a single broad ligament that extends obliquely from dorsoproximal on the radius to its palmarodistal attachment on the radial carpal bone (Fig. 32-1). The angle between the longitudinal axis of the radius and the medial collateral ligament is approximately 100°. Due to its oblique course, the medial collateral ligament not only counteracts valgus stress, but it also prevents dislocation of the carpal bones in a palmar direction (1). The straight superficial part of the medial collateral ligament, which is present in the dog, is absent in cats. The lateral collateral ligament has a similar arrangement as described for dogs (2).

The distal radius and ulna are connected to each other by the joint capsule of the radioulnar joint and the radioulnar ligament (2). The radioulnar joint allows rotational movement between the distal radius and ulna, allowing for supination and pronation of the paw, both important functions of the antebrachium in cats.

32.2 Diagnosis and treatment options

Carpal injuries include ligament sprains resulting in instability or luxation, and fractures of the carpal bones (Table

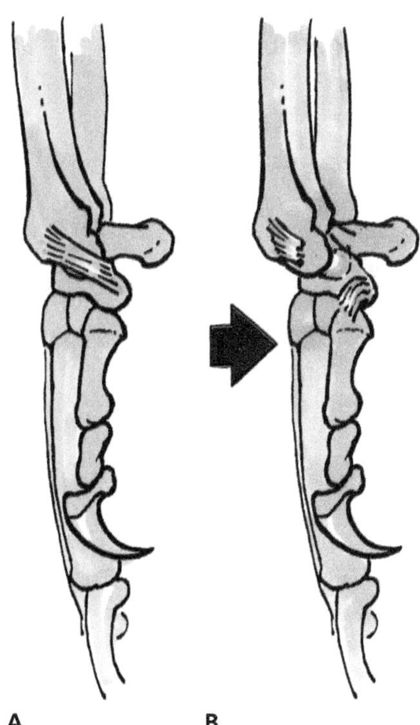

Figure 32-1 Diagram illustrating anatomy and function of the feline medial collateral ligament. (**A**) The angle between the longitudinal axis of the radius and the medial collateral ligament is approximately 100°. (**B**) Rupture of the medial collateral ligament results in palmar dislocation of the antebrachiocarpal joint, similar to a drawer motion. (Reproduced with permission from: Voss K, Geyer H, Montavon PM. Antebrachiocarpal luxation in a cat. A case report and anatomical study of the medial collateral ligament. Vet Comp Orthop Traumatol 2003;16:268.)

Localization of lesion	Type of lesion	Treatment options
Antebrachiocarpal joint instability/luxation	Medial collateral ligament sprain (medial instability)	Ligament prosthesis External coaptation
	Antebrachiocarpal luxation	Primary repair Pancarpal arthrodesis
	Luxation of the radial carpal bone	Primary repair
	Hyperextension injury	External coaptation Pancarpal arthrodesis
Middle carpal joint instability/luxation	Instability or luxation	External coaptation Partial carpal arthrodesis
	Hyperextension injury	Partial carpal arthrodesis
Carpometacarpal joint instability/luxation	Hyperextension injury	Partial carpal arthrodesis
	Dorsal, medial or lateral instability with intact palmar ligaments	Dorsal plate or internal fixator (adaptation function) Screw and wire technique Partial carpal arthrodesis
Fractures of carpal bones	Fractures of the accessory carpal bone	External coaptation Removal of fragment
	Fractures of the ulnar styloid process	External coaptation Tension band repair

Table 32-1. Carpal injuries and possible treatment options. Antebrachiocarpal instability and luxation and carpometacarpal hyperextension are the most common injuries

32-1). Fractures of the distal radius and ulna (Chapter 31) and fractures of the proximal aspect of the metacarpal bones (Chapter 33) may also affect the carpal joint. Cats with carpal injuries often present with non-weight-bearing lameness. The carpal area is swollen, and instability and/or crepitation may be felt. Comparison to the contralateral side can be useful to detect mild periarticular swelling. Septic or immune-mediated arthritis should be considered as differential diagnoses in cases with carpal effusion and periarticular swelling (Chapters 5 and 14).

Thorough palpation of a painful carpal joint often necessitates sedation or a short general anesthetic. The presence of crepitus is suggestive of fractures, luxations, or severe arthritis. Joint stability is evaluated by manipulation of the carpus in all directions. The normal degree of carpal extension differs between individual cats, ranging from 10° to 25°, so the contralateral side should be used as a reference point. Hyperextension can be present after injury to the palmar ligamentous support. Valgus and varus stress are applied to the extended carpal joint to detect medial or lateral instability. Avoid pronating or supinating the antebrachium while applying these mediolateral stresses. Finally, dorsopalmar stability should also be tested to evaluate fully the integrity of the medial collateral ligament (Fig. 32-1).

Mediolateral and dorsopalmar radiographs of the carpus are obtained to diagnose or rule out luxations and fractures. Stress radiographs in hyperextension, valgus, and varus stress are performed if ligament damage is suspected from clinical findings. Hyperextension stress views determine the level of palmar instability at the radiocarpal, the middle carpal, or the carpometacarpal joint level (see section on hyperextension injury, below). Interpretation of valgus and varus stress radiographs is difficult due to the small size of bones and the oblique course of the medial collateral ligament in cats. The normal appearance of valgus and varus stress radiographs of the feline carpus is shown in Figure 32-2. Medial opening of

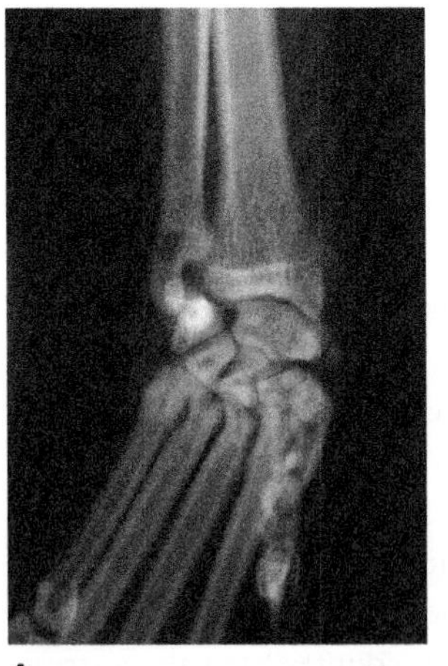

A

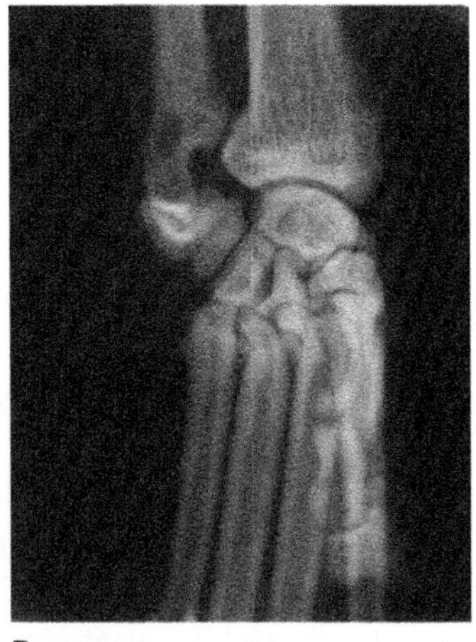

B

Figure 32-2 (**A**) Valgus and (**B**) and varus dorsopalmar stress radiographs of an extended normal feline carpus. Note the large physiological range of motion in valgus stress.

the antebrachiocarpal joint in valgus stress is not as pronounced as in dogs in the presence of medial collateral ligament sprain (see below). More commonly, varus stress causes the radial carpal bone to dislodge in a mediopalmar direction (Fig. 32-3).

32.3 Approaches to the carpal joints

A medial approach to the carpal joint is made for most procedures. The medial approach allows repair of medial collateral ligament ruptures, luxation of the radial carpal bone, and pancarpal or partial carpal arthrodesis with a medial plate or internal fixator. The skin is incised along the craniomedial border of the distal radius and carpal joint. The incision is extended distally just cranial to the first digit, if the distal carpal rows have to be approached. The antebrachial fascia is then incised and the tendon of the abductor pollicis longus muscle identified. It covers part of the medial collateral ligament close to its proximal attachment, before inserting at the base of the metacarpal bone I. The tendon is spared but can be retracted to visualize the medial collateral ligament. Incision of the radiocarpal joint capsule is performed in a longitudinal direction, cranial to the medial collateral ligament, if necessary.

A dorsal approach to the carpal joints is performed for partial carpal arthrodesis by the pin fixation method, and for pancarpal arthrodesis with a dorsal plate (3). The extensor tendons are retracted laterally or medially without damaging them. If partial carpal arthrodesis is performed, the dorsal joint capsule of the radiocarpal joint can be left intact.

32.4 Antebrachiocarpal instability and luxation

Injuries to the ligamentous support of the antebrachiocarpal joint include medial collateral ligament sprain, antebrachiocarpal luxation, luxation of the radial carpal bone, and antebrachiocarpal hyperextension injury (Table 32-1). Medial collateral ligament sprains and antebrachiocarpal luxations are the most frequently diagnosed injuries at the antebrachiocarpal level. Luxation of the radial carpal bone and antebrachiocarpal hyperextension are rare. Whereas medial collateral ligament rupture and radiocarpal luxation are more commonly caused by motor vehicle accidents, hyperextension injury is almost invariably seen after falls from a height. Motor vehicle accidents may also result in degloving and open antebrachiocarpal joint injuries. Treatment of open joint injuries is described in Chapter 14.

32.4.1 Medial collateral ligament sprain

Sprain of the medial collateral ligament is a common cause of antebrachiocarpal instability. Medial collateral ligament rupture results in both medial instability and palmar subluxation of the radiocarpal joint (Fig. 32-3). It may even lead to complete palmar radiocarpal luxation if the dorsal joint capsule is also ruptured (see next section).

Primary surgical reconstruction is the treatment of choice for medial collateral ligament sprains resulting in either marked subluxation or luxation (Box 32-1). Conservative treatment with a splinted bandage can be tried for minor instability. In the presence of radiocarpal joint luxation it is imperative also to evaluate the integrity of the palmar ligamentous support before surgery (see section on hyperextension injury, below). Primary repair should be attempted before arthrodesis is considered, if the palmar ligaments are intact.

32.4.2 Antebrachiocarpal luxation

Complete antebrachiocarpal luxation in a palmar or dorsal direction is occasionally encountered. Palmar antebrachiocarpal luxation is more common than dorsal luxation in cats. Palmar luxation is often caused by rupture of the medial collateral ligament and the dorsal joint capsule (Fig. 32-5). Dorsomedial luxation of the antebrachiocarpal joint was associated with disruption of the radioulnar ligament and a grade II medial collateral ligament strain in one report (2). The enhanced mobility of the distal ulna with respect to the

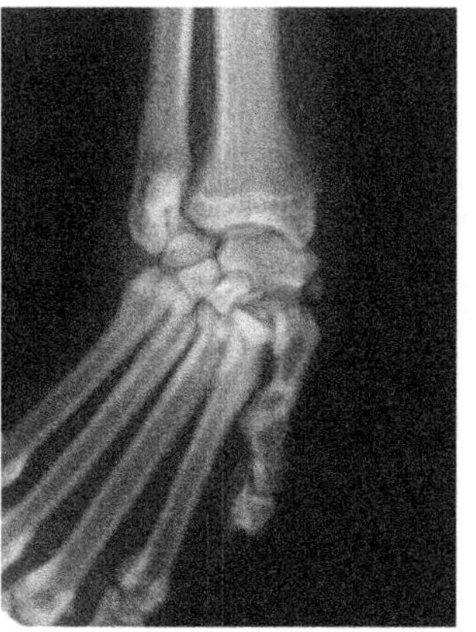

A

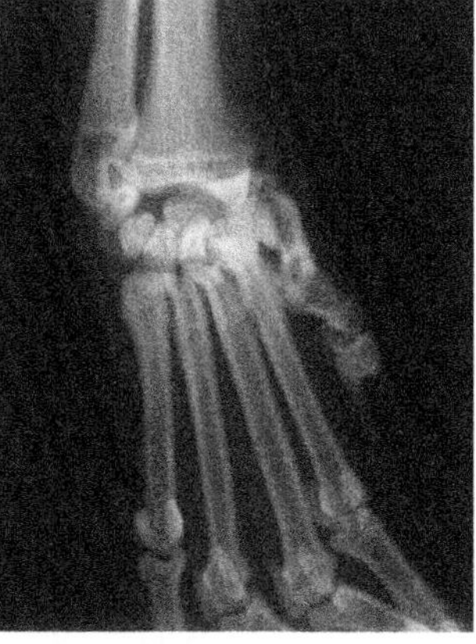

B

Figure 32-3 (**A**) Valgus and (**B**) varus stress radiographs of a cat with medial collateral ligament sprain. Valgus stress radiographs do not necessarily result in excessive opening of the medial radiocarpal joint. Varus stress causes palmaromedial subluxation of the radiocarpal joint, as identified by the abnormal radiocarpal joint space.

Box 32-1. Medial collateral ligament prosthesis

A medial approach to the carpal joint is performed as described above. The ligament ends are identified below the tendon of the abductor pollicis longus muscle, and are sutured with a locking-loop suture if possible. A ligament prosthesis is applied to protect the primary ligament repair. The prosthesis must mimic the physiological course of the ligament (Fig. 32-4). A 1.5-mm screw is placed in the radial epiphysis in a dorsomedial to palmarolateral direction. Avoid penetrating the ulna with the screw tip, as this would impede supination and pronation movements. A second 1.5-mm screw is inserted palmar to the tendon of the abductor pollicis longus muscle into the radial carpal bone. A figure-of-eight suture is anchored around the screw heads below the tendon of the abductor pollicis muscle. Flexion, extension, supination, and pronation are tested after the suture has been tightened. Impaired range of motion or dorsal subluxation can occur if the suture is too tight. Instability will persist if it is left too loose.

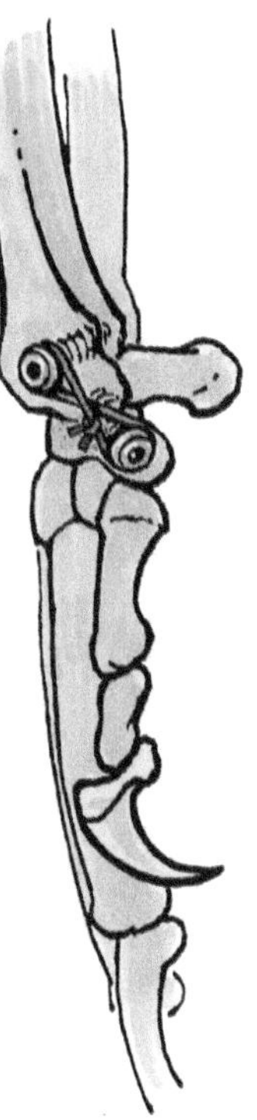

Figure 32-4 The screws are positioned at the insertion sites of the medial collateral ligament. The ligament prosthesis mimics the anatomic course of the ligament, and prevents both medial opening of the joint and palmar (sub)luxation of the radial carpal bone.

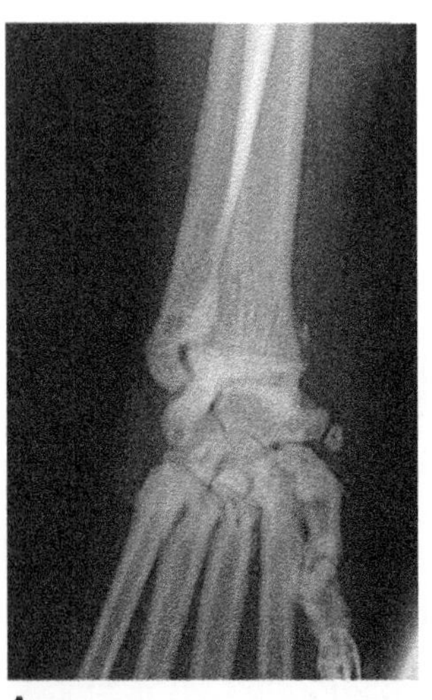

A

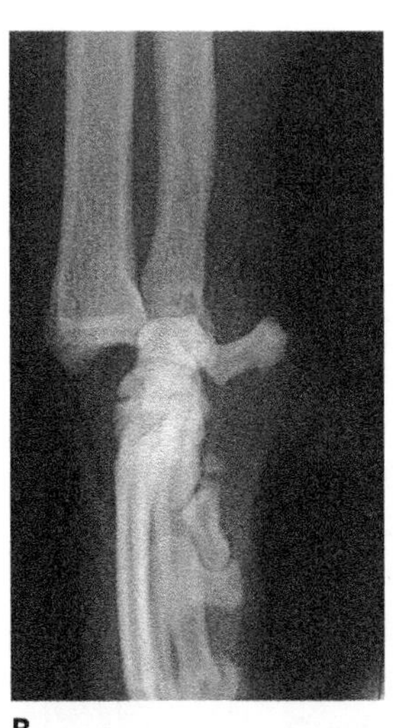

B

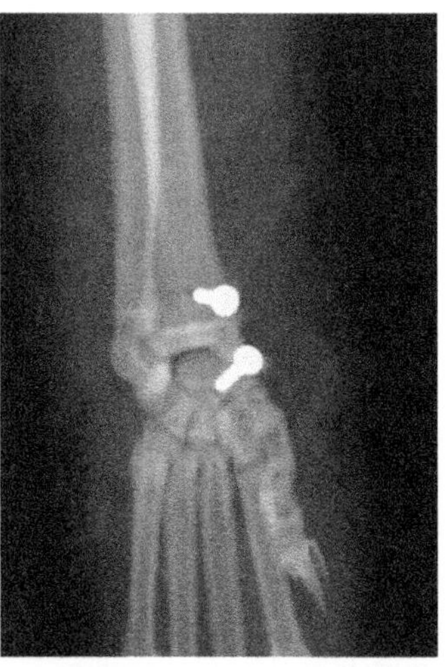

C

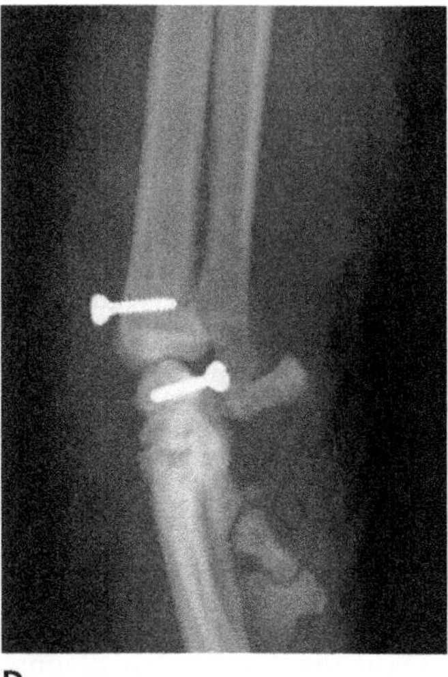

D

Figure 32-5 (**A, B**) Preoperative and (**C, D**) postoperative radiographs of the carpal joint of a cat with palmar radiocarpal luxation, caused by medial collateral ligament sprain and rupture of the dorsal joint capsule. Avulsion fragments are seen at the insertion site of the medial collateral ligament at the distal radius (**A**). The radiocarpal joint is luxated towards palmar (**B**). Note the reciprocal directions of the two 1.5-mm screws used for anchorage of the prosthesis on the postoperative radiographs (**C, D**).

radius, caused by radioulnar joint disruption, resulted in lateral instability of the antebrachiocarpal joint, despite an intact lateral collateral ligament (2).

Stress radiographs are performed when closed reduction of the luxation is feasible to evaluate integrity of the collateral ligaments and the palmar ligamentous support. Evaluation of joint structures can also be done during surgery, especially in cases where closed reduction and preoperative stress radiographs were not feasible.

Antebrachiocarpal luxation is not necessarily associated with palmar ligament damage in cats, and primary repair of ruptured ligaments should be attempted if the palmar ligaments are intact (1, 2). Pancarpal arthrodesis is indicated when anatomic reduction and stable primary repair are not possible. Further indications for pancarpal arthrodesis are severe degloving injuries with loss of bone and/or prolonged septic arthritis.

Primary repair involves apposition of and suturing the ruptured joint capsule and ligaments when possible. A medial collateral ligament prosthesis is additionally applied in the presence of medial collateral ligament rupture (Fig. 32-5 and Box 32-1). Instability of the radioulnar joint can be treated with a temporary screw or pin inserted from the distal ulna into the distal radius to allow fibrous healing of the joint capsule and radioulnar ligament (2). This implant is removed after 4–6 weeks, because it restricts pronation and supination of the antebrachium.

32.4.3 Luxation of the radial carpal bone

Luxation of the radial carpal bone is an uncommon injury that has only been described in one cat (4). The radial carpal bone is luxated in a palmar direction with the proximal articular aspect of the radial carpal bone coming to lie facing dorsally (Fig. 32-6). The injury is associated with rupture of the dorsal joint capsule, the intercarpal ligament, which connects the radial and ulnar carpal bones, and the medial collateral ligament (4). The mechanism of injury in dogs is thought to be hyperextension combined with pronation, followed by supination of the foot, as may occur during a fall. Open reduction using a dorsomedial approach to the radiocarpal joint and internal fixation is the treatment of choice. The radial carpal bone is secured to the ulnar carpal bone with a 1.5-mm screw or small Kirschner wire, and the medial collateral ligament is reconstructed (Fig. 32-6). The repair is protected with a splinted bandage or a transarticular external skeletal fixator for 2–3 weeks. The prognosis is favorable.

32.5 Hyperextension injury

The palmar ligaments and fibrocartilage are the main structures that resist carpal hyperextension. Carpal hyperextension injuries in cats result from a fall from a height, where large tensile forces are generated on the palmar side of the

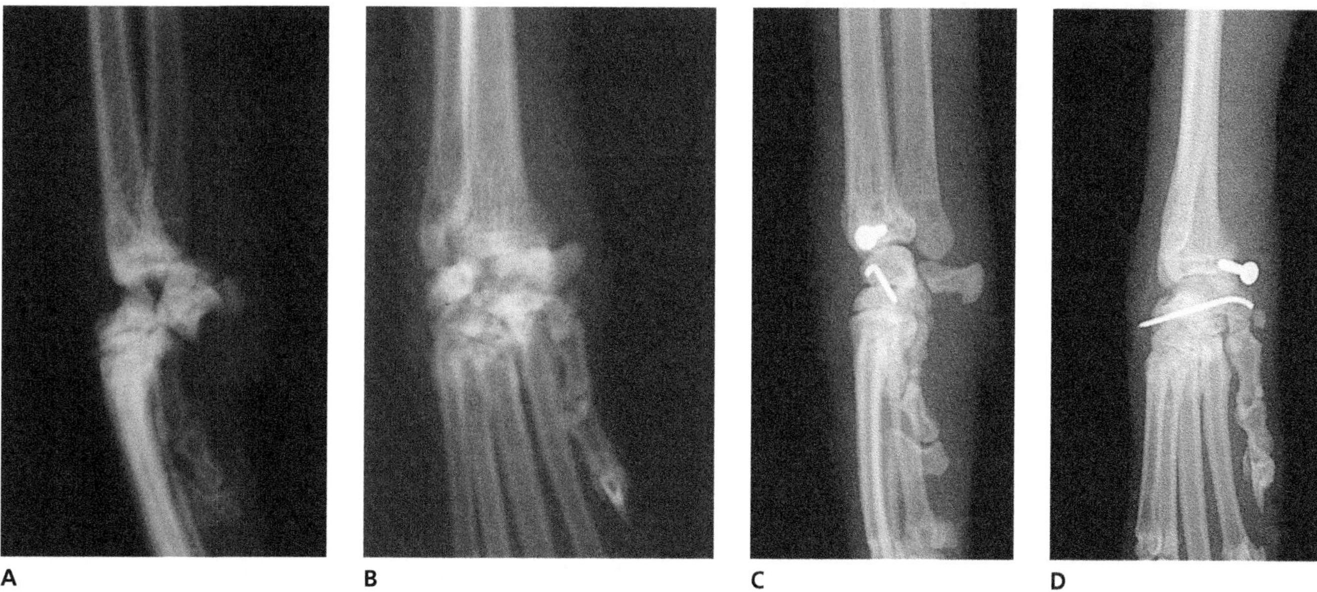

Figure 32-6 A cat with luxation of the radial carpal bone. (**A, B**) The preoperative radiographs show the luxated and rotated radial carpal bone. Its proximal articular surface is located dorsally. (**C, D**) The radial carpal bone was reduced and stabilized to the ulnar carpal bone with a 1.0-mm Kirschner wire. The medial collateral ligament was sutured, and a ligament prosthesis was placed between the 1.5-mm screw in the radius and around the bent pin end.

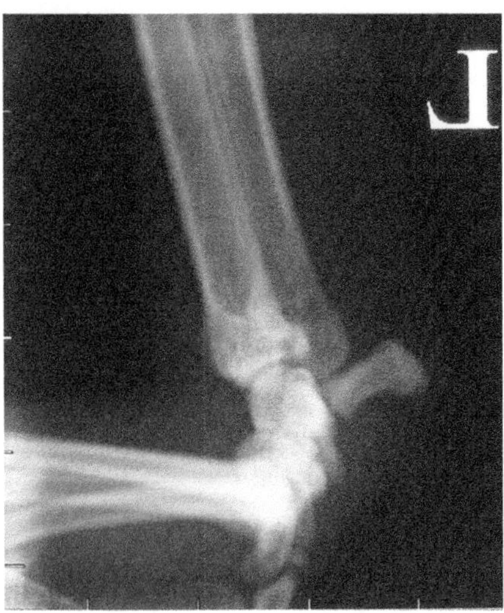

Figure 32-7 Mediolateral stress radiograph of a cat with carpometacarpal hyperextension injury. The metacarpal bones are angled in a dorsal direction in relation to the distal row of carpal bones. The antebrachiocarpal joint is intact. The treatment of choice is partial carpal arthrodesis.

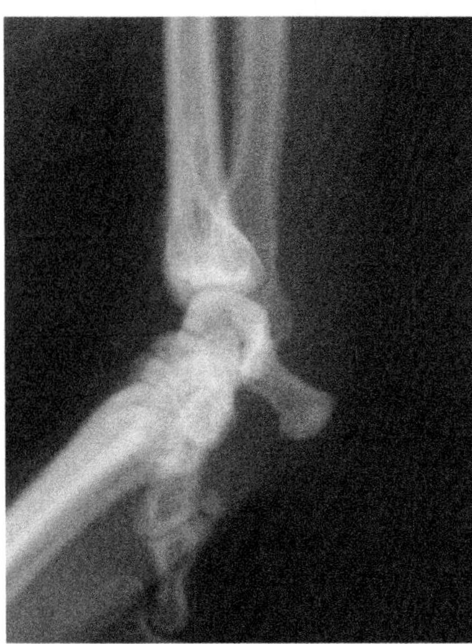

Figure 32-8 Mediolateral stress radiograph of a cat with antebrachiocarpal hyperextension. The increased antebrachiocarpal joint angle and the angle between the radius and the accessory carpal bone larger than 90° indicate either instability at the level of the antebrachiocarpal joint or disruption or dysfunction of the flexor carpi ulnaris tendon. Pancarpal arthrodesis is performed if lameness and/or a palmigrade stance persists after conservative treatment.

carpus during impact on the ground. The carpometacarpal joint is affected in the majority of cases (Fig. 32-7). Radiocarpal and intercarpal hyperextension injuries are infrequent (Fig. 32-8). Although cats may be able to walk after fibrous healing of the palmar ligaments following conservative treatment or primary ligament reconstruction, clinical results are unsatisfactory because a palmigrade stance persists. Arthrodesis is therefore the treatment of choice (5, 6). Partial carpal arthrodesis is performed for intercarpal and carpometacarpal hyperextension injuries (5–8). Hyperextension injuries involving the antebrachiocarpal joint necessitate pancarpal arthrodesis. A cat with atraumatic hyperextension at the antebrachiocarpal joint level should be screened for diabetes mellitus. A conservative treatment trial usually precedes the decision to perform pancarpal arthrodesis in cases with minor palmar instability at the antebrachiocarpal joint level. External immobilization with the carpal joint in slight flexion may allow fibrous healing of the ligaments and result in acceptable function. Partial carpal arthrodesis and pancarpal arthrodesis are described at the end of this chapter.

32.6 Rare carpal injuries

Intercarpal or carpometacarpal instabilities other than hyperextension injury can occur after rupture of the short intercarpal and carpometacarpal ligaments. The exact site of instability is difficult to diagnose radiographically, and these lesions are usually treated by partial carpal arthrodesis. For isolated dorsal instabilities at the intercarpal or carpometacarpal joint levels, a dorsally applied internal fixator or miniplate in adaptation function, or dorsal fixation using two screws and a figure-of-eight suture, are used to allow fibrous healing of the dorsal ligaments. The techniques for repair of short dorsal ligaments are similar to those described in Chapter 40 for the more frequent dorsal instabilities of intertarsal joints.

Fractures of the carpal bones are exceptionally rare in cats, and mostly affect the accessory carpal bone (Fig. 32-9). Fractures of the accessory carpal bone have been classified into five types in racing greyhounds (9). Accessory bone fracture types seen by the authors in cats include type I, distal basilar fractures, and type V, comminuted fractures. Type I injuries may be associated with hyperextension injury due to avulsion of the accessoroulnar ligaments. Treatment usually consists of external coaptation with the carpus immobilized in 20° of flexion for a time period of around 4 weeks, as the fragments of the small accessory bone are too small to be reattached with a lag screw. Removal of the fragment, partial carpal arthrodesis, or pancarpal arthrodesis may be indicated if lameness persists.

32.7 Partial carpal arthrodesis

Partial carpal arthrodesis is indicated for the treatment of carpometacarpal and intercarpal hyperextension injuries, comminuted fractures of the distal joint levels, and other non-reconstructable injuries at the intercarpal and carpo-

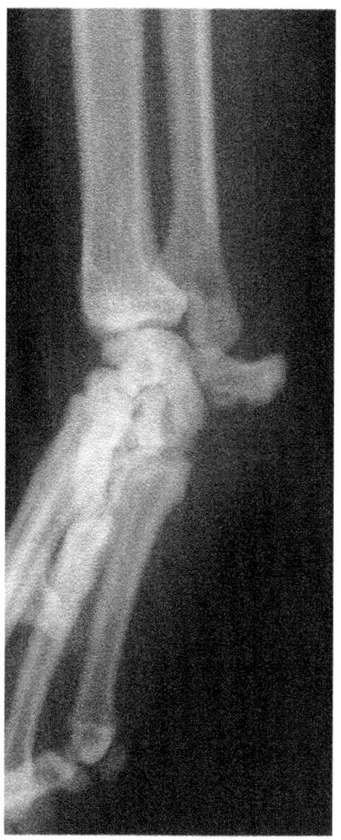

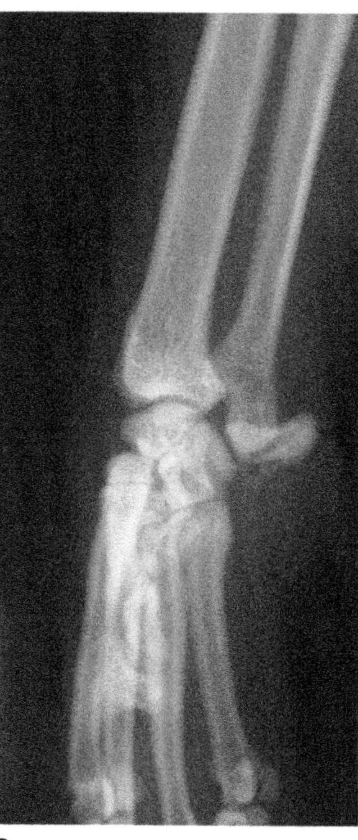

A B

Figure 32-9 Examples of accessory carpal bone fractures. Both cats were treated conservatively with a splinted bandage.
(**A**) A distal basilar fracture of the accessory carpal bone.
(**B**) A mildly comminuted fracture of the accessory carpal bone.

metacarpal joint levels. The advantage of partial carpal arthrodesis is the preservation of functional mobility of the antebrachiocarpal joint. To our knowledge, partial carpal arthrodesis has not been published in cats. In dogs, a pinning technique, cross pinning, and dorsal application of a T-plate have been described (5–8).

The pin fixation technique works well in cats (Box 32-2), and has the advantage of not requiring any specialized equipment or implants (Fig. 32-11). The pins are inserted from the metacarpal bones II and III so the tips can be seated in the radial carpal bone. Pin insertion can be hazardous due to the small diameter of the medullary cavity at the base of the metacarpals and the hard quality of the carpal bones.

Dorsal plating is not feasible in cats, because the small size of the radial carpal bone would result in irritation of the radiocarpal joint and distal radius from impingement of the proximal end of the plate. Instead, partial carpal arthrodesis can be performed with a medially applied plate (Box 32-2). A small plate, such as the 1.3-mm compact hand plate or a 1.5-mm miniplate, can be used, because the medial side of the carpus is under tension during weight-bearing, and the plate is more stable against bending along its broad axis. A 2.0-mm internal fixator could also be applied medially, although the 2.0-mm screws are relatively large for insertion into the thin metacarpal bones.

32.8 Pancarpal arthrodesis

Pancarpal arthrodesis is indicated for treatment of antebrachiocarpal injuries with damage to the palmar ligamentous support, comminuted fractures involving the radiocarpal joint surfaces, abrasion injuries with severe damage to the joint surface, and other non-reconstructable injuries of the radiocarpal joint. Infrequent indications are joint destruction by septic or immune-mediated arthritis. Pancarpal arthrodesis relieves pain and restores stability of the limb to allow weight-bearing, but it causes noticeable functional deficits and gait disturbances. The functional abnormalities are more disabling for cats as compared to dogs due to the restriction of pronation and supination motion. The carpus should be fused in about 15–20° of extension; the exact angle chosen should be dependent on comparative measurements of the weight-bearing contralateral carpus.

Pancarpal arthrodesis may also be performed in cats with radial nerve paralysis and an inability to extend the carpal joint and toes. The carpal joint should be fused in 20–30° of extension in such cases to prevent trauma to the toes (10). Patients must be selected carefully, as partial carpal arthrodesis only gives functional results if the function of the triceps muscle is preserved. It can help to observe the gait of the cat with the carpal joint stabilized in an extended position by an external splint prior to performing surgery.

Cross pinning (10), dorsal plating (11), and external skeletal fixation (12) have been suggested for panarthrodesis of the carpus in cats. Only the dorsal plating technique has been described in detail, including an anatomic study to evaluate suitable plate and screw size (11). Screw size is restricted by the size of the metacarpal bones and the authors suggested using a 1.5-mm miniplate (11). Screws with a diameter of 1.5 mm can also be inserted through a 2.0-mm dynamic compression plate (DCP) or a 1.5/2.0-mm veterinary cuttable plate. Cross pinning is a less stable fixation, carrying the risks of implant loosening and delayed fusion. Prolonged external coaptation is necessary if this method is chosen. Panarthrodesis with external skeletal fixation is a useful option, especially in the presence of open injuries.

Medial plating for pancarpal arthrodesis has recently been described in dogs (13), and can also be performed in cats. Medial plating has the advantage of the plate being less subject to bending forces and therefore less liable to break. More stability is achieved because the screws engage more bone material. Screw loosening is even less likely when an internal fixator is used, compared to a conventional 2.0-mm DCP. The 2.0-mm Unilock plate is a reconstruction plate

Box 32-2. Partial carpal arthrodesis

Adequate preparation of all intercarpal and carpometacarpal joint spaces is needed to achieve fusion, regardless of which stabilization method is used. Preparation of the joint spaces involves complete debridement of the articular cartilage and application of a bone graft. See Chapter 13 for grafting techniques and Chapter 14 for principles of arthrodesis.

Pinning technique: A dorsal approach to the carpal joints and metacarpal bones is used with a skin incision over the third metacarpal bone. The extensor carpi radialis tendon is preserved and the joint capsule of the antebrachiocarpal joint remains intact. Slots are drilled or burred into the mid- to distal diaphyseal area of metacarpus II and III. The slots have to be long enough to introduce 0.8–1.0-mm Kirschner wires into the medullary cavity and avoid inadvertent penetration of the transcortex. The Kirschner wires are advanced while the carpus is held in flexion until their tips emerge in the carpometacarpal joint. The medullary cavity of the metacarpal bones can be opened proximally by predrilling a hole from the proximal joint surface prior to pin insertion, which helps directing the pins. Cancellous bone graft is packed into the joints. The carpus is reduced, and the pins are advanced until they come to lie in the radial carpal bone, just below the radiocarpal joint surface (Fig. 32-10A). Position of the pins is verified by comparing the length of pin inserted with another pin of the same length. Curved mosquito forceps can be introduced into the antebrachiocarpal joint through a small incision in the joint capsule to feel for protruding pin tips if in doubt. The distal ends of the pins are bent and cut short.

Medial plating: A dorsomedial approach to the carpometacarpal joints and metacarpus II is performed. A five- or six-hole miniplate or internal fixator is contoured to the medial surface of the carpal bones and metacarpal bone II. The medial collateral ligament and the abductor pollicis longus tendon are preserved. The proximal phalanx of the first digit can be removed if it interferes with plate position, and part of it can be used as bone graft. The first screw is inserted into the radial carpal bone. The distal carpal joints are reduced and a screw is inserted into the base of the metacarpal bones. Distraction between the metacarpal bones must be avoided during insertion of the first screw. One screw should engage the distal row of carpal bones. The distal holes of the plate overlying the second metacarpal bone are filled, aiming the screws slightly towards dorsal (Fig. 32-10B).

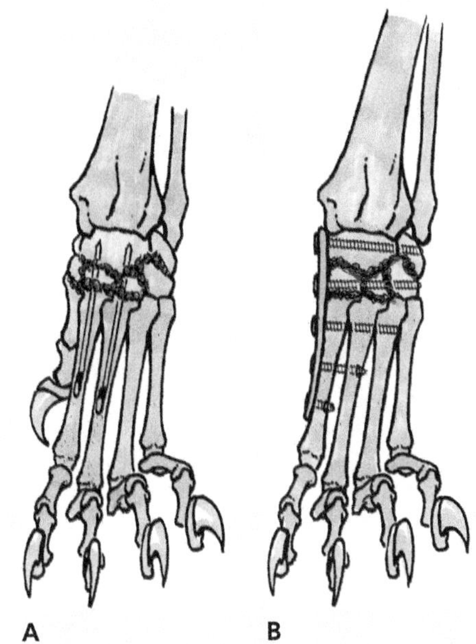

Figure 32-10 Two techniques for partial carpal arthrodesis. (**A**) Partial carpal arthrodesis with the pinning technique. The pins are inserted into the metacarpal bones II and III. Their tips engage the radial carpal bone, and are ideally located just below the proximal joint surface of the radial carpal bone. (**B**) Partial carpal arthrodesis with a medially applied 1.5-mm miniplate. One screw is inserted into the radial carpal bone, one is inserted into the distal row of carpal bones, and three screws engage the metacarpals.

which facilitates contouring to the carpus. The advantage of using a 2.0-mm DCP is that 1.5-mm screws can be inserted into the small metacarpal bones and the radial diaphysis (Fig. 32-12).

Techniques for pancarpal arthrodesis in cats are described in Box 32-3.

32.9 Postoperative treatment and prognosis

External coaptation of the carpus is necessary in the postoperative period after primary repair of carpal injuries, and after partial or pancarpal arthrodesis. Techniques for apply-

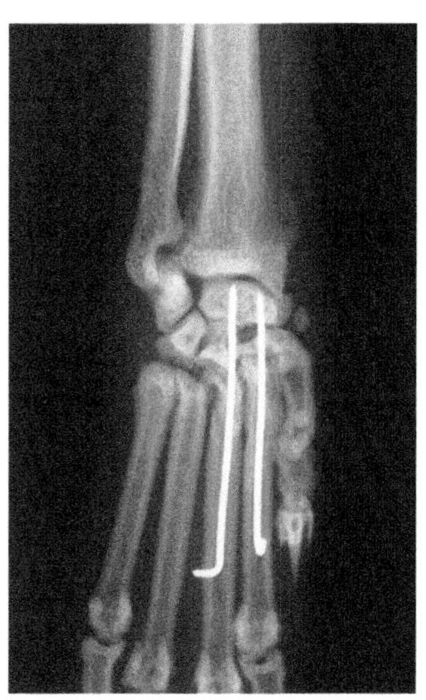

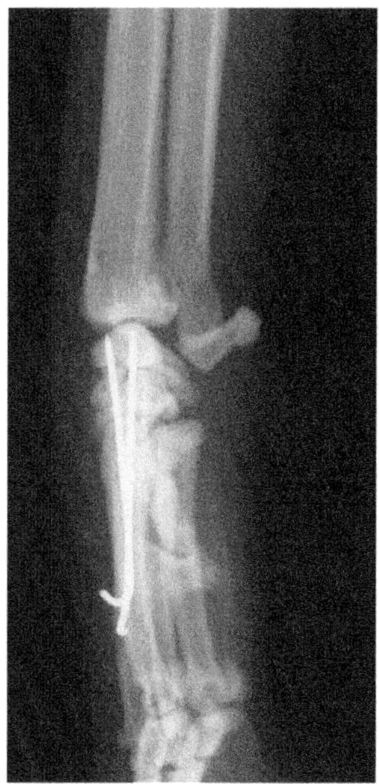

A B

Figure 32-11 (**A**) Dorsopalmar and (**B**) mediolateral radiographs following partial carpal arthrodesis of the cat in Figure 32-7 with carpometacarpal hyperextension injury. The tips of the 0.8-mm pins are nicely seated in the radial carpal bone.

ing bandages and splints are described in Chapter 22. Bandages and splints should be changed weekly to be able to check for the development of pressure sores and skin irritation.

32.9.1 Primary repair of carpal injuries

The healing of ligaments is slow. It takes several weeks until the resistance to tensional forces is sufficient to withstand full weight-bearing. External coaptation is used to protect the surgical repair of ruptured ligaments, until periarticular scar tissue has been built up sufficiently to provide some intrinsic stability. The duration of external coaptation depends on stability achieved during surgery and postoperative activity of the cat and anticipated healing time. After surgical repair of medial collateral ligament sprains, 2–3 weeks of external immobilization is usually adequate. After repair of complex carpal injuries, such as complete antebrachiocarpal luxation and luxation of the radial carpal bone, 3–4 weeks are needed. Although a splinted bandage does not provide absolute immobilization, it usually provides sufficient stability. A transarticular external skeletal fixator (Fig. 32-14) can be used if rigid immobilization is deemed necessary, and is also helpful in the presence of degloving wounds, when frequent bandage changes are necessary. The carpus should be immobilized for no longer than 4 weeks.

Carpal range of motion in flexion will be reduced after immobilization. Early passive physiotherapy is beneficial to preserve carpal range of motion. Physiotherapy can be conducted during bandage changes, and after the external coaptation has been removed. Some degree of carpal osteoarthritis is likely to develop after all injuries of the carpal joint, but functional outcome can be expected to be good after adequate reduction and stabilization of the joint (1, 2).

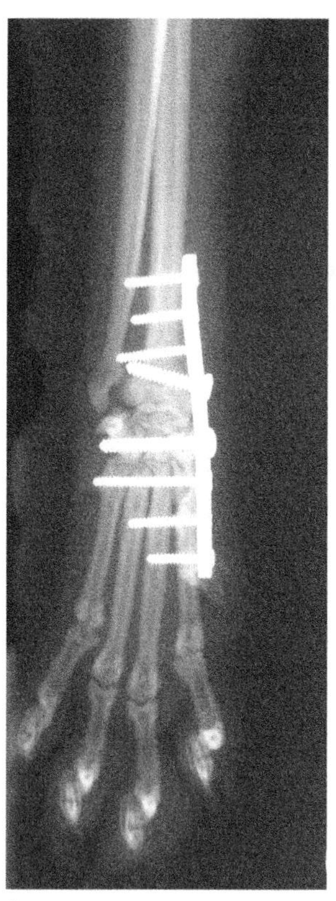

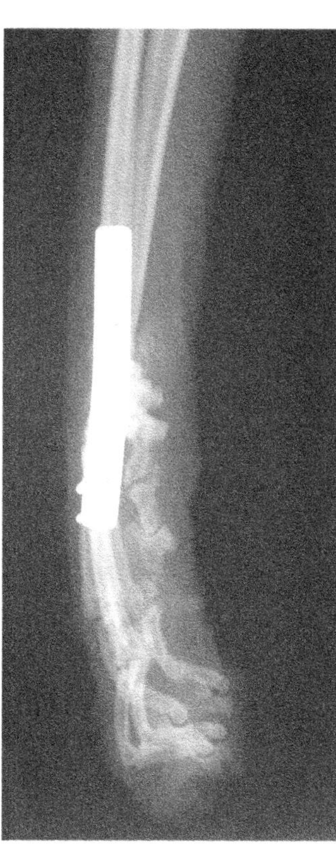

A B

Figure 32-12 (**A**) Example of a cat with pancarpal arthrodesis performed with a medially applied 2.0-mm dynamic compression plate, using both 2.0- and 1.5-mm screws. (**B**) The carpus could not be fused in more extension in this case due to contracture of the flexor muscles. Also note the slight radioulnar distraction due to the screw tips pushing the ulna away.

32.9.2 Partial carpal and pancarpal arthrodesis

External coaptation is provided with a splinted bandage for 4 weeks after partial carpal arthrodesis. Kirschner wires can be left in place if they are not migrating or causing other problems. It may be advantageous to remove plates used for partial carpal arthrodesis after fusion has occurred to minimize irritation of the medial aspect of the radiocarpal joint and periarticular structures.

Loss of range of motion in flexion is expected after partial carpal arthrodesis. The incidence of development of secondary radiocarpal degenerative joint disease is not known in cats, but around 15–30% of dogs develop degenerative joint disease in the radiocarpal joint (6, 7). Despite this, functional outcome seems good in most cases.

Box 32-3. Pancarpal arthrodesis

Successful pancarpal fusion requires preparation of all joint levels. The articular cartilage is completely debrided, and cancellous bone graft is inserted into the joint spaces. Cancellous or corticocancellous graft is additionally packed on to the dorsal joint surface and around the implants before wound closure. Grafting techniques are covered in Chapter 13, and principles of arthrodesis are further described in Chapter 14.

Dorsal plating: A dorsal approach to the carpal joint is used, and the extensor tendons are spared. After debridement of the joint surfaces, an eight-hole internal fixator or plate is contoured to the dorsal surface of the radius and the third metacarpal bone to give 15–20° of extension to the joint: 2.0-mm screws are used in the radial metaphysis and the radial carpal bone, and 1.5-mm screws distal to that. The first screw is inserted into the radial carpal bone, followed by one screw in the third metacarpal bone and one in the distal radius. If alignment is satisfactory, the other screw holes are filled (Fig. 32-13A).

Medial plating: A medial approach to the carpal joint is performed. The proximal phalanx of the first digit is removed to achieve a flat surface for plate application. It can be used as additional bone graft. The articular cartilage is debrided from all joints. An eight-hole internal fixator or plate is bent 10° longitudinally and contoured to the medial surface. Twisting the plate proximally and distally to apply it on the caudomedial surface of the radius and metacarpal bones, respectively, gives additional degrees of carpal extension. A 2.0-mm screw is inserted first into the radial carpal bone, ideally also engaging the ulnar carpal bone. The plate is then secured to the radius and the metacarpal bones with one screw each. If alignment is considered appropriate, the remaining screw holes are filled (Fig. 32-13B). Then 2.0-mm screws can be

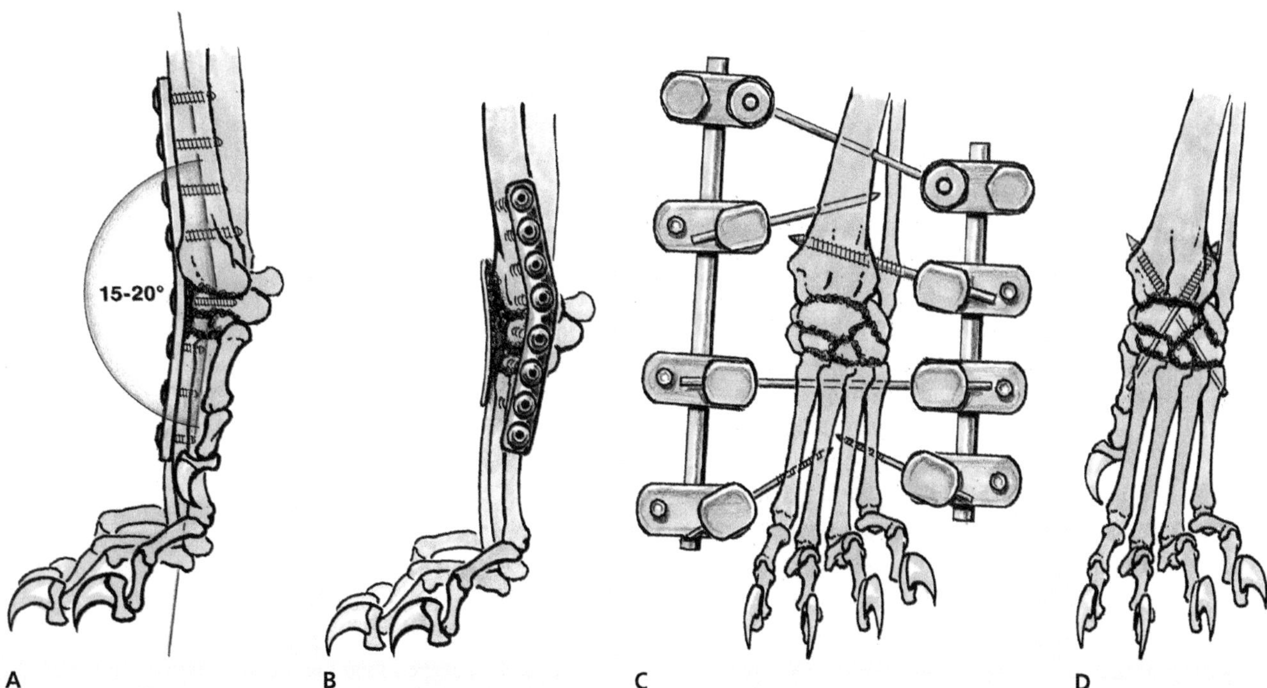

Figure 32-13 Different techniques for pancarpal arthrodesis.
(**A**) Pancarpal arthrodesis with a dorsally applied eight-hole 2.0-mm dynamic compression plate (DCP): 1.5-mm screws are used in the metacarpal bones. The carpal joint is fused with 15–20° of extension.
(**B**) Pancarpal arthrodesis with a medially applied eight-hole 2.0-mm DCP: 1.5-mm screws are inserted into the metacarpal bones and the radial diaphysis in a slight dorsal direction.
(**C**) Pancarpal arthrodesis with external skeletal fixation. Full pins are placed across the radius and base of the metacarpal bones. At least two additional small half pins are added both proximally and distally.
(**D**) Pancarpal arthrodesis with cross pins. Positive-threaded 1.6-mm pins can be used in large cats. The pins must cross each other distal to the radiocarpal joint surface to give enough rotational stability.

inserted into the radial metaphysis, and 1.5-mm screws are used for the radial diaphysis and the metacarpal bones. The screws are directed in a slight cranial and dorsal direction. The ulna should not be engaged with the screws to allow movement of the radioulnar joint, necessary for pronation and supination.

External skeletal fixator: Panarthrodesis of the carpus using external skeletal fixation is indicated in the presence of open and contaminated carpal injuries. A type II frame is applied to the distal radius and metacarpal bones after preparation of the joint surfaces (Fig. 32-13C). One full pin is inserted into the radius, and one across the base of the metacarpal bones. Additional transfixation pins are added once the external bars have been connected to the full pins, holding the carpal joint in 15–20° of extension. Non-threaded pins are angled 70° to the long axis of the bones.

Cross pinning: After joint preparation and reduction, two 1.1–1.4-mm Kirschner wires are drilled from the base of both metacarpus II and IV into the distal radial metaphysis in cross-pinning fashion (Fig. 32-13D). Aiming devices help in directing the pins. Care is taken not to lose reduction during insertion of the pins. The pins should cross below the antebrachiocarpal joint level to achieve rotational stability. The pins should not enter the ulna, as rotational movement between the radius and ulna can cause pin loosening.

External coaptation is provided for 4–6 weeks after pancarpal arthrodesis. Plates can be removed once fusion of the carpal joint is completed in order to prevent iatrogenic fractures of the metacarpal bones or the radius at the plate ends (Fig. 32-15). Functional outcome for walking and running is good if an appropriate carpal position is achieved, and if the radioulnar joint has not been fused. However, some gait abnormalities may be noted and cats are restricted in their climbing and hunting activities.

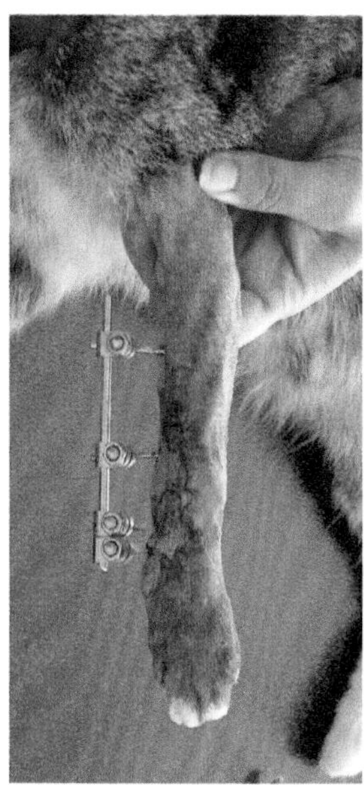

Figure 32-14 Photograph showing a medially applied transarticular external fixator immobilizing the carpus after primary repair of an antebrachiocarpal luxation. The fixator was left in place for 3 weeks.

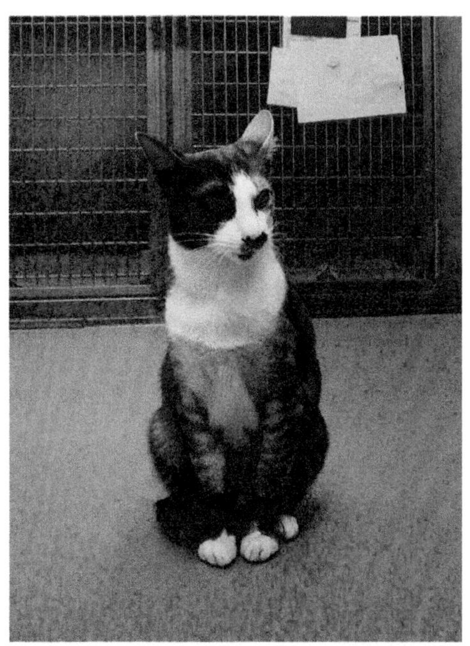

A

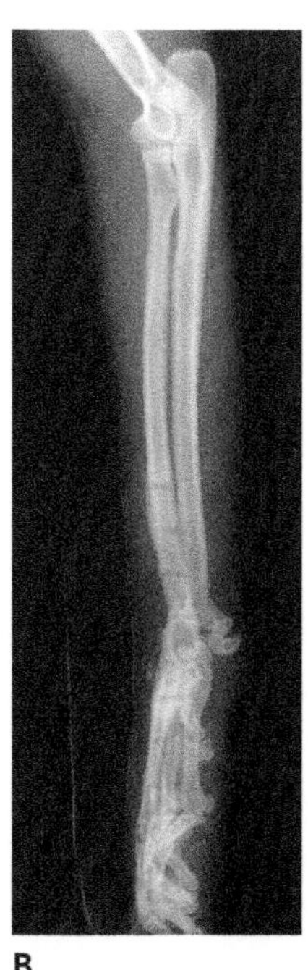

B

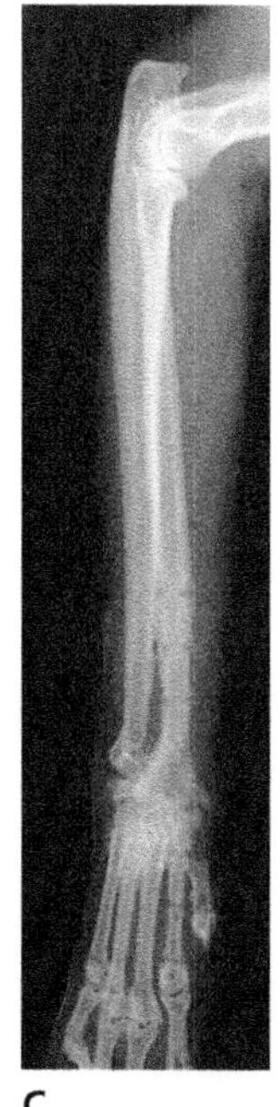

C

Figure 32-15 A cat 6 months after left pancarpal arthrodesis with a medial 2.0-mm Unilock plate.
(**A**) The cat before plate removal. The cat had good function of the limb with minimal gait abnormality.
(**B**) Mediolateral radiograph after plate removal. Arthrodesis is complete in all carpal joints.
(**C**) Dorsopalmar radiograph after plate removal. Note that the radioulnar joint is not fused, allowing some pronation and supination motion.

References and further reading

1. Voss K, et al. Antebrachiocarpal luxation in a cat: a case report and anatomical study of the medial collateral ligament. Vet Comp Orthop Traumatol 2003;16:266–270.
2. Shales CJ, Langley-Hobbs SJ. Dorso-medial antebrachiocarpal luxation with radio-ulna luxation in a domestic shorthair. J Feline Med Surg 2006;8:197–202.
3. Piermattei DL, Johnson KA. An atlas of surgical approaches to the bones and joints of the dog and the cat, 4th edn. Philadelphia: WB Saunders; 2004.
4. Pitcher GD. Luxation of the radial carpal bone in a cat. J Small Anim Pract 1996;37:292–295.
5. Piermattei DL, Flo GL. Fractures and other orthopedic conditions of the carpus, metacarpus, and phalanges. In: Piermattei DL, Flo GL (eds) Small animal orthopedics and fracture repair. Philadelphia: WB Saunders; 1997: pp. 344–389.
6. Willer RL, et al. Partial carpal arthrodesis for third degree carpal sprains – a review of 45 carpi. Vet Surg 1990;19:334–340.
7. Haburjak JJ, et al. Treatment of carpometacarpal and middle carpal joint hyperextension injuries with partial carpal arthrodesis using a cross pin technique: 21 cases. Vet Comp Orthop Traumatol 2003;16:105–111.
8. Slocum B, Devine T. Partial carpal fusion in the dog. J Am Vet Med Assoc 1982;180:1204–1208.
9. Johnson KA. Accessory carpal bone fractures in the racing greyhound: classification and pathology. Vet Surg 1987;16:60–64.
10. Denny HR, Butterworth S. A guide to canine and feline orthopedic surgery, 4th edn. London: Blackwell Scientific Publications; 2000.
11. Simpson D, Goldsmith S. Pancarpal arthrodesis in a cat: a case report and anatomical study. Vet Comp Orthop Traumatol 1994;7:45–50.
12. Kapatkin AS, Matthiesen DT. Feline high-rise syndrome. Compend Continuing Educ 1991;13:1389–1394.
13. Guerrero TG, Montavon PM. Medial plating for carpal panarthrodesis. Vet Surg 2005;34:153–158.

33 Metacarpus, metatarsus, and phalanges

S.J. Langley-Hobbs, K. Voss, P.M. Montavon

Metacarpal and metatarsal fractures account for only 2% of feline fractures (1). Motor vehicle accidents and falls from a height are the most common causes. Concurrent soft-tissue injuries are often encountered. Motor vehicle accidents can cause degloving injuries, and encounters with lawnmowers and harvesting machinery often result in grade III open fractures and luxations, or even traumatic amputation of parts of the digits. Such injuries can be severe enough to result in critical disruption of the vascularity of the foot. The treatment of degloving injuries is described in Chapter 16. Fractures or luxations of toes can also occur after minor injury.

External coaptation is a commonly used and adequate method for the treatment of selected metacarpal, metatarsal, and phalangeal fractures, but internal fixation is preferred in some cases. Miniaturized implants are necessary to stabilize the tiny bones. Amputation of a digit is a useful salvage procedure if other treatments fail to achieve a functional outcome (Chapter 41).

The paws may also be affected by diseases of the claws, clawbeds, or footpads. These conditions are summarized in Chapter 7.

33.1 Surgical anatomy

The metacarpal, metatarsal, and phalangeal bones and joints are highly functional despite their small size. They are numbered I–V from medial to lateral. Only digits II–V are weight-bearing. Digit I is missing on the hindlimb, where it is only present as a small rudimentary piece of bone. The third digit is the longest one in the forelimb in cats. The metacarpal and metatarsal bones articulate with the distal carpal bones and distal tarsal bones proximally, and with the proximal phalanges distally. They have a growth plate distally, which closes between 29 and 40 weeks of age (2). The growth plates of the phalangeal bones close between 16 and 22 weeks of age (2). The distal phalanx (P3) ends in the claw. The claws of the second to fifth toe are retracted into the skin fold and are positioned dorsolateral to the middle phalanx when the cat is standing. This is caused by a special elastic ligament, which runs from the lateral surface of the middle phalanx to the extensory process of the distal phalanx.

The metacarpophalangeal, metatarsophalangeal, and interphalangeal joints have collateral ligaments that are important for joint stability. Paired sesamoid bones are present at the palmar and plantar surface of the metacarpophalangeal and metatarsophalangeal joints II–V. These serve as a gliding and pressure bed for the digital flexor tendons. Small cartilaginous bodies are located in the dorsal joint capsule of the metacarpophalangeal, metatarsophalangeal, and interphalangeal joints. Those of the metacarpophalangeal and metatarsophalangeal joint can ossify and are then visible on radiographs.

33.2 Stabilization techniques

Metacarpal, metatarsal, and phalangeal fractures can be treated with either external coaptation alone or with internal stabilization, often combined with external coaptation. The decision on what method to use to stabilize metacarpal, metatarsal, and phalangeal fractures depends on how many digits are fractured, and on fracture configuration and location. Table 33-1 provides a general overview on possible fixation techniques. No strict rules exist for the choice of whether to use conservative or surgical treatment, but, as a general rule, fractures of more than two metacarpi, metatarsi, or phalanges and grossly displaced fractures are treated surgically.

The presence of open wounds or extensive soft-tissue bruising and swelling also has an influence on treatment choice. Severe soft-tissue injuries can markedly complicate treatment and postoperative care, and often prolong hospitalization time and treatment costs. If viability of one or several toes is questionable at the time of admission, the wounds are minimally debrided, flushed, and treated with wet-to-dry splinted bandages, until demarcation of devitalized tissue is obvious, allowing definitive debridement and selective excision of dead tissue (Chapter 16). Care has to be taken not to bandage too tightly to keep blood vessels patent, and avoid pressure necrosis. In some cases, a small external skeletal fixator can be applied to provide temporary stability, until definitive repair can be performed. Survival of the footpads is essential for function of the digits or paw. Necrosis of the footpads or entire toe often requires amputation of the affected digit. Amputation of the toes is described in Chapter 41.

33.2.1 Intramedullary pinning

Intramedullary pinning of fractures of the metacarpal and metatarsal bones is commonly used, as implants are

Table 33-1. Fractures and luxations occurring in the metacarpi, metatarsi, and phalanges, and possible treatment options

Localization of lesion	Type of lesion	Treatment options
Metacarpal and metatarsal fractures	Base of metacarpus and metatarsus	Conservative Tension band repair (II or V)
	Diaphysis	Conservative IM pin Miniplate
	Supracondylar and physeal	Conservative Cross pins
	Intercondylar	Transcondylar lag screw Conservative (if reconstruction is not possible) Amputation (if lameness persists)
Phalangeal fractures	Non-articular	Conservative Cross pin Miniplate
	Articular	Transcondylar lag screw Conservative (if reconstruction is not possible) Amputation (if lameness persists)
Metatarsophalangeal, metacarpophalangeal, and interphalangeal	Luxation	Closed reduction Open reduction and ligament prosthesis

IM pin, intramedullary pin.

inexpensive and readily available. Intramedullary pins provide bending stability, but no axial compression or rotational stability. They are used to repair simple fractures, where the fracture ends prevent axial collapse of the bone. Rotational stability is not as essential as in other long bones, because the adjacent digits help restrict movement. Small pins must be used because of the narrow intramedullary canal, especially at the base of the metacarpals. Small pins are also more flexible, facilitating pin insertion. Kirschner wires with a diameter of 0.8 or 0.9 mm are generally appropriate for metacarpal bones, and 0.9–1.2-mm pins can be used in the metatarsal bones. The abaxial metatarsal bones (II and V) are narrower than the axial bones (III and IV) so different-sized pins should be used to obtain the optimal diameter pin for each bone.

The intramedullary pins can be inserted in two ways: either normograde, from distal to proximal (Fig. 33-1), or as toggle pins (Fig. 33-2). The entry point for normograde insertion is at the dorsal and distal aspect of the metacarpus or metatarsus, just proximal to the condyle and at least 5 mm away from the fracture line. The pins have to be inserted as parallel as possible to the intramedullary canal to avoid penetration of the transcortex and inadvertent exit caudally. This is facilitated by burring a longitudinal slot into the dorsal cortex for the pin entry point, and by bending the tip of the pin slightly towards dorsal (Fig. 33-1). The pin is then advanced proximally across the fracture until it is seated in the base of the bone.

An alternative technique is toggle pinning, or intramedullary pinning with distraction (3) (Fig. 33-2). It is technically easier and faster to perform than conventional intramedullary pinning, and is mainly used for distally located fractures. The pins are left completely encased in bone and are therefore difficult to retrieve if this became necessary. The pin is first placed into the proximal intramedullary canal. It is then cut, with about 0.5–1.5 cm left protruding from the medullary canal, depending on the length of the distal fragment. The fracture is distracted and the distal fragment is carefully levered on to the protruding pin tip (Fig. 33-2). If it is not possible to reduce the fracture on to the pin, then the pin can be gradually shortened until this is possible. It is important not to force the end of the bone on to the pin, as fissuring can occur. The careful use of a small mosquito hemostat as a bone holder can facilitate fracture reduction.

33.2.2 Screws and plates

Isolated screws are rarely used, except when they are applied as lag screws across oblique fractures or condylar fractures. The small size of the metacarpal and metatarsal bones only allows insertion of screw sizes of 1.5 mm or smaller.

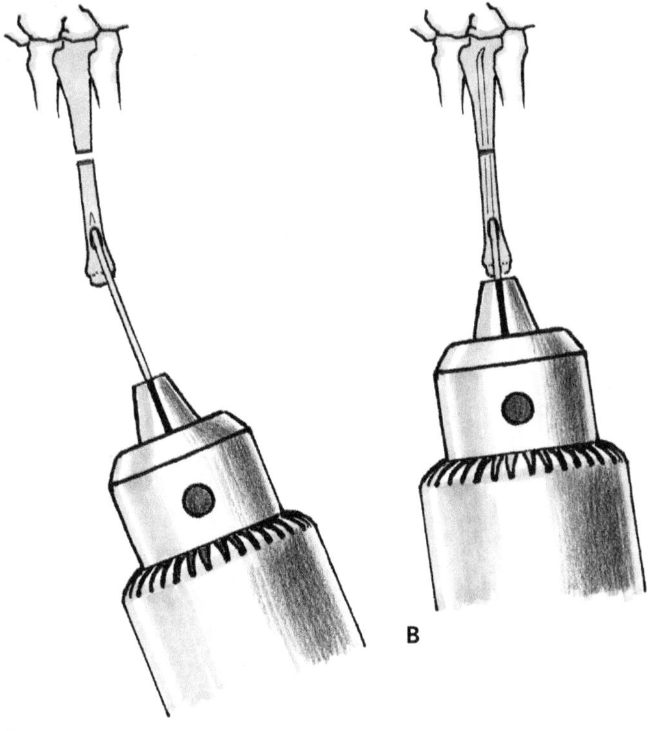

Figure 33-1 Normograde intramedullary pinning of a metacarpal or metatarsal bone.
(**A**) A slot can be burred into the dorsal cortex of the metacarpus or metatarsus to facilitate insertion of the pin. The entry point of the pin is at least 5 mm, but preferably further away from the fracture site. The tip of the pin is slightly bent towards dorsal before insertion.
(**B**) The tip of the pin is advanced across the fracture and is seated in the base of the metacarpal or metatarsal bone. The pin is cut short.

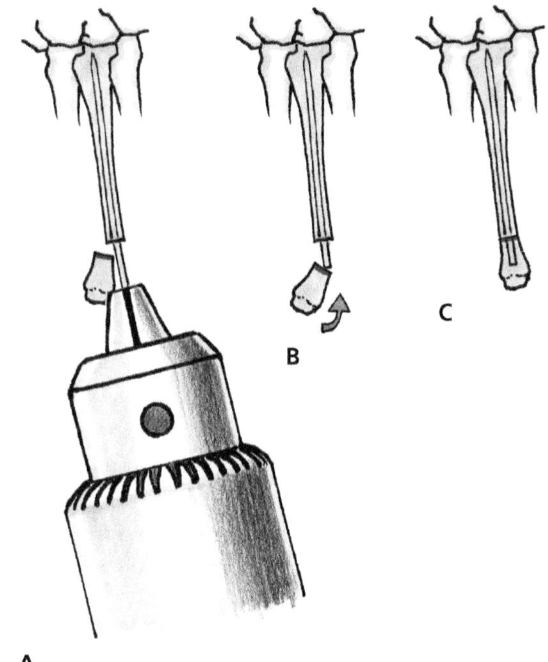

Figure 33-2 Toggle pinning of a distal metacarpal or metatarsal fracture.
(**A**) The pin is inserted into the proximal medullary canal.
(**B**) The protruding pin is cut to a length of approximately 5 mm. The distal fragment is carefully levered on to the protruding pin tip using traction on the digits. Mosquito forceps can be used as bone holders on the proximal and distal bone fragments.
(**C**) Completed toggle pin.

Plate osteosynthesis can be used for simple and comminuted diaphyseal fractures of the metacarpus and metatarsus. Miniaturized plate systems, such as the 1.5-mm miniplate, the 1.3-mm compact hand plate, and the 1.0-mm maxillofacial miniplate can be applied (Chapter 24). The plates are applied dorsally on the flat surface of the bone. At least two screws must be inserted per fragment. Plate positioning on the dorsal side has the disadvantage of the plate being located on the compression side of the bone. The weak 1.0-mm maxillofacial miniplates are therefore only suitable for simple and anatomically reduced fractures. Stabilization of comminuted fractures is performed with the 1.3- or 1.5-mm plates.

33.3 Fractures of the metacarpal and metatarsal bones

Fractures of the metacarpus and metatarsus can be classified into fractures of the base, the diaphysis, and the head. Fractures of the base usually affect the metacarpus or metatarsus II or V. Fractures of the diaphysis and/or head tend to involve several or even all four weight-bearing bones. Fracture of all four bones is also called a serial metacarpal or metatarsal fracture.

33.3.1 Approaches to the metacarpal and metatarsal bones

The bones are usually approached via a straight or curved dorsal skin incision. The skin edges can be retracted medially and laterally to access adjacent metacarpal bones. The extensor tendons are spared and carefully retracted. A more localized incision is made over the affected bone if only one bone is fractured. When plates are used, it is preferable that the skin incision is not directly located over the implant to minimize the chance of wound dehiscence.

33.3.2 Fractures of the base of metacarpals and metatarsals II or V

The bases of the metacarpals and metatarsals II and V are the insertion sites for the short medial and lateral carpometacarpal and tarsometatarsal ligaments, and the tendon of the lateral ulnar muscle, and peroneus brevis muscle, respec-

Box 33-1. Stabilization of an avulsion fracture of the base of metacarpus and metatarsus II or V

A lateral or medial approach to the base of metacarpus or metatarsus II or V is performed. The avulsed fragment is reduced and stability of the joint is assessed with the fragment in reduction.

Tension band fixation: A 0.8–1.0-mm Kirschner wire is inserted from the proximal aspect of the avulsed base into the medullary canal of the diaphysis. A 0.5- or 0.6-mm piece of orthopedic wire is then placed in a figure-of-eight wire pattern around the protruding proximal pin end, and through a hole drilled into the shaft. The protruding end of the Kirschner wire is bent over to avoid migration, and is cut short (Fig. 33-3A).

Lag screw: A 1.5-mm lag screw is inserted from the avulsed fragment, perpendicular to the fracture, into the transcortex (Fig. 33-3B). Two metacarpal or metatarsal bones can be incorporated to enhance pull-out resistance. With small fragments, it may be safer to use pointed reduction forceps to achieve reduction and compression, and then place a positional screw. This avoids the need to drill the larger glide hole for the lag screw.

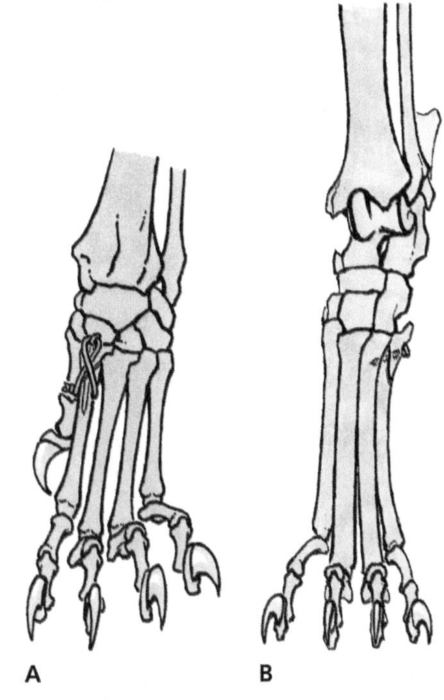

Figure 33-3 Stabilization of fractures of the base of metacarpal or metatarsal bone II or V.
(**A**) Tension band fixation of an avulsion fracture of the second metacarpal bone.
(**B**) Screw stabilization of an avulsion fracture of the fifth metatarsal bone.

tively. Avulsion fractures of the base of metacarpus or netatarsus II and V are therefore often associated with joint instability. Such injuries are rare in cats, and occur more commonly in the hindlimb. Undisplaced fractures with a stable joint can be treated conservatively with a splinted bandage. Displacement of the avulsed fragment and concurrent carpometacarpal or tarsometatarsal instability are indications for surgical stabilization. A tension band fixation or a 1.5-mm lag screw can be used to reattach larger fragments (Box 33-1). A partial carpal or tarsal arthrodesis needs to be performed if the fragment is too small to be reattached, and joint instability is present (Chapters 32 and 40).

33.3.3 Fractures of the shaft

Diaphyseal fractures of only one or two metacarpal or metatarsal bones are usually treated conservatively. The adjacent intact bones allow weight-bearing, and act as an internal splint. If possible, the fractures are reduced in a closed manner when displaced, and a splinted bandage is applied to the level of the distal third of the radius or tibia. The splint is usually required for 3–4 weeks, depending on fracture type and stability, and age of the cat. Principles and techniques for application of a splinted bandage are described in Chapter 22. Open reduction and internal fixation are indicated if there is significant fragment displacement, and closed reduction is not possible.

Although no difference in healing rates between conservative and surgical treatment was reported in dogs (4, 5), surgery is usually preferred if three or all four metacarpal or metatarsal bones are fractured. Fractures of all four bones are unstable injuries, and have a tendency for fracture union disorders, and malunion in a valgus position if not treated surgically (4, 6). Distal and mid-diaphyseal fractures as opposed to proximal fractures are more likely to be displaced and to heal with malunion (Fig. 33-4), so the level of the fracture should also be considered when deciding whether to treat surgically (4).

It is not always necessary to stabilize all four bones, but at least two of the bones should be treated to allow weight-bearing. In older cats with slower fracture healing, or if other limbs are also traumatized, it is advantageous to perform internal fixation of three or all of the bones. The decision on which and how many bones to stabilize depends on fracture types and soft-tissue trauma. If both simple and comminuted fractures are present, it is easier, less invasive, and provides more stability to stabilize the simple fractures, and leave the comminuted metacarpals or metatarsals. Internal implants should also be avoided in fractures in areas with open wounds.

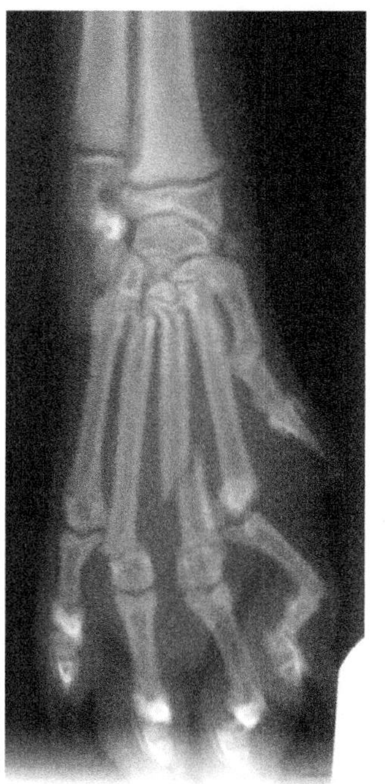

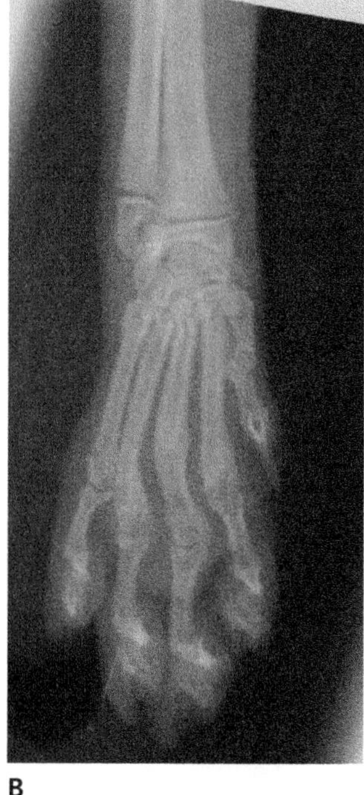

A B

Figure 33-4 (**A**) Radiographs of a 7-month-old cat with distal fractures of metacarpals III, IV, and V, treated with a splinted bandage for 4 weeks. (**B**) There is good fracture healing after 4 weeks with functional malunion.

Intramedullary pinning is most commonly used for simple fractures (Figs 33-5 and 33-6). Miniplates can be applied to the dorsal surface of the metacarpal bones for both simple and comminuted fractures. The small size of the bones only allows insertion of 1.5-mm or smaller screws. Plating of metatarsal fractures is easier than plating of metacarpal fractures, due to their larger size and flat dorsal surface (Fig. 33-7). Simple long oblique fractures can also be stabilized with 1.5-mm lag or positional screws. The surgical techniques are described in Box 33-2.

33.3.4 Fractures of the metacarpal and metatarsal heads

Fractures of the head of the metacarpal or metatarsal bones can be supracondylar, unicondylar, or comminuted. Salter and Harris fractures may occur in immature cats. Salter and Harris type I and II fractures are treated with cross pins. Cross pins can also be used for supracondylar fractures with a small distal fragment, but toggle pinning (Fig. 33-2) is preferred if the distal fragment is large enough to seat the pin.

Condylar fractures cause incongruity and instability of the metacarpophalangeal joints and should be treated surgically. They are stabilized with a 1.5-mm transcondylar screw in order to restore joint congruity. Although a lag screw is usually used for this purpose, it is safer to insert a positional

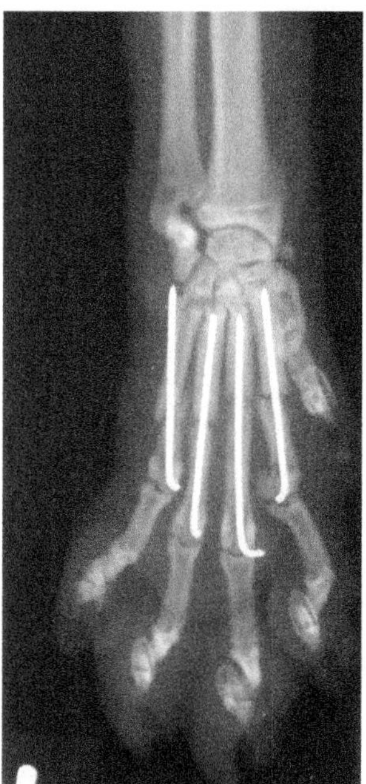

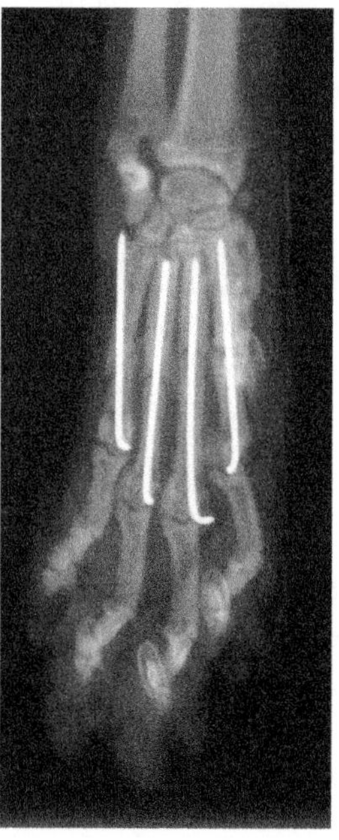

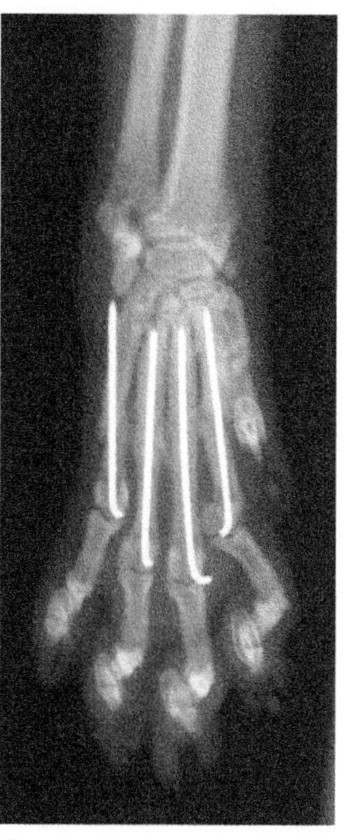

A B C

Figure 33-5 Radiographs of metacarpal non-unions in a 4-year-old cat with serial fractures that had been treated with external coaptation for 6 weeks. (**A**) Immediate postoperative film showing normograde intramedullary pinning of all four bones; the pin in metacarpal V inadvertently exited the bone in the proximal fragment. (**B**) At 4 weeks postoperatively, there is evidence of fracture healing and remodeling of the fracture sites in all four bones. (**C**) The 8-week postoperative films show that fracture healing is now nearly complete.

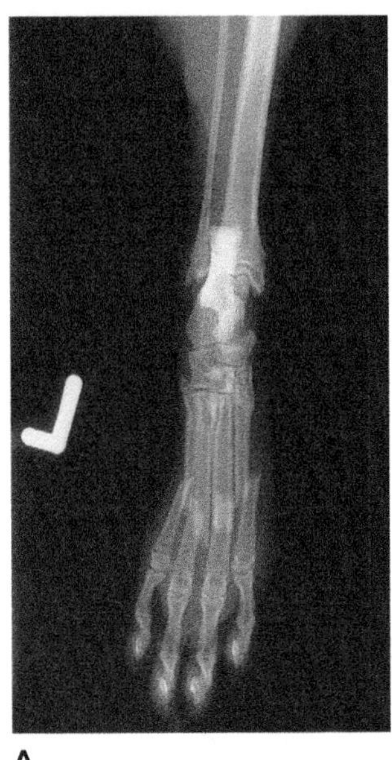
A

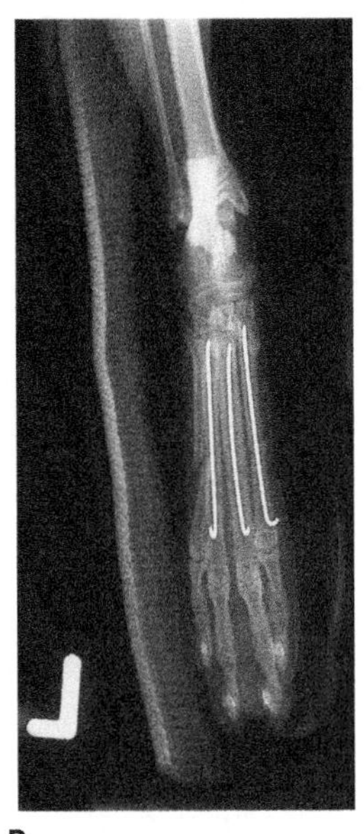
B

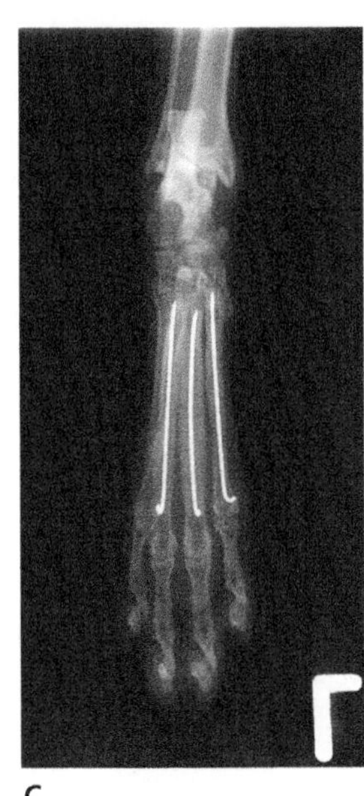
C

Figure 33-6 Example of intramedullary pinning of the metatarsal bones.
(**A**) Preoperative radiographs showing a serial fracture of the metatarsal diaphysis in an immature cat.
(**B**) Radiographs after intramedullary pinning of the metatarsal bones II–IV. Note that the pins enter the intramedullary cavity proximal to the growth plates.
(**C**) Follow-up radiograph 6 weeks later. All fractures are healed.

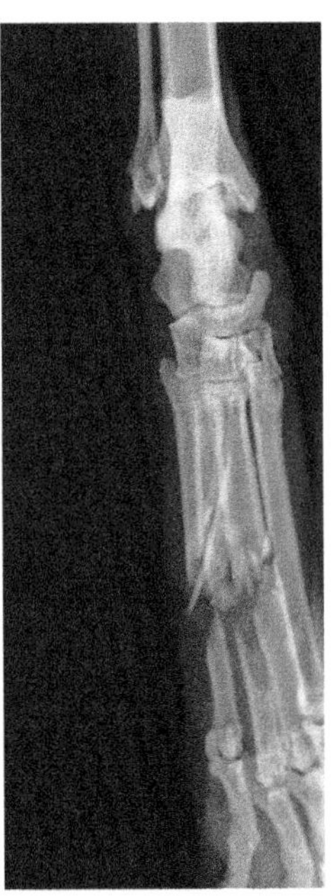
A

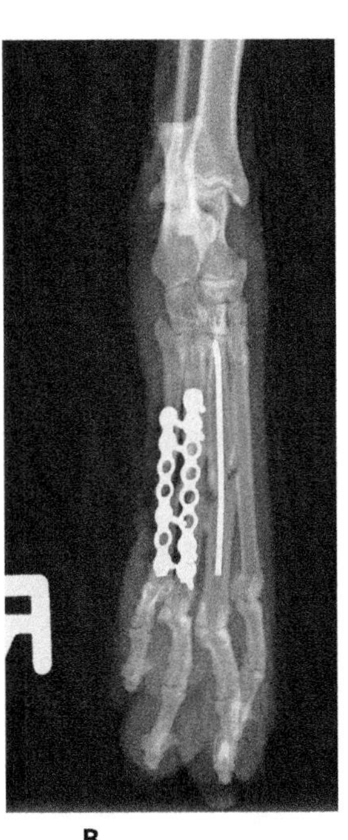
B

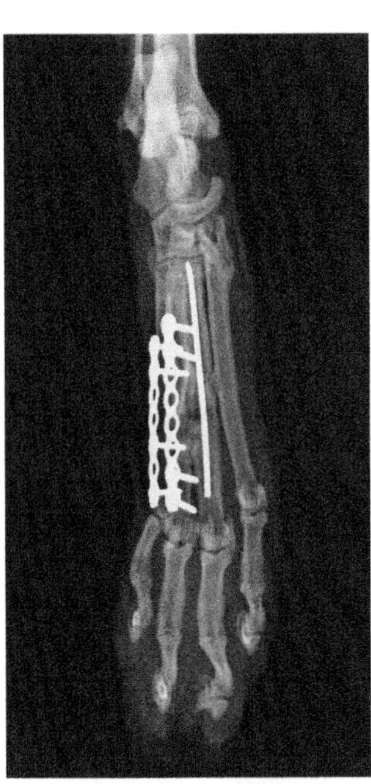
C

Figure 33-7 Radiographs of a cat with grade III open fractures of metatarsal (MT) bones III–V.
(**A**) The wound was treated with wet-to-dry bandages, and surgery was delayed until the area was covered with granulation tissue.
(**B**) MT III was stabilized with a toggle pin, MT IV and V with 1.3-mm compact hand plates. Cancellous bone graft was inserted in the gaps where bone was missing.
(**C**) The 4-week postoperative radiograph shows advanced fracture healing of MT III and IV. MT V went into atrophic non-union, but limb function was good.

screw after anatomic reduction and application of a small bone reduction forceps, to avoid iatrogenic fractures of the tiny piece of bone. A transcondylar screw is also used in comminuted intracondylar fractures, if possible. The supracondylar part can be left to heal with external coaptation when stabilization with cross pins is not feasible. Nonreconstructable comminuted joint fractures may necessitate amputation of the affected digit (Chapter 41). The surgical techniques are described in Box 33-3.

33.4 Fractures of the phalanges

Most fractures of the phalanges can be treated with external coaptation, because it is unusual for more than two digits to be affected. Open reduction and surgical stabilization are indicated for condylar fractures, and involve screw fixation as described above (Box 33-3). Displaced fractures of the phalangeal shaft may also benefit from internal stabilization. Mini screws and plates from the 1.0-mm maxillofacial or the

Box 33-2. Stabilization of diaphyseal metacarpal or metatarsal fractures

A dorsal approach is performed, and the skin and extensor tendons are retracted as needed. It may not be necessary to stabilize all fractured bones surgically, but at least two, and preferably three, metacarpals should be intact or stabilized. Displaced, simple, and axial fractures are preferentially stabilized. Comminuted fractures should be minimally handled to maintain the blood supply. Implants are avoided in areas with open wounds.

Intramedullary pinning: Normograde intramedullary pinning is used for simple mid-diaphyseal fractures of the metacarpals or metatarsals (Fig. 33-8A). A slot can be burred into the dorsal cortex of the distal metacarpus or metatarsus to facilitate insertion of the pin (Fig. 33-1). The entry point of the Kirschner wire is at least 5 mm away from the fracture site. A useful landmark site for pin placement is the small depression in the bone just proximal to the distal condyle. The tips of small flexible Kirschner wires can be bent or curved slightly, which aids pin placement up the medullary canal. When the pin exits the medullary canal at the fracture site, the fracture is reduced and the pin is advanced across the fracture and seated in the base of the metacarpus or metatarsus. The pin is cut short or is bent at the distal edge of the slot to prevent migration.

Toggle pinning: Toggle pinning is most useful for distal or proximal metacarpal and metatarsal fractures (Fig. 33-8B). The pin is inserted into the proximal medullary canal and seated in the base of the bone. The protruding end is cut short to 0.5–1.0 cm. The distal or proximal fragment is then gently levered on to the protruding pin tip using traction (Fig. 33-2).

Plating: Plating allows stabilization of both simple and comminuted fractures, but is more commonly used for comminuted fractures. The metatarsal bones are slightly broader than the metacarpal bones, so it is preferable to use 1.5-mm miniplates for the metatarsi; 1.3-mm compact hand plates can be used for the metacarpi (Fig. 33-8C and 33-8D). The plates are applied to the dorsal surface of the bones. At least two, and preferably three, screws should be inserted into the proximal and distal fragments.

Lag screw: A 1.5-mm lag screw can be used to treat a simple oblique fracture (Fig. 33-8D). Lag screw fixation does not provide much dorsopalmar bending stability, and is only used if other metacarpal bones are intact or stabilized with other implants.

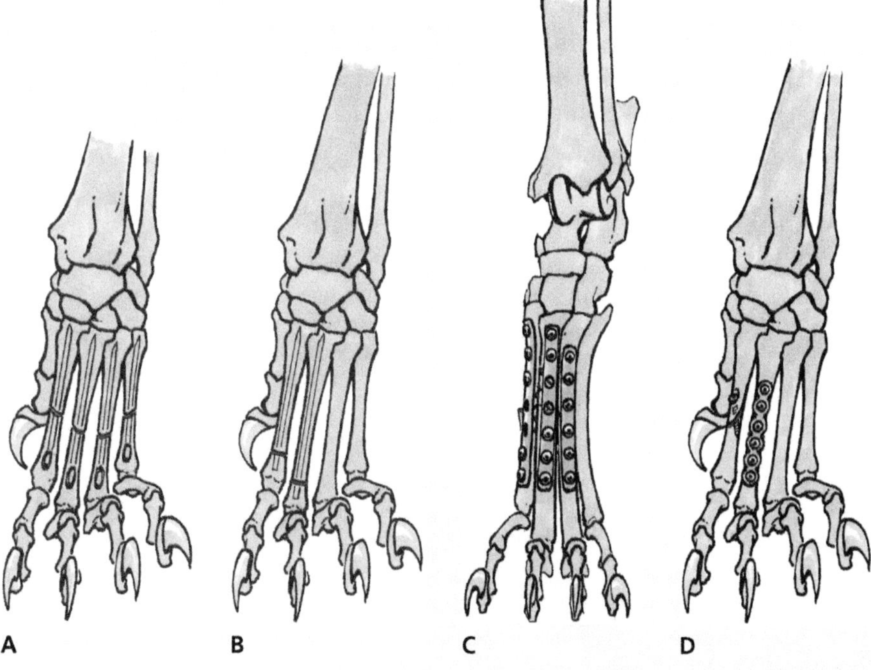

Figure 33-8 Options for stabilizing metacarpal and metatarsal fractures.
(**A**) Normograde intramedullary pinning of simple transverse mid-diaphyseal metacarpal fractures.
(**B**) Toggle pinning of simple transverse distal metacarpal fractures.
(**C**) Plate osteosynthesis of both simple and comminuted metatarsal fractures, using 1.5-mm miniplates.
(**D**) Screw fixation of a simple oblique fracture of the second metacarpal bone. The third metacarpal bone was stabilized with a 1.3-mm miniplate.

Box 33-3. Stabilization of fractures of the metacarpal, metatarsal, and phalangeal heads

A dorsal approach is performed, the joint capsule is opened longitudinally, and the fracture is reduced anatomically.

Cross pinning of Salter and Harris I and II or supracondylar fractures: The fracture is held in reduction manually. Two 0.6-mm Kirschner wires are inserted from the medial and the lateral condyle in a cross-pin fashion (Fig. 33-9A). Their ends are cut short.

Transcondylar screw for intercondylar fractures: The intercondylar fracture is temporarily compressed with small pointed bone reduction forceps in anatomic reduction. A 1.5-mm intercondylar positional screw is inserted (Fig. 33-9B).

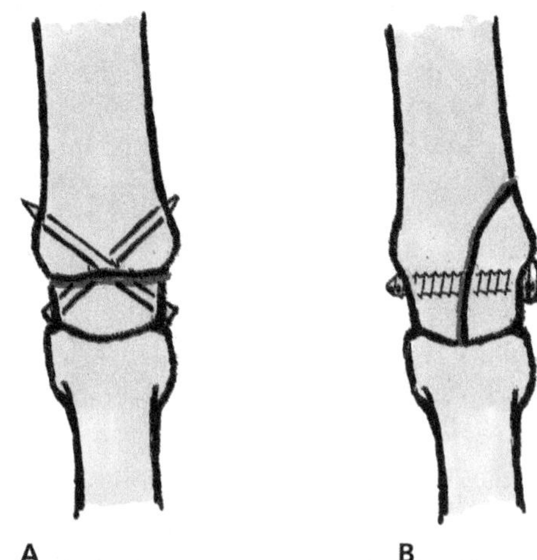

Figure 33-9 Stabilization of fractures of the metacarpal, metatarsal, or phalangeal head.
(**A**) Cross pinning of a Salter and Harris type I fracture.
(**B**) Fixation of a unicondylar fracture with a 1.5-mm positional screw.

1.3-mm compact hand system are used for the small fracture fragments. Amputation of the digit is a salvage procedure if fracture healing and pain-free function cannot be achieved by either conservative or surgical treatment (Chapter 41).

33.5 Metacarpophalangeal, metatarsophalangeal, and interphalangeal luxation

Metacarpophalangeal, metatarsophalangeal, and interphalangeal joint luxations are occasionally encountered, and can be accompanied by other fractures or joint injuries of the paw. Clinically, they should be suspected if pain and local swelling of one or more joints are detected. A pathological position of the affected toe is sometimes also seen (Fig. 33-10). Closed reduction and external coaptation are successful in most cases (Fig. 33-11). Surgical stabilization is indicated if closed reduction is not feasible, or if reluxation occurs. Surgery includes imbrication sutures of the joint capsule and ruptured collateral ligaments. A suture sling can be applied as a ligament prosthesis if the periarticular structures are impossible to suture, or if insufficient stability is achieved (Box 33-4).

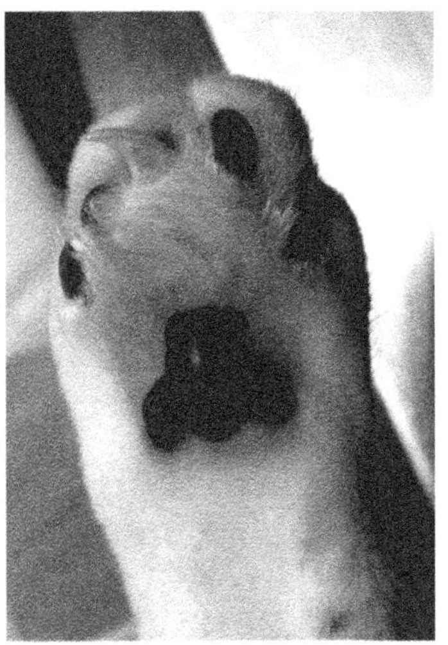

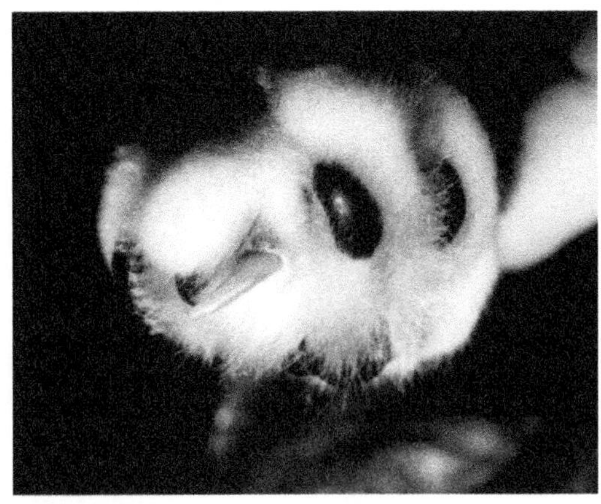

Figure 33-10 The foot of a cat with a P2/3 luxation. Note the 90° rotation of nail, visible from both the palmar (**A**) and the distal aspect (**B**). The joint was stable after closed reduction.

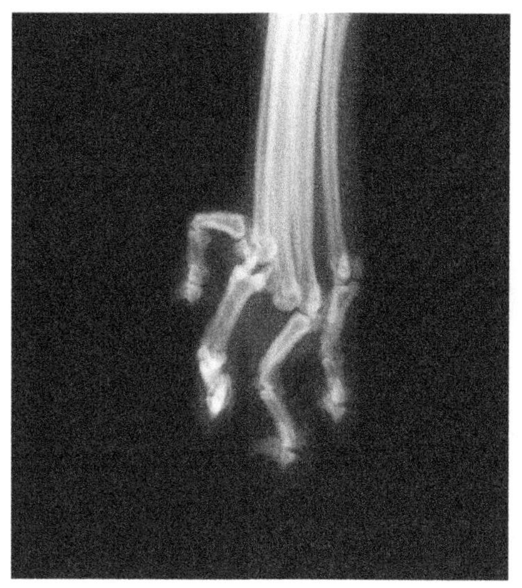
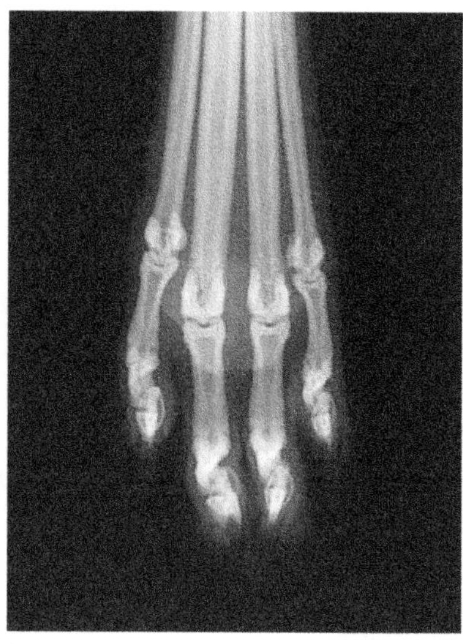

A B

Figure 33-11 (**A**) Radiographs of the left hindpaw of a cat with metatarsophalangeal luxation of the second and third digits. The joints were reduced in a closed manner, and a splinted bandage was applied for 10 days. (**B**) Follow-up radiographs 4 weeks later show maintenance of reduction.

33.6 Postoperative treatment and prognosis

The implants used for stabilization of metacarpal, metatarsal, and phalangeal fractures are too weak to allow early weight-bearing. A splinted bandage is therefore necessary in the postoperative period after most types of fracture fixation. The duration for external coaptation depends on the fixation stability achieved with surgery and on progression of healing, but usually ranges between 2 and 6 weeks: 2 weeks in young cats with stable fractures, 6 weeks in older cats with unstable fractures, such as comminuted metacarpal or metatarsal serial fractures. The presence of open wounds, such as degloving injuries, may markedly complicate postoperative treatment and enhance costs. Please also see Chapter 16 for treatment of concurrent soft-tissue injuries.

Progressive fracture healing usually occurs irrespective of stabilization method, if the surrounding soft tissues are not severely traumatized and avascular. More than 80% of metacarpal or metatarsal fractures treated with toggle pinning healed without complications in a recent study (3). Complications are most likely to occur with conservative treatment of fractures of three or all four metacarpal bones, and include delayed union or non-union (Fig. 33-13), and malunion. Non-unions need to be treated surgically with stable internal fixation and application of a bone graft. Malunions tend to occur in a valgus position. They do not require revision if functional outcome is good (Fig. 33-4). Fracture alignment was consistently improved by open reduction and internal fixation of acute fractures with bone plates in dogs (4).

Box 33-4. Ligament prosthesis for metacarpophalangeal, metatarsophalangeal, and interphalageal joint luxation

A dorsal approach to the affected joint is performed. Holes are drilled through the articular condyles with a small drill bit or Kirschner wire. A size 2-0 or 0 nonabsorbable suture is inserted through the holes. Hypodermic needles can be helpful to guide the suture through the bone. The joint is reduced and, if feasible, the joint capsule is sutured. The ligament prosthesis is tightened (Fig. 33-12).

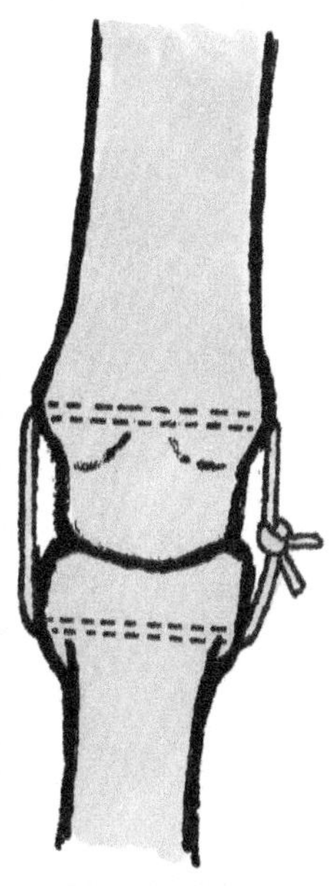

Figure 33-12 Appearance of a ligament prosthesis for stabilization of a metacarpophalangeal, metatarsophalangeal, or interphalangeal luxation.

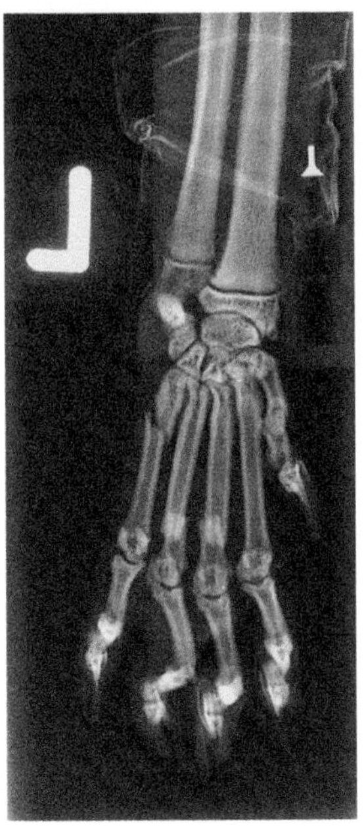

A

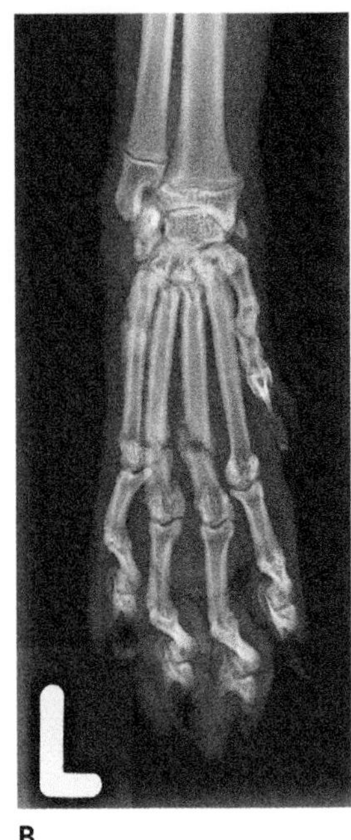

B

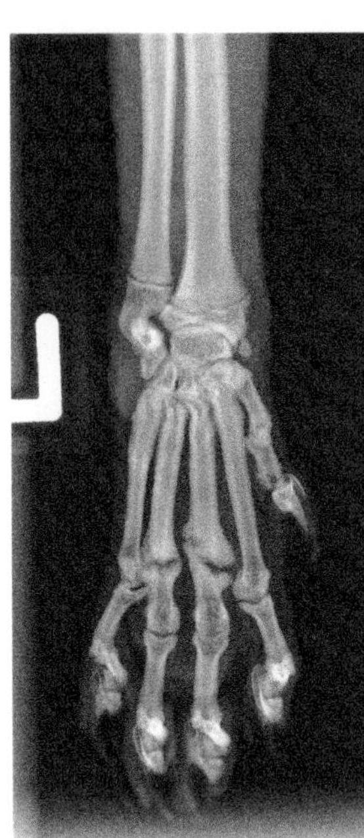

C

Figure 33-13 (**A–C**) Serial radiographs of a 9-month-old cat with fractures of metacarpals III, IV, and V, treated with a splinted bandage. Metacarpus V was healed well after 6 weeks, but hypertrophic non-unions developed in the metacarpal bones III and IV, indicating instability (**C**). Internal stabilization with toggle pins for these distal fractures would have been a better option.

References and further reading

1. Hill FWG. A survey of bone fractures in the cat. J Small Anim Pract 1977;18:457–463.
2. Smith RN. Fusion of ossification centres in the cat. J Small Anim Pract 1969;10:523–530.
3. Degasperi B, et al. Intramedullary pinning of metacarpal and metatarsal fractures in cats using a simple distraction technique. Vet Surg 2007;36:382–388.
4. Muir P, Norris JL. Metacarpal and metatarsal fractures in dogs. J Small Anim Pract 1997;38:344–348.
5. Kapatkin AS, et al. Conservative versus surgical treatment of metacarpal and metatarsal fractures in dogs. Vet Comp Orthop Traumatol 2000;3:123–127.
6. Piermattei DL, Flo GL. Fractures and other orthopedic conditions of the carpus, metacarpus, and phalanges. In: Piermattei DL, Flo GL (eds) Small animal orthopedics and fracture repair. Philadelphia: WB Saunders; 1997: pp. 344–389.

34 The spine

K. Voss, P.M. Montavon

Surgical conditions of the spine include spinal fractures and luxations, disc disease, spinal tumors, and miscellaneous conditions such as subarachnoid cysts or epidural empyema. Spinal fractures and luxations may be due to motor vehicle accidents, falls from a height, dog bites, and gunshot injury. Around half of cats with spinal injuries have concomitant trauma to other body systems and must undergo a thorough general clinical and radiological examination. Spinal injuries were negatively correlated with survival in one study evaluating radiographs of 100 consecutively traumatized cats (1). Although spinal stabilization procedures often have to be performed on an emergency basis, the patients should be well hydrated before induction of anesthesia. Careful evaluation and monitoring of cardiovascular and respiratory function are necessary in the peri- and postoperative period to avoid death of the patient (2, 3).

This chapter focuses mainly on the surgical treatment of spinal fractures and luxations. Decompressive procedures are also described. Interpretation of the neurological examination and diagnostic procedures are covered in Chapters 1 and 2 of this book. Diseases of the spine are summarized in Chapter 6. The reader is also referred to Chapter 15, where decision-making processes and principles of spinal surgery are described.

34.1 Surgical anatomy

The spine has seven cervical, 13 thoracic, seven lumbar vertebrae, the sacrum, and a variable number of coccygeal vertebrae. Cats have long and slender vertebral bodies with a thin and fragile dorsal and lateral lamina. With the exception of the atlantoaxial joint, an intervertebral disc is located between all the vertebral bodies. The spinous processes are connected to each other by the supra- and interspinous ligaments. These ligaments act as tension bands and contribute to spinal stability. They should be preserved during surgery.

The spinal cord consists of eight cervical, 13 thoracic, seven lumbar, three sacral, and approximately seven caudal segments. The spinal segments are located slightly cranial to their corresponding vertebrae, especially in the caudal lumbar spine, although the ascensus medullae is not as pronounced in cats as it is in dogs. The medullary cone of the spinal cord extends as far caudally as S1 in most cats (4, 5). Spinal nerves L7 and S1 originate at the level of the vertebral body of L5 or the L5–L6 junction, and spinal nerves S2 and S3 at the L5–L6 junction or at the level of L6 (4).

The spinal cord is wider at the cervical and lumbar intumescences, where the nerve roots for the front and hindlimbs arise. The nerve roots of C6–T2 form the brachial plexus supplying the front limbs, and the nerve roots of L4–S3 form the pelvic plexus supplying the hindlimbs, the bladder, the rectum, and the perineal region. The nerve roots exit the spinal canal at the cranial aspect of their corresponding foramen.

Vessels to preserve during surgery include the vertebral artery, running through the foramina of the transverse processes of the cervical spine, and the venous plexus, located bilaterally on the floor of the spinal canal. The venous plexus is a thin-walled vein, which is easily damaged during surgery.

34.2 Diagnosis and general considerations

The diagnosis of spinal diseases and injuries requires a thorough neurological examination, spinal radiographs, and often additional diagnostic imaging procedures. The clinical neurological examination should provide information on localization and severity of the lesion, therefore guiding the clinician as to which areas to focus on for imaging (Chapter 1). Diagnostic imaging procedures are required to confirm or diagnose specific diseases or injuries (Chapter 2). It should be remembered that it is not the radiological appearance of a spinal injury or disease but the severity of the preoperative neurological deficits that is relevant for the prognosis. Diseases of the spine and spinal cord are described in Chapter 6, and basic information on spinal injuries is covered in Chapter 15 of this book. The reader is also referred to Chapter 15 for radiological interpretation of spinal fractures and luxations.

Many cats with spinal fractures and luxations have sustained additional soft-tissue or orthopedic injuries (3). A thorough clinical examination of the thorax and abdomen and the skeletal system is necessary to diagnose these injuries. Life-threatening injuries are treated before addressing the spinal injury, but spinal surgery is performed as soon as possible to prevent further damage to the spinal cord.

34.3 Decompressive procedures

Decompressive procedures in general include dorsal laminectomy, hemilaminectomy, pediculectomy, ventral slot, and

Decompression procedure	Localization	Indications	Comments
Ventral slot	Cervical	Cervical disc	Creates instability; stabilization is advised
Hemilaminectomy	Cervical Thoracolumbar	Cervical disc Thoracolumbar disc Exploration of spinal canal after fractures/luxations Tumors	May cause instability with concurrent injury of the ventral compartment, requiring surgical stabilization
Pediculectomy	Thoracolumbar	Exploration of spinal canal after fractures/luxations Thoracolumbar disc	Does not create instability; limited exposure of spinal canal
Dorsal laminectomy	Lumbosacral Thoracolumbar	Lumbosacral disc Compression fractures of dorsal compartment Tumors	Facet joints are left intact At least one facet joint is left intact; surgical stabilization should be considered with fractures
Durotomy	Thoracolumbar	Diagnosis of myelomalacia Additional decompression in patients with severe deficits Intradural or subdural tumors	A wide hemilaminectomy is needed to perform a durotomy

Table 34-1. Spinal cord decompression techniques and their indications

durotomy. Localization of the lesion and type of spinal cord compression dictate the type of decompression surgery performed (Table 34-1). The most common indications for decompressive procedures in cats are intervertebral disc extrusion and neoplasia.

Anatomic reduction and stabilization of fractures and luxations often result in indirect decompression of the spinal cord by restoring the integrity of the spinal canal. A decompressive procedure is then only required if fracture fragments or disc material remain, compressing the spinal cord after reduction. Decompression as a single measure is only recommended for compression fractures of the dorsal or lateral lamina without additional injuries. The reader is also referred to Chapter 6 on diseases of the feline spine, and Chapter 15 on injuries of the feline spine, for further information.

34.4 Stabilization of spinal fractures/luxations

Surgical stabilization of spinal injuries is indicated in cats with neurological deficits, and cats with spinal instability. Conservative treatment should be reserved for patients without neurological deficits and with stable fractures. Stability of the spine can be difficult to judge on radiographs, but, in general, fractures with involvement of both the dorsal and ventral compartment and fractures with vertebral displacement should be considered unstable. Please also see Chapter 15 for further information on interpretation of radiographs.

The most common localization for spinal fractures and luxations in cats is the sacrococcygeal area (1). The lumbar spine is the next most commonly affected area, followed by the thoracolumbar junction (2, 3). Fractures and luxations involving the lumbosacral segment are less common, and fractures and luxations of the cervical spine are rare.

Dorsal stabilization methods with small and flexible pins and cerclage wire can be used for most spinal fractures, except for the cervical spine, where ventral stabilization with an internal fixator, plates or pins and bone cement is used (Table 34-2). Internal fixators or pins and bone cement can also be useful for stabilizing fractures in the lumbosacral area of the spine, where the small spinous processes render dorsal stabilization methods difficult.

34.5 Surgical conditions of the cervical spine

Surgical conditions of the cervical spine are rare in cats. They mainly include cervical disc disease, cervical spinal fractures and luxations, and possibly tumors of the cervical spine. See Chapter 6 for more information on diseases of the spine and spinal cord.

34.5.1 Approaches to the cervical spine

The cervical spine can be approached from dorsally, laterally, and ventrally, depending on the type of surgery to be performed. The ventral approach to the vertebral bodies and

Table 34-2. Localization and types of spinal fractures and luxations, and stabilization methods

Localization of lesion	Type of lesion	Treatment options
Cervical spine	All unstable fracture/luxations	Ventral internal fixator Ventral plate Screws and PMMA
Thoracolumbar spine	All unstable fracture/luxations	Spinal stapling Tension band repair Dorsal internal fixator
Lumbar spine	All unstable fracture/luxations	Tension band repair Dorsal internal fixator
Lumbosacral spine	L7 fractures	Transilial pin Dorsal internal fixator External skeletal fixator
	Lumbosacral luxation	Dorsal suture sling
Sacrococcygeal spine	S2/S3 fracture	Dorsal hemicerclage wire
	Endplate fracture of S3 and sacroccocygeal luxation	Dorsal suture sling

PMMA, polymethyl methacrylate.

intervertebral discs is most often used (6). It gives access for performing ventral slots, and stabilization of cervical fractures/luxations. The lateral approach can be used to perform a hemilaminectomy between C3–C4, C4–C5, or C5–C6 to remove lateral disc extrusions (6).

34.5.2 Decompression of the cervical spinal cord

A ventral slot or a hemilaminectomy is used to decompress the cervical spinal cord. A ventral slot is a partial corpectomy of two adjacent vertebral bodies and the corresponding intervertebral disc to gain access to the ventral spinal canal (Box 34-1). Ventral slots are performed in the cervical spine to treat centrally located intervertebral disc herniation. The slender vertebral bodies in cats make this technique demanding, and visibility is limited. Some degree of spinal instability is created and stabilization of the affected segments should be considered after having performed a ventral slot. Cervical hemilaminectomy is a good alternative for the treatment of lateralized intervertebral disc extrusions (Box 34-2).

34.5.3 Fractures and luxations of the cervical spine

Cervical spinal fractures and luxations are rarely encountered in cats. Clinical signs include neck pain, possibly accompanied by tetraparesis or tetraplegia. Unstable lesions are stabilized surgically to reduce the risk of further spinal cord damage, diminish pain, and to facilitate anatomic healing. Ventral stabilization methods are used in dogs to treat cervical spinal fractures and luxations (7), and can be applied in cats as well.

A ventral midline approach to the cervical spine is performed. Fracture reduction is aided by having an assistant apply manual traction to the head, with the atlantoaxial joint held in flexion. The feline vertebrae are very slender and do not offer much bone purchase. Miniaturized implants must therefore be used. Size 1.5- or 2.0-mm internal fixators or plates, or 1.5- to 2.0-mm screws or pins embedded in polymethyl methacrylate (PMMA), are possible options.

Internal fixators are especially useful to repair cervical spinal fractures, because interlocking of the screw heads in the plate enhances overall stability, and reduces the risk for pull-out of the screws compared to conventional plates (Fig. 34-3) (8, 9). Two 2.0-mm internal fixator plates are contoured and placed along the left and right borders of the ventral surface of the two vertebral bodies adjacent to the lesion (10). One or two screws are inserted bilaterally in each vertebra adjacent to the lesion. The maximum screw length is evaluated from laterolateral radiographs to avoid penetration into the spinal canal. Care is taken not to injure the vertebral arteries.

34.6 Surgical conditions of the thoracolumbar spine

Indications for surgery of the thoracolumbar spine include thoracolumbar fractures and luxations, disc disease, tumors, and rare diseases such as subarachnoid cysts. Diseases of the spine and spinal cord are described in Chapter 6.

Box 34-1. Ventral slot

The cat is positioned in dorsal recumbency, with the neck extended and supported dorsally, and the front legs retracted and tied backwards. A ventral midline approach is performed. The prominent transverse processes of C6 and the C1–C2 junction serve as landmarks for localizing the affected disc space.

The ventral tubercle cranial to the disc space is removed with rongeurs, and the central portion of the ventral annulus is excised with a scalpel blade. A very small-size high-speed pneumatic drill or power bur is then used to create the slot. The disc spaces are oriented at a caudal to cranial angle, so the center of the slot is located cranial to the disc space (Fig. 34-1A). The extent of the slot should not exceed half the length of the vertebral bodies, and half their width (Fig. 34-1B). Care is taken while drilling the inner cortical layer with the bur, and once the inner cortical layer is penetrated, the thin remaining bone is removed with small bone curettes or scrapers. The dorsal anulus and protruded disc material are removed with fine rongeurs. The dorsal longitudinal ligament is then visible and can be partially excised if necessary. Avoid injuring the venous sinuses once the vertebral canal is opened. Instability is created, especially if the slot is wide. Ventral stabilization, using internal fixators or screws and bone cement, should be performed if the affected segment is considered unstable at the end of surgery.

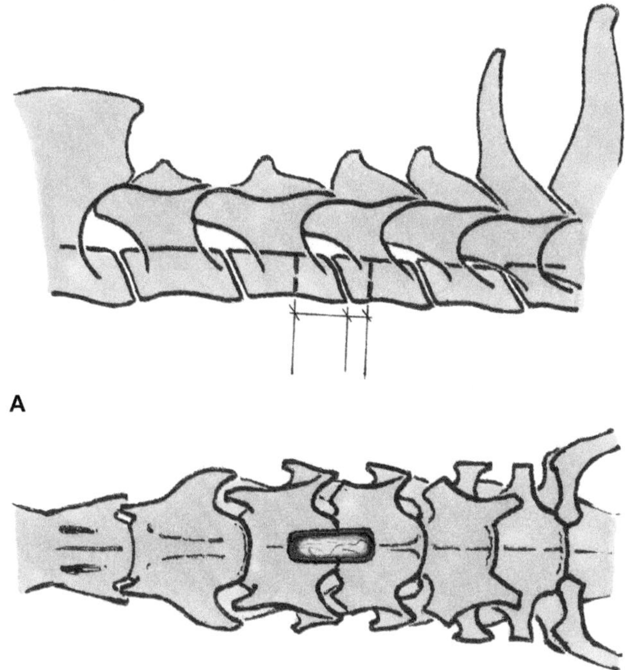

Figure 34-1 Creating a ventral slot.
(**A**) The slot should be started from a slightly cranial position to center it over the dorsal anulus fibrosus because of the caudal to cranial angle of the disc space
(**B**) The extent of the slot should not exceed half the length or half the width of the vertebral bodies.

34.6.1 Approaches to the thoracolumbar spine

A dorsal approach to the thoracolumbar spine is used for dorsal stabilization techniques (6). The skin incision extends from three vertebrae cranial to three vertebrae caudal to the lesion. The dorsal fascia is incised bilaterally on each side of the four spinous processes centered over the lesion, and the epaxial musculature is elevated from the dorsal lamina, while sparing the supraspinous and interspinous ligaments between the spinous processes.

Muscular attachments on the mamillary and accessory processes can be preserved if no decompressive procedure is required. To perform a hemilaminectomy, the multifidus muscles are incised and elevated from their attachment on the mamillary processes. The small tendons of the longissimus muscle are also incised at their attachment on the accessory processes to access the most ventral aspect of the spinal canal by either hemilaminectomy or pediculectomy.

34.6.2 Decompression of the thoracolumbar spinal cord

Decompression procedures of the thoracolumbar spine include hemilaminectomy and pediculectomy. Hemilaminectomy is the unilateral removal of the dorsolateral lamina with the facet joint (Box 34-3). It is most commonly performed to treat

Box 34-2. Cervical hemilaminectomy

The cat is positioned in ventral recumbency with the neck slightly rotated away from the surgeon to ease visualization of the lateral aspects of the spinal cord. The neck is gently flexed and supported. The prominent transverse processes of C6 and the spinous process and the alar wings of C2 are important landmarks for localizing the affected intervertebral space.

The approach is slightly different depending on whether the lesion is in the cranial or caudal cervical spine. The skin, subcutis, and platysma muscle are incised for an approach to the cranial cervical spine. The brachiocephalic muscle is then incised or bluntly dissected over the corresponding articular facets. If a caudal cervical approach is performed, the serratus ventralis cervicis muscle is retracted caudally, and the splenius muscle dorsally. The articular facets are exposed, by creating a plane of dissection between the overlying muscles.

Once the desired articular facets are freed of musculature, a high-speed bur and rongeurs are used to perform a hemilaminectomy (Fig. 34-2). After opening the cervical spinal canal, extruded disc material is removed with probes, fine rongeurs, or mosquito forceps, avoiding damage to the internal vertebral venous plexus.

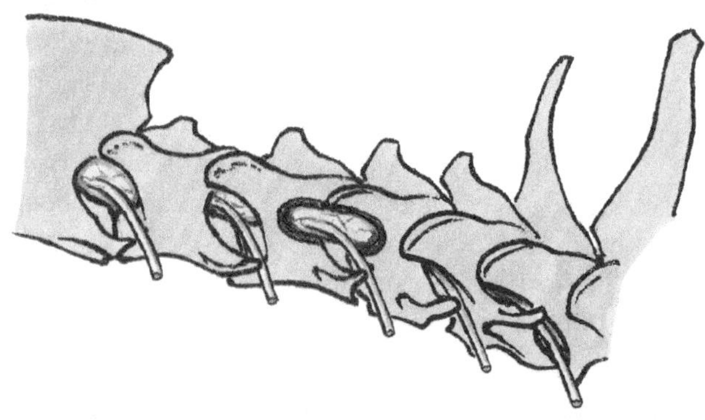

Figure 34-2 Appearance of a cervical hemilaminectomy.

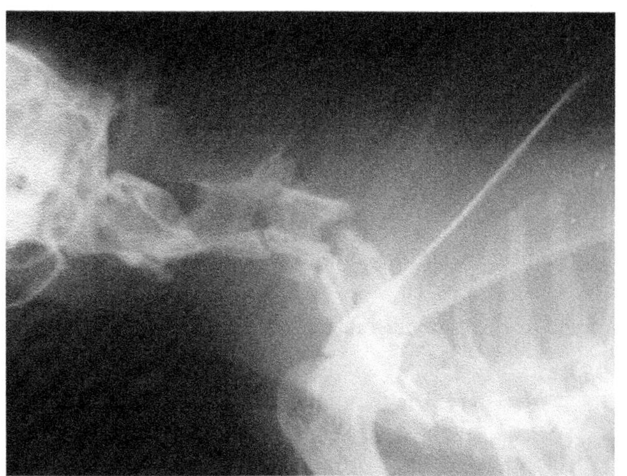

A

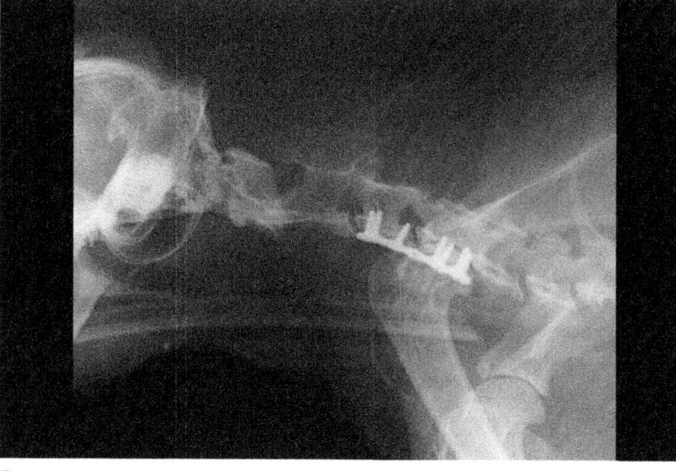

B

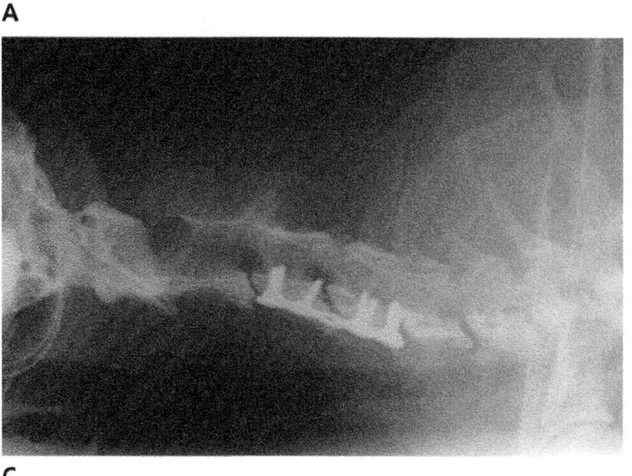

C

Figure 34-3 Radiographs of a cat with a vertebral body fracture of C3 (**A**) preoperatively, (**B**) postoperatively after stabilization with an internal fixator, and (**C**) at follow-up 6 weeks postoperatively. The cat had a non-ambulatory tetraparesis and regained full function after surgery. (Reproduced with permission from: Voss K, Steffen F, Montavon PM. Use of the ComPact UniLock system for ventral stabilization procedures of the cervical spine. A retrospective study. Vet Comp Orthop Traumatol 2006;19:24.)

Box 34-3. Thoracolumbar hemilaminectomy

The cat is positioned in ventral recumbency, with the abdomen supported and slightly elevated. The last rib is used to localize T13 for orientation. A dorsal midline approach or a paramedian approach is performed. The articular processes are removed with rongeurs. The hemilaminectomy can then be performed with rongeurs or with a high-speed pneumatic drill.

For a hemilaminectomy with rongeurs, an assistant uses small Kocher forceps to elevate the dorsal spinous processes, which opens the intervertebral foramen and facilitates insertion of a small rongeur into the spinal canal at the level of the accessory process (see pediculectomy). The opening is then enlarged cranially and caudally with fine rongeurs (Fig. 34-4).

If a high-speed pneumatic drill is used, a rectangular portion of bone is selected and burred, extending from ventral to the accessory process to dorsal to the articular facets. Care is taken when drilling the inner cortical layer and entering the spinal canal. The thin bone of the inner cortical layer is removed with curettes or rongeurs.

The spinal cord and spinal canal are explored and compressive lesions are carefully removed. The epidural space is narrow in cats and care is taken not to compress or injure the spinal cord with the instruments or to injure the venous sinus and the nerve roots. If necessary, the nerve roots are retracted out of the way in a cranial direction.

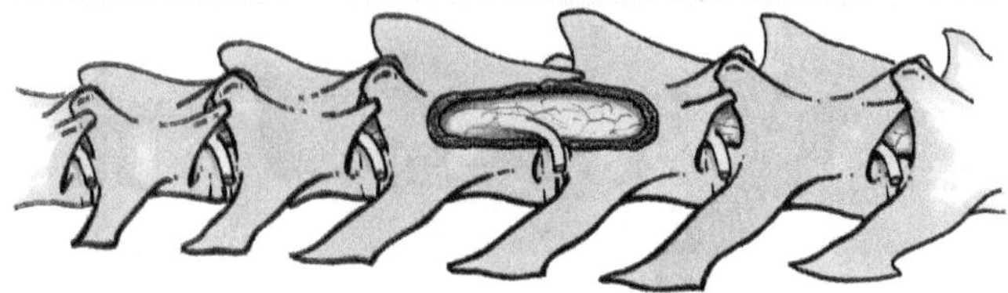

Figure 34-4 Appearance of a thoracolumbar hemilaminectomy. It extends from ventral to the accessory process to the dorsal border of the articular facets. The spinal cord and the nerve root are clearly visible.

thoracolumbar disc disease. Hemilaminectomy generates a wide opening of the spinal canal, which allows good visualization of the spinal canal and spinal cord, and achieves good decompression, but it creates a degree of instability by removing one articular facet joint. Although hemilaminectomy was shown not to affect bending strength of the spine (11), rotational instability does occur if fenestration is combined with unilateral facetectomy (12). Patients with fractures/luxations commonly have partially ruptured discs or other injuries of the ventral compartment, and hemilaminectomy may worsen instability. Surgical stabilization is then required.

Pediculectomy is the unilateral removal of the laminar pedicle while preserving the facet joint (Box 34-4). Significant decompression is not achieved, and the small opening created may lead to difficulties in exploration of the dorsal spinal canal. Pediculectomy is especially indicated for exploration of the ventral spinal canal after thoracolumbar fractures and luxations, because spinal stability is unaltered.

Durotomy can be used in addition to a hemilaminectomy as a diagnostic or therapeutic procedure. A wide and long hemilaminectomy is necessary to perform a durotomy. Durotomy allows direct inspection of the spinal cord and helps in the intraoperative diagnosis of myelomalacia. Myelomalacia should be suspected in patients suffering acute spinal cord compression with grade 5 neurological deficits (2). Patients with intraoperative findings suggestive for myelomalacia have a grave prognosis and euthanasia should be suggested to the owners. Durotomy may also help in releasing pressure on the spinal cord, as the dura mater is a relatively inelastic structure which restricts expansion of the spinal cord in the presence of severe spinal cord swelling.

The cranial and caudal aspects of the durotomy incision should extend to within a few millimeters of the ends of the hemilaminectomy. The dura can be incised with a number 11 scalpel blade or a small-gauge hypodermic needle. The cutting edge of either a scalpel blade or a hypodermic needle is reversed towards the surgeon and is held parallel to the spinal cord while performing the incision. The spinal cord is discolored or hemorrhagic, swollen, and significantly softer in the presence of myelomalacia. In severe cases it may even flow out of the durotomy incision.

34.6.3 Fractures and luxations of the thoracolumbar spine

Fractures of the thoracic and lumbar spine are common in cats. Approximately 50% of cats with spinal fractures/luxations suffer from concurrent injuries (3). These injuries include thoracic trauma, abdominal trauma, head trauma, and orthopedic or neurological injuries at other sites. Scapular fractures, which are otherwise rare in cats, were observed in two out of 16 cats with spinal fractures in one study (3).

Whereas in dogs most of the fractures occur around the thoracolumbar junction, the second to sixth lumbar vertebrae seem to be predisposed to fractures/luxations in cats (2, 3). The most common type of injury in cats is fracture of the endplate with vertebral subluxation (2). Vertebral subluxation and luxation are less common (2). Comminuted fractures of the vertebral bodies seem to occur less commonly than in dogs.

Box 34-4. Pediculectomy

The cat is positioned in ventral recumbency and a dorsal approach is performed as for a thoracolumbar hemilaminectomy. The articular facets are left intact.

An assistant elevates the spinous processes with Kocher forceps to open the intervertebral foramen. A small rongeur is inserted over the accessory process into the spinal canal, taking care to stay close to bone with the inner blade. The accessory process is removed in total with this first bite. The opening is then carefully enlarged with fine rongeurs in a cranial and caudal direction, but staying below the articular facets (Fig. 34-5). The pediculectomy can be transformed into a hemilaminectomy if visualization remains insufficient.

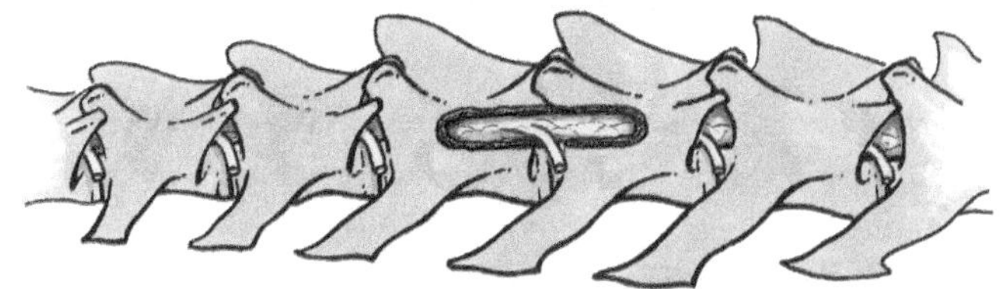

Figure 34-5 A pediculectomy is centered over the accessory process and stays below the articular facets. It allows visualization of the ventral aspect of the spinal canal and spinal cord.

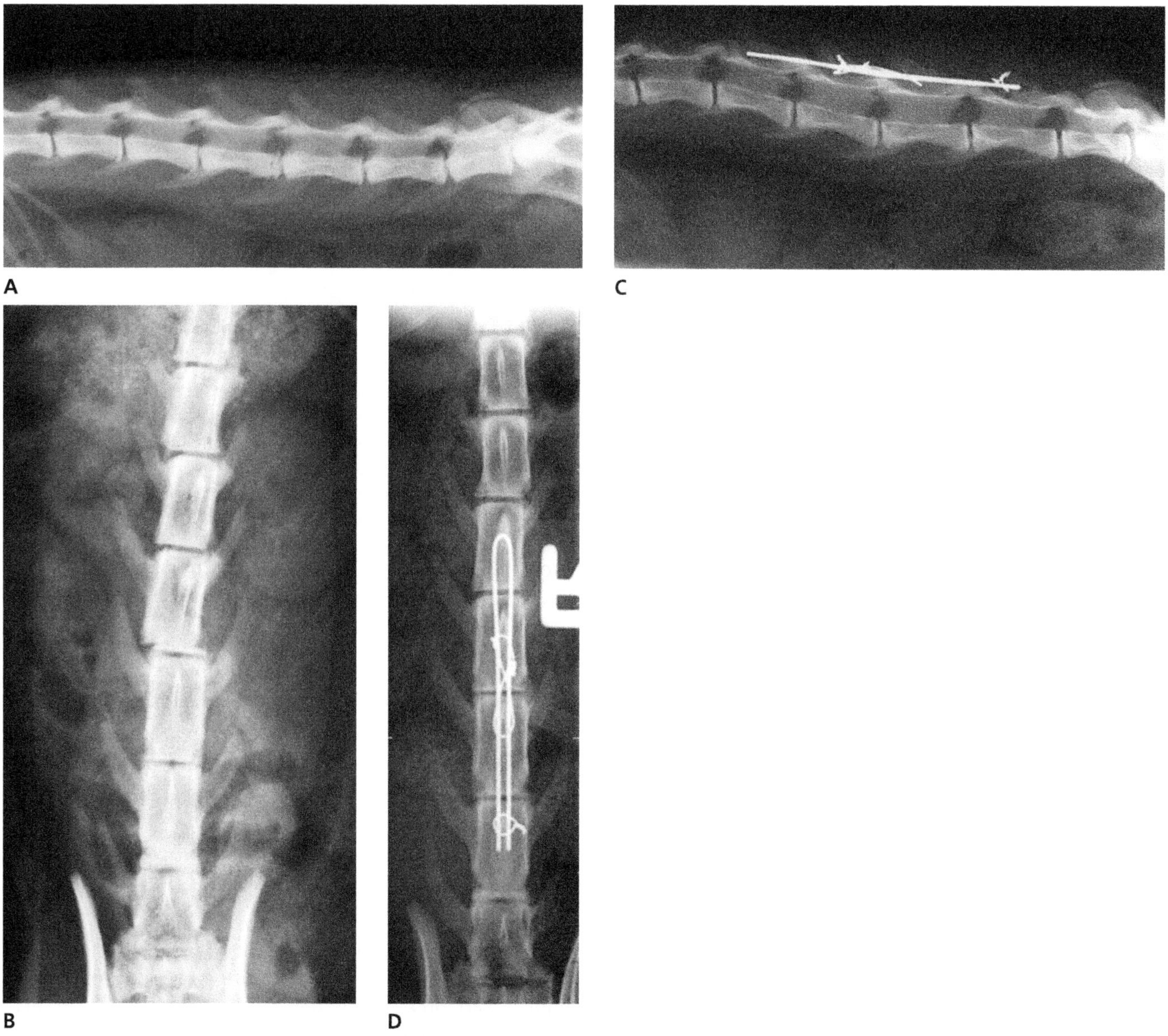

A

C

B

D

Figure 34-6 Cat with a fracture of L4.
(**A**, **B**) Preoperative radiographs showing a fracture of the caudal endplate of L4, which is not displaced on the laterolateral view, but is displaced on the ventrodorsal view.
(**C**, **D**) Postoperative radiographs. The fracture was reduced and stabilized with the dorsal tension band technique.

Box 34-5. Stabilization of thoracolumbar spinal fractures and luxations with a tension band fixation

After elevation of the epaxial musculature as described above, a 1.0–1.25-mm Kirschner wire is inserted through the base of the largest spinous process cranial or caudal to the fracture just dorsal to an imaginary curved line between two adjacent articular processes to avoid penetration of the spinal canal. To be able to insert it perpendicularly, it can be passed through the soft tissues initially before being redirected above the epaxial musculature. Once the Kirschner wire is inserted to its midpoint, it is bent into a U shape with bending pliers (Fig. 34-7A), and is then positioned bilaterally along the dorsal lamina in the groove between the spinous and articular processes of four vertebrae. The fracture is reduced and the free ends of the Kirschner wire are secured to the spinous process with a 0.6-mm hemicerclage wire (Fig. 34-7B). Holes are drilled ventral to the Kirschner wire through the bases of the spinous processes on each side of the lesion. A 0.6–0.8-mm orthopedic wire is passed through the holes and placed over the U-shaped Kirschner wire, and below the supraspinous and interspinous ligaments in a figure-of-eight fashion (Fig. 34-7C). The wire is tightened bilaterally under visual control to ensure correct positioning of the articular facets. Correct reduction depends on adequate positioning of the U-shaped Kirschner wire along the groove between spinous processes and articular facets.

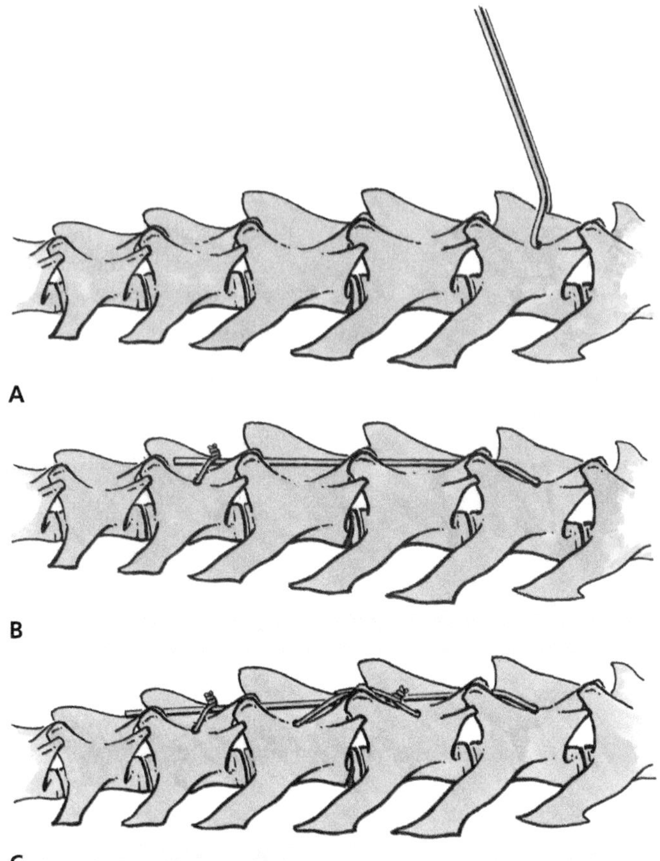

Figure 34-7 Tension band fixation of a thoracolumbar fracture. (**A**) A Kirschner wire is inserted into the largest spinous process adjacent to the affected segment, and is bent into a U shape. (**B**) The Kirschner wire is then adapted to the groove between the spinous and articular processes. Its free ends are secured to the spinous process on the opposite side of the affected segment with a hemicerclage wire. (**C**) The figure-of-eight wire is centered over the lesion. The vertebrae are pulled towards the Kirschner wire while it is tightened.

Multiple methods have been described for stabilization of thoracolumbar fractures in dogs (7). The small size of the vertebrae in cats precludes performing some of these techniques. Dorsal stabilization methods using pins and orthopedic wire are therefore commonly used in cats. Spinal stapling offers adequate strength in small patients, and is a biomechanically sound technique because the implants are positioned on the tension side of the spine (13). A modification of spinal stapling, using a figure-of-eight wire as a tension band, has been shown to be an effective surgical technique for stabilization of thoracolumbar fractures/luxations in cats (Fig. 34-6 and Box 34-5). No implant-related complications were seen with this technique in 16 cats with thoracolumbar spinal fractures/luxations (3). The tension band technique is most appropriate for fractures located between T12 and L6 with an intact dorsal lamina. Fractures cranial to T12 are mostly stabilized with the classical spinal stapling technique.

Fracture stabilization is also possible with internal fixators, applied to the dorsal or lateral lamina, or the vertebral bodies. The 2.0-mm Unilock mandible locking system (Chapter 24) is an adequate internal fixator to be used in cats (Fig. 34-8). It is mainly indicated for fractures of the sixth or seventh lumbar vertebrae, where dorsal stabilization methods may offer insufficient stability because of the small spinous process of L7.

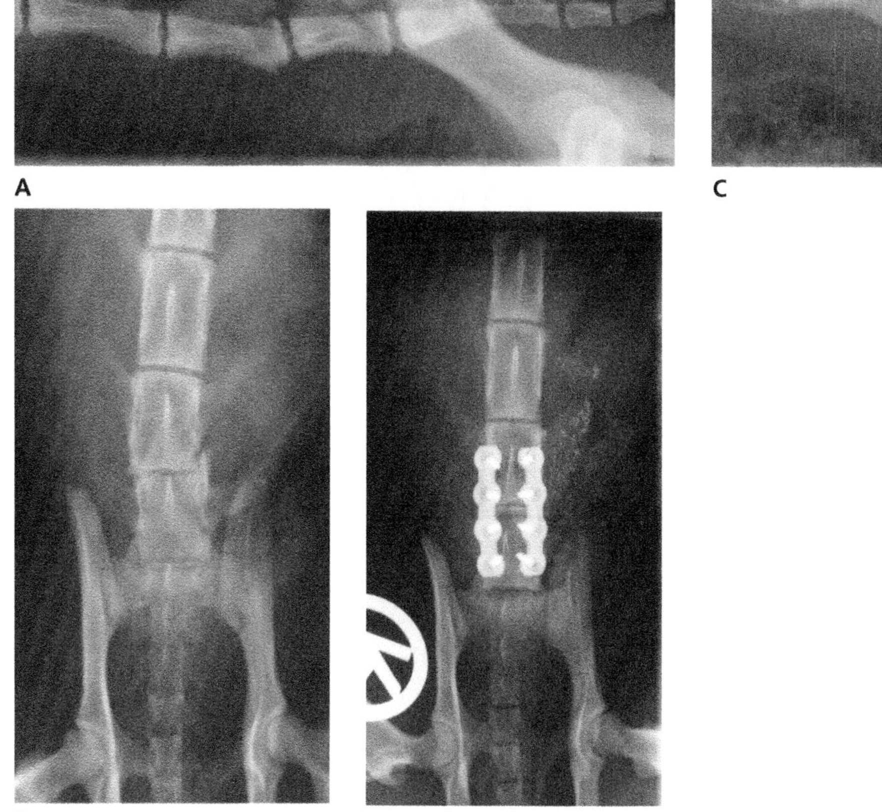

Figure 34-8 Cat with a fracture of L6.
(**A, B**) Preoperative radiographs showing an endplate fracture and fracture of the dorsal lamina of L6 with L6–L7 dislocation.
(**C, D**) Postoperative radiographs. The fracture was stabilized with two 2.0-mm Unilock plates applied to the vertebral bodies of L6–L7 using a ventroabdominal approach. (Courtesy of Urs Weber.)

34.7 Surgical conditions of the lumbosacral spine

Surgery of the lumbosacral spine is most commonly performed to treat fractures and luxations. The most common lesion in this area is fracture of the seventh lumbar vertebra. Luxations between the seventh lumbar vertebra and the sacrum also occur in cats (14). Decompression can be indicated in cases with lumbosacral disc disease or spinal empyema (Chapter 6).

34.7.1 Approaches to the lumbosacral spine

The most commonly used approach to the lumbosacral area is the dorsal approach to the seventh lumbar vertebra and the sacrum (6). It is used for all dorsal decompression and stabilization techniques. A ventral abdominal approach (6) can be used for ventral stabilization of fractures.

34.7.2 Decompression of the lumbosacral spinal cord and nerve roots

The spinal cord and nerve roots at the lumbosacral junction are decompressed by dorsal laminectomy (Box 34-6). Dorsal laminectomy is removal of the dorsal lamina, with or without the facet joints. Removal of both facet joints creates significant spinal instability and is discouraged. Dorsal laminectomy is rarely performed in cats. The most common indication would be protrusion of the lumbosacral disc. Decompression is usually only performed indirectly by open reduction and internal fixation in the presence of fractures or luxations.

34.7.3 Fractures and luxations of the lumbosacral spine

Trauma to the lumbosacral spine may result in fractures of the seventh lumbar vertebra, luxation of the lumbosacral joint, and fractures of the sacrum.

Box 34-6. Dorsal laminectomy

The cat is placed in ventral recumbency with the hind legs in a frog position. The abdomen is supported. A dorsal midline approach is performed. The caudal half of the spinous process of L7 and the spinous process of S1 are removed with rongeurs. The laminectomy is started, by removing a rectangular piece of bone with a high-speed power bur. The lateral extent of the dorsal laminectomy is restricted by the facet joints, which are left intact (Fig. 34-9). Care is taken while burring the inner cortex. The ligamentum flavum between L7 and S1 is removed with a scalpel blade when only a thin shelf of bone is left. The thin bone shelf is then elevated and removed with fine curettes or rongeurs. The cone of the medullary canal and its nerve roots can be retracted sideways with a nerve hook to explore the dorsal anulus fibrosus and the L7 nerve root.

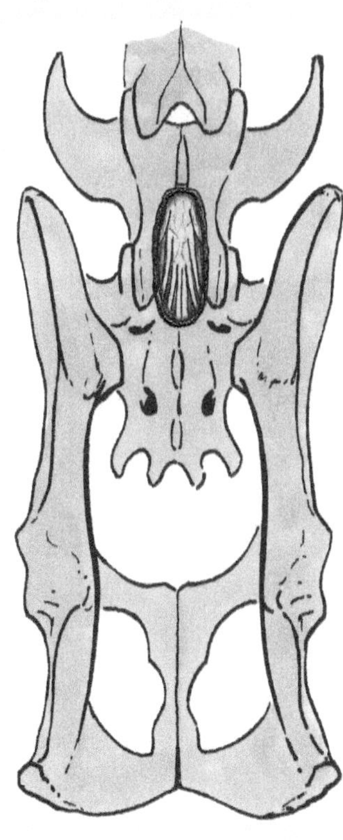

Figure 34-9 Diagram showing the extent of a lumbosacral dorsal laminectomy. The facet joints have been preserved.

Fractures of L7 often show marked cranioventral displacement of the caudal segment due to the pull of the iliopsoas musculature ventrally, causing significant narrowing or even obliteration of the spinal canal (Fig. 34-10). Besides neurological dysfunction of the sciatic nerve, bladder and anus paralysis may result from pudendal and pelvic nerve injury. Stable fixation of these fractures is difficult due to the high mobility and force transmission in this area. Transilial pinning is a method for stabilization of these fractures, but correct pin placement is crucial to achieve adequate fixation stability (Box 34-7). The pin must lie in close contact with the dorsal lamina of L7, cranial to the fracture, to be able to prevent ventral dislodgment of the caudal fracture segment. A certain degree of axial compression and shortening of the L7 vertebral body is seen during healing, even with correctly placed pins. External skeletal fixation combined with internal dorsal stabilization has been described in dogs and is considered more stable than transilial pinning (15). It may be potentially applicable in cats if small implants are used. The use of internal fixators or pins and PMMA are other treatment options. Internal fixators can also be applied to the ventral surface of L7 and the sacrum, using an abdominal approach, in addition to a transilial pin.

Traumatic lumbosacral luxation is occasionally observed in cats (14). Radiographic features include subluxation on laterolateral radiographs and rotational malalignment of the spinous processes on dorsoventral radiographs (Fig. 34-12). A dorsal midline approach to the lumbosacral junction is performed. The articular facets are usually both luxated but not fractured. Reduction of the articular facets is achieved by distracting the articular facets while flexing the lumbosacral joint. This is done with the help of pointed bone reduction forceps, one positioned at the base of the spinous process of L7 and another one placed lateral to the articular facets of the sacrum. The lesion appears stable after reduction. A suture sling is anchored between the spinous processes of L7 and S2 in order to prevent hyperflexion and reluxation in the recovery period. A small tension band repair should be considered in the presence of fractured articular facets.

Fractures of the sacrum occur commonly in cats. Most often they are avulsion fractures of the craniolateral edge of the sacral wing in conjunction with sacroiliac luxation, and pelvic fractures. These are usually stabilized with sacroiliac screw fixation (Chapter 35). Other sacral fractures, such as foraminal and transverse fractures (see Chapter 13 for classification of sacral fractures), are also treated surgically in the

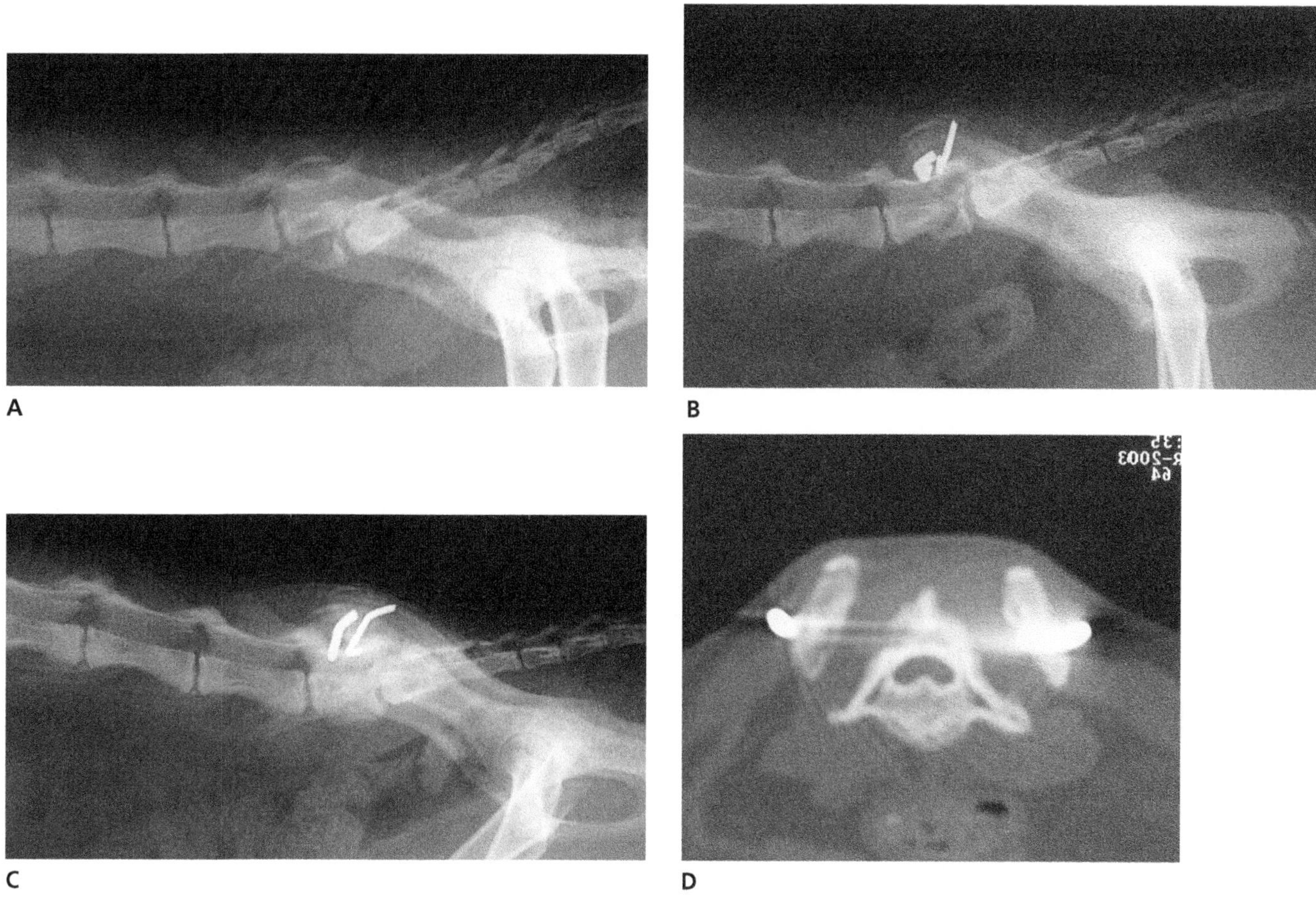

Figure 34-10 A cat with a fracture of L7.
(**A**) Preoperative radiographs. The caudal fragment is dislocated cranioventrally due to the pull of the iliopsoas musculature.
(**B**) Reduction and fixation with two transilial pins resulted in satisfactory realignment of the spinal canal.
(**C**) Healing in axial compression and shortening of L7 is seen on 6-week follow-up radiographs. The cat regained the ability to walk, but had residual tibial nerve and voiding deficits.
(**D**) Transverse computed tomography view of the transilial pin. The tuber coxae are used to anchor the pin in the pelvis. Close contact of the pin with the dorsal lamina of L7 cranial to the fracture prevents the caudal part of the spine and the pelvis displacing ventrally.

Box 34-7. Transilial pinning of L7 fractures

A dorsal approach to the dorsal lamina of L7 and the iliosacral joint is performed. A 1.6–2.0-mm Kirschner wire is inserted through the tuber coxae on one side, using a mini intergluteal approach. The entrance site is aimed so that the pin will be located at the level of the roof of L7, cranial to the fracture. The caudal part of the spinous process can be removed with rongeurs if necessary. It is crucial that the pin comes to lie in close contact to the dorsal lamina of L7 (Figs 34-10D and 34-11). Only then is it able to prevent cranial dislocation of the caudal fragment. The fracture is reduced, and the pin is then advanced along the dorsal lamina of L7 until it has penetrated the contralateral tuber coxae. The pin ends can be bent bilaterally prior to cutting them to avoid migration (Fig. 34-11).

Transilial pinning can be also used as an auxillary stabilization method for repair of sacroiliac luxations (Chapter 35).

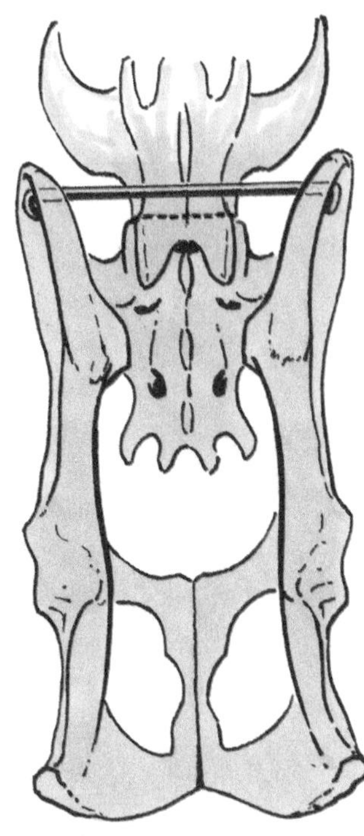

Figure 34-11 Transilial pinning for an L7 fracture. The pin is anchored in the tuber coxae bilaterally and lies on the dorsal lamina of L7, cranial to the fracture (also see Figure 34-10D).

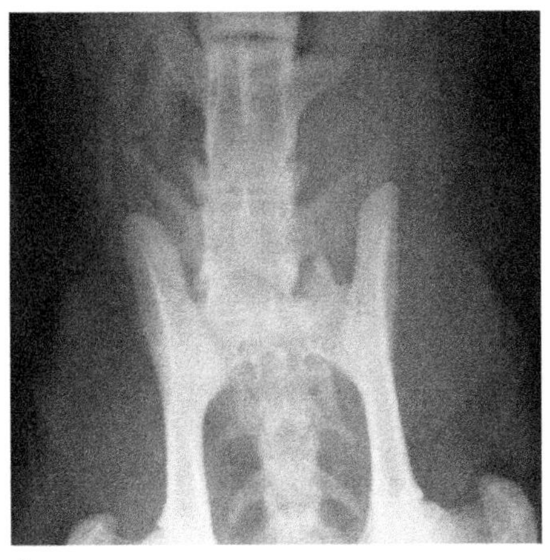

A

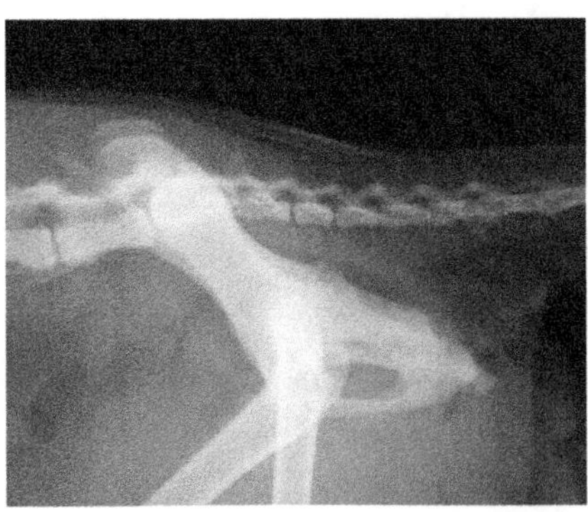

B

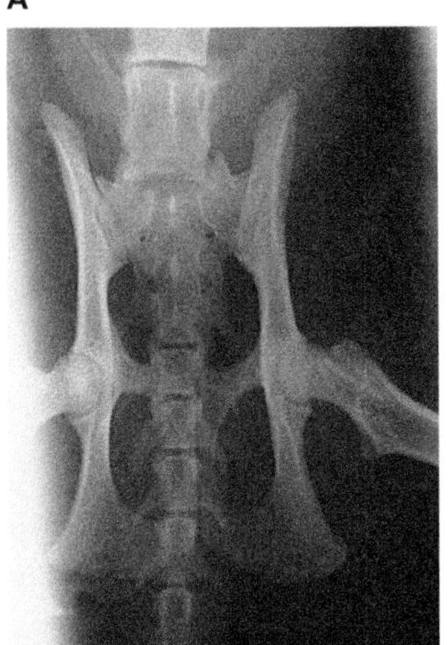

C

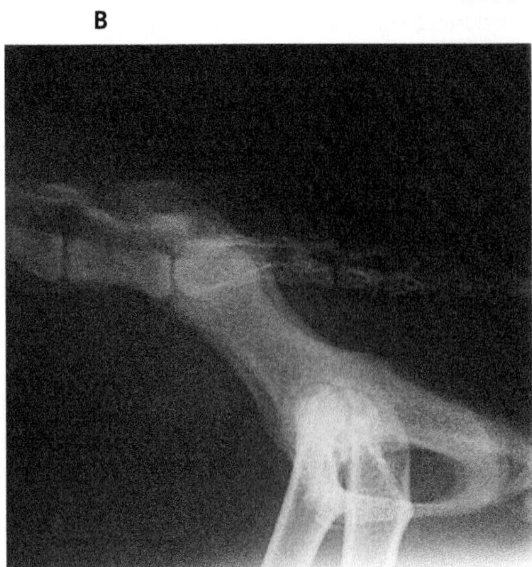

D

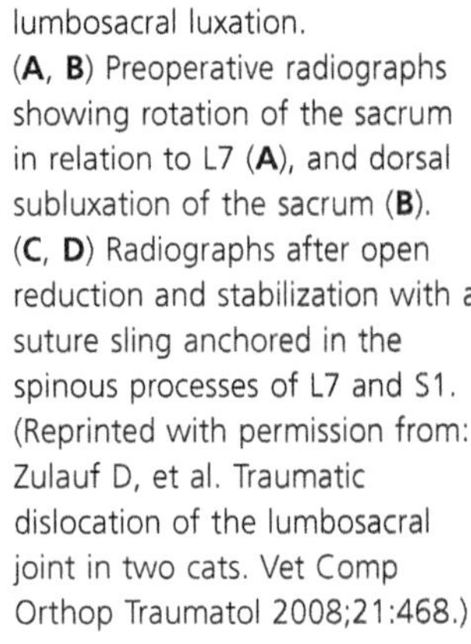

Figure 34-12 A cat with lumbosacral luxation. (**A**, **B**) Preoperative radiographs showing rotation of the sacrum in relation to L7 (**A**), and dorsal subluxation of the sacrum (**B**). (**C**, **D**) Radiographs after open reduction and stabilization with a suture sling anchored in the spinous processes of L7 and S1. (Reprinted with permission from: Zulauf D, et al. Traumatic dislocation of the lumbosacral joint in two cats. Vet Comp Orthop Traumatol 2008;21:468.)

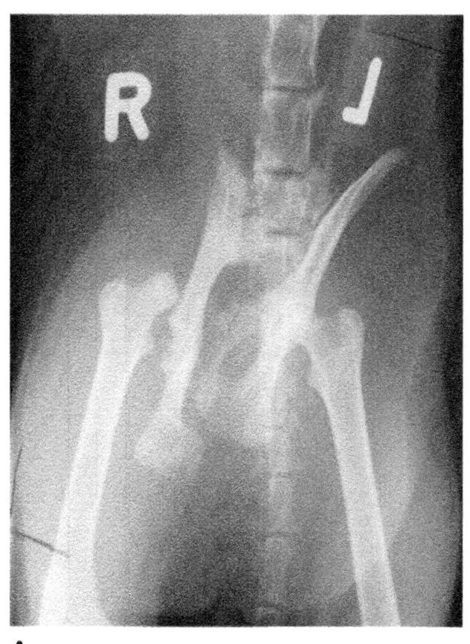

A

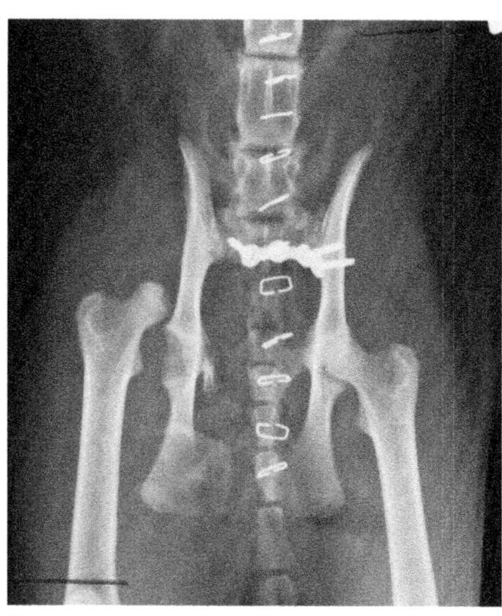

B

Figure 34-13 A cat with pelvic fractures, hip luxation, and a foraminal fracture of the sacrum. (**A**) Preoperative radiographs showing cranial displacement of the left hemipelvis. The fractured part of the sacral wing is attached to the sacroiliac joint. (**B**) A 2.0-mm Unilock plate was applied on to the ventral aspect of the sacral body and the ilial wing after reduction. The luxated hip was treated at a later date.

presence of neurological deficits and fracture displacement. Foraminal fractures are best stabilized with internal fixators or plates using a ventroabdominal approach (Fig. 34-13). Dorsal stabilization methods can be used for transverse fractures.

34.8 Surgical conditions of the sacrococcygeal spine

Sacrococcygeal fractures or luxations are the most common spinal injuries in feline patients. These injuries are a result of traction to the tail, resulting in fractures or luxations at the tail base, often accompanied by damage to the nerves of the tail, bladder, perineum, and anus. They are usually caused by motor vehicle accidents, when the tail is trapped under a wheel. Concurrent injuries of the pelvis and/or hindlimbs are common.

34.8.1 Approach to the sacrococcygeal spine

The sacrococcygeal spine is approached from dorsally (6). In some cases the nerve roots have been torn out of the vertebral canal, and can be located dorsal to the spine. They can be manipulated carefully, but no traction should be applied.

34.8.2 Fractures and luxations of the sacrococcygeal spine

Sacrococcygeal fractures or luxations include three different types of injury: sacrococcygeal luxation, a fracture between the second and third sacral segment, or an endplate fracture of the third sacral bone (Fig. 34-14). The sacral growth plates close around 18 months of age and seem to be a predilection site for fractures in younger cats (16). Regardless of the type of injury, the traction exerted on the sacral and coccygeal nerve roots during trauma results in damage to the nerve roots themselves, and can also cause myelomalacia of the sacral and caudal lumbar spinal cord segments (17). Important nerves involved are the coccygeal nerves, the pudendal nerve, and the pelvic nerve (Chapter 1). Many cats with sacrococcygeal fracture/luxation suffer from concurrent pelvic fractures or other injuries of the hindlimbs.

Symptoms depend on the severity of neurological involvement, but include local hyperesthesia, flaccid tail paralysis, swelling around the tail base, and dribbling of urine. The neurological examination should include assessment of motor and sensory function of the tail. Sensory and motor function of the pudendal nerve is assessed by testing perineal reflex activity. The presence or absence of anal tone reflects motor function of the pudendal nerve. Inability to urinate and the presence of residual urine after micturition are usually caused by pelvic nerve dysfunction. A classification system of the severity of neurological deficits suggested by Smeak and Olmstead (18) is shown in Table 34-3.

Although cats with only tail paralysis frequently recover after both conservative and surgical stabilization, surgical stabilization of the lesion may have some benefits. Surgical stabilization restores the pelvic diaphragm, and prevents further neurological damage due to traction on the nerve roots during the healing period. Persistent hyperesthesia has been described in some cats after conservative treatment (16, 18). Surgically treated patients had no evidence of hyperesthesia, and a larger number of cats regained motor function of the tail than patients treated conservatively in one study (16). From current knowledge, surgery does not seem to have a significant effect on regaining the ability to urinate. A simple technique for surgical stabilization is the dorsoventral suture sling (16) (Box 34-8). Significant undermining of the

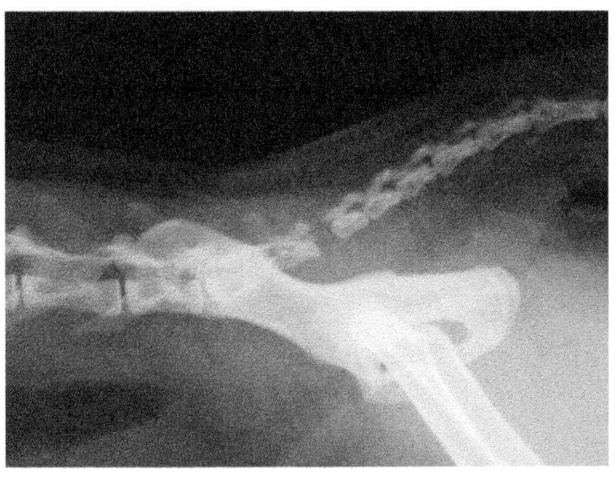

A

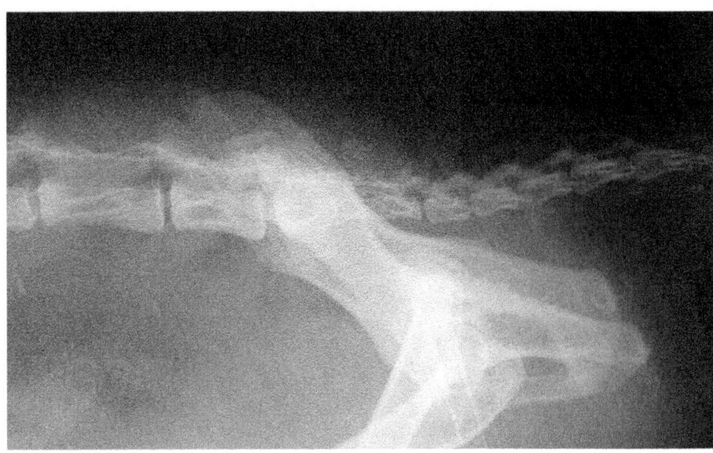

B

Figure 34-14 (**A**) Preoperative and (**B**) postoperative radiographs of a cat with a sacrococcygeal luxation.

Table 34-3. Classification of cats with sacrococcygeal fracture/luxation based on neurological signs and prognosis

Grade	Neurological signs	Nerves	Prognosis for ability to urinate
Grade 1	Hyperesthesia only		Excellent
Grade 2	Flaccid tail paralysis	Coccygeal nerves	Excellent
Grade 3	Flaccid tail paralysis	Coccygeal nerves	Good in most cases
	Some residual urine	Pelvic nerve	
Grade 4	Flaccid tail paralysis	Coccygeal nerves	<75% recovery rate
	Residual urine	Pelvic nerve	
	Perineal reflex and anal tone reduced	Pudendal nerve	
	Urethral tone normal (bladder hard to express)	Reflex dyssynergia	
Grade 5	Flaccid tail paralysis	Coccygeal nerves	<50% recovery rate
	Residual urine	Pelvic nerve	
	Absent perineal reflex and anal tone	Pudendal nerve	
	Urethral tone diminished or absent (bladder easy to express)	Pudendal nerve	

Adapted from Smeak DD, Olmstead ML. Fracture/luxations of the sacrococcygeal area in the cat. A retrospective study of 51 cases. Vet Surg 1985;14:319–324.

skin from avulsion of subcutaneous tissue can be present around the tail base, necessitating drainage.

Tail amputation should also be considered in the cat with a paralyzed tail. If this is done early it may relieve distraction and the pendulum effect by the weight of the limp tail. Alternatively it can be done after 6 weeks if motor and sensory function is not regained. The tail is usually amputated distal to the level of the injury, thereby leaving the cat with a small stump and minimizing further disruption and disturbance to the pelvic diaphragm musculature. Tail amputation is also necessary in cats developing skin necrosis of the tail. For further details on tail amputation see Chapter 41.

34.9 Postoperative treatment and prognosis of spinal fractures and luxations

Postoperative treatment depends on the neurological function of the patient. Basic principles for the postoperative

Box 34-8. Stabilization of sacrococcygeal fractures and luxations

The cat is positioned in ventral recumbency with the tail prepared surgically to allow free manipulation. A dorsal approach is performed over the lesion. The dorsal fascia is incised paramedian, sparing the interspinous ligaments. After elevation of the epaxial musculature, the lesion and the articular facets are visible. The coccygeal nerves are often swollen and protrude through the lesion. If reduction of the lesion compresses the nerve roots, a small dorsal laminectomy can be performed with a fine rongeur.

Sacrococcygeal luxation and endplate fractures: A hole is drilled manually through the base of the spinous process of S2 with a 0.8-mm Kirschner wire. A suture sling is then placed around the transverse processes of the first coccygeal vertebra and through the hole in C2 bilaterally (Fig. 34-15A). Non-resorbable monofilament suture material size 2-0 is used. Reduction is achieved by careful manipulation of the tail, before the sutures are tightened using sliding knots. Over-reduction and entrapment of nerve roots should be avoided.

Transverse fracture between S2 and S3: A dorsal suture sling can be anchored between the bases of the dorsal spinous processes of S2 and S3 to repair these fractures (Fig. 34-15B). Care is taken not to break the fragile dorsal spinous process of S3. Non-resorbable monofilament suture material is used.

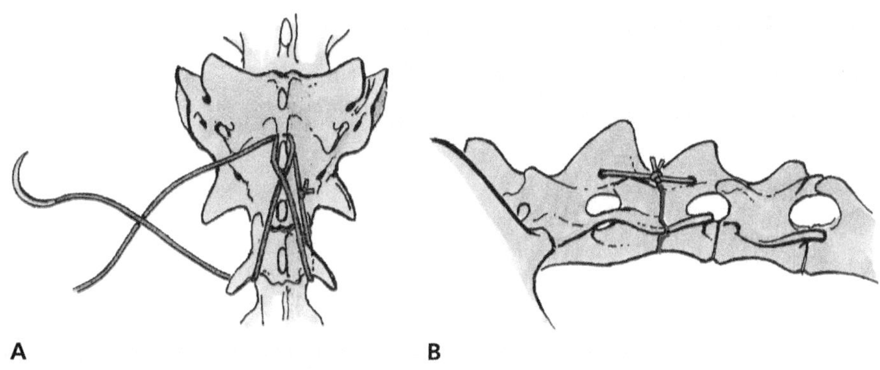

Figure 34-15 Repair of sacrococcygeal fractures and luxations.
(**A**) A dorsal suture sling between the transverse processes of C1 and the dorsal spinous process of S2 is used to stabilize sacrococcygeal luxations and fractures of the endplate of the sacrum.
(**B**) A dorsal suture sling between the spinous processes of S2 and S3 is used for stabilization of transverse sacral fractures between S2 and S3.

treatment of neurological disorders are also described in Chapter 20.

34.9.1 Cervical and thoracolumbar fractures/luxations

Cats should be confined to a cage for at least 10 days after surgical repair of cervical and thoracolumbar spinal fractures. Activity is further restricted by keeping the cat indoors for another 6 weeks. Ancillary external stabilization with splints is not used by the authors. Control radiographs are usually performed after 3–4 weeks. Radiographs must be taken prior to this to detect potential fixation failure, if neurological recovery is inadequate, or if a sudden worsening of the neurological status occurs.

Prognosis after spinal cord injury depends on the preoperative neurological state of the cat, and on the type and presence of concurrent injuries. Overall, only 50% of cats that presented with traumatic spinal lesions survived in one study (2). Forty percent of patients died or were euthanized within 4 days after the injury, due to severe neurological deficits, intraoperative evidence of myelomalacia, postoperative cardiovascular complications, and owner's decision (2). Ten percent of treated cats did not recover satisfactory restoration of gait or ability to urinate and had to be euthanized during the treatment period (2). In another study, evaluating outcome of surgically stabilized spinal fractures and locations in dogs and cats, 79% of patients regained satisfactory or complete neurological recovery (3). Cats with preoperative grade 1–3 neurological deficits treated surgically had a good to excellent outcome (3). Around one-third of cats with grade 4 deficits did not regain satisfactory function of gait or ability to urinate, and were euthanized during the treatment period (3). No cats with grade 5 deficits recovered (2, 3).

In summary, cats with spinal fractures and luxations and grade 1–3 neurological deficits have a good to excellent prognosis, especially after surgical stabilization. Cats with grade 4 deficits seem to have a more guarded prognosis. Cats with grade 5 neurological deficits have a poor prognosis due to the high likelihood of spinal cord disruption and/or myelomalacia.

34.9.2 Sacrococcygeal fractures/luxations

Postoperative treatment mainly depends on the ability to urinate. In the absence of normal micturition, the bladder has to be emptied 3–4 times daily by manual expression or by catheterization if the bladder is hard to express. A urinary catheter, connected to a closed suction system, is a good method to avoid the stress and microtrauma associated with repeated catheterization. Although most bladders are easy to express due to lower motor neuron lesions of the pudendal nerve, some cats show normal sphincter tone or reflex dyssynergia. Detrusor muscle function can be assisted pharmacologically (Chapter 20).

Prognosis depends on the neurological deficits present and is summarized in Table 34-3. Motor function of the tail returns in around 50% of patients (16–18), although in some cases only the proximal third of the tail recovers. Mean time to recovery has been described as 1 month (18), but it may take significantly longer. If the tail remains completely paralyzed, it should be amputated to avoid self-trauma and soiling. Recovery of urinary function is the most important factor for survival of affected cats. If the ability for voiding returns, it usually does so within 1 month (18). The chance for recovery is poor after that time, and most cats are euthanized.

One complication occasionally encountered after sacrococcygeal fractures and luxations is necrosis of the tail. It can be encountered after both surgical and conservative therapy (16) and necessitates tail amputation. Fecal incontinence is rarely a problem, due to functional intrinsic innervation of the colon and rectum (18). Constipation is occasionally seen, but can usually be managed by dietary means, laxatives, and enemas.

References and further reading

1. Zulauf D, et al. Radiographic examination and outcome in consecutive feline trauma patients. Vet Comp Orthop Traumatol 2008;21:36–40.
2. Grasmueck S, Steffen F. Survival rates and outcomes in cats with thoracic and lumbar spinal cord injuries due to external trauma. J Small Anim Pract 2004;45:284–288.
3. Voss K, Montavon PM. Tension band stabilization of fractures and luxations of the thoracolumbar spine in dogs and cats: 38 cases (1993–2002). J Am Vet Med Assoc 2004;225:78–83.
4. Kot W, et al. Anatomical survey of the cat's lumbosacral spinal cord. Prog Vet Neurol 1994;5:162–166.
5. Frewein J, Vollmerhaus B. Anatomie von Hund und Katze. Berlin: Blackwell; 1994.
6. Piermattei DL, Johnson KA. An atlas of surgical approaches to the bones and joints of the dog and the cat, 4th edn. Philadelphia: WB Saunders; 2004.
7. Wheeler SJ, Sharp NJ. Small animal spinal disorders. London: Mosby-Wolfe; 2005.
8. Smith SA, et al. An in-vitro biomechanical comparison of the Orosco and AO locking plates for anterior cervical spine fixation. J Spinal Disorders 1995;8:220–223.
9. Richman JD, et al. Biomechanical evaluation of cervical spine stabilization methods using a porcine model. Spine 1995;20:2192–2197.
10. Voss K, et al. Use of the ComPact UniLock system for ventral stabilization procedures of the cervical spine: a retrospective study. Vet Comp Orthop Traumatol 2006;19:21–28.
11. Smith GK, Walter MC. Spinal decompressive procedures and dorsal compartment injuries: comparative biomechanical study in canine cadavers. Am J Vet Res 1988;49:266–273.
12. Shires PK, et al. A biomechanical study of rotational instability in unaltered and surgically altered canine thoracolumbar vertebral motion units. Prog Vet Neurol 1991;2:6–14.
13. Gage ED. A new method of spinal fixation in the dog (a preliminary report). Vet Med Small Anim Clin 1969;64:295–303.
14. Zulauf D, et al. Traumatic dislocation of the lumbosacral joint in two cats. Vet Comp Orthop Traumatol 2008;21:467–470.
15. Shores A, et al. Combined Kirschner-Ehmer device and dorsal spinal plate fixation technique for caudal lumbar fractures in dogs. J Am Vet Med Assoc 1989;195:335–339.
16. Bernasconi C, et al. Simple techniques for the internal stabilization of fractures and luxations in the sacrococcygeal region in cats and dogs. Schweiz Arch Tierheilk 2001;143:269–303.
17. Lautersack O, et al. About the avulsion of the tail in the cat. Tieräztl Prax 2002;30:41–49.
18. Smeak DD, Olmstead ML. Fracture/luxations of the sacrococcygeal area in the cat. A retrospective study of 51 cases. Vet Surg 1985;14:319–324.

35 Pelvis

K. Voss, S.J. Langley-Hobbs, L. Borer, P.M. Montavon

Pelvic fractures are a common complaint in feline orthopedics, accounting for 22–32% of fractures (1, 2). Motor vehicle trauma is the most frequent cause for pelvic injuries. Many cats with pelvic fractures have sustained additional injury of other bones, organs, or nerves, which may influence treatment decisions, costs, and prognosis. Fracture categories include sacroiliac luxations, ilial body fractures, acetabular fractures, pelvic floor fractures, and fractures of the pelvic margin (3). The pelvic floor is the most commonly fractured region of the pelvis in cats, followed by sacroiliac fracture/luxations, ilial fractures, and ischial fractures (1).

35.1 Surgical anatomy

The pelvis is a ring-like structure consisting of the two os coxae and the sacrum. The os coxae each consist of the os ilium, the os ischium, and the os pubis. In kittens there is a small bone, the os acetabulae, which fuses to the other bones to form the acetabular fossa. All four bones form part of the acetabulum. The acetabulum, the ilium, and the sacroiliac joint are the weight-bearing structures of the pelvis. The main load-bearing area of the acetabular fossa is the caudal and central thirds (4).

Palpable bony prominences are the tuber coxae and tuber sacrale of the ilial wing, and the tuber ischiadicum of the os ischium. The ilium is slimmer and straighter in cats than in dogs. The body of the ilium has a relatively thick cortical shell, but the ilial wing is mainly composed of cancellous bone (Fig. 35-1) (5). The ilium articulates medially with the sacral wings. The sacroiliac joint has both a fibrocartilaginous and a synovial part. The synovial part is covered with hyaline cartilage and is visible as a crescent-shaped structure on the sacral wing with the concave side facing craniodorsally. The ischial bone and the pubic bone unite ventrally at the pubic symphysis.

The lumbosacral plexus and the sciatic nerve are important structures coursing close to the pelvic bones. They are at risk of being damaged during pelvic trauma or surgery. The lumbosacral plexus is composed of the sixth and seventh lumbar, and the first and second sacral nerve roots. The resulting nerves course ventrolateral to the sacrum, and along the medial surface of the ilium, from where the sciatic nerve separates to leave the pelvic canal caudodorsal to the hip joint.

35.2 Diagnosis and general considerations

Around 60% of cats with pelvic fractures are unable to bear weight on the pelvic limbs at admission (5). A thorough neurological examination is necessary to rule out neurological injury, especially of the sciatic, the pudendal, and coccygeal nerves. Sciatic nerve dysfunction occurs in 11% of cats with pelvic fractures (1). The nerve deficits were associated with ilial body fractures in around 70%, and with sacroiliac luxations in approximately 30% of cases (1). Craniomedial displacement of ilial fractures and cranial displacement of sacroiliac luxations enhance the risk for damage to the lumbosacral plexus (6). Injury to the pudendal and coccygeal nerves is common with concurrent sacrococcygeal fractures or luxations.

Radiographs are performed to identify and classify the injuries (Chapter 13). Because the pelvis is ring-shaped, at least two different fracture/luxations will occur simultaneously. The pelvis was broken at three or more sites in 76% of dogs and cats in one study (3). A total of 160 possible combinations of fractures was observed in the same study.

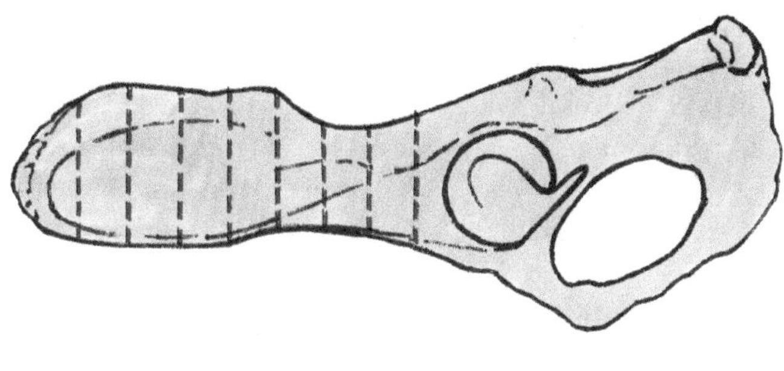

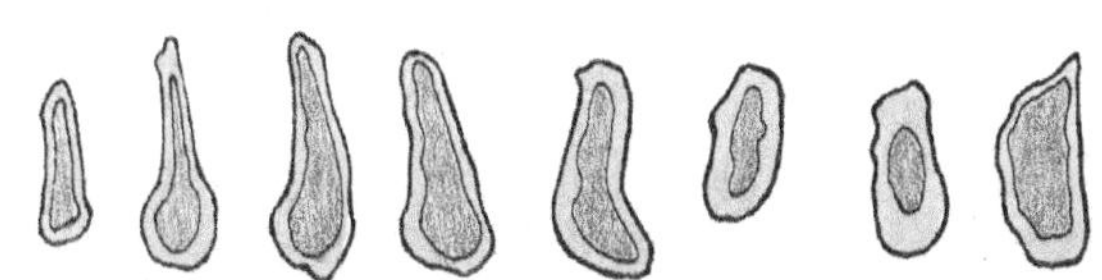

Figure 35-1 Cross-sectional views of the ilium. The ilial body is a tubular structure with a relatively thick cortex. The ilial wing is mainly composed of cancellous bone. Its thickest area is at the ventral aspect. (Adapted from Böhmer E. Beckenfrakturen und -luxationen bei der Katze. Munich: Ludwig-Maximilians-Universität; 1985.)

Box 35-1. The most common combinations of feline pelvic fractures

Ilial body and pelvic floor fracture
Ilial body fracture and contralateral sacroiliac luxation, with/without pelvic floor fracture
Unilateral sacroiliac luxation and pelvic floor fracture
Bilateral sacroiliac luxation, with/without pelvic floor fracture

Common combinations of pelvic fracture/luxations are listed in Box 35-1.

Significant trauma is necessary to cause fracture of the pelvic bones, which are well protected by musculature, and as many as 74% of cats with pelvic fractures have extrapelvic injuries (1). These occur mainly in the caudal body of the cat and include sacrococcygeal fracture/luxation, coxofemoral luxation, femoral fractures, sciatic nerve injury, and caudal body wall hernias. Thoracic trauma is also common. In one study urinary tract trauma occurred in more than 30% of dogs with pelvic fractures (7). Surprisingly, this was described to be far less common in cats (1).

Hematuria is a common clinical finding in cats with pelvic fractures. It can be caused by injury to any part of the urinary system, but is often due to lesions of the urinary bladder mucosa. Other possible injuries to consider include kidney trauma, and rupture of the ureters, urinary bladder, and urethra. Plain radiographs, ultrasonography, abdominocentesis, and contrast radiography may confirm or rule out clinically significant urinary tract trauma (Chapter 12). Hematuria caused by mucosal lesions of the urinary bladder is usually self-limiting after 2–3 days and no specific treatment is necessary. However, cats may lose a significant amount of blood and should be monitored for anemia.

35.3 Stabilization techniques

Fractures or luxations of the pelvic ring are classified into sacroiliac luxation, fractures of the ilium, acetabular fractures, pelvic floor fractures, and fractures of the pelvic margin (Chapter 13) (1, 3). The most common combinations of pelvic fractures in cats are listed in Box 35-1. The decision for conservative or surgical treatment mainly depends on whether the acetabulum or other weight-bearing parts of the pelvis are fractured, and on the presence of neurological injury and degree of pelvic canal narrowing.

Fractures of the non-weight-bearing elements of the pelvis, that is the pelvic floor, the ilial wing, and the ischium, can often be treated conservatively. However, surgical stabilization of these fractures can be beneficial if there is marked instability, displacement, and pain. Conservative treatment of pelvic fractures consists of providing analgesia, controlling and monitoring urination and defecation, and cage confinement for 2–4 weeks.

Fractures of the weight-bearing elements of the pelvis, that is, the acetabulum, the ilial body, and the sacroiliac joint, are usually repaired surgically to allow early return to function, and to prevent malunion, delayed union, and pelvic canal narrowing. Pelvic canal narrowing of more than 45% is likely to result in obstipation or constipation (8). Extreme pain and the presence of neurological deficits are also indications to perform exploratory surgery because these signs could be caused by entrapment of nerves between the fracture fragments. Box 35-2 provides a summary of indications for surgery. Fractures of the weight-bearing parts of the pelvis often occur bilaterally.

The two hemipelves are connected to each other by the pelvic floor. Fracture reduction and stabilization of one hemipelvis should automatically result in adequate reduction of the contralateral side, provided that the pelvic floor has remained intact. However, the pelvic floor is fractured in 90% of cases (1), and bilateral injuries with concurrent fractures of the pelvic floor result in marked instability of both hemipelves, often necessitating bilateral fracture/luxation repair. Either bilateral surgical repair, or unilateral repair and stabilization of the pelvic floor, may be necessary in these cases. If bilateral surgery is to be performed, the side where anatomic reduction is more important, for example an acetabular fracture, should be operated first. If unilateral nerve deficits are present, the affected side should also be operated first to prevent nerve entrapment during manipulation of fragments affecting the other hemipelvis.

Surgical stabilization of pelvic fractures is most commonly performed with plate osteosynthesis. Screw fixation and pin and wire techniques also have some indications. The use of an oscillating drill mode reduces the risk of iatrogenic damage to the nerves of the lumbosacral plexus and sciatic nerve while drilling screw holes or inserting pins (9). If available it should be used, especially for sacroiliac luxation repair, and for osteosynthesis of the ilium. Treatment options for the different fracture types are listed in Table 35-1.

35.3.1 Pins and wires

Pins and wires are rarely used for the repair of pelvic fractures. Temporary interfragmentary insertion of a small Kirschner wire can help maintain fracture reduction while a plate is contoured and applied. This is especially helpful for repair of acetabular fractures. Orthopedic wire can be applied to repair symphyseal pubic fractures with hemicerclage or cerclage wiring. Skewer pins with a figure-of-eight cerclage

Box 35-2. Indications for surgical stabilization of pelvic fractures

Acetabular fractures
Fractures of the ilial body
Sacroiliac dislocation (if >50% displaced)
Pelvic canal narrowing (if >40% narrowing)
Extreme pain
Nerve deficits
Pelvic floor fractures (if widely displaced or unstable or abdominal wall avulsion)
Fractures of the ischial tuberosity (if clinically disabling)

wire can be used to stabilize long oblique fractures of the ilial body, but the fracture line must be long enough to allow application of at least two skewer pins.

35.3.2 Screws

Screw fixation is mainly used for stabilization of sacroiliac luxations (see corresponding section). Screws with a diameter of 2.0–2.7 mm are appropriately sized.

Long oblique fractures of the ilial body are another indication for screw fixation. Lag screw stabilization of long oblique ilial fractures has been shown to be biomechanically superior to lateral plating in dogs (10). A minimum of two 2.0-mm lag screws are inserted perpendicular to the fracture line and parallel to each other.

Table 35-1. Treatment options for the different fracture types. Treatment decisions also depend on the combination of the different lesions

Fracture localization	Fracture type	Treatment options
Sacroiliac joint	Unilateral luxation	Conservative Screw fixation Repair of pelvic floor
	Bilateral luxation	Conservative Unilateral screw fixation if pelvic floor intact Bilateral screw fixation if pelvic floor broken Unilateral screw fixation and repair of pelvic floor (if broken) Transilial pin/bolt
Ilium	Simple transverse	Lateral or dorsal plate or internal fixator
	Simple long oblique	Lag screws Skewer pins Lateral or dorsal plate or internal fixator
	Comminuted	Lateral plate(s) or internal fixator(s)
Acetabulum	Simple	Plate Internal fixator Tension band repair
	Comminuted	Plate Internal fixator Femoral head and neck resection
Pelvic floor	Symphysis	Conservative Hemicerclage wires Plate Internal fixator
	Other	Plate Internal fixator
Pelvic margin	Ilial wing	Conservative
	Ischial tuberosity	Conservative Divergent pins Tension band

35.3.3 Plating

Plate osteosynthesis is the most commonly used method for surgical repair of pelvic fractures. It is indicated to stabilize ilial body fractures, acetabular fractures, and fractures of the pelvic floor. Short plates are often used for the small size of the pelvic bones, because they are more easily contoured to the curved bone surfaces compared to longer plates. A minimum of two screws must be inserted per fragment, but three or four screws are preferable in the thin bone of the ilial wing. Meticulous technique should be applied to prevent stripping of the screws, especially in the ilial wing with its thin cortical shell. The screws can be inserted without tapping a thread in areas that are predominantly composed of cancellous bone.

Useful plates for repair of ilial fractures include the 2.0-mm dynamic compression plate (DCP), the 2.4-mm limited contact-DCP (LC-DCP), and the 1.5/2.0-mm or 2.0/2.7-mm veterinary cuttable plate (VCP). Plates are most often applied to the lateral surface of the ilium, although it does not offer much bone purchase for the screws, especially in the thin ilial wing. For lateral plating, the implants are best applied along the ventral border of the ilial wing where the bone is thicker (5). Dorsal plating is possible for fractures of the ilial body, and has the advantage of being able to insert longer screws compared to lateral plating (8).

Acetabular fractures are often repaired with 2.0-mm reconstruction plates, which allow more accurate contouring to the curved bone surface compared to conventional plates. The reconstruction plates are weak and should be applied dorsally, which is the tension side of the acetabulum. A short 2.0-mm DCP or a 1.5/2.0-mm VCP can also be used. These stronger plates are beneficial for the repair of comminuted fractures. Specifically designed 2.0-mm acetabular plates are also available.

If pelvic floor fractures are to be stabilized surgically, miniature implants are best suited, such as the 1.5-mm miniplates, and the 1.3-mm compact hand plates. The different plates are described in Chapter 24.

35.3.4 Internal fixators

Internal fixators are good implants to use in pelvic fractures, because they offer superior stability in the soft and thin bone of the pelvis and render screw loosening less likely. Two locking screws per fragment are generally sufficient. Another advantage of using locking plates is that, because the plate is not pressed on to the bone while the screws are tightened, secondary loss of reduction does not occur, even if the plate is not contoured perfectly. This especially facilitates repair of acetabular fractures. The 2.0-mm Unilock mandible locking plates (Chapter 24) are a suitable size for the feline pelvis.

35.4 Sacroiliac fracture/luxation

Approximately 60% of cats with pelvic fractures have sustained a sacroiliac luxation or fracture/luxation (1). Sacroiliac fracture/luxations can occur uni- or bilaterally, and are accompanied by a variety of possible pelvic fracture combinations. Bilateral luxation occurred in 37% of cats in one study (11). Common fracture combinations are unilateral sacroiliac luxation with pelvic floor fracture, bilateral sacroiliac luxation with and without pelvic floor fracture, and unilateral sacroiliac luxation with contralateral ilium fracture, with or without pelvic floor fracture (Box 35-1).

Sacroiliac fracture/luxations are best identified on ventrodorsal pelvic radiographs (Fig. 35-2). Sacroiliac luxation and sacroiliac luxation with an avulsion fracture of the cranial part of the sacral wing are the two most commonly seen injuries. The nerve roots of the sixth and seventh lumbar nerves and the obturator nerve course ventromedial to the sacroiliac joint, and are at risk of damage, especially in cranial and ventral luxations. The sacral nerve roots can also be torn during sacroiliac luxation. Neurological deficits of the sciatic nerve and voiding dysfunction are observed in approximately 20% of cats with sacroiliac luxation (11).

Minimally displaced sacroiliac luxations can be treated conservatively, especially if unilateral. A general rule is that displacement of less than 50% of the length of the joint allows conservative treatment. Although cats seem to recover well after conservative treatment, many will develop ankylosis of one or both sacroiliac joint, as well as degenerative changes in the lumbosacral joint (5). In cases with a contralateral fracture of the ilium and an intact pelvic floor, repair of the ilium will result in indirect reduction of the sacroiliac joint (Fig. 35-3).

Indications for surgical repair are pain and lameness, bilateral injuries (Fig. 35-2), neurological deficits, and displacement exceeding 50% of the length of the joint surface. Severe pain and neurological deficits indicate nerve entrapment or damage. The classical and commonly used stabilization method is insertion of a lag screw from the lateral aspect of the ilial wing across the sacroiliac joint into the sacral body (Fig. 35-2). Alternatively, a positional screw can be inserted across the joint using a ventroabdominal approach (12). The ventroabdominal approach can also be used to repair concurrent fractures of the sacrum with a ventrally applied internal fixator or miniplate (Chapter 34). The use of a transsacral screw has been described for bilateral sacroiliac fracture/luxations for use in both dogs and cats (13), and a tension band wire technique has also been reported in 18 cats (14). The lateral and ventral screw methods are described in Boxes 35-3 and 35-4.

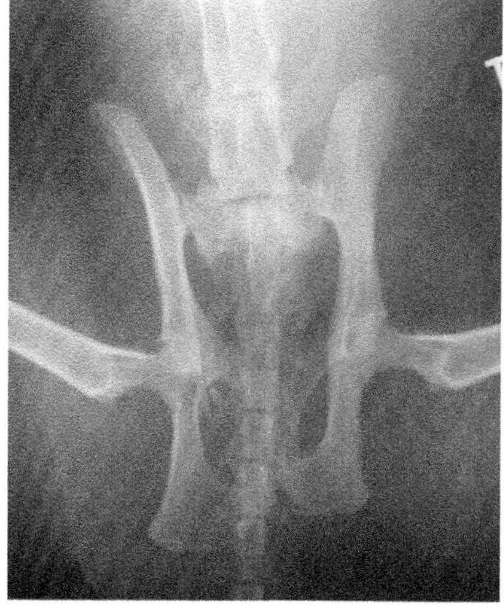

A

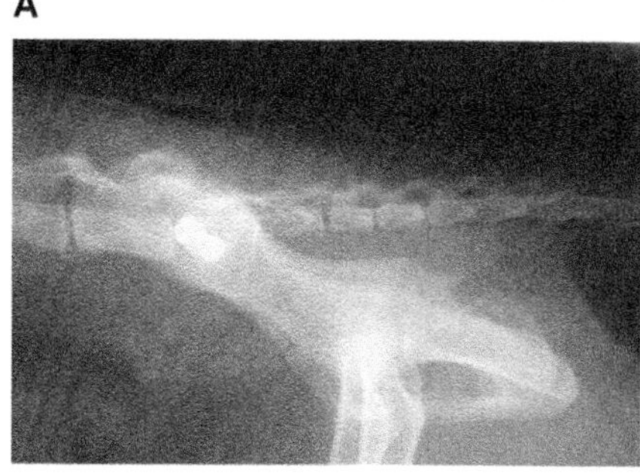

C

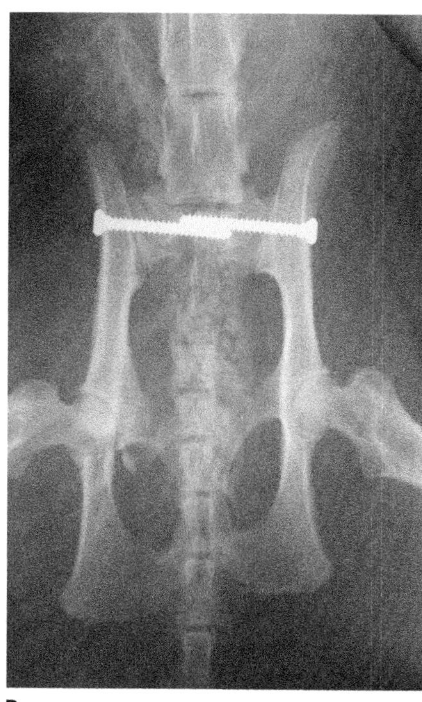

B

Figure 35-2 A cat with bilateral sacroiliac luxation.
(**A**) Ventrodorsal radiograph showing bilateral sacroiliac luxation, fractures of the pelvic floor, and an ischial/caudal acetabular fracture.
(**B**) The sacroiliac joints were stabilized bilaterally with 2.7-mm lag screws inserted from lateral. Reduction and screw position and length are good.
(**C**) Laterolateral postoperative radiograph showing correct position of the screws in the body of the sacrum.

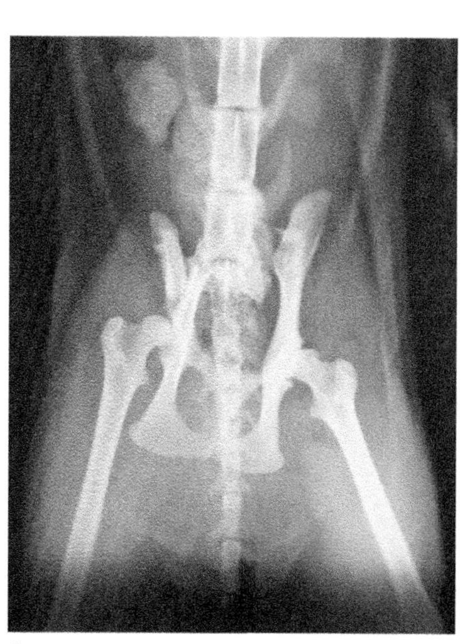

A

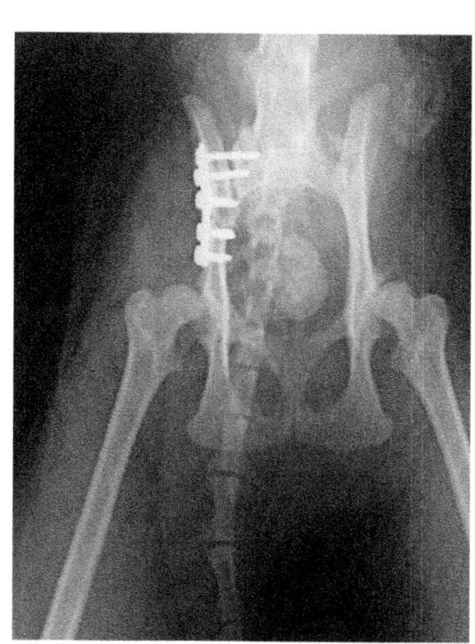

B

Figure 35-3 A cat with an ilial fracture and contralateral sacroiliac luxation.
(**A**) Preoperative radiograph showing a fracture of the left ilium with contralateral sacroiliac luxation. Note that the cat also has hip dysplasia.
(**B**) Stabilization of the ilial fracture with a five-hole plate resulted in indirect reduction of the sacroiliac joint because the pelvic floor was intact.

Box 35-3. Lag screw fixation of sacroiliac luxation using a dorsolateral approach

The cat can be placed in either lateral or sternal recumbency for unilateral injury. If bilateral stabilization is necessary, the cat should be positioned in sternal recumbency. A dorsolateral approach to the sacroiliac joint is performed. A 2.0- or 2.7-mm lag screw is used for stabilization.

A thread hole is drilled into the sacral body after visualization of the luxation. The entrance point is located just cranial to the crescent-shaped hyaline cartilage, and slightly dorsal to the geometric center of the sacroiliac joint (Fig. 35-4A). The hole is drilled perpendicular to the long axis of the sacrum, across at least 60% of the sacral width (Fig. 35-4C). Drilling perpendicular to the joint space would aim the screw into the lumbosacral disc space, because of the craniocaudal inclination angle of the sacral wing. The thread is cut.

A gliding hole is then drilled from lateral to medial through the ilial wing. The hole is located slightly ventral to the center of the ilial wing height, and at a distance of about 60–70% of the sacral tuber length. The hole is usually located on the ventral gluteal line, a small bony crest on the lateral surface of the ilial wing (Fig. 35-4B).

Screw length is premeasured from ventrodorsal radiographs to be 60% of sacral width (Fig. 35-4C). It is usually around 20–24 mm. The screw is inserted from lateral into the ilial wing until it emerges on the medial ilial surface. The fracture/luxation is then reduced under visual control. Reduction is helped by manipulating the ilium with bone-holding forceps, and by using a small Hohmann retractor on the caudal aspect of the sacral wing when reduction is difficult. The screw is advanced into the predrilled hole in the sacral body.

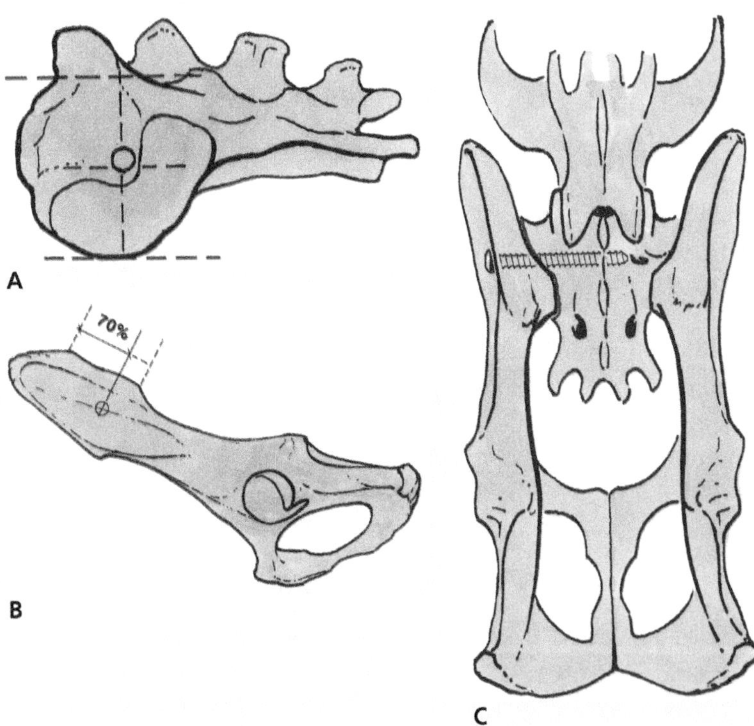

Figure 35-4 Insertion of a sacroiliac lag screw from lateral. (**A**) Entry point of the thread hole into the sacral body. (**B**) Entry point of the gliding hole on the lateral surface of the ilium at a distance of about 70% of the sacral tuber length. The hole is usually located on the ventral gluteal line. (**C**) Correct position of the sacroiliac lag screw, incorporating 60% of sacral body width. Note the screw is inserted perpendicular to the long axis of the sacrum, not perpendicular to the joint surface.

35.4.1 Approaches to the sacroiliac joint

Approaches to the sacroiliac joint include a dorsolateral approach to the sacrum and the wing of the ilium (15), a ventrolateral approach to the ventral aspect of the sacroiliac joint (15), and a ventroabdominal approach to the ventral aspect of the sacrum and sacroiliac joint (12).

The dorsolateral approach to the sacrum and ilial wing or the ventrolateral approach is used to insert a lag screw through the lateral aspect of the ilial body for treatment of sacroiliac luxations. Visualization of the sacroiliac joint is better with the dorsolateral approach. The ventrolateral approach only allows digital palpation of reduction, but facilitates screw placement in correct reduction (16).

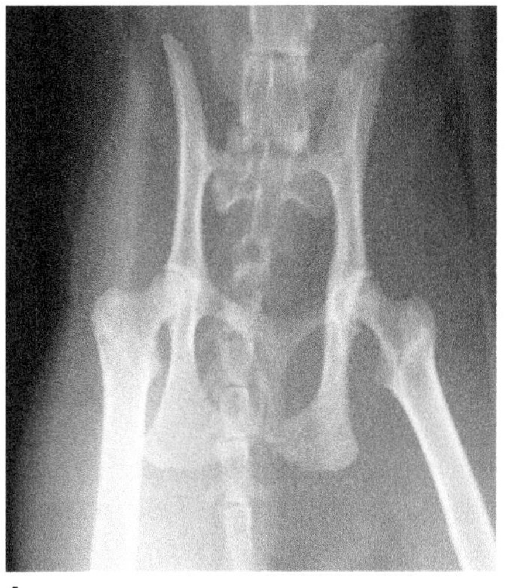

A

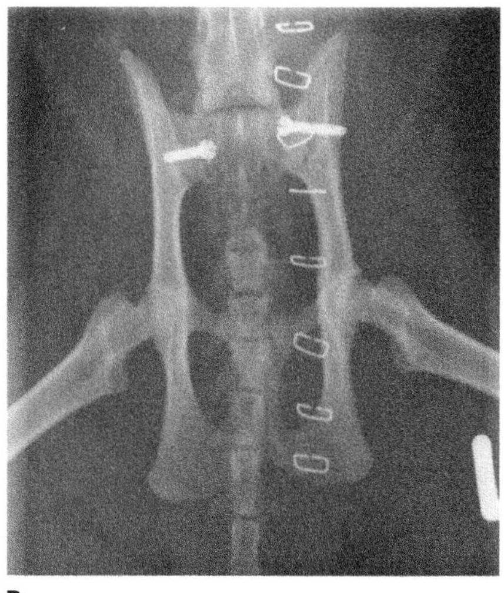

B

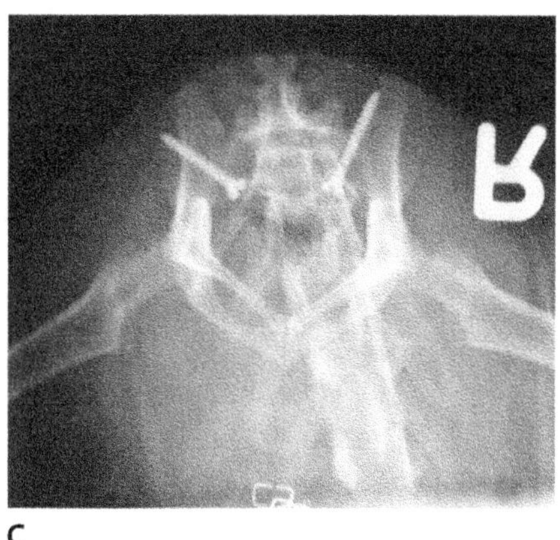

C

Figure 35-5 Sacroiliac screw placement using a ventroabdominal approach.
(**A**) Preoperative radiograph of a cat with bilateral sacroiliac luxation.
(**B**) Postoperative ventrodorsal radiograph, showing good reduction and stabilization of both sacroiliac joints with positional screws inserted via a ventroabdominal approach.
(**C**) Intrapelvic radiographs can be used to further evaluate screw positioning. The left screw is placed correctly. The right screw should have been inserted at a slightly greater angle to obtain more bone purchase in the ilial wing.

A ventroabdominal approach to the iliosacral joint can be performed for screw insertion in a medioventral to laterodorsal direction. The ventroabdominal approach allows simultaneous treatment of bilateral luxations, repair of sacral wing fractures, identification of nerve damage, and repair of concurrent injuries of the pelvic floor and abdominal cavity (12). Screw placement is less likely to result in malpositioning of the screw into the spinal canal or disc space as compared to screw insertion from lateral, but reduction of the luxation can be more difficult.

35.4.2 Fixation of sacroiliac fracture/luxation using a dorsolateral approach

Knowledge of regional anatomy and correct positioning of the screw are required for this fixation method. The sacroiliac lag screw should penetrate at least 50–60% of the width of the sacrum to prevent screw loosening (11, 17). Correct reduction was also shown to enhance fixation stability of the repair (17). Anatomic guidelines have been published for correct screw placement in the cat (18). These are described in Box 35-3. The size of the area for safe screw insertion is smaller than 0.5 cm^2 (18), but correct positioning of the screws was achieved in all clinical cases, and anatomic reduction in 80% of cases, when the described guidelines where respected (11). Screw loosening was not observed. Figure 35-2 shows the radiographic appearance of correct screw positioning.

35.4.3 Fixation of sacroiliac fracture/luxation using a ventroabdominal approach

The insertion of transarticular screws is also possible via a ventroabdominal approach (Box 35-4) (12). Positional screws are aimed from the ventral surface of the sacral wing, across the iliosacral joint, into the ilial wing. The radiological appearance of screw positioning using the ventroabdominal approach is shown in Figure 35-5. Most uni- or bilateral sacroiliac luxations are accompanied by fractures of the pelvic floor. The ventroabdominal approach has the advantage of the surgeon being able to stabilize bilateral sacroiliac fracture/luxations via a single approach. The approach can also be extended caudally to repair concurrent fractures of the pelvic floor. Intra-abdominal injuries could also be addressed with the same approach.

The ventral nerve roots of the sixth and seventh lumbar segments form the main part of the sciatic nerve. Both these nerve roots and the obturator nerve can be directly visualized as they course ventromedially close to the sacroiliac joint. The authors have seen impingement or disruption of these nerves in a handful of cases using this approach. The nerves and associated vessels have to be carefully retracted during surgery.

Box 35-4. Screw fixation of sacroiliac luxation using a ventroabdominal approach

The cat is placed in dorsal recumbency with the abdomen and both the hind legs surgically prepared and draped within the surgical field. A caudal celiotomy is performed extending from the umbilicus to the pelvic floor. Intra-abdominal organs are retracted cranially, and the bladder and colon are retracted to the unaffected side. The tendon of the psoas minor muscle and the promontory of the sacrum are localized. The retroperitoneal fat is bluntly dissected away from the psoas minor muscle at the level of the promontory, without damaging the ureters, and the external iliac artery and vein. The psoas minor muscle is retracted laterally, and dissection is continued medial to it for exposure of the ventral surface of the sacroiliac joint. The ventral nerve roots of L6 and L7 and the obturator nerve are visualized at this point ventral and medial to the sacroiliac joint. They are carefully retracted medially.

Reduction of the sacroiliac joint is best achieved by placing Kocher forceps cranially on the ilial wing and/or by manipulation of the aseptically prepared unbound hindlimbs. Reduction is facilitated if the limbs are pulled cranially, thus flexing the hip joints. A small temporary Kirschner wire can be inserted across the sacroiliac joint to hold reduction during oscillatory drilling and insertion of a 2.0- or 2.4-mm positional screw. The use of a self-tapping screw is beneficial to avoid the risk of losing reduction during tapping. The entry point of the screw hole is located just medial to the sacral wing, with the drill bit angled 45° or more to the median plane in a transverse direction (Fig. 35-6). The length of the hole is measured, and an appropriate screw is inserted. Screw length is usually around 16–18 mm.

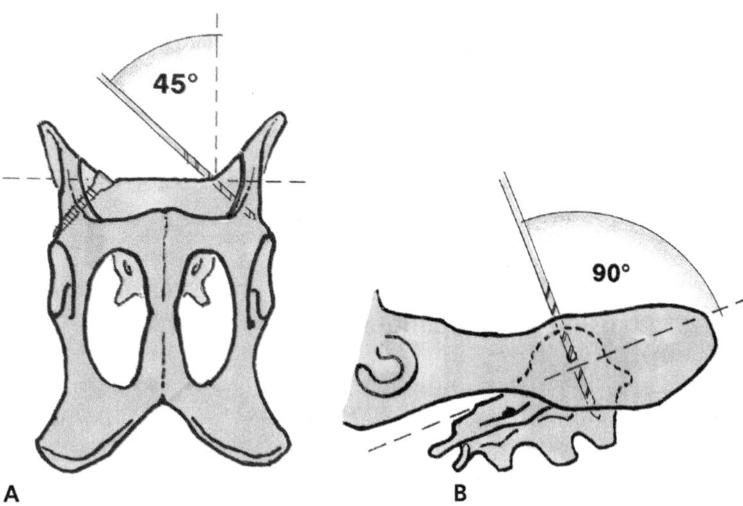

Figure 35-6 Diagrams showing the angles for insertion of a sacroiliac positional screw via a ventroabdominal approach. (**A**) The entry point of the positional screw is located just medial to the sacral wing. The screw is angled laterally, 90° to the long axis of the spine (**B**), and 45° to the median plane (**A**).

35.4.4 Ancillary fixation of sacroiliac fracture/luxation

Ancillary fixation of a sacroiliac fracture/luxation may be advantageous in certain cases, and can be performed using a transilial pin, or a bolt. This technique is usually done in combination with the lateral sacroiliac lag screw or in conjunction with sacral fracture repair. With significant medial displacement of the hemipelvis, the addition of a transilial implant through the ilial wings can increase stability of the fracture repair, and help lateralize the hemipelvis. The technique of transilial pinning can also be applied for repair of fractures of the seventh lumbar vertebra, and is described in Chapter 34, Box 34-7. The technique is described using a Kirschner wire. Alternativel, a customized transilial bolt and two nuts can be used.

35.5 Fractures of the ilium

Fractures of the ilium can be classified into simple transverse, long oblique, and comminuted fractures. Long oblique and comminuted fractures are most common. The caudal fracture fragment has a tendency to displace medially and ventrally. The nerves of the lumbosacral plexus and the sciatic nerve course along the medial surface of the ilium and may be damaged during trauma, during manipulation of the fracture fragments, or while screw holes are drilled. Surgical exploration of the pelvic trunk and sciatic nerve is indicated if significant neurological deficits and severe pain indicate nerve entrapment (6).

Lateral plating of fractures of the ilium is associated with a high incidence of screw loosening (8, 19), with more than half of the cats having loose screws with varying degrees of pelvic canal narrowing in one study (8). The high incidence of screw loosening is likely to be due to suboptimal screw-holding power in the thin cortices of the ilium, especially the ilial wing. Plates should therefore be positioned along the ventral border of the ilial wing, where the bone is slightly thicker (5) (Fig. 35-1). Cranially located screws can also be inserted across the sacroiliac joint into the sacral wing to enhance fixation stability.

A recent study showed that screw loosening and subsequent incidence and degree of pelvic canal collapse are less common when the plate is applied along the dorsal rim of the ilium (8). It is likely that a better screw purchase is achieved with dorsal plating, because longer screws can be inserted.

35.5.1 Approaches to the ilium

A lateral approach to the ilium with a roll-up of the gluteal muscles is suitable for osteosynthesis of most ilial body fractures, specifically for lateral plating, and insertion of lag screws or skewer pins (14). A dorsal or lateral approach to the wing of the ilium can be used for dorsal plating (14). Fractures located close to the acetabulum may be approached by a cranial approach to the hip joint (14).

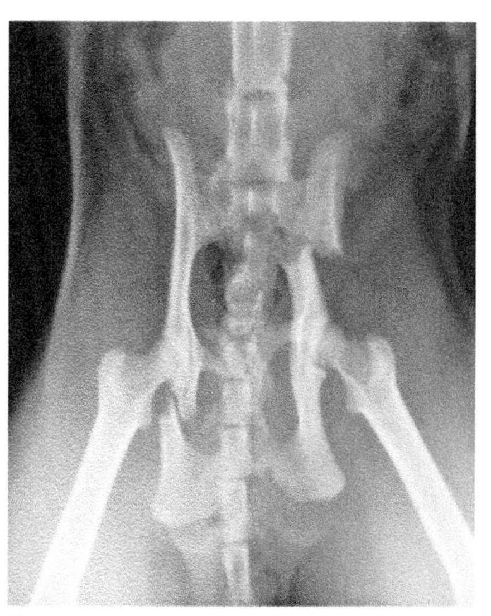
A

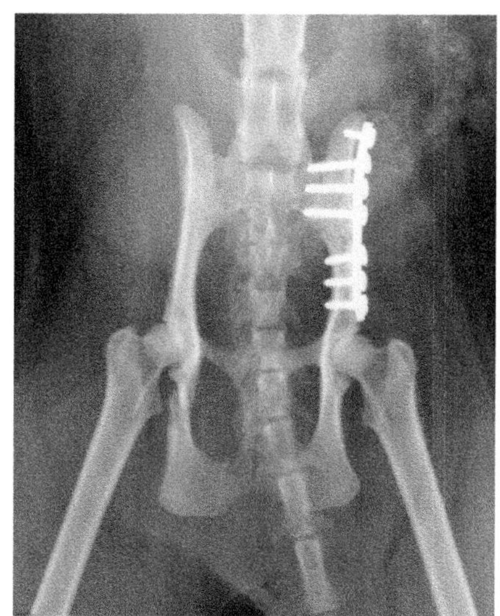
B

Figure 35-7 Stabilization of an ilial fracture with a lateral plate. (**A**) Preoperative and (**B**) postoperative radiographs of a cat with a transverse ilial and contralateral ischial fracture. The ilial fracture was stabilized with a lateral plate, with three of the cranial screws engaging the sacral wing. Engagement of the sacral wing compensates for the thin bone and cancellous nature of the ilial wing, but screws crossing the sacroiliac joint have an increased risk for screw loosening.

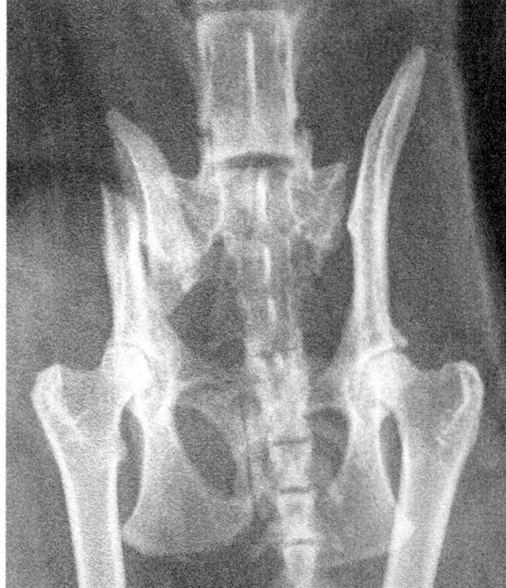
A

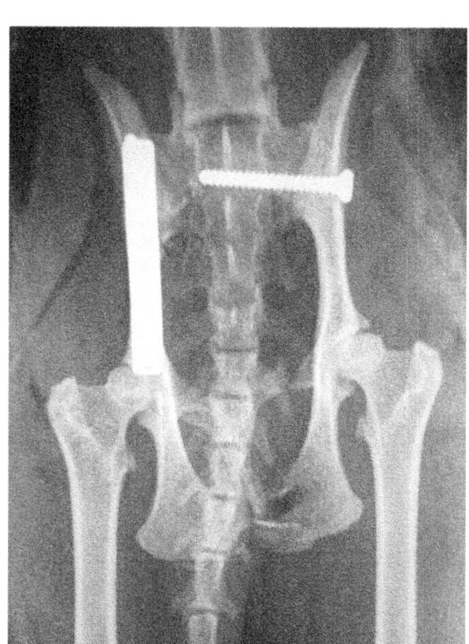
B

Figure 35-8 Stabilization of an ilial fracture with a dorsal plate. (**A**) Preoperative and (**B**) postoperative radiographs of a cat with a transverse ilial fracture, and concurrent contralateral sacroiliac luxation and fractures of the pelvic floor and ischium. Longer screws can be inserted in the dorsoventral plane than in the lateromedial plane. The contralateral sacroiliac luxation was stabilized with a lag screw.

Box 35-5. Stabilization of simple transverse and comminuted fractures of the ilium

A lateral approach to the ilium is performed for lateral plating. A dorsal or lateral approach is used for dorsal plating. The caudal fragment usually has to be levered up in a lateral and dorsal direction. A finger Hohmann retractor, carefully placed between the fragments, is useful in levering the caudal fragment laterally. Bone reduction forceps can also be placed on the greater trochanter or ischial tuberosity to help bring the caudal fragment laterally and dorsally.

Lateral plating: The plate is contoured to the lateral surface of the ilium and is positioned along its ventrolateral border (Fig. 35-9A). It is overbent slightly more concave than necessary to help restore the pelvic canal width. Preferably, a minimum of three screws is inserted into both the caudal and cranial fragments. An L- or T-plate can be used if the caudal fragment is too small for insertion of a sufficient number of screws without compromising the hip joint (Fig. 35-9B). Once the plate is secured to the caudal fragment, it can be used to help lever the fracture into reduction. The screws inserted cranially into the ilial wing may be aimed to cross the sacroiliac joint if additional bone stock of the sacral body is deemed necessary for fixation stability.

Lateral double plating: Double plating is used for comminuted fractures, or for simple fractures if screw purchase seems insufficient by numbers or holding power. The first plate is applied to the ventrolateral surface of the ilium as described above. A second plate is then positioned parallel and dorsal to the first one (Fig. 35-9C). Each plate should be anchored to the bone, giving a combined total of at least four screws in the caudal fragment, and four to six screws in the cranial fragment.

Dorsal plating: The fracture is partially reduced with the assistance of bone holders and a Hohmann retractor. A plate of appropriate length to allow at least three screws in the caudal and cranial fragment is selected and contoured with a slight concave bend to it (Fig. 35-9D). The plate is then applied to the caudal fracture fragment. When placing screws over the acetabulum, the drill bit should be aimed to exit the medial cortex of the pelvis. The fracture is then reduced and further screws inserted into the cranial fragment. Drilling the holes for the screws can be done with a C-guide or by careful aiming through the medullary canal of the ilial body and wing. Care should be taken to ensure that the drill bit or screw does not deviate medial to the ilial wing, which could cause damage to the lumbosacral plexus.

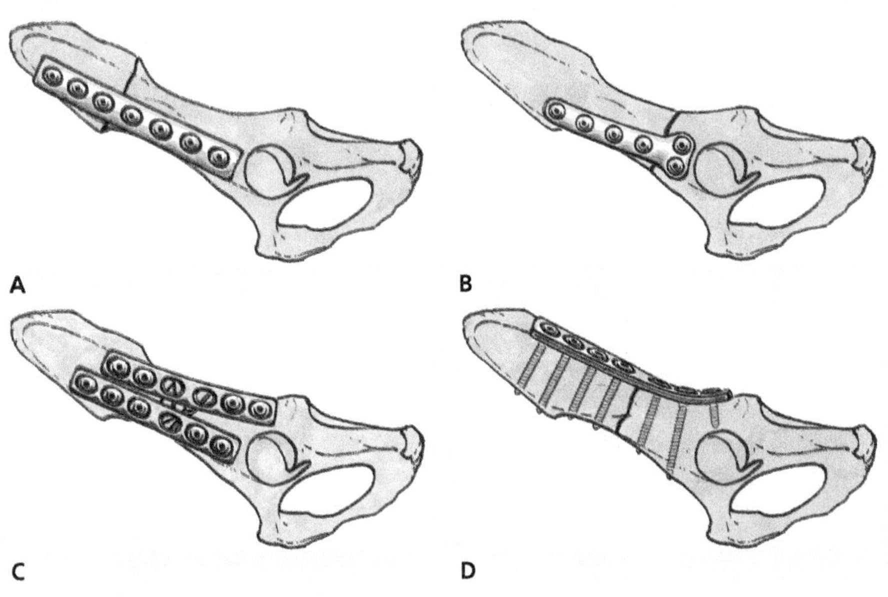

Figure 35-9 Options for plate osteosynthesis of simple transverse and comminuted fractures of the ilium.
(A) Simple transverse fracture of the ilium, stabilized with a lateral plate positioned along the ventral border of the ilium.
(B) A lateral T-plate for a caudally located simple transverse fracture of the ilium.
(C) Double plating for the repair of a comminuted fracture of the ilium.
(D) Dorsal plating for the repair of a transverse fracture of the ilium.

35.5.2 Simple transverse and comminuted fractures

Comminuted fractures are more common than simple transverse fractures. Even fractures that appear simple on the radiograph often have fissuring of the fracture fragments or avulsion of larger cortical fracture fragments, especially in young cats. The 2.0-mm DCP is the most commonly used plate for repairing fractures of the ilium, but a 1.5/2.0-mm VCP can also be applied. The use of a DCP allows interfragmentary compression in the presence of a simple transverse fracture.

Simple transverse fractures can be repaired with a laterally or dorsally applied plate (Figs 35-7 and 35-8). Double plating is also possible, and may be chosen if the screws inserted into the cranial fragment do not hold sufficiently in the thin cancellous bone of the ilial wing, or if the fracture line is close to the acetabulum, with the caudal fragment too small to allow insertion of at least two screws. The use of T- or L-plates is another option to enable insertion of a sufficient number of screws in a fracture located close to the acetabulum.

A lateral or dorsal plate may also result in sufficient stability for the repair of comminuted fractures, provided that three good screws can be inserted per main fragment. However, screw-holding power is often poor in the ilial wing, and application of two plates parallel to each other on the lateral surface of the ilium enhances fixation stability. Plating techniques for simple transverse and comminuted fractures of the ilium are described in Box 35-5.

Internal fixators are also useful for the repair of ilial fractures, and are used similarly to conventional plates. They provide superior stability than conventional plates, especially if only two screws can be inserted in a fragment (20), and screw loosing is less likely (Chapter 24).

35.5.3 Long oblique fractures

Long oblique fractures of the ilium are relatively common. They usually course in a cranioventral to caudodorsal direction. Long oblique fractures with a fracture length equal or larger than twice the dorsoventral measurement of the ilium are best stabilized with interfragmentary screws or skewer pins (Figs 35-10 and 35-11 and Box 35-6). This type of fixation compresses the fracture and counteracts the tendency of the caudal fragment to displace and rotate distally. Interfragmentary lag screw fixation of long oblique ilial fractures has been shown to result in a stronger and stiffer fixation in torsion, axial compression, and bending compared to lateral

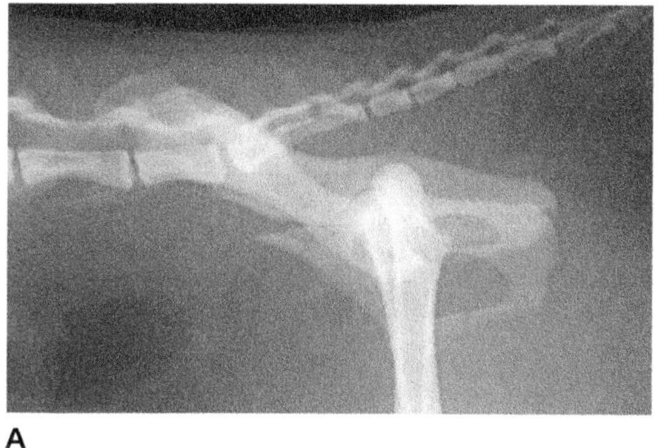

A

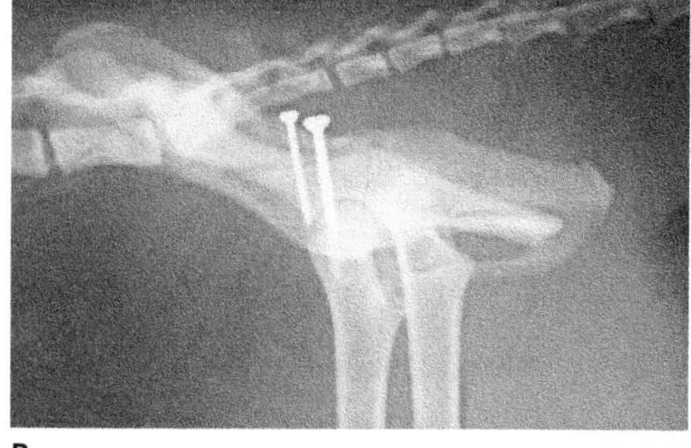

B

Figure 35-10 (**A**) Preoperative and (**B**) postoperative radiographs of the pelvis of a cat with a long oblique fracture of the ilium, stabilized with a 2.0-mm and a 1.5-mm interfragmentary lag screw.

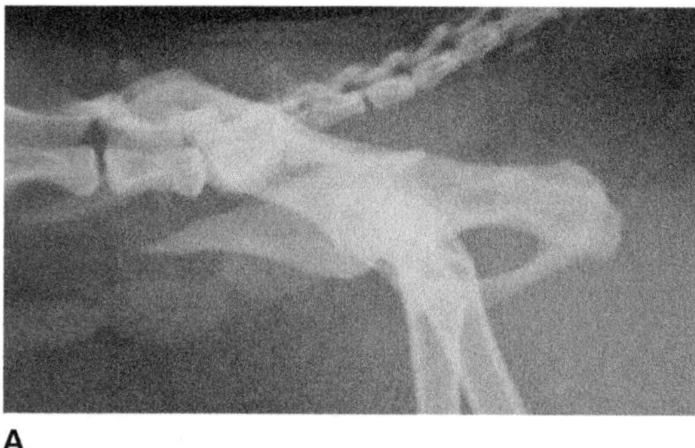

A

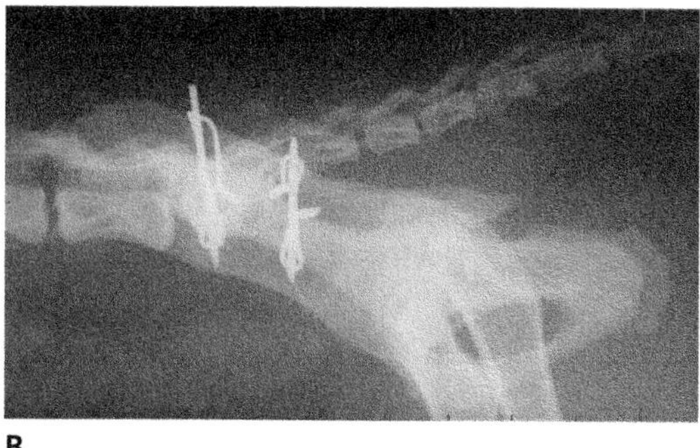

B

Figure 35-11 (**A**) Preoperative and (**B**) postoperative radiographs of the pelvis of a cat with a long oblique fracture of the ilium, stabilized with two skewer pins and figure-of-eight wires.

Box 35-6. Stabilization of long oblique fractures of the ilium

A lateral approach to the ilium is performed. The fracture is reduced anatomically, and is maintained in reduction with one or two pointed reduction forceps placed perpendicular to the fracture line.

Screw fixation: Two or three 2.0-mm positional or lag screws are inserted perpendicular to the fracture line, equally distributed over the length of the fracture line (Fig. 35-12A). The drill sleeve with the drill bit is gently pushed from dorsal through the gluteal musculature to be able to drill the holes in the axis of the ilium. The thread is cut in a similar manner, protected with a drill sleeve. Screws can be inserted without cutting a thread in young cats with soft bone.

Skewer pins: Two Kirschner wires are inserted from the dorsal to the ventral edge of the ilium, perpendicular to the fracture line, and equally distributed along the length of the fracture line (Fig. 35-12B). They are inserted through the gluteal musculature, which is protected with a drill sleeve. The Kirschner wires are cut dorsally, leaving 2 or 3 mm of a protruding tip. A figure-of-eight wire is then placed around both ends of each pin and tightened laterally. Tightening of the wire around the pins results in interfragmentary compression.

Dorsal plating: Dorsal plating, as described in Box 35-5, can also be used.

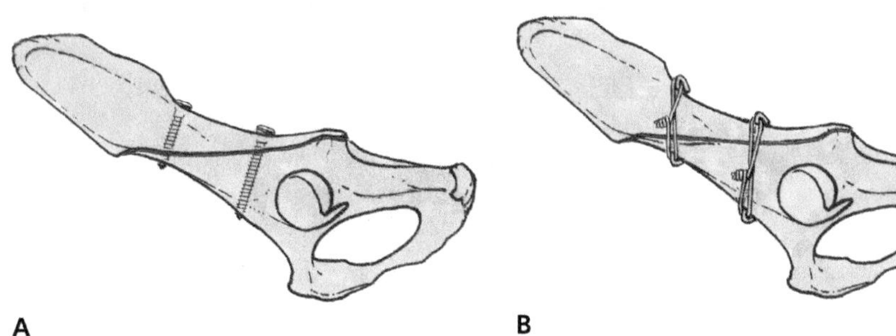

Figure 35-12 Options for stabilization of long oblique fractures of the ilium. (**A**) Stabilization using two positional or lag screws. (**B**) Stabilization with two skewer pins with a figure-of-eight wire.

plating in dogs (10). Positional screws may be used instead of lag screws after the fracture has been reduced and temporarily stabilized with pointed bone reduction forceps.

Interfragmentary compression with lag screws or skewer pins may not be possible in some cases with presence of cortical damage or fissuring of the fracture ends. Dorsal or lateral plating is then used, but dorsal plating is more suitable for long oblique fractures (Box 35-5).

35.6 Acetabular fractures

Most acetabular fractures have to be reduced and stabilized surgically to restore hip joint congruity, and prevent the development of severe degenerative joint disease and chronic pain. Conservative treatment can be indicated in immature cats with non-displaced acetabular fractures. These cats are confined to a cage for approximately 2–3 weeks, after which control radiographs are performed. However, surgery in these young cats is associated with excellent results and may give a quicker return to function (21).

In general, surgical fracture stabilization is indicated in all acetabular fractures, where anatomic reduction and stable fixation are deemed possible. The main load transmission in cats occurs in the central and caudal thirds of the acetabulum, not in the cranial part, as in humans (4). Fractures in this area should therefore also be repaired surgically, although conservative treatment of fractures of the caudal acetabulum is sometimes suggested. Plate osteosynthesis is the most widely applied stabilization method for all fracture types. Other techniques, such as screw or tension band fixation, are only indicated for specific fracture types.

Anatomic reconstruction of the joint surface and restoration of stability may be impossible in severely comminuted fractures. Femoral head and neck excision is performed in these cases as a salvage procedure. Cats have an acceptable, although not normal, limb function after femoral head and neck excision (Chapter 36). It can be difficult to evaluate on preoperative radiographs if the fracture is reducible or not, and the decision for femoral head and neck excision is often taken intraoperatively. This should be discussed with the owners prior to surgery.

35.6.1 Approaches to the acetabulum

Several approaches to the acetabulum may be chosen. A craniodorsal approach to the hip joint is usually adequate for simple acetabular fractures located in the cranial third of the acetabular fossa (15). A dorsal intergluteal approach to the acetabulum is sufficient to apply a short plate or pin and tension band for simple fractures of the middle or caudal acetabulum (15). An approach to the hip joint using a trochanteric osteotomy or gluteal tenotomies gives the best exposure of the whole acetabulum (15). This approach is chosen for comminuted fractures or where a wider exposure is useful. The greater trochanter is reattached at the end of surgery using a tension band fixation, a lag screw, or divergent Kirschner wires (Chapter 37).

35.6.2 Reducible fractures in adult cats

Reducible fractures include simple transverse fractures, simple oblique fractures, and reducible multifragmentary fractures. The latter is rare in cats, because the fragments are often too small to allow insertion of implants. Fracture reduction is often the most challenging part of surgery. The caudal fragment is usually dislocated or rotated ventrally due to the pull of the hamstring muscles. Placing a Kirschner wire in or small Kern bone-holding forceps on the ischial tuberosity helps to manipulate the caudal fragment. Manipulation of the greater trochanter and hip joint also helps to achieve reduction if the caudal fragment is attached to the round ligament. A nerve hook placed in the obturator foramen can also help in fracture reduction. Pointed reduction forceps or a temporary or permanent Kirschner wire inserted across the fracture helps to maintain reduction while other implants are applied.

Different plates can be used depending on fracture location and type. These include the 2.0-mm DCP, 2.0-mm acetabular plate, and 2.0-mm reconstruction plates. Perfect plate contouring is necessary to obtain anatomic reduction. This is best done preoperatively with the help of the pelvic bone of a skeleton. The plate is positioned dorsally on the tension side of the fracture (Fig. 35-13). Short plates with only two screws in each fragment can be used in simple transverse fractures. Application of short plates facilitates plate contouring and carries less risk for secondary loss of reduction during plate application. Longer plates are chosen for oblique and multifragmentary reducible fractures.

Internal fixators, such as the 2.0-mm Unilock plate, are a valuable alternative to use instead of conventional plates. Their advantages include better stability with only two screws

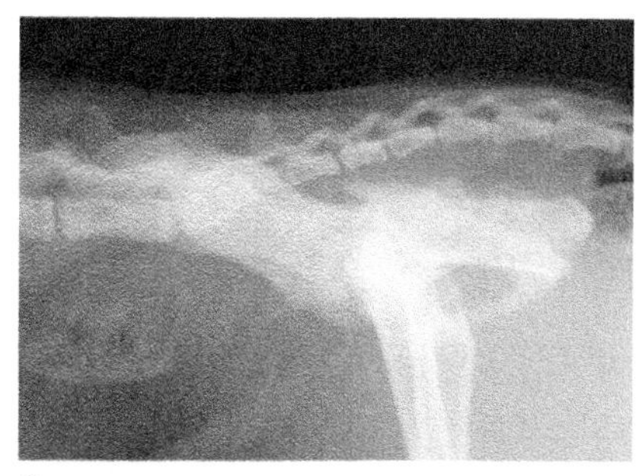
A

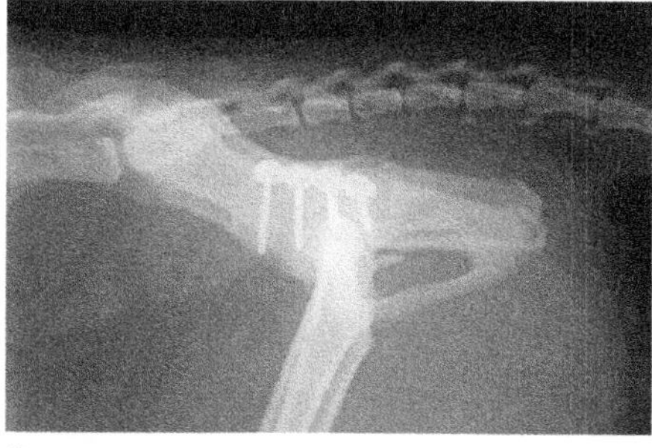
C

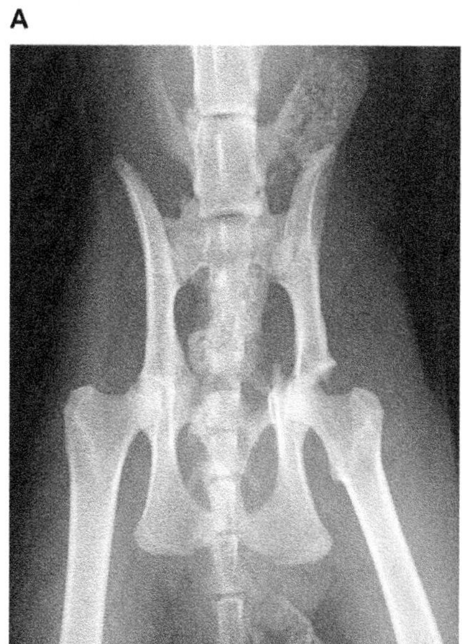
B

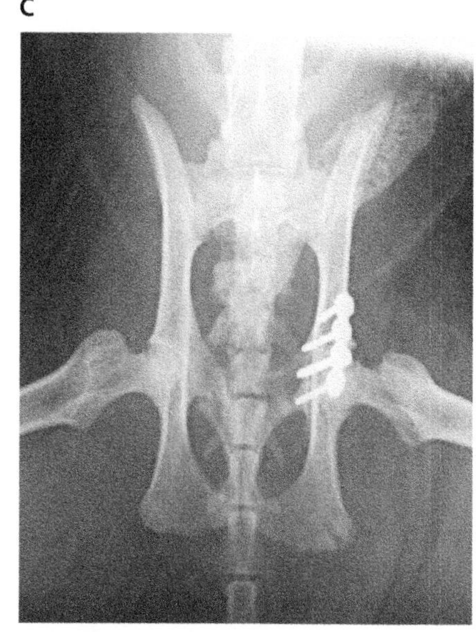
D

Figure 35-13 (**A**, **B**) Preoperative and (**C**, **D**) postoperative radiographs showing a simple oblique acetabular fracture in a 1-year-old cat. The fracture was anatomically reduced and stabilized with a dorsolaterally applied 2.0-mm Unilock plate.

Box 35-7. Stabilization of acetabular fractures

A craniolateral approach, caudal intermuscular approach, trochanteric osteotomy, or gluteal tenotomies are performed to visualize the fracture. The fracture is reduced anatomically as described above, and the hip joint is cleared of debris.

Plating: The plate is positioned as dorsal as possible to achieve a tension band function, and to reduce the risk of screw insertion into the joint. Exact plate contouring is essential in order to maintain reduction. The dorsal aspect of the feline pelvis is fairly flat, and both a straight 2.0-mm dynamic compression plate and 2.0-mm reconstruction plate can be successfully used for simple transverse fractures (Fig. 35-14A). Insertion of two screws cranial and caudal to the fracture is sufficient in simple fractures, because the plate is applied in tension band function. Longer plates with three screws must be used for oblique and multifragmentary fractures. Screw penetration into the hip joint is avoided.

Internal fixator: An internal fixator with two locking screws per fragment is applied at the same location as a plate. Secondary loss of reduction does not occur with internal fixators, so plate contouring is less critical. Screws can be inserted monocortically to avoid the hip joint. If screws need to be angled to avoid the hip joint, a non-locking screw has to be used.

Tension band repair: The tension band repair can be used for physeal fractures or simple transverse fractures with inherent stability. One or two small Kirschner wires may be inserted across the fracture to aid maintenance of reduction. A 1.5–2.0-mm screw is then inserted into both cranial and caudal fracture fragments. Both screws need to be placed at the same distance from the acetabular rim to avoid shear and loss of fracture reduction as the intervening wire is tightened (Fig. 35-14B). Stainless-steel washers can be used under the screw heads to decrease the chance of the figure-of-eight wire slipping off. The screw heads are connected with a figure-of-eight wire using 0.4–0.8-mm orthopedic wire. A small bleb of sterile polymethyl methacrylate can be used on top of the implants to decrease implant loosening and increase stability of the construct. Early implant removal should be considered to reduce the chance of premature closure in very young kittens.

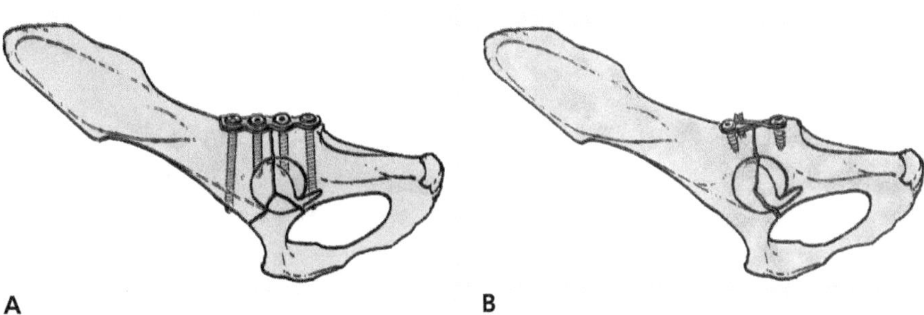

Figure 35-14 Stabilization options for acetabular fractures. (**A**) Simple transverse fracture stabilized with a 2.0-mm plate in tension band function. (**B**) Tension band repair of a physeal fracture.

in each fragment (20), the possibility of using monocortical screws, and that there is no risk for secondary loss of reduction, because the plate is not compressed down on to the bone during screw insertion.

Lag screw fixation can rarely be chosen for simple oblique fractures through the cranial or caudal acetabulum. At least two lag screws are placed perpendicular to the fracture line. Tension band repair is also possible in some simple transverse fractures with inherent stability. An interfragmentary pin may need to be inserted additionally to prevent shearing motion. The repair is less stable than plate osteosynthesis, but technically easier, and there may be less chance of loss of fracture reduction. The techniques for repair of acetabular fractures are described in Box 35-7.

35.6.3 Acetabular physeal fractures

The acetabulum can fracture through the acetabular physis in immature cats. These can be repaired using a screw and tension band technique (21) (Fig. 35-15). In kittens younger than 12 weeks, there is a possibility of premature fusion of the acetabular bone, resulting in development of a deformed, shallow acetabulum and hip subluxation. Early implant removal in such young kittens may decrease the severity of deformity caused by premature physeal closure. In kittens of 16 weeks or older, the prognosis is good for normal acetabular development, and implant removal is not necessary. Four kittens treated in this manner had an excellent outcome and full limb use following fracture repair (21).

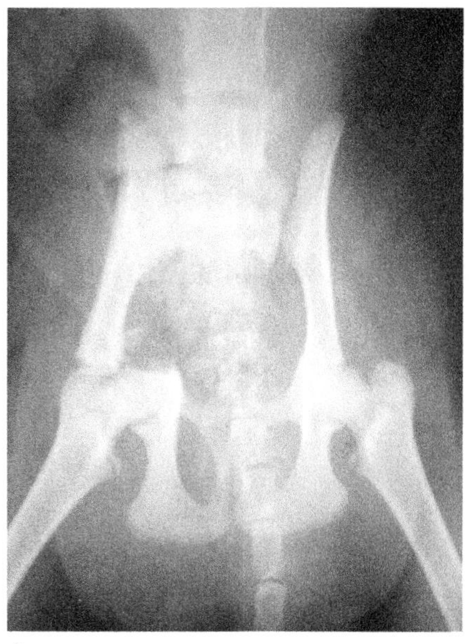

A

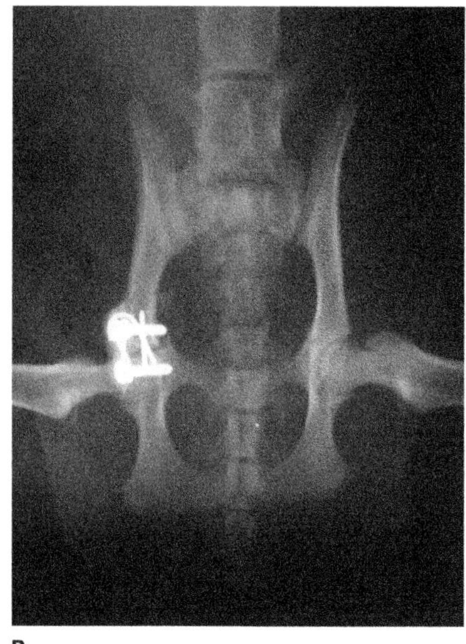

B

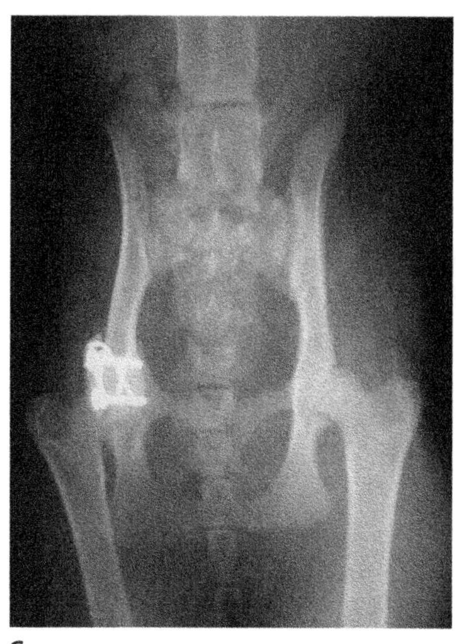

C

Figure 35-15 Kitten with an acetabular physeal fracture.
(**A**) Preoperative radiograph of a 14-week-old kitten with a displaced mildly comminuted physeal fracture and sacroiliac subluxation after falling off a wardrobe.
(**B**) The fracture was reduced and stabilized with small crossed Kirschner wires, two 2.0-mm screws, a 0.8-mm figure-of-eight tension band wire, and a small bleb of sterile bone cement.
(**C**) Follow-up radiograph at 8 weeks shows fracture healing. (Reproduced with permission from: Langley-Hobbs SJ, et al. Tension band stabilisation of acetabular physeal fractures in four kittens. J Feline Med Surg 2007;9:177–178.)

35.7 Fractures of the pelvic floor

The pelvic floor is fractured in 90% of cats with pelvic fractures (1). Most of the pelvic floor fractures are accompanied by uni- or bilateral sacroiliac joint luxation, or fractures of the ilial body. Fractures of the pelvic floor may be classified as symphyseal separations, and uni- or bilateral fractures of the pubic body or ramus, and/or ischial ramus. Fractures of the pelvic floor may result in loss of ability to adduct the hindlimbs, when one or both hemipelves are unstable due to concurrent lesions. Affected cats may be unable to stand and walk.

Stabilization of concurrent fracture/luxations of the weight-bearing parts of the pelvic ring often results in sufficient stability and allows healing of the pelvic floor without specific treatment. A hobble sling may be applied to prevent abduction of the hind legs (Chapter 22).

However, there are some indications where stabilization of pelvic floor fractures is advantageous. Bilateral sacroiliac luxations or sacroiliac luxation with a contralateral ilial fracture render both hemipelves markedly unstable, when associated with pelvic floor fractures (Fig. 35-16). Surgical repair of the pelvic floor re-establishes the shape of the pelvic ring, prevents collapse of the pelvic canal, and reduces the risk of implant loosening of sacroiliac screws and ilial plates in severely unstable lesions.

It is most practical to stabilize pelvic floor fractures surgically if an approach to the area has to be performed for other reasons. Examples include repair of sacroiliac joint luxations with a ventroabdominal approach (Box 35-4), and if an abdominal approach is performed for repair of body wall hernias or other abdominal injuries. Symphyseal separations can be repaired with hemicerclage wires or cerclage wires through the obturator foramen. Plate osteosynthesis is required to stabilize fractures of the pubic body and ramus (Box 35-8).

35.8 Fractures of the pelvic margin

Fractures of the pelvic margin include fractures of the ilial wing and ischial tuberosity. These fractures are caused by avulsion of muscle insertion sites and may be significantly displaced. Avulsion fractures of the ischial tuberosity are frequently seen in cats (Fig. 35-18). They accompany other pelvic fractures and injuries of other parts of the hindlimbs, or occur as an isolated injury. Most of these fractures can be treated conservatively. Reattachment will provide a more rapid and functional healing if the avulsed fragment is large, grossly displaced, and/or very painful. Divergent threaded pins or a pin and tension band technique can be used to repair these avulsion fractures.

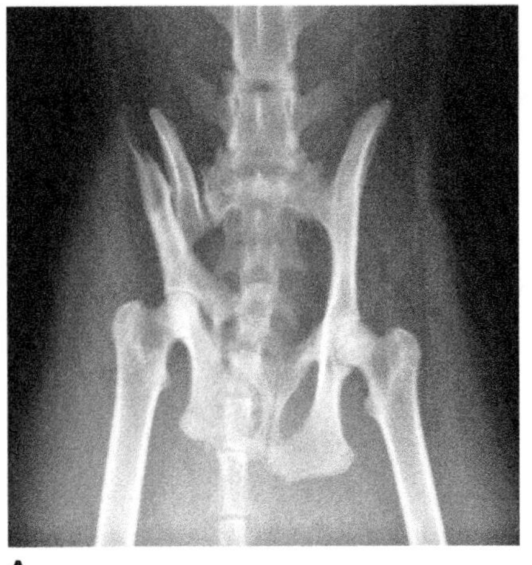
A

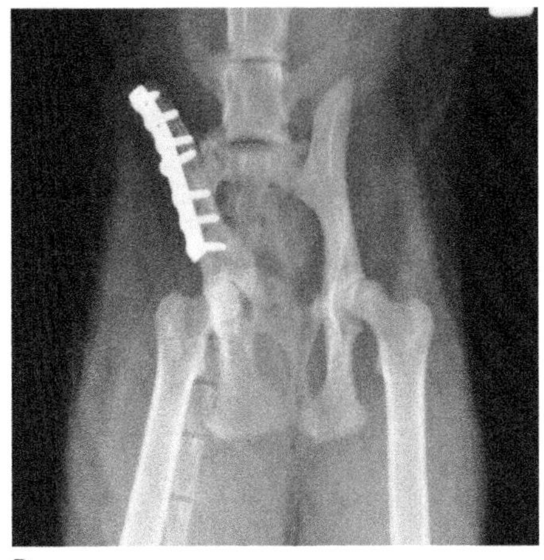
B

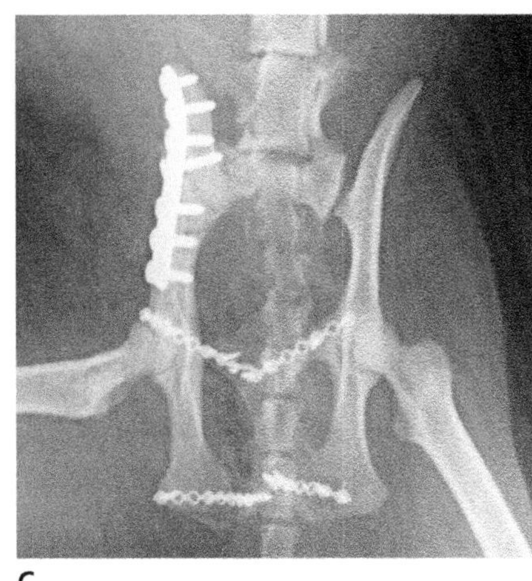
C

Figure 35-16 Repair of the pelvic floor indicated by pelvic canal narrowing.
(**A**) Radiograph of a cat with an ilial fracture, and bilateral pubic and ischial fractures.
(**B**) The ilial fracture was stabilized with a plate. On postoperative radiographs a sacral wing fracture was visible (not seen on the preoperative films), which resulted in medial displacement of the hemipelvis.
(**C**) Reduction and stabilization of the pelvic floor with miniplates allowed restoration of the width of the pelvic canal.

Box 35-8. Stabilization of fractures of the pelvic floor

A ventral approach to the pelvic floor is performed. Intrapelvic organs must be protected during reduction and implant placement. Anatomic reduction of the pelvic floor may not be possible if surgical repair of a sacroiliac luxation or ilial fracture has already been performed imperfectly. It is then stabilized as is.

Hemicerclages: One or two holes are predrilled bilateral to the symphysis, and a piece of 0.6-mm orthopedic wire is passed through the holes prior to reduction, taking care not to injure intrapelvic soft-tissue structures. The symphysis is reduced and the wires are tightened (Fig. 35-17A). Alternatively, the wires can be placed through the obturator foramen as cerclage wires. Care must be taken not to overtighten the wire, which could cause overlap of the symphysis.

Plates: Small plates, such as 1.0-mm maxillofacial plates, 1.3-mm hand plates, or 1.5-mm miniplates, are used to stabilize fractures of the pubic body and ramus (Fig. 35-17B). The pubic ramus is very thin and the screws must be well centered to prevent stripping. Two screws should be inserted per fragment. The screws in the pubic ramus are angled cranially to avoid the acetabular fossa. Miniplates can additionally be applied on the ventral surface of the ischium, as shown in Figure 35-16.

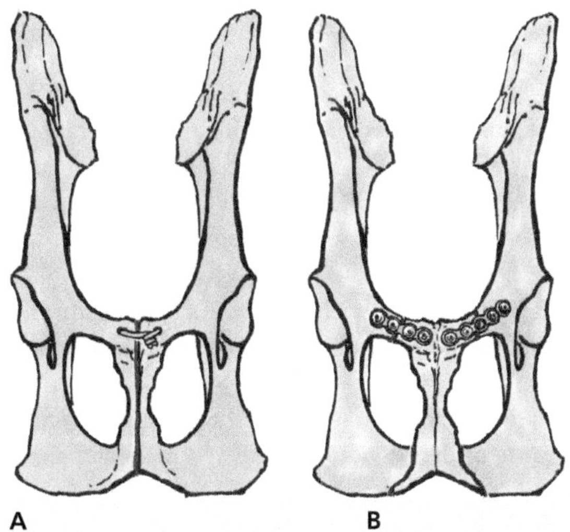

Figure 35-17 Options for stabilizing fractures of the pelvic floor.
(**A**) Stabilization of a symphyseal separation with hemicerclage wire.
(**B**) Plate osteosynthesis of a fracture of the pelvic floor, using miniplates. Care is taken to avoid the acetabular fossa with the most lateral screws.

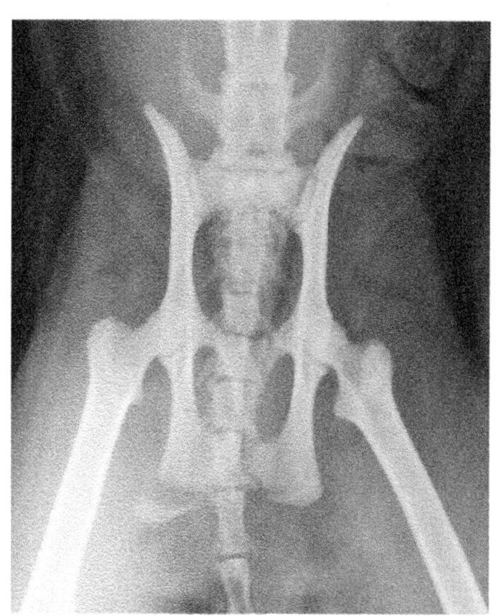

Figure 35-18 Radiograph of a cat with an isolated avulsion fracture of the ischial tuberosity. The cat was presented with an acute onset of lameness, which resolved with cage rest.

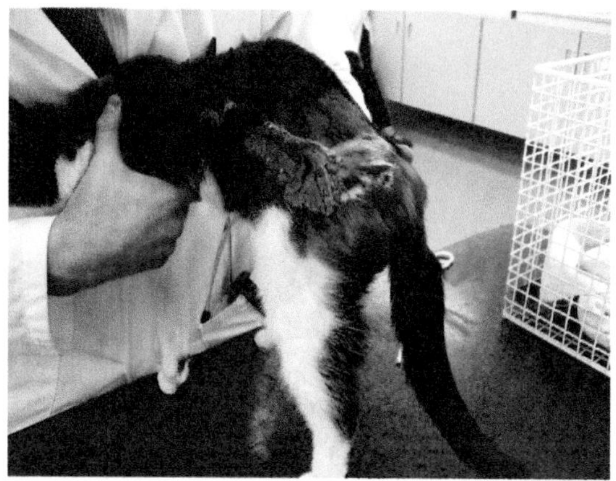

Figure 35-19 Skin necrosis after pelvic fracture in a 2-year-old cat. The skin over the lateral abdominal and pelvic area progressively formed a hard black eschar several days after the accident. Six weeks postoperatively (picture) the contracted skin had formed a scab, which was then removed. Delayed primary closure and placement of a closed suction drain were necessary to close the wound completely.

35.9 Postoperative treatment and prognosis

Postoperative treatment of pelvic fractures consists of cage confinement for 2–4 weeks, and restriction of activity to indoors for another 3–6 weeks. An appropriate analgesic protocol is necessary in the immediate postoperative period to improve overall well-being and food and water intake, and promote early weight-bearing. Intravenous infusions are provided until the patient starts to eat. Inability or unwillingness to stand up or move can result in urinary retention and obstipation. Gentle manual expression of the bladder or placement of an indwelling urinary catheter and application of enemas may be required.

A number of complications can be encountered after pelvic fractures. Avascular necrosis of the skin around the perineum, back, and tail sometimes develops due to skin avulsion at the original trauma (22). The skin can be left until it has formed a scab (Fig. 35-19). The scab is then removed or resected with the remaining contracted underlying lesion treated as an open wound. Antibiotics are administered until a healthy granulation bed has formed. Delayed wound closure or a skin graft can then be performed.

Cats with pelvic canal narrowing of more than 40% are likely to develop chronic constipation and obstipation (Fig. 35-20) (8). Medical management may be sufficient in mild cases. It includes oral administration of stool softeners, a high-fiber diet, and application of enemas. Phosphate enemas are contraindicated in cats because of toxicity (23). Cases which cannot be managed conservatively, and in which clinical signs have persisted for less than 6 months, should undergo surgical widening of the pelvic canal (23). Long-standing constipation and dilation of the colon result in irreversible neuromuscular damage of the intestinal wall. Subtotal colectomy is therefore indicated if clinical signs have been present for longer than 6 months (23, 24).

35.9.1 Sacroiliac luxation

Overall, the prognosis is good after sacroiliac luxation if no neurological deficits are present and the implants were placed correctly. However, numerous complications can occur. These including malpositioning of the screw in the lumbosacral intervertebral space or, less commonly in the spinal canal, postoperative nerve deficits, malreduction, generally concurrent with medial displacement of the caudal hemipelvis, and screw loosening in the postoperative period. Residual lameness was described to occur in 9–33% of cats with sacroiliac luxation repaired with a lateral lag screw (11). The incidence was lower if screw positioning was correct (11).

Sacroiliac fracture repair with a lag screw was the most common reason for sciatic injury in one study (25). Three of the cats had tibial nerve palsy, and one tibial and peroneal nerve deficits. All four cats regained neurological function within 6 months.

35.9.2 Ilium fractures

The prognosis for fractures of the ilium is good, providing that adequate stability is achieved and no nerve deficits are present. Fracture-healing disorders such as malunion, nonunion, and exuberant callus formation enhance the risk for entrapment of the sciatic nerve (26). Lateral plating of fractures of the ilium is associated with a high incidence of screw loosening (8, 19). More than half of the cats had loose screws

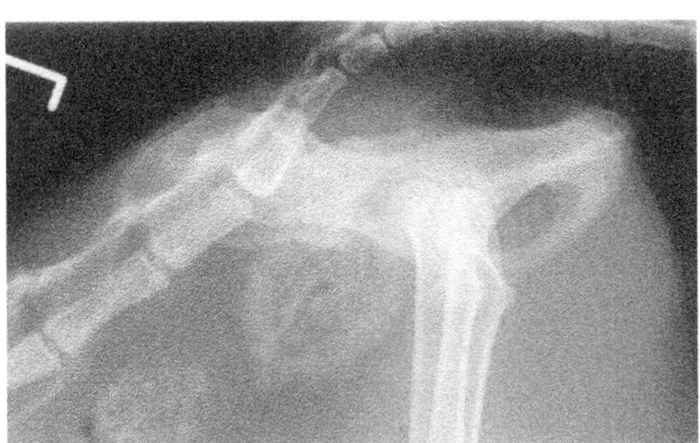

A

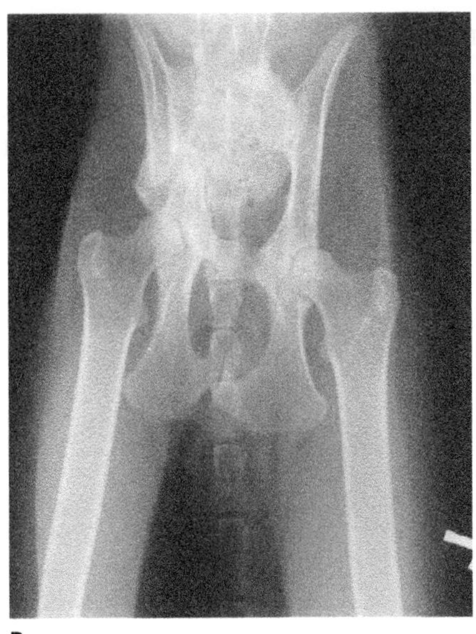

B

Figure 35-20 (**A**) Radiographs of a cat with constipation (**B**) secondary to pelvic canal narrowing.

with varying degrees of pelvic canal narrowing in one study (8). Screw loosening is less likely with dorsal plating. The prognosis for return of neurological function depends on the severity of nerve damage. Cats with loss of deep pain sensation of the sciatic dermatomes have a guarded prognosis. Overall, around 80% of dogs and cats with sciatic nerve paresis associated with pelvic fractures are likely to regain good to excellent limb function (6). Regeneration of peripheral nerves does take time, but if no improvement is seen after 3 months, the prognosis is poor.

35.9.3 Acetabular fractures

Most cats seem to regain good function after acetabular fracture repair; however, a variable degree of degenerative joint disease must be expected, mainly dependent on the reduction achieved of the severity of the original fracture. In the study on acetabular physeal fractures in four kittens the outcome was excellent with no clinical signs of lameness in any of the cases, despite radiographic evidence of degenerative joint disease (21). Iatrogenic sciatic nerve injury has been described in two cats after acetabular fracture repair, one of which regained neurological function (25).

References and further reading

1. Bookbinder PF, Flanders JA. Characteristics of pelvic fracture in the cat. Vet Comp Orthop Traumatol 1992;5:122–127.
2. Hill FWG. A survey of bone fractures in the cat. J Small Anim Pract 1977;18:457–463.
3. Messmer M, Montavon PM. Pelvic fractures in the dog and cat: a classification system and review of 556 cases. Vet Comp Orthop Traumatol 2004;4:167–173.
4. Beck AL, et al. Regional load bearing of the feline acetabulum. J Biomech 2005;38:427–432.
5. Böhmer E. Beckenfrakturen und -luxationen bei der Katze. München: Ludwig-Maximilians-Universität; 1985.
6. Jacobson A, Schrader SC. Peripheral nerve injury associated with fracture or fracture-dislocation of the pelvis in dogs and cats: 34 cases (1978–1982). J Am Vet Med Assoc 1987;190: 569–572.
7. Selcer BA. Urinary tract trauma associated with pelvic trauma. J Am Anim Hosp Assoc 1982;19:785.
8. Hamilton MH, et al. A review of feline ilial fractures repaired by lateral plating and the use of a dorsal plate as an alternative method of repair. Proceedings of the ECVS meeting 2006; Seville, Spain; pp. 314–317.
9. Damur DM, Montavon PM. Comparison of the conventional versus the oscillating drilling mode in pelvic surgery in dogs. BSAVA Congress 2001; Birmingham, England.
10. VanGrundy TE, et al. Mechanical evaluation of two canine iliac fracture fixation systems. Vet Surg 1988;17:321–327.
11. Burger M, et al. Sacroiliac luxation in the cat. Part 2: cases and results. Kleintierpraxis 2005;50:281–348.
12. Borer LR, et al. Ventral abdominal approach for screw fixation of sacroiliac luxation in clinically affected cats. Am J Vet Res 2008;69:549–556.
13. Kaderly RE. Stabilization of bilateral sacroiliac fracture-luxations in small animals with a single transsacral screw. Vet Surg 1991;20:91–96.
14. Raffan PJ, et al. A tension band technique for stabilisation of sacroiliac separations in cats. J Small Anim Pract 2002;43: 255–260.
15. Piermattei DL, Johnson KA. An atlas of surgical approaches to the bones and joints of the dog and the cat, 4th edn. Philadelphia: WB Saunders; 2004.
16. Montavon PM, et al. Ventrolateral approach for repair of sacroiliac fracture-dislocation in the dog and cat. J Am Vet Med Assoc 1985;186:1198–1201.
17. DeCamp CE, Braden TD. Sacroiliac fracture-separation in the dog: a study of 92 cases. Vet Surg 1985;14:127–130.

18. Burger M, et al. Surgical anatomy of the feline sacroiliac joint for lag screw fixation of sacroiliac fracture-luxation. Vet Comp Orthop Traumatol 2004;17:146–151.
19. Roush JK, Manley PA. Mini plate failure after repair of ilial and acetabular fractures in nine small dogs and one cat. J Am Anim Hosp Assoc 1992;28:112–118.
20. Sikes JW, et al. Comparison of fixation strengths of locking head and conventional screws, in fracture and reconstruction models. J Oral Maxillofac Surg 1998;56:468–473.
21. Langley-Hobbs SJ, et al. Tension band stabilisation of acetabular physeal fractures in four kittens. J Feline Med Surg 2007;9:177–187.
22. Declercq J. Alopecia and dermatopathy of the lower back following pelvic fractures in three cats. Vet Dermatol 2004;15: 42–46.
23. Colopy-Poulsen SA, et al. Managing feline obstipation secondary to pelvic fractures. Compend Continuing Educ 2005:27: 662–669.
24. Washabau RJ, Holt D. Pathogenesis, diagnosis, and therapy of feline idiopathic megacolon. Vet Clin North Am Small Anim Pract 1999;29:589–603.
25. Forterre F. Iatrogenic sciatic nerve injury in eighteen dogs and nine cats. Vet Surg 2007;36:464–471.
26. Chambers JN, Hardie EM. Localization and management of sciatic nerve injury due to ischial or acetabular fracture. J Am Anim Hosp Assoc 1986;22:539–544.

36 Hip joint

K. Voss, S.J. Langley-Hobbs, P.M. Montavon

The feline hip joint is commonly injured. Injuries include luxations, fractures of the femoral head and neck, and acetabular fractures. Fractures of the femoral head and neck are described in Chapter 37, and fractures of the acetabulum are covered in Chapter 35. The present chapter focuses on the treatment of coxofemoral luxations.

The most common diseases of the hip joint are hip dysplasia and coxarthrosis. Hip dysplasia has been recognized to occur with a higher frequency than what would be expected from the number of cats with clinical signs due to dysplasia seen in veterinary clinics. Other diseases involving the hip joint in cats are slipped capital physes or femoral neck metaphyseal osteopathy. These are also described in this chapter.

36.1 Surgical anatomy

The hip joint consists of the acetabular fossa and the femoral head. The acetabulum in cats is shallower than in dogs. The most important stabilizers of the hip joint are the teres ligament, the joint capsule, and the transverse ligament, which completes the acetabular fossa ventrally. The teres or round ligament originates from the acetabular fossa and inserts on the fovea capitis of the femur. The joint capsule extends from the acetabular rim to the base of the femoral neck, enclosing the femoral neck and the proximal capital physis in growing animals. The blood supply to the hip joint is derived from four different arteries: the medial and lateral circumflex femoral arteries: the caudal gluteal artery, and the iliolumbar artery (1). These arteries form a ring-like vascular net around the femoral neck. They supply the greater trochanter, the femoral neck, and the femoral head in adult cats. In young cats the femoral head is also supplied by a branch of the medial circumflex femoral artery, which courses from the acetabulum via the round ligament into the femoral head. This branch disappears after 7 months of age (1).

36.2 Diagnosis and treatment options

Trauma to the hip joint can result in coxofemoral luxation, acetabular fractures, and fractures of the femoral head and neck. An acute often non-weight-bearing lameness results. Clinical examination findings for all of these conditions are pain and crepitation on manipulation of the hip joint and a reduction in the range of motion.

The hip joint usually luxates in a craniodorsal or caudodorsal direction. Affected cats hold the hindlimb in adduction and external rotation, and the affected limb appears to be shorter than the contralateral one. Comparing leg length or the distance between the bony protuberances of the pelvis and the greater trochanter between the injured and the normal limb is an easy test to detect hip joint luxation in cats (Fig. 36-1). Radiographs are necessary to confirm the diagnosis and to detect concurrent abnormalities or fractures. Laterolateral radiographs are the best views to take to confirm coxofemoral luxation. Orthogonal ventrodorsal extended and/or frog-leg radiographs should also be taken for detection of fractures of the dorsal rim of the acetabulum, avulsion fractures of the teres ligament, and concurrent fractures of the greater trochanter. The goal of treatment is to reduce the hip joint and to stabilize it sufficiently to allow fibrous healing of the joint capsule and surrounding tissue, resulting in a stable and functional joint. Treatment options include either closed reduction or open reduction with internal stabilization of the hip joint. Several procedures have been described, some of which are summarized in Table 36-1.

Cats with diseases of the hip joint, such as hip dysplasia and coxarthrosis, and diseases of the femoral head and neck are usually presented with a more chronic insidious-onset lameness, reluctance to move or jump, and muscle atrophy. Diagnosis is best obtained from ventrodorsal radiographs.

36.3 Approaches to the hip joint

The craniolateral approach is most commonly performed, and is used for repair of coxofemoral luxations, and for femoral head and neck excision (2). A partial incision of the tendon of the deep gluteal muscle is performed approximately 3 mm away from its insertion on the greater trochanter. The tendon is reconstructed with a tendon suture (Chapter 16). Caudodistal retraction of the greater trochanter with a small Meyerding retractor improves visualization of the acetabular fossa.

The hip joint can also be approached through a ventral incision, with the cat in dorsal recumbency and the limbs abducted (2). Care has to be taken not to injure the femoral

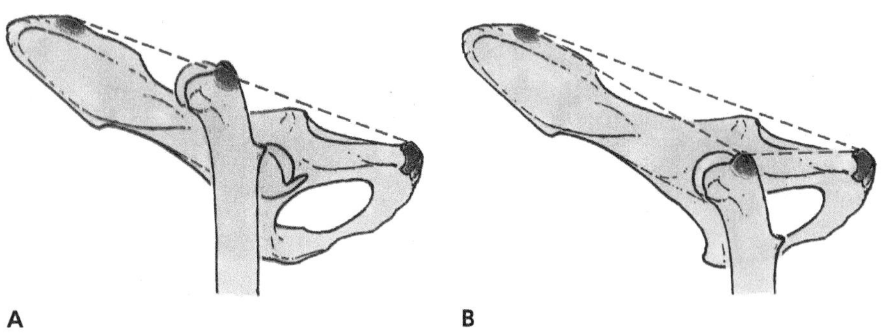

Figure 36-1 The greater trochanter is displaced dorsally and cranially with craniodorsal luxation of the hip joint. The distance between the tuber ischium and the greater trochanter is therefore longer on the affected side (**A**) than on the contralateral side (**B**).

Table 36-1. A summary of treatment options for conditions of the hip joint.

Type of lesion	Further classification	Treatment options
Hip dysplasia and coxarthrosis		Conservative FHNE or THR if pain persists
Conditions of the femoral head and neck	Slipped capital femoral physis Femoral neck metaphyseal osteopathy	FHNE Parallel pinning in very early cases? THR?
Craniodorsal or caudodorsal hip luxation	Normal configuration of hip joint and absence of avulsion fractures	Closed reduction Open reduction and capsular suture Iliofemoral suture sling Transarticular pinning Other techniques
	Avulsion fractures	Open reduction and transarticular pinning FHNE if fracture fragments are large
	Severe hip dysplasia	FHNE or THR
Ventral hip luxation		Closed reduction Open reduction and ventral stabilization

FHNE, femoral head and neck excision; THR, total hip replacement.

artery and vein, the saphenous nerve, and the medial circumflex femoral artery and vein during dissection. This approach can be used for femoral head and neck excisions, and for pin stabilization of femoral head or neck fractures (Chapter 37).

36.4 Hip dysplasia

Hip dysplasia is an inherited disease that is well documented in several species. Feline hip dysplasia was first described in the 1970s (3, 4), and surprisingly high radiographic incidences have been reported since, ranging from 7% to 32% (5, 6). The wide variation in the reported frequency of hip dysplasia may be due to more systematic screening, different criteria used for radiographic evaluation of the hip joints, and differences in breeds examined. Purebred cats have a higher incidence of hip dysplasia compared to domestic short-hair cats. The prevalence for hip dysplasia in domestic short-hair cats was 6% versus 12% in purebred cats in one report (5). Breeds reported or suspected to have a high prevalence for hip dysplasia include the Maine Coon, Himalayan, Siamese,

Abyssinian, Devon Rex, and Persian cats (5, 6). The mode of inheritance is not yet clear, but seems to follow a multifactorial pattern.

Despite the high frequency of hip dysplasia in radiological studies, few reports exist of cats with clinical problems due to hip dysplasia (4, 7). Clinical signs are often more discrete and awareness of feline hip dysplasia is lower when compared to dogs, probably leading to underdiagnosis of the disease. Clinical signs of feline hip dysplasia and/or coxarthrosis include inactivity, lameness, reluctance to jump and climb stairs, muscle atrophy, and crepitation and pain on manipulation of the hip joint. Some cats with hip dysplasia have been reported to suffer from patellar luxation concurrently (4–9).

Radiographic features of hip dysplasia and coxarthrosis in the cat are somewhat different from in the dog. The most obvious radiological findings of hip dysplasia are a shallow acetabulum and subluxation of the femoral head (5, 7) (Fig. 36-2). Degenerative changes seem to develop later and to a lesser extent than in dogs. The most extensive proliferative and remodeling changes involve the craniodorsal aspect of the acetabulum. Remodeling of the femoral head and neck is usually absent or mild (Fig. 36-3). When evaluating feline hip joints it should be taken into account that the normal acetabulum of cats is generally shallower than in dogs. However, less than 50% coverage of the femoral head is commonly, but not necessarily, associated with the development of coxarthrosis (5).

The relationship between objective radiographic measurements and development of coxarthrosis has been evaluated in 78 cats (6). In this study the Norberg angle and distraction indices were compared between cats with and without coxofemoral degenerative joint disease. The Norberg angle is the angle between a line drawn from the center of the femoral head to the cranial acetabular edge, and a line drawn between the centers of the two femoral heads. The Norberg angle of normal cats was 95°, which is lower than in dogs. This difference reflects the shallower acetabulum in cats. All but one cat with an angle larger than 93° were free of degenerative joint disease. The mean Norberg angle of cats with degenerative joint disease was 84°, which is significantly lower than in cats without degenerative joint changes. The distraction index is used to measure passive coxofemoral laxity. The distraction index also differed between cats with and without degenerative joint disease. Cats with a distraction index lower than 0.4 did not have signs of degenerative joint disease, whereas cats with degenerative changes had a mean distraction index of 0.6. The distraction index of normal cats seems to be higher than in normal dogs, indicating that cats have more normal passive laxity in their coxofemoral joints than dogs.

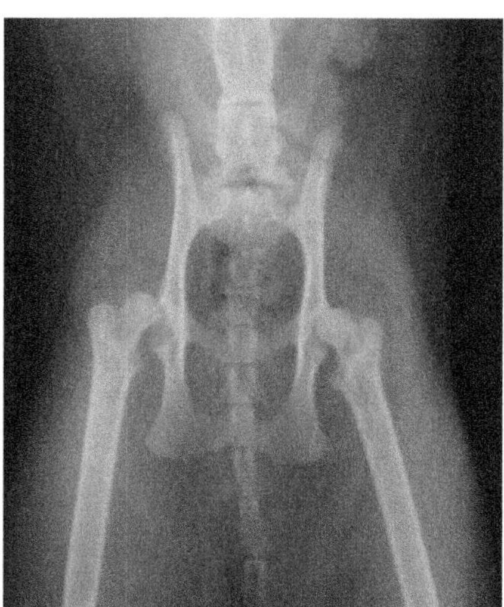

Figure 36-2 A 1-year-old Devon Rex cat with bilateral hip dysplasia. The acetabula seem shallow. There is a marked subluxation of the right, and a less pronounced subluxation of the left hip joint. The cat also had bilateral patellar luxation.

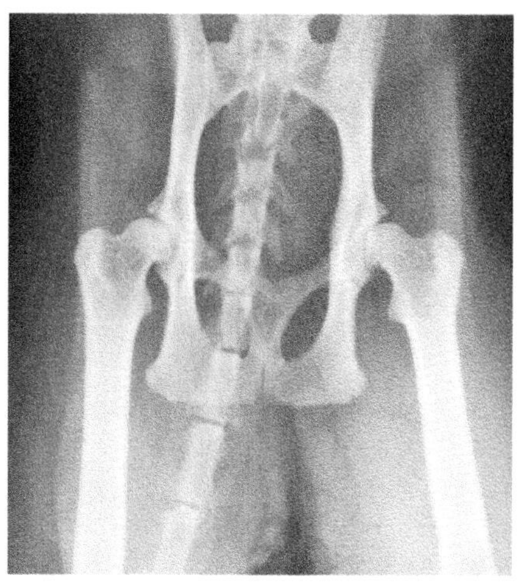

Figure 36-3 Radiograph of a 3-year-old cat with coxarthrosis secondary to hip dysplasia. The cat was presented for reluctance to jump. Note the shallow acetabula, and degenerative joint changes most evident at the cranial border of the acetabula.

Although many cats with coxarthrosis do not display clinical signs, severe degenerative changes of the hip joint will lead to pain and discomfort. Breeders of the affected purebred cats should be aware of that potential, and cats with obvious changes should not be used for breeding, even in the absence of conclusive criteria for exclusion of cats from breeding programs. It appears that cats with a Norberg angle of 84° and lower, and a distraction index of 0.6 or higher, are likely to develop degenerative joint disease (6). These cats should be excluded from breeding, or at least be rechecked to monitor for the development of degenerative changes.

Conservative treatment of hip dysplasia and coxarthrosis is often successful in cats and includes weight reduction, pain medication, and the long-term application of slow-acting disease-modifying agents (Chapter 5). Surgical treatment options should be considered if conservative treatment fails.

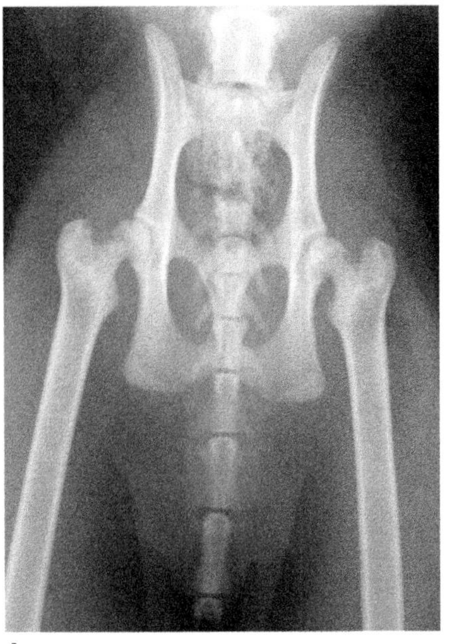
A

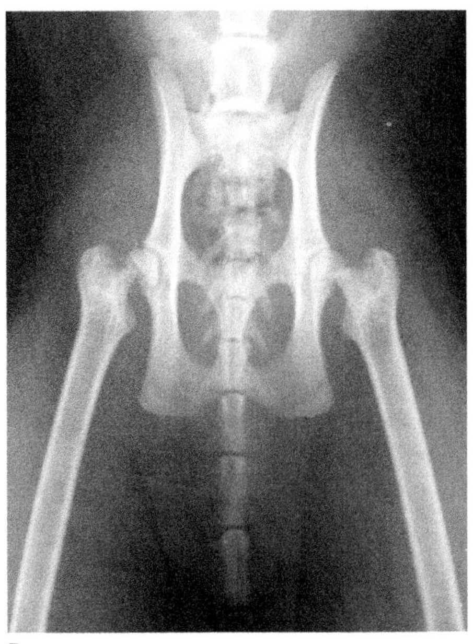
B

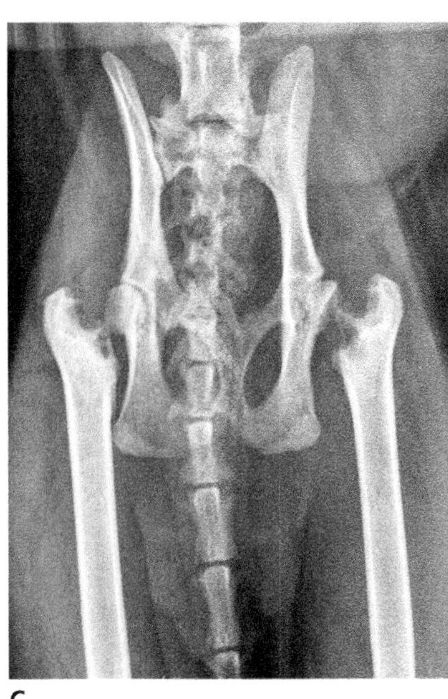
C

Figure 36-4 A 1.5-year-old male castrated cat with bilateral slipped capital femoral physes/femoral neck metaphyseal osteopathy. (**A–C**) The radiographs were taken 3 weeks apart from each other. The main feature in this cat is a rapidly progressing resorption of the femoral necks. Slippage of the physes is less pronounced. Frog leg radiographs could have been performed to further evaluate physeal stability. (Courtesy of B. Peirone.)

Tenectomy of the pectineus muscle was performed successfully in one cat with hip dysplasia (3). Although the use of tenectomy or myectomy of the pectineus muscle in cats cannot be extrapolated from a single case report, the technique may have advantages over femoral head and neck excision in some cases. It can easily be performed bilaterally, may reduce pain and dorsal subluxation of the femoral head, and femoral head and neck excision is still possible at a later date if necessary. Tenotomy of the iliopsoas and neurectomy of the ventral joint capsule could also be combined with pectineus myectomy as described for dogs (10).

Femoral head and neck excision is a salvage treatment option, reserved for cats with disabling clinical problems. Although it is generally thought that cats function well after femoral head and neck excision, around one-third of cats remain slightly lame and have pain on hip manipulation (11, 12). Prosthetic hips have recently been developed for cats, and may be the salvage option of choice in the future, although the limited depth of the acetabulum may make a stable acetabular implantation difficult. Clinical experience with total hip prosthesis in cats is very limited at present.

36.5 Conditions of the femoral head and neck

Conditions of the femoral head and neck occur predominantly in young male, adult cats. Both sides are usually affected. Radiographic changes include spontaneous fractures of the femoral capital physes, pathological fractures of the femoral neck, and bone remodeling and deformation. Two entities have been described: spontaneous capital femoral fractures and femoral neck metaphyseal osteopathy. Considering the similarities between the two, it is also possible that the conditions reflect the same disease at a different stage of chronicity.

36.5.1 Spontaneous femoral capital physeal fractures

Spontaneous separation of the proximal femoral physis without evidence of trauma has been observed in a number of cats. The condition has been termed feline capital physeal dysplasia syndrome, slipped capital femoral epiphysis, or spontaneous femoral capital physeal fracture (13–16). Most of the affected cats are castrated males and they usually present at the clinic between 1 and 2 years of age with clinical signs of hindlimb lameness, weakness, or inability to jump. The disease may be unilateral or bilateral. Bilaterally affected cats have marked problems when trying to walk and jump, and show muscle hypotrophy. Overweight cats are at greater risk of developing spontaneous capital physeal fractures (13, 15). Siamese cats had a higher risk for physeal dysplasia in one study (15). Diagnosis is based on radiographic signs, which include capital physeal incongruity, displacement of the femoral epiphysis, and femoral neck resorption, osteolysis, and sclerosis (13, 16) (Fig. 36-4).

The etiology of the disease is unclear. Histopathologically, the growth plate contains irregular clusters of chondrocytes, instead of the normal columnar arrangement, with abundant cartilaginous matrix. These changes may be consistent with delayed physeal closure or may reflect physeal dysplasia. The bone of both the epiphysis and femoral neck is viable (13, 15). The proximal femoral physis closes between 30 and 40 weeks of age in intact cats (17), but castration before that age delays physeal closure significantly (18, 19). This delay in closure might predispose castrated cats to spontaneous capital physeal fractures due to prolonged loading of the physis. Obesity possibly also results in higher forces across the growth plate and may contribute to the disease.

The osteolytic and sclerotic changes in the metaphyseal bone increase with time and pseudarthrosis develops (13). Not enough cases have been described to suggest a specific therapy. In mildly or acutely affected animals without evidence of much metaphyseal bone resorption and lysis, stabilization of the capital physeal fracture with small Kirschner wires may be an option. However, the disease is frequently diagnosed in an advanced stage with marked bony changes, and femoral head and neck excision is then the treatment of choice. Significant improvement of clinical signs can be expected after femoral head and neck excision. Total hip replacement may be another treatment option.

36.5.2 Femoral neck metaphyseal osteopathy

A disease similar to the capital physeal dysplasia syndrome was described in 17 cats (20). As with physeal dysplasia, most of the cats were castrated males and presented with similar clinical signs at an age younger than 2 years. About half of the cases had bilateral disease, although sometimes the problem developed in the second limb at a later date. Radiographically, severe bone lysis of the femoral neck is evident and pathological fractures through the physis may also be observed (Fig. 36-4). Histopathology showed bone necrosis, hemorrhage, vascular congestion, and the presence of reactive fibrous tissue (20). The authors suggested that primary bone loss, similar to Legg–Calvé–Perthes disease in dogs, resulted in secondary pathological fractures of the femoral neck. The epiphysis is not affected, in contrast to Legg–Calvé–Perthes disease in dogs, but cats have a substantial blood supply to the epiphysis through the round ligament, which may preclude the epiphysis from avascular changes. Treatment of femoral neck metaphyseal osteopathy is by femoral head and neck excision or, possibly, total hip replacement.

36.6 Coxofemoral luxation

Coxofemoral luxations often result from motor vehicle accidents (21, 22) and many cats with hip joint luxation have sustained concurrent orthopedic injury (23). The degree of local soft-tissue injuries varies, but parts of the joint capsule and the round ligament are always ruptured. The gluteal muscles are torn or lacerated in severe cases. Concomitant regional fractures can also be present, including fracture of the dorsal rim of the acetabulum, avulsion fractures at the attachment of the round ligament on the femoral head, and trochanteric fractures. Trochanteric fractures mainly occur in immature animals.

Hip joint luxations are classified according to the direction that the femoral head has moved in relation to the acetabulum. It should be considered, though, that the position of the femoral head on radiographs does not necessarily match the initial direction of luxation or the location of the capsular tears. Craniodorsal luxations are most commonly seen, accounting for 72% of luxations (21). Caudodorsal luxations also occur with some frequency. Ventral luxations are exceedingly rare (21).

36.6.1 Craniodorsal and caudodorsal coxofemoral luxation

Closed reduction and conservative treatment

Closed reduction is recommended as the first treatment option for cats with acute craniodorsal and caudodorsal hip joint luxations (Box 36-1). However, reluxation is common and appropriate case selection is necessary to improve success rates. Reluxation has been reported to occur in approximately 50% of cats after closed reduction (23, 24). The most likely reason for reluxation after closed reduction is that soft tissues such as blood clots, swollen round ligament stumps, and joint capsule remain in the acetabular fossa, preventing a tight fit. The location and severity of joint capsule damage are also important for stability after closed reduction. Avulsion of the joint capsule at the acetabular rim results in unstable joints, because the fibrous labrum of the acetabulum is missing (25). Cats with avulsion fractures of the dorsal acetabular rim or femoral head and cats with hip dysplasia are also at high risk for reluxation (Fig. 36-6). Consequently, closed reduction is reserved for cases with an acute hip joint luxation, without concurrent fractures, and with a normal hip joint conformation (Fig. 36-7).

Application of an Ehmer sling after closed reduction does not seem to influence the reluxation rate in cats (22). The slings often are not tolerated well, and they tend to slip because the skin is very mobile in cats (26). Confinement of the cat to a cage for the first 10 days may therefore be more appropriate than relying on an Ehmer sling, which is difficult to apply and maintain appropriately. However, if it is felt after closed reduction that the hip joint is stable in inward

Box 36-1. Closed reduction of a craniodorsal coxofemoral luxation

Closed reduction of a luxated hip joint is performed under general anesthesia. The cat is placed in lateral recumbency. The aim of the manipulation is to bring the femoral head across the acetabular rim and back into the acetabular fossa without causing additional iatrogenic damage (Fig. 36-5). The femoral head is first externally rotated, and pulled caudally and ventrally by exerting manual traction on the femoral condyle. Once the femoral head is assumed to be located at the level of the acetabulum, it is internally rotated. A satisfying clunk should occur if closed reduction is successful.

Correct reduction is confirmed on a laterolateral radiograph. The femoral head is then pressed into the acetabular fossa with the thumb, and the hip joint is manipulated carefully, through a full range of motion, to aid removal of soft tissue out of the acetabular fossa. The leg is held in inward rotation during these manipulations. Stability is tested after this by putting the hip joint through its range of motion. Excessive outward rotation of the hip and adduction of the leg are avoided, as they will cause reluxation in most cases.

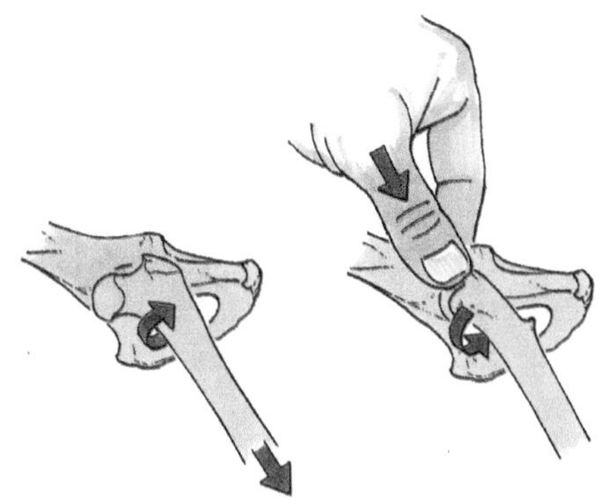

Figure 36-5 Closed reduction of a craniodorsal hip joint luxation. The femoral head is first rotated outwards (arrow) by grasping the distal femur. The femur is then pulled in a caudodistal direction (arrow). Once the femoral head is located over the acetabular fossa, the femoral head is rotated inwards (arrow) until it snaps back into the acetabular fossa, while digital pressure is applied on the greater trochanter (arrow).

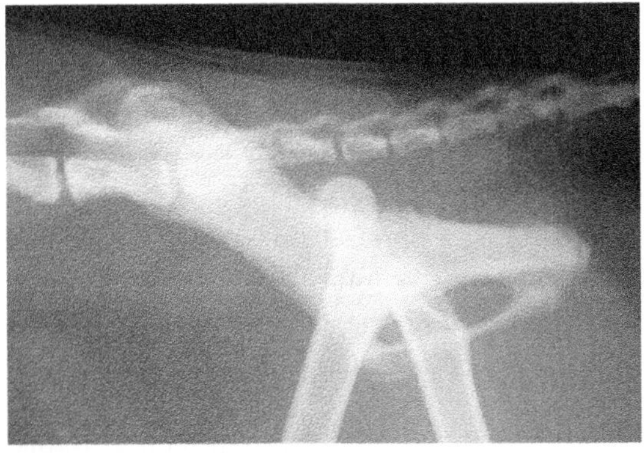

A

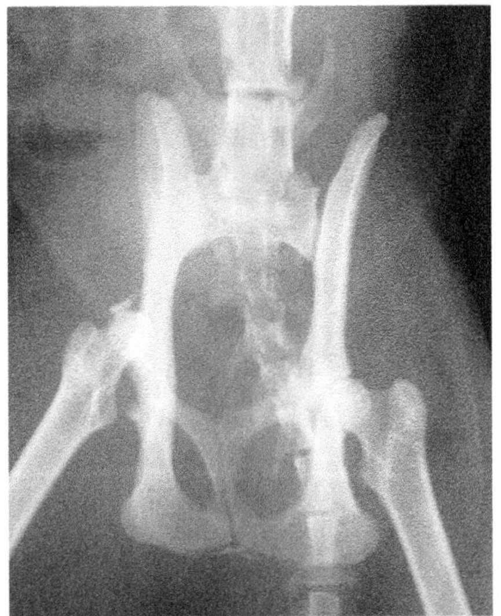

B

Figure 36-6 (**A**) Laterolateral and (**B**) ventrodorsal radiographs of a cat with craniodorsal hip luxation. Note the avulsed fragment from the dorsal acetabular rim, visible on both the laterolateral and ventrodorsal radiographs. Closed reduction is not recommended for these cases, and even with surgical stabilization there is a high risk for reluxation.

rotation and unstable in outward rotation, an Ehmer sling as described in Chapter 22 can be tried.

Open reduction and internal stabilization

Open reduction and internal stabilization are indicated if the hip joint remains unstable after closed reduction, if reluxation occurs, or if closed reduction is not possible. Cats with injuries to other limbs should also be treated surgically.

Numerous surgical stabilization methods have been described. These include suturing of the joint capsule, prosthetic capsular enhancement, De Vita pinning, transarticular pinning, and an iliofemoral suture technique (21, 22, 25,

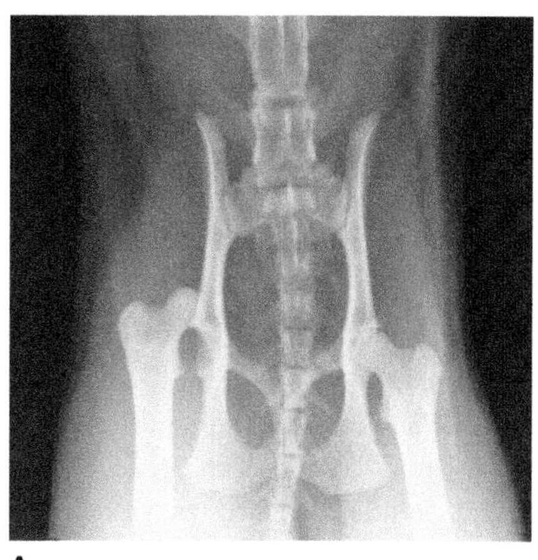

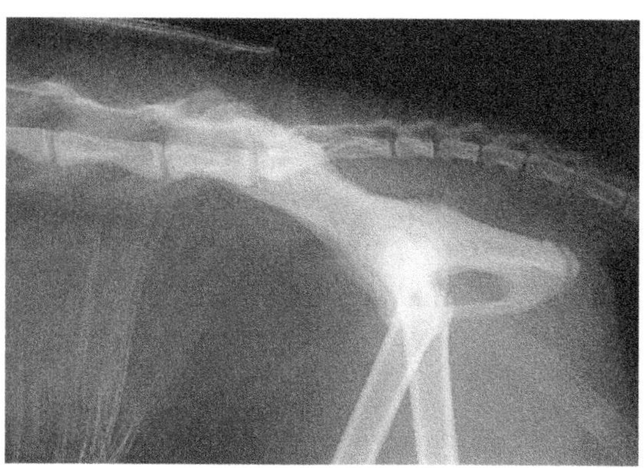

A B

Figure 36-7 Radiographs of a cat with craniodorsal hip luxation, treated successfully with closed reduction.
(**A**) Prereduction ventrodorsal radiograph revealing a normal configuration of the luxated hip with absence of concurrent fractures.
(**B**) Postreduction laterolateral radiograph showing the reduced hip joint. A modified Ehmer sling was used for 10 days in this cat.

27–29). A technique using a stainless-steel rope, similar to toggle pinning but inserted via a ventral approach to the hip joint, was also described (30). All methods of treatment bear some risk for reluxation, and conclusive evidence on which of the methods is best is lacking. Reluxation rates range around 10–20% for most techniques (23, 29, 30). Internal fixation of the luxated hip joint with suturing of the joint capsule and an iliofemoral suture technique or transarticular pinning are the techniques preferred by the authors. The De Vita pins should not be used due to the risk of sciatic nerve damage, and the difficulty in anchoring the pin in the straight ilial wing of cats.

The iliofemoral suture technique consists of a suture sling, which prevents reluxation by holding the femur in internal rotation, adduction, and ventromedial compression (31) (Box 36-2). The technique should only be performed in the absence of avulsion fractures, and if the hip does not reluxate intraoperatively when holding the femur in internal rotation and applying axial compression (31). Cases in which the dorsal joint capsule can be sutured have a greater chance of success. Braided suture material seems to be advantageous over monofilament suture material, because it is less likely to break. Polyglactin 910 (Vicryl) has an excellent initial size to strength ratio, and was used successfully in dogs (32).

Temporary transarticular pinning for hip dislocation involves placement of a small K wire across the reduced hip joint, in a similar position to the teres ligament (Fig. 36-9 and Box 36-2). It was originally described for dogs (33) and can also be used in cats (29). Selection of pin sizes used in the feline study was based on recommendations previously made for transarticular pinning in dogs (33). The pin is removed after 2–3 weeks once sufficient soft-tissue healing has occurred. The technique is particularly indicated for cases with other orthopedic injuries, as it allows early weight-bearing, yet the movement in the hip joint is necessarily restricted. It is also useful as a salvage technique when other options have failed, and in the presence of small avulsion fragments of the dorsal acetabular rim.

36.6.2 Ventral coxofemoral luxation

Ventral coxofemoral luxations are exceedingly rare. The femoral head is displaced ventral to the acetabulum, and may become entrapped in the obturator foramen. Ventral coxofemoral luxation carries the risk of sciatic and obturator nerve damage. Closed reduction is achieved by pulling the affected leg in a distal direction to remove the femoral head from the obturator foramen, followed by lateral pressure on the medial aspect of the femur. The femoral head should also be pushed in a cranial direction to minimize sciatic nerve damage during reduction. The hip joint is likely to be stable after reduction. A hobble sling (Chapter 22) can be applied for 10 days to avoid abduction of the leg, and reluxation of the hip joint.

36.7 Femoral head and neck excision

Femoral head and neck excision is a salvage procedure used in hip joint conditions where other treatment modalities are unable to relieve pain or to provide acceptable clinical function. Indications include chronic hip luxations, clinically debilitating coxarthrosis, comminuted acetabular fractures, non-unions of femoral neck and proximal physeal fractures, and diseases of the femoral neck. The femoral head and neck can be excised via a craniolateral or a ventral approach to the hip joint (Box 36-3). The craniolateral approach is preferred, particularly in the presence of a luxated hip.

Box 36-2. Internal stabilization of craniodorsal or caudodorsal hip joint luxation

A craniodorsal approach to the hip joint is performed. If possible, the hip joint is reduced beforehand because dissection is easier with the hip joint in place. The joint capsule needs to be preserved for later suturing. The acetabular fossa and the femoral head are cleared of fibrin, blood clot, and remnants of the round ligament.

Iliofemoral suture sling: Two holes are drilled through the greater trochanter in a caudal to cranial direction with a 1.2-mm pin or 1.5-mm drill bit. The pins should exit in the area of the base of the neck. Another hole is drilled in the ventral rim of the ilium, just cranial to the acetabulum. This hole should be positioned as ventrally and as close to the acetabulum as possible to be able to place the sling in a cranioventral to caudodorsal direction (Fig. 36-8A). Two or three strands of 2-0 polyglactin sutures, or other suture material of similar strength, are preplaced through the holes in a figure-of-eight fashion and are left untied. Every attempt is made to suture the joint capsule with 4-0 polydioxanone because this will markedly improve joint stability. The iliofemoral sling is then tied while an assistant holds the leg in slight inward rotation and abduction. Stability is tested by moving the hip through its full range of motion, and by applying axial compression.

Temporary transarticular pinning: Pin sizes range from 1.4 to 2.0 mm, but a 1.6-mm pin is appropriate for most cats. If a 1.6-mm pin is going to be inserted, a 1.5-mm hole is drilled in a retrograde fashion from the fovea capitis towards the third trochanter or in a normograde fashion from the third trochanter. Using a C drill guide is advisable for normograde drilling to ensure that the hole exits through the fovea capitis. The pin is inserted until the tip is just visible at the fovea capitis. The hip joint is then reduced and held slightly abducted and internally rotated. The pin is then carefully driven through the acetabulum using a hand-held Jacobs chuck a maximum of 5 mm into the pelvic canal (Fig. 36-8B). The pin is cut short and the end bent over, taking care not to lever on the hip and pull it out of the acetabulum. The pin is removed after 2–3 weeks.

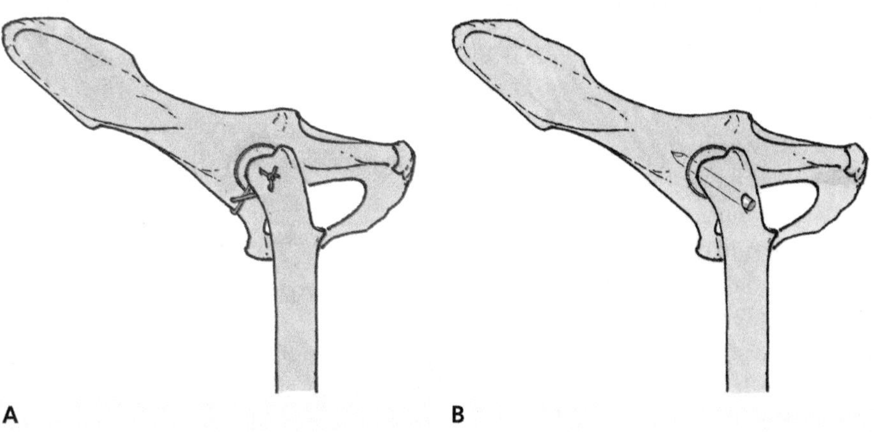

Figure 36-8 Surgical methods for stabilizing a luxated hip joint. (**A**) The iliofemoral suture sling should course in a ventromedial to dorsolateral direction. It therefore mimics the course of the round ligament and holds the femoral head and neck in internal rotation to prevent reluxation. (**B**) Temporary transarticular pinning allows limited motion around the axis of the pin, but limits rotation, abduction, or adduction of the hip and allows fibrosis and healing of the surrounding soft tissues.

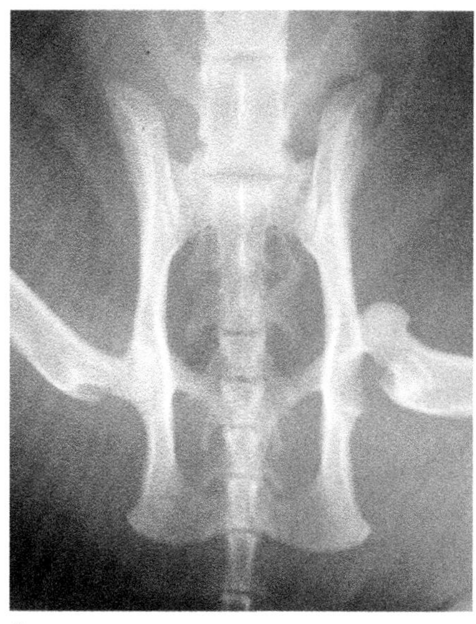
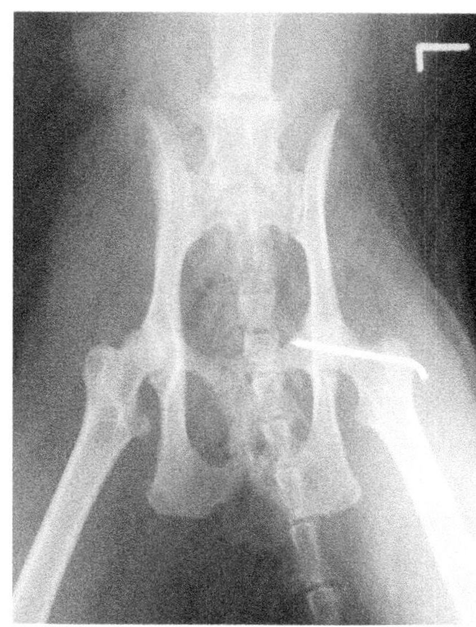

A B

Figure 36-9 (**A**) Preoperative and (**B**) postoperative radiographs after use of a 1.6-mm temporary transarticular pin in a cat with a left craniodorsal hip luxation.

A fibrous connection will develop between the proximal femur and the acetabulum following resection of the femoral head and neck, allowing weight-bearing and motion (Fig. 36-11). It is important to inform the owners that although many cats function well after excision of the femoral head and neck, complications such as chronic lameness, muscle atrophy, shortening of the leg, periarticular mineralization deposition, and a reduced range of motion are common (see postoperative treatment and prognosis, below).

36.8 Total hip replacement

A cemented total hip prosthesis is now available for use in cats (Biomedtrix). Indications for total hip replacement are basically the same as for femoral head and neck excision, although an intact femoral neck is necessary for the collar of the implant to rest on. The cat has a relatively shallow acetabulum, making positioning and seating of the acetabular prosthesis technically more difficult than in the dog. Total hip replacement in the cat is a novel technique and there are currently no published reports in the literature.

36.9 Postoperative treatment and prognosis

36.9.1 Coxofemoral luxation

An Ehmer sling is often applied postoperatively in dogs, but these slings are not well tolerated by cats, and have a tendency to slip. Reluxation rate does not seem to be influenced by the use of an Ehmer sling (22). Cats are therefore usually only cage-rested for 10 days postoperatively after having sutured the joint capsule and performed an iliofemoral suture sling. A clinical and radiological check-up should be performed after 10–14 days to confirm maintenance of reduction. Activity is then restricted for another 3 weeks by keeping the cat indoors, and avoiding playing and jumping activities.

After transarticular pinning the cat is also confined to a cage. Control radiographs are taken after 2–3 weeks when the pin is removed. In simple luxations with no other injuries, 2 weeks is sufficient; if other legs are injured or if there are neurological deficits, it is safer to leave the pin for 3 to maximally 4 weeks.

The success rate for maintaining reduction after internal fixation of coxofemoral luxations with capsular sutures, augmentation of the dorsal joint capsule, or iliofemoral suture sling was around 80–85% in one study, at the time when the cats were released from hospital (23). However, long-term results suggest a worse prognosis. Lameness and coxarthosis or neoarthrosis were seen in 42% of cases (23) (Fig. 36-12). In a long-term follow-up of 13 cats treated with transarticular pinning, there were two reluxations, one in a cat with bilateral injuries (29).

36.9.2 Femoral head and neck excision

Pain management and immediate physiotherapy are important in the immediate postoperative period to encourage early weight-bearing and preservation of range of motion. The mean time to full recovery has been described to be around 4–5 weeks (11, 12).

Good to excellent clinical outcome is reported in most studies for cats after femoral head and neck excision (11, 34), but functional deficits were found in many, and chronic pain

Box 36-3. Excision of the femoral head and neck

Using a craniolateral approach to the hip joint: A craniolateral approach to the hip joint is performed with the cat in lateral recumbency, and the joint capsule is incised in an inverted T-pattern. The joint capsule is elevated from the femoral neck. The femur is externally rotated by 90° to perform the osteotomy (Fig. 36-10A). Two mosquito forceps or small Hohmann retractors are placed cranial and caudal around the femoral neck for soft-tissue retraction and protection of surrounding tissues. The osteotomy follows an imaginary line between the proximal ends of the greater and lesser trochanter to remove as much bone as possible without damaging muscle insertions (Fig. 36-10A). An osteotome and mallet, an oscillating saw, bone cutters or rongeurs can be used. After removal of the femoral head and neck, the osteotomy surface of the femoral neck is checked digitally, and any leftover sharp ends are removed with rongeurs or a rasp until the surface feels smooth and crepitation is not palpable during manipulation of the hip joint through its normal range of motion. Efforts are made to suture the joint capsule and tendon of the deep gluteal muscle during closure of the incision.

Using a medial approach to the hip joint: The medial approach allows bilateral femoral head and neck excisions without repositioning the cat. Anatomic orientation is difficult in luxated hips, and the approach is therefore only used for unluxated hips. The cat is placed in dorsal recumbency, the approach is performed, and the joint capsule is incised and dissected away from the femoral neck. Two mosquito forceps are positioned cranial and caudal to the femoral neck for protection of soft tissues. An osteotome or oscillating saw is positioned at an angle of 45° with the femoral shaft, and the osteotomy is started at the level of the lesser trochanter (Fig. 36-10B). Leftover sharp edges of the femoral neck are removed before wound closure.

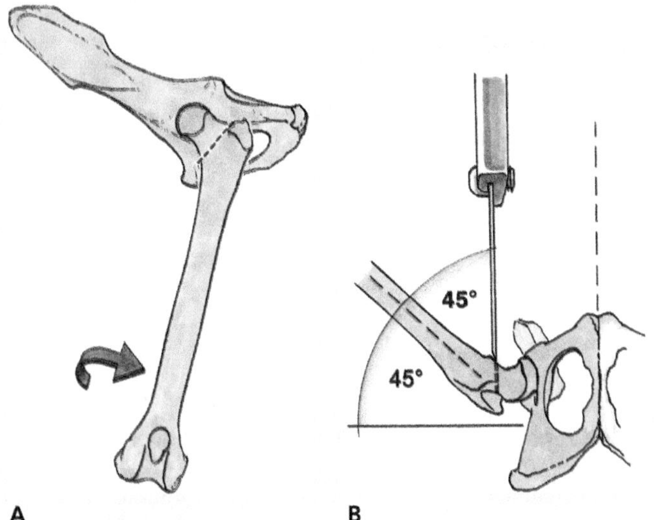

Figure 36-10 Possible options for excision of the femoral head and neck.
(**A**) Femoral head and neck excision using a craniolateral approach. The limb is externally rotated before the osteotomy is performed.
(**B**) Femoral head and neck excision using a ventral approach. The osteotomy is performed at an angle of 45° with the femoral shaft.

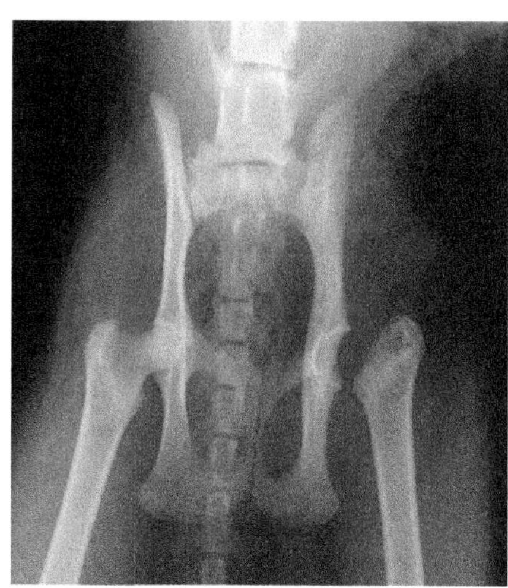

Figure 36-11 Postoperative radiograph of a cat after excision of the right femoral head and neck because of reluxation of the hip after internal stabilization. The excision is correctly performed through an imaginary line between the greater and lesser trochanter.

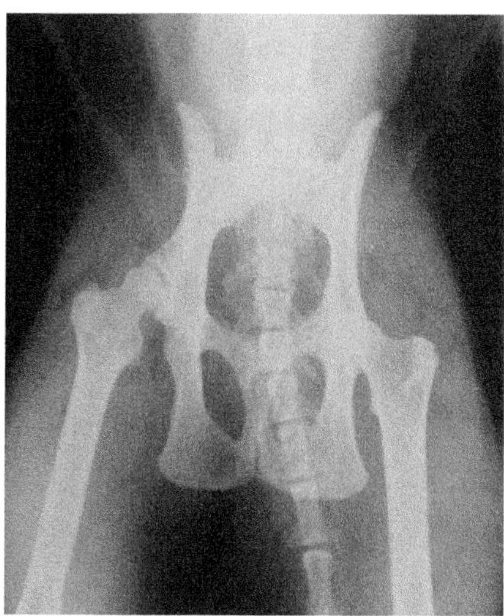

Figure 36-12 Radiograph of a cat with chronic hip joint luxation. A false joint (neoarthrosis) has developed craniodorsal to the original acetabular fossa. The cat had a chronic low-grade lameness.

in some cats of another study (12). Out of 15 cats with a follow-up period of up to 12 years, five showed a mild lameness at home, 13 had shortening of the leg due to proximal displacement of the femur, seven had muscle atrophy, 11 had restricted range of motion, and four exhibited pain on manipulation of the hip joint (12).

Unsatisfactory function is often due to inadequate excision of the ventral part of the femoral neck, causing bone-to-bone contact (Fig. 36-13) (34). The duration of clinical signs prior to surgery has also been shown to have an effect on outcome (11). Animals with clinical signs for more than 6 months prior to surgery had a worse outcome than animals with only a short duration of clinical signs.

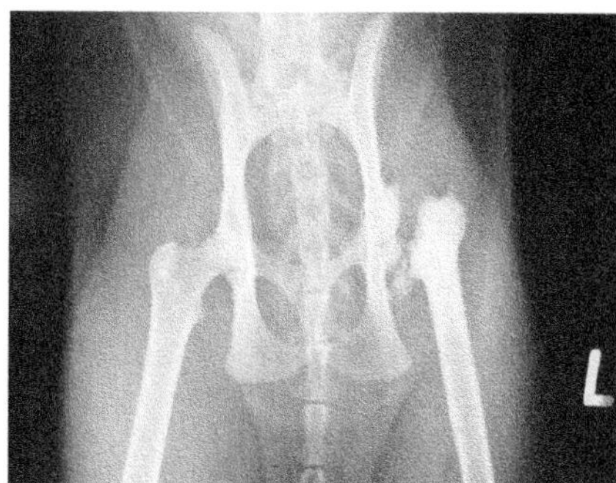

Figure 36-13 Ventrodorsal radiograph of the pelvis of a cat with a femoral head and neck excision, performed years ago, presented for hindlimb lameness. The cat had a reduced range of motion, pain, and crepitation of the left hip joint.

References and further reading

1. Pohlmeyer K. Arteries of the articulatio coxae and the proximal end of the femur in cats. Anat Histol Embryol 1981;10:246–256.
2. Piermattei DL, Johnson KA. An atlas of surgical approaches to the bones and joints of the dog and the cat, 4th edn. Philadelphia: WB Saunders; 2004.
3. Kolde DL. Pectineus tenectomy for treatment of hip dysplasia in a domestic cat. J Am Anim Hosp Assoc 1974;10:564–565.
4. Hayes HM, et al. Feline hip dysplasia. J Am Anim Hosp Assoc 1979;15:447–448.
5. Keller GG, et al. Hip dysplasia: a feline population study. Vet Radiol Ultrasound 1999;40:460–464.
6. Langenbach A, et al. Relationship between degenerative joint disease and hip joint laxity by use of distraction index and Norberg angle measurement in a group of cats. J Am Vet Med Assoc 1998;213:1439–1443.
7. Patsikas MN, et al. Hip dysplasia in the cat: a report of three cases. J Small Anim Pract 1998;39:290–294.
8. Houlton JEF, Meynink E. Medial patellar luxation in the cat. J Small Anim Pract 1989;30:349–352.
9. Smith GK, et al. Evaluation of the association between medial patellar luxation and hip dysplasia in cats. J Am Vet Med Assoc 1999;1:40–45.
10. Ballinari U, et al. Pectineus myectomy, tenotomy of the iliopsoas and neurectomy of the articular capsule as a symptomatic treatment for coxarthrosis in the dog. Schweiz Arch Tierheilkd 1995;137:251–257.
11. Gendreau C, Cawley AJ. Excision of the femoral head and neck: the long term results of 35 operations. J Am Anim Hosp Assoc 1977;13:605–608.
12. Off W, Matis U. Excision arthroplasty of the hip joint in dogs and cats. Clinical, radiographic and gait analysis findings at the surgical veterinary clinic of the Ludwig Maximilians University of Munich. Tierarztl Prax 1997;25:379–387.
13. McNicholas WT, et al. Spontaneous femoral capital physeal fractures in adult cats: 26 cases (1996–2001). J Am Vet Med Assoc 2002;221:1731–1736.
14. Steger H, et al. Bilateral idiopathic slipped capital femoral epiphysis in a cat. Schweiz Arch Tierheilkd 1999;141:47–52.

15. Craig LE. Physeal dysplasia with slipped capital femoral epiphysis in 13 cats. Vet Pathol 2001;38:92–97.
16. Forrest LJ, et al. Feline capital physeal dysplasia syndrome. Am J Vet Res 1999;40:672.
17. Smith RN. Fusion of ossification centers in the cat. J Small Anim Pract 1969;10:523–530.
18. May C, et al. Delayed physeal closure associated with castration in cats. J Small Anim Pract 1991;32:326–328.
19. Root MV, et al. The effect of prepubertal and postpubertal gonadectomy on radial physeal closure in male and female domestic cats. Vet Radiol Ultrasound 1997;38:42–47.
20. Queen J, et al. Femoral neck metaphyseal osteopathy in the cat. Vet Rec 1998;142:159–162.
21. Basher AWP, et al. Coxofemoral luxation in the dog and cat. Vet Surg 1986;15:356.
22. Duff SRI, Bennett D. Hip luxation in small animals: an evaluation of some methods of treatment. Vet Rec 1982;111:140–143.
23. Böhmer H. Zur Luxatio ossis femoris traumatica bei der Katze. Munich: Ludwig-Maximilians-Universität; 1987.
24. Wildgoose WH. Hip dislocation and the use of the De Vita pin in the cat. J Small Anim Pract 1983;24:261–268.
25. Piermattei DL, Flo GL. The hip joint. In: Piermattei DL, Flo GL (eds) Small animal orthopedics and fracture repair. Philadelphia: WB Saunders; 1997: pp. 422–468.
26. Fry PD. Observations on the surgical treatment of hip dislocation in the dog and cat. J Small Anim Pract 1974;15:661–670.
27. Meij BP, et al. Results of extra-articular stabilisation following open reduction of coxofemoral luxations in dogs and cats. J Small Anim Pract 1992;33:320–326.
28. Ablin LW, Gambardella PC. Orthopedics of the feline hip. Compend Continuing Educ 1991;13:1379–1388.
29. Sissener TR, et al. Transarticular pinning of the coxofemoral joint in cats. Poster. World Veterinary Orthopedic Congress; Keystone, Colorado; 2006.
30. Kawamata T, et al. Open reduction and stabilisation of coxofemoral joint luxation in dogs and cats, using a stainless steel rope inserted via a ventral approach to the hip joint. Aust Vet J 1996;74:460–464.
31. Slocum B, Slocum TD. Single-suture technique for a dislocated hip. In: Bojrab MJ (ed.) Current techniques in veterinary surgery, 4th edn. Baltimore: Williams & Wilkins; 1997: pp. 1183–1185.
32. Martini FM, et al. Extra-articular absorbable suture stabilization of coxofemoral luxation in dogs. Vet Surg 2001;30:468–475.
33. Hunt CA, Henry Jr WB. Transarticular pinning for repair of hip dislocation in the dog: a retrospective study of 40 cases. J Am Vet Med Assoc 1985;8:828–833.
34. Berzon JL, et al. A retrospective study of the efficacy of femoral head and neck excision in 94 dogs and cats. Vet Surg 1980;9:88–92.

37 Femur

K. Voss, S.J. Langley-Hobbs, P.M. Montavon

The femur is the most commonly fractured bone in cats, accounting for more than 30% of feline fractures (1, 2). Fractures of the femur can be divided into those involving the proximal femur, diaphysis, and distal femur. The shaft and distal femur are most frequently fractured (3). Femoral fractures are usually the result of motor vehicle accidents or falls from a height. Such high-velocity trauma commonly causes concurrent injury, such as pelvic or spinal fractures and abdominal injury. A thorough clinical and orthopedic examination is necessary to rule out these concurrent injuries. Surgical repair of femoral fractures should not be overly delayed, as quadriceps contracture can develop, especially following diaphyseal fractures, and in the presence of muscle contusion or laceration.

37.1 Surgical anatomy

The shaft of the femur is round and almost straight in cats. The femoral neck is angled approximately 130° from the femoral shaft and has an anteversion angle of around 30° (4). Blood supply to the femoral head mainly depends on vessels from an extracapsular vascular ring surrounding the femoral neck. In contrast to dogs, a substantial blood supply to the femoral epiphysis is also derived from a vessel in the round ligament in young cats (5), but this vessel disappears in cats older than 7 months (6). Meticulous surgical technique is required during operations on the femoral head and neck to minimize vascular injury.

The femoral condyle has less caudal bowing when compared to dogs. The distal growth plate is located within the joint capsule of the stifle joint and a stifle arthrotomy is necessary for repair of distal Salter and Harris fractures. Four bony protuberances on the metaphyseal side of the physis match corresponding depressions on the epiphyseal side. This interdigitation helps in fracture stability after reduction of distal Salter and Harris type I and II fractures.

37.2 Stabilization techniques

Femoral fractures should be surgically stabilized, with the exception of greenstick fractures in very young cats, which can heal with cage rest alone. The straight nature of the feline femoral diaphysis makes it especially suitable for plate osteosynthesis, and intramedullary pinning or nailing. External skeletal fixation of femoral fractures is also well tolerated in the cat. A summary of feline femoral fractures and possible stabilization methods for each fracture type is provided in Table 37-1.

37.2.1 Intramedullary pinning

Intramedullary pinning of the femur is especially helpful for comminuted fractures, because the position of the pin in the neutral axis of the bone enhances bending stability in the absence of a medial buttress, and the pin can be used to facilitate alignment of the main fragments. Intramedullary pins should be nearly always used in conjunction with some kind of antirotational implants, such as cerclage or hemicerclage wires, plates, or external skeletal fixators.

The diameter of an intramedullary pin should not exceed 30–40% of the diameter of the bone marrow cavity if it is used in conjunction with a plate or an external skeletal fixator. The mean medullary canal diameter is 5–6 mm in most cats, so Kirschner wires of a diameter of 1.4–2.0 mm are usually used. Thicker pins, comprising around 70% of the bone marrow cavity, are required if they are only combined with cerclage wires.

Normo- and retrograde pinning is possible in the femur (Figs 37-1 and 37-2). Normograde pinning is recommended, as retrograde pinning is associated with a higher risk of iatrogenic trauma to the sciatic nerve. Sciatic nerve injury may occur either during pin placement or postoperatively from motion or migration of the protruding pin tip in the proximity of the nerve. The incidence of sciatic nerve paresis after intramedullary pinning of the femur in cats was as high as 23% in one study (7). Retrograde pinning, a medial position of the proximal pin end, and excessive length of the protruding pin end were considered causative factors (7). Normograde pinning allows better control of the position of the proximal pin to end in a more lateral position. The proximal pin end is either cut short or bent laterally to be tied in to an external skeletal fixator.

37.2.2 Interlocking nailing

The interlocking nail has been used with more frequency in the femur when compared to all the other long bones in the cat (8–10). The femur is an ideally shaped bone for

Table 37-1. Fracture types and their possible stabilization methods

Fracture localization	Fracture type	Stabilization methods
Proximal femur	Femoral neck fracture	Parallel pinning Lag screw and antirotational pin
	Capital physeal fracture	Parallel pinning Ventral cross pinning
	Avulsion of greater trochanter	Tension band fixation Diverging pins
	Simple subtrochanteric fracture	Compression plate Internal fixator
	Comminuted subtrochanteric fracture	Buttress plate and IM pin Internal fixator and IM pin ESF and IM pin
Diaphysis	Simple transverse or short oblique	Compression plate Internal fixator IM pin and ESF Interlocking nail
	Simple long oblique and multifragmentary reducible	Lag screw and neutralization plate Lag screw and internal fixator IM pin and ESF IM pin and cerclage or hemicerclage wires Interlocking nail
	Comminuted	Buttress plate ± IM pin Internal fixator ± IM pin ESF ± IM pin Interlocking nail
Distal femur	Supracondylar simple	Lateral plate ± IM pin Double plating
	Supracondylar comminuted	Double plating or internal fixators IM pin and lateral plate or internal fixator ESF ± IM pin
	Intracondylar and Salter and Harris type III and IV	Transcondylar lag screw and Kirschner wire
	Condylar T or Y	Transcondylar lag screw and: - dynamic pins - single or double plate - single or double internal fixator - ESF
	Salter and Harris type I and II	Cross pinning Dynamic intramedullary pinning

IM pin, intramedullary pin; ESF, external skeletal fixator.

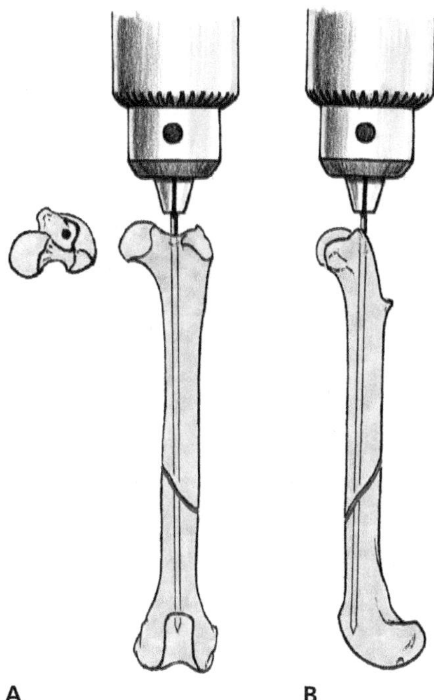

Figure 37-1 Normograde insertion of an intramedullary pin. The pin is started at the most craniolateral aspect of the trochanteric fossa. It is carefully advanced down the medullary canal, until its tip is at the level of the fracture. The fracture is reduced, and the pin is further advanced into the distal fragment while maintaining axial alignment of the bone in both the mediolateral (**A**) and craniolateral (**B**) axes.

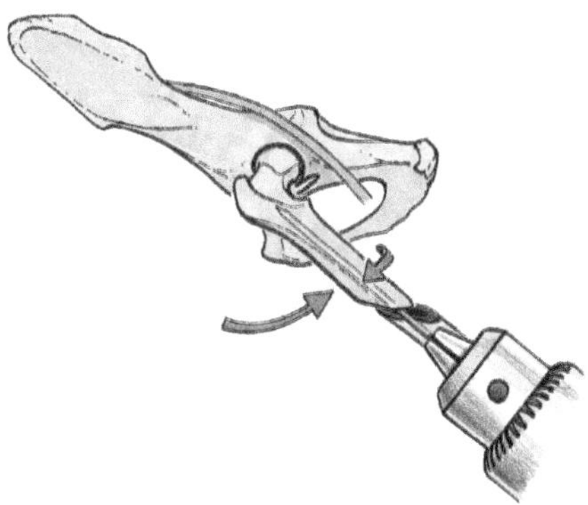

Figure 37-2 Retrograde insertion of an intramedullary pin. A pin with trocar tips on both ends is used. Holding the leg in adduction, slight inward rotation (short arrow), and extension (long arrow) directs the nail away from the sciatic nerve. The pin is aimed to exit laterally in the trochanteric fossa.

interlocking nails, being straight and having a fairly uniform diameter from distal to proximal. The most common length of interlocking nail used in the cat was 91 mm, with a range from 79 to 101 mm (9). The 4.7-mm nail was used in 11, and the 4.0-mm nail in one of the cats, but it was considered significantly easier to place the 4.0-mm nail compared to the 4.7-mm nail when the isthmus was intact, so the latter may be a better option for the average-sized cat (9). Only one implant complication occurred in this series: this involved a broken proximal screw, resulting in a functional non-union (9).

The length of the nail to be used is determined by using the templates and the preoperative radiographs of the intact contralateral limb. Normograde placement of the nail is recommended (see above). The nail should be aimed down the middle of the medullary canal with the point ending level to the proximal aspect of the patella. The proximal aspect of the femoral nail should be buried in the intertrochanteric fossa to prevent muscle irritation, seroma formation, and potential sciatic neuropathy.

A 3.5-mm titanium nail has recently been developed for retrograde insertion from the intercondylar notch (11). It was used successfully in 24 cats with supracondylar and diaphyseal fractures. No implant-related problems occurred. Stifle osteoarthritis was seen in only one cat with a pre-existing sciatic neuropathy.

37.2.3 External skeletal fixation

Only type I and modified type II external skeletal fixators can be used in the femur, because of the proximity of the bone to the abdominal wall. Type I external skeletal fixators are appropriate for most fractures (12). The main indication for modified type II constructs is a comminuted fracture of the distal femoral diaphysis or metaphysis, where there is only room for insertion of one or two pins in the distal fragment. External skeletal fixators in the femur are commonly combined with an intramedullary pin. The tie-in configuration enhances fixator strength (13), and is therefore ideal for severely comminuted fractures or in immature cats with soft bone, where transosseus pins may be at risk for pull-out (14). Additionally, the tie-in configuration seems to cause less soft-tissue morbidity than when the protruding tip of the pin is not connected to the external skeletal fixator (13). Closed reduction of femoral fractures is difficult due to the overlying muscle mass, so a minimally invasive approach and indirect reduction techniques are used. Insertion of an intramedullary pin prior to application of the external skeletal fixator facilitates fracture reduction and spatial alignment of the main fragments, without necessitating extensive soft-tissue dissection.

Transosseous pin size should not exceed 20–25% of the bone diameter to prevent iatrogenic fractures. Positive- or negative-threaded 2.0-mm pins are appropriately sized for most feline femurs. Smaller pins, such as 1.6-mm positive-threaded or smooth pins, may have to be used to pass an intramedullary pin. All pins are inserted just caudal to the belly of the vastus lateralis muscle, through separate skin incisions. The number of transosseous pins inserted per fragment depends on fracture type and location, ancillary implants used, and age of the cat. As a rule of thumb, three pins should be inserted per fragment if both rotational and axial stability must be counteracted. Two pins are sufficient to neutralize rotational forces.

37.2.4 Plating

Femoral fractures are most often stabilized with 2.7-mm dynamic compression plates (DCP) or 2.0/2.7-mm veterinary cuttable plates (VCP), the latter being applied alone or in sandwich function. The 2.4-mm limited contact-DCP (LC-DCP) can also be used. The straight shape of the femoral shaft renders plate contouring easier when compared to dogs. Long plates have to be contoured to the shape of the greater trochanter proximally, and to the lateral aspect of the femoral condyle distally. Special plates, such as condylar or reconstruction plates, may be used for fractures in the supracondylar region.

For treatment of comminuted fractures the plates should be contoured before surgery, with the aid of radiographs and a bone specimen. In general, a DCP is applied in compression function for simple transverse fractures, in neutralization function for oblique or reducible multifragmentary fractures, and in buttress function for comminuted fractures (Chapter 13). The plate and rod system provides additional stability in fractures with absence of a medial buttress, and has been applied successfully in clinical cases (15).

37.2.5 Internal fixators

Internal fixators have some indications in the repair of femoral fractures despite the higher implant costs. They can be used as neutralization or buttress implants for femoral diaphyseal fractures, but the main indications are distal diaphyseal and supracondylar fractures, where there is little bone stock available for screw placement. The 2.0-mm Unilock mandible locking plates (Chapter 24) have been found to be a versatile implant for fractures of the distal femur. Both monocortical and bicortical screws can be used, and the insertion of only two screws into the distal fragment results in sufficient stability. Bilateral application of an internal fixator is also possible, and is a useful technique for repairing comminuted supracondylar fractures.

The 2.4-mm Unilock mandible locking plates (Chapter 24) have been successfully used for the treatment of femoral diaphyseal fractures. Iatrogenic fissures or fractures have been observed by the authors when using the 2.4-mm system with bicortical screws in the femoral diaphysis in older cats. In elderly cats it is therefore recommended to use bicortical screws only at the proximal and distal plate end, and monocortical screws in the middle. Bicortical screws can be used if deemed necessary in young cats with softer bones. Internal fixators can be combined with an intramedullary pin, but care should be taken that the screws do not come into contact with the pin, as iatrogenic fissures/fractures could occur.

37.3 Fractures of the proximal femur

Fractures of the proximal femur include fractures of the femoral head, fractures through the capital femoral physis, femoral neck fractures, avulsion fractures of the greater trochanter, and subtrochanteric fractures. With the exception of subtrochanteric fractures, these are all usually seen in cats less than 1 year of age. Although affected cats often present with non-weight-bearing lameness, some cats with fractures of the femoral head and neck exhibit less obvious clinical signs, and a thorough orthopedic examination is necessary to make the diagnosis. Manipulation of the hip joint reveals pain, reduced range of motion, and crepitus. Definitive diagnosis is based on radiographic findings.

37.3.1 Approaches to the proximal femur

The femoral head and neck are most commonly approached via a craniolateral approach to the hip joint (16). The craniolateral approach is used for repair of proximal physeal fractures, and femoral neck fractures. The tendon of the deep gluteal muscle has to be partially incised for improved visualization. The tenotomy is performed in the tendinous part of the muscle, approximately 3 mm away from its insertion on the greater trochanter in order to allow reconstruction later. Tendon sutures are described in Chapter 16. The joint capsule is incised longitudinally to the femoral neck to access capital physeal fractures, and femoral neck fractures that are located within the capsule.

As an alternative, the femoral head and neck can be approached through a ventral incision, with the cat in dorsal recumbency and the limbs abducted (16). The ventral approach is used for repair of avulsion fractures of the femoral head, and also allows repair of proximal physeal femoral fractures. The approach can be performed with or without pectineomyectomy. Care has to be taken not to injure the femoral artery and vein, the saphenous nerve, and the medial circumflex femoral artery and vein during dissection.

The greater trochanter and the subtrochanteric region of the femur are easily accessed via a lateral approach (16). After incising the fascia lata the biceps femoris muscle is retracted caudally. The sciatic nerve is located below the biceps femoris muscle, and must be identified and protected.

37.3.2 Proximal physeal fractures and fractures of the femoral neck

Fractures of the capital physis and the femoral neck occur frequently in the cat (Fig. 37-3). Traumatic femoral neck

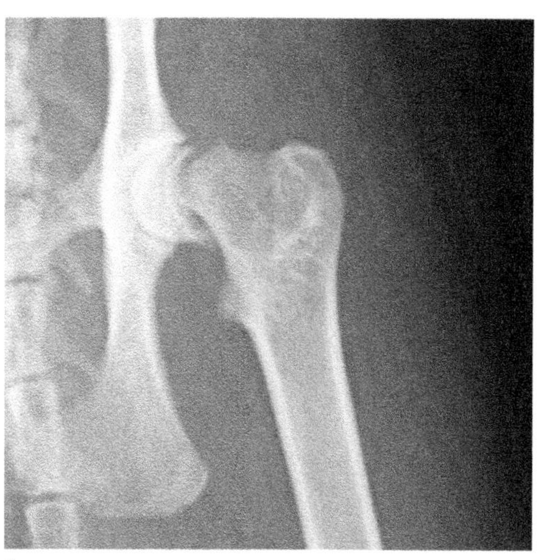
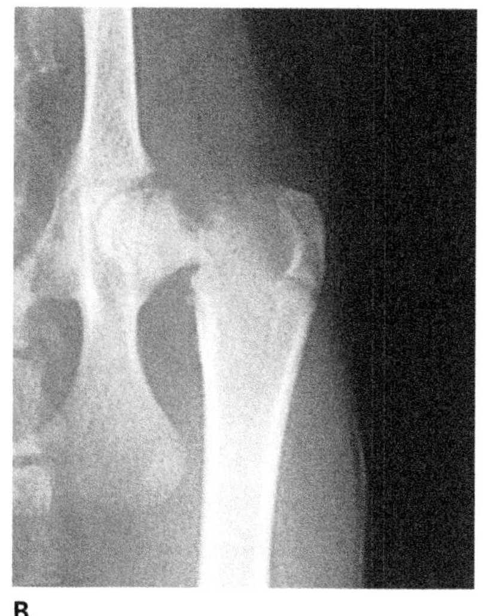
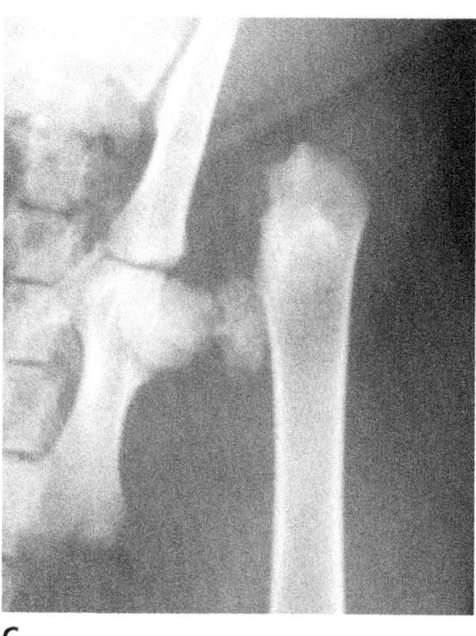

A B C

Figure 37-3 Examples of different fractures of the proximal femur in young cats.
(**A**) Proximal physeal fracture in a 10-month-old cat.
(**B**) Fracture through the femoral neck in a 4-month-old cat.
(**C**) Fracture through the femoral neck with concurrent avulsion fracture of the greater trochanter in a 3-month-old cat.

fractures are more common than fractures through the proximal growth plate in very young cats (17, 18). Femoral neck fractures predominate in cats up to 6 months of age; both lesions occur with an equal frequency between 6 and 12 months, and the incidence of both types of fractures drops after 12 months (18). The capital femoral physis closes between 30 and 40 weeks in intact cats (19), but closure is delayed in gonadectomized cats. Physeal fractures therefore can occur in cats markedly older than 1 year.

Besides traumatic fractures, spontaneous fractures of the femoral capital physis and pathological fractures secondary to femoral neck metaphyseal osteopathy have been described in felines (20–23) (Chapter 36). These conditions must be differentiated from traumatically induced fractures. Cats with a traumatic fracture are usually presented with an acute unilateral lameness, whereas cats with non-traumatic fractures may present with a progressive lameness, which may be bilateral. The signalment of the cat is also an important differentiating factor, as traumatic fractures usually occur in cats younger than 1 year, whereas spontaneous capital physeal fractures and femoral neck osteopathy generally affect male castrated cats older than 1 year.

Conservative treatment of femoral neck and physeal fractures almost invariably results in hypertrophic pseudarthroses (17, 18). Healing after surgical repair seems to be better in cats than in dogs (5, 24, 25), and surgical stabilization is the treatment of choice in acute fractures. Femoral head and neck excision should be reserved for comminuted fractures of the femoral neck, and for long-standing fractures with rounded and fibrotic fracture ends.

Both traumatic capital physeal fractures and femoral neck fractures are usually stabilized with two small Kirschner wires (Fig. 37-4 and Box 37-1). In adult cats a lag screw can be used with an antirotational pin. Biomechanical comparison between parallel and divergent pin placement suggested parallel pinning to be stronger (26). The pins can be inserted retrograde or antegrade. Retrograde pinning facilitates pin placement, but normograde pinning is preferred, because less manipulation of the fracture fragments is needed, and less vascular damage is caused. An applecore appearance of the femoral neck is sometimes observed after parallel pinning of capital femoral physeal fractures, indicating devascularization. As an alternative, femoral capital physeal fractures can be stabilized with pins using a ventral approach (27) (Box 37-1). The ventral approach to the hip joint requires less soft-tissue dissection, and may preserve the blood supply derived from the joint capsule better.

37.3.3 Avulsion fractures of the greater trochanter

Avulsion fractures through the physis of the greater trochanter occur in young cats, often in conjunction with coxofemoral luxation or fractures of the capital femoral physis or femoral neck (Fig. 37-4). Three out of 19 cats with fractures of the capital femoral physis or femoral neck and one out of 19 cats with coxofemoral luxation had simultaneous separation of the greater trochanter in one study (17). The pull of the gluteus musculature causes proximal displacement of the avulsed fragment. The fracture is not always easily detectable

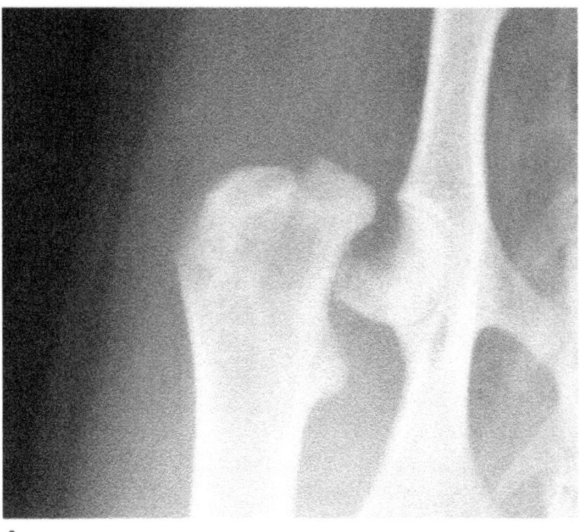

A

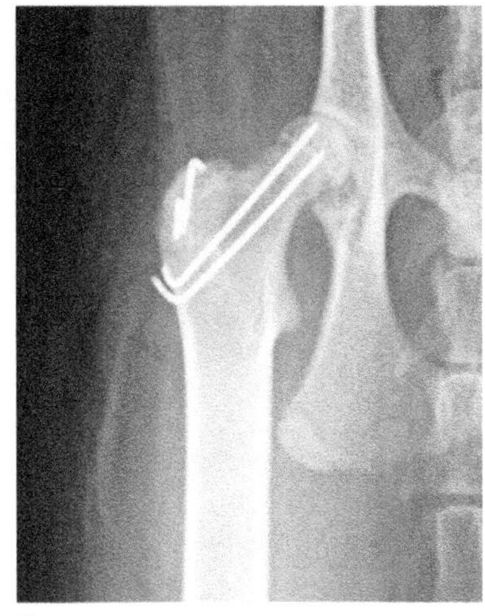

B

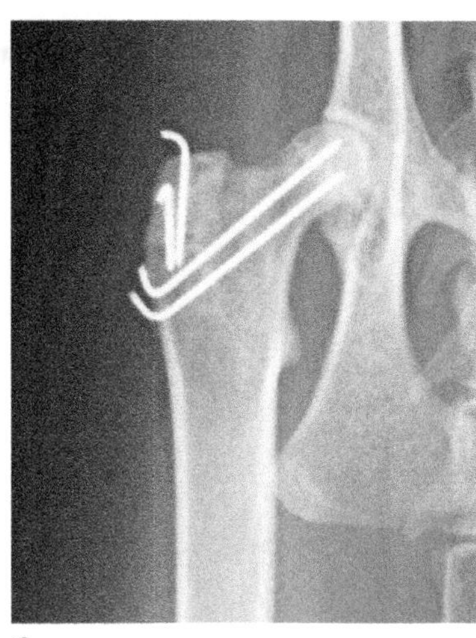

C

Figure 37-4 Parallel pinning of a capital physeal fracture.
(**A**) Preoperative radiograph of an 8-month-old cat with a capital physeal and trochanteric fracture.
(**B**) The physeal fracture was stabilized using two parallel Kirschner wires. The trochanter was reattached with two diverging pins.
(**C**) Uncomplicated healing is visible on the 4-week postoperative radiographs.

on radiographs, and laterolateral, ventrodorsal, and frog-leg views should be taken. Surgical stabilization with a tension band is indicated to restore function of the gluteal musculature and to enhance stability of the hip joint (Box 37-2). The tension band fixation is also used after trochanteric osteotomy for approach to the hip joint (Chapter 36).

37.3.4 Subtrochanteric fractures

Subtrochanteric fractures are rare in cats, and are generally part of a comminuted diaphyseal fracture. They are treated similarly to diaphyseal fractures, as described in the following sections. Both plate osteosynthesis and external skeletal fixation can be used. The main challenge in repairing these fractures is to insert a sufficient number of implants into the small proximal fragment. An additional intramedullary pin helps to reduce the number of screws or pins required in the proximal fragment. Screw engagement in four cortices per fragment is sufficient with the plate and rod technique, and two transosseous pins per fragment are also usually adequate with an external skeletal fixator tie-in configuration (12).

37.4 Diaphyseal fractures of the femur

Many diaphyseal femoral fractures are comminuted. Diaphyseal femoral fractures always require surgical stabilization, with the rare exception of greenstick or undisplaced fractures in kittens. The choice of implants is based on fracture type, age of the animal, clinical factors, and surgeon preference (Chapter 13). The straight form of the femoral diaphysis in cats makes it especially suitable for plate osteosynthesis and intramedullary pinning or interlocking nailing procedures. External skeletal fixation is used mainly for comminuted femoral fractures, where other fixation methods are less practical, and in immature cats. The disadvantage of external skeletal fixation of the femur is the morbidity associated with the pins interfering with the muscles of the thigh, especially near the stifle joint.

Open reduction is usually necessary for repair of femoral fractures, because the surrounding muscles render closed reduction difficult. The quadriceps muscle is inspected for lacerations, and/or intrafascial hemorrage and edema. Hemorrhage and edema can elevate intrafascial pressure, resulting in quadriceps fibrosis. Small fascial incisions, and leaving the fascia lata open after surgery, can relieve intrafascial pressure (Chapter 16).

37.4.1 Approach to the femoral diaphysis

A lateral approach to the femoral shaft is used for all stabilization procedures (16).

37.4.2 Simple transverse and short oblique fractures

Simple transverse and short oblique fractures seem more common in young cats than in older cats. They can be stabilized with an intramedullary pin and a type I external skeletal

Box 37-1. Stabilization of capital physeal and femoral neck fractures

Femoral neck fractures are stabilized with parallel pins using a craniolateral approach. Femoral capital physeal fractures can be repaired with the same technique, or with cross pins inserted via a ventromedial approach. Meticulous surgical technique is used to preserve as much of the blood supply as possible if the craniolateral approach is used.

Parallel pinning of capital physeal and femoral neck fractures: A craniolateral or caudolateral approach to the hip joint is performed, and the joint capsule is incised longitudinally to the femoral neck for fracture visualization. The femoral head remains within the acetabulum due to its attachment to the round ligament, and the femoral neck is usually displaced dorsally and slightly cranially. Two 0.8–1.0-mm Kirschner wires are driven from the caudolateral aspect of the third trochanter into the femoral neck. The pin tips are advanced until they are flush with the fracture surface. The fracture is manually reduced using caudodistal traction. The hip joint is then placed in internal rotation to hold fracture reduction during further pin insertion by applying digital pressure on the greater trochanter. The pins are advanced until they are seated in the femoral epiphysis (Figs 37-5A and 37-5B). Inadvertent pin placement into the hip joint is checked visually or by palpation of the articular surface with a small pair of curved mosquito forceps. The joint is moved through its range of motion. No crepitation should be noted. The pins are carefully bent over and cut short.

Cross pinning of capital physeal fractures: A ventral approach to the hip joint is performed. Care is taken not to disrupt the round ligament. Two divergent small threaded Kirschner wires are inserted in a retrograde fashion from the cranial aspect of the neck in a proximolateral direction into the epiphysis (Fig. 37-5C). The pins are cut short.

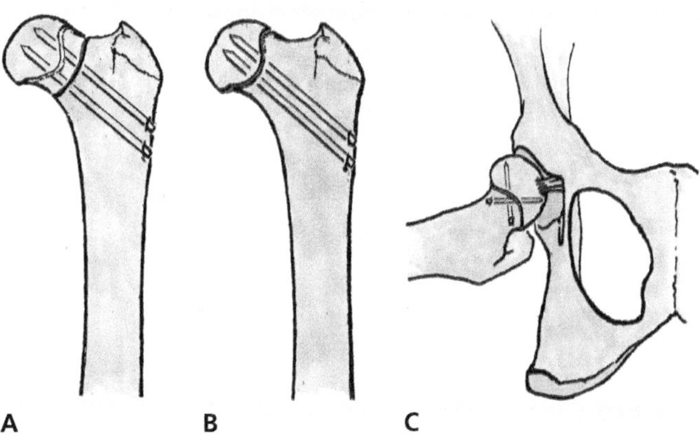

Figure 37-5 Options for stabilization of capital physeal and femoral neck fractures. (**A**) Stabilization of a femoral neck fracture with parallel pins. (**B**) Stabilization of a capital physeal fracture with parallel pins. (**C**) Stabilization of a capital physeal fracture with divergent cross pins inserted from ventrally.

fixator, with an interlocking nail or with a plate in compression function. Intramedullary pinning and external skeletal fixation are useful in immature cats with soft bone quality and fast healing times (Fig. 37-7). Plate osteosynthesis or interlocking nailing is usually preferred in adult cats. The techniques are described in Box 37-3.

Internal fixators could also be applied in both young and older cats, but their advantages over other implants are not huge for the stabilization of simple fractures, and may not justify the higher implant costs.

37.4.3 Long oblique and reducible multifragmentary fractures

Long oblique and some reducible multifragmentary fractures can be reduced anatomically and stabilized under compression. Long oblique fractures in young cats may be treated with an intramedullary pin and cerclage or hemicerclage wires. A relatively thick intramedullary nail, comprising about 70% of the diameter of the medullary canal, is used to provide sufficient bending and axial stability. Although this technique provides less stability than others, good results can be achieved with appropriate case selection and good surgical technique (Fig. 37-9). Hemicerclage wires (Chapter 24) can be used as an alternative to cerclage wires, especially in shorter oblique fractures, but care must be taken not to cause fissuring of the bone when placing and tightening them. Hemicerclage wires are preplaced prior to full insertion of the intramedullary pin.

Stabilizing long oblique fractures with a lag screw and a neutralization plate provides more stability (Box 37-4). A 2.7-mm DCP, 2.4-mm LC-DCP or a 2.0/2.7-mm VCP can be

Box 37-2. Tension band fixation of the greater trochanter

A lateral approach to the greater trochanter is performed and the avulsed fragment is reattached with a tension band fixation (Fig. 37-6). Depending on the size of the cat, two parallel 0.6–1.0-mm Kirschner wires are inserted from the proximal aspect of the greater trochanter, across the fracture/osteotomy line, and into the medial cortex. A 0.6- or 0.8-mm piece of orthopedic wire is then applied in a figure-of-eight pattern through a predrilled hole in the caudal aspect of the proximal femur and around the pin ends. The distance between the hole in the femur and the fracture line should approximate the distance between the fracture line and the protruding pin tips proximally. The pin ends are carefully bent over and cut short.

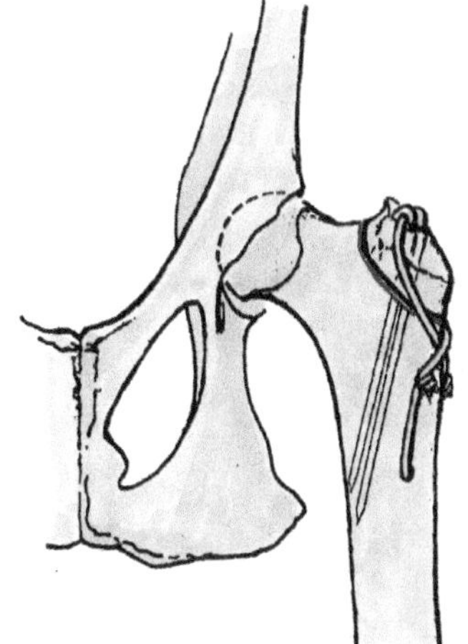

Figure 37-6 Tension band fixation of an avulsion fracture or an osteotomy of the greater trochanter.

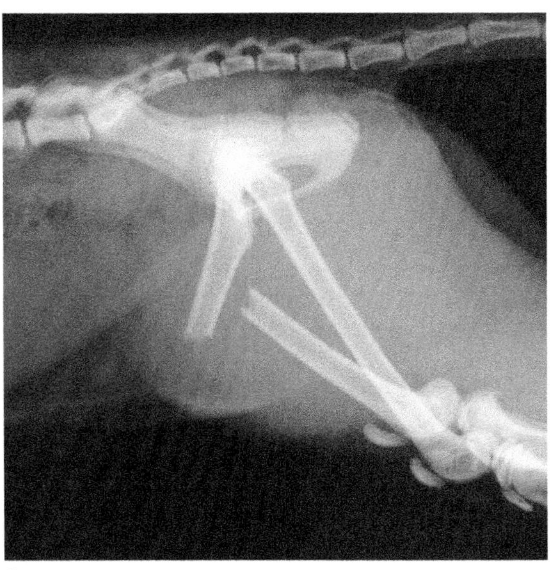

A

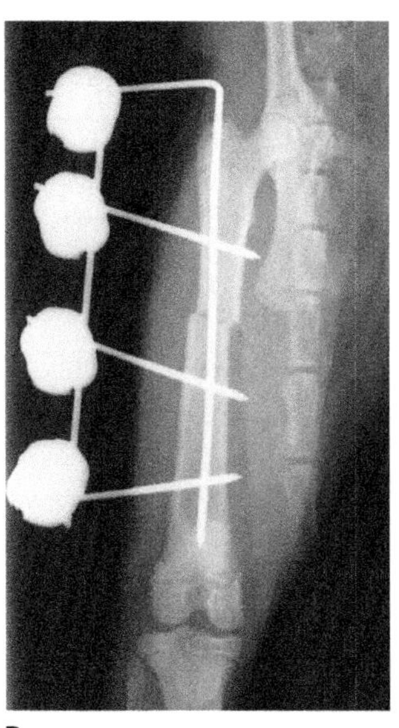

B

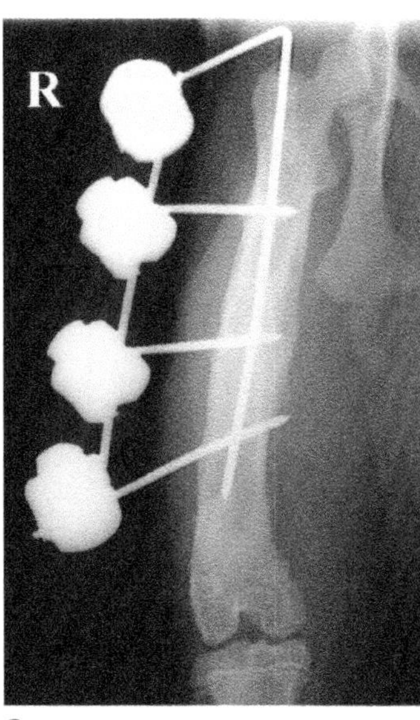

C

Figure 37-7 Simple transverse fracture of a femoral fracture in a 7-month-old cat.

(**A**) Preoperative radiograph showing a simple transverse mid-diaphyseal fracture.

(**B**) The fracture was stabilized with an external skeletal fixator in a tie-in configuration. The transosseous pins mainly serve to counteract rotational forces, although the intramedullary pin is rather small.

(**C**) Follow-up radiographs at 2 months show a completely healed fracture with good callus formation.

Box 37-3. Stabilization of a simple transverse or short oblique fracture of the femoral diaphysis

A lateral approach to the femoral diaphysis is performed for fracture reduction. Only a small approach is necessary for intramedullary pinning and interlocking nailing.

Interlocking nail: A 4.0- or 4.7-mm interlocking nail is inserted in a normograde fashion, using a small surgical approach for reduction. The fracture is anatomically reduced before the interlocking nail is secured to the femoral cortex with two bolts or two screws per fragment (Fig. 37-8A).

Intramedullary pin and type I external skeletal fixator: A 1.4–2.4-mm intramedullary pin is inserted in a normograde fashion. A small surgical approach is made for directing the pin into the distal fragment. At least one, but preferably two, 1.4–2.0-mm transosseous pins are inserted per fragment, depending on the age of the cat. If smooth pins are used, they are angled 70° to the long axis of the bone to enhance stability, and to prevent pull-out (Fig. 37-8B).

Compression plate: The fracture is anatomically reduced and stabilized with a 2.4-mm limited contact-dynamic compression plate or a 2.7-mm dynamic compression plate applied in compression function. At least three screws are inserted in the proximal and distal fragment. It is advisable to use a longer plate and not fill all screw holes, rather than selecting the shortest plate possible (Fig. 37-8C). One screw proximal and one distal are inserted eccentrically to achieve interfragmentary compression.

A 2.7/2.0-mm veterinary cuttable plate can also be used, but interfragmentary compression is not possible.

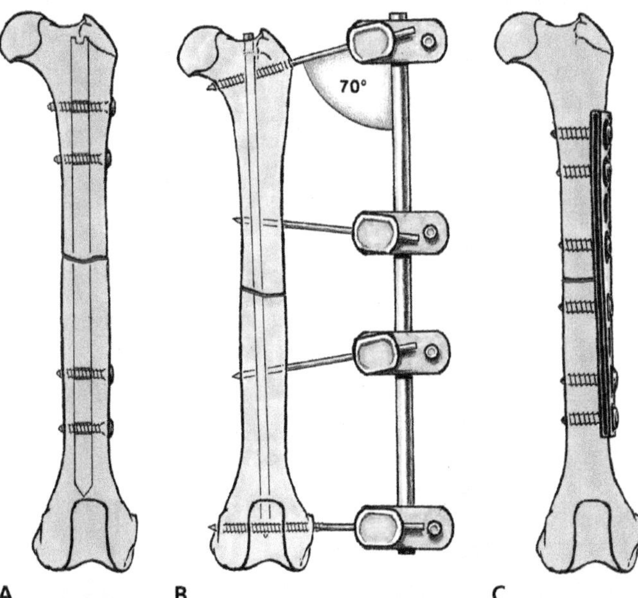

Figure 37-8 Options for treatment of simple transverse and short oblique fractures of the femoral shaft.
(**A**) Fixation of a short oblique fracture of the mid-shaft with a 4.0-mm interlocking nail.
(**B**) Stabilization of a transverse fracture with an intramedullary pin, and a type I external skeletal fixator to prevent rotation.
(**C**) Stabilization of a simple transverse fracture with an eight-hole 2.7-mm dynamic compression plate in compression function with three screws proximal and distal.

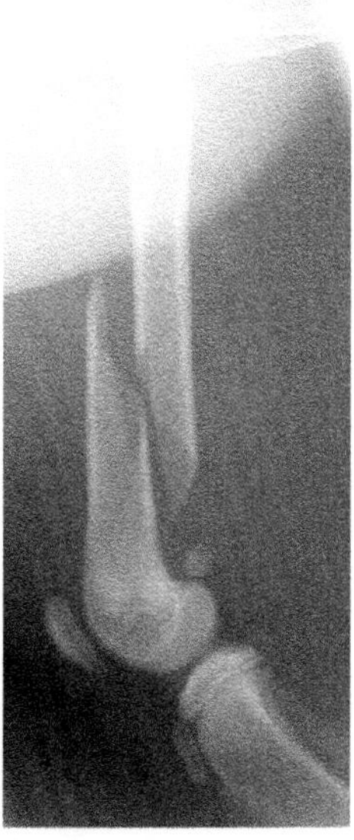
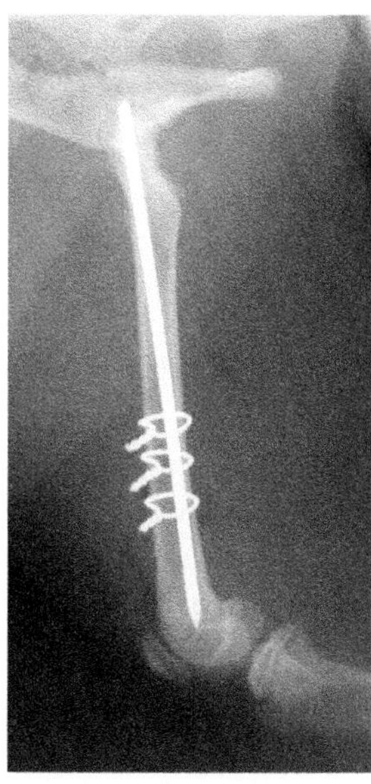
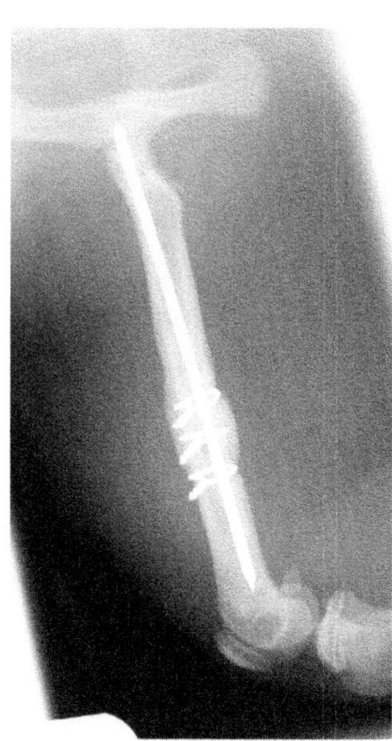

A B C

Figure 37-9 Correct indication and application of cerclage wires. (**A**) Preoperative radiograph of a long oblique fracture in a 6-month-old cat. (**B**) Postoperative radiograph. The fracture has been stabilized with a 1.6-mm normograde intramedullary pin and three 0.8-mm cerclage wires. (**C**) The fracture is healed with good callus formation after 4 weeks.

Box 37-4. Stabilization of long oblique and reducible multifragmentary fractures

A lateral approach to the femoral shaft is conducted.

Intramedullary pin and cerclage wires: A 1.6–3.0-mm intramedullary pin is inserted in a normograde fashion. Two or three 0.8-mm pieces of orthopedic wire are applied, using a wire passer, at least 5 mm away from the proximal and distal ends of the fracture line. The cerclage wires are twisted and tightened (Fig. 37-10A). Care is taken not to engage soft tissues between the bone and wires.

Intramedullary pin and type I external skeletal fixator: This type of fixation is especially useful for immature cats. A 1.4–2.4-mm intramedullary pin is inserted. The external skeletal fixator comprises two 1.4–2.0-mm transosseous pins per main fragment, angled 70° to the long axis of the bone if smooth pins are used (Fig. 37-10B).

Lag screw(s) and neutralization plate: The main fracture fragments are anatomically reduced and the fracture line is temporarily compressed with pointed reduction forceps. One or two 2.0–2.7-mm lag screws are inserted perpendicular to the fracture line. A plate is then applied in neutralization function (Fig. 37-10C). The lag screws can also be inserted through the plate if fracture configuration allows.

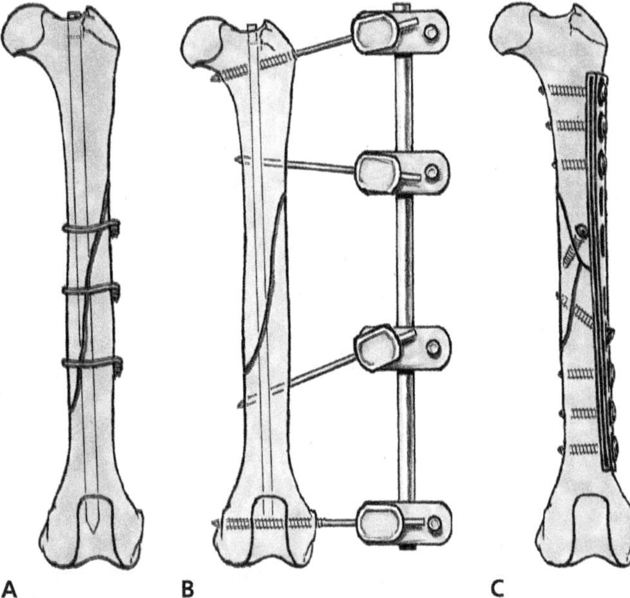

Figure 37-10 Options for stabilization of simple oblique or reducible multifragmentary fractures of the femoral diaphysis. (**A**) Stabilization of a long oblique fracture with an intramedullary pin and three cerclage wires. (**B**) Stabilization of a long oblique fracture with an intramedullary pin and a type I external skeletal fixator. (**C**) Stabilization of a butterfly fracture with lag screws and a plate in neutralization function.

used. Reducible multifragmentary fractures, such as fractures with a large butterfly fragment, can also be repaired with lag screws and a neutralization plate. Anatomic repair of fractures requires extensive dissection of soft tissues, and should only be attempted if anatomic reduction seems possible from preoperative radiographs. If the fragments are too small to be stabilized with interfragmentary compression, these fractures are better treated as comminuted fractures with a minimally invasive approach and stabilization of only the main fragments (see section below).

Plating is not an ideal stabilization method in immature cats because the periosteal blood supply is disrupted, and the bone is soft. These fracture are best treated with an intramedullary pin and a type I external skeletal fixator. Although this type of fixation does not provide interfragmentary compression, fracture healing is expected to be fast due to the preservation of periosteal blood supply. Alternatively, an internal fixator can be used.

37.4.4 Comminuted fractures

Interlocking nails, external skeletal fixators, and plates or internal fixators in buttress function are possible choices of treatment for comminuted fractures of the femoral diaphysis (Box 37-5). The advantages and disadvantages of internal stabilization methods should be weighed against those of external skeletal fixation. Although application of an external skeletal fixator is a versatile method and causes the least disturbance of the fracture area, some morbidity from the pin tracts should be expected, especially near the stifle joint.

Box 37-5. Stabilization of a comminuted fracture of the femoral diaphysis

A lateral approach is made to the femoral diaphysis. A small approach is sufficient for intramedullary pinning and interlocking nailing. An open but do-not-touch approach is used for plate fixation. Comminuted fractures are reduced with indirect reduction techniques in order not to disturb the local blood supply. Insertion of an intramedullary pin can help the reduction by providing axial alignment of the main fragments. Large medial fragments remaining disconnected from the reduced shaft may be brought closer using a resorbable suture as a cerclage.

Interlocking nail: A 4.0- or 4.7-mm interlocking nail is inserted in a normograde fashion. The fracture is checked for rotational malalignment prior to stabilizing it with two screws proximally and distally (Fig. 37-11A). One or two cerclage wires can be placed in the presence of fissures if they will improve fracture stability.

External skeletal fixation: Type I external skeletal fixators are normally used with an intramedullary pin. A 1.4–2.0-mm intramedullary pin is placed first to provide axial alignment. Two to three 1.6–2.0-mm transosseous pins are then inserted per fragment. The proximal end of the intramedullary pin is either cut as short as possible, or is bent laterally to be tied in to the connecting bar (Fig 37-11B). Three to four pins are inserted per fragment in the absence of an intramedullary pin (Fig 37-11C). A external fixator system with a large connecting bar or a double bar should be used for severely comminuted fractures to enhance bending stability.

Buttress plate/internal fixator: A long 2.7-mm dynamic compression plate (DCP), 2.4-mm limited contact-DCP (LC-DCP) or a sandwiched 2.7/2.0-mm veterinary cuttable plate (VCP) is precontoured from the radiographs of the contralateral limb and/or a bone specimen to achieve correct spatial alignment of the main fragments. The plate is secured first to the proximal fragment, and is then used to aid reduction by pulling the distal fragment to the plate. At least six cortices must be engaged with the screws, proximally and distally.

Plate and rod: A 2.7-mm DCP, 2.4-mm LC-DCP or a 2.0/2.7-mm VCP in sandwich fashion is combined with a 1.4–2.0-mm intramedullary pin (Fig. 37-11D). The pin is inserted first to align the main proximal and distal fragments. Four cortices of screw purchase per main fragment are sufficient with the plate and rod technique. Monocortical screws are inserted if the drill bit engages the intramedullary pin. If the fracture extends proximally into the subtrochanteric area screws can be angled into the femoral neck area for extra purchase (Fig. 37-11D).

Internal fixator: A 2.4-mm Unilock plate is used similar to a buttress plate, but plate contouring is not as critical as the locking plate does not need to be in close contact with the bone. Bicortical screws are inserted at the proximal and distal plate end into the wider metaphyseal bone, and monocortical screws are used in the narrower diaphysis. At least four cortices should be engaged with screws, in both the proximal and distal main fragment.

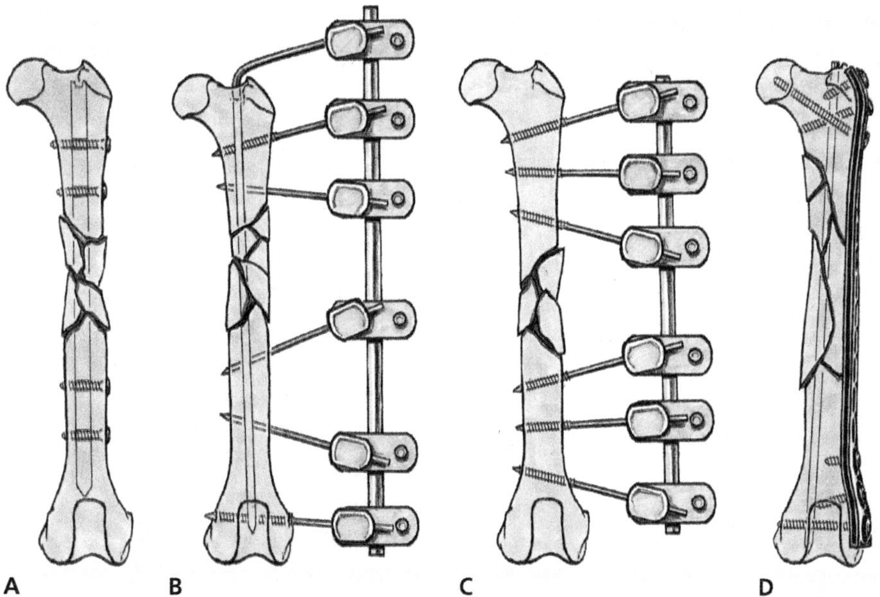

Figure 37-11 Stabilization options for comminuted fractures of the femoral shaft.
(**A**) An interlocking nail used to stabilize a comminuted mid-diaphyseal fracture.
(**B**) Stabilization of a comminuted fracture of the middle and proximal diaphysis using an external skeletal fixator in tie-in configuration.
(**C**) Stabilization of a mildly comminuted femoral fracture with a type I external skeletal fixator, using three pins per fragment.
(**D**) Plate and rod stabilization of a comminuted femoral fracture extending into the subtrochanteric area. The proximal screws are angled as shown to achieve sufficient bone purchase.

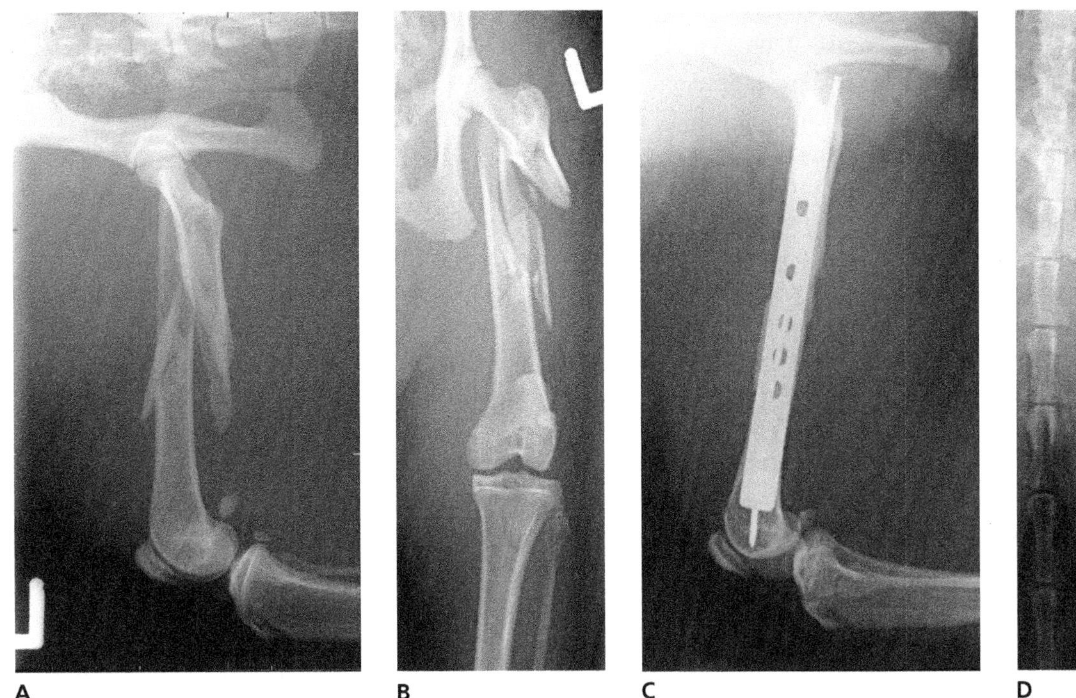

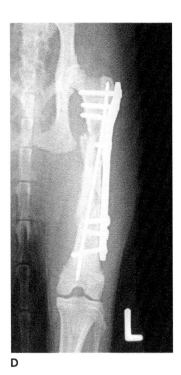

Figure 37-12 Plate and rod stabilization of a comminuted femoral fracture.
(**A, B**) Preoperative radiographs show a comminuted fracture of the proximal half of the femoral diaphysis in a 2-year-old cat.
(**C, D**) Radiographs 3 weeks after fracture stabilization with a plate and rod technique. The intramedullary pin was placed first to help align the main fragments. The plate was then applied to the main fragments with three screws each. One additional monocortical screw was used to stabilize the large lateral cortical fragment. Fracture healing is in progress.

An intramedullary pin is often used together with an external skeletal fixator or a plate (Fig. 37-12). This is especially useful in fractures that extend far proximally or distally, leaving insufficient room for the insertion of three transosseous pins or screws. Pin or screw engagement into four cortices per fragment provides adequate stability in the presence of an intramedullary pin. The intramedullary pin also facilitates fracture reduction.

Rotational malalignment is a common mistake after reduction and stabilization of femoral diaphyseal fractures. Femoral fractures in cats have a tendency to be stabilized with retroversion of the femoral head and neck. Rotational alignment can be assessed by visualization of the linea aspera at the caudolateral aspect of the femoral shaft, or it may be controlled by evaluation of the range of motion of the hip joint. An internal rotation of the hip joint of approximately 45° and an outward rotation of approximately 90° is physiological.

Application of a bone graft is not normally necessary in femoral fractures. Even severely comminuted fractures tend to heal if the bone fragments have soft-tissue attachments and an adequate blood supply. Large cortical fracture gaps that allow soft-tissue invasion should be grafted.

37.5 Fractures of the distal femur

Distal femoral fractures are common in cats, and most of them are Salter and Harris type I or II fractures of the distal femoral physis. Supracondylar fractures, and simple or comminuted fractures of the femoral condyle and/or trochlea, are occasionally seen in adult cats. Distal femoral fractures are often caused by falls from a height. Clinically, it can be difficult to differentiate between stifle joint instability and distal femoral fractures, but careful palpation of the patellar ligament and patella often helps reveals the site of injury.

37.5.1 Approaches to the distal femur

Most of the fractures of the distal femur are located within the joint capsule of the stifle joint, and are accessed by a craniolateral parapatellar approach to the stifle joint (16). Supracondylar fractures proximal to the joint capsule are approached via a lateral approach to the distal femoral shaft. Repair of some fractures requires an approach to both the medial and the lateral side of the distal femur. It is therefore advantageous to position the cat in dorsal recumbency, which will allow a medial parapatellar approach to the stifle joint if necessary (16).

A tibial tuberosity osteotomy can be performed for maximal visibility; this can be advantageous for repairing intracondylar fractures. The tibial tuberosity is reattached with pins and a tension band wire.

37.5.2 Supracondylar fractures

Supracondylar fractures can be a surgical challenge, especially if comminuted. Even simple supracondylar fractures do not have inherent rotational and shearing stability after reduction, and consequently must be rigidly stabilized with a plate or external skeletal fixator. The main challenge is to insert a sufficient number of screws or transfixation pins into the distal fragment.

The use of non-standard plates should be considered to facilitate insertion of two or three bicortical screws into the distal fragment plates. Reconstruction plates can be adapted to the caudal curvature of the distal femur, permitting placement of one screw more when compared to straight plates (28). Another plate to be considered is the recently introduced 2.0-mm condylar plate (29). These plates match the anatomic form of the femoral condyles and are available for the left and right leg. They have three round holes distally, and four oval holes proximally. Another plate, the supracondylar distal femoral plate, has 11 holes in total and is cuttable to the required length (Chapter 24). Anatomic fracture reduction is mandatory if only two screws are inserted in the distal fragment. Additional measures are needed if this cannot be achieved. An intramedullary pin can usually be inserted distal enough to enhance fixation stability (Fig. 37-13). Some fracture configurations make placement of an interfragmentary screw possible.

Bilateral plating is another option for severely comminuted fractures, or in cats with more than one traumatized limb (Box 37-6). Internal fixators are ideal for double plating, because the screws can be inserted monocortically. They also have the advantage of providing superior stability to conventional plates when only two screws can be inserted per fragment (30). The 2.0-mm plates from the Unilock mandibular locking plate system (Chapter 24) are a suitable size for the distal femur.

External skeletal fixators can also be used for stabilization of supracondylar fractures, but may cause some morbidity associated with the pin tracts due to the mobile soft tissue and skin around the stifle joint. A modified type II external skeletal fixator (31), and hybrid constructs with the IMEX mini circular external fixator (32), have been described.

37.5.3 Fractures through the femoral condyle

Fractures of the femoral condyle may be simple intracondylar fractures, affecting only the medial or lateral aspect of the condyle, or T- or Y-fracture where both the medial and lateral aspects of the condyle are separated from the diaphysis.

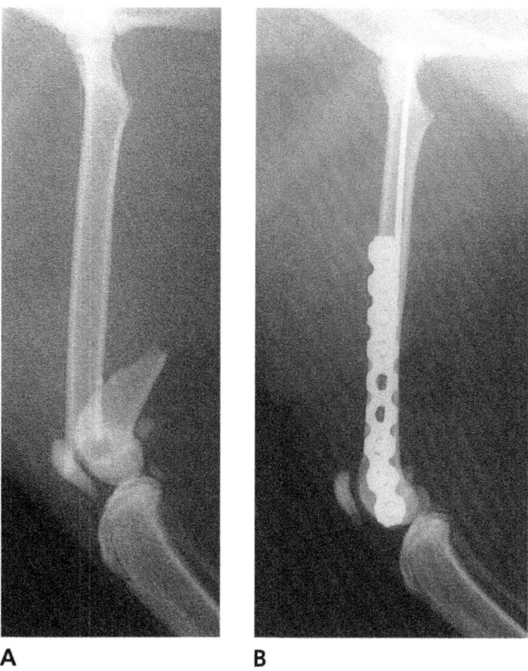

Figure 37-13 (**A**) A distal oblique supracondylar fracture in an adult cat (**B**) stabilized with a reconstruction Unilock plate and an intramedullary pin.

The medial aspect of the femoral condyle is affected more often than the lateral. Fractures of the medial part are usually only minimally displaced, because the fracture fragment is held in place by the caudal cruciate ligament and the medial collateral ligament. Anatomic reconstruction and stable fracture fixation with a lag screw are necessary to maintain joint function and prevent degenerative joint disease (Box 37-7).

Fracture of both the medial and lateral aspects of the condyle often have a T- or Y-configuration, but the supracondylar part of the fracture may be comminuted (Fig. 37-15). Anatomic reduction of the joint surfaces and stable fixation of the fracture fragments are challenging. The intra-articular fracture fragments are first stabilized with a lag screw, prior to addressing the supracondylar part of the fracture. Reconstruction plates, condylar plates, or internal fixators are best used for stabilization of the supracondylar part of the fracture (Box 37-8). Dynamic intramedullary pinning or Kirschner wires provide less stability, but can be sufficient in simple reducible fractures in young cats.

Condylar femoral fractures that differ from the standard condylar fracture patterns, and that involve the femoral trochlea, have been described in cats (33). These fractures are often comminuted, and one or several fracture lines cross the trochlea in a transverse or oblique direction. Avulsed frag-

Box 37-6. Stabilization of supracondylar femoral fractures

A lateral approach to the distal femur and stifle joint is performed and the fracture is anatomically reduced if possible. An additional medial approach is performed for bilateral plating. The stifle joint should be held in flexion to maintain the achieved reduction in place. Bone graft should be applied for comminuted fractures to enhance fracture healing.

Plating: A 2.0-mm dynamic compression plate, a 2.7-mm reconstruction plate or a 2.0-mm condylar plate (Fig. 37-14A) can be used. Simple fractures are anatomically reduced prior to application of the plate. At least two, and preferably three, bicortical screws must be inserted into the distal fragment with conventional plates. Additional insertion of an intramedullary pin is recommended if fewer than three screws can be inserted (Fig. 37-14B).

Internal fixator: Internal fixators are especially useful for comminuted fractures. A 2.0-mm locking plate can either be applied in conjunction with an intramedullary pin as described above, or one plate is applied medially and one laterally (Fig 37-14C). Screws can be inserted monocortically, but bicortical screw placement is advisable in the epiphyseal bone with its thin cortex.

External skeletal fixation: External fixators are mainly indicated for comminuted fractures. A modified type II configuration is commonly used, with or without an intramedullary pin (Fig. 37-14D). A transcondylar 2.0-mm centrally threaded transfixation pin is inserted across the femoral condyle. One half pin is inserted into the proximal fragment and the lateral bar connected between the two pins. One or two more half pins are then inserted into the distal and proximal fragment. The medial aspect of the transcondylar pin is connected with a curved bar to the lateral connecting bar. An intramedullary pin tie-in configuration can be used additionally, particularly if the distal fragment is too small for insertion of a second pin.

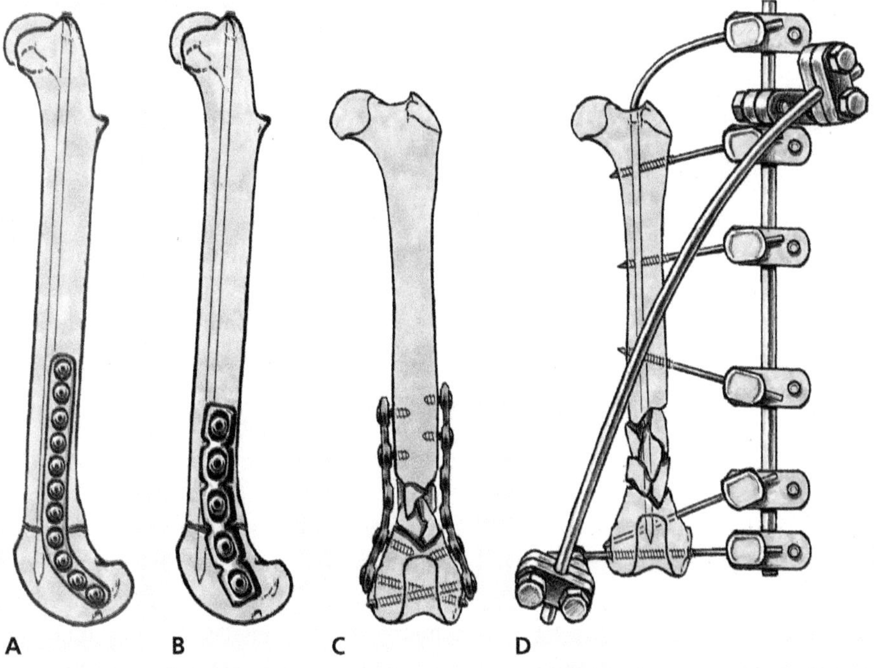

Figure 37-14 Options for stabilization of supracondylar fractures.
(**A**) Reconstruction of a simple supracondylar fracture with an intramedullary pin and a condylar plate.
(**B**) Stabilization of a simple supracondylar fracture with an intramedullary pin and 2.7-mm reconstruction plate.
(**C**) Fixation of a comminuted supracondylar fracture with bilateral 2.0-mm Unilock plates.
(**D**) Stabilization of a comminuted supracondylar fracture with a modified type II external skeletal fixator.

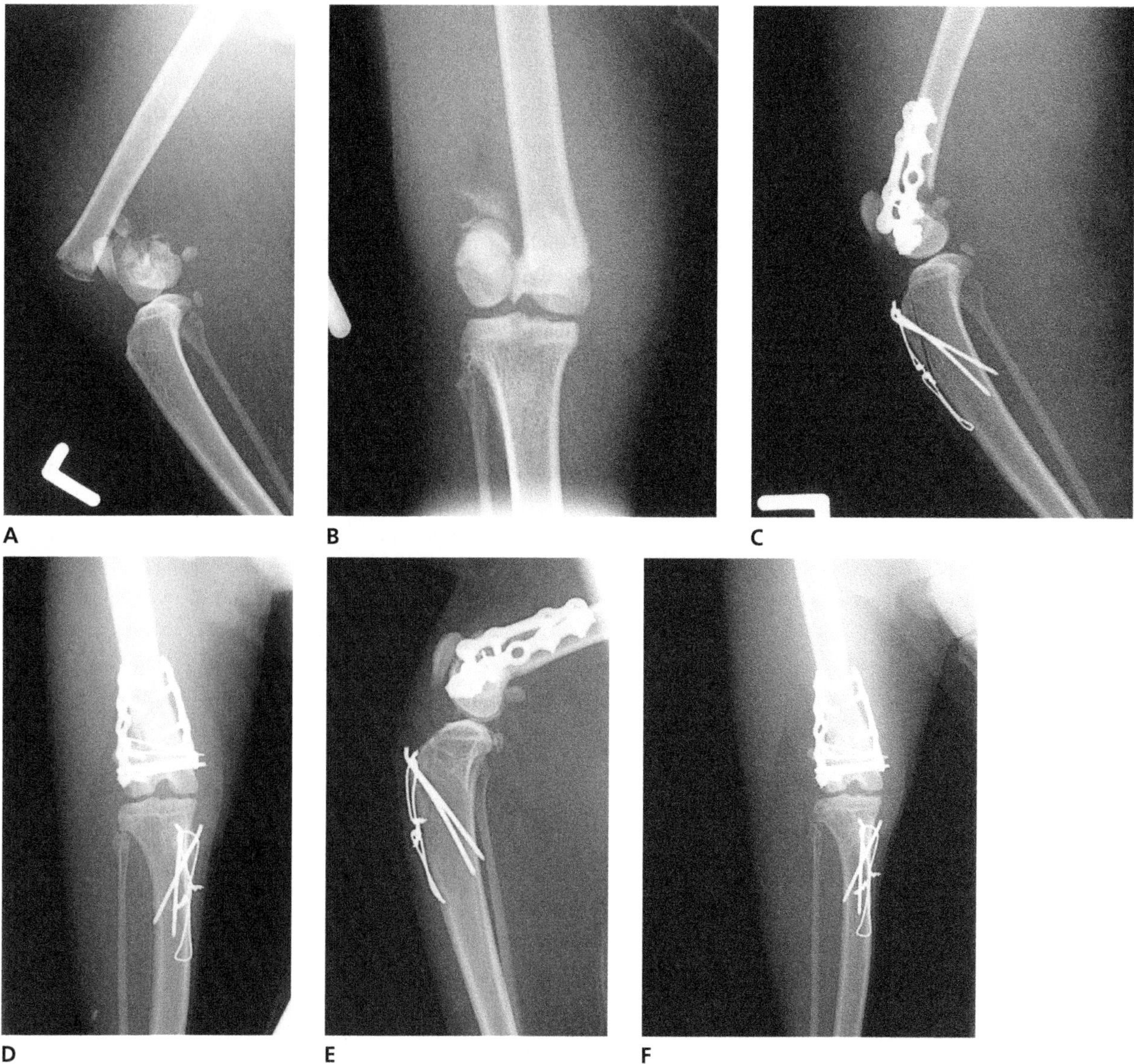

Figure 37-15 A 2-year-old cat with a intracondylar T-fracture of the femur. (**A**, **B**) Preoperative radiographs show an intracondylar T-fracture with mild comminution of the supracondylar part of the fracture. (**C**, **D**) The intracondylar fracture part was stabilized with a 2.0-mm lag screw, and the supracondylar part of the fracture was addressed with a medial and lateral 2.0-mm Unilock plate. An osteotomy of the tibial tuberosity enabled reflection of the patellar ligament, and therefore enhanced visualization of the articular surface during reduction. (**E**, **F**) The fracture and the osteotomy have healed after 3.5 months.

ments from the trochlea are reattached with small screws or pins, depending on fragment size.

37.5.4 Salter and Harris fractures

Fractures of the distal femoral physis are common injuries in cats, and are usually Salter and Harris type I or II fractures (34, 35). The average age of cats with Salter I fractures is 9.5 months, and 6.5 months in cats with Salter II fractures (34). The distal femoral physis closes between 54 and 76 weeks in intact cats (19), but early neutering delays physeal closure and therefore young adult cats can also sustain distal femoral physeal fractures. The distal fragment is often displaced caudally because of the pull of the hamstring and gastrocnemius muscles (Fig. 37-18). Correct fracture alignment is necessary to restore stifle joint conformation and to achieve fixation stability. The metaphyseal fragment has four bony protuberances that fit into corresponding depressions in the epiphysis. This shape aids control and maintenance of reduction, and provides stability against rotational and shear forces once the fracture is reduced. Cross pinning, dynamic intramedullary pinning, or conventional intramedullary pinning are all

Box 37-7. Stabilization of a fracture of the medial aspect of the femoral condyle

A medial approach to the stifle joint is performed. The fracture fragment is reduced anatomically, and is temporarily stabilized to the condyle with pointed bone reduction forceps. A 2.0- or 2.7-mm lag screw is then inserted from the medial epicondyle across the fracture line into the lateral condyle. Anatomic reduction of the joint surface is critical for a satisfactory outcome. The lag screw is only fully tightened after insertion of a 0.8-mm Kirschner wire from the medial epicondyle into the lateral cortex of the femoral metaphysis as an antirotational implant (Fig. 37-16).

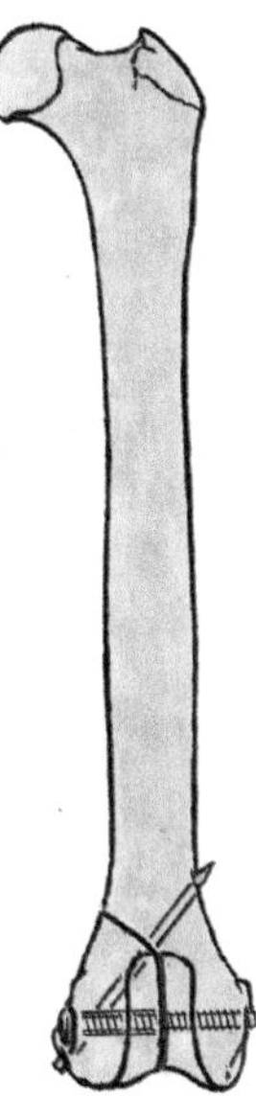

Figure 37-16 Lag screw and Kirschner wire fixation of a fracture of the medial aspect of the femoral condyle.

reported methods used for fracture stabilization (35). Intramedullary pinning as a sole fixation method is only possible due to the inherent rotational stability. Cross pinning is the technique most widely used (Box 37-9).

Salter and Harris type IV fractures of the distal femur are rarely encountered. They are treated like simple condylar fractures, as described above.

37.6 Postoperative treatment and prognosis

Postoperative treatment depends on fixation stability achieved, and implants used, but usually involves confinement to the house for 6 weeks. Cage rest is employed if deemed necessary to reduce activity during the first 1–2 weeks. Control radiographs are performed after 4–6 weeks in adult cats, and after 2–3 weeks in immature cats. Early gentle physical therapy is indicated if the patient is not using the leg to prevent development of quadriceps contracture.

Uneventful fracture healing is reported in several studies on feline capital physeal and femoral neck fractures (5, 24, 25). Cats can be expected to be sound after 4–8 weeks (24, 25) and functional results are also good at long term (36). An applecore appearance of the femoral neck, shortening of the femoral neck, and osteoarthritis of the hip joint are sometimes observed radiologically.

Postoperative treatment of diaphyseal fractures depends on the fixation method chosen. External skeletal fixation requires frequent check-ups and monitoring of the pin–skin interface. Intramedullary pins may migrate proximally and cause soft-tissue irritation if not connected to an external skeletal fixator. Clinical signs of pin migration include worsening of the lameness, soft-tissue swelling medial to the greater trochanter, pain on hip manipulation, and sciatic nerve deficits in the worst-affected cases. Most of the femoral diaphyseal fractures in cats heal without complications if adequately treated and cats can be expected to return to full function (12). Fracture union disorders and osteomyelitis are only rarely encountered. The common incidence of non-unions in the older literature was due to the fact that most femoral fractures were stabilized with an intramedullary pin alone and were therefore lacking rotational stability. Rotational malunion can occur particularly with comminuted or older fractures where the hip is stabilized in retroversion. This can cause a functional gait abnormality and lateral patellar luxation.

The prognosis for fractures of the distal femur is also good. A return to full function can be expected in cats with distal femoral physeal fractures if correctly aligned and stabilized (35), although osteoarthritis and/or meniscal calcification is likely to develop (36). As most of the fractures occur in cats between 6.5 and 9.5 months of age (34), significant shortening of the femur is not common.

The prognosis for supracondylar fractures is also good to excellent after adequate fracture alignment and stabilization. Lameness and loss of stifle range of motion were observed in 2 of 10 cats in one study (29). Condylar and trochlear fractures carry a good prognosis if the stifle joint is reconstructed anatomically. Despite the severity of comminuted trochlear fractures, satisfactory or good clinical outcome was reported in 85% of cases (33). Because implants have to be placed close or inside the stifle joint, they could interfere with the joint capsule and cause irritation, and it may be beneficial to remove them after the fracture has healed.

Box 37-8. Stabilization of an intracondylar T- or Y-fracture

Both a medial and lateral approach is often necessary to reduce and stabilize T- or Y-fractures of the distal femur. Osteotomy of the tibial tuberosity provides excellent visualization for the reduction of the condylar fragments.

The femoral condyle is first reduced and stabilized anatomically using a 2.0-mm transcondylar lag screw, The metaphyseal part of the fracture is repaired afterwards. Cross pinning or dynamic intramedullary pinning using two small-diameter Kirschner wires can be used in simple Y- or T-fractures in young cats (Fig. 37-17A), but better stability is provided with lateral or bilateral plates or internal fixators, as described for supracondylar fractures (Fig. 37-17B).

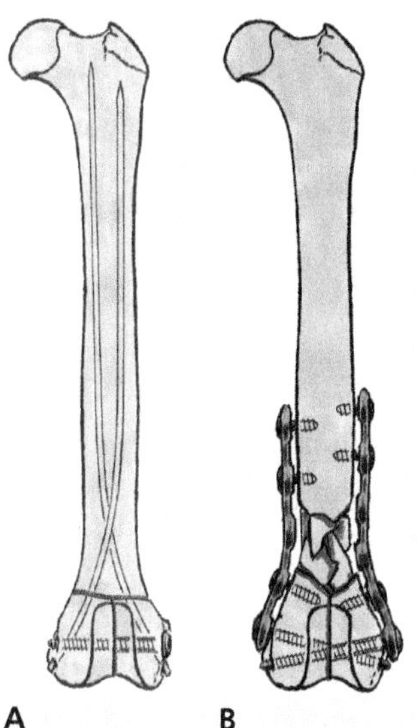

Figure 37-17 Stabilization of combined intra- and supracondylar femoral fractures.
(**A**) Stabilization of a simple T-fracture with a transcondylar lag screws and dynamic pinning.
(**B**) Stabilization of an intracondylar fracture with supracondylar comminution using a transcondylar lag screws and a medial and lateral 2.0-mm internal fixator.

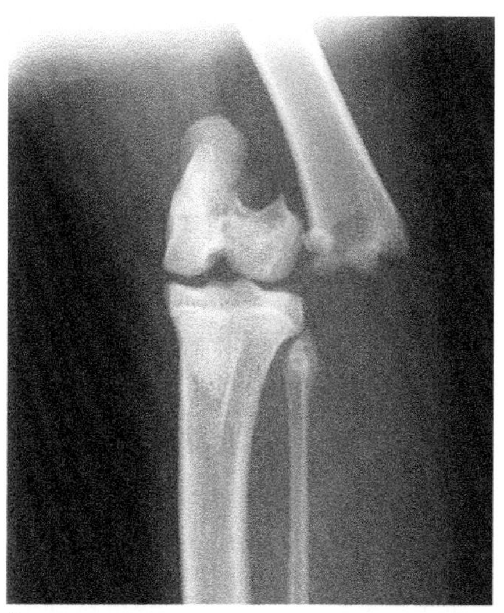

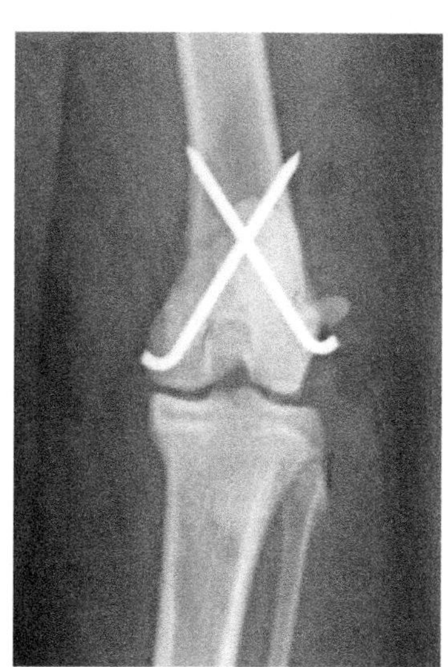

Figure 37-18 Preoperative radiograph (**A**) of a Salter and Harris type II fracture of the distal femur, stabilized with cross pins (**B**).

Box 37-9. Stabilization of Salter and Harris type I and II fractures

A lateral parapatellar approach to the stifle joint is performed. A small medial parapatellar approach is also necessary to insert the medial Kirschner wire. The epiphysis in young animals consists of very soft bone, and the fracture fragments should be manipulated very carefully. In fractures less than 2–3 days old, manual fracture reduction is usually possible. The fracture should be over-reduced rather than under-reduced. Blood clots or fibrous tissue in between the fracture gap are removed before reduction. Reduction is more difficult in older fractures due to fibrosis and new bone formation, which is most evident caudally. The epiphyseal fragment is carefully dissected from the fibrous tissue with a periosteal elevator until it can be manipulated sufficiently. With the stifle joint in extension, a large pointed reduction forceps may be carefully placed between the intercondylar notch and a small hole drilled in the cranial metaphysis of the femur both to aid fracture reduction and to prevent distraction of the fragments during pin insertion.

Cross pinning: The 1.2–1.6-mm Kirschner wires are inserted from just cranial to the lateral and medial collateral ligament, and are aimed towards proximal to engage the contralateral cortex of the femoral shaft segment. It is important that the pins are started distal enough in the epiphyseal fragment, and that they cross above the fracture line to enhance rotational stability (Fig. 37-19A).

Dynamic intramedullary pinning: The technique is similar to cross pinning, and is used if the Kirschner wires are being inserted at a steep angle, which avoids penetration of the transcortex. The pins will then glide along the endosteal surface of the intramedullary canal (Fig. 37-19B). The pins do not need to be repositioned if this occurs inadvertently, but they should be inserted further proximal into the medullary cavity, up to the level of the greater trochanter.

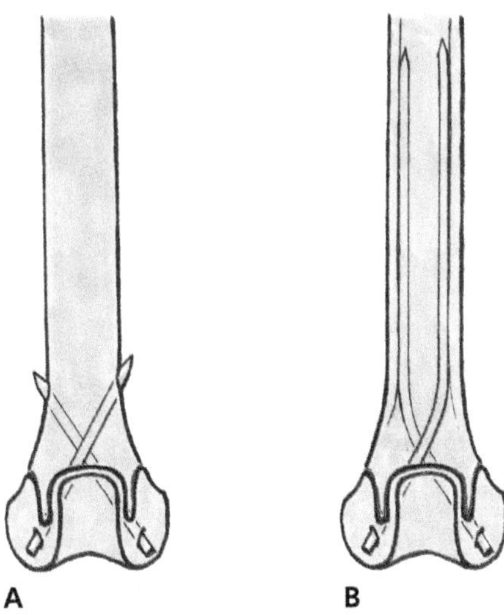

Figure 37-19 Options for stabilization of Salter and Harris type I and II fractures of the distal femur.
(A) Fixation of a distal physeal fracture with cross pins.
(B) Fixation of a distal physeal fracture with dynamic intramedullary pins.

References and further reading

1. Hill FWG. A survey of bone fractures in the cat. J Small Anim Pract 1977;18:457–463.
2. Bookbinder PF, Flanders JA. Characteristics of pelvic fracture in the cat. Vet Comp Orthop Traumatol 1992;5:122–127.
3. Lidbetter DA, Glyde MR. Supracondylar femoral fractures in adult animals. Compend Continuing Educ 2000;22: 1041–1049.
4. Frewein J, Vollmerhaus B. Anatomie von Hund und Katze. Berlin: Blackwell; 1994.
5. Culvenor JA, et al. Repair of femoral capital physeal injuries in cats – 14 cases. Vet Comp Orthop Traumatol 1996;9:182–185.
6. Pohlmeyer K. Arteries of the articulatio coxae and the proximal end of the femur in cats (*Felis catus*). Anat Histol Embryol 1981;10:246–256.
7. Fanton JW, et al. Sciatic nerve injury as a complication of intramedullary pin fixation of femoral fractures. J Am Anim Hosp Assoc 1982;19:687–694.
8. Endo K, et al. Interlocking intramedullary nail method for the treatment of femoral and tibial fractures in cats and small dogs. J Vet Med Sci 1998;60:119–122.
9. Larin A, et al. Repair of diaphyseal femoral fractures in cats using interlocking intramedullary nails: 12 cases (1996–2000). J Am Vet Med Assoc 2001;219:1098–1104.
10. Duhautois B. Use of veterinary interlocking nails for diaphyseal fractures in dogs and cats: 121 cases. Vet Surg 2003;32:8–20.
11. Scotti SA, et al. Retrograde placement of a novel 3.5 mm titanium interlocking nail for supracondylar and diaphyseal femoral fractures in cats. Vet Comp Orthop Traumatol 2007;20: 211–218.
12. Langley-Hobbs SJ, et al. Use of external skeletal fixators in the repair of femoral fractures in cats. J Small Anim Pract 1996;37:95–101.
13. Aron DN, et al. Experimental and clinical experience with an IM pin external skeletal fixator tie-in configuration. Vet Comp Orthop Traumatol 1991;4:86–94.
14. Peirone B, et al. Femoral and humeral fracture treatment with an intramedullary pin/external fixator tie-in configuration in

growing dogs and cats. Vet Comp Orthop Traumatol 2002;15: 85–91.
15. Reems MR, et al. Use of a plate-rod construct and principles of biological osteosynthesis for repair of diaphyseal fractures in dogs and cats. J Am Vet Med Assoc 2003;223:330–335.
16. Piermattei DL, Johnson KA. An atlas of surgical approaches to the bones and joints of the dog and the cat, 4th edn. Philadelphia: WB Saunders, 2004.
17. Bennett D. Orthopedic disease affecting the pelvic region of the cat. J Small Anim Pract 1975;16:723–738.
18. Perez-Aparicio FJ, Fjeld TO. Femoral neck fractures and capital epiphyseal separations in cats. J Small Anim Pract 1993;34: 445–449.
19. Smith RN. Fusion of ossification centres in the cat. J Small Anim Pract 1969;10:523–530.
20. Queen J, et al. Femoral neck metaphyseal osteopathy in the cat. Vet Rec 1998;142:159–162.
21. Craig LE. Physeal dysplasia with slipped capital femoral epiphysis in 13 cats. Vet Pathol 2001;38:92–97.
22. McNicholas WT Jr, et al. Spontaneous femoral capital physeal fractures in adult cats: 26 cases (1996–2001). J Am Vet Med Assoc 2002;221:1731–1736.
23. Forrest LJ, et al. Feline capital physeal dysplasia syndrome. Vet Radiol Ultrasound 1999;40:672.
24. Jeffery ND. Internal fixation of femoral head and neck fractures in the cat. J Small Anim Pract 1989;30:674–677.
25. Fischer HR, et al. Surgical reduction and stabilization for repair of femoral capital physeal fractures in cats: 13 cases (1998–2002). J Am Vet Med Assoc 2004;224:1478–1482.
26. Lambrechts N, et al. Internal fixation of femoral neck fractures in the dog – an in vitro study. Vet Comp Orthop Traumatol 1993;6:188.
27. Guerrero TG, et al. Fixation of a proximal femoral physeal fracture in a dog using a ventral approach and two Kirschner wires. Vet Comp Orthop Traumatol 2005;18:110–114.
28. Lewis DD, et al. Use of reconstruction plates for stabilization of fractures and osteotomies involving the supracondylar region of the femur. J Am Anim Hosp Assoc 1993;29:171–178.
29. Forterre F. A new condylar plate for supracondylar fractures in cats. Kleintierpraxis 2005;50:299–304.
30. Sikes JW, et al. Comparison of fixation strengths of locking head and conventional screws, in fracture and reconstruction models. J Oral Maxillofac Surg 1998;56:468–473.
31. Klause SE, et al. A modification of the unilateral type 1 ESF configuration for primary or secondary support of supracondylar humeral or femoral fractures. Vet Comp Orthop Traumatol 1990;3:130–134.
32. Farese JP, et al. Use of IMEX SK-circular external fixator hybrid constructs for fracture stabilization in dogs and cats. J Am Anim Hosp Assoc 2002;38:279–289.
33. Chico AC, et al. Trochlear femoral fractures in cats: results of seven cases. Vet Comp Orthop Traumatol 2001;14:51–55.
34. Grauer GF, et al. Incidence and mechanisms of distal femoral physeal fractures in the dog and cat. J Am Anim Hosp Assoc 1981;17:579–586.
35. Hardie EM, Chambers JN. Factors influencing the outcome of distal femoral physeal fracture fixation: a retrospective study. J Am Anim Hosp Assoc 1984;20:927–931.
36. Strodl S. Spätergebnisse nach intraartikulären und gelenknahen Frakturen des Hüft- und Kniegelenkes von Hund und Katze. Munich: Ludwig-Maximilians-Universität; 2000.

38 Stifle joint

K. Voss, S.J. Langley-Hobbs, P.M. Montavon

Most surgical conditions of the feline stifle joint are caused by ligament injuries. Rupture of the cranial cruciate ligament is the most commonly encountered surgical condition of the stifle joint. Stifle joint disruption or luxation is also common, and is seen more frequently in cats than in dogs. Isolated ruptures of the caudal cruciate ligament and the medial collateral ligament occur rarely.

Other differential diagnoses to be considered in a cat with a stifle joint problem include articular fractures, patellar luxation, patellar fractures, meniscal calcification, degenerative joint disease, osteochondrosis, and patellar tendon injury. Degenerative joint disease is mostly found in older cats, and may be secondary to cranial cruciate ligament tears or other injuries. Patellar fractures can occur spontaneously and cause an acute lameness. Diagnosis and treatment of the most frequent stifle joint disorders are described in the following sections.

38.1 Surgical anatomy

The stifle joint consist of the femorotibial and the femoropatellar articulations. The cruciate ligaments and the medial and lateral collateral ligament are the primary stabilizing structures. Secondary stabilizers are the joint capsule, the menisci, and the muscles and tendons that span the joint.

The cranial cruciate ligament prevents stifle hyperextension, excessive internal rotation, and cranial translation of the tibia. The caudal cruciate ligament prevents caudal translation of the tibia. The cranial cruciate ligament is stronger than the caudal cruciate ligament in cats (1), which may explain why isolated caudal cruciate ligament ruptures are occasionally seen. The collateral ligaments mainly provide stability against valgus and varus deviation of the stifle joint.

Four sesamoid bones are present in the vicinity of the stifle joint: the patella, the medial and lateral fabella, and the popliteal sesamoid bone. Whereas the lateral fabella is consistently ossified and visible on radiographs, the medial fabella is often not visible on radiographs in many cats. Radiolucent medial fabellas consist of fibrocartilage histologically (2). Non-pedigree cats have a higher prevalence of radiolucent medial fabellas compared to pedigree cats (2). The popliteal sesamoid bone is a small oval bone located within the tendon of the popliteal muscle.

38.2 Diagnosis and treatment options

The diagnosis of stifle joint disorders is based mainly on clinical examination findings. A summary list of the potential diseases and injuries of the stifle joint and the treatment options is provided in Table 38-1.

Cats with acute traumatic cranial cruciate ligament ruptures will show a sudden-onset moderate to high-grade lameness, pain on extension of the stifle, and a joint effusion. A positive cranial drawer sign confirms rupture of the cranial cruciate ligament. Young cats especially can have some normal craniocaudal laxity in their stifle joints, and stability of the affected joint should always be compared with the contralateral side. Chronic degenerative joint disease may precede cranial cruciate ligament rupture, especially in older cats. These patients tend to have a history of inactivity or chronic low-grade lameness.

A caudal drawer sign can be elicited with isolated ruptures of the caudal cruciate ligament. Lameness and pain are usually less pronounced with caudal cruciate ligament rupture. Rupture of the medial collateral ligament causes valgus instability, and rupture of the lateral collateral ligament causes varus instability.

Cats with stifle joint disruption are presented with non-weight-bearing lameness, extensive soft-tissue swelling, conformational changes, and obvious instability or luxation of the stifle joint. Cranial and caudal drawer tests and medial and lateral stability are affected. These tests should be performed after closed reduction of the stifle joint to evaluate which of the anatomic structures are damaged, but stifle reduction and the manipulations are painful and best performed under sedation or general anesthesia after cardiovascular and respiratory stabilization of the patient.

The patella should be palpated and manipulated to detect patellar luxation or patellar fractures. A grading system for patellar luxation is provided in Table 38-2. Cats have a relatively large flat patella, and more normal laxity than dogs.

Radiographs of the stifle joint are performed to confirm the clinical diagnosis and to exclude periarticular or articular fractures. Valgus and varus stressed radiographs can be performed under general anesthesia to evaluate integrity of the collateral ligaments.

Table 38-1. Summary of injuries and diseases of the feline stifle joint and possible surgical treatment options

Type of lesion	Further classification	Treatment options
Stifle joint instability	Cranial cruciate ligament rupture	Conservative Extracapsular stabilization TTA/TPLO
	Caudal cruciate ligament rupture	Conservative
	Collateral ligament sprain	Conservative Collateral ligament prosthesis
Stifle joint luxation	Dependent on the ligaments involved	Surgical repair of damaged ligaments + external coaptation + TESF + transarticular pin
Patellar fracture	Fatigue stress fracture	Conservative Encircling wire ± tibial quadriceps wire ± protection Partial patellectomy
	Traumatic fracture	Tension band repair ± protection Partial patellectomy
Patellar luxation	Different grades	Transposition of tibial tuberosity Sulcoplasty Soft-tissue correction
Tendon injury (Chapter 16)	Avulsion of the tendon of the long digital extensor muscle	Surgical reattachment to femur or tibia
	Quadriceps tendon rupture	Surgical repair and protection

TTA, tibial tuberosity advancement; TPLO, tibial plateau leveling osteotomy; TESF, transarticular external skeletal fixator.

Grade	Clinical features
A	Patella can be completely luxated with digital pressure, but immediately returns into position after pressure is released
B	Patella can be completely luxated with digital pressure and remains temporarily luxated once the pressure is released
C	Patella luxates when the tibia is internally rotated, without exerting direct digital pressure
D	Patella is temporarily or permanently luxated without any manipulation

Table 38-2. Suggestion for a grading system of patellar luxation in cats

38.3 Approaches to the stifle joint

The stifle joint can be approached through either a lateral (3) or a medial (3) incision. The lateral parapatellar approach is most commonly used and is indicated for exploration and debridement of the joint, for application of lateral imbrication sutures for the treatment of cranial cruciate ligament ruptures, for repair of lateral collateral ligament sprains, and for treatment of patellar luxation. Care is taken not to injure the tendon of the long digital extensor muscle, which originates in an intra-articular location on the lateral femoral condyle.

The medial approach to the stifle joint is used for repair of medial collateral ligament injuries, for surgery of the tibial tuberosity, such as lateralization of the tibial tuberosity for treatment of patellar luxations or cranialization of the tibial

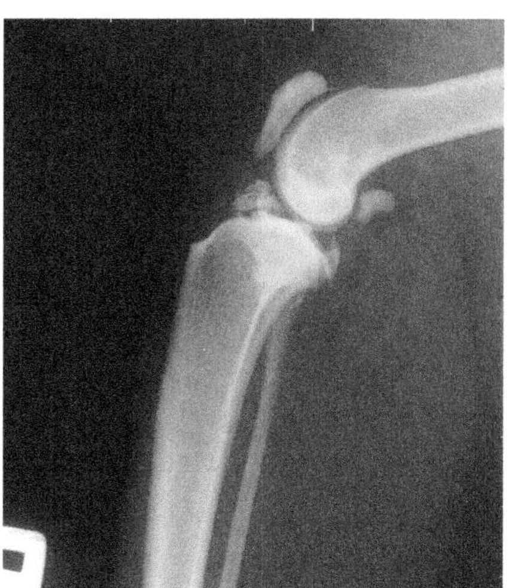

Figure 38-1 Mediolateral radiograph of the stifle joint of a 12-year-old cat with a large mineralized body located in the cranial aspect of the joint, and degenerative joint changes. A rupture of the cranial cruciate ligament was diagnosed clinically.

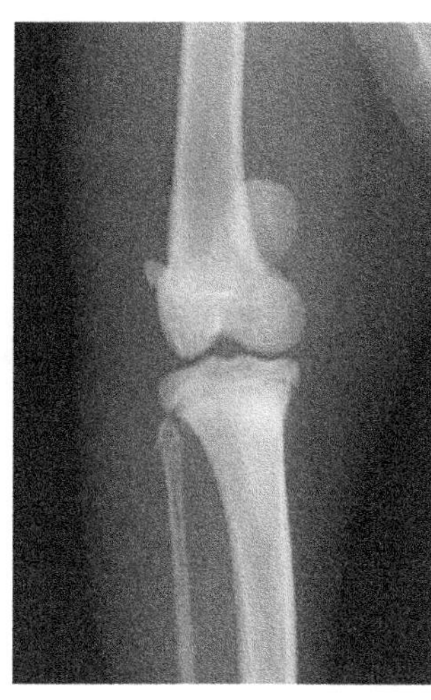

Figure 38-2 Caudocranial radiograph of the left stifle joint of a 7-month-old domestic short-hair cat with medial patellar luxation.

tuberosity or tibial plateau leveling osteotomy (TPLO) for treatment of cranial cruciate disease.

38.4 Meniscal mineralization

Meniscal mineralization has only been described in a small number of cats (4, 5) but is a frequent feature in feline practice. These calcifications or ossifications are generally thought to occur in the cranial horn of the medial or lateral meniscus, but the authors have also seen areas of mineralization in the cranial attachment of the cranial cruciate ligament, the synovial membrane, and the infrapatellar fat pad. They are visible radiographically as one or several radiodense bodies located in the cranial aspect of the joint (Fig. 38-1). Most affected cats are elderly, many have concurrent gonarthrosis, and the lesions often occur bilaterally. Evidence suggests that the mineralization is associated with cranial cruciate ligament rupture, either occurring secondary to cranial cruciate ligament disease, or preceding it (4–6). In one study, 12 out of 14 cats with cranial cruciate ligament disease developed radiodense bodies in the stifle joint visible on follow-up radiographs (6). These findings implied that meniscal calcification occurs as a sequel to cranial cruciate ligament rupture, although preoperative radiographs were not taken in the majority of cats in this series. In contrast, in another study, five out of six cats with meniscal mineralization suffered concurrent cranial cruciate ligament rupture, and two out of six cats with bilateral lesions later developed cranial cruciate ligament disease in the contralateral leg (5). The authors hypothesized that a mineralized meniscus loses its normal compliance and predisposes the joint to cranial cruciate ligament rupture (5).

Clinical signs associated with the abnormal meniscus are not recognized in many cats. Joint stability should be carefully assessed in order to rule out concurrent rupture of the cranial cruciate ligament when lameness and clinical signs are present. Clinical signs were relieved after excision of the calcified meniscus in one cat without rupture of the cranial cruciate ligament (5).

38.5 Disorders of the patella

Disorders of the patella include patellar luxation and patellar fractures. Patellar luxation is more common. Patellar fractures in cats are often stress fractures, unassociated with external trauma (7). Patellar aplasia has also been described (8).

38.5.1 Patellar luxation

Patellar luxation is less common in cats than in dogs. Patellar luxation can be traumatic in origin or occurring as a sequel to the conformational changes in the limb after femoral or tibial fractures, but most of the cases seen are developmental (9, 10). Certain breeds, such as Abyssinian and Devon Rex cats, have been reported to have a higher prevalence for patellar luxation (11–13), but other breeds and non-pedigree cats are affected as well (9, 10). As many as 38% of Abyssinian cats had loose patellas during palpation in one study (11). The condition has also been documented in two British shorthair littermates (14). Patellar luxation seems to have a hereditary component, but the exact mode of inheritance is unclear. Prevalence and grade of luxation are thought to be modified by several factors, implicating a polygenetic trait, as in dogs (11). Patellar luxation can also be associated with hip dysplasia (10, 13, 15, 16).

The patella usually luxates medially, and both stifle joints are often affected (Fig. 38-2). Affected cats are usually relatively young at the time of presentation (9). One study, however, reported a median age of 3.3 years, which is con-

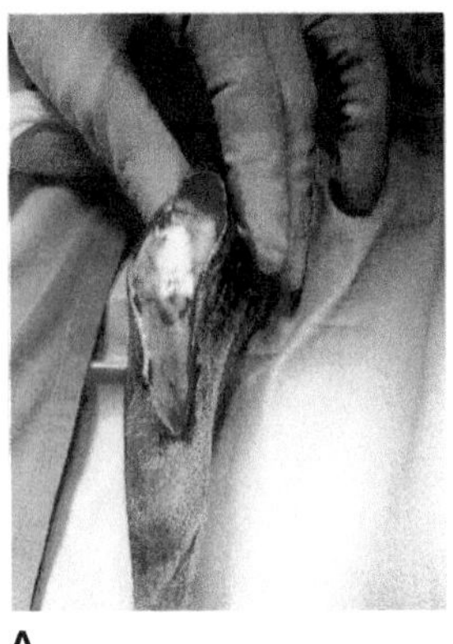
A

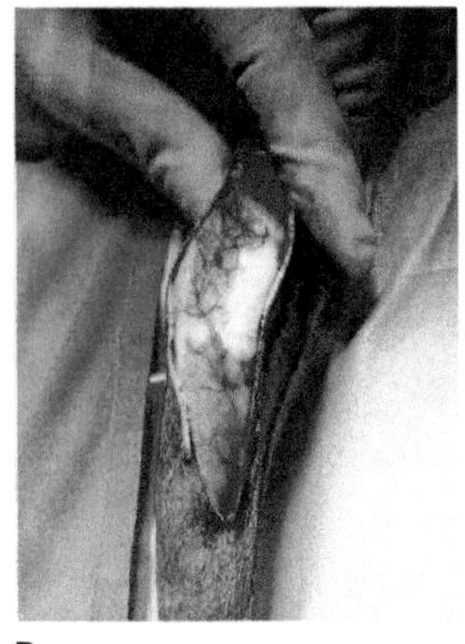
B

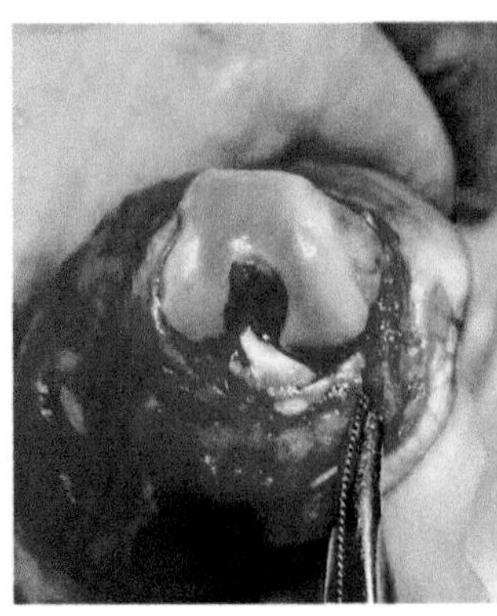
C

Figure 38-3 A cat with developmental medial patellar luxation.
(**A**) View after incision of the skin. The patella is in situ.
(**B**) Minimal lateral digital pressure on the quadriceps muscle causes the patella to luxate medially.
(**C**) The patella is luxated medially after a lateral parapatellar approach. Cartilage erosions are often seen on the medial condylar crest and on the retropatellar surface. The trochlear groove is flat.

siderably older than the median age for dogs presenting with patellar luxation (17). Cats have a larger patella and a higher physiological laxity of the patella than dogs, and the patella can be manually moved on to the trochlear ridge of the femoral condyles in many normal cats. Therefore, grading systems developed for dogs should be used with caution. Table 38-2 provides a classification system for patellar luxation in the cat. Most of the cats have grade A and B luxations; grade D luxations are rare in cats (17). Anatomic changes include a shallow trochlear groove and medial displacement of the tibial tuberosity. Gross conformational changes are generally not present. Secondary osteoarthritis is often absent or mild, but older cats especially can have more severe degenerative changes in their stifle joints (17). Cartilage erosions may be seen retropatellar and on the medial condylar crest (Fig. 38-3).

Laxity of the patella is always interpreted in conjunction with clinical signs. Common clinical complaints are a crouched gait, inactivity, and inability to jump. Some cats show intermittent lameness or sudden-onset distress with vocalization and unwillingness to use the affected leg. These signs are likely to be due to sudden dislocation of the patella. Acute lameness can also occur if a cranial cruciate ligament rupture occurs in conjunction with patellar luxation. Traumatic patellar luxations will also have an acute onset.

Surgical correction of the condition is indicated in cats that show clinical signs associated with patellar luxation. The aim of surgery is to restore normal patellar position and improve femoropatellar joint function. Several procedures, used alone or in combination, clinically improve patellar function in most cats (10, 17). The techniques include tibial crest transposition, sulcoplasty, and soft-tissue corrections. Soft tissues are secondary stabilizing structures of the joint and their correction alone rarely leads to sufficient and long-term restoration of functional anatomic relationships. An indication to use only soft-tissue correction methods is in the rare case of an acute traumatic patellar luxation, caused by rupture of the lateral or medial retinaculum (Fig. 38-4).

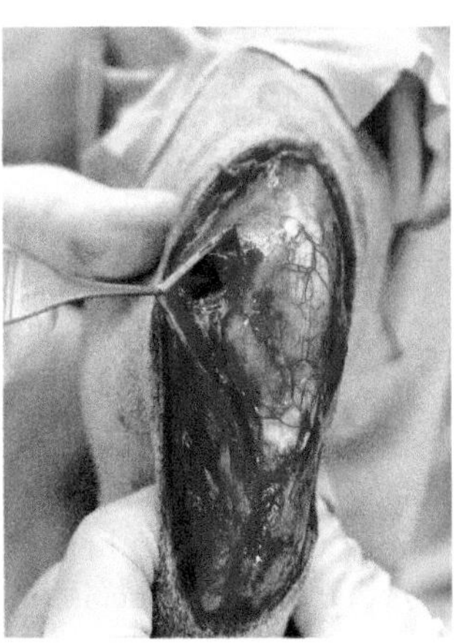
Figure 38-4 A cat with traumatic lateral patellar luxation, caused by rupture of the medial retinaculum and joint capsule.

Transposition of the tibial crest, or a combination of transposition of the tibial crest with sulcoplasty, yields more reliable results in non-traumatic patellar luxation (10). Transposition of the tibial crest towards lateral restores the normal axis of the quadriceps/patellar tendon mechanism in medial patellar luxation. Lateralization of the tibial crest can be combined with cranialization to reduce retropatellar pressure and pain (18) (Box 38-1). Medial transposition is performed for lateral patellar luxation. Transposition of the tibial tuberosity is avoided in immature cats to avoid damaging the tibial tuberosity growth plate. Sulcoplasty deepens the abnormally flat patellar groove, and is usually performed in conjunction with transposition of the tibial crest.

38.5.2 Patellar fractures

Patellar fractures may occur spontaneously or may be caused by trauma. Three cases of non-traumatic patellar fracture have been described in the literature (7) and data on a further 34 cases are in preparation for publication (19). Spontaneous patellar fractures usually occur in both stifle joints with some delay between the left and right limb and with no evidence of trauma (Fig. 38-6). They are therefore likely to be fatigue

Box 38-1. Correction of a medial patellar luxation

A lateral or medial parapatellar approach is performed, according to surgeon preference. The stifle joint is explored for concurrent pathologies.

Sulcoplasty: The depth of the trochlear groove is assessed, and a sulcoplasty is performed if deemed necessary. In cats having a tibial tuberosity transposition, the sulcoplasty is performed after the osteotomy, but before reattachment of the tibial tuberosity. A wedge sulcoplasty is usually chosen (Fig. 38-5A). Cats have a relatively wider patella than dogs, so it is important to ensure the wedge is made wide enough to accommodate this.

Lateralization and cranialization of the tibial tuberosity: An osteotomy of the tibial tuberosity is performed with an oscillating saw or with a hand-held saw (Fig. 38-5B). If using a hand saw, the cranial tibial muscle must be partially elevated from the lateral aspect of the proximal tibia before making the cut with the saw inserted caudal to the patellar ligament. The tibial crest is cut in a slight oblique direction, extending from just cranial to the medial meniscus medially, to just cranial to the long digital extensor tendon laterally (Fig. 38-5B). The tibial crest is transposed laterally and stabilized in its new position. A carefully placed pair of pointed reduction forceps can be used to maintain the position of the tibial tuberosity during insertion of the pins. Two 0.8- or 1.1-mm Kirschner wires are driven from just distal to the insertion of the patellar tendon through the tibial tuberosity in a distocaudal and medial direction, until the pin ends engage or just penetrate the caudal cortex of the tibia. A 0.6- or 0.8-mm figure-of-eight cerclage wire is anchored around the proximal pin ends and through a hole drilled through the cranial aspect of the tibia distal to the cut (Fig. 38-5C). The wire should not cross exactly over the distal aspect of the osteotomy. Great care is taken not to strangulate the distal aspect of the patellar tendon with the wire, as this may result in avascular necrosis and tendon rupture.

Soft-tissue correction: For medial patellar luxation, the lateral joint capsule and fascia is imbricated during closure. In severe cases, such as grade 3 and 4 luxations, the medial fascia might have to be released to reduce its medial pull on the patella. The position of the patella is evaluated again in extension, flexion, and inward and outward rotation before closure of the skin.

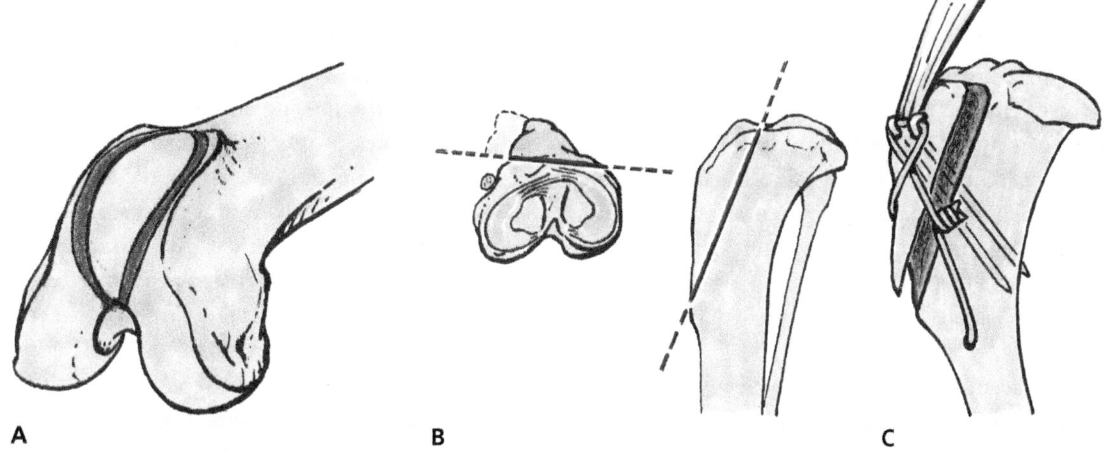

Figure 38-5 Surgical techniques for treatment of a medial patellar luxation.
(**A**) Wedge sulcoplasty. Ensure the wedge is wide enough to accommodate the patella.
(**B**) Tibial tuberosity transposition. Diagrams showing position of the osteotomy. The cut is made from just cranial to the medial meniscus to just cranial to the long digital extensor tendon. Due to the slight oblique course of the osteotomy, lateralization of the tibial tuberosity also results in a degree of cranialization.
(**C**) Stabilization of the osteotomized tibial tuberosity in its new position with a tension band fixation. Care is taken not to strangulate the distal aspect of the patellar tendon.

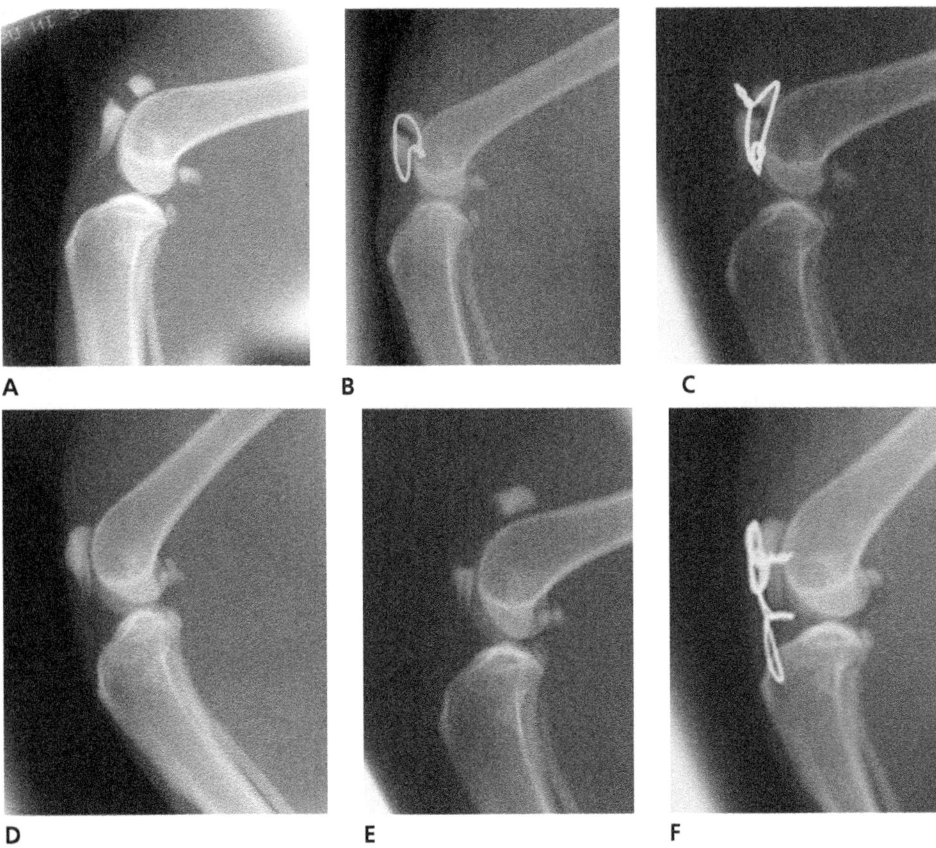

Figure 38-6 (**A**) Spontaneous stress fractures of the patellae in a 3-year-old indoor female spayed Russian Blue cat that presented with sudden-onset left-hindlimb lameness. A fatigue fracture of the left patella was diagnosed and (**B**) treated with an encircling wire. (**C**) The 3-month postoperative radiograph of the left patella has a functional non-union. (**D**) The right patella had a sclerotic appearance at first presentation. (**E**) The right patella spontaneously fractured 3 months later. (**F**) The bone was stabilized with an encircling wire and tibial quadriceps wire. (With permission from: Langley-Hobbs SJ. Survey of 52 fractures of the patella in 34 cats. Vet Rec 2009;164:80–86.)

fractures, secondary to internal stresses. Most of them are simple transverse fractures occurring at the level of the proximal third of the bone (7). Clinical findings commonly include a sudden onset of lameness, and pain and swelling around the patella, although some cases may be asymptomatic (7). The contralateral leg should be radiographed if a patellar fracture is diagnosed. Evidence of bone remodeling can be seen in the normal patella prior to its subsequent fracture (Fig. 38-6).

Minimally displaced and chronic fractures with minimal lameness can be treated conservatively. In contrast to traumatically induced patellar fractures, the soft tissue around the patella may stay intact with stress fractures, and help in counteracting the tensile forces exerted by the quadriceps muscle. Radiographic features of a non-treated idiopathic patellar fracture did not change over a time period of 18 months (7). Surgical treatment of spontaneous patellar fractures is often unrewarding because of a high likelihood of non-union and implant failure (Fig. 38-6). Non-union occurred in two cats with surgical stabilization of stress fractures, and was not necessarily associated with degenerative joint disease and a poor outcome (7). Pin and tension band wire fixation of stress fractures of the patella was consistently unsuccessful, often resulting in further fragmentation of the brittle bone and requiring additional surgical procedures for revision or removal of broken implants (19).

Surgical repair should be attempted if the fragments are widely displaced and lameness is marked, using an encircling wire around the patella and a tibial quadriceps wire (Fig. 38-6) or a transarticular external skeletal fixator. Tears of the quadriceps and parapatellar cartilages should be sutured with appropriate suture patterns to restore integrity to the quadriceps. Partial patellectomy is a salvage procedure and is conducted when internal fixation fails or is not possible, and if clinical problems persist. Complete patellectomy should not be done in cats.

True traumatic patellar fractures are rare. They are usually diagnosed in association with distal femoral or proximal tibial fractures, cruciate ruptures, and patellar luxation. The fracture fragments can be removed by partial patellectomy if they are small. Larger fragments should be stabilized surgically to restore function of the quadriceps mechanism. Surgical stabilization of patellar fractures is difficult, as the bone is small and hard, and the large tensile forces exerted by the quadriceps muscle must be counteracted with small implants. The implants should be applied in a tension band fashion.

Possible treatment options include insertion of a skewer pin and figure-of-eight orthopedic wire, multiple pinning, or an encircling wire and a tibial quadriceps wire as described for spontaneous fractures. Anatomic repair is necessary to achieve joint congruity. Transarticular stabilization may be applied additionally.

38.6 Tendon injury

38.6.1 Quadriceps tendon rupture

Rupture of the quadriceps tendon, or patellar ligament, is an uncommon problem in the cat (20), but results in severe disability due to inability to maintain the stifle joint in extension. Radiographs show proximal displacement of the patella. Flexed and extended views of the lateral stifle can be taken to demonstrate the loss of quadriceps tendon integrity, if in doubt (Fig. 38-7). The tendon can be sutured with a three-loop pulley suture (Chapter 16). Postoperative protection with a tibial quadriceps wire, external coaptation and splint, or a transarticular external fixator, or a combination of the above is required. The prognosis is guarded, and breakdown and postoperative complications are common.

38.6.2 Avulsion of the origin of the long digital extensor tendon

Traumatic avulsion of the origin of the long digital extensor tendon is a condition occasionally encountered in young large-breed dogs. Affected patients are lame and show stifle joint effusion. Radiographically, a radiodense body, which is the avulsed origin of the tendon, is frequently seen in the craniolateral compartment of the femorotibial joint. Avulsion of the origin of the long digital extensor tendon has been described in one cat (21). Reapposition of the avulsed fragment with two small Kirschner wires resulted in complete recovery. If it is impossible to reattach the origin of the tendon to its physiological position, it may be sutured to the surrounding soft tissue at the level of the proximal tibia. Postoperatively, the limb is immobilized with the stifle joint in an extended position for 3 weeks.

38.7 Ligament injuries

Cranial and caudal cruciate ligament ruptures, collateral ligament sprains, and stifle joint disruption with the corresponding surgical stabilization techniques are described in the following sections.

38.7.1 Rupture of the cranial cruciate ligament

Cranial cruciate ligament rupture in cats is generally thought to be traumatic in origin. Falls from a height seem to be the most common cause. A positive cranial drawer sign can be elicited, and radiographs show joint effusion and cranial dislocation of the tibia (Fig. 38-8). A small bony fragment may be seen at the tibial insertion site of the cranial cruciate ligament in cases of ligament avulsion (22).

However, trauma is not always observed, and it is suspected in some cases that, similar to the condition in dogs, ligament degeneration may precede rupture of the cranial cruciate ligament (23). Reasons for this assumption are: cats with cranial cruciate ligament rupture are usually older than

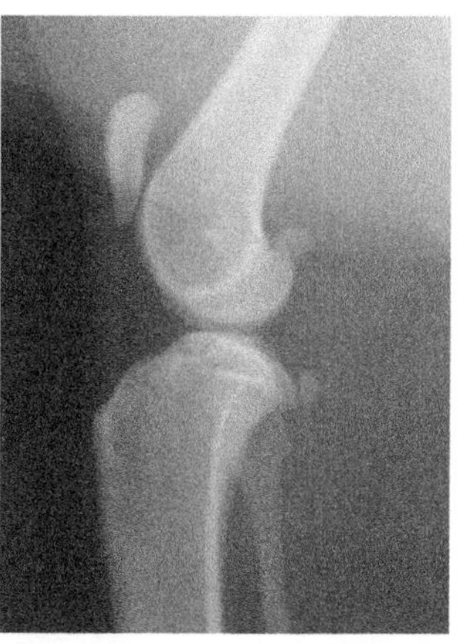

A

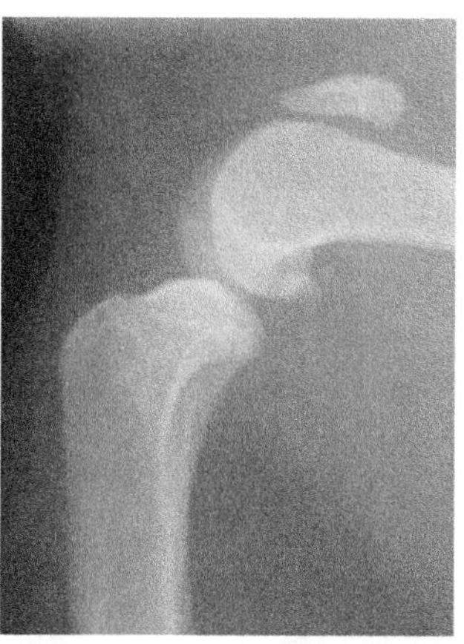

B

Figure 38-7 Cat with quadriceps tendon rupture. (**A**) A mediolateral radiograph with the stifle extended shows slight proximal displacement of the patella. (**B**) The radiograph with the stifle flexed demonstrates a quadriceps tendon disruption. A small radiopaque fragment is visible; this is an avulsion fracture of the distal patella.

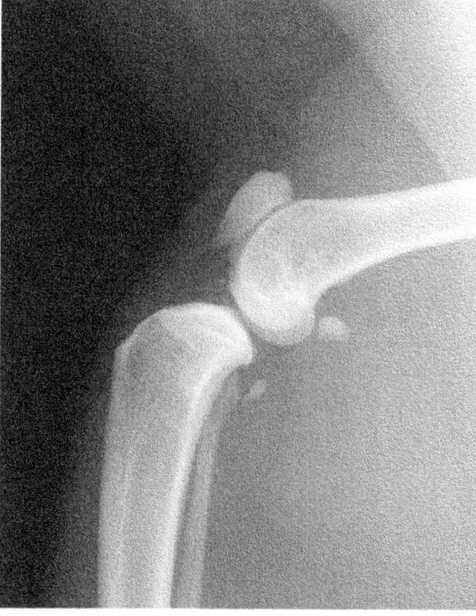

Figure 38-8 Mediolateral radiograph of a cat with traumatic rupture of the cranial cruciate ligament after a fall from a height. Note the cranial subluxation of the tibia. Joint effusion and an avulsion fragment, possibly from the tibial attachment of the cranial cruciate ligament, are also seen.

cats with other types of trauma, with published mean ages of 7.4–8.5 years (6, 23). Some cats presenting with an acute lameness in conjunction with clinical signs of cranial cruciate rupture already have degenerative joint changes and meniscal calcification on radiographs (Fig. 38-1). Also, as in the dog, cranial cruciate ligament rupture has been described as occurring more often in overweight cats (23, 24).

The incidence and significance of meniscal injury after cranial cruciate ligament rupture or disease are unknown in cats, but lesions of the medial meniscus have been observed in cats after experimental transection of the cranial cruciate ligament (25). Osteoarthritic changes in unstable feline stifle joints seem to progress at a slower rate than in dogs (25), but osteophytes are apparent 3 months after transection of the cranial cruciate ligament, and degeneration of the stifle joint continues over a 1-year period. Osteophytes form at the proximal end of the patella, the proximal patellar groove, and the mediodorsal border of the tibia (26) (Chapter 5).

Both conservative treatment and surgical stabilization have been described as treatment options. Conservative therapy consists of weight reduction where necessary, and confining the cat indoors to avoid strenuous activity. A short course of non-steroidal anti-inflammatory drugs, and long-term administration of disease-modifying agents, can also be prescribed (Chapter 5). Complete restoration of normal gait was visually observed at 5 weeks postoperatively in a clinical study on 16 cats with cranial cruciate ligament rupture (6). Results from experimental studies using force plate analysis suggest that it takes 3–4 months until cats return to normal or near-normal limb loading after transection of the cranial cruciate ligament (25, 26). Even after 1 year, peak forces remained slightly lower than normal, although this was not statistically significant (26). A cranial drawer sign persisted in nearly all cats after conservative treatment (6, 26).

No direct comparison between conservative and surgical treatment of cranial cruciate disease has been made, and the choice of treatment is based on surgeon preference. Return to normal function was 2–4 weeks in clinical studies on cats with extracapsular repair of cranial cruciate ligament rupture, comparing favorably with conservative treatment (23, 27). Surgical stabilization of a stifle joint with cranial cruciate ligament rupture may reduce or slow down the progression of degenerative joint disease. Stabilization of the stifle joint also improves proprioceptive abilities, when compared to non-reconstruction (28).

Overall, surgical stabilization seems to be beneficial, although not absolutely necessary. We advise surgical stabilization in obese cats, in young and active cats, if other legs are injured concurrently, or if lameness has not subsided after 3–4 weeks of conservative treatment. The lateral retinacular imbrication technique is most commonly performed in cats. Corrective osteotomy techniques, such as TPLO (Fig. 38-9) and tibial tuberosity advancement (TTA) (Fig. 38-10), are believed to be superior to extracapsular stabilization techniques in dogs, but have not been clinically evaluated in large numbers of cats. One cat with cranial cruciate ligament rupture and malformation of the proximal tibia was successfully treated using TPLO and cranial closing wedge osteotomy (29). TTA has been used successfully by the authors. Corrective osteotomy techniques may be superior to extracapsular techniques in obese cats, and in cases with chronic cranial cruciate ligament ruptures with concurrent gonarthrosis, but this remains to be evaluated. Lateral retinacular suture imbrication is described in Box 38-2.

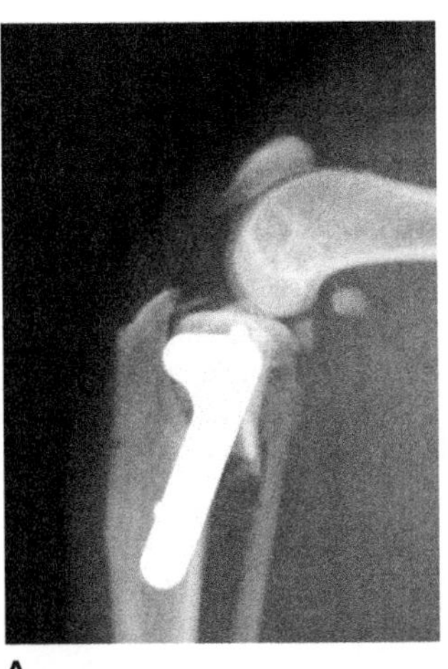
A

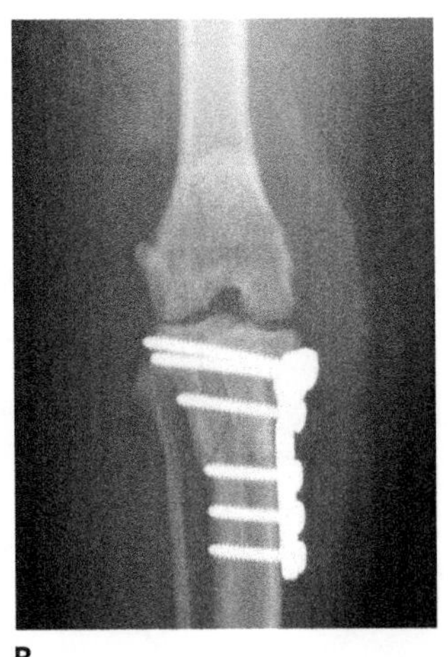
B

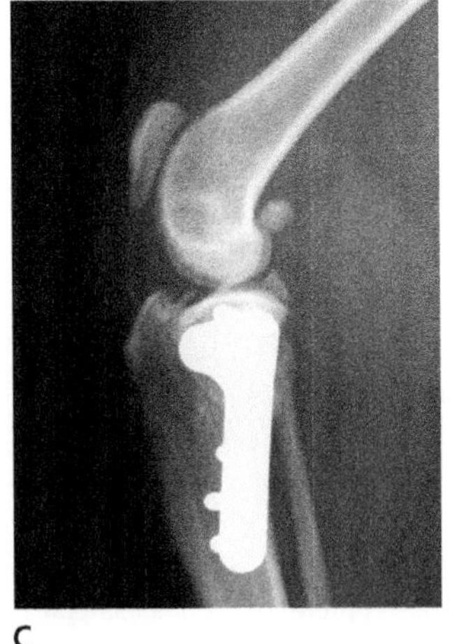
C

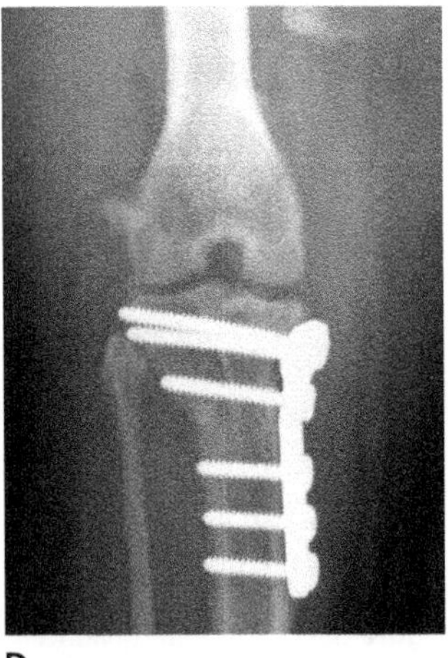
D

Figure 38-9 (**A, B**) Postoperative and (**C, D**) 3-month follow-up radiographs of the stifle joint of a cat with cranial cruciate ligament rupture, treated with tibial plateau leveling osteotomy (TPLO). A 2.0-mm TPLO plate was used to stabilize the osteotomized proximal tibia. (Courtesy of Prof. U. Matis, copyright.)

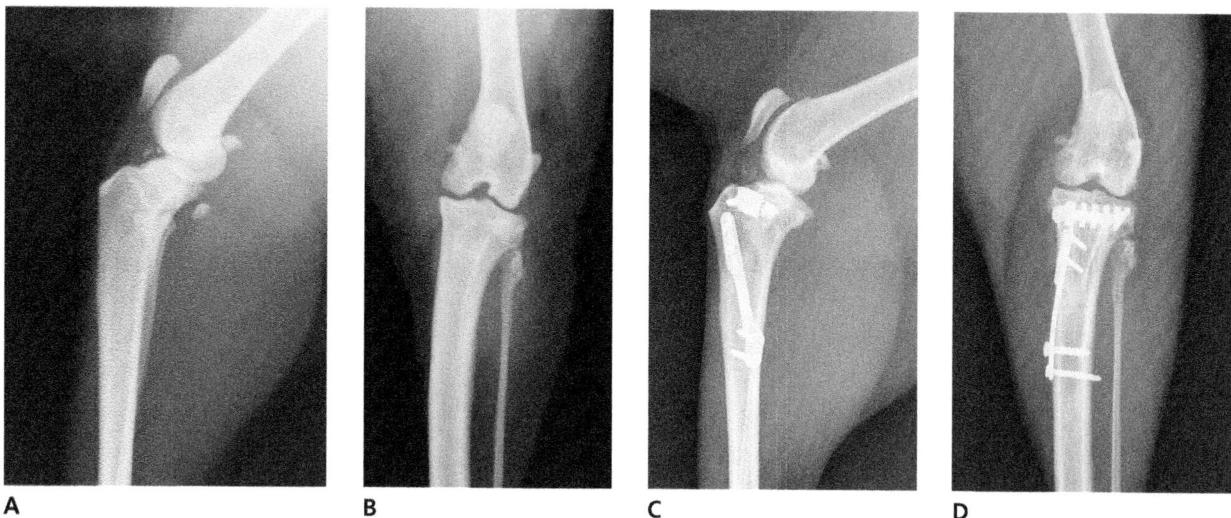

Figure 38-10 (**A**, **B**) Preoperative and (**C**, **D**) 8-month follow-up radiographs of the stifle joint of a 11-year-old overweight cat with cranial cruciate ligament rupture, treated with tibial tuberosity advancement (TTA). Note that the cat has varus deformity of the distal femur, and valgus deformity of the distal tibia, which is rarely seen.

Box 38-2. Lateral retinacular suture imbrication

After a lateral parapatellar approach to the stifle joint, the joint is explored and meniscal lesions are treated by partial meniscectomy. Remnants of the ruptured cranial cruciate ligament are carefully removed, taking care not to injure the cranial intermeniscal ligament. The joint capsule is closed and an extracapsular suture is placed through a hole in the cranioproximal aspect of the tibial tuberosity, and around the lateral fabella (Fig. 38-11). Either a size 0 monofilament non-absorbable suture material or 50-lb (23-kg) breaking-strain nylon leader line is used for the suture. Care has to be taken to avoid pressure over the patellar ligament, and to avoid injury of the peroneal nerve. The stifle joint is held in moderate flexion and slight outward rotation as the knot is tied. The lateral fascia is then closed over the suture in an imbricating suture pattern, and the subcutaneous tissue and skin are closed routinely.

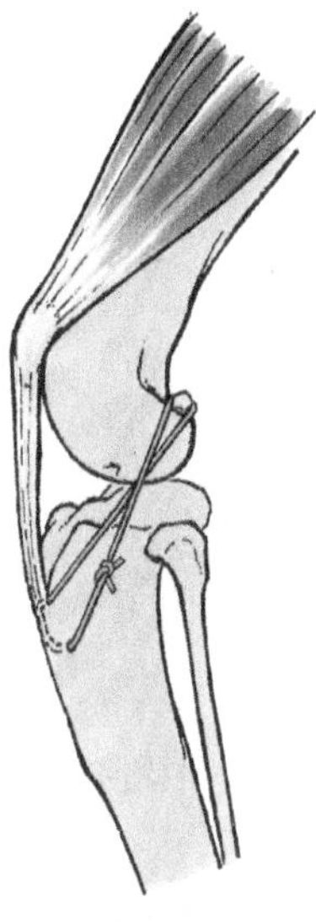

Figure 38-11 Diagram showing the position of the lateral retinacular suture for stabilization of a cranial cruciate ligament rupture.

38.7.2 Rupture of the caudal cruciate ligament

Isolated rupture of the caudal cruciate ligament is rare in cats. A caudal drawer sign can be elicited, and radiographs may reveal caudal displacement of the tibia (Fig. 38-12). Outcome seems to be good with conservative therapy in most cases. Surgical stabilization should be considered if lameness does not resolve after 3–4 weeks of activity restriction (Box 38-3). Repair of the caudal cruciate ligament is also undertaken if there is concurrent damage to the cranial cruciate and/or collateral ligaments in cats with stifle joint disruption.

38.7.3 Collateral ligament sprain

Isolated collateral ligament injuries occur occasionally, but collateral ligament damage is more often associated with stifle joint disruption (see below). The medial collateral ligament is damaged more often than the lateral collateral ligament. Grade 1 ligament sprains cause minimal clinical signs and are rarely diagnosed. Soft-tissue swelling is present over the area of the affected ligament in grade 2 and 3 sprains. Grade 3 sprains also cause palpable valgus or varus instability. Stress radiographs reveal opening of the joint space on the affected side (Fig. 38-14). Avulsion fragments may be seen at the ligament insertion sites.

Conservative treatment can be used in cases with grade 1 and 2 injuries and minor instability. Activity is restricted by keeping the cat in a cage for 10 days to allow fibrous healing of the periarticular structures, followed by a gradual return

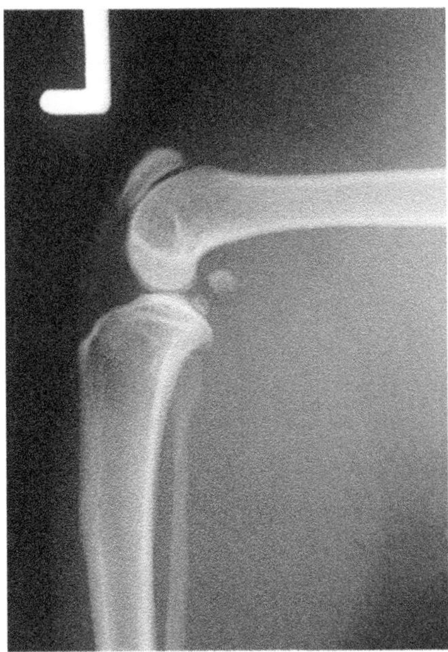

Figure 38-12 Mediolateral radiograph of the stifle joint of a cat after a fall from a height. Caudal subluxation of the tibia is evident, indicating rupture of the caudal cruciate ligament.

Box 38-3. Stabilization of caudal cruciate ligament ruptures

A lateral parapatellar approach to the stifle joint is conducted. A suture sling is anchored around the fibular head and through the proximal aspect of the patellar tendon, using monofilament non-absorbable or slowly absorbable suture material (Fig. 38-13). The suture should not be overtightened. Visualization and retraction of the peroneal nerve are necessary while the suture is placed around the fibular head.

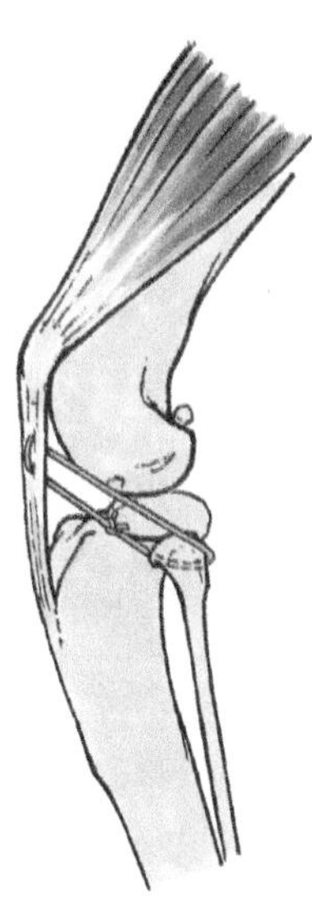

Figure 38-13 Diagram showing a fibulopatellar tendon suture sling for extra-articular augmentation of a rupture of the caudal cruciate ligament.

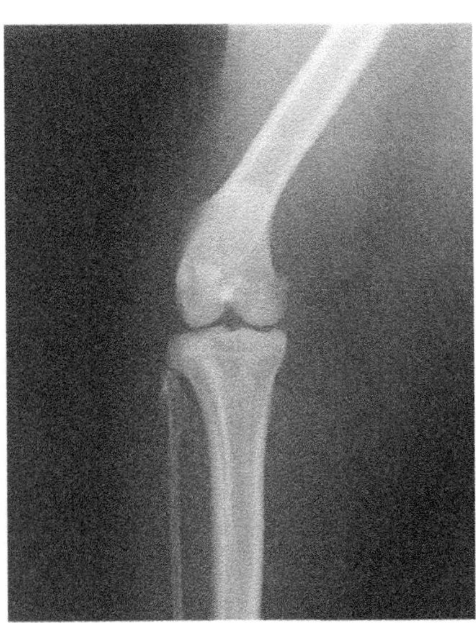

A

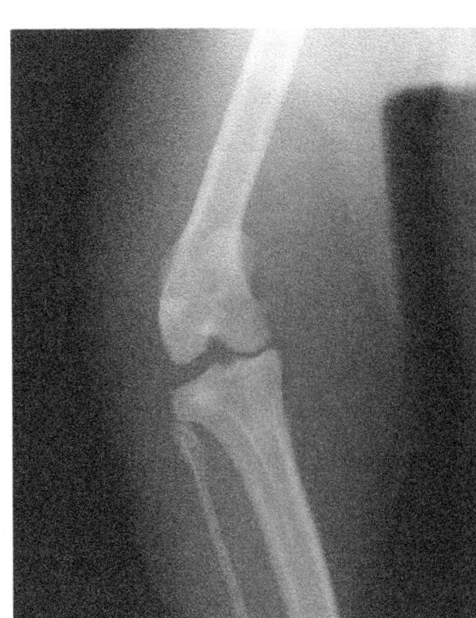

B

Figure 38-14 (**A**) Valgus and (**B**) varus stress radiographs of a cat with grade 2–3 lateral collateral ligament sprain. Note the increased opening of the lateral femorotibial joint space with the leg positioned in varus. The cat also has grade A medial patellar luxation.

Box 38-4. Collateral ligament prosthesis

The medial collateral ligament is approached via a medial approach, and the lateral collateral ligament from a lateral approach. The stifle joint is explored for concurrent injuries. The joint capsule and the ligament ends are sutured with a locking-loop suture pattern, using 4-0 monofilament slowly absorbable suture material. This may not always be possible due to shredding of the ligament. A size 0 monofilament non-absorbable or slowly absorbable suture material is usually used for the ligament prosthesis. Range of joint motion and joint stability are checked before closure of the wound.

Medial collateral ligament prosthesis: One 2.0-mm screw or suture anchor is inserted at the insertion site of the medial collateral ligament on the femoral condyle, and one 2.0-mm screw is positioned in the proximal tibia (Fig. 38-15A). The tibial screw can be directed in a slightly proximal direction, which will prevent slipping of the suture from the screw head. The use of smooth 2.0-mm stainless-steel washers also helps to prevent suture slipping. The suture is anchored around the screw heads in a figure-of-eight fashion before the screws are tightened.

Lateral collateral ligament prosthesis: One 2.0-mm screw is inserted into the lateral femoral epicondyle at the insertion site of the lateral collateral ligament. The suture is then passed between the fibular head and tibia (Fig. 38-15B) or, alternatively, a second screw is directed from the fibular head into the tibia. A 1.5-mm screw should be used here due to the small size of the fibular head. A figure-of-eight suture is then applied as described above.

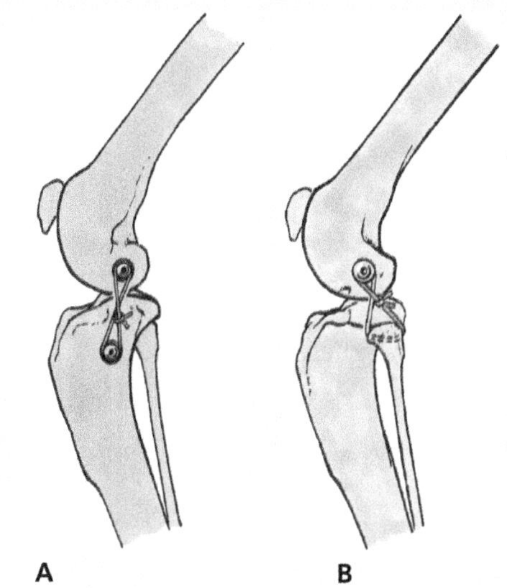

Figure 38-15 Diagrams showing medial and lateral collateral ligament prostheses.
(**A**) Medial collateral ligament prosthesis, anchored around two screws.
(**B**) Lateral collateral ligament prosthesis, anchored around a screw in the femoral condyle, and the fibular head.

to activity over 4 weeks. Surgical stabilization is performed in cases with unstable grade 2 or 3 injuries (Box 38-4). Surgical stabilization is likely to slow down the development of degenerative joint changes secondary to prolonged instability. The ruptured ligament ends are sutured if possible, and ligament prostheses are applied. In cases with avulsion of a larger bone fragment, the fragment can be reattached with a small lag screw, with or without washer.

38.8 Stifle joint disruption

Stifle joint disruption is a severe injury, resulting in complete dislocation of the tibiofemoral joint and severe instability (Fig. 38-16). This injury is caused by rupture of several of the ligamentous joint stabilizers, including the collateral ligaments, cruciate ligaments, and joint capsule. Several combinations of ligament sprains can cause stifle joint disruption, but the most common combination of injuries is rupture of the cranial and caudal cruciate ligaments, and the medial collateral ligament (30). Concurrent meniscal injury is present in nearly all cases. Peripheral avulsions are most common (30).

Although preoperative stress radiographs can be taken, the radiographs can be difficult to interpret, and the exact extent of injuries is usually more easily diagnosed by careful palpation of the anesthetized cat, and during surgical exploration of the joint. Both a medial and lateral parapatellar approach are often necessary to evaluate the joint fully. The goal of surgery is to repair or replace all ruptured structures, and to achieve anatomic joint reduction with adequate stability. Temporary immobilization of the stifle joint is necessary to protect the primary repair during the first 2–3 weeks, and to allow periarticular fibrosis to develop without losing joint reduction. External splints or casts do not provide rigid immobilization of the stifle joint, so a transarticular external skeletal fixator or a transarticular pin is commonly used (Fig. 38-16 and Box 38-5).

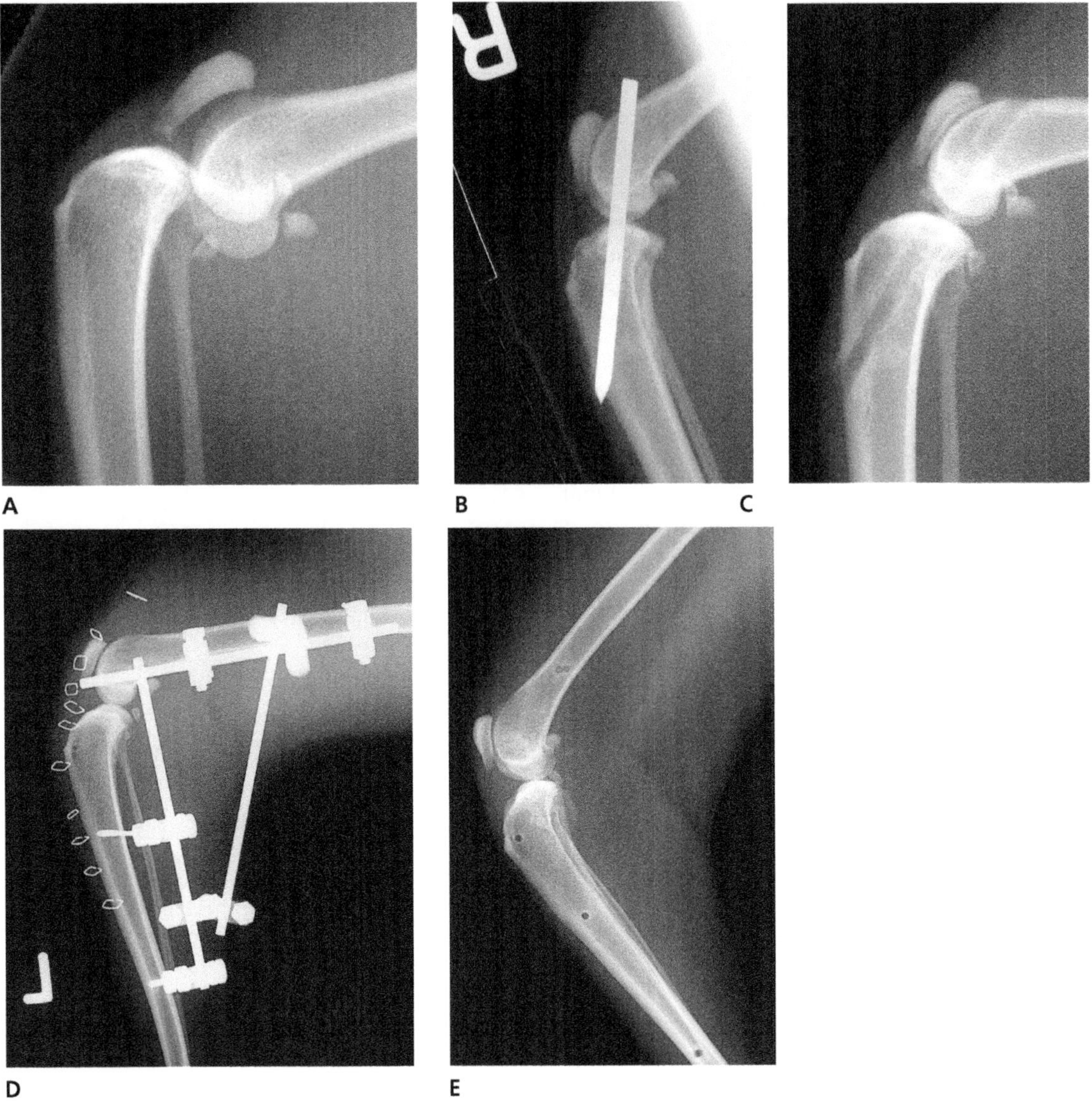

Figure 38-16 Two options for postoperative immobilization of a disrupted stifle joint.
(**A**) Preoperative radiograph showing a cranially luxated stifle joint.
(**B**) Postoperative radiograph of the stifle joint, temporarily stabilized with a 3.0-mm transarticular pin.
(**C**) Radiograph after removal of transarticular pin, 3 weeks after the injury.
(**D**) Another disrupted stifle joint has been stabilized with a transarticular external fixator after repair of the medial collateral and cranial cruciate ligament.
(**E**) Radiograph 3 weeks postoperatively after removal of the external skeletal fixator.

Transarticular pinning combined with a lateral splint for 3 weeks was performed in seven cats with stifle luxations (31). These cats had an arthrotomy and debridement but no attempt was made to repair the damaged ligaments. The cats had an average weight of 4.7 kg, and pins with a size range of 2.4–3.5 mm were used (average 3.0 mm). Complications included loosening, migration, and bending of the pin, which may have been the result of using too small a pin or inadequate external coaptation. Long-term outcome was reported as excellent in four, fair in one, and poor in one cat.

Transarticular external fixation provides rigid fixation, but can be associated with a number of complications, such as pin loosening, pin breakage, or iatrogenic fractures through the most proximal or distal pin holes (30). Positive-threaded pins lower the incidence of pin loosening and pin breakage. Placing the most proximal pin in the proximal third of the femur, and the most distal pin in the distal third of the tibia, is recommended to reduce the risk of iatrogenic fractures (30). Correct pin insertion techniques, avoidance of damage of the cranial or caudal cortex, and the use of

Box 38-5. Stabilization of a disrupted stifle joint

A medial parapatellar approach is performed in cases with suspected rupture of the medial collateral ligament. The lateral collateral ligament can be exposed with a lateral parapatellar approach if necessary. The collateral ligaments, joint capsule, and intra-articular structures are explored.

Repair of structures and debridement of the joint: Meniscal lesions are treated first, either by reattaching peripheral avulsions to the joint capsule, or by partial or total meniscectomy. The joint is flushed and the joint capsule is sutured. The next step involves suturing the collateral ligaments and application of a ligament prosthesis, as described in Box 38-4. Extracapsular sutures are then placed to stabilize the cranial and caudal cruciate ligaments, as shown in Boxes 38-2 and 38-3. The sutures are tied carefully to avoid overcorrection and subsequent subluxation. Range of motion and joint stability are tested before wound closure. In severely unstable joints it can be advantageous to place a temporary transarticular pin as described below prior to reconstruction of the ligaments, which helps to hold the stifle in reduction during tightening of the sutures.

Ancillary temporary transarticular stabilization is necessary in most cases.

Temporary immobilization with a transarticular external fixator: A type I transarticular external fixator using 2.0-mm positive-threaded pins in the femur, and 1.6–2.0-mm positive-threaded pins in the tibia is applied laterally (Fig. 38-17A). The most proximal pin should be located in the proximal third of the femur, and the most distal pin in the distal third of the tibia. It is important not to damage the cranial or caudal cortex as these pins are inserted. An external bar is bent to hold the stifle joint in a slightly overflexed standing angle. The external fixator is removed after 2–3 weeks.

Temporary immobilization with a transarticular pin: A size 2.4–3.2-mm transarticular pin is placed from just proximal to the trochlear groove, across the stifle joint to exit the tibia on the cranial aspect, with the joint held at a normal or slightly overflexed standing angle. The pins are left slightly long for easy retrieval (Fig. 38-17B). The pin is removed through a small stab incision over the tibia or femur approximately 3 weeks after placement.

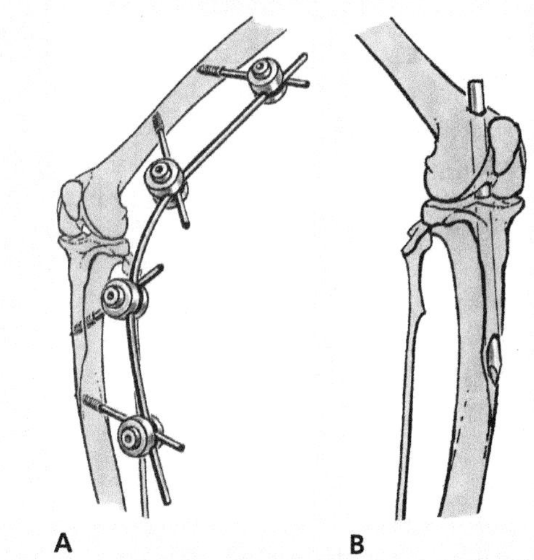

Figure 38-17 Options for temporary immobilization of the stifle joint. (**A**) A lateral type I transarticular external fixator for temporary immobilization of the stifle joint.
(**B**) Position of a transarticular pin for temporary immobilization of the stifle joint.

pins not exceeding 25% of the bone diameter are also important.

38.9 Arthrodesis

Arthrodesis of the stifle joint is a salvage treatment option if joint function cannot be preserved with other methods. Arthrodesis will leave the cat with significant gait alterations, and careful consideration should be made before electing for this option. Amputation of the limb may also be selected in certain cases. Indications for arthrodesis include crippling degenerative joint disease, for example after sepsis or badly managed deranged stifles, unreconstructable fractures, quadriceps contracture, or genu recurvatum (Fig. 38-18).

The angle of fusion is estimated from the standing angle of the contralateral limb, and is around 110°. It is best to fuse the joint in a slightly more flexed angle, rather than too straight, because the cat may find use of an extended leg cumbersome, particularly during a crouched gait. Strict attention should be paid to surgical technique to avoid complications. These tend to occur because of the long lever arm created, which can result in fracture of the femur or tibia at the implant–bone junction. Implants should end in metaphyseal areas and not over the narrowest part of the diaphysis to avoid this complication. Leaving the distal and proximal plate holes empty or use of a monocortical screw in these sites may also help decrease the stress riser effects. The surgical technique is described in Box 38-6.

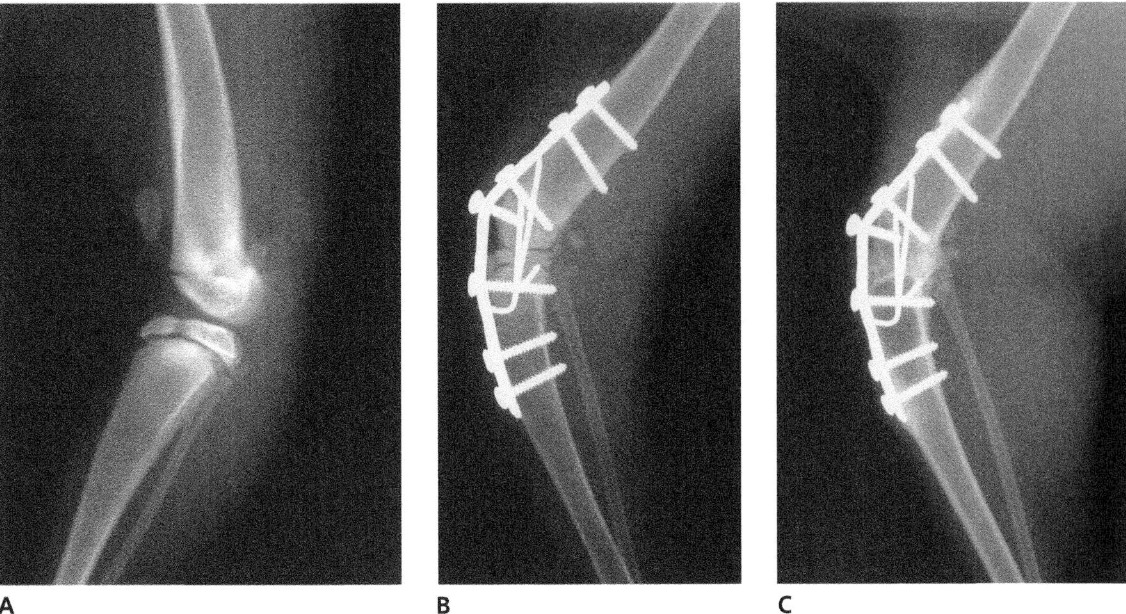

Figure 38-18 Cat with stifle arthrodesis.
(**A**) Preoperative radiograph of a 4-month-old kitten with congenital genu recurvatum.
(**B**) Stifle arthrodesis using cross pins and a 2.0-mm dynamic compression plate and 2.0-mm screws.
(**C**) Note the arthrodesis healing and bone remodeling at the proximal and distal aspects of the plate 4 weeks after surgery. (Reproduced with permission from Houlton JEF, et al. (eds) BSAVA manual of canine and feline musculoskeletal disorders. Cheltenham: BSAVA; 2006.)

38.10 Postoperative treatment and prognosis

Postoperative treatment and prognosis depend on the type and severity of the injury. Prognosis is usually good even for severe injuries with early intervention, but poor if treatment is delayed.

38.10.1 Isolated ligament injuries

Activity is restricted by keeping the cat indoors or caged for 4 weeks after repair of single ligament injuries, such as cranial or caudal cruciate ligament rupture or isolated collateral ligament rupture. A splinted bandage may be applied after repair of collateral ligament sprains for the first 10 postoperative days. Jumping on or off elevated objects should be prevented. Prognosis for return to normal function is good to excellent, although some degree of degenerative joint disease is likely to develop. Stiffness after rest and slight residual lameness were observed in cats with degenerative disease after extracapsular stabilization (23). Death due to cardiomyopathy was described in three cats after cranial cruciate ligament surgery (32).

38.10.2 Stifle joint disruption

Stability of the stifle joint depends mainly on the integrity of the soft-tissue structures and external immobilization is essential after repair of grossly unstable stifle joint injuries. A transarticular external skeletal fixator or a transarticular pin is left in place for approximately 2–3 weeks, and cats are strictly confined during that time. Joint stability is tested clinically after removal of the devices.

Range of motion is usually markedly reduced after 3 weeks of immobilization, but will rapidly improve when the cat resumes activity. The owners should be advised to restrict activity of the cat markedly and prevent jumping in the first 2 weeks after removal of the transarticular pin or external fixator to allow gradual reorganization and remodeling of the fibrous scar tissue, and to prevent iatrogenic fractures through the external skeletor fixator pin holes. Cats are kept indoors for 2–3 months. Despite the severity of the injury, the prognosis for return to satisfactory function is good, although thickening and decreased range of motion and degenerative joint disease are likely to occur (30, 31). Possible complications are loosening, bending or breakage of the transarticular or external skeletal fixator pins, and femoral or tibial fractures through pin holes, with secondary loss of reduction (30). Transarticular pinning may also cause damage to intra-articular structures during insertion of the pin.

38.10.3 Patellar luxation

The limb is placed in a soft bandage for a couple of days after surgery. For medial patellar luxation the bandage is applied

Box 38-6. Stifle arthrodesis

Stifle arthrodeses can be stabilized by application of a cranial plate or an external skeletal fixator after appropriate cartilage debridement and bone grafting. A lateral skin incision is made with the cat in dorsal recumbency, and the stifle joint is approached from both laterally and medially.

Preparation of the stifle joint: After elevation of the cranial tibial muscle from the lateral aspect of the proximal tibia, an osteotomy of the tibial tuberosity is performed. Elevation of the tibial tuberosity towards proximal gives excellent access to the whole stifle joint. The cranial cruciate ligaments and menisci are resected carefully with a sharp scalpel blade. With an oscillating saw, the proximal tibial plateau cartilage and subchondral bone are removed perpendicular to the long axis of the tibia (Fig. 38-19A). The distal femur is cut parallel to the cut of the proximal tibia, while the stifle joint is held in the predetermined arthrodesis angle (Fig. 38-19A). A prebent K wire can be laid on the tibia and femur as a guide. Further cartilage can be removed from the trochlear ridges and trochlea. Cancellous or corticocancellous graft is harvested from the osteotomized bone fragments and the iliac crest, and is placed at the arthrodesis site. The femur and tibia are anatomically reduced and the angle is checked prior to immobilization with two crossing K wires of 1.1–1.4-mm diameter.

Plate fixation: A 2.7- or 2.0-mm dynamic compression plate or a 2.0/2.7 (stacked) veterinary cuttable plate is contoured and applied to the cranial aspect of the femur and tibia with at least three bicortical screws in each bone. The length of plate selected should ensure that the implant ends in metaphyseal areas and not over the narrowest part of the diaphysis. One screw can be inserted across the stifle joint, either through a plate hole or separate from the plate, as a lag screw (Fig. 38-19B). The distal and proximal plate holes are left empty or are filled with monocortical screws to decrease the stress riser effects (Fig. 38-19C). The tibial tuberosity needs to be reattached to the tibia, lateral or medial of the plate (Fig. 38-19D). A lag screw or a tension band fixation can be used.

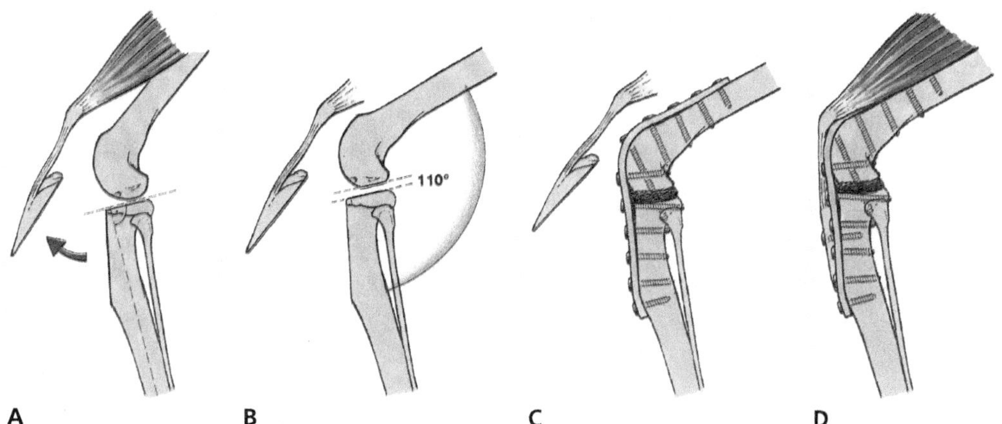

Figure 38-19 Arthrodesis of the stifle joint.
(**A**) The tibial tuberosity was osteotomized and retracted cranially. The osteotomy of the tibial plateau is made perpendicular to the long axis of the bone.
(**B**) The osteotomy of the distal femur is made parallel to the proximal tibial cut while the stifle joint is held in the desired flexion angle (usually 110°).
(**C**) Stifle arthrodesis using an interfragmentary lag screw and a cranial plate. Note that the most proximal and distal holes are only filled with monocortical screws.
(**D**) The tibial tuberosity is reattached to the tibia, adjacent to the plate.

in outward rotation. The cats are confined indoors for at least 3–4 weeks until control radiographs confirm healing of the osteotomy. Good function can be expected in 90% of cats treated surgically, whereas conservative management of the disease fails to lead to improvement (10).

38.10.4 Arthrodesis

After surgery the cat needs to be exercise-restricted by confining it to a cage or small room where it is unable to jump or climb. Radiographs are taken after 4 weeks in an adult cat, and exercise is gradually increased by enlarging the size of the exercise area dependent on the appearance of the radiograph and degree of healing. Prognosis is guarded for a full return to function. Cats will have a circumducting gait, and they may encounter difficulty when walking with a crouching gait and when jumping or climbing. Possible post-operative complications include fracture of the tibia or femur at the bone–implant junction, non-union, and infection.

References and further reading

1. McLaughlin RM. Surgical diseases of the feline stifle joint. Vet Clin North Am Small Anim Pract 2002;32:963–982.
2. Arnbjerg J, Heye NI. Fabellae and popliteal sesamoid bones in cats. J Small Anim Pract 1993;34:95–98.
3. Piermattei DL, Johnson KA. An atlas of surgical approaches to the bones and joints of the dog and the cat, 4th edn. Philadelphia: WB Saunders; 2004.
4. Whiting PG, Pool RR. Intrameniscal calcification and ossification in the stifle joints of three domestic cats. J Am Anim Hosp Assoc 1985;21:579–584.
5. Reinke J, Mughannam A. Meniscal calcification and ossification in six cats and two dogs. J Am Anim Hosp Assoc 1994; 30:145–152.
6. Scavelli TD, Schrader SC. Nonsurgical management of rupture of the cranial cruciate ligament in 18 cats. J Am Anim Hosp Assoc 1987;23:337–340.
7. Arnbjerg J, Bindseil E. Patella fracture in cats. Feline Pract 1994;22:31–35.
8. Milovancev M, Ralphs SC. Congenital patellar aplasia in a family of cats. Vet Comp Orthop Traumatol 2004;17:9–11.
9. Johnson ME. Feline patellar luxation: a retrospective case study. J Am Anim Hosp Assoc 1986;22:835–838.
10. Houlton JEF, Meynink SE. Medial patellar luxation in the cat. J Small Anim Pract 1989;30:349–352.
11. Engvall PD, Bushnell N. Patellar luxation in Abyssinian cats. Feline Pract 1990;18:20–22.
12. Flecknell PA, Gruffydd-Jones TJ. Congenital luxation of the patella in the cat. Feline Pract 1979;9:18–20.
13. Smith GK, et al. Evaluation of the association between medial patellar luxation and hip dysplasia in cats. J Am Vet Med Assoc 1999;215:40–45.
14. Davies M, Gill I. Congenital patellar luxation in the cat. Vet Rec 1987;121:474–475.
15. Hayes HM, et al. Feline hip dysplasia. J Am Anim Hosp Assoc 1979;15:447–448.
16. Patsikas MN, et al. Hip dysplasia in the cat: a report of three cases. J Small Anim Pract 1998;39:290–294.
17. Loughlin CA, et al. Clinical signs and results of treatment in cats with patellar luxation: 42 cases. J Am Vet Med Assoc 2006; 228:1370–1375.
18. L'Eplattenier H, Montavon PM. Patellar luxation in dogs and cats: pathogenesis and diagnosis. Compend Continuing Educ 2002;24:234–298.
19. Langley-Hobbs SJ. Surgery of 52 fractures of the patella in 34 cats. Vet Rec 2009;164:80–86.
20. Brunnberg L, et al. Injury to the patella and the patella ligaments in dogs and cats II: rupture of the patellar ligament. Eur J Comp Anim Pract 1993;3:69–73.
21. Voorhout G, et al. Avulsion fracture of the tendon of origin of the long extensor muscle of the toe in a horse and a cat. Tijdschr Diergeneeskd 1986;111:1225–1228.
22. Campos AG, et al. What is your diagnosis? Intra-articular avulsion fracture at the tibial insertion of the cranial cruciate ligament. J Am Vet Med Assoc 2005;227:883–884.
23. Harasen GLG. Feline cranial cruciate rupture. 17 cases and a review of the literature. Vet Comp Orthop Traumatol 2005;4: 254–257.
24. Umphlet RC. Feline stifle disease. Vet Clin North Am Small Anim Pract 1993;23:897–913.
25. Herzog W, et al. Hindlimb loading, morphology and biochemistry of articular cartilage in the ACL-deficient cat knee. Osteoarthritis Cartilage 1993;1:243–251.
26. Suter E, et al. One-year changes in hind limb kinematics. Ground reaction forces and knee stability in an experimental model of osteoarthritis. J Biomechanics 1998;31:511–517.
27. Alexander JW, et al. Anterior cruciate ligament rupture. Feline Pract 1977;July:38–39.
28. Gomez-Barrena E, et al. Anterior cruciate ligament reconstruction affects proprioception in the cat's knee. Acta Orthop Scand 1999;70:185–193.
29. Hoots EA, Petersen SW. Tibial plateau leveling osteotomy and cranial closing wedge ostectomy in a cat with cranial cruciate ligament rupture. J Am Anim Hosp Assoc 2005;41:395–399.
30. Bruce WJ. Stifle joint luxation in the cat: treatment using trans-articular external skeletal fixation. J Small Anim Pract 1999; 40:482–488.
31. Welches CD, Scavelli TD. Transarticular pinning to repair luxation of the stifle joint in dogs and cats: a retrospective study of 10 cases. J Am Anim Hosp Assoc 1990;26:207–214.
32. Janssens LAA, et al. Anterior cruciate ligament rupture associated with cardiomyopathy in three cats. Vet Comp Orthop Traumatol 1991;4:35–37.

39 Tibia and fibula

K. Voss, S.J. Langley-Hobbs, P.M. Montavon

Fractures of the tibia and/or fibula are common, accounting for about 10–20% of fractures in cats (1, 2). Usually both the tibia and fibula are fractured. The fractures are often caused by falls from a height, but may occur after any type of trauma (3–5). Most of the fractures of the feline tibia involve the middle and distal diaphysis (2–4). The diaphysis of the tibia is surrounded by minimal soft tissue, and many tibial fractures are comminuted and/or open. The incidence of open fractures of the tibial diaphysis has been reported to be as high as 21–46% (3, 4). Cats with high-rise syndrome sustain open fractures more commonly than cats with other causes of trauma (4). The high incidence of comminuted and open fractures, and the limited extraosseous blood supply and soft-tissue envelope, is likely to account for the higher rate of complications, such as delayed union, non-union, and osteomyelitis, when compared to fractures of other bones.

39.1 Surgical anatomy

The tibia is a straight bone with a triangular shape in the proximal third and a round to oval shape in the distal two-thirds. The fibula is very thin in cats and does not contribute to weight-bearing, but it is important for stifle and tarsal joint stability because it serves as the attachment site for the lateral collateral ligaments of both joints. The distal fibula has a ligamentous connection to the tibia, the inferior tibiofibular ligament. This ligament is important for stability of the tarsal joint, because the medial and lateral malleolus are not only the sites of origin of the tarsal collateral ligaments but also serve as a medial and lateral restraint for the trochlea of the talus (Chapter 40).

39.2 Stabilization techniques

Many stabilization methods can be used to treat tibial fractures. The reader is referred to Chapters 13 and 24 to review the factors influencing the choice of treatment and implants for different fracture types. External coaptation with a cast is successful for stabilization of certain tibial fractures in young cats, such as greenstick, simple transverse fractures, and tibial fractures with an intact fibula. Indications and application techniques for external coaptation are described in Chapter 22. The tibia is the ideal bone for closed reduction and external skeletal fixation, because it is surrounded by minimal soft tissue. This technique is most useful for comminuted and open fractures. Fracture types occurring in the proximal tibia, the diaphysis, and the distal bone, and possible options for treating them are summarized in Table 39-1.

39.2.1 Intramedullary pinning

Although the straight form of the tibia is ideal for inserting intramedullary pins, they are not used as commonly in the tibia, as compared to the humerus and femur. Intramedullary pins should always be inserted in a normograde fashion into the tibia because retrograde pinning in cats invariably results in penetration of the patellar tendon (6). Intramedullary pins must be used in conjunction with implants resistant to rotation and axial compression, dependent on the fracture type. The size of the pin is selected according to the smallest diameter of the distal medullary cavity. If the pin is combined with a plate or an external fixator, the size selected should be around 30% of the diameter of the distal medullary canal to leave room for insertion of the screws or pins. Selecting too large a pin and then trying to pass pins or screws past the pin can result in cortical fissures. Kirschner wires of a diameter of 1.2–2.0 mm are usually adequate.

A medial parapatellar approach to the stifle is performed for normograde intramedullary pin insertion. The pin entry point is located on the medial aspect of the tibial plateau, between the insertion of the patellar tendon and medial collateral ligament, cranial to the intermeniscal ligament (Fig. 39-1). Holding the stifle joint in 90° of flexion facilitates insertion of the pin. The pin is then advanced along the medial cortex using a Jacobs chuck until its tip is located close to the fracture. The fracture is reduced, and the pin is further advanced until resistance is felt at the distal epiphysis. The distal tibial epiphysis is a short piece of bone, so great care must be taken not to push the pin into the tibiotarsal joint. The proximal end of the pin is cut as short as possible to avoid irritation of the patellar tendon and parapatellar tissue.

39.2.2 Interlocking nailing

The use of an interlocking nail for stabilization of feline tibial fractures has been described as part of a large

Table 39-1. A summary of feline tibial fractures and selected treatment options

Fracture localization	Fracture type	Stabilization methods
Proximal tibia	Salter and Harris type II	Parallel or cross pinning IM pin and antirotational K wire Lag screw and antirotational K wire External coaptation
	Simple metaphyseal	IM pin and: – ESF – plate – internal fixator Plate and tension band Internal fixator and tension band
	Comminuted metaphyseal	IM pin and: – ESF – plate – internal fixator
Diaphysis	Simple transverse or short oblique	IM pin and ESF Compression plate Internal fixator External coaptation
	Simple long oblique and reducible multifragmentary	Lag screw and neutralization plate Lag screw and internal fixator IM pin and ESF IM pin and cerclage wire
	Comminuted	ESF (closed reduction) ESF ± IM pin Buttress plate Internal fixator Interlocking nail
Distal tibia	Simple metaphyseal	ESF and IM pin Plate ± IM pin Internal fixator ± IM pin
	Comminuted metaphyseal	IM pin and: – ESF – plate – internal fixator
	Salter and Harris type I	Cross pinning

IM pin, intramedullary pin; ESF, external skeletal fixator.

retrospective study involving nail use in dogs and cats (7). The interlocking nail was applied infrequently in the tibia in the cat, when compared to other long bones, but from the information obtained from the study no complications occurred with its use. With the current range of interlocking nail sizes, the nail can only be used in large cats with fractures involving the mid to proximal third of the tibial diaphysis.

The 4.0-mm nail with 2.0-mm screws or bolts is the most appropriate size to use, and the length of the nail is determined by using the templates and the preoperative radiographs of the intact contralateral limb. The nail is inserted in a normograde fashion, as described in Figure 39-1. A small medial approach is made to the tibial diaphysis for fracture reduction and directing the nail into the distal bone. The distal tibial epiphysis in the cat is very short and there is a risk of inadvertent penetration of the tibiotarsal joint while seating the nail in the distal metaphyseal bone. Removing the sharp point from the end of the nail and therefore making a blunter end can help prevent penetration.

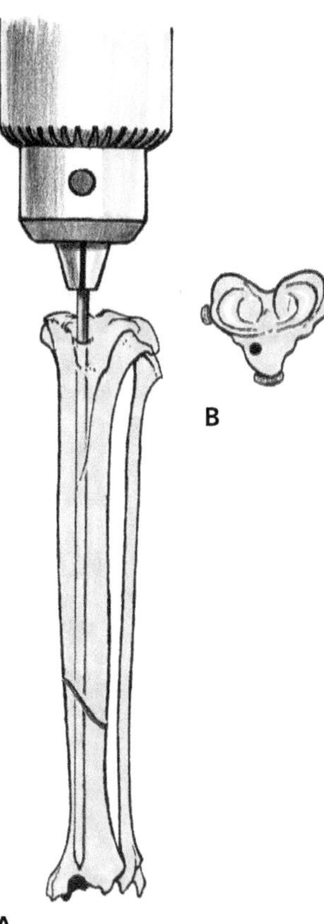

Figure 39-1 (**A**) Normograde pinning of the tibia. (**B**) The pin entry point on the medial edge of the tibial plateau is reached through a small medial parapatellar incision, and the pin is inserted along the medial cortex of the tibia.

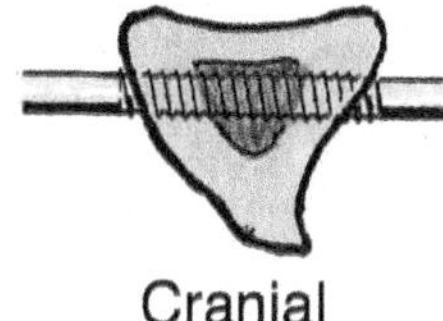

Figure 39-2 Diagram showing positioning of a centrally threaded transosseous pin in the caudal aspect of the triangular-shaped proximal tibia. Screws are also inserted in this position.

39.2.3 External skeletal fixation

The main indications for external skeletal fixation are comminuted and open fractures, and fractures located in the distal diaphysis or metaphysis. Either a closed or an open reduction can be used. If open reduction is chosen, only a minimal approach should be performed to preserve the blood supply. Closed reduction and application of external fixation is the treatment of choice for comminuted fractures with significant soft-tissue damage, and for open fractures. Closed reduction and external skeletal fixation were associated with a higher rate of malunion compared to closed reduction in one study (4), so care has to be taken to align the main fragments adequately.

Older cats can have brittle bones, and iatrogenic fractures could be created if oversized transosseous pins, especially positive-threaded pins, or incorrect insertion techniques are applied. Pin size is usually 2.0 mm for the proximal tibia, and 1.6 mm for the distal tibia. Because the proximal tibia has a triangular shape, transosseous pins are inserted into the broader caudal aspect of the proximal tibia to obtain more bone purchase (Fig. 39-2).

Both type I and type II configurations can be used. A type I external fixator applied on the medial side of the bone is the best choice, as the pins only penetrate the skin and do not interfere with the laterally located extensor muscles. A type I configuration provides sufficient stability for moderately comminuted fractures, and fractures in younger cats. Stability of a type I external skeletal fixator can be improved by using fixator systems with large connecting bars, or by using a double bar. The tubular external fixator is a valuable implant for distally located fractures (Chapter 24).

A type II external fixator is applied for severely comminuted or open fractures with longer anticipated healing times. Its configuration provides more stability, and reduces the risk of premature failure. Positive-threaded pins and the employment of a correct pin insertion technique (Chapter 24) are also crucial for prevention of premature pin loosening. Type II external fixators, or very occasionally type III fixators, are also indicated if the size of the proximal or distal fragment only allows insertion of one or two pins. The type III fixator frame has the advantage of allowing insertion of additional pins from a different direction.

39.2.4 Plating

Bone plates can be applied to repair closed fractures of the tibial diaphysis. Plates are positioned along the caudomedial border of the proximal tibia, because its triangular shape allows more bone purchase caudally (Fig. 39-2). The 2.7/2.0-mm veterinary cuttable plate (VCP) and the 2.7-mm dynamic compression plate (DCP) are often used, although 2.7-mm screws are at the upper range of size for the feline tibia, especially in the distal diaphysis. A thick 2.0-mm DCP or a 2.0/2.7 VCP with 2.0-mm screws is more appropriate for the diameter of the distal tibia in cats. However, the 2.0-mm DCP has a limited length, which is often insufficient, and the VCP is relatively weak, unless applied in a stacked fashion (8). Another useful plate for the tibia is the 2.4-mm limited contact-DCP (LC-DCP).

In summary, simple transverse fractures are anatomically reduced and stabilized with a DCP or LC-DCP applied in compression function, or with a single VCP. Long oblique fractures are reduced and stabilized with lag screws, before applying a plate in neutralization function. A plate applied in buttress function is used to treat comminuted fractures. The 2.0/2.7-mm VCP should be stacked for this purpose. A minimally invasive approach is performed without disturbing the soft-tissue attachment of the fragments in the comminuted area. The plate and rod technique is also feasible in cats, if a small intramedullary pin and 2.0-mm screws are used.

Comminuted tibial fractures are also amenable to minimally invasive plate osteosynthesis (MIPO), in which the fracture site is not approached at all (9). Two small skin incisions are made over the medial proximal and distal metaphysis. A precontoured plate is inserted through the proximal incision and is slid along the medial surface of the bone towards distally. It is first fixed to the proximal main fragment through the local incision. The main fragments are aligned, and the plate is secured to the distal main fragment. Care is taken to avoid outward rotation.

39.2.5 Internal fixators

Internal fixators can be used in neutralization or buttress function instead of conventional plates to repair fractures of the tibial diaphysis. When used for diaphyseal fractures, the main advantage is the preservation of the periosteal blood supply, and the prevention of cortical necrosis, which is most beneficial in the treatment of comminuted fractures with poor vascularity. Another good indication for internal fixators are fractures near the stifle or tarsal joint, where the size of the proximal or distal main fragment only allows insertion of two screws. The 2.4-mm Unilock mandible locking plates (Chapter 24) are of sufficient strength for the tibial diaphysis. The thick 2.0-mm plates can be applied to repair distal tibial fractures, where there is little room for screw insertion. The 2.0-mm plates should be combined with an intramedullary nail if used in buttress function.

39.3 Fractures of the proximal tibia and fibula

Fractures of the proximal tibia and fibula are rare. They include Salter and Harris fractures of the proximal tibial physis in immature animals, or fractures of the tibial metaphysis in adult cats. Other fractures are exceedingly rare, but avulsion fractures of the tibial tuberosity or metaphyseal fractures extending into the stifle joint can occur.

39.3.1 Approaches to the proximal tibia and fibula

The proximal tibia is approached through a medial incision (10). The combined fascia of the sartorius, gracilis, and semitendinosus muscles is sharply incised medial to the patellar ligament along the craniomedial tibial crest, and elevated from the medial aspect of the proximal tibia in a caudal direction. Care is taken not to damage the medial collateral ligament of the stifle joint.

39.3.2 Salter and Harris fractures

The immature proximal tibia has two separate growth plates, one for the proximal epiphysis and one for the tibial tuberosity. These two growth plates fuse to each other between 36 and 44 weeks of age, forming a cap that sits on the metaphysis (11). This combined growth center then fuses to the

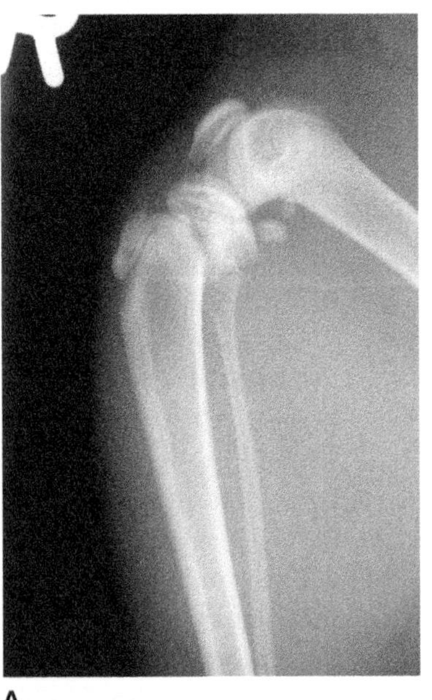
A

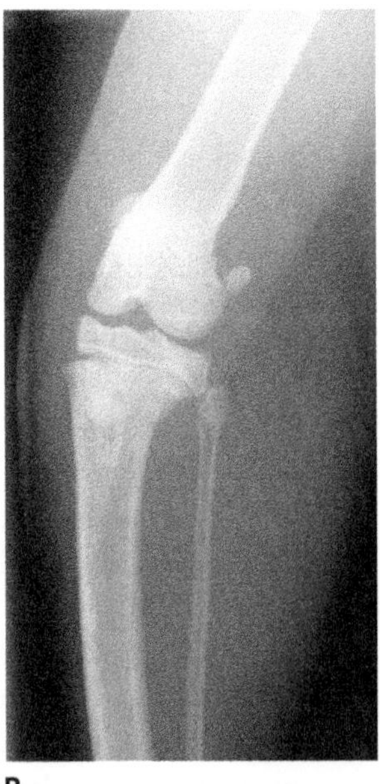
B

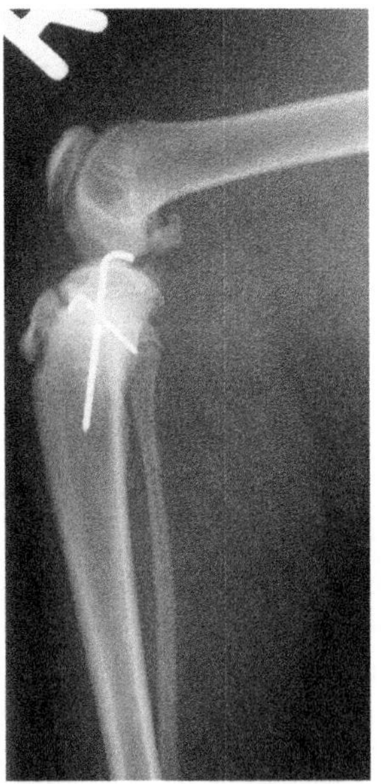
C

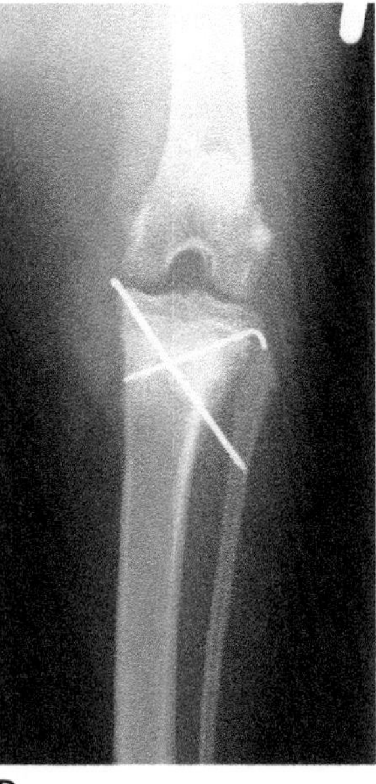
D

Figure 39-3 (**A**, **B**) Preoperative and (**C**, **D**) 4-week follow-up radiographs of a 5-month-old cat with a Salter and Harris type II fracture of the proximal tibial physis. The fracture was repaired with cross pins.

Box 39-1. Stabilization of Salter and Harris type I, II, and III fractures of the proximal tibia

A medial approach to the proximal tibia is performed. Fracture reduction is assisted by holding the stifle joint in extension. The proximal fracture fragment is levered forward and medially with the help of a periosteal elevator or a mini Hohmann retractor. Delicate handling of the epiphyseal fragment is mandatory to prevent iatrogenic damage of the small bone fragment and the growth plate. A small local lateral approach is needed for insertion of Kirschner wires from the lateral side.

Cross pinning: A 0.8–1.2-mm Kirschner wire is inserted from the medial edge of the tibial plateau, and is advanced in a distolateral direction to penetrate the lateral cortex. A second Kirschner wire is inserted from the lateral edge of the tibial plateau into the medial cortex (Fig. 39-4A). Unless the bone is very soft, the pin ends should be bent over to prevent pin migration.

Intramedullary nail and antirotational Kirschner wire: This technique may be advantageous in Salter and Harris type II fractures with a large lateral metaphyseal fragment. The intramedullary nail is inserted first, as described above. A small Kirschner wire is then driven from the lateral edge of the tibial tuberosity across the fracture in a distomedial direction, until it engages the medial cortex (Fig. 39-4B).

An additional tension band or a positional screw can be applied across the tibial tuberosity physis into the caudal cortex in Salter and Harris type I and II fractures with either technique. This should only be performed in cats without further growth potential.

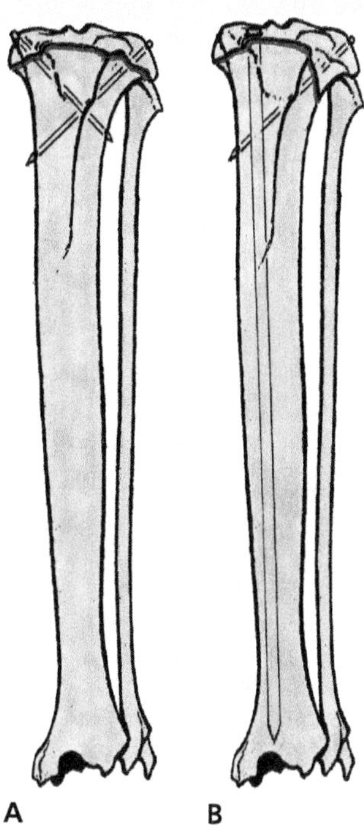

Figure 39-4 Options for stabilization of Salter and Harris type I and II fractures of the proximal tibia. (**A**) Repair of a Salter and Harris type I fracture with cross pins. (**B**) Internal fixation of a Salter and Harris type II fracture with an intramedullary pin and Kirschner wire, inserted from lateral.

metaphysis between 50 and 76 weeks of age (11). Before fusion of the two growth centers has taken place, the two physes can fracture individually, and a Salter and Harris type I or II fracture of the proximal epiphysis (Fig. 39-3) or an avulsion fracture of the tibial tuberosity can result. Fractures occurring after fusion of the two growth centers are also classified as Salter and Harris type I or II fractures.

The proximal epiphyseal fragment has a tendency to displace in a caudolateral direction relative to the tibia. The resulting change in angle of the tibial plateau compromises biomechanics of the stifle joint, and impairs its function if left untreated. The majority of cases therefore require open reduction and internal stabilization. Possible repair options for Salter and Harris type I, II, and III fractures include cross pinning (Fig. 39-3) or combining an intramedullary pin with an antirotational pin (Box 39-1).

Fixation stability can be enhanced by placing an additional tension band wire across the tibial tuberosity in Salter and Harris type I and II fractures. The tension band should only be applied in older cats without further growth potential. Undisplaced proximal physeal fractures are occasionally encountered, and can be treated with external coaptation.

39.3.3 Metaphyseal fractures

Metaphyseal fractures of the proximal tibia usually occur in adult cats, and are more frequent than Salter and Harris fractures (3). The proximal fragment has a tendency to tilt in a proximocranial direction because of the tension exerted by the patellar tendon. The main surgical challenge lies in being able to insert a sufficient number of screws or pins into the small proximal fragment.

Treatment options for simple transverse fractures include an intramedullary pin and a simple external skeletal fixator, or a medial plate (Box 39-2). T- or L-plates allow insertion of two screws even in very small proximal fragments (Fig. 39-6). A cranial tension band fixation is added in cases with marked distraction of the cranial aspect of the fracture.

Comminuted fractures usually extend into the tibial diaphysis and are treated like comminuted diaphyseal fractures, which are described later. Type II or III external skeletal fixators are advisable if the size of the proximal fragment only allows insertion of one or two pins.

One author has seen several proximal transverse tibial fractures in older cats with concurrent chronic patellar fractures.

Box 39-2. Stabilization of a simple transverse fracture of the proximal tibial metaphysis

A medial approach to the proximal metaphysis is performed. The approach is extended proximally, parallel to the patellar tendon if an intramedullary pin is inserted.

Intramedullary pin and type I external skeletal fixator: This repair is preferred in young cats. A 1.4–1.6-mm intramedullary pin is inserted in a normograde manner. For the medially applied external skeletal fixator, 1.4–2.0-mm transosseous pins are driven into the proximal fragment, and 1.4–1.6-mm pins are used in the distal tibial shaft (Fig. 39-5A). Smooth pins should be angled 70° to the long axis of the bone to enhance pull-out resistance. A cranial tension band wire as described in Figure 39-5B can also be applied.

Plate and tension band repair: This repair is preferred in older cats. A 2.0-mm T-plate or dynamic compression plate in compression function can be used if the proximal fragment allows insertion of three screws. The plate is applied at the caudomedial edge of the tibia in order to benefit from the increased bone purchase. A 0.6–0.8-mm figure-of-eight wire is positioned across the cranial fracture line as a tension band (Fig. 39-5B). A 2.0-mm internal fixator is a good alternative if only two screws can be inserted into the proximal fragment.

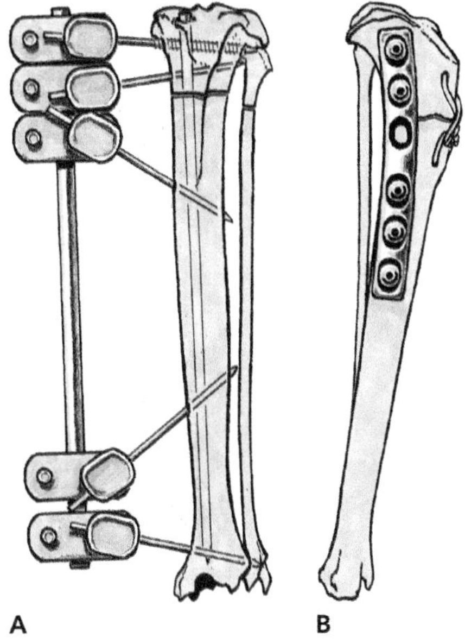

Figure 39-5 Options for stabilization of a simple transverse fracture of the proximal tibial metaphysis. (**A**) Repair of a simple proximal transverse fracture with an intramedullary pin and a medial type I external skeletal fixator. (**B**) Stabilization of a simple proximal transverse fracture using a six-hole plate and a cranial tension band wire.

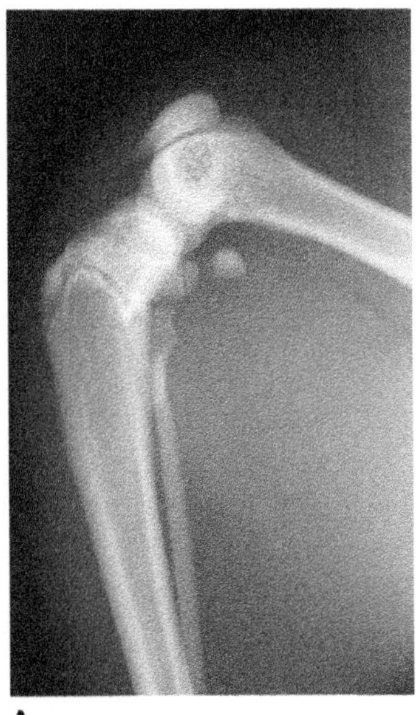

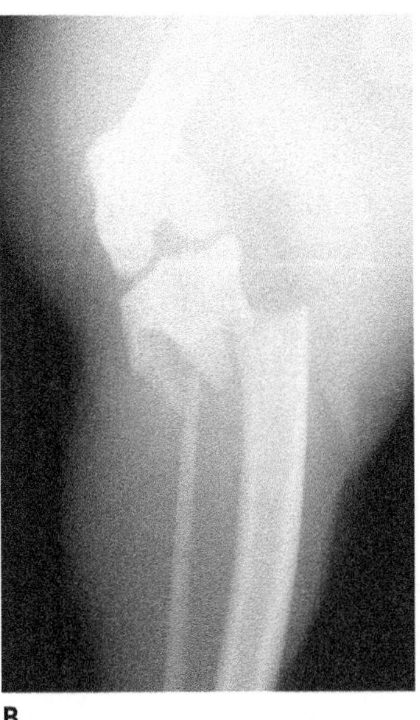

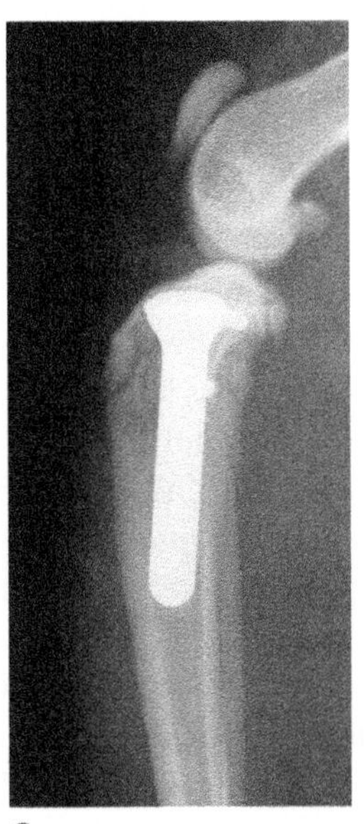

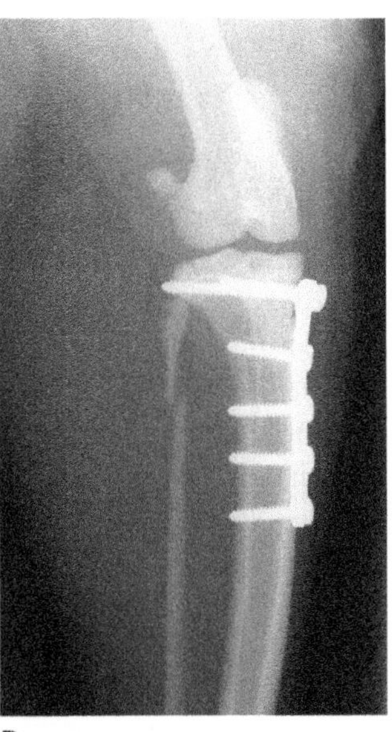

Figure 39-6 (**A, B**) Preoperative and (**C, D**) postoperative radiographs of a 2-year-old cat with a proximal metaphyseal tibial fracture. Use of a 2.0-mm T-plate allowed insertion of two screws into the proximal fragment.

These fractures showed remodeling of the cranial cortex of the tibia, and are thought to be stress fractures related to decreased flexion in the stifle joint, resulting in the bending force in the hindlimb being transferred to the proximal tibia. Fractures will often occur bilaterally several months apart, and most cats have a history of other non-traumatic fractures of the acetabulum, ischium, or humeral condyle. An underlying bone abnormality is suspected but unproven. The tibial fractures in these cats seem to heal best when repaired with a pin and tension band, or plate and screw and tension band technique.

39.4 Diaphyseal fractures of the tibia and fibula

Fracture healing of diaphyseal tibial fractures tends to be slow, probably caused by the lack of surrounding soft tissue and the sparse blood supply. Careful tissue handling, preservation of blood supply, and respecting the principles of osteosynthesis are crucial for success. The choice of treatment for diaphyseal tibia and fibula fractures is mainly based on fracture severity and location, age, body weight, temperament of the patient, and implants available (Chapters 13 and 24). The various implant systems have their own advantages and disadvantages. Closed reduction and external skeletal fixation of severe tibial fractures seem to reduce the incidence of osteomyelitis, when compared to open reduction and internal fixation methods (4). It is therefore often the method of choice for severely comminuted and open fractures. Plate osteosynthesis has the advantage of easier postoperative management compared to external skeletal fixation, making it more suitable for cats that are difficult to handle. On the other hand, plate osteosynthesis causes more iatrogenic damage to the sparse blood supply, and tibial fractures stabilized with bone plates had the longest healing times in two studies (2, 4).

39.4.1 Approach to the tibial diaphysis

The tibial diaphysis is approached via a medial skin incision. The saphenous vein is spared. It can be gently dissected free and retracted with a Penrose drain.

39.4.2 Simple transverse and short oblique fractures

Simple transverse and short oblique fractures may be treated with a cast after reduction. Tibial fractures with an intact fibula are also amenable to be treated with external coaptation because the fibula acts as an internal splint. The disadvantage of external coaptation is the prolonged immobilization of adjacent joints, which can cause cartilage degeneration, periarticular fibrosis, and muscle contractures. Therefore, only fractures expected to have achieved clinical union within 4 weeks should be treated with external coaptation. Incomplete and undisplaced fractures in very young kittens may be treated with a splinted bandage. For complete fractures and fractures in older cats a full cast provides more stability. Application and maintenance of bandages and casts are described in Chapter 22. It is important to immobilize the tarsus in a flexed position to prevent contracture of the gastrocnemius muscle. Contraction of the gastrocnemius muscle can occur within days in immature cats.

Internal stabilization or external skeletal fixation results in faster return to function and allows immediate weight-bearing and motion of adjacent joints. Simple fractures of both the tibia and fibula in adult cats are therefore usually treated surgically. A type I external skeletal fixator, with or without intramedullary pin, a medially applied 2.7- or 2.0-mm DCP in compression function, a single 2.0/2.7-mm VCP, or a 2.4-mm LC-DCP are all implants that could be used (Box 39-3). Open fractures are treated with external skeletal fixation.

39.4.3 Long oblique and multifragmentary reducible fractures

Simple long oblique or reducible multifragment fractures of the tibia are not very common. They are usually treated with anatomic reduction and stable internal fixation. Anatomic fracture reduction enhances fixation stability by creating load sharing of the cortex, but has the disadvantage of causing soft-tissue trauma and bone devascularization. It should only be attempted in long oblique fractures, and fractures with one large reducible butterfly fragment. If it seems questionable from preoperative radiographs that anatomic reduction is possible, the fracture is treated as a comminuted fracture (section below).

Intramedullary pinning and cerclage wires, and interfragmentary lag screws with a neutralization plate, are treatment options for anatomic reduction of long oblique fractures. Stabilization with a lag screw and a neutralization plate is preferred over fixation with an intramedullary pin and cerclage wires in the tibia (Fig. 39-8 and Box 39-4). Application of cerclage wires around the tibia requires additional soft-tissue dissection between the tibia and fibula, and has the potential for further diminution of the blood supply.

Long oblique fractures can also be stabilized with an intramedullary pin and external skeletal fixator (Box 39-4). The intramedullary pin enhances bending stability, and the external skeletal fixation pins prevent axial collapse and rotation. This type of fixation does not provide interfragmentary compression, but fracture healing should be faster because of preservation of local blood supply. Open fractures are also treated with external skeletal fixation.

Box 39-3. Stabilization of a simple transverse or short oblique fracture of the tibial diaphysis

Simple fractures treated with intramedullary pin and external skeletal fixator can be reduced and stabilized in a closed manner. A medial approach to the tibial shaft is performed for plate osteosynthesis. The fracture is anatomically reduced.

Intramedullary pin and type I external skeletal fixator: This combination is commonly used to treat simple fractures of the tibia in young cats. An intramedullary pin is inserted in a normograde manner to align the fracture fragments. Two transosseous pins are then placed in each fracture fragment to provide rotational stability (Fig. 39-7A). Usually, 1.4–2.0-mm pins are used in the proximal tibia, and 1.4–1.6-mm pins in the distal tibia.

Plate osteosynthesis: The plate is applied to the medial tibial surface. Interfragmentary compression is exerted if a dynamic compression plate (DCP) or limited contact-DCP (LC-DCP) is used. One screw on each side of the fracture is applied eccentrically for interfragmentary compression. Overall, at least three screws are required per fragment. It is advisable to select a longer plate and leave some holes empty, rather than taking a short plate and filling all holes (Fig. 39-7B). Care must be taken not to leave a single empty plate hole at the level of the fracture.

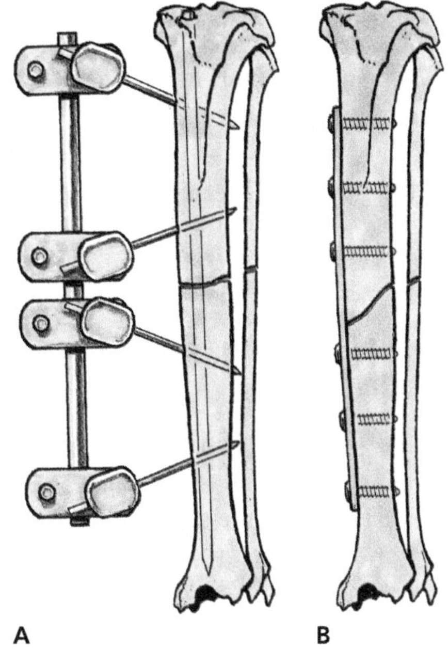

Figure 39-7 Options for stabilization of simple transverse or short oblique fractures of the tibial diaphysis.
(**A**) Repair of a transverse diaphyseal tibial fracture with an intramedullary pin and a type I external skeletal fixator.
(**B**) Internal fixation of a short oblique tibial fracture with a medially applied plate. Anatomic reduction is important.

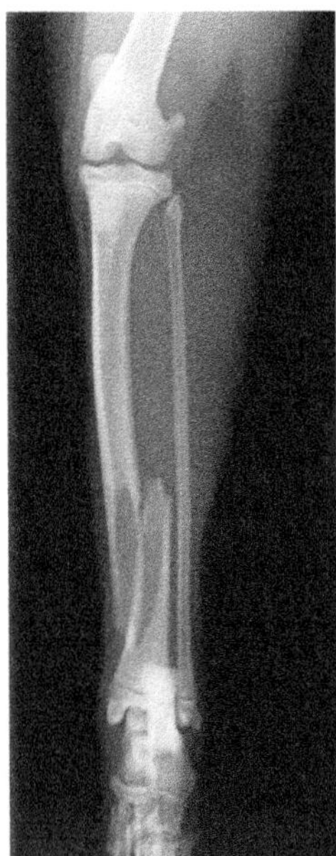

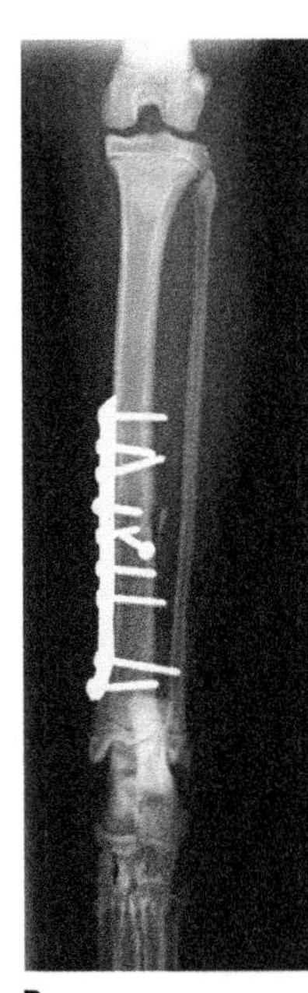

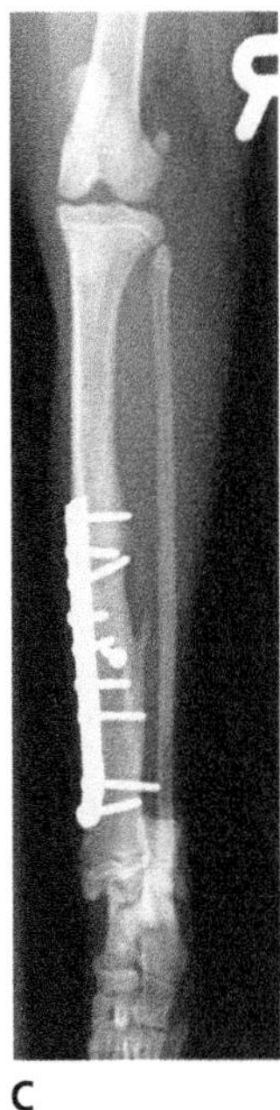

Figure 39-8 A 10-month-old cat with a long oblique fracture of the tibia.
(**A**) Preoperative radiograph showing a long oblique fracture of the distal tibial shaft.
(**B**) The fracture was stabilized with a 2.0-mm lag screw and a 1.5/2.0-mm veterinary cuttable plate in neutralization function. This relatively weak and short plate could be used because the fibula was intact.
(**C**) The fracture was healed after 5 weeks.

Spiral fractures of the tibia with an intact fibula can be successfully treated with external coaptation in immature cats (12). External coaptation for long oblique fractures is not recommended in adult cats.

39.4.4 Comminuted fractures

Comminuted and open fractures of the tibia are common. Open fractures are commonly located in the distal diaphysis. Closed, mildly comminuted fractures can be treated with a plate in buttress function, if the main fragments allow insertion of a sufficient number of screws. Internal fixators can also be used as buttress implants, and have the advantage of preserving cortical blood supply and requiring only two screws per fragment (Fig. 39-10).

External skeletal fixation is the treatment of choice for open fractures and is also commonly used to stabilize comminuted fractures. A type I or II external skeletal fixator is used depending on fracture location and severity. A type I external skeletal fixator with three transosseous pins per fragment is adequate for mild to moderate comminuted fractures in younger cats. Healing can take several months in severely comminuted and open tibia fractures (4) (Fig. 39-11), and

Box 39-4. Stabilization of long oblique or reducible butterfly fractures of the tibial diaphysis

A medial approach to the tibial shaft is performed if anatomic fracture reduction and interfragmentary compression are planned. Closed reduction or a minimally invasive approach can be used for external skeletal fixation.

Lag screws and neutralization plate: The fracture is anatomically reduced and reduction is maintained with pointed reduction forceps. One or two 2.0-mm lag screws are inserted perpendicular to the fracture line(s). A long plate is then applied in neutralization function (Fig. 39-9A). At least three screws should be inserted proximal and distal to the limit of the fracture. If fracture configuration allows, the lag screws can also be inserted directly through the plate.

Intramedullary pin and external skeletal fixator: An intramedullary pin is inserted normograde. The fracture can be held in reduction with pointed reduction forceps while transosseous pins are inserted. Two to three transosseus pins are inserted per fragment (Fig. 39-9B). Size 2.0-mm pins are usually used in the proximal metaphysis, and 1.4–1.6-mm pins in the diaphysis and distal metaphysis.

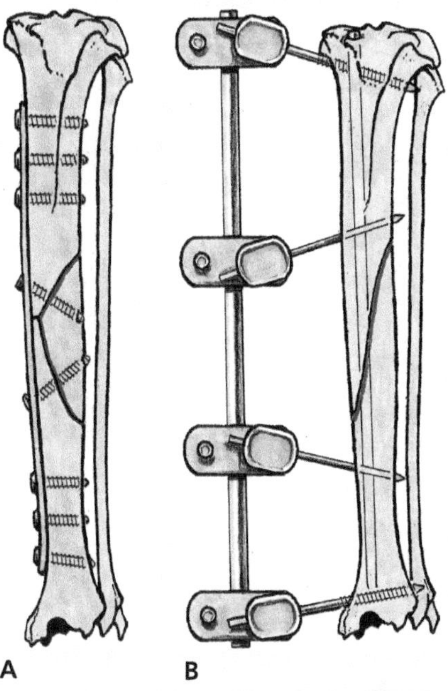

Figure 39-9 Options for stabilization of long oblique fractures, or reducible fractures with a butterfly fragment, of the tibial diaphysis. (**A**) Stabilization of a tibial fracture with a butterfly fragment with lag screws and a neutralization plate.
(**B**) Repair of a long oblique fracture in the tibial shaft with an intramedullary pin and a type I external skeletal fixator.

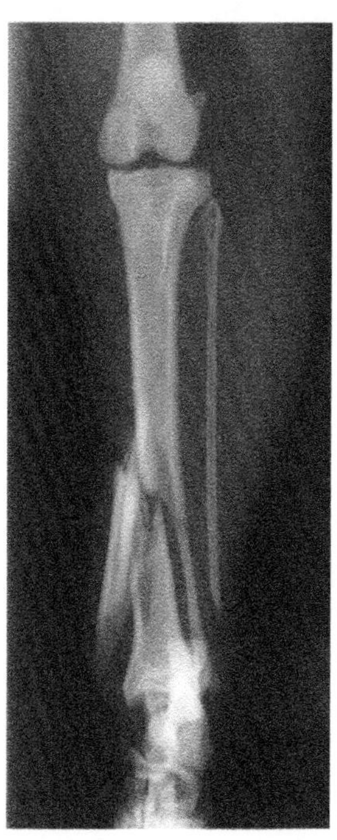
A

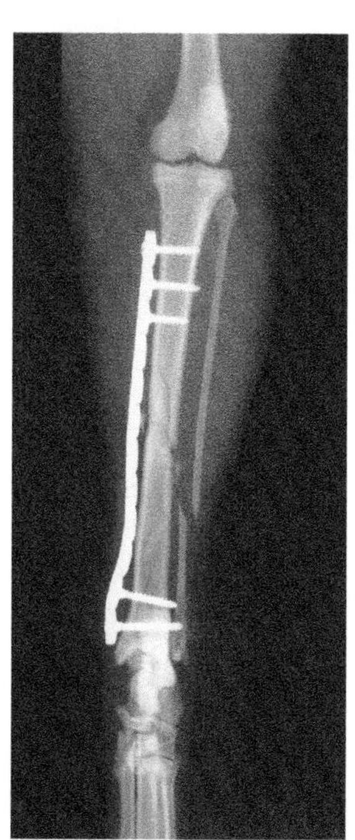
B

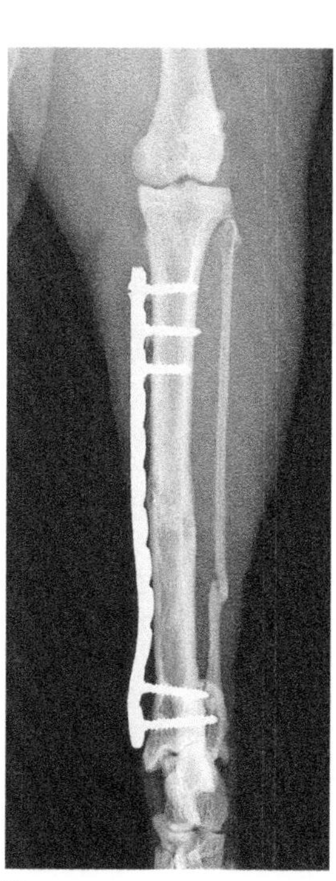
C

Figure 39-10 (**A**) Preoperative, (**B**) postoperative, and (**C**) 1-year follow-up radiographs of a cat with a comminuted fracture of the distal shaft of the tibia, stabilized with an internal fixator (2.4-mm Unilock plate). Note the small gap between plate and bone, and that only two screws were inserted in the small distal fragment.

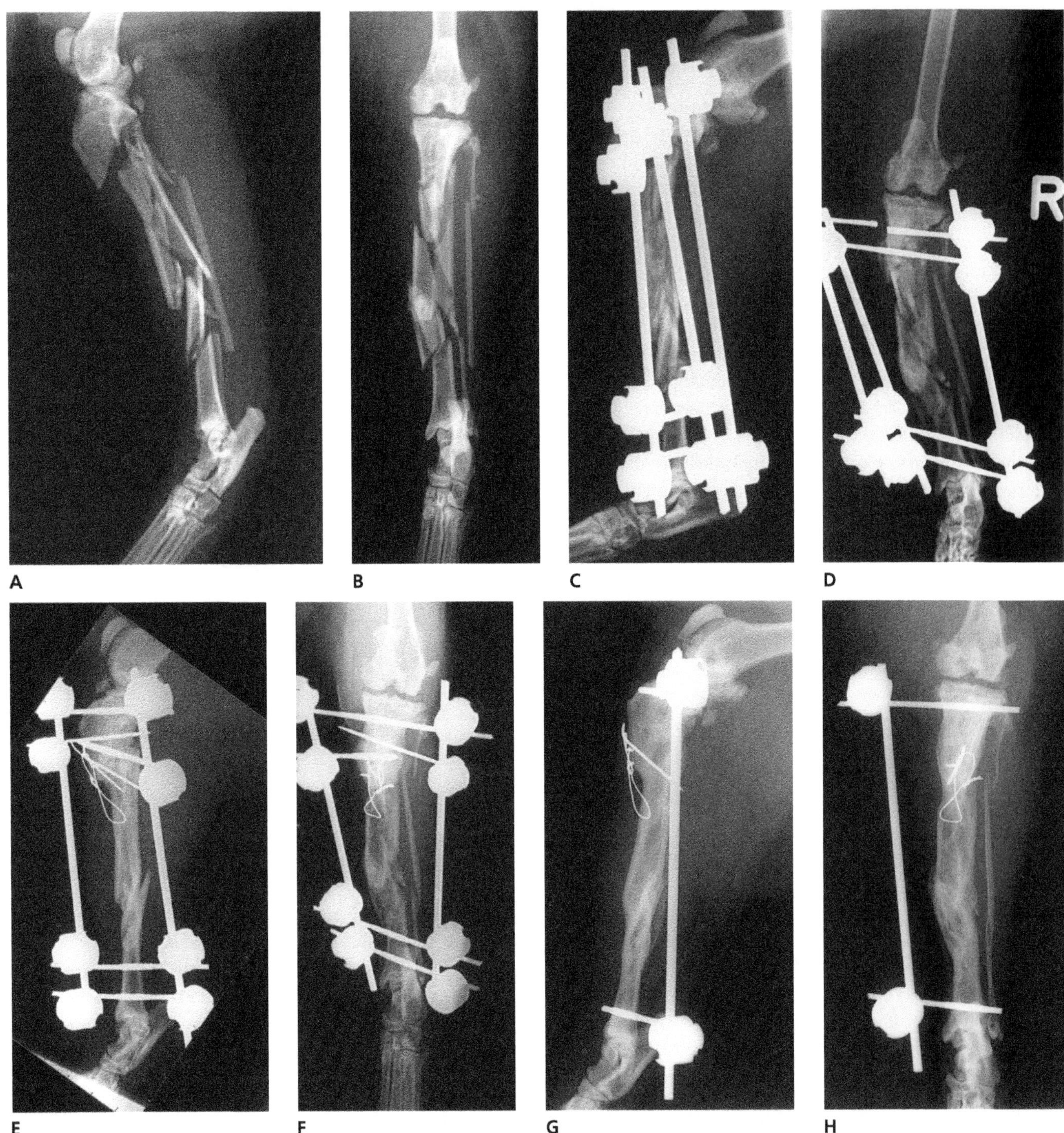

Figure 39-11 Delayed healing of a comminuted fracture of the tibia.
(**A**, **B**) Preoperative radiographs show a highly comminuted fracture.
(**C**, **D**) Radiographs taken 3 months after closed reduction and stabilization with a type II external skeletal fixator. The most proximal pin is broken, there is a non-union of the most proximal part of the fracture, and the proximal fragment is tilted cranially.
(**E**, **F**) Radiographs taken another 3 months after replacement of proximal pins, insertion of a cancellous bone graft, and application of a tension band to pull the proximal fragment distally and caudally. Callus formation is now evident.
(**G**, **H**) Radiographs after 11 months finally show healing. The type I external skeletal fixator was left in place for another month.

Box 39-5. Stabilization of comminuted fractures of the tibial diaphysis

Closed reduction can be used to apply an external skeletal fixator. A surgical approach is usually performed for plating, but care is taken to disturb the soft-tissue attachments of the fragments and local blood supply minimally. The least invasive approach to apply a plate is the minimally invasive plate osteosynthesis (MIPO) technique. Bone grafting is indicated if large fracture gaps or devitalized fracture fragments are present.

External skeletal fixation: Type I and II external fixators are mostly used with 2.0-mm transosseous pins proximally, and 1.6-mm pins distally. The most proximal and most distal positive-threaded transosseous pins are inserted first, parallel to the stifle and tarsal joint. These pins are end-threaded for a type I fixator (Fig. 39-12A), and centrally threaded for a type II fixator (Fig. 39-12B). The fracture is reduced indirectly by bringing the two pins parallel to each other, and connecting them with the external bar. This relies on accurate pin positioning, and overall alignment should also be checked by flexing and extending the hock and stifle to ensure that they are bending in the same plane. Care is taken to avoid valgus, outward rotation, craniocaudal malalignment, and overdistraction of the main fragments. Two additional positive end-threaded or smooth pins are then added from medial per main fragment as half pins.

Buttress plate: A 2.7-mm dynamic compression plate (DCP), a 2.4-mm limited contact-DCP (LC-DCP) or a stacked 2.0/2.7-mm veterinary cuttable plate can be used. The plate should span the whole length of the tibia, and should allow insertion of at least three screws proximally and distally (Fig. 39-12C). Minimal plate contouring is necessary. The plate is fixed to the proximal fragment first. Then reduction is achieved by securing the distal fragment to the plate. The intervening fracture fragments are not manipulated. An intramedullary pin can give additional bending stability, especially if the proximal or distal fragments are too short to allow insertion of three screws. The intramedullary pin is inserted prior to plate application, and helps in obtaining alignment. The disadvantage is that it may be difficult to pass the screws in the narrow distal diaphysis.

Internal fixator: An internal fixator, for example the 2.4-mm Unilock plate, can be applied in buttress function, as shown in the radiographs of Figure 39-10.

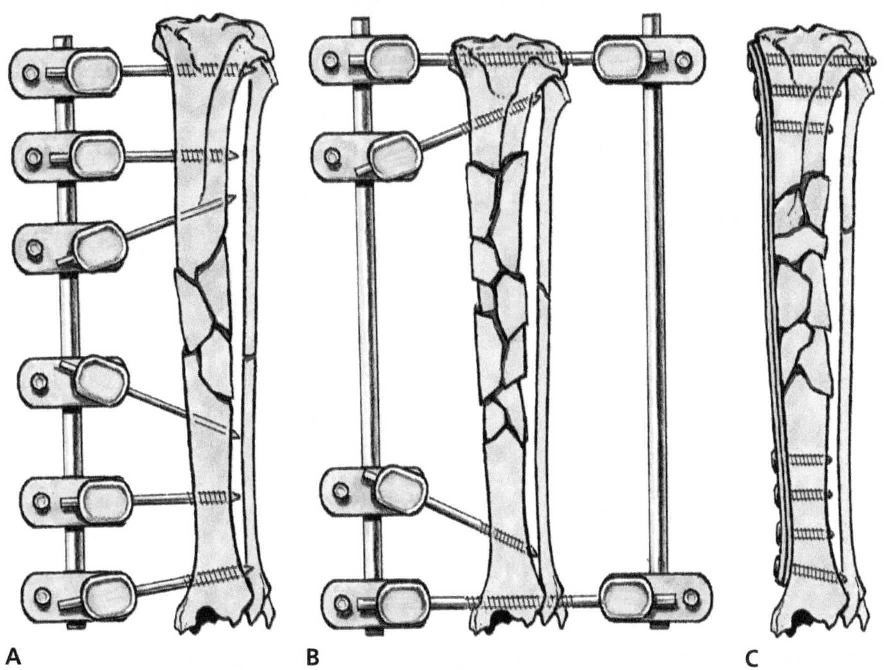

Figure 39-12 Options for stabilization of comminuted fractures of the tibial shaft. (**A**) Stabilization of a mildly comminuted mid diaphyseal fracture with a type I external skeletal fixator. Three transosseous pins are inserted per fragment. (**B**) Repair of a severely comminuted fracture of the tibia with a type II external skeletal fixator. At least two pins should be inserted per fragment. (**C**) Internal fixation of a comminuted fracture using a buttress plate.

pin loosening is likely to occur during such long healing times if simple frames are used. Severely comminuted fractures, especially in older cats, are therefore best stabilized with a type II configuration. A type II or even type III configuration is also used if a small proximal or distal metaphyseal segment only allows insertion of the minimum number of pins from two sides or planes (Box 39-5).

An interlocking nail is another treatment option for comminuted fractures in the proximal or mid diaphyseal area in larger cats. The tibia and its intramedullary canal

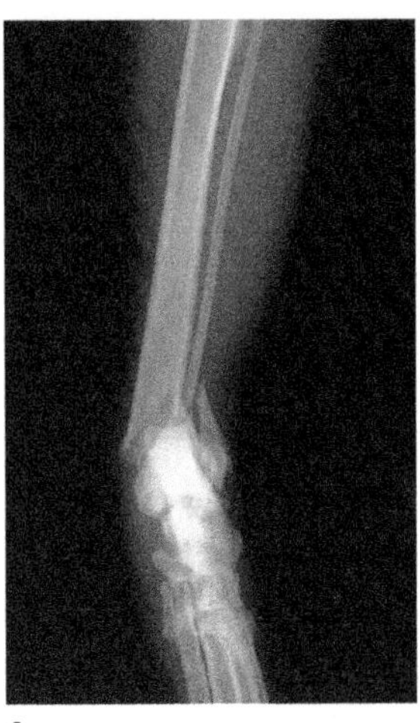

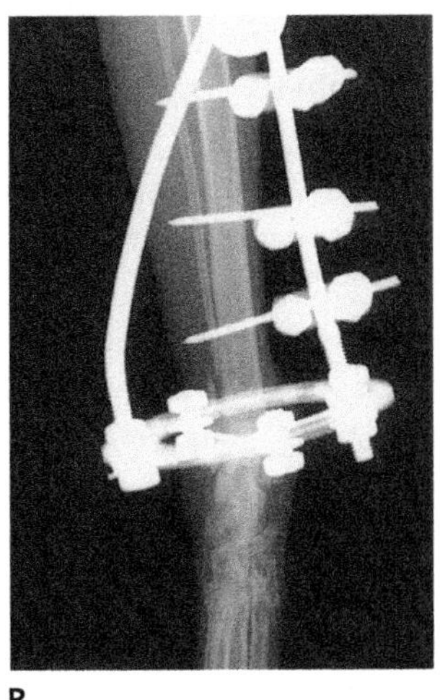

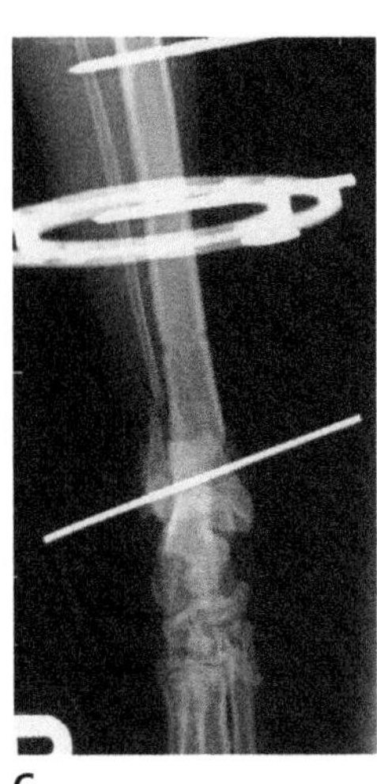

Figure 39-13 (**A**) Preoperative, (**B**) postoperative, and (**C**) 3-month follow-up radiographs of a cat with a very distal oblique metaphyseal fracture of the tibia and fibula. A hybrid circular external fixator was used for stabilization. The fracture had healed 3 months after surgery.

narrow distally, so with the current range of interlocking nail sizes, the nail can only be used in large cats with fractures involving the mid to proximal third diaphysis (7).

Fractures with devitalized fracture fragments and fractures with large fracture gaps are at risk of developing non-union and should be grafted. Excessive distraction of the main fragments creating large fracture gaps should be avoided during external skeletal fixation repair. Cancellous bone grafting has been shown to be capable of preventing non-unions of the tibia in the presence of large fracture gaps (13). Autogenous or allogenous cancellous bone graft, or a combination of the two, can be used. Open fractures may require delay of the grafting until the wound is considered to be free of infection.

39.5 Fractures of the distal tibia and fibula

Distal fractures of the tibia and fibula include metaphyseal fractures in adult cats, Salter and Harris fractures in growing cats, and tarsal joint fractures. Lateral and medial malleolar fractures are common distal tibial and fibular fractures, and are associated with tarsal instability.

39.5.1 Approaches to the distal tibia and fibula

A medial approach is used to access the distal tibial diaphysis and the medial malleolus. The fibula is approached from laterally.

39.5.2 Metaphyseal fractures of the distal tibia

Distal metaphyseal tibial fractures occur commonly in cats, and the incidence of open fractures is relatively high. Closed fractures can be stabilized with plate osteosynthesis or external skeletal fixation. The treatment of choice for open fractures is an external skeletal fixator. The small size of the distal fragment can make it difficult to insert a sufficient number of screws or transosseous pins.

External skeletal fixators can often be used after closed reduction. The tubular external skeletal fixator is especially suitable for distal metaphyseal fractures because it allows insertion of a larger number of transosseous pins over a small distance than other external skeletal fixator systems (14) (Chapter 24). A hybrid construct with a circular external skeletal fixator (15, 16) (Fig. 39-13) or a fixator with an acrylic bar also allows fixation of very small fragments, and is useful for distally located fractures.

The small distal fragment does not usually allow insertion of a sufficient number of screws with a 2.7-mm DCP. A 2.0-mm thick DCP or a 2.0/2.7 or 1.5/2.0 VCP are therefore used. To compensate for the lower stability of these shorter and weaker plates, an intramedullary pin can be inserted prior to plate application if there is concern about construct stability. The cuttable plate can be used in sandwich function to enhance bending stability. Internal fixators can also be used in fractures close to joints where it is only possible to insert two screws per fragment (Box 39-6).

39.5.3 Salter and Harris fractures

The distal physis of the tibia closes between 40 and 52 weeks of age in intact cats (11). Fractures of the distal tibia are usually Salter and Harris type I or II fractures (Fig. 39-15). Salter and Harris type III fractures have also been reported (17). Salter and Harris type I and II fractures are best stabilized with cross pins (Box 39-7). Conservative treatment with a cast is an option in undisplaced Salter and Harris type I or II fractures, particularly in young kittens. Cats younger than 6 or 7 months with further growth potential are at risk of development of growth disturbances if premature physeal closure occurs.

Box 39-6. Stabilization of metaphyseal fractures of the distal tibia

Although closed reduction is possible with external skeletal fixation, a small medial approach to the distal fragment is often performed for ease of pin positioning. A medial approach is also used for plate application.

Tubular external skeletal fixator: The distal transosseous pin is inserted first, close to and perpendicular to the tarsal joint. A 1.6-mm, or maximally a 2.0 positive end-threaded pin, is used. The direction of this first pin is critical, as it will determine the position of the connecting tube, perpendicular to the pin. A 6.0-mm tube is secured to the pin. The fracture is reduced and a transosseous pin is inserted into the proximal fragment. If the distal pin is placed correctly, the tube will be positioned parallel to the long axis of the tibia. At least three pins are inserted into the proximal fragment, and at least two or three are inserted into the distal fragment (Fig. 39-14A). If an intramedullary pin is also used it is inserted prior to application of the fixator.

Intramedullary pin and plate: An intramedullary pin, comprising approximately 30% of the diameter of the distal medullary canal, is inserted in a normograde fashion. A long 2.0-mm dynamic compression plate or a 1.5/2.0 veterinary cuttable plate (VCP) is then applied in neutralization or buttress function. If used in buttress function, consider stacking or sandwiching the VCP. Screws must engage at least four cortices in the distal and proximal fragment (Fig. 39-14B), but six or even eight cortices are preferred, especially in the proximal bone.

Internal fixator: A 2.0-mm locking plate can be used as a neutralization or buttress implant, with two screws in the distal fragment, and three in the proximal fragment.

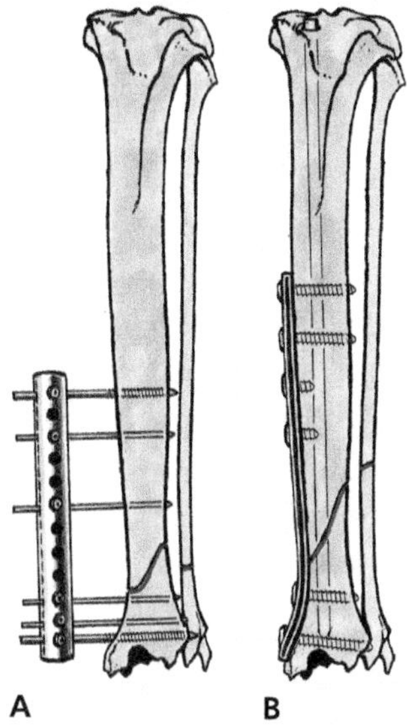

Figure 39-14 Stabilization options for distal metaphyseal fractures of the tibia.
(**A**) Repair of a simple transverse fracture with a 6.0-mm tubular external skeletal fixator.
(**B**) Internal fixation of an oblique fracture with an intramedullary pin and a 12-hole 2.0-mm dynamic compression plate.

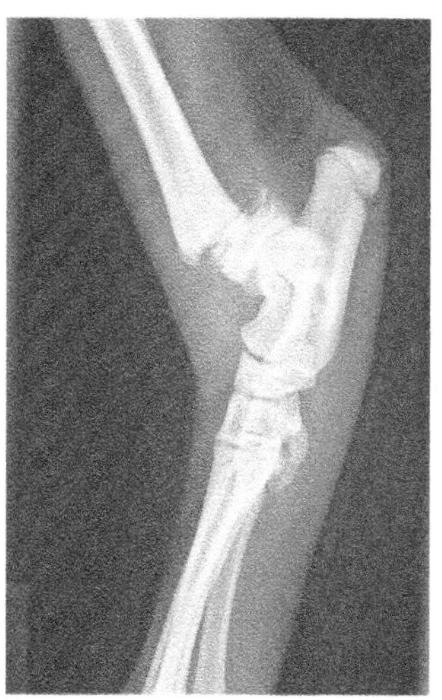
A

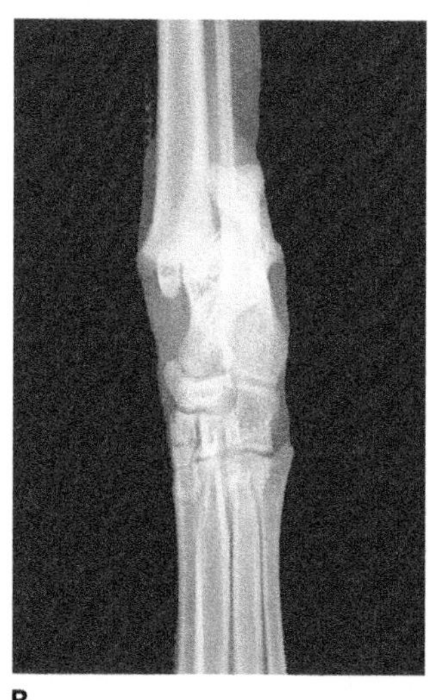
B

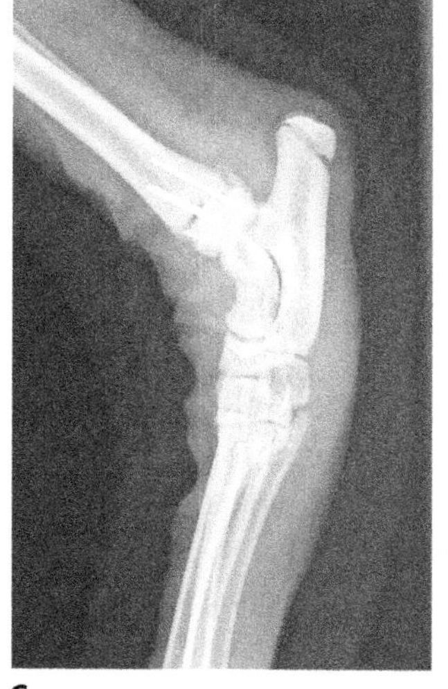
C

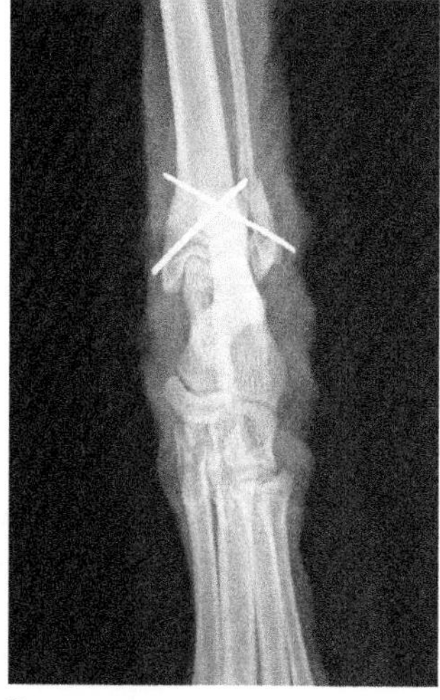
D

Figure 39-15 (**A, B**) A 5-month-old cat with a Salter and Harris type I fracture of the distal tibia, and a fracture of the distal fibula. (**C, D**) Postoperative radiographs show reduction and stabilization with two Kirschner wires inserted as cross pins.

Box 39-7. Stabilization of Salter and Harris type I and II fractures of the distal tibia

An approach to the distal tibia and medial malleolus is performed. The fracture is carefully reduced, using distal traction on the flexed tarsus and manipulation of the foot and careful levering with a freer periosteal elevator. Anatomic reduction is mandatory for fixation stability. A 0.9–1.2-mm Kirschner wire is driven from the medial malleolus in a proximolateral direction to be seated in the lateral cortex of the distal tibia. Care has to be taken not to enter the tibiotarsal joint. A second Kirschner wire is then inserted from the distal fibula across the tibia, exiting through the medial cortex (Fig. 39-16). A separate lateral skin incision is required for pin placement. It is important that both pins are securely engaged in the distal tibial fragment. If one or both pins are inserted subperiostally, loss of reduction and instability may occur.

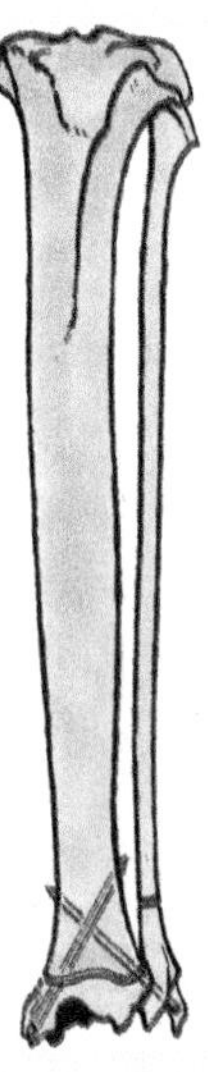

Figure 39-16 Cross pinning of a Salter and Harris type II fracture of the distal tibia with one pin inserted from the medial malleolus, and one from the lateral malleolus.

39.5.4 Fractures of the distal tibia involving the tarsal joint

Epiphyseal fractures include malleolar fractures, cranial slab fractures, and complex articular fractures. Fractures of the lateral or medial malleolus are the most common type of distal tibia and fibula fractures. The malleoli serve as a medial and lateral restraint to the talus, and they are the insertion sites for the tarsal collateral ligaments. Malleolar fractures result in talocrural instability, and are covered in Chapter 40.

Cranial slab fractures of the distal tibia are encountered occasionally in cats. These fractures cause tarsal instability, because the dorsal rim of the tibia is part of the insertion of the joint capsule. If the fragment is large enough, it is stabilized with a small lag screw or a small threaded pin to restore congruity of the joint surface and joint stability. If the fragment is too small to be reattached, it is probably best removed, followed by external immobilization of the tarsus for 2–3 weeks in order to allow healing of the insertion of the joint capsule.

Fortunately, complex fractures of the epiphysis of the tibia are rare, but they may occur after falls and gunshot wounds. If comminution precludes anatomic and stable repair of the tibiotalar joint surface, pantarsal arthrodesis is the only treatment option (Chapter 40).

39.6 Postoperative treatment and prognosis

External coaptation is usually not necessary after stable fixation of metaphyseal and diaphyseal fractures. Follow-up radiographs are generally performed after 4–6 weeks.

Fractures of the tibial diaphysis are more prone to develop complications than fractures of other bones, possibly due to the high incidence of comminuted and open fractures, and the poor soft-tissue covering. Both fracture-healing disorders and osteomyelitis can occur. Fracture healing is slower for comminuted and high-grade open fractures (4), and some severely comminuted fractures may take several months to heal. The tibia has been reported to be predisposed to non-unions, with an incidence of approximately 15% (18). Non-unions are most likely to develop after comminuted fractures and open fractures, in older and overweight cats (18). Osteomyelitis occurs in up to 15% of tibial diaphyseal fractures (2, 4). Predisposing factors include wound contamination or infection in the presence of open fractures, and poor vascularity caused by soft-tissue trauma.

Proximal and distal physeal fractures are expected to heal rapidly, but a splinted bandage should be applied for approximately 2 weeks to protect the repair. Radiographs are performed after 2–3 weeks to detect premature physeal closure, and to evaluate fixation stability. The Kirschner wire ends may cause irritation of periarticular structures, and should be removed in the presence of local swelling, seroma formation, or radiographic evidence of implant migration.

Prognosis after distal tibial fractures depends mainly on the ability to achieve anatomic reduction of the fragments and a stable fracture repair. Malalignment or instability will cause dysfunction and degenerative joint disease of the tibiotarsal joint. One study reported a suboptimal outcome in 18% of distal physeal fractures, perceptible as continued lameness, malunion, and reduced range of motion of the tarsal joint (3).

References and further reading

1. Hill FWG. A survey of bone fractures in the cat. J Small Anim Pract 1977;18:457–463.
2. Boone EG, et al. Fractures of the tibial diaphysis in dogs and cats. J Am Vet Med Assoc 1986;188:41–45.
3. Brunnberg L. Tibia and fibular fractures in the cat. Kleintierpraxis 2003;48:9–23.
4. Richardson EF, Thacher CW. Tibial fractures in cats. Compend Continuing Educ 1993;15:383–394.
5. Whitney WO, Mehlhaff CJ. High-rise syndrome in cats. J Am Vet Med Assoc 1987;191:1399–1403.
6. Payne J, et al. Comparison of normograde and retrograde intramedullary pinning of feline tibias. J Am Anim Hosp Assoc 2005;41:56–60.
7. Duhautois B. Use of veterinary interlocking nails for diaphyseal fractures in dogs and cats: 121 cases. Vet Surg 2003;32:8–20.
8. Fruchter AM, Holmberg DL. Mechanical analysis of veterinary cuttable plate. Compend Continuing Educ 1991;4:116–119.
9. Schmökel HG, et al. Percutaneous plating of tibial fractures in two dogs. Vet Comp Orthop Traumatol 2003;16:191–195.
10. Piermattei DL, Johnson KA. An atlas of surgical approaches to the bones and joints of the dog and the cat, 4th edn. Philadelphia: WB Saunders; 2004.
11. Smith RN. Fusion of ossification centres in the cat. J Small Anim Pract 1969;10:523–530.
12. Zaal MD, Hazewinkel HAW. Treatment of isolated tibial fractures in cats and dogs. Vet Q 1997;119:191–194.
13. Toombs JP, Wallace LJ. Evaluation of autogeneic and allogeneic cortical chip grafting in a feline tibial nonunion model. Am J Vet Res 1985;46:519–528.
14. Haas B, et al. Use of the tubular external fixator in the treatment of distal radial and ulnar fractures in small dogs and cats. Vet Comp Orthop Traumatol 2003;16:132–137.
15. Farese JP, et al. Use of IMEX SK-circular external fixator hybrid constructs for fracture stabilization in dogs and cats. J Am Anim Hosp Assoc 2002;38:279–289.
16. Clarke SP, Carmichael S. Treatment of distal diaphyseal fractures using hybrid external skeletal fixation in three dogs. J Small Anim Pract 2006;47:98–103.
17. Boone EG, et al. Distal tibial fractures in dogs and cats. J Am Vet Med Assoc 1986;188:36–40.
18. Nolte DM, et al. Incidence of and predisposing factors for nonunion of fractures involving the appendicular skeleton in cats: 18 cases (1998–2002). J Am Vet Med Assoc 2005;226:77–82.

40 Tarsal joint

K. Voss, S.J. Langley-Hobbs, P.M. Montavon

Injuries of the tarsal joint are common in cats and include ligament sprains resulting in instability or luxation and fractures of the tarsal bones. Injury of the Achilles tendon also affects function of the tarsal joint. Tarsal injury usually results from motor vehicle accidents and falls from a height. Ligament injuries can affect the tarsocrural joint, the proximal and distal intertarsal joints, and the tarsometatarsal joints. Instability and luxation of the tarsocrural joint are the most common tarsal injuries in cats (1). Ligament injuries at the joint levels distal to the tarsocrural joint are also frequently seen. Knowledge of regional anatomy and a thorough clinical and radiological examination are required to diagnose the exact site of ligament sprain, and to choose the appropriate treatment.

Tarsal injuries are often associated with open wounds, either caused from internal penetration of the skin by displaced bones, or more commonly from shear or degloving injury. General treatment of open joint injuries is described in Chapter 14, and treatment of skin defects is described in Chapter 16.

40.1 Surgical anatomy

The distal tibia and fibula are connected to each other via the inferior tibiofibular ligament (Fig. 40-1). Both the medial and lateral malleolus enclose the trochlea tali and thus prevent mediolateral displacement. The malleoli are also the insertion sites for the collateral ligaments. In contrast to dogs, cats only have short collateral ligaments (2). The medial and lateral collateral ligaments each consist of straight and oblique branches (Fig. 40-1). The oblique tibiotalar part of the ligament on the medial side and the talofibular part on the lateral side are hidden below the malleoli, and are difficult to access surgically.

The tarsus is composed of seven tarsal bones. The articulations between the bones are known as the tarsocrural, talocentral, calcaneoquartal, centrodistal and the tarsometatarsal joints. The distal tibia, the distal fibula, and the talus contribute to the tarsocrural joint. Axial force transmission is through the distal tibia and the talus.

An intertarsal joint is the articulation between adjacent tarsal bones, some of which have specific names. For ease of description, although not technically correct, the talocentral and calcaneoquartal joints are often referred to as the proximal intertarsal joint. The joints between the small tarsal bones are generally considered joints with low mobility, but some functional motion is present, especially in the talocentral, calcaneoquartal, and talocalcaneal joint. The centrodistal and tarsometatarsal joints are tighter joints, with less motion.

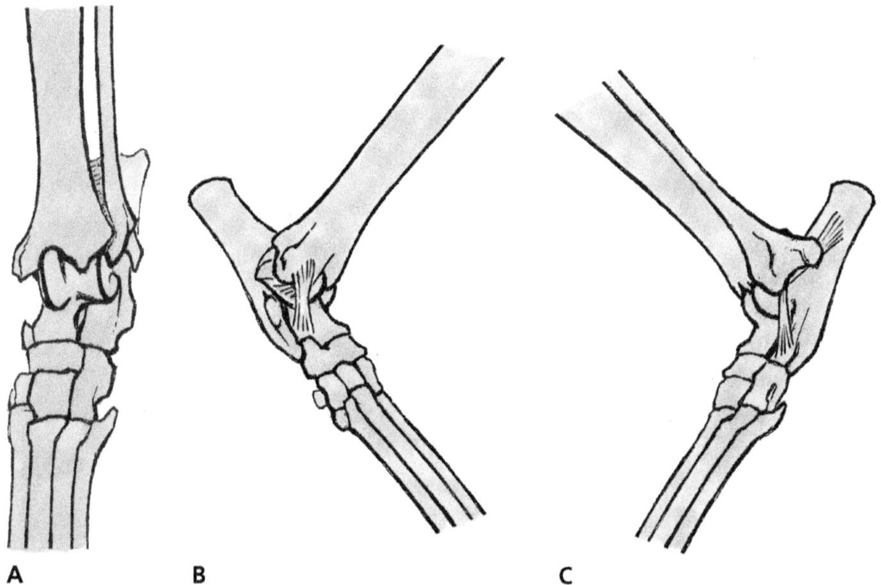

Figure 40-1 Important ligaments of the tarsocrural joint. (**A**) The tibiofibular ligament complex is responsible for the tight connection between the distal tibia and fibula. (**B**) The short medial collateral ligament consists of a straight tibiocentral and an oblique tibiotalar part. The tibiotalar part is partially hidden under the malleolus. (**C**) The short lateral collateral ligament has a calcaneofibular part, and a talofibular part. The calcaneofibular part of the lateral collateral ligament has an oblique and a straight branch.

Numerous short ligaments span the small bones of the tarsus. For functional reasons they can be divided into short dorsal and plantar ligaments, and short medial and lateral ligaments. The plantar ligaments are located on the tension side of the limb and are therefore subject to large tensile forces. A long ligament is present at the plantar side of the tarsus extending from the distal end of the calcaneus to both the fourth tarsal bone and the base of the fourth metatarsal bone.

40.2 Diagnosis and treatment options

Tarsal injuries usually cause obvious clinical signs, such as lameness, swelling, pain, and crepitus. Crepitus can be present with both instability and fractures. The integrity of the tarsal ligaments is assessed in hyperextension, hyperflexion, valgus, and varus stress.

Valgus and varus instability is usually caused by rupture of the tarsocrural collateral ligaments, but also may be present at the level of the talocentral, calcaneoquartal, centrodistal, or tarsometatarsal joints. Rupture of the short dorsal ligaments results in hyperextension at the affected level, whereas rupture of the plantar ligaments causes hyperflexion. Cats have more normal joint laxity than dogs, and comparison of the range of motion of the contralateral normal joint helps when examining cases with minor instability.

Although the area of instability – dorsal, plantar, medial, or lateral – is usually easy to palpate, obtaining an exact anatomic location of the injury is difficult by palpation alone, and radiographs should be taken in an attempt to obtain a specific diagnosis. Routine radiographs are performed to diagnose or rule out fractures. Stress radiographs are obtained in valgus and varus stress for medial and lateral instability, and in hyperflexion and hyperextension for plantar or dorsal instabilities.

The possibility of a tendon injury should also be considered, especially in cats with a plantigrade stance. The common calcaneal tendon is palpated to detect tendon swelling, avulsion fractures, or rupture. Luxation of the superficial digital flexor tendon is rare but has been described in one cat (3).

Arthritis is another potential differential diagnosis to consider in the presence of swollen and painful tarsal joints. Immune-mediated polyarthritis frequently manifests in the tarsal joints (Chapter 5), and cat bite wounds or other open injuries can cause a septic monoarthropathy (Chapter 14). Common tarsal injuries and their treatment options are listed in Table 40-1.

40.3 Approaches to the tarsal joint

A medial approach to the tarsocrural joint (4) is used to explore the medial malleolus, the medial collateral ligament,

Location of lesion	Type of lesion	Treatment options
Achilles tendon rupture	Tendon rupture, avulsion	Tendon sutures and transarticular stabilization
Tarsocrural joint	Medial collateral ligament sprain	Ligament prosthesis Conservative treatment
	Fracture of the distal fibula	Tension band repair Divergent pins
	Tarsocrural luxation	Surgical repair and transarticular external skeletal fixation
Talocentral and calcaneoquartal joint	Dorsal instability Plantar instability	Adaptation plate Partial tarsal arthrodesis
Talocalcaneal and talocentral joint	Talocalcaneal luxation	Adaptation plate Talocalcaneal screw
Centrodistal and tarsometatarsal joints	Dorsal instability	Adaptation plate Dorsal tension band
	Plantar instability	Partial tarsal arthrodesis
Talus	Simple reducible fracture	Screw or pin stabilization
	Extra-articular comminuted fracture	Transarticular external skeletal fixator
	Intra-articular comminuted fracture	Pantarsal arthrodesis
Calcaneus	Fracture	Tension band repair
	Distal fracture with plantar instability	Partial tarsal arthrodesis

Table 40-1. Feline tarsal injuries and their treatment options

and the craniomedial aspect of the joint. The joint capsule is incised dorsal and parallel to the medial collateral ligament. A medial approach using a malleolar osteotomy (4) is rarely necessary, but can improve visualization, for example to repair a fracture of the proximomedial aspect of the talus. The lateral approach to the tarsocrural joint (4) is mainly used to stabilize lateral malleolar fractures. Care is taken not to injure the peroneus tendons during incision of the fascia and extensor retinaculum.

The medial and dorsomedial aspect of the tarsal bones is accessed by incising the fascia dorsal to the tendon of the cranial tibial muscle (4). The tendon is retracted medially. This approach is used for dorsal stabilization of intertarsal and tarsometatarsal instabilities, and for stabilization of talocalcaneal luxation. A lateral approach to the calcaneus and lateral and plantarolateral aspect of the tarsal bones is often used for partial tarsal arthrodesis (4).

The calcaneus and the Achilles tendon are approached from laterally (4). The fascial incision is made along the lateral border of the superficial digital flexor tendon, and is continued along the caudolateral border of the calcaneus. The approach can be extended distally to the lateral or caudal aspect of the bones of the tarsus (4).

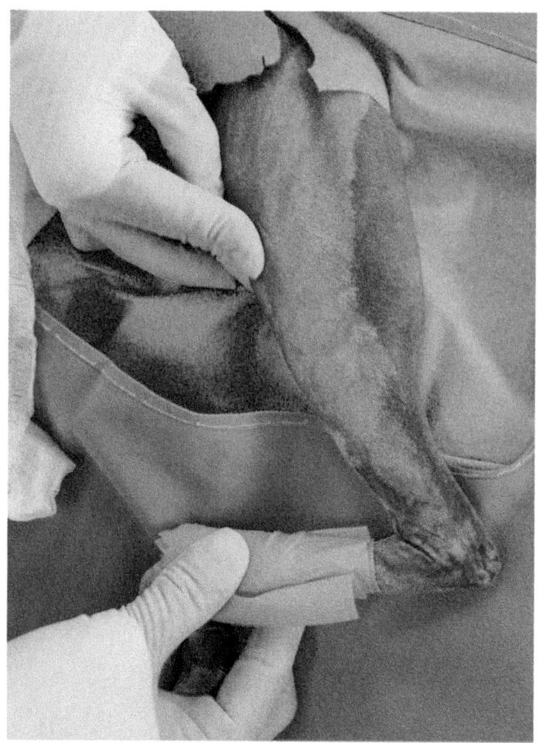

Figure 40-2 A cat with rupture of the Achilles tendon. The tarsal joint can be flexed while the stifle joint is held in extension.

40.4 Rupture or avulsion of the Achilles tendon

The Achilles tendon mechanism is composed of three separate tendons: the tendon of the gastrocnemius muscle; the common tendon of the semitendinosus, gracilis, and biceps femoris muscles; and the tendon of the superficial digital flexor muscle. The superficial digital flexor tendon courses over the calcaneus to insert on the plantar aspect of the middle phalanges of the second to fifth digits. In cats, an additional muscle, the soleus muscle, has a small tendon joining the Achilles tendon laterally (2). The muscles and tendons of the Achilles mechanism extend the tarsal joint and flex the toes.

Disruption of the Achilles tendon mechanism is relatively rare in cats. Based on clinical impressions, most injuries are closed ruptures or avulsions of the tendons from the tuber calcanei. Cats with acute rupture of the Achilles tendon mechanism usually present with a non-weight-bearing lameness and hyperflexion of the hock. Palpation of the Achilles tendon reveals loss of continuity of the tendon, thickening, swelling, and pain. Skin wounds are present when the tendon has been lacerated with a sharp object. Diagnosis of functional deficits of the Achilles tendon mechanism is confirmed if the tarsal joint can be flexed while the stifle joint is held in extension (Fig. 40-2). If the superficial digital flexor tendon is intact, the toes flex simultaneously.

With chronic injuries the cat may bear weight on the affected leg but with a plantigrade stance. Causes such as a diabetic neuromyopathy or neurological lesions such as injury of the tibial nerve have to be considered as differential diagnoses for a plantigrade stance. Bilateral chronic sprains of the Achilles tendon can occur (Fig. 40-3), but the underlying pathology has not been described (Chapter 7).

Radiographs are obtained to detect avulsion fractures of the insertion of the tendons on the tuber calcaneus, and local soft-tissue swelling. Radiographs of the whole crus should be obtained to evaluate the position of the fabellas. Ultrasonography can also be used to confirm the diagnosis, and to specify further the degree and localization of the lesion (Chapter 2).

Surgical treatment is indicated in most cases because of disabling functional deficits. A longitudinal skin incision is performed over the caudolateral surface of the tendon. The individual tendons are identified if possible. The proximal ends may be displaced quite far proximally. Debridement of blood clots and excision of excessively frayed tendon ends may be necessary. The tendons are then individually sutured with a locking-loop or a three-loop pulley pattern, using monofilament non-absorbable suture material (Chapter 16). The sutures can be anchored through a bone tunnel in the calcaneus, if insufficient tendon remains distally. It may not be possible to identify the individual tendons in chronic inju-

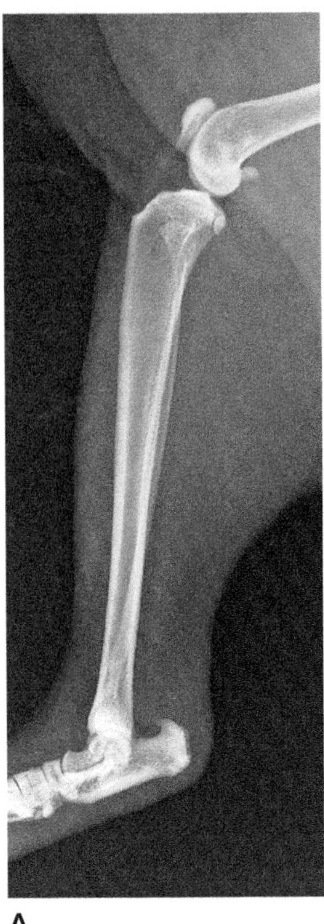

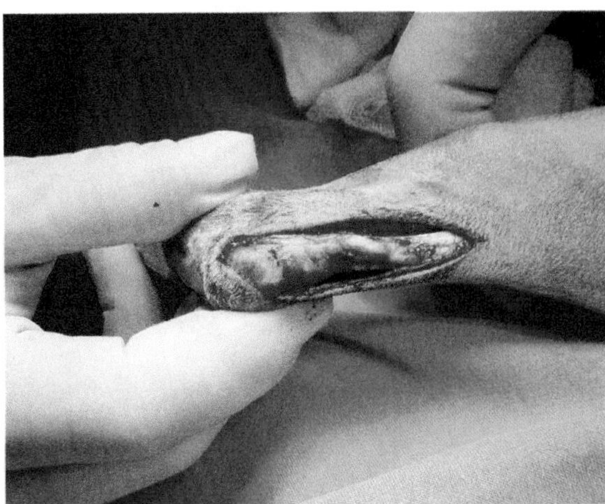

A B

Figure 40-3 (**A**) Mediolateral radiograph of the right crus, and (**B**) intraoperative appearance of a cat with bilateral rupture of the gastrocnemius tendon. Periosteal proliferations are present at the tuber calcaneus, indicating a chronic process, and the gastrocnemius tendon is thickened and avulsed from the tuber calcaneus. The cat suffered from hyperthyroidism.

ries, so the tendons are sutured as one. Care should be taken to obtain adequate functional tension, because the tendons tend to elongate during the healing process.

Postoperatively, a transarticular external fixator is usually applied for 3–4 weeks to immobilize the tarsal joint and allow formation of a fibrous scar. After removal of the external skeletal fixator a splinted bandage is applied for another 2 weeks. The splint does not restrict motion and tension completely, which allows maturation of the scar and longitudinal orientation of the collagen fibers. Tendon healing should have resulted in strong enough tissue to sustain weight-bearing forces after 6 weeks. Cats are kept indoors for approximately 3–4 months to avoid strenuous activity and the possibility of re-rupture.

40.5 Luxation of the superficial digital flexor tendon

The superficial digital flexor tendon crosses the tuber calcaneus during its distal course. Spontaneous or traumatic rupture of the retinaculum may cause luxation of the tendon, which is well reported in the dog (5–8). Lateral luxation of the superficial digital flexor tendon has been described in a 9-year-old, obese, neutered female Siamese cat, presented for chronic lameness (3). Clinical symptoms included swelling over the right calcaneal tendon, and the superficial digital flexor tendon could be subluxated laterally. At surgery the medial retinaculum was found to be edematous and the bursa below the tendon was distended. Treatment consisted of incising the medial retinaculum, and reapposing it to the medial edge of the superficial flexor tendon with non-absorbable suture material (3). The tendon remained in position in the cat described, and clinical outcome was excellent (3).

40.6 Tarsocrural instability and luxation

Tarsocrural instability or luxation results from various combinations of medial and lateral collateral ligament sprain, malleolar or fibular fractures, and disruption of the inferior tibiofibular ligament. Complete luxation is only possible if several of the above-mentioned structures are damaged. This severe injury is common in cats (1).

40.6.1 Collateral ligament sprain

Functional impairment of either the medial or lateral collateral ligament apparatus results in tarsocrural instability on the affected side. Collateral ligament sprains are more common than avulsion fractures of the ligament insertion sites at the malleoli. Degloving injuries can result in partial or complete abrasion of both the soft-tissue support and the malleoli on the affected side.

Collateral ligament sprains occur most commonly on the medial side, resulting in medial or valgus instability. Stress radiographs are performed to confirm the diagnosis (Fig. 40-4). Caudal subluxation of the talus is also seen occasionally, and is probably caused by rupture of the oblique parts of the collateral ligaments.

Surgical repair is advised for grades II and III ligament sprains causing clinical and radiographic instability. The torn ligaments are identified. Primary apposition and suturing are attempted, but may not be possible as the ligaments are short and often shredded. A ligament prosthesis should also be applied to protect the primary repair (Box 40-1). Although ideally the ligament prosthesis is performed to imitate both the straight tibiocentral and the oblique tibiotalar ligament,

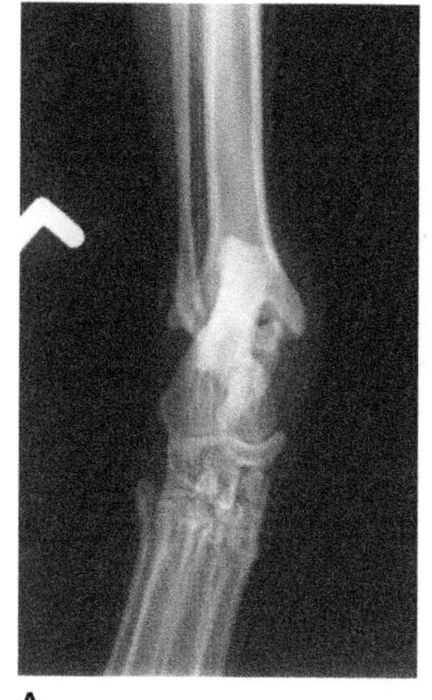

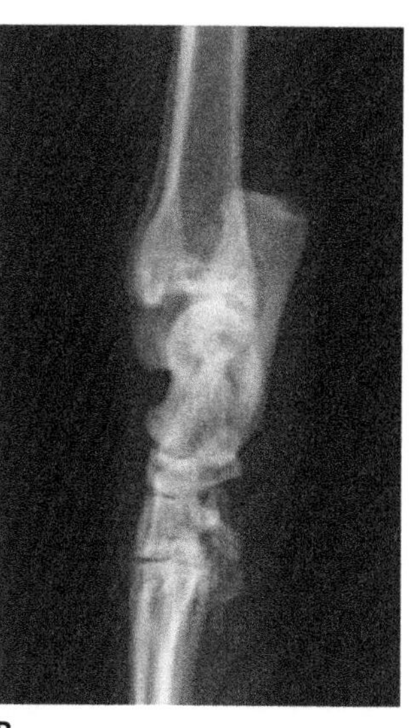

A B

Figure 40-4 (**A**) Valgus and (**B**) hyperextension stressed radiographs of a cat with a medial collateral ligament sprain. Note the opening of the medial aspect of the tibiotalar joint (**A**), and the caudal subluxation of the talus (**B**).

Box 40-1. Medial collateral ligament prosthesis

A medial approach to the talocrural joint is performed. The joint and periarticular structures are explored, and the joint is flushed. The accessible ligaments and joint capsule are sutured with 4-0 monofilament slowly absorbable suture material in a locking-loop or mattress pattern.

Ligament prosthesis using screws or suture anchors: For replacement of the straight tibiocentral ligament, one 1.5-mm screw or a small suture anchor is inserted in the medial malleolus, and one into the base of the talus or into the central tarsal bone. A figure-of-eight suture is preplaced around the screw heads, using 2-0 or 0 monofilament non-absorbable suture material (Fig. 40-5A). A washer is used if the suture tends to slip off the screw heads. The screws are fully inserted and the figure-of-eight suture is tightened. If instability persists, a ligament prosthesis can be added to mimic the oblique course of the tibiotalar ligament. An additional 1.5-mm screw is inserted into the calcaneus, close to the caudodistal edge of the malleolus. A figure-of-eight suture is applied around this screw and the screw in the malleolus (Fig. 40-5B).

Ligament prosthesis using the tunnel technique: Bone tunnels are drilled through the medial malleolus and through the base of the talus with a 1.1–1.5-mm drill bit or a small Kirschner wire. A 2.0 or 0 non-absorbable suture is passed through the tunnels in a figure-of-eight pattern, and is tightened.

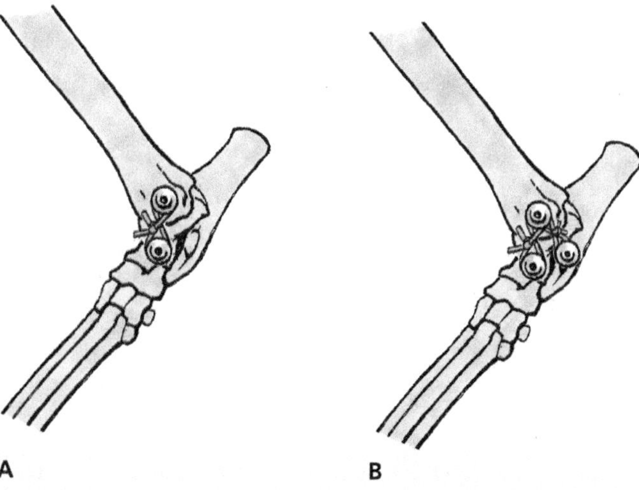

Figure 40-5 Options for application of a medial ligament prosthesis for the talocrural joint. (**A**) Prosthetic replacement of the straight tibiocentral ligament by applying a figure-of-eight suture around a screw in the malleolus and a screw in the base of the talus.
(**B**) Prosthetic replacement of both the straight tibiocentral and oblique tibiotalar ligament.

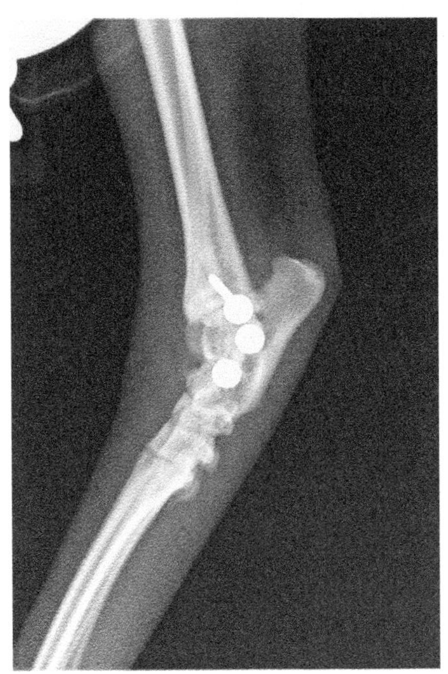

A

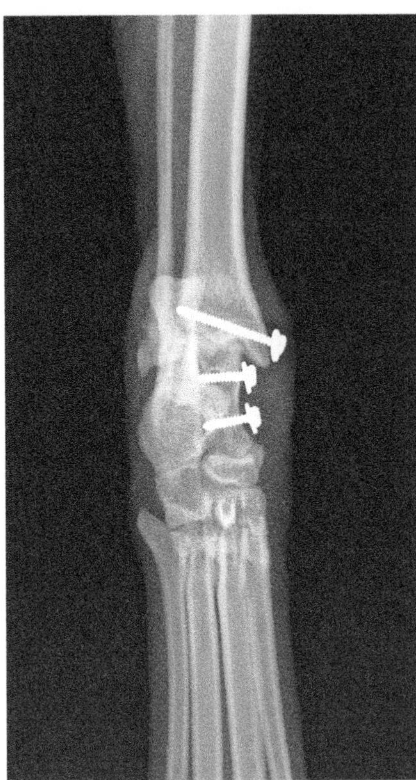

B

Figure 40-6 (**A**) Mediolateral and (**B**) dorsoplantar radiographs of a cat with medial collateral ligament rupture, 4 weeks after surgical repair. Both the straight and oblique portions of the medial collateral ligament were stabilized in this case.

this is difficult in cats because the tibiotalar part of the medial collateral ligament is hidden under the malleolus. The straight tibiocentral ligament is replaced by insertion of one screw into the medial malleolus, and one screw into the base of the talus (Box 40-1). In cases where instability persists after replacement of the straight portion of the ligament, the oblique tibiotalar portion can be stabilized additionally by the insertion of a second screw into the calcaneus (Fig. 40-6).

As an alternative technique, the suture can be placed through bone tunnels drilled into the tibia and the head of the talus. The anatomic course of the ligaments is not fully respected with this technique, but the repair provides protection against valgus deviation.

In cases with avulsion fractures, the avulsed fragment is reattached to the tibia or malleolus with tension band fixation or a small screw. A mattress suture anchoring the ligament through a small tunnel in the malleolus can be used for very small fragments.

Postoperative immobilization is required after any type of repair. A splinted bandage is usually sufficient.

Surgical stabilization is often delayed in cats with degloving injuries. Temporary joint immobilization is performed with a splinted bandage or preferably a transarticular external fixator. The wound is managed appropriately until the presence of healthy granulation tissue indicates the wound to be free of infection (Chapter 16). Fibrous periarticular tissue, which is formed during immobilization by a transarticular external skeletal fixator, can result in sufficient joint stability to obviate the need for specific ligament replacement.

40.6.2 Fractures of the distal fibula

Instability of the lateral side of the tarsocrural joint is usually caused by fracture of the distal fibula. Fibular fractures often occur concurrent with disruptions of the tibiofibular ligament complex if they are located proximal to this connection. The loss of connection between fibula and tibia allows the fractured part of the fibula to displace laterally and distally, resulting in functional deficiency of the lateral collateral ligament complex (Fig. 40-7). The lateral restraint of the talus by the lateral malleolus is also lost. Surgical repair is always indicated to restore stability. A tension band fixation or two divergent pins can be used (Box 40-2). This injury may occur alone, but is commonly seen with tarsocrural luxation. Postoperative immobilization with a splinted bandage is sufficient in isolated injuries. In conjunction with tarsocrural luxation, a transarticular external skeletal fixator provides more stability (Box 40-3).

Avulsion fractures of the lateral malleolus distal to the tibiofibular ligament complex are rare, but also cause dysfunction of the lateral collateral ligament complex. A tension

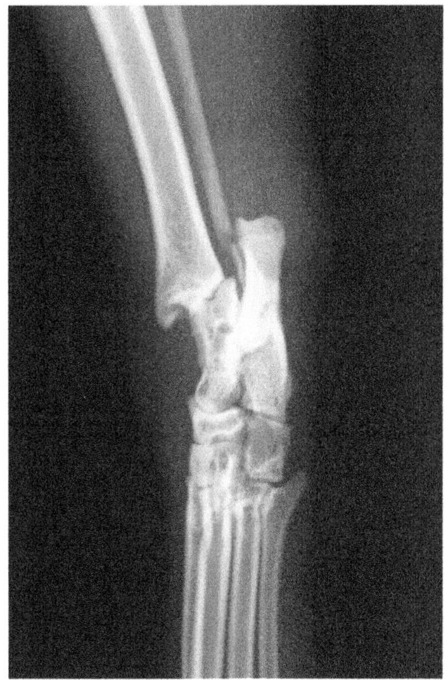

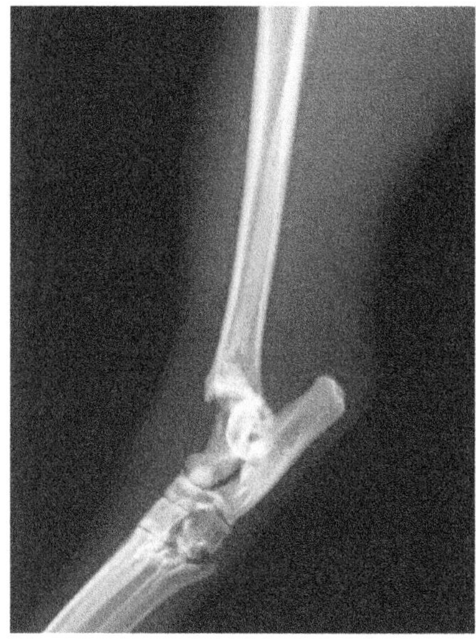

Figure 40-7 (**A**) Dorsoplantar and (**B**) mediolateral radiographs of the tarsus of a cat with a fracture of the distal fibula and disruption of the tibiofibular ligament complex. Note the displacement of the distal part of the fibula away from the tibia on the dorsoplantar view (**A**), and the tibiotalar subluxation on the mediolateral view (**B**).

Box 40-2. Stabilization of fractures of the distal fibula with disruption of the tibiofibular ligament complex

A lateral approach to the distal fibula and the talocrural joint is performed. The distal part of the fibula is anatomically reduced and carefully stabilized to the tibia with pointed reduction forceps. Reduction is also checked at the fracture site.

Divergent pins: Two 0.6–0.8-mm Kirschner wires are driven carefully from the distal end of the malleolus into the tibia. The pins have to be angled towards proximal to avoid entering the talocrural joint (Fig. 40-8A). Insertion of two well-seated divergent pins often results in sufficient pull-out resistance and stability. Pull-out resistance can be enhanced by using 1.0-mm negative-threaded pins in cases with a large-enough fragment. The pins are cut short after insertion.

Tension band fixation: A tension band wire should be placed additionally if the pins were inserted parallel to each other, or if only one pin could be used due to the small fragment size. A 0.5- or 0.6-mm piece of orthopedic wire is passed in a figure-of-eight fashion around the distal pin ends and through a hole drilled into the tibia, and tightened (Fig. 40-8B).

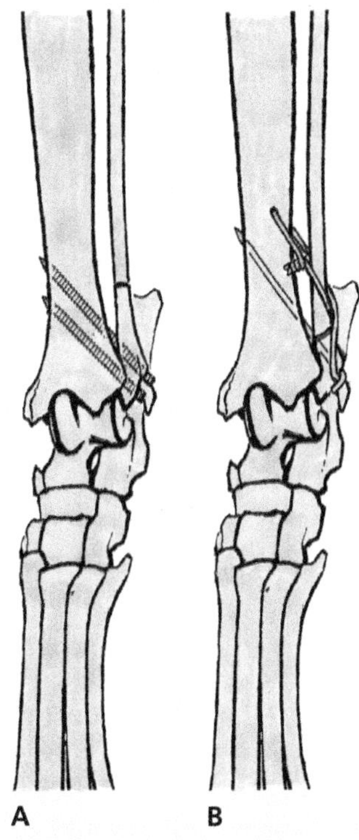

Figure 40-8 Options for repair of a distal fibular fracture.
(**A**) Stabilization of the distal fibula to the tibia with two divergent threaded pins.
(**B**) Tension band repair of a more distally located fracture using a single Kirschner wire and a figure-of-eight wire anchored to the tibia.

Box 40-3. Stabilization of tarsocrural luxations and application of a transarticular external skeletal fixator

Both a lateral and medial approach to the tarsocrural joint are necessary to stabilize the fractured fibula, and the ruptured medial collateral ligaments. The lateral approach is performed first and the joint is explored. A transarticular external skeletal fixator is often applied for postoperative immobilization.

Primary repair of structures: If the fibula is broken and the inferior tibiofibular ligament complex is ruptured, the fibula is attached to the tibia with two divergent pins or a tension band fixation as the first step (Box 40-2). Anatomic reduction of the lateral malleolus is required to restore normal joint congruity and stability. Avulsion fractures of the fibula distal to the inferior tibiofibular ligament are reattached with a small tension band fixation. The second step involves repair of medial collateral ligament ruptures, as described in Box 40-1. The joint is flushed, and the joint capsule is sutured. Range of motion and stability of the repair are assessed prior to wound closure.

Transarticular external fixator: A type II transarticular external fixator is used for postoperative immobilization if considered necessary to maintain stability. Several variations of fixator configuration can be used with the KE, SK, Meynard, or APEF systems. Two possible frame types are described.

Option 1 (Fig. 40-9A) – a 1.6-mm positive centrally threaded full pin is inserted into the proximal tibia, and 1.4–1.6-mm smooth or Ellis pin into the proximal metatarsi, medially and laterally. These pins are angled in a slightly dorsal direction to gain purchase of at least two metatarsal bones. Two connecting bars are bent to stabilize the tarsus at an angle of approximately 100–110°, and are connected to the transosseus pins. An additional 1.6-mm smooth, negative- or positive-threaded half pin is inserted into the distal tibia, avoiding placement through open wounds. Two more 1.2–1.4-mm pins are inserted distally into the proximal third of the metatarsal bones.

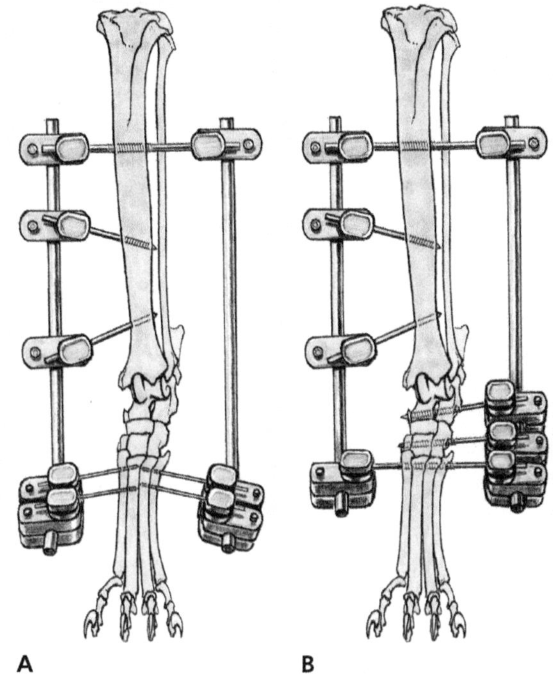

Figure 40-9 Two examples of transarticular external fixator configurations for temporary immobilization of the tarsus are shown.
(**A**) Type II transarticular external fixator with pins in the tibia and proximal metatarsi.
(**B**) Type II transarticular external fixator with pins in the tibia, tarsal bones, and proximal metatarsi.

Option 2 (Fig. 40-9B) – a pin is inserted into the proximal tibia as described above. A 1.2–1.4-mm smooth pin, or in larger cats a 1.6-mm smooth or centrally positive threaded pin is inserted as a full pin, through the base of the metatarsi. The pins are connected bilaterally with connecting rods, prebent to the standing angle of 100–110°. Additional 1.6-mm pins are inserted into the distal tibia, and across the tarsal bones.

band repair is used if the avulsed fragment is large enough. Otherwise, a collateral ligament prosthesis is performed.

40.6.3 Tarsocrural luxation

The medial and collateral ligament support and the inferior tibiofibular ligament are usually damaged in complete tarsocrural luxations. A classification for tarsocrural luxations based on human literature was suggested for cats (Table 40-2) (9). Type C is the most common type of luxation (Fig. 40-10). Type B luxations occur occasionally, and type A luxations are rare. Tarsocrural luxations are severe injuries, but satisfactory to good functional results can be achieved in many cats with restoration and repair of all damaged structures. The tarsocrural joint is reduced under general anesthesia, and stabilized in a splinted bandage until surgery is performed to minimize discomfort and prevent further cartilage damage. Surgery usually involves repair of the medial collateral ligament (Box 40-1), and stabilization of the fractured fibula to the tibia (Box 40-2).

In the presence of open tarsal luxations, early and aggressive cleaning of the wound and flushing of the joint are

Luxation type	Injuries	Tibiofibular ligament complex
Type A	Rupture of lateral collateral ligament or avulsion fracture of malleolus below the level of the tibiofibular joint Rupture or avulsion of the medial collateral ligament	Intact
Type B	Fracture of the distal fibula at the level of the tibiofibular ligament complex Rupture or avulsion of the medial collateral ligament	Partially disrupted
Type C	Fracture of the fibula proximal to the tibiofibular ligament complex Rupture or avulsion of the medial collateral ligament	Disrupted, resulting in dislocation of the distal fibula from the tibia

Table 40-2. Classification of tarsocrural luxations according to R. Vannini (9)

imperative to prevent joint infection. The wound is usually left to heal by second intention, because most of the wounds have to be considered dirty (Chapter 16). Open-wound treatment is conducted until healthy granulation tissue is present, allowing internal stabilization, as described above. The tarsocrural joint is best immobilized with a transarticular external skeletal fixator (Box 40-3) while the open injuries granulate. Further repair of the ruptured ligaments is often unnecessary in cases with severe soft-tissue loss, because, as the granulation tissue turns into fibrous and scar tissue, sufficient periarticular stability results.

A transarticular external fixator is also commonly used for postoperative joint immobilization (Box 40-3). These fixators are especially indicated in cases where postoperative stability seems insufficient, in heavy cats, and if other legs are injured. Type II constructs are used, because premature loosening of the distal pins was found to be a problem with type I transarticular fixators (10). External splints may be sufficient for postoperative stability in some cases. The external splint or external skeletal fixator is usually left in place for approximately of 3 weeks or until wound healing has advanced sufficiently.

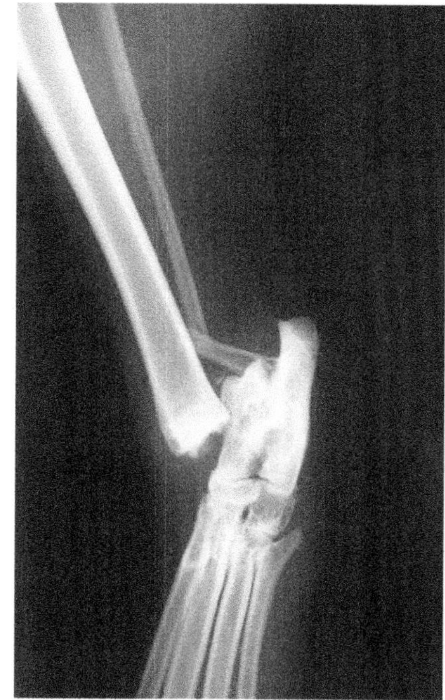

Figure 40-10 Cat with type C tarsocrural luxation. Note the displacement of the distal part of the fractured fibula away from the tibia, indicating disruption of the tibiofibular ligaments.

40.7 Intertarsal and tarsometatarsal instability

Intertarsal and tarsometatarsal instabilities result from disruption of the short ligaments spanning the individual joints. For simplicity, the talocentral and calcaneoquartal joints are referred to as the proximal intertarsal joint in the following text.

Three basic types of injuries can be encountered in the intertarsal or tarsometatarsal area: dorsal instabilities at one of the joint levels, talocalcaneal luxation, and plantar instabilities at one of the joint levels. Plantar intertarsal or tarsometatarsal ligament injuries are more disabling than dorsal ligament injuries, because the plantar side is under tension during weight-bearing and the dorsal side is under compression. Dorsal intertarsal and tarsometatarsal instabilities occur more commonly than plantar instabilities in the feline patient (11).

40.7.1 Dorsal intertarsal and tarsometatarsal instabilities

Rupture of the short dorsal ligaments is caused by hyperextension of the tarsal joints. Dorsal instabilities occur most commonly at the proximal intertarsal (Fig. 40-11) and the tarsometatarsal joint level. The centrodistal joint is rarely involved. Most patients have additional medial or lateral instability at the affected joint (11). The tarsometatarsal joint is completely luxated in some cases (Fig. 40-12). Concurrent

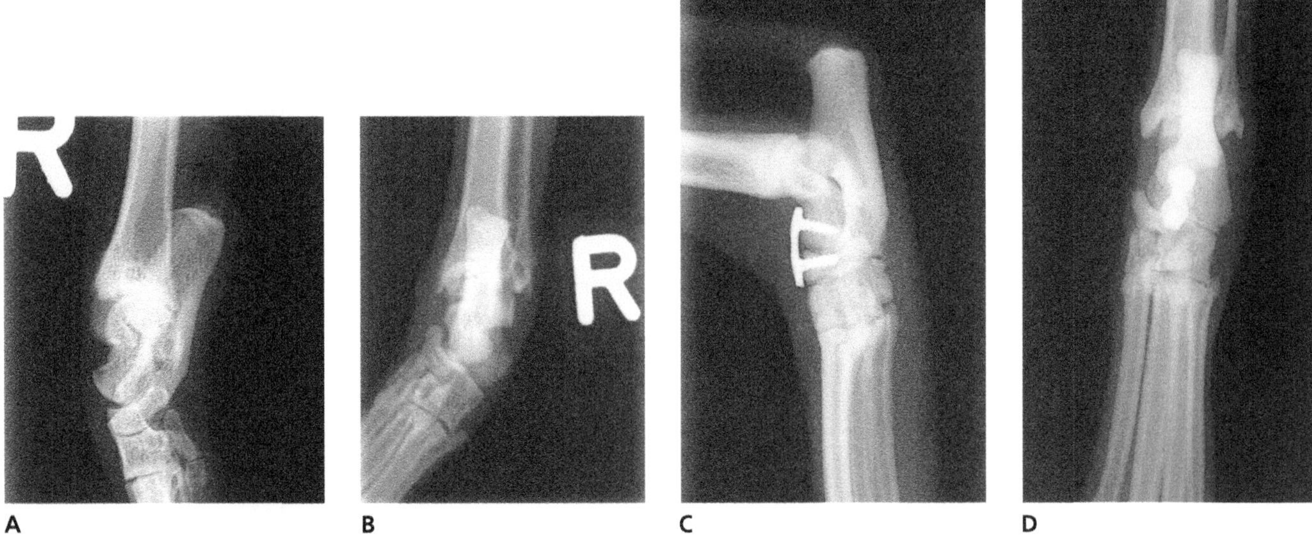

Figure 40-11 A cat with a dorsomedial proximal intertarsal instability.
(**A**, **B**) Preoperative hyperextension and valgus stress radiographs. Note the opening of the talocentral joint dorsally. Only minimal medial instability is present at the same level.
(**C**, **D**) The lesion was stabilized with a 2.0-mm Unilock plate with one screw inserted into the base of the talus, and one screw into the central tarsal bone.

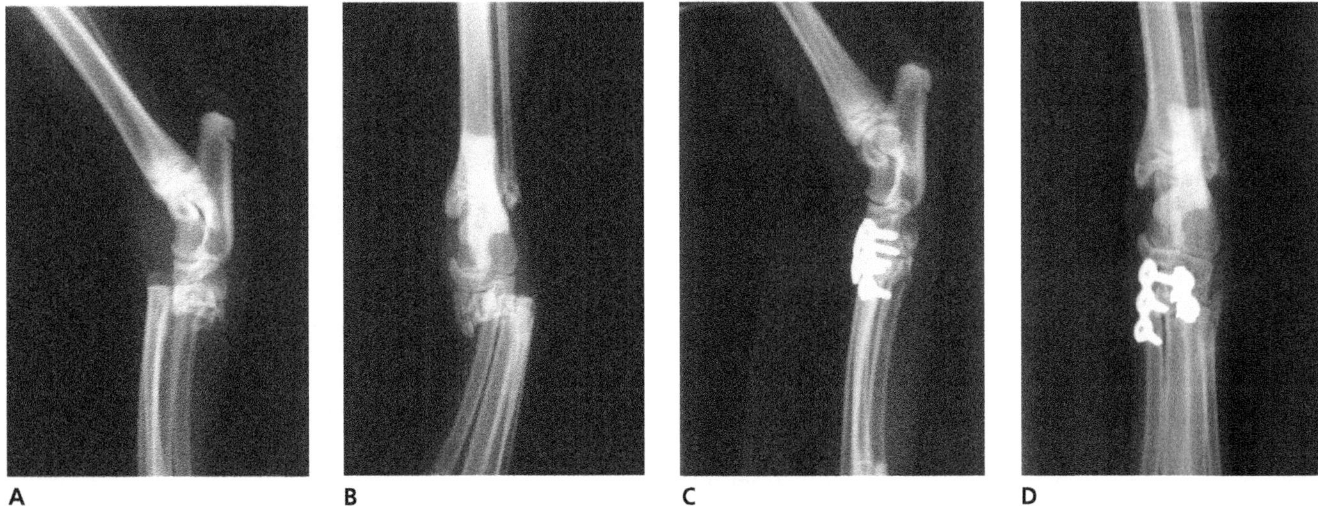

Figure 40-12 A cat with tarsometatarsal luxation.
(**A**, **B**) Mediolateral and dorsoplantar radiographs showing dorsal luxation of the tarsometatarsal joint. The plantar ligaments were considered stable on palpation after the joint had been reduced.
(**C**, **D**) Two short 2.0-mm Unilock plates were applied across the tarsometatarsal joints to prevent reluxation and to allow healing of the dorsal ligaments.

Box 40-4. Stabilization of dorsal intertarsal and tarsometatarsal instabilities

A dorsal approach is made over the affected area. The affected joint space is explored, flushed, and reduced. The implants are positioned over the area of instability. They may have to be applied in parallel if significant medial or lateral instability is present concurrently, and for tarsometatarsal instabilities.

Internal fixator: Internal fixators can be used for all types and levels of dorsal instabilities. One or two two-hole 2.0-mm locking plates are contoured if necessary and are applied across the lesion. One locking screw is inserted into the tarsal bone proximal, and one into the tarsal bone distal to the lesion for intertarsal instabilities (Fig. 40-13A). For tarsometatarsal instabilities, two screws are usually used in the metatarsal bone, and the application of a second plate is advantageous to improve stability (Fig. 40-12).

Miniplate: This type of repair can be used for dorsomedial instabilities at all levels, but has the disadvantage of bridging several joint rows. A 1.3- or 1.5-mm plate is contoured to match the dorsomedial aspect of the tarsus, from the neck of the talus to metatarsus II. One or two screws are inserted into the base and neck of the talus, one screw is inserted into the central tarsal bone, and two screws into the proximal metatarsal II (Fig. 40-13B).

Tension band repair: A tension band repair provides less stability than locking plates or the miniplate. One 1.5-mm screw is placed into the tarsal bone proximal and one distal to the lesion. A 0.5–0.6-mm orthopedic wire or a strong non-absorbable suture is positioned and tensioned around the screw heads in a figure-of-eight fashion (Fig. 40-13C).

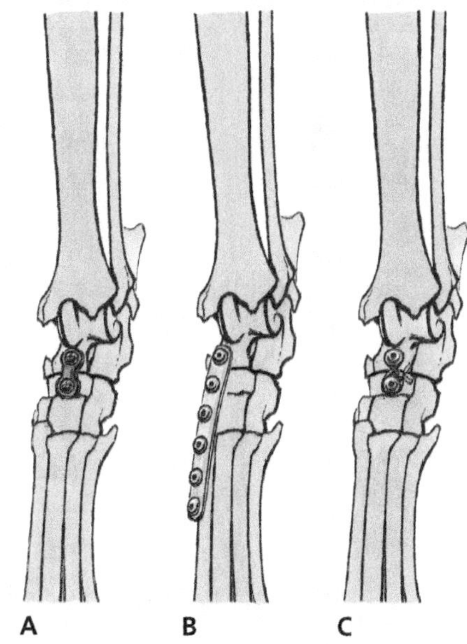

Figure 40-13 Options for stabilization of dorsal intertarsal and tarsometatarsal instability.
(**A**) Stabilization of a dorsal proximal intertarsal instability using a locking plate, with one screw in the base of the talus and one screw in the central tarsal bone.
(**B**) Stabilization of a dorsomedial proximal intertarsal instability with a 1.5-mm miniplate. A longer plate has to be used to provide sufficient stability.
(**C**) Tension band repair of a dorsal proximal intertarsal instability.

phalangeal fractures or luxations can occur and the radiographs need to be carefully scrutinized for these.

Because the short dorsal ligaments are not under tensile stress during weight-bearing, fibrous healing of the periarticular tissue results in restoration of functional joint stability if the affected joint is immobilized. Partial tarsal arthrodesis is not necessary. Minor instability of the dorsal aspect of the proximal intertarsal joint that is strictly limited to the dorsal aspect can be treated with a splinted bandage for 3 weeks. Significant dorsal instability and instability that also involves the medial or lateral intertarsal ligaments need to be treated surgically. Tarsometatarsal instability is always treated surgically.

The affected joint space is splinted with implants to allow fibrous tissue healing (Box 40-4). Locking plates are ideal implants for internal immobilization of dorsal intertarsal and tarsometatarsal instabilities (11). Due to the locking mechanism between the plate hole and the screw head, placement of only one screw proximal and one distal to the lesion results in stable fixation, allowing selective stabilization of only one joint level (Figs 40-11 and 40-12). Two short plates may have to be used in the presence of additional medial or lateral instability.

An alternative method to plating is tension band fixation using screws or pins and a figure-of-eight wire across the lesion (12). Miniplates can also be applied, but at least two screws are needed proximally and distally (13). The increase in plate length has the disadvantage that several joint rows have to be incorporated.

The implants can be removed after a time period of 4–6 weeks to avoid ankylosis of the affected joints. However, most owners decline implant removal because of the good clinical function of their animal (11).

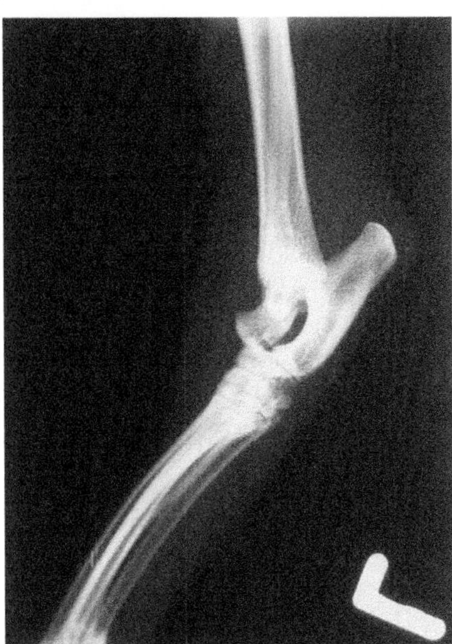

Figure 40-14 Mediolateral radiograph of a cat with a dorsal talocalcaneal luxation. The talocalcaneal ligaments are ruptured in addition to the talocentral ligament.

40.7.2 Talocalcaneal luxation

The talocalcaneal joint is a tight joint, but some rotational movement between the talus and the calcaneus is normal (14). Talocalcaneal luxation occurs if the talocalcaneal ligaments rupture. The most common form seen in cats is dorsal luxation of the base of the talus (Fig. 40-14). With this injury both the talocalcaneal and the talocentral ligaments are disrupted, allowing the base of the talus to slide along the central tarsal bone in a dorsal direction. The injury is thought to result from blunt trauma causing hyperextension and axial compression. Plantar talocalcaneal luxation rarely occurs.

Luxation of the base of the talus is a debilitating injury if left untreated because the weight-bearing axis from the talus to the central tarsal bone is lost. These injuries have an excellent prognosis with internal splinting using locking plates or miniplates (11, 15). The dorsally applied plates act as a buttress by preventing dorsal subluxation of the talus, and simultaneously stabilize the talocentral joint. The surgical technique is the same as described for proximal intertarsal instabilities (Box 40-4).

An alternative technique is insertion of a positional screw from the base of the talus into the calaneus (Box 40-5) (12, 14). A concern with this technique is early screw breakage due to residual motion in the talocalcaneal joint (14), but the technique seems to provide sufficient stability in cats.

40.7.3 Plantar intertarsal and tarsometatarsal instabilities

Plantar intertarsal and tarsometatarsal instabilities result from trauma causing excessive tensile stress on the plantar side of the tarsus. The calcaneoquartal joint and the tarsometatarsal joints are affected most commonly. Stress radiographs are used to diagnose the lesion (Fig. 40-16). Complete luxation at the affected joint level occurs in some cases.

Rupture of the plantar ligaments is a more severe injury than rupture of the dorsal ligaments, because loss of the plantar ligament support prevents weight-bearing, and the large tensile forces do not allow healing of the ligaments. Plantar instabilities are therefore treated by partial tarsal arthrodesis (Box 40-6).

40.8 Fractures of the tarsal bones

Fracture of the talus is the most common fracture type (1). Calcaneal fractures are occasionally encountered, whereas fractures of other tarsal bones are rare.

40.8.1 Fractures of the talus

Fractures of the talus are classified into intra-articular and extra-articular fractures. Intra-articular fractures extend into the tibiotalar joint, and include chip fractures along the lateral or medial trochlear ridge, and transverse and comminuted talar fractures. Extra-articular fractures include fractures of the talar body, neck, or head.

Chip fractures of the trochlear ridge are reattached with small countersunk Kirschner wires if the fragment is large enough (Fig. 40-18). Small fragments can be removed and the prognosis is good (1). Transverse intra-articular fractures can be repaired with a small lag screw and an antirotational pin, taking care to restore the joint surface anatomically. Unfortunately, most of the intra-articular talar fractures are comminuted, rendering restoration of the joint impossible. Pantarsal arthrodesis is then the only treatment option (Box 40-7).

Simple fractures of the talar body or neck can be stabilized with cross pins or with a dorsally applied 1.5-mm miniplate or 2.0-mm locking plate, as described in Box 40-4. Application of a temporary transarticular external fixator for about 3 weeks is advisable to protect the primary repair (Box 40-3). Indirect stabilization of talar neck fractures in five cats with a transarticular external skeletal fixator alone for a time period of 8–12 weeks was also described (16). However, prolonged joint immobilization is likely to reduce range of motion of the joint, cause cartilage degeneration, and promote degenerative joint disease.

Box 40-5. Stabilization of a talocalcaneal luxation

A dorsomedial approach to the talocentral joint is performed. The head of the talus is reduced, using digital pressure.

Internal fixator: A 2.0-mm locking plate is applied across the talocentral joint, using one screw proximal, and one distal to it, as described in Box 40-4.

Positional screw: A pair of pointed reduction forceps is placed between the talus and calcaneus to hold the reduction. A 1.5-mm drill hole is made from the talus into the calcaneus. An appropriate-length positional screw is inserted across the two bones after tapping the thread (Fig. 40-15).

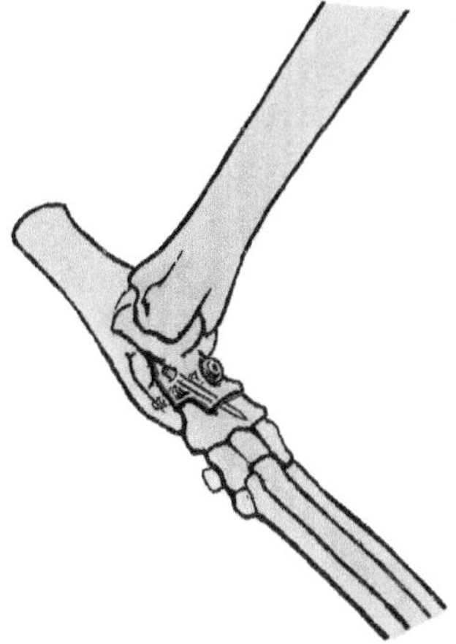

Figure 40-15 Stabilization of a talocalcaneal luxation using a 2.0-mm positional screw, inserted across the talocalcaneal joint. Additional insertion of a small pin across the talocentral joint may improve stability.

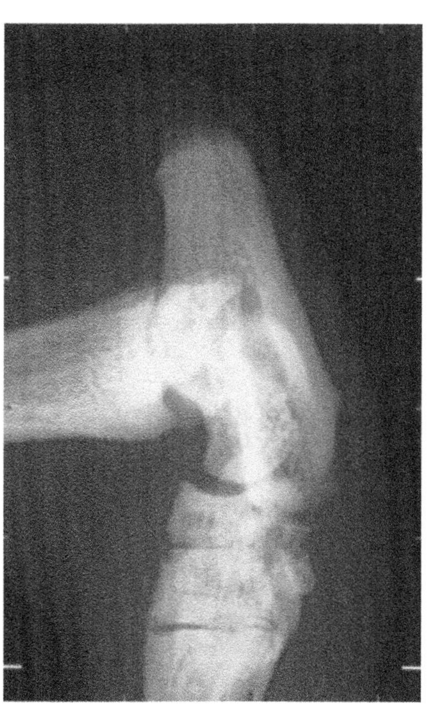

A

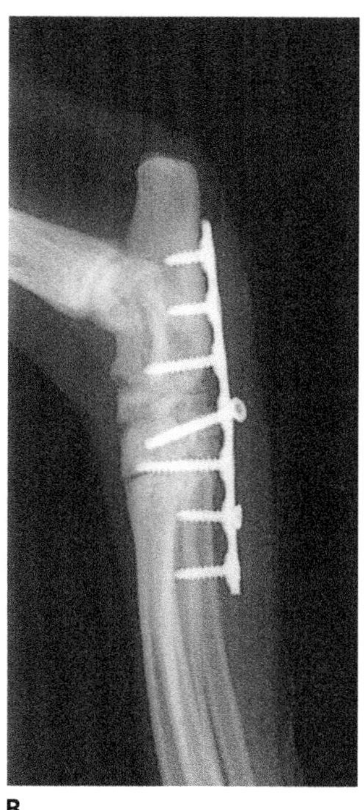

B

Figure 40-16 A cat with plantar calcaneoquartal instability. (**A**) Preoperative stress radiographs showing plantar instability. (**B**) Follow-up radiographs 1 month after partial arthrodesis with a 2.0-mm locking plate positioned on the plantar aspect of the tarsus.

40.8.2 Fractures of the calcaneus

Fractures of the calcaneus are rare but disabling injuries, because the calcaneus is subject to large tensile forces. It serves as the insertion site for the Achilles tendon and acts as a fulcrum for the superficial digital flexor tendon. Calcaneal fractures may involve the tuber calcanei, the shaft, or the base.

Fractures of the tuber or shaft are best treated by tension band fixation. Shaft fractures can be stabilized with a plate applied to the lateral or plantar surface of the calcaneus.

Avulsion fractures of the base of the calcaneus are often associated with plantar intertarsal instability because the plantar calcaneoquartal ligaments insert at the base of the calcaneus. Although lag screw fixation of larger fragments is

Box 40-6. Partial tarsal arthrodesis

The surgical approach is selected according to the method of arthrodesis to be used. The cartilage in the affected joint spaces is removed with small bone curettes or a power bur. Cancellous bone graft is packed into the joint spaces, and at the end of surgery any remaining graft is placed adjacent to the joints.

Calcaneoquartal arthrodesis with a pin and tension band wire: A caudolateral approach to the calcaneus and fourth tarsal bone is performed. A 1.2–2.6-mm Kirschner wire is driven into the calcaneus from its proximal end and directed towards its base. Once the pin emerges in the calcaneoquartal joint, the joint is reduced. The Kirschner wire is then further advanced into the distal aspect of the fourth tarsal bone. It is cut short proximally. A 0.8-mm orthopedic wire is passed through predrilled holes in the calcaneus and fourth tarsal bone in a figure-of-eight fashion, and is tightened bilaterally (Fig. 40-17A). Passing the wire dorsal to the pin as shown proximally reduces risk of wire pull-out.

Calcaneoquartal arthrodesis with a lateral plate: A caudolateral approach to the calcaneus, intertarsal and tarsometatarsal joints, and fifth metatarsal bone is performed. Several types of plates or internal fixators can be used, including a 2.0-mm dynamic compression plate (DCP), a 1.5/2.0-mm veterinary cuttable plate, or a 2.0-mm Unilock plate. The selected plate is contoured to the plantarolateral surface of the calcaneus, fourth tarsal bone, and fifth metacarpal bone. Two or three screws are placed in the calcaneus, one or two screws are inserted into the fourth tarsal bone, and two screws are placed in the fifth metatarsal bone (Fig. 40-17B). A plantar figure-of-eight wire can also be applied.

Tarsometatarsal arthrodesis with a laterally and/or medially applied plate: A 2.0-mm DCP, 1.5/2.0-mm veterinary cuttable plate, or a 2.0-mm internal fixator can be used. A lateral plate is applied in a similar manner to that described for calcaneoquartal arthrodesis, with three screws inserted distal and three proximal to the tarsometatarsal joints (Fig. 40-17C). For medial plating, a medial approach is made to the talus, intertarsal and metatarsal joints. The plate is contoured to the medial surface of the talus, central tarsal bone, and second metatarsal bone (Fig. 40-17D). One to two screws are placed into the talus, one screw into the central tarsal bone, and three screws in the second metatarsal bone.

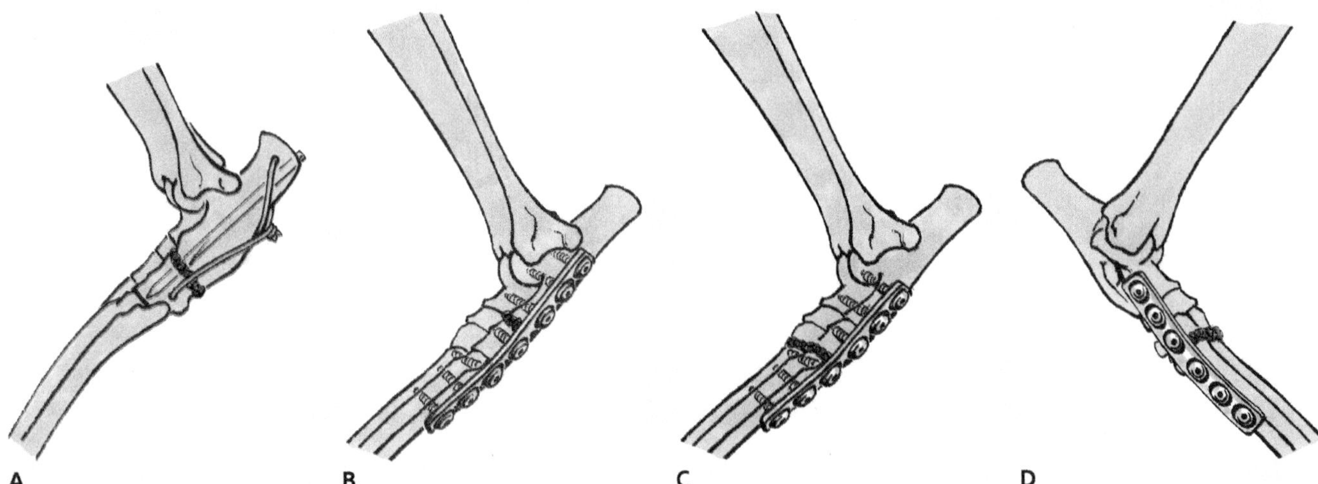

Figure 40-17 Options for partial tarsal arthrodesis.
(**A**) Calcaneoquartal arthrodesis for stabilization of a plantar proximal intertarsal instability using a pin and plantar tension band technique.
(**B**) Calcaneoquartal arthrodesis with a laterally applied plate. A plantar tension band wire can be used in addition.
(**C**) Tarsometatarsal arthrodesis with a laterally applied plate.
(**D**) Tarsometatarsal arthrodesis with a medially applied plate.

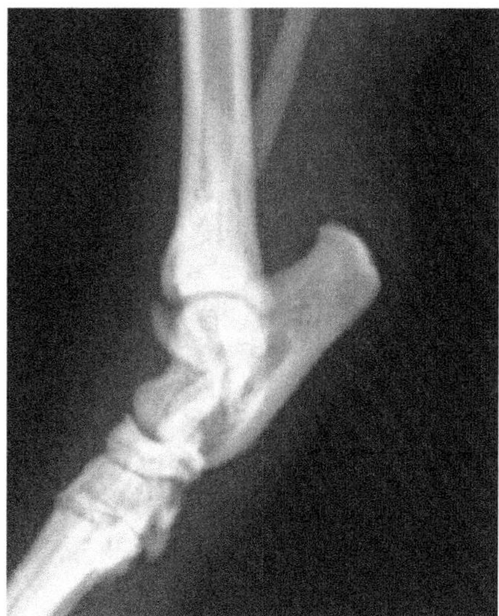
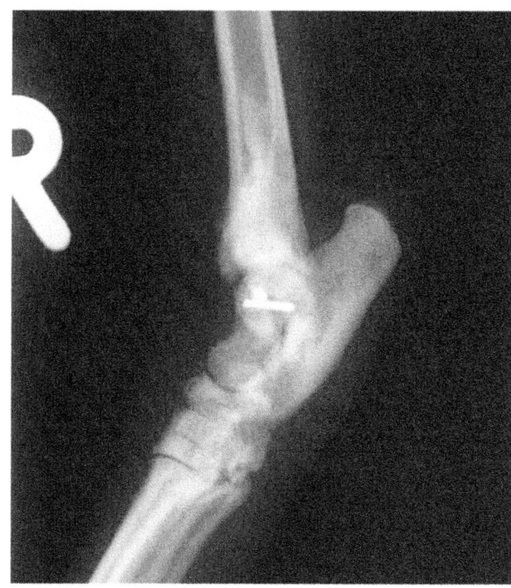

A B

Figure 40-18 A cat with a talar fracture. (**A**) Preoperative laterolateral radiograph showing a small fracture fragment off the cranial part of the lateral trochlear ridge, which is displaced dorsally. (**B**) The fragment was reattached in anatomic reduction using a 1.0-mm miniscrew and a small pin.

described for dogs, the avulsed fragment is likely to be too small for primary stabilization in cats, and partial tarsal arthrodesis as described for plantar ligament injuries is usually necessary (Box 40-6).

40.9 Partial tarsal arthrodesis

Partial tarsal arthrodesis is performed for conditions of the proximal intertarsal to tarsometatarsal joint levels, where pain-free normal joint function cannot be restored by other means. The main indications are plantar ligament instability (Fig. 40-16), luxations, and comminuted fractures of the distal rows of tarsal bones. Concurrent trauma of the tarsocrural joint has to be ruled out before partial tarsal arthrodesis is performed. Several methods have been described for partial tarsal arthrodesis in dogs, some of which can also be used in the cat.

Arthrodesis of the calcaneoquartal joint can be performed with a pin and tension band technique or with a plate (17) (Box 40-6). Although neither was proven superior, the pin and tension band technique should only be used for plantar calcaneoquartal instabilities. In the presence of concurrent fractures, plating is preferred. Plates can be applied to the lateral or plantar surface of the calcaneus and distal tarsus.

Arthrodesis of the tarsometatarsal joints is best achieved with a laterally or medially applied plate (18, 19) (Box 40-6). A Steinmann pin and cross-pinning technique and the use of a type II external skeletal fixator with acrylic bars have also been described (20, 21). Transarticular external skeletal fixators are mainly indicated in the presence of open injuries. Care must be taken to ensure that the foot does not become externally rotated when inserting screws into the metatarsal bones.

Regardless of the method used, the affected joint spaces have to be debrided of cartilage and cancellous or corticocancellous bone graft is used to facilitate bony fusion (Chapter 14). Inadequate preparation of the joints carries the risk of delayed union and subsequent implant failure.

40.10 Pantarsal arthrodesis

Pantarsal arthrodesis is indicated for stabilization of the tarsus after injuries or disease involving the tarsocrural joint that cannot be treated by other means. These include comminuted articular distal tibial fractures, comminuted articular talar fractures (Fig. 40-20), unreconstructable tarsocrural luxations, and joint destruction after severely debilitating degenerative or inflammatory joint disease (22). Arthrodesis of the talocrural joint alone has been shown to be associated with a poorer functional outcome than panarthrodesis in dogs (23). Panarthrodesis is therefore preferred by most surgeons, even if only the tarsocrural joint is affected.

Pantarsal arthrodesis is most commonly performed with a dorsally applied plate. However, dorsal plating is less than ideal from a biomechanical point of view, because the plate is positioned on the compression side of the joint, and is subject to large bending forces. Implant loosening and plate breakage are common consequences (24). Adequate preparation of the joint surfaces, correct screw positioning, and bone grafting are necessary to obtain good results if this technique is used. The addition of an intramedullary pin placed from the tibia across the tibiotalar joint has been shown to improve stability when compared to dorsal plating alone (25). A common cause for poor functional results and complications is inadequate incorporation and stabilization of the calcaneus in the arthrodesis. This is thought to result from residual

Box 40-7. Pantarsal arthrodesis

The standing angle of the tarsus is measured preoperatively on the contralateral leg. It is often between 90 and 110°. It is usually better to stabilize the tarsus in a slightly more flexed, rather than extended, angle. The surgical approach is selected according to the method of arthrodesis to be used. Regardless of the surgical stabilization technique, the joint cartilage is removed from the tibiotalar, and the proximal, distal, and tarsometatarsal joints. Osteostixis is performed in avascular bone to create channels for vascular ingrowth. Cancellous bone graft is packed into the joint spaces to shorten healing time. Cancellous or corticocancellous graft is additionally placed around the joints at the end of surgery. An intramedullary pin, inserted from the proximal tibia (Chapter 39) into the talus, can be used in addition to dorsal or medial plating.

Pantarsal arthrodesis with a dorsal plate: A dorsal approach to the distal tibia, tarsus, and third metatarsal bone is performed. A 1.5/2.0-mm stacked veterinary cuttable plate, a 2.7/2.0-mm pancarpal arthrodesis plate, a 2.4-mm limited contact-dynamic compression plate, or a 2.4-mm Unilock plate is prebent to achieve the desired flexion angle of the tarsus. The plate is first secured to the third metatarsal bone with three or four 1.5–2.4-mm bone screws, depending on which plate is used. The plate is then attached to the tibia with a bone clamp, and the angle and alignment are checked. If alignment is considered correct, four screws are inserted into the tibia. Ideally, the most distal of those screws should incorporate the distal margin of the tibia, the talus, and the calcaneus. The two remaining screw holes are then filled, with the screws aimed to go through both the talus and the calcaneus (Fig. 40-19A).

Pantarsal arthrodesis with a medial plate: A dorsomedial approach to the distal tibia, tarsal bones, and second metatarsal bone is performed. After debridement of all joints, the tibiotarsal joint is temporarily stabilized with an intramedullary nail or with cross pins at the desired angle and alignment. Angle and alignment are checked. A customized pantarsal arthrodesis plate or a 2.0- or 2.4-mm Unilock plate can be used. The Unilock plates are contoured as necessary along their broad axis to obtain the correct flexion angle. When using the customized pantarsal arthrodesis plate no contouring is necessary, but the medial malleolus and proximal metatarsal bone should be removed to form a smooth flat surface for the bone to lie against.

The first screws are inserted into the metatarsal bone, then into the tibia, and finally into the talus. The screw through the talus should also engage the calcaneus. Care must be taken that the foot does not become externally rotated. Altogether, at least three screws should be inserted into the tibia: one into the talus and calcaneus, one into the distal tarsal bones, and two or three into the metatarsal bones V and IV (Fig. 40-19B). The intramedullary nail or cross pins used for initial stabilization can be left in place if they seem to add to stability; otherwise they are removed.

Pantarsal arthrodesis with an external skeletal fixator: A dorsal approach is used to prepare the joint spaces and insert the bone graft. A type II external skeletal fixator is applied, as described in Box 40-3. Angle of the joint and alignment of the limb are checked when the curved external bars have been fixed to the first pins bilaterally.

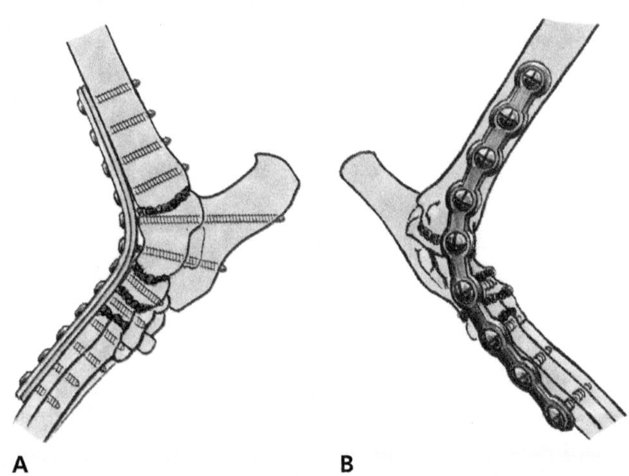

Figure 40-19 Options for performing a pantarsal arthrodesis. (**A**) Arthrodesis with a dorsally applied plate. It is important to engage the calcaneus with one or two screws. (**B**) Arthrodesis with a medially applied Unilock plate.

motion in the talocalcaneal and calcaneoquartal joints due to the pull of the Achilles tendon, so at least two screws must incorporate the calcaneus (26).

Pantarsal arthrodesis can also be performed with a medially or laterally applied plate (27). Customized plates are available from Veterinary Instrumentation (Sheffield, UK) for this indication. Alternatively, the 2.0- or 2.4-mm Unilock mandible-locking plates can be used. Pantarsal arthrodesis using a type II external skeletal fixator is another good alternative for panarthrodesis of the tarsus in cats. The main indication for this technique is the presence of open or infected tarsal injuries (Figs 40-19 and 40-21).

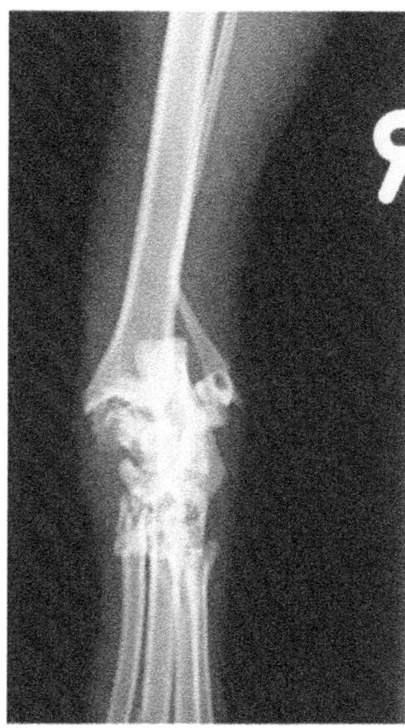

Figure 40-20 Radiograph of a cat with tibiotarsal luxation and a comminuted talar fracture. Pantarsal arthrodesis is the only suitable treatment option for such cases.

40.11 Postoperative treatment and prognosis

40.11.1 Tarsocrural instability

External immobilization of the tarsus is provided with a splinted bandage after surgical repair of medial collateral ligament sprains. The splint is usually left in place for 2–3 weeks. Care is taken to avoid pressure sores, especially over the tuber calcanei. Activity is restricted by keeping the cat indoors for another 1–2 months. Radiographs are usually taken before removal of the splinted bandage to check for evidence of joint subluxation and maintenance of position of the screws or suture anchors. Screws may have to be removed if they migrate or cause other problems due to their close vicinity to the joint. The prognosis for return to full function is good.

A transarticular external fixator may be used instead of a splinted bandage in the presence of large degloving injuries, or if difficulties are anticipated in keeping a splint in place. The external fixator provides rigid immobilization during bandage changes, and facilitates wound healing or skin graft incorporation. The prognosis for degloving injuries is generally good (28), but a risk of joint infection and restriction of range of motion due to scar tissue formation and wound contracture remains.

40.11.2 Tarsocrural luxation

Postoperative immobilization is always required after tarsocrural luxation. Temporary immobilization with a transarticular external skeletal fixator provides the best stability,

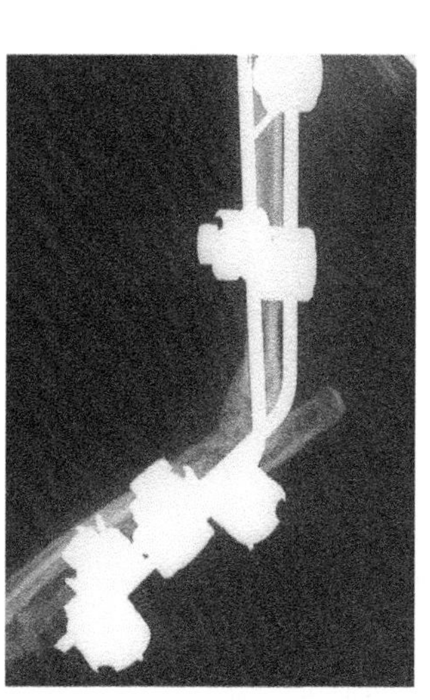

A

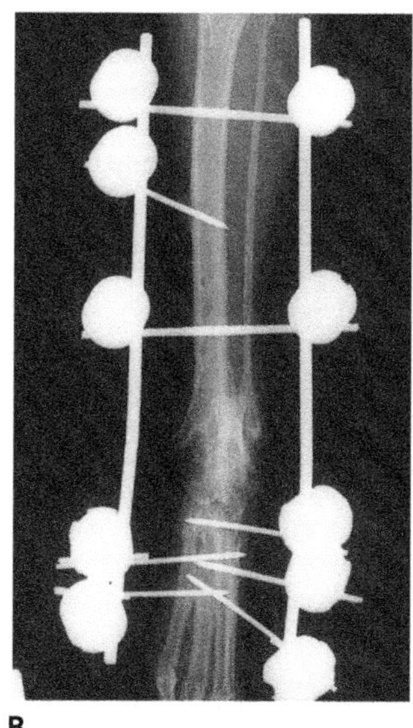

B

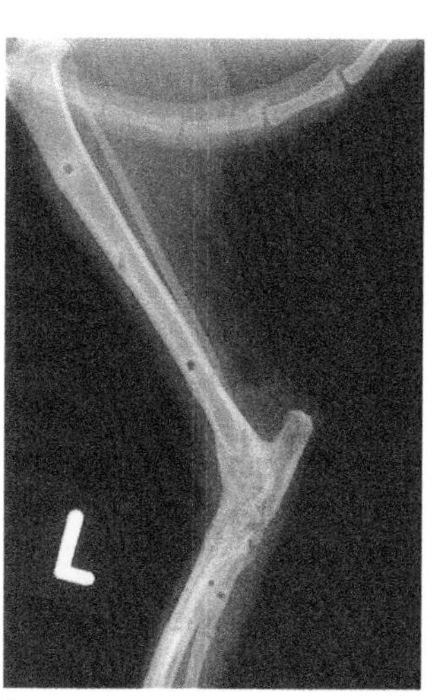

C

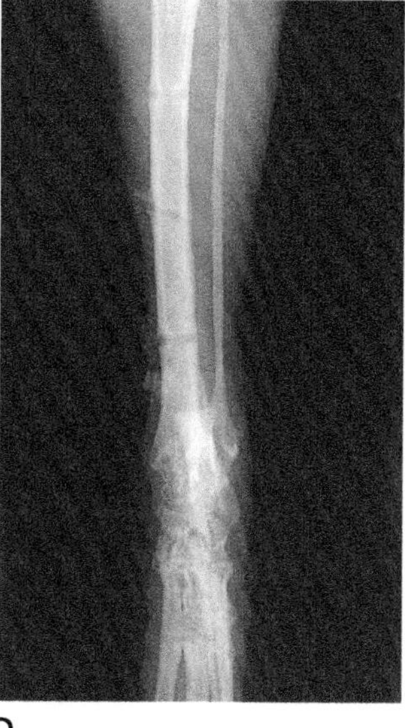

D

Figure 40-21 Pantarsal arthrodesis using a type II external skeletal fixator.
(**A, B**) The fixator was applied 1 month earlier to revise an infected arthrodesis. The screw holes of the dorsal plate are still visible.
(**C, D**) Radiographs after removal of the external skeletal fixator 4 months later. All joint rows are well bridged with bone.

but a cast or a splint could also be used. Although the tarsus is often immobilized for a time period of 3–4 weeks, earlier mobilization may be preferred in some cases. Cats with a cast or splint for only 10 days and early physiotherapy tended to have a better outcome than cats with a splint for 3–4 weeks in a study on nine cats with tarsocrural luxation (29). Early removal of the external immobilization device after 10 days requires absolute stability of the surgical repair and is only used if the surgeon feels confident with fixation stability. If stability of the repair is considered to be suboptimal, it is safer to leave the external fixation device for a longer period.

Activity of the cat must be strictly restricted for 4 weeks after early removal of the external immobilization device. Overall, cats are confined to the house for 3 months.

Degenerative joint disease will develop in all cats with tarsocrural luxation, and can be quite severe. Intermittent or permanent lameness may result in some cats. In a study of nine cats clinical outcome was unsatisfactory in one cat, moderate in four cats, and good to excellent in four cats (29). Chronic low-grade joint infection should be ruled out in cats with less than ideal function, especially if the initial injury was open. A course of antibiotics is administered if infection is suspected or diagnosed (Chapters 13 and 14). Treatment of degenerative joint disease is described in Chapter 5. Pantarsal arthrodesis can be performed as a salvage procedure in patients with chronic pain and clinical dysfunction.

40.11.3 Dorsal intertarsal and tarsometatarsal instabilities

External support is not necessary after stable internal immobilization of dorsal intertarsal and tarsometatarsal instabilities with plates or internal fixators, but the cats should be confined indoors with restricted activity for 3–4 weeks. External immobilization with a splinted bandage may be chosen for 10 days after having used a tension band technique with screws and wire.

The implants can be removed after 4–6 weeks to prevent unwanted joint fusion secondary to prolonged immobilization (11). However, signs of impeding ankylosis did not seem to affect clinical function. Return to function is fast, and the prognosis is excellent for cats with dorsomedial or dorsolateral intertarsal and tarsometatarsal injuries, stabilized with Unilock plates (11).

40.11.4 Partial and pantarsal arthrodeses

Postoperative immobilization of the joint is recommended after both partial tarsal and pantarsal arthrodesis. Immobilization should not exceed 4 weeks after partial tarsal arthrodesis to preserve function and mobility of the tarsocrural joint. Healing of an arthrodesis takes at least 3 months, and cats should be confined indoors until radiographic healing is evident. Control radiographs are usually performed after 6 weeks and 3 months. Partial tarsal arthrodesis usually results in excellent limb function and is associated with few complications, but delayed healing, implant failure, or bandage-related complications can occur.

Pantarsal arthrodesis is a less benign surgical procedure, although the final functional outcome is usually good to excellent. Possible complications include osteomyelitis, malalignment, delayed fusion, implant loosening or breakage, and bandage complications (17, 24). A dorsally applied 2.7-mm DCP broke in a cat 4 months after surgery (24). Cats are especially prone to develop pressure necrosis of the skin if both large implants and a bandage are applied. Correct bandaging techniques and regular rechecks and bandage changes are necessary to avoid these complications.

The plate can be removed after healing has taken place, to reduce the risk of iatrogenic fractures at the proximal or distal plate end, but this should not be performed earlier than 6 months after surgery. Plates should always be removed if a low-grade osteomyelitis is suspected from radiographic findings and/or poor clinical function.

References and further reading

1. Schmökel HG, et al. Tarsal injuries in the cat: a retrospective study of 21 cases. J Small Anim Pract 1994;35:156–162.
2. Frewein J, Vollmerhaus B. Anatomie von Hund und Katze. Berlin: Blackwell; 1994.
3. McNicholas WT Jr, et al. Luxation of the superficial digital flexor tendon in a cat. J Am Anim Hosp Assoc 2000;36: 174–176.
4. Piermattei DL, Johnson KA. An atlas of surgical approaches to the bones and joints of the dog and the cat, 4th edn. Philadelphia: WB Saunders; 2004.
5. Vaughan LC, Faull WB. Correction of a luxated superficial digital flexor tendon in a greyhound dog. Vet Rec 1955;59: 335–336.
6. Mauterer JV, Prata RG. Displacement of the tendon of the superficial digital flexor muscle in dogs: 10 cases. J Am Vet Med Assoc 1993;203:1162–1165.
7. Reinke J, et al. Lateral luxation of the superficial digital flexor tendon in 12 dogs. J Am Anim Hosp Assoc 1993;29:303–309.
8. Damur DM, Montavon PM. Die chirurgische Behandlung der Luxation des oberflächlichen Zehenbeugers mittels einer Drahtschlinge bei zwei Hunden. Kleintierpraxis 2001;46: 805–809.
9. Vannini R. Tarsal luxations in cats. AO Vet Course 2002; Davos, Switzerland; pp. 56–57.
10. Owen MA. Use of contoured bar transhock external fixators in 17 cats. J Small Anim Pract 2000;41:440–446.
11. Voss K, et al. Internal splinting of dorsal intertarsal and tarsometatarsal instabilities in dogs and cats with the ComPact UniLock 2.0/2.4 System. Vet Comp Orthop Traumatol 2004;17: 125–130.

12. Piermattei DL, Flo GL. Fractures and other orthopedic injuries of the tarsus, metatarsus, and phalanges. In: Piermattei DL, Flo GL (eds) Small animal orthopedics and fracture repair. Philadelphia: WB Saunders; 1997: pp. 607–655.
13. Von Werthern CJ, Bernasconi CE. Application of the maxillofacial mini-plate Compact 1.0 in the fracture repair of 12 cats/2 dogs. Vet Comp Orthop Traumatol 2000;13:92–96.
14. Gorse MJ, et al. Talocalcaneal luxation: an anatomic and clinical study. Vet Surg 1990;19:429–434.
15. Montavon PM, et al. The mini instrument and implant set and its clinical application. Vet Comp Orthop Traumatol 1988;1: 44–51.
16. McCartney WT, Carmichael S. Talar neck fractures in five cats. J Small Anim Pract 2000;41:204–206.
17. Allen MJ, et al. Calcaneoquartal arthrodesis in the dog. J Small Anim Pract 1993;34:205–210.
18. Muir P, Norris L. Tarsometatarsal subluxation in dogs: partial arthrodesis by plate fixation. J Am Anim Hosp Assoc 1999;35: 155–162.
19. Dyce J, et al. Arthrodesis of the tarsometatarsal joint using a laterally applied plate in 10 dogs. J Small Anim Pract 1998;39: 19–22.
20. Penwick RC, Clark DM. A simple technique for tarsometatarsal arthrodesis in small animals. J Am Anim Hosp Assoc 1988;24: 183–188.
21. Shanil J, et al. Arthrodesis of the tarsometatarsal joint, using type II ESF with acrylic connecting bars in four dogs. Vet Comp Orthop Traumatol 2006;19:61–63.
22. Mathews KG, et al. Resolution of lameness associated with Scottish fold osteodystrophy following bilateral ostectomies and pantarsal arthrodeses: a case report. J Am Anim Hosp Assoc 1995;31:280–288.
23. Gorse MJ, et al. Tarsocrural arthrodesis: long-term functional results. J Am Anim Hosp Assoc 1991;27:231–235.
24. DeCamp C, et al. Pantarsal arthrodesis in dogs and a cat: 11 cases. J Am Vet Med Assoc 1993;203:1705–1707.
25. Kirsch JA, et al. In vitro mechanical evaluation on the use of an intramedullary pin-plate combination for pantarsal arthrodesis in dogs. Am J Vet Res 2005;66:125–131.
26. Vannini R. Tarsal panarthrodesis. BSAVA meeting 1998; Birmingham, England.
27. McKee WM, et al. Pantarsal arthrodesis with a customized medial or lateral bone plate in 13 dogs. Vet Rec 2004;154: 165–170.
28. Beardsley SL, Schrader SC. Treatment of dogs with wounds of the limbs caused by shearing forces: 98 cases (1975–1993). J Am Vet Med Assoc 1995;207:1071–1075.
29. Schmökel HG, Ehrismann G. The surgical treatment of talocrural luxation in nine cats. Vet Comp Orthop Traumatol 2001; 14:46–50.

41 Amputations

S.J. Langley-Hobbs, K. Voss, P.M. Montavon

Amputation may be necessary in cats with severe irreparable fractures and disturbed vasculature of the distal limb, for chronic unremitting pain in the high-motion joints like the elbow or stifle when arthrodesis is not the preferred treatment option, for congenital or acquired deformity, for severe infection unresponsive to treatment, and for excision of tumors and irreversible neurological deficits.

Cats cope very well with the loss of a limb or appendage, such as a tail or digit. They may function better with an amputation than with preservation of a functionally abnormal or painful leg. However, except for treatment for neoplasia, amputation should be considered a last-resort salvage option, only to be performed if limb function cannot be preserved.

In one study it was shown that many owners were reluctant to consider amputation for their pet, but after surgery they were satisfied with the mobility and appearance of their animals (1). In another study, only two out of 22 cats showed a marked reduction of quality of life after forelimb or hindlimb amputation according to owner assessment. Quality of life remained unchanged or only slightly reduced in all of the others. The most common minor problems were difficulties when jumping on high objects, and when grooming or scratching (2).

41.1 Preoperative evaluation

An amputation is rarely an emergency procedure and the patient should be stable prior to surgery. Amputation is a major procedure and a complete physical examination should be done prior to surgery. Blood loss is possible and baseline packed cell volume and plasma proteins should be assessed preoperatively. The other limbs are carefully examined preoperatively to rule out orthopedic and/or neurological disease. Severe disease in another limb may make an animal a poor candidate for amputation. In the presence of neoplasia, the tumor should be staged to check for local extent and distant metastasis (Chapter 8).

Neurological dysfunction such as brachial plexus avulsion or sciatic neuropathy is confirmed and monitored by physical examination and electromyography (Chapter 2). In select cases the limb can be salvaged by the use of muscle relocation techniques and/or arthrodesis. Reinnervation can occur but is often slow, and if owners are unwilling or unable to perform the necessary physical therapy in the intervening period to prevent muscle contracture, amputation is justified.

41.2 General principles of amputation

The surgical site should be widely clipped from the carpus or hock to the dorsal and ventral midline, extending far enough cranially and caudally to allow adequate aseptic preparation. The whole leg should be draped out to permit full manipulation. Open infected wounds distal to the amputation site should be covered if possible.

The skin incision should be made distal enough to allow for sufficient skin to close without tension. Excess skin can be trimmed later as necessary. The lateral skin on the limbs and dorsal skin on the tail should be retained where possible, and more removed from the thinner and less densely haired skin of the groin, axilla, or ventral tail. The surgery should involve systematic and meticulous dissection and transection of muscles. Muscles are transected at their tendinous insertion sites if possible to reduce hemorrhage. The use of cutting diathermy reduces hemorrhage from muscle bellies. The muscles contract once cut, so ensure they are cut sufficiently distally when it is desired that the remaining tissue stumps will provide some protective cover to the cut bone ends. Avoid undermining skin to minimize dead space.

Arteries and veins are ligated separately to avoid the formation of arteriovenous fistulae (3). Arteries and major veins should be double-ligated. Silk or a braided absorbable suture material, such as Vicryl, are appropriate suture materials. Nerves should be handled gently and are sharply severed with a sharp scalpel blade. The nerve can be splash blocked with lidocaine prior to transection.

Bone should be cut neatly with a handsaw, power-driven saw, or Gigli wire. The use of bone cutters in diaphyseal bone should be avoided in adult cats as the bone is brittle and will tend to fissure or crack, resulting in an uneven or spiky stump. After disarticulation of the hip or shoulder, no special treatment is required for the articular surface.

Box 41-1. Forequarter amputation

The cat is placed in lateral recumbency. An inverted Y-shaped skin incision is made, extending from the dorsal spine of the scapula to the acromion. Then the incision is extended cranially over the greater tubercle, and medially in the axilla curving round at the axillary fold to meet the lateral incision at the level of the acromion (Fig. 41-1A).

The axillobrachial and omobrachial veins are ligated and severed proximal to the greater tubercle. The cephalic vein is ligated and severed distal to the cleidobrachialis muscle. The brachiocephalicus muscle is transected just proximal to the clavicle. The omotransversarius and trapezius muscles are severed along the cranial edge of the spine of the scapula (Fig. 41-1B). The latissimus dorsi muscle is separated from the teres major and severed close to its insertion on the humerus.

The scapula is then elevated and the insertions of the rhomboideus and serratus muscles are severed close to the medial aspect of the scapula. The suprascapular and the nerves of the brachial plexus are severed. The axillary lymph node can be removed at this time if necessary. The axillary vein and artery are double ligated and severed (Fig. 41-1C). The superficial and deep pectoral muscles are transected at their attachment on the humerus to complete the removal of the limb.

The cut ends of the muscle bellies are inverted and apposed with mattress sutures. The lateral fascial sheaths of the latissimus dorsi muscle, omotransversarius, and trapezius are sutured to the lateral fascial sheaths of the pectoral muscle. Subcutaneous tissues and skin are closed routinely, taking care to close down dead space and remove excess tissue from the medial axillary flap, so more of the thicker lateral brachial skin is preserved, to achieve a cosmetic result (Fig. 41-1D).

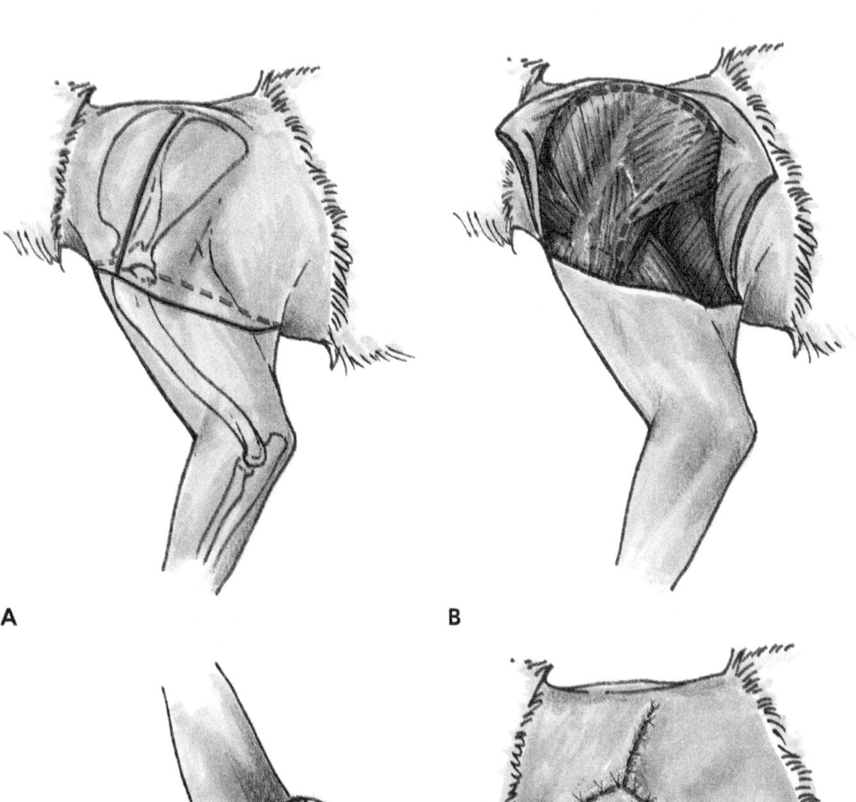

Figure 41-1 Forequarter amputation.
(**A**) T-shaped skin incision for forequarter amputation.
(**B**) Muscles are transected along the scapula.
(**C**) The scapula is retracted laterally, and the medial muscles are elevated from the bone. The brachial plexus nerves are cut, and the axillary artery and vein are ligated. The remaining muscles are cut to release the scapula.
(**D**) Muscles are apposed to minimize dead space, and the subcutis and skin are closed.

When amputating for neoplasia, the site of amputation must be sufficiently proximal to give a clean margin. Veins should be ligated first to prevent possible spread of tumor cells during manipulation. The amputated leg is submitted for histopathological analysis to confirm tumor type and to check for clean margins.

Muscles are apposed to close down dead space and cover bone ends by inverting the cut edges with absorbable mattress sutures. Subcutaneous sutures and skin sutures are used to obtain a cosmetic closure. Excess skin may need to be trimmed to avoid dog ears at the wound edges.

The decision as to what level to amputate and whether to disarticulate the joint or amputate by cutting through bone is open to debate. However, there is concern that the remaining cartilage will not atrophy and could promote complications such as seroma and infection. Conversely, amputations performed by cutting through bone and leaving a stump can be more painful, the skin over the stump can ulcerate, and overgrowth of the bone can occur in young animals (4, 5). The procedure of choice must be the one that works best for each individual patient and veterinary surgeon.

41.3 Forelimb amputation

Indications for amputation of the forelimb include neoplasia, severe degloving injuries of the distal limb, brachial plexus avulsions, muscle contractures, fracture disease, and chronic debilitating joint conditions, and where finances may not permit an attempt at surgical repair (Box 41-1).

Amputation of the forelimb can be performed at the level of the proximal humerus, by disarticulation of the scapulohumeral joint or by removal of the whole limb including the scapula – a forequarter amputation. Foreleg amputation through the proximal humerus is an easy procedure, but is restricted to cases where the abnormality is located distal to the elbow joint (6). Abrasion and ulceration of the overlying skin may occur if the humeral stump is left with insufficient soft-tissue coverage or if the humerus is left too long. The scapula is preserved with both disarticulation of the scapulohumeral joint and amputation through the proximal humerus, and atrophy of the adjacent muscles can lead to a prominent scapular spine and acromion process, which may be disturbing to some owners (Box 41-2). The scapular spine can be partially removed during surgery to prevent this.

Amputation by removal of the whole forelimb including the scapula (forequarter amputation) gives a better cosmetic result and is the preference of the authors, although it involves slightly more dissection (7). Major blood vessels and nerves are easily visualized, bone-cutting equipment is not required, and no prominent scapular spine is left behind (8).

For some tumors involving the proximal half of the scapula it may be possible to preserve the limb function by just removing the affected portion of the scapula with adequate margins (9).

41.4 Hindlimb amputation

Indications for amputation of the hindlimb include neoplasia, sciatic neuropathy, irreparable fractures, non-unions or chronic unremitting osteomyelitis, quadriceps contracture, and end-stage stifle conditions where arthrodesis is not an option.

The hindlimb can be amputated at the level of the proximal femur (Box 41-3) or by coxofemoral disarticulation (Box 41-4). The area of soft-tissue or bony lesion determines which of the removal techniques is indicated. Amputation by cutting through the proximal femur is easier to perform than coxofemoral amputation, and will give better cosmetic results by leaving the proximal aspect of the femur with its associated musculature (10). It is appropriate for most cases, except for neoplasia of the femur, where excision of the whole femur is required. Partial or total hemipelvectomy can be done for tumors involving the pelvis or coxofemoral joint, where a wider margin of tissue needs to be excised (11).

41.5 Tail amputation

Indications for tail amputation include degloving injuries, skin necrosis, tumors, and paralysis. The most common reason for amputation of the tail in cats is paralysis following tail pull injuries after road traffic accidents (Box 41-5).

41.6 Metacarpal, metatarsal, and phalangeal amputation

Indications for amputation of digits and associated metacarpal and metatarsal bones include neoplasia, chronic osteomyelitis, and severe trauma. The level of amputation is not as critical as with an entire limb amputation. When removing the fifth or second metacarpal and metatarsal bones the proximal aspects should be preserved along with their ligaments, otherwise instability can result (Box 41-6).

Disarticulation through the distal interphalangeal joint is the commonest type of amputation in cats (12). Elective feline onychectomy or declaw procedure is unethical or illegal in most countries when performed to prevent scratching of furniture, but there may be some medical indications such as for treatment or biopsy of nail bed disease, or to remove a previously damaged claw that is growing in an abnormal direction. It is usually performed under tourniquet and it is essential to remove all the germinative tissue in the ungual crest to prevent regrowth. Either the entire third phalanx can be dissected out and removed or a small palmar portion of the third phalanx can be retained. Following oncychectomy,

Box 41-2. Forelimb amputation at the level of the proximal humerus

The cat is placed in lateral recumbency. The curved skin incision is made from cranial to the shoulder, extending distally across the distal humerus, and curving back up to the axillary fold. A straighter incision is made medially, not extending as far distally, so the lateral skin flap can later be used to cover the stump (Fig. 41-2A).

The superficial cleidobrachialis and brachiocephalic muscles are transected craniomedially. The brachial artery, located caudal to the biceps muscle on the medial aspect of the limb, is double ligated and transected proximally. The brachial vein is ligated separately at the same level. The median, ulnar, and musculocutaneous nerves are sharply divided. The tendon of the triceps muscle, and the brachial and biceps muscles are transected close to their insertion sites around the elbow joint to minimize bleeding (Fig. 41-2B).

The cephalic vein is ligated on the lateral aspect of the limb. The radial nerve is identified and sharply dissected. Both structures are severed at their proximal aspect. Remaining lateral muscle attachments are transected close to the elbow joint (Fig. 41-2C). The attachment of the brachiocephalic muscle along the humeral shaft is elevated from the bone from distal to proximal, until the deltoid tuberosity in the proximal third of the humerus is reached.

The humeral shaft is transected in its proximal third with a handsaw, oscillating saw or Gigli wire just distal to the deltoid tuberosity (Fig. 41-2D). Meticulous hemostasis is performed before closure. The stump of the humerus is well covered by suturing the brachial and biceps brachii muscles to the triceps muscle. The bone needs to be well covered with muscles, especially over the cranial aspect of the stump. During closure of the subcutaneous tissues, preserve as much lateral skin as possible as this is thicker with a denser hair coat, which will give a better cosmetic result. Take care to avoid dead space (Fig. 41-2D).

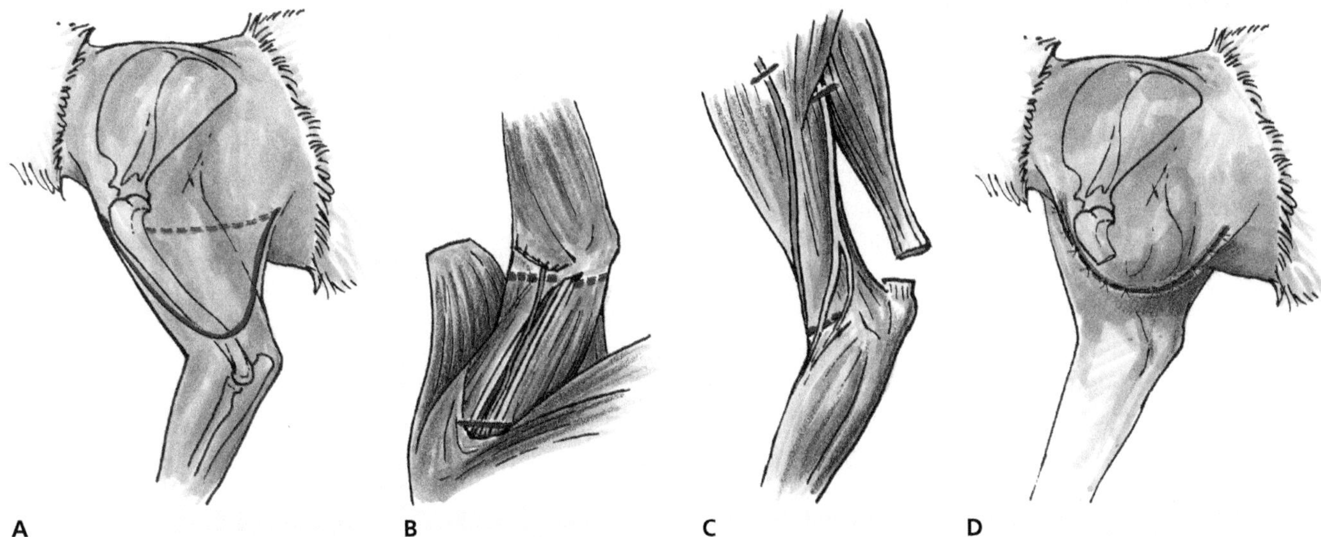

Figure 41-2 Forelimb amputation at the level of the proximal humerus.
(**A**) Skin incision with the lateral curve extending to the distal humerus.
(**B**) The forelimb is reflected to reach the medial side. Vessels are ligated, and vessels and nerves are transected proximally; muscles are transected close to the elbow joint.
(**C**) Laterally, the radial nerve is transected, and the cephalic vein ligated and transected proximally; muscles are transected close to the elbow joint.
(**D**) The humerus is cut through at the proximal metaphyseal region, muscles are apposed to minimize dead space, and subcutis and skin are closed.

Box 41-3. Hindlimb amputation at the level of the proximal third of the femur

The cat is placed in lateral recumbency. The skin incision is centered just proximal to the stifle, curving from the fold of the flank to the caudal thigh and meeting medially distal to the inguinal crease (Fig. 41-3A). The medial skin incision should be at mid femoral level, the longer lateral flap serves to hide the scar on the medial part of the leg and protects the stump, as the lateral skin is much thicker than the medial.

The leg is elevated to reach its medial aspect, and the femoral artery is double ligated just proximal to the proximal caudal femoral artery (Fig. 41-3B). The femoral vein is ligated at a similar level. The cranial part of the sartorius, tensor fascia lata, quadriceps and biceps femoris muscles are severed at the level of the distal femur. The quadriceps muscle is transected just proximal to the patella (Fig. 41-3B).

The caudolateral muscles are reflected proximally and the sciatic nerve is transected (Fig. 41-3C). The semimembranosus and semitendinosus muscles are transected at the caudomedial aspect of the stifle. The leg is elevated and the gracilis and pectineus muscles and caudal sartorius are transected through their tendinous bellies at their insertions on the tibia (Fig. 41-3C).

Caudally, the adductor is elevated off the bone to expose the proximal third of the femur. The muscles are reflected and the femur is transected between the proximal and mid thirds (Fig. 41-3D), using a handsaw, Gigli wire or oscillating bone. Hemorrhage from the bone can be controlled with absorbable gelatin sponge. The site is closed by apposing the sartorius, quadriceps, and biceps femoris muscles to the semitendinosus, semimembranosus, and gracilis muscles with mattress sutures, to cover the remaining bone. Subcutis and skin are closed while taking care to avoid leaving dead space.

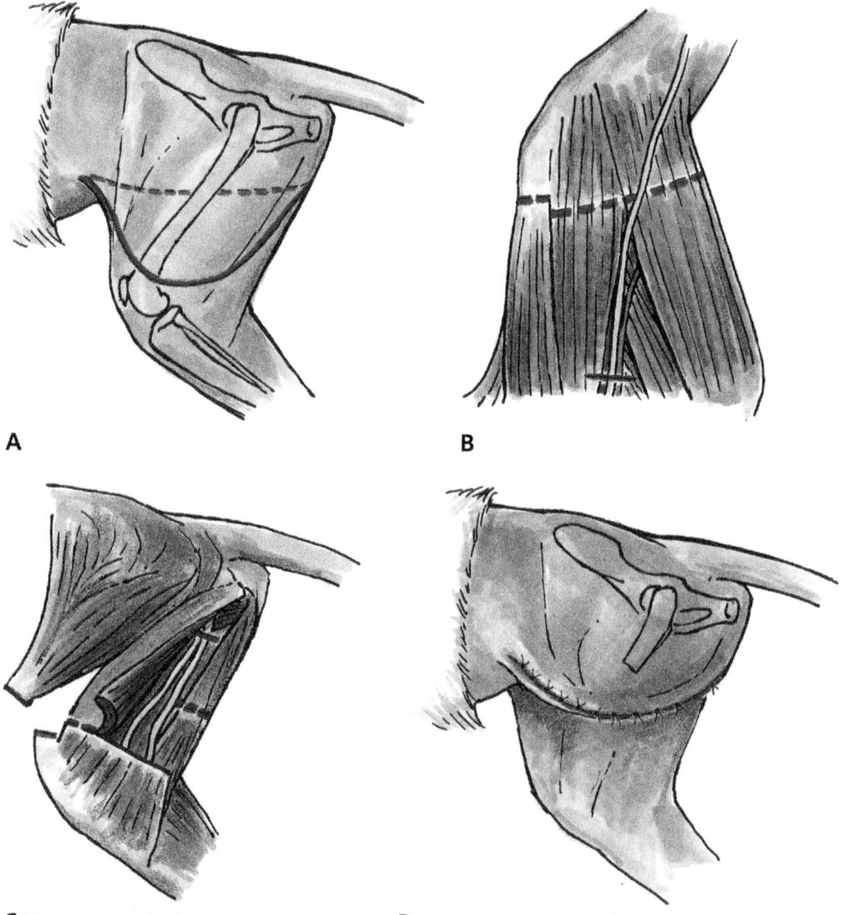

Figure 41-3 Hindlimb amputation at the level of the proximal femur.
(**A**) Skin incision with the lateral curve extending to the distal femur.
(**B**) The femur is reflected laterally, the femoral vessels are ligated proximally, and the femoral nerve is transected at the same level. Muscles are cut through their tendinous insertions close to the stifle joint.
(**C**) On the lateral side, the sciatic nerve is transected proximally, and the lateral and caudal muscles are dissected close to the stifle joint.
(**D**) The bone is cut at its proximal third, muscle are closed over the bone stump, and subcutis and skin are closed.

Box 41-4. Hindlimb amputation by coxofemoral disarticulation and removal of the thigh muscles

The cat is placed in lateral recumbency with the affected leg uppermost and quadrant draped. A curved skin incision is made from the fold of the flank across at the level of the midshaft of the femur to the ischial tuberosity. The medial skin incision is made at a similar level (Fig. 41-4A).

The leg is elevated and the femoral artery and vein identified in the femoral triangle, which is bordered cranially by the sartorius muscles and caudally by the pectineus. The femoral artery is double ligated and severed proximal to the superficial circumflex iliac artery and lateral circumflex iliac artery branches (Fig. 41-4B). The femoral vein is ligated at a similar level. With the leg still elevated, the caudal muscle bellies are first elevated. The pectineus is elevated from the iliopectineal eminence. The gracilis, adductor longus and adductor magnus et brevis are then elevated from the pubic symphysis. Then the semimembranosus and semitendinosus are removed from the tuber ischium. The proximal part of the pectineus is reflected, exposing the medial circumflex.

The lateral skin incision is then undermined to the level of the greater trochanter to reach the musculature close to the coxofemoral joint (Fig. 41-4C). The tensor fascia lata and biceps femoris muscles are dissected free from the sacrotuberous ligament and lateral aspect of the tuber ischii. The sciatic nerve is exposed as the biceps is reflected distally and it is transected. The vastus lateralis, medialis, and intermedius are not severed but are removed with the femur. The muscles of the femoral neck are removed next. The gluteal muscles are transected at their insertions on the greater trochanter and third trochanter and are reflected dorsally and cranially. The tendons of insertion of the

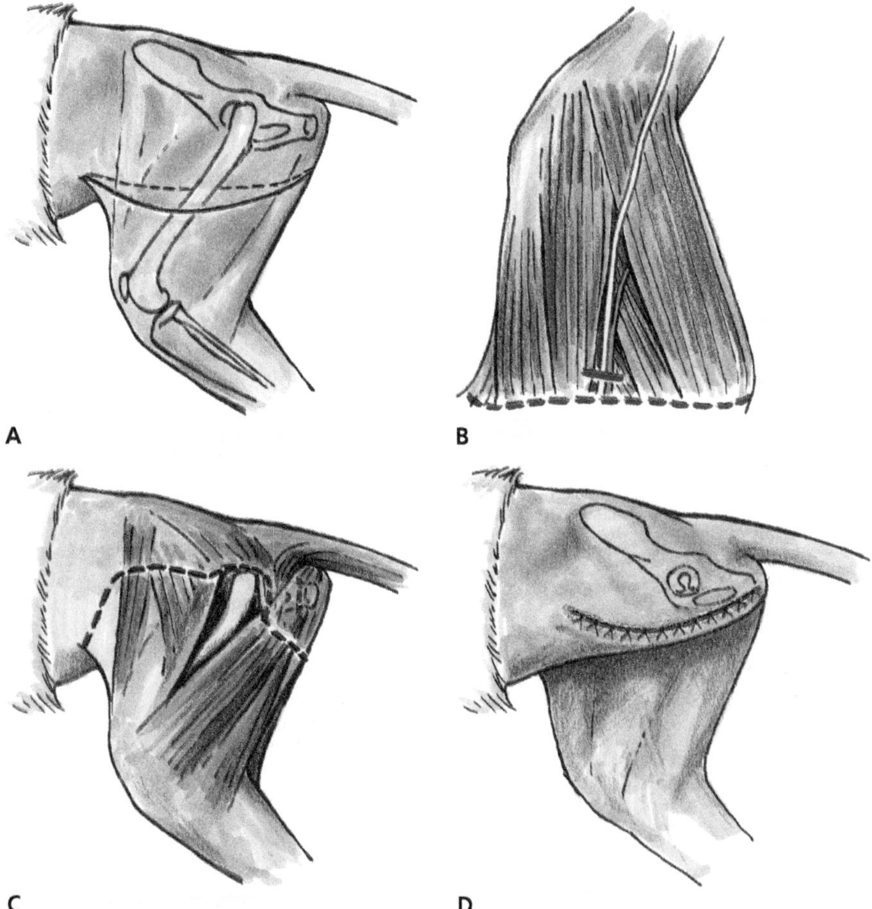

Figure 41-4 Hindlimb amputation by coxofemoral disarticulation.
(**A**) Skin incision for hindlimb amputation for coxofemoral disarticulation.
(**B**) The leg is elevated, the femoral artery and vein are ligated proximally, and the vessels and femoral nerve are transected. The medial muscles are cut.
(**C**) Muscles are transected close to the coxofemoral joint laterally. The sciatic nerve is sharply divided.
(**D**) The coxofemoral joint is disarticulated and the leg removed. Muscles are apposed over the acetabulum to minimize dead space, and the subcutis and skin are closed.

gemelli, internal obturator, and quadratus femoris muscles are transected at their insertions on the trochanteric fossa. The cranial thigh muscles are dealt with next. The tensor fascia lata is dissected from its combined origin on the tuber coxae and aponeurosis with the gluteal muscles and reflected distally. The cranial and caudal bellies of the sartorius muscle are freed from the iliac crest and lumbodorsal fascia and reflected distally. The rectus femoris tendon, the only component of the quadriceps group to cross the coxofemoral joint, is transected close to its tuberosity on the pelvis. The only remaining connecting muscle, the iliopsoas, is then freed from its insertion on the lesser trochanter.

To remove the limb, the joint capsule is incised circumferentially and the coxofemoral joint is disarticulated after transecting the teres ligament from the medial side of the joint (Fig. 41-4D). Hemostasis is performed, and the remaining muscles are sutured together with mattress sutures. Apposition of these muscles should result in coverage of the acetabulum. As there has been extensive removal of muscle the use of drains should be considered. Closed suction drains are preferable. If open drains such as Penrose are used they should be placed to exit cranially, and are covered with a sterile dressing. A pressure bandage should be applied if no drain is used.

Box 41-5. Tail amputation

Two semicircular incisions are made dorsally and ventrally, creating two skin flaps (Fig. 41-5). The skin incision is made distal to the planned point of transection, and the skin is then pushed proximally to allow further dissection. The two lateral caudal vessels and the median caudal vessels are ligated or cauterized and severed. Skin flaps are retracted cranially, coccygeal muscles are transected, and the coccygeal vertebrae is cut through with a pair of bone cutters or disarticulated according to personal preference. The dorsal skin flap is pulled over the stump and sutured to the ventral skin flap.

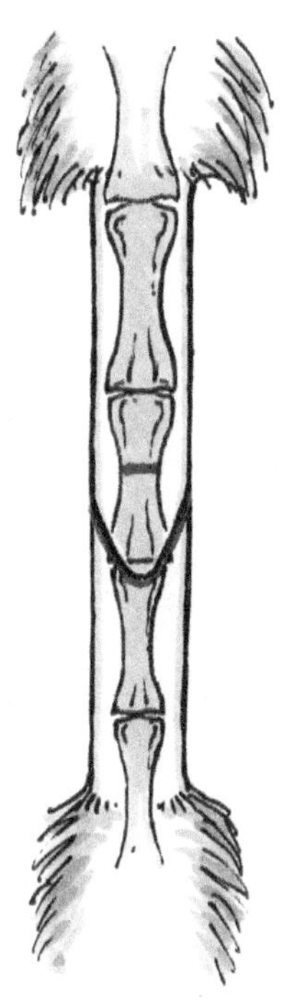

Figure 41-5 Diagram showing the skin incision for tail amputation, and a line indicating the more proximal cut through the coccygeal vertebral body.

the second phalanx should be inspected and any overlapping remnants of the third phalanx resected.

41.7 Postoperative treatment and complications

Drains are not usually required if adequate attention is paid to hemostasis and atraumatic surgical technique. A padded bandage can be applied to the thorax to minimize swelling and eliminate dead space. The bandage may be resented by the cat, and must not be applied too tightly to compromise respiration.

After surgery, the patient is monitored for pain, hypothermia, and bleeding. Please see Chapter 18 for information on perioperative pain management. Postoperative hemorrhage can occur as a slow ooze and swelling under the wound or as a sudden catastrophic bleed. If the amount of blood loss is minimal, a pressure bandage should be applied if possible.

Box 41-6. Metacarpal, metatarsal, and phalangeal amputation

Depending on the level of amputation a variety of incisions are used (Fig. 41-6). Adequate skin must be preserved for closure over the stump. The area to be removed is exposed and the arterial supply ligated or cauterized. The bones are removed at the required level either by disarticulation or by cutting through the bone. Closure entails suturing the deep fascia and subcutaneous tissue to close dead space, followed by routine skin closure.

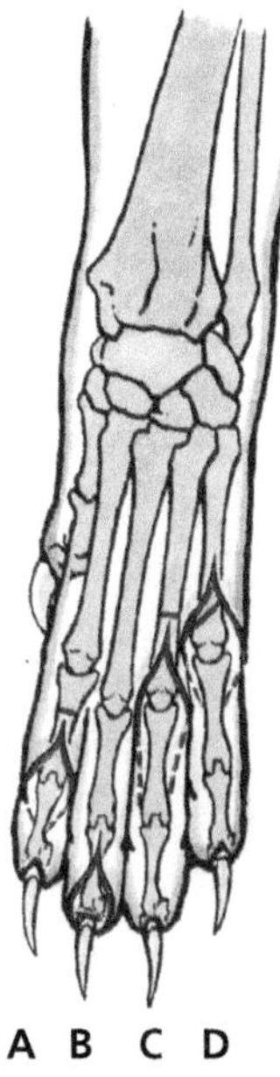

Figure 41-6 Examples of levels for amputation of a digit.
(**A**) Amputation of phalanges 3 and 2 of digit II by cutting through phalanx 1.
(**B**) Amputation of phalanx 3 of digit III by disarticulation or removal of the whole ungual crest. The digital pad must be retained.
(**C**) Amputation of digit IV by cutting through the distal metacarpal bone.
(**D**) Amputation of digit V by oblique osteotomy through the metacarpal bone

A large or continuous amount of hemorrhage indicates a bleeding vessel and the operative incision should be opened and the vessel ligated.

Skin ulceration may be caused by inaccurate skin apposition, inadequate drainage, circulatory impairment due to too tight a closure, or too long a stump of bone rubbing under the skin. Ulcerations are treated with excision of ulcerated tissue and wound closure without tension. It may be necessary to resect bone at a more proximal level to allow tension-free closure, if the stump was left too long initially. Phantom-limb pain has been reported in one cat (13). This cat had an iatrogenic sciatic nerve injury and subsequent hindlimb amputation. Multimodal analgesic therapy resulted in resolution of signs of pain.

References and further reading

1. Carberry CA, Harvey HJ. Owner satisfaction with limb amputation in dogs and cats. J Am Anim Hosp Assoc 1987;23: 227–232.
2. Von Werthern C, et al. Limb amputation in dogs and cats: owner response. Kleintierpraxis 1999; 44:169–176.
3. Muir P, Pead MJ. Chronic lameness after digit amputation in three dogs. Vet Rec 1998;143:549–550.
4. Abraham E, et al. Stump overgrowth in juvenile amputees. J Pediatr Orthop 1986;6:66–71.
5. Weigel JP. Amputations. In: Slatter D (ed.) Textbook of small animal surgery, 2nd edn. Philadelphia: WB Saunders; 1993: pp. 1901–1910.
6. Trout NJ, et al. Partial scapulectomy for management of sarcomas in three dogs and two cats. J Am Vet Med Assoc 1995;207: 585–587.
7. Straw RC, et al. Partial or hemipelvectomy in the management of sarcomas in nine dogs and two cats. Vet Surg 1992;21: 183–188.
8. Swalec-Tobias K. Feline onychectomy at a teaching institution: a retrospective study of 163 cases. Vet Surg 1994;23:274–280.
9. O'Hagan BJ. Neuropathic pain in a cat post-amputation. Aust Vet J 2006;84:83–86.
10. Budsberg SC. Amputations. In: Olmstead ML (ed.) Small animal orthopaedics, Missouri: Mosby Year Book; 1995: pp. 531–548.
11. Daly WR. Amputation of the forelimb. In: Bojrab MJ (ed.) Current techniques in small animal surgery, 3rd edn. Philadelphia: Lea and Febiger; 1990: pp. 802–806.
12. Harvey CE. Complete forequarter amputation in the dog and cat. J Am Anim Hosp Assoc 1974;10:25–30.
13. Knapp DW. Amputation and disarticulation of the rear leg. In: Bojrab MJ (ed.) Current techniques in small animal surgery, 3rd edn. Philadelphia: Lea and Febiger; 1990: pp. 730–735.
14. Montavon PM. Voss K. [Amputations]. In: Horzinek MC, Schmidt V, Lutz H (eds) Krankheiten der Katze, 3rd edn. Stuttgart: Enke Verlag; 2003: pp. 720–723.

42 Bloopers

P.M. Montavon

We were often wrong, but never in doubt
(Steven Birchard)

Introduction

Empirical knowledge of surgery is acquired by seeing or doing, and it is sometimes difficult to cover it in a book. Surgery is not an exact science and only experience and observation allow us to perform what can be done, although not always achieving our desire of perfection. According to *Webster's Dictionary*, a blooper in baseball is hitting a ball in a low arc, so that it falls between the fielders. We have selected a few clinical cases to illustrate situations we underestimated, scenarios we neglected, or outcomes or eventualities which resulted from unexpected conditions. These situations depict both lucky and unlucky surgical circumstances in our world of small-animal veterinary surgeons. The experience of such cases and the successful resolution should help the surgeon to perform in a better manner the next time. No written theory can ever fully teach us everything.

Knowing when to cut (Fig. 42-1)

A 5-year-old female cat was admitted to the clinic at 4 a.m. in shock, and recumbent. After intravenous perfusion, radiographs were taken (Fig. 42-1A and 42-1B). The heart was small and displaced cranially with the pulmonary parenchyma; the thoracic vessels were small. A dorsal rupture of the diaphragm was present, with the stomach and a large part of the duodenum displaced into the thorax. A calculus was visible in the urinary bladder, and mineralizations were present in the left stifle. The cat was placed in an oxygen cage and given intravenous fluids at shock rates to stabilize it prior to surgery. She died 90 minutes later due to further distension of the stomach. Only an immediate surgical intervention, decompressing the stomach or replacing it in the abdomen and treating the rupture of the diaphragm, might have saved this cat.

Recognizing the difference between cats and dogs (Fig. 42-2)

An 11-month-old female cat was presented after a fall from a height. A closed Monteggia fracture with comminution of the proximal ulna and luxation of the head of the radius was present (Fig. 42-2A). The immediate postoperative radiographs showed inaccurate reduction of the proximal ulnar fracture, resulting in abnormal articular congruence of the elbow joint. The surgeon had not realized that the proximal

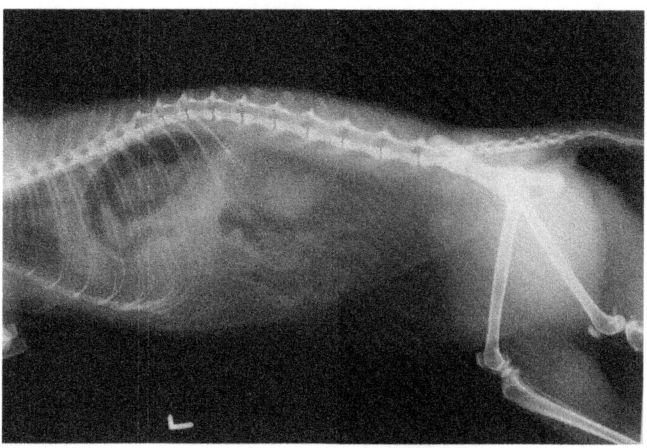

A

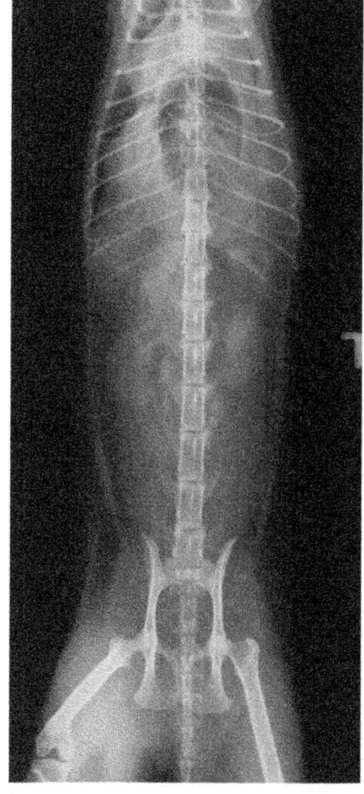

B

Figure 42-1 A 5-year-old female cat was admitted in the early morning to the clinic recumbent and in shock. (**A**) The laterolateral chest view shows a small heart displaced cranially with small thoracic vessels. (**B**) The ventrodorsal view confirms a rupture of the diagram with the stomach displaced into the thorax.

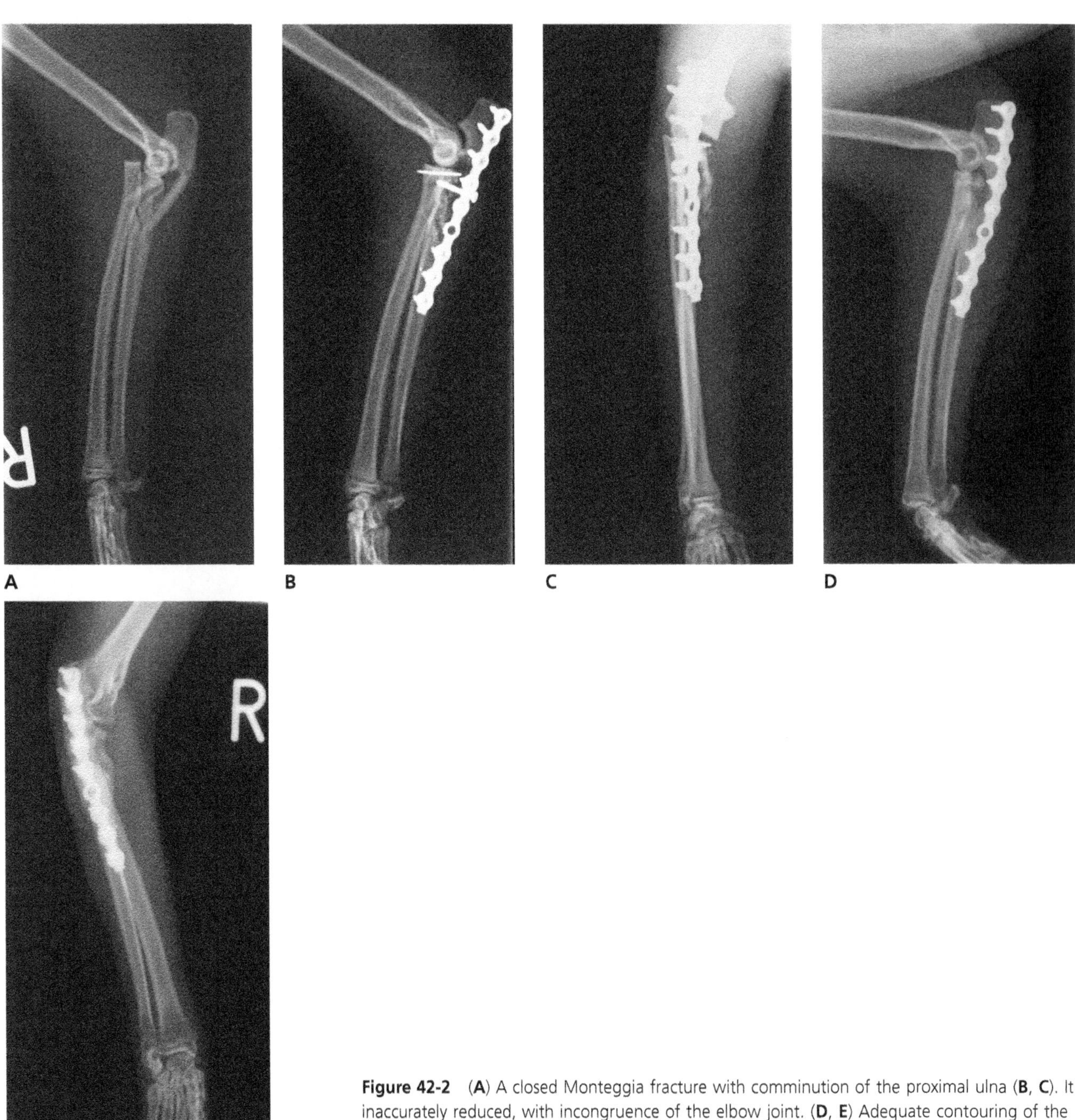

Figure 42-2 (**A**) A closed Monteggia fracture with comminution of the proximal ulna (**B**, **C**). It was inaccurately reduced, with incongruence of the elbow joint. (**D**, **E**) Adequate contouring of the proximal area of the plate and removal of the two implants causing disruption improved the reduction.

ulna has a different shape in cats compared to dogs. Immediate revision surgery was performed (Fig. 42-2B and 42-2C). Accurate contouring of the same plate to the caudal edge of the ulna and removal of two implants that were causing disruption was performed during this second surgery (Fig. 42-2D and 42-2E). The cat is walking without lameness at this time.

The perils of a weaker plate (Fig. 42-3)

A 2-year-old male cat had an automobile accident and sustained a comminuted tibial fracture (Fig. 42-3A and 42-3B). He was treated with a 2.4-mm locking compression plate, used for human hand surgery, with 2.7-mm screws. The fracture was reduced with a mild valgus deviation, but

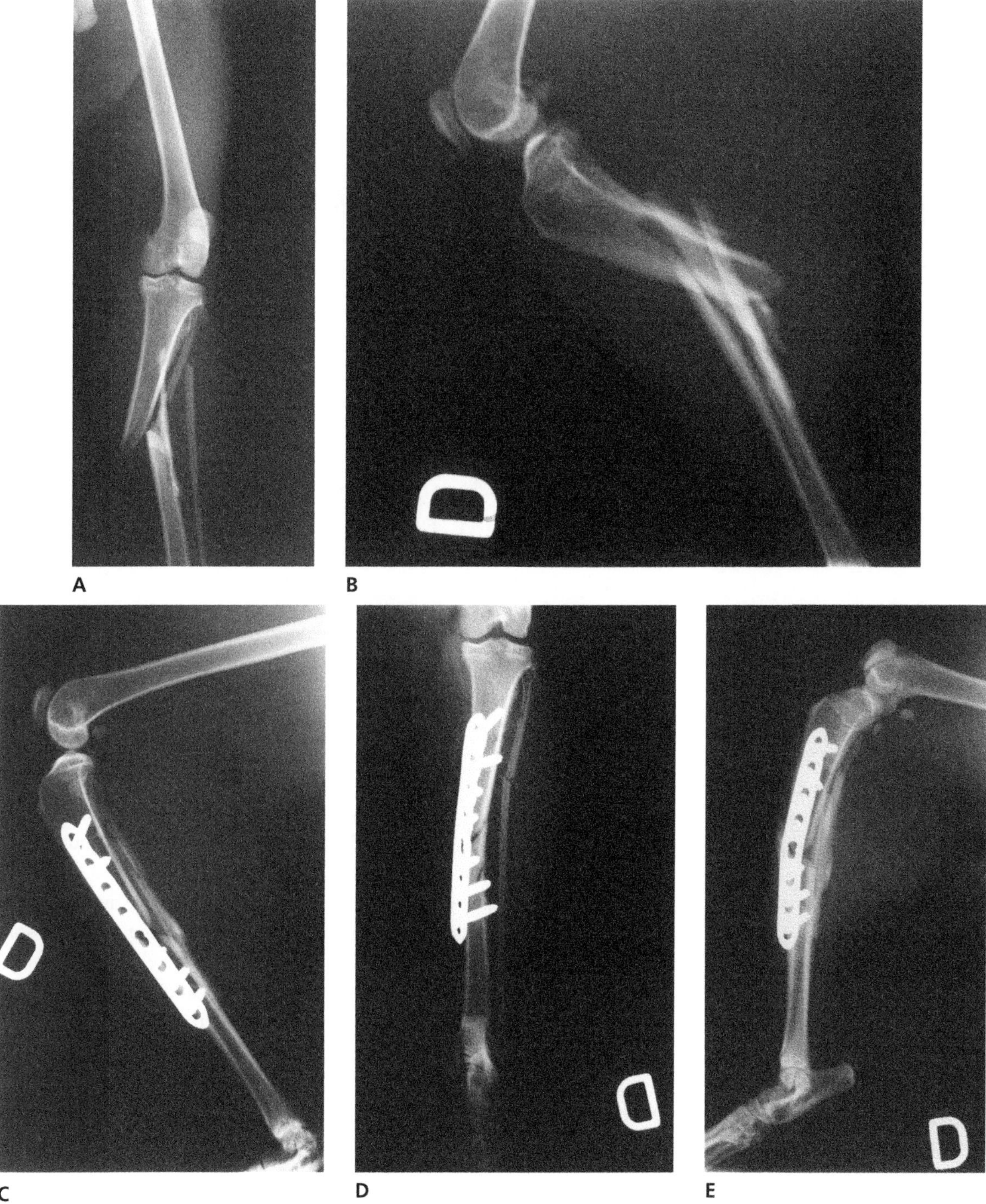

Figure 42-3 (**A**, **B**) A comminuted fracture of the tibia was present in this cat, after an automobile accident. (**C**, **D**) It was adequately reduced and stabilized with a locking compression plate in buttress function and 2.7-mm screws. (**E**, **F**) The plate bent at the level of the fracture one week postoperatively. (**G**, **H**) It was replaced with a longer 14-hole 2.0-mm dynamic compression plate in a more varus position. A wave plate (Fig. 13-23) also could have been applied.

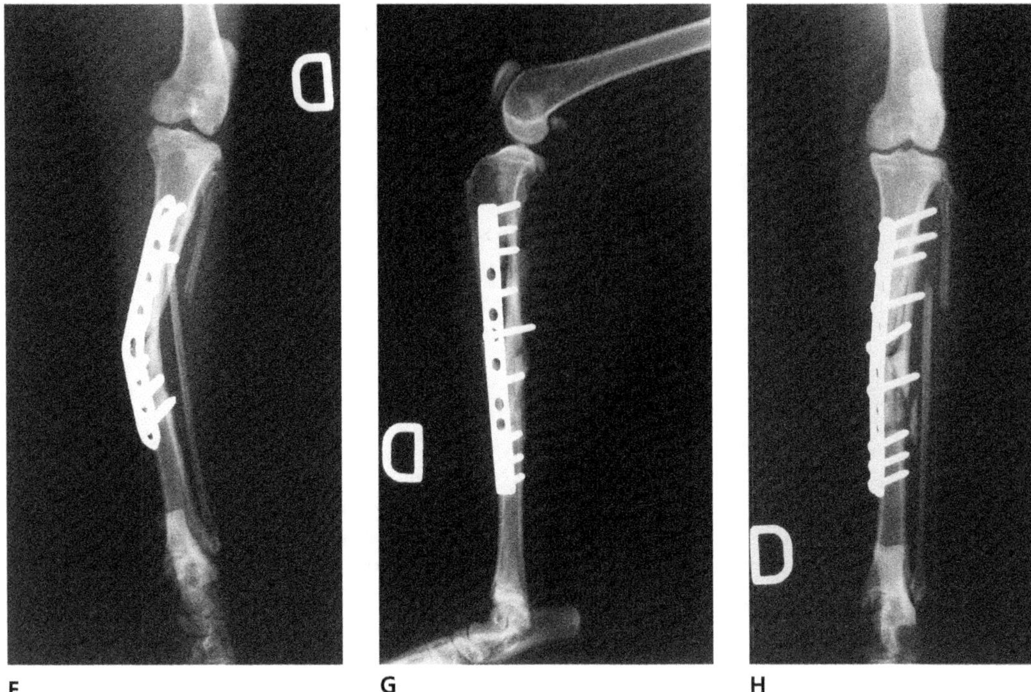

Figure 42-3 *Continued*

otherwise appeared adequate (Fig. 42-3C and 42-3D). At 1 week postoperatively, the plate used for fixation was bent at the fracture site, at the level of the empty hole. The locking compression plate, with its new more flexible design involving less metal, was not strong enough to be used in buttress function (Fig. 42-3E and 42-3F). It was successfully replaced with a 14-hole 2.0-mm dynamic compression plate (Fig. 42-3G and 42-3H). Another technique could have been the use of a second short plate, placed perpendicularly to give additional axial stability to the initial plate. A wave plate (see Fig. 13-23) could have been applied to treat the non-union.

Three small screws can be better then two big ones (Fig. 42-4)

The mid-diaphyseal humeral fracture of a young cat was treated with a laterally applied 2.7-mm dynamic compression plate. The distal part of the repair failed a short time after surgery (Fig. 42-4A and 42-4B). On the mediolateral view, one can see that only two screws were applied in the distal fragment, with the proximal one very close to the fracture. A fissure developed between the two screws. A cranial veterinary cuttable plate in sandwich was used for revision, which allowed reinforcement of the distal aspect with a larger number of smaller screws directed from cranially to caudally (Fig. 42-4C). This judicious revision surgery was sufficiently stable and led to healing of the fracture.

Avoid overdistraction (Fig. 42-5)

A male cat was 3.5 years old when he had a car accident and sustained a fracture of the fibula, and a communited fracture of the tibia (Fig. 42-5A and 42-5B). A 2.7-mm dynamic compression plate, including the use of two monocortical screws, was applied for the fracture stabilization (Fig. 42-5C and 42-5D). A relatively large defect remained at the fracture site. This can allow invasion or collapse of muscle and soft tissues into the fracture site and can contribute to delayed fracture healing in this situation. In this cat, union took over 10 months (Fig. 42-5E and 42-5F). Radiographically discrete evidence of healing is occurring at the extremities of the fracture site but a large cortical defect is still present under the plate. The fracture was stable at this time. Unfortunately, this cat was then killed in another accident.

This type of situation is not rare after surgery on the tibia; overdistraction can also occur if the bone is forcibly reduced with extension of the tarsus, creating a large fracture gap with plate or external skeletal fixation. Overdistraction of the fracture fragments, combined with the minimal soft tissue around the distal tibia, can cause delayed or non-unions with tibial fractures. The situation might be improved by placing an absorbable suture as a cerclage around the butterfly fragment in selected fractures, to reduce its distracted position.

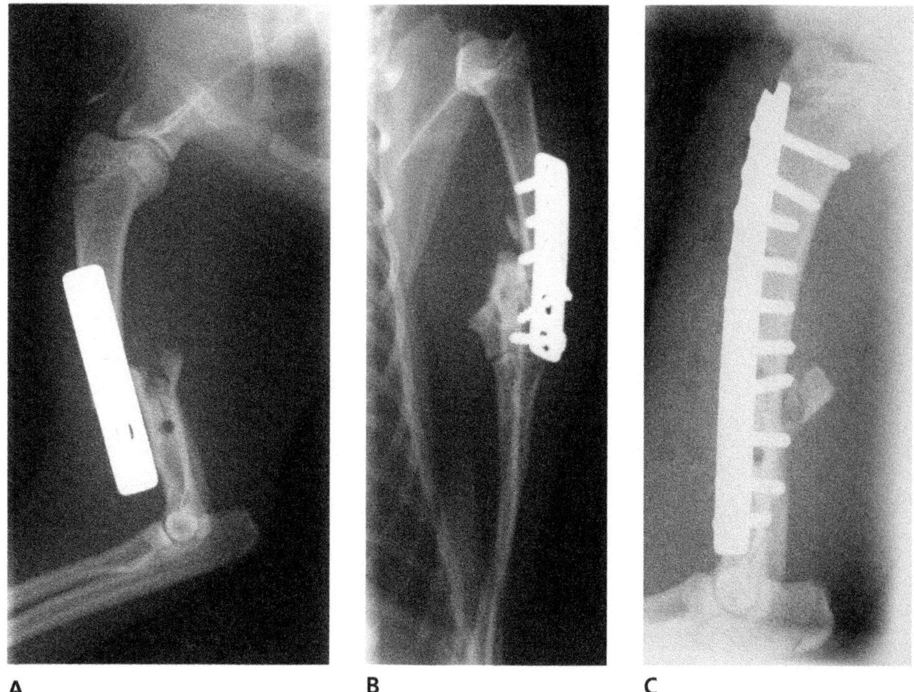

Figure 42-4 (**A**, **B**) The transverse humeral fracture was repaired with a 2.7-mm dynamic compression plate with only 2 screws in the distal fragment and the third proximal screw very close to the fracture. (**A**) A fissure developed between the two distal screws and the repair collapsed. (**C**) Two cranial veterinary cuttable plates sandwiched with a larger number of screws was a judicious successful revision.

The consequences of surgery in a young growing cat (Fig. 42-6)

A 6-month-old female cat, with potential for further growth, was presented with a medial patellar luxation of grade C and a mild varus deformity of the distal femur (Fig. 42-6A and 42-6B). The tibial tuberosity was transposed too distally during the initial surgery (Fig. 42-6C and 42-6D). A mid-diaphyseal fracture of the femur occurred 14 months later. The combination of securing the tibial tuberosity too distally and tuberosity drift occurring from premature closure of the tuberosity and continued growth of the tibial plateau have resulted in deformity of the proximal tibia (Fig. 42-6E and 42-6F). Plating of the femur and proximal reposition of the tibial tuberosity were indicated. This case shows the problems of performing an osteotomy on a young growing animal, and especially if it has been neutered, when the physes remain active for longer. A better technique for a cat of this age would have been a sulcus recession, and delaying transposition of the tibial osteotomy if it was warranted.

Insufficient stability of a small fragment near a high-motion joint (Fig. 42-7)

A 3-month-old male European short-hair cat had a car accident. One elbow sustained an intracondylar fracture (Fig. 42-7A and 42-7B). The fracture was stabilized with a 1.5-mm screw and a large intramedullary pin was placed, but was not seated well into the distal epicondyle. Additional stabilization against rotation was provided with the tubular external skeletal fixator (FESSA) system, but only with very limited anchorage. The humeral reduction was poor, resulting in a varus deviation (Fig. 42-7C and 42-7D). Fixation failure occurred 1 week after surgery (Fig. 42-7E and 42-7F) and the system was revised and improved by using a larger intracondylar screw, a thinner intramedullary pin tied in to an external skeletal fixator, and several small Kirschner wires crossing through the distal fragment (Fig. 42-7G and 42-7H). Eight weeks later, the fracture was healed and the implants removed, just leaving the intracondylar screw (Fig. 42-7I and 42-7J).

Too large pins and a transarticular fixator (Fig. 42-8)

A 9-year-old castrated male cat presented with a disrupted stifle (Fig. 42-8A and 42-8B) including rupture of the cranial cruciate ligament, damage to the medial meniscus, and avulsion of the medial collateral ligament. Articular structures were repaired, with prosthetic replacement of the medial collateral ligament. A transarticular external fixator was placed, using too large pins and double connecting bars, somewhat too big and positioned too far from the bones and at the extremities of the external fixator (Fig. 42-8C and

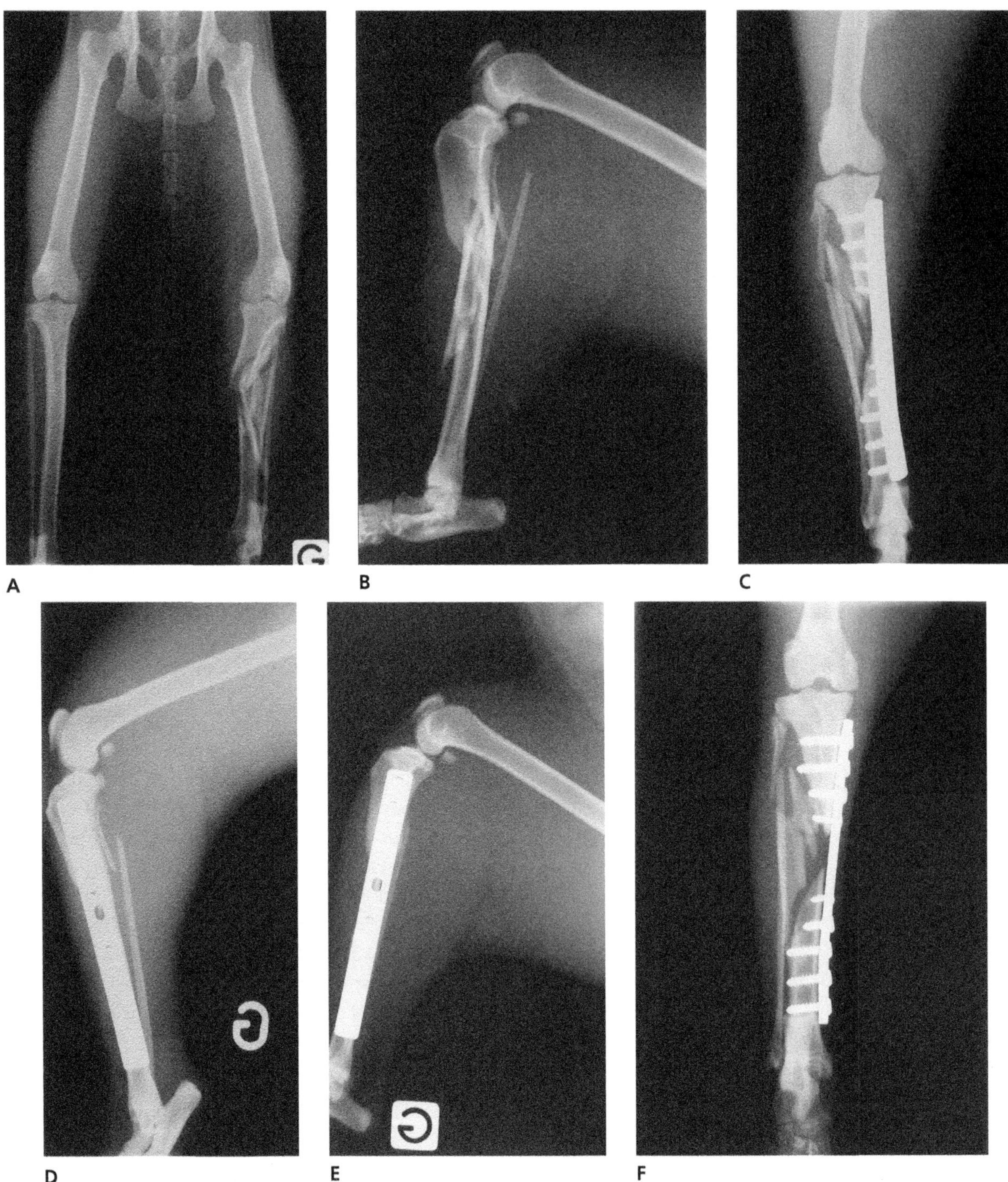

Figure 42-5 (**A**, **B**) This comminuted fracture of the tibia with fracture of the fibula was repaired with a 2.7-mm dynamic compression plate (**C**, **D**). The main fragments of the tibia remained distracted and a large defect was present at the fracture site. (**E**, **F**) Discrete evidence of healing is present at 10 months, but the large cortical defect is still present under the plate. The cat was unfortunately killed in another accident so there was no further follow up.

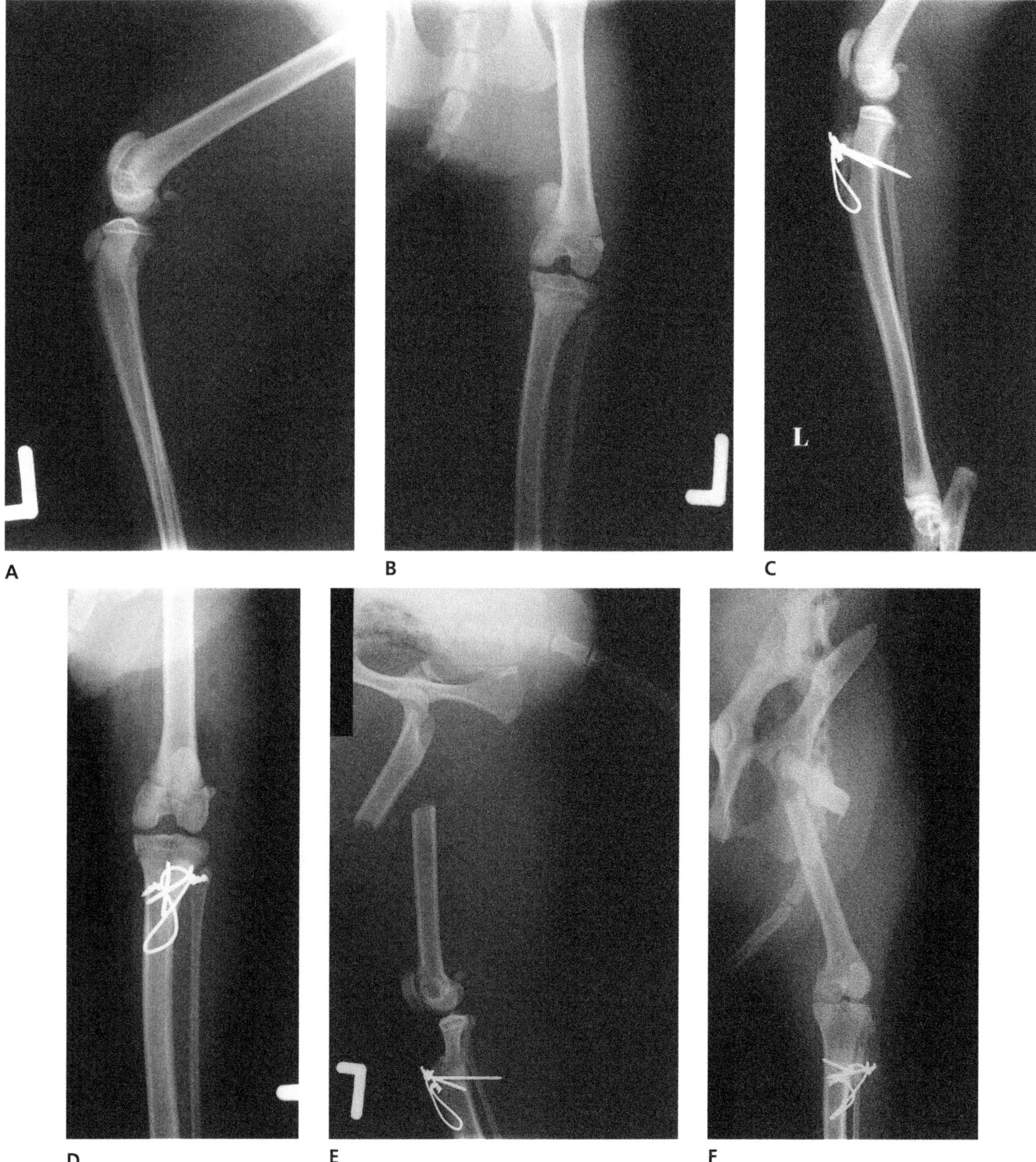

Figure 42-6 (**A**, **B**) A 6-month-old female cat with potential for further growth was presented with medial patellar luxation. (**C**, **D**) The tibial tuberosity was transposed too distally during the initial surgery. (**E**, **F**) Tibial plateau deformity occurred with tuberosity drift leading to a mid-diaphyseal femoral fracture. Plating of the femur with repositioning of the tibial tuberosity was indicated. A better technique for this immature cat would have been a sulcus recession, delaying the transposition of the tibial deformity until the cat was skeletally mature, if it was still necessary at that time.

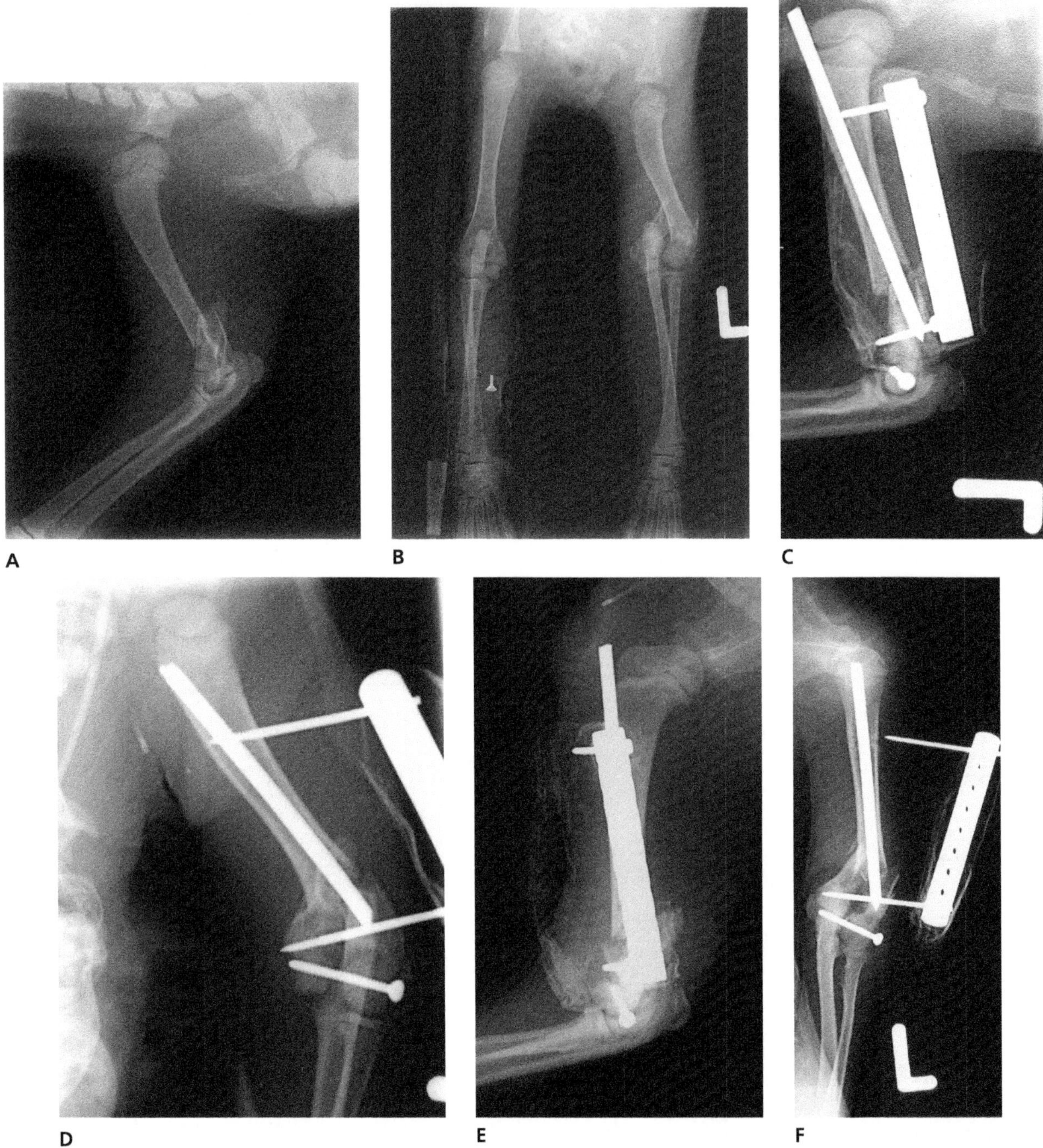

Figure 42-7 (**A**, **B**) An intracondylar fracture was diagnosed in a 3-month old cat. (**C**, **D**) The fracture was stabilized with an intracondylar screw, a large intramedullary pin, poorly seated in the distal fragment, and a tubular external skeletal fixation with limited anchorage of two pins, placed to provide resistance against rotation. (**E**, **F**) Failure of the fixation occurred after one week. (**G**, **H**) Revision was with a larger intracondylar screw and a thinner intramedullary pin tied-in to an external skeletal fixator, with more pins included in the distal fragment. (**I**, **J**) The fracture healed and the external skeletal fixation was removed after two months.

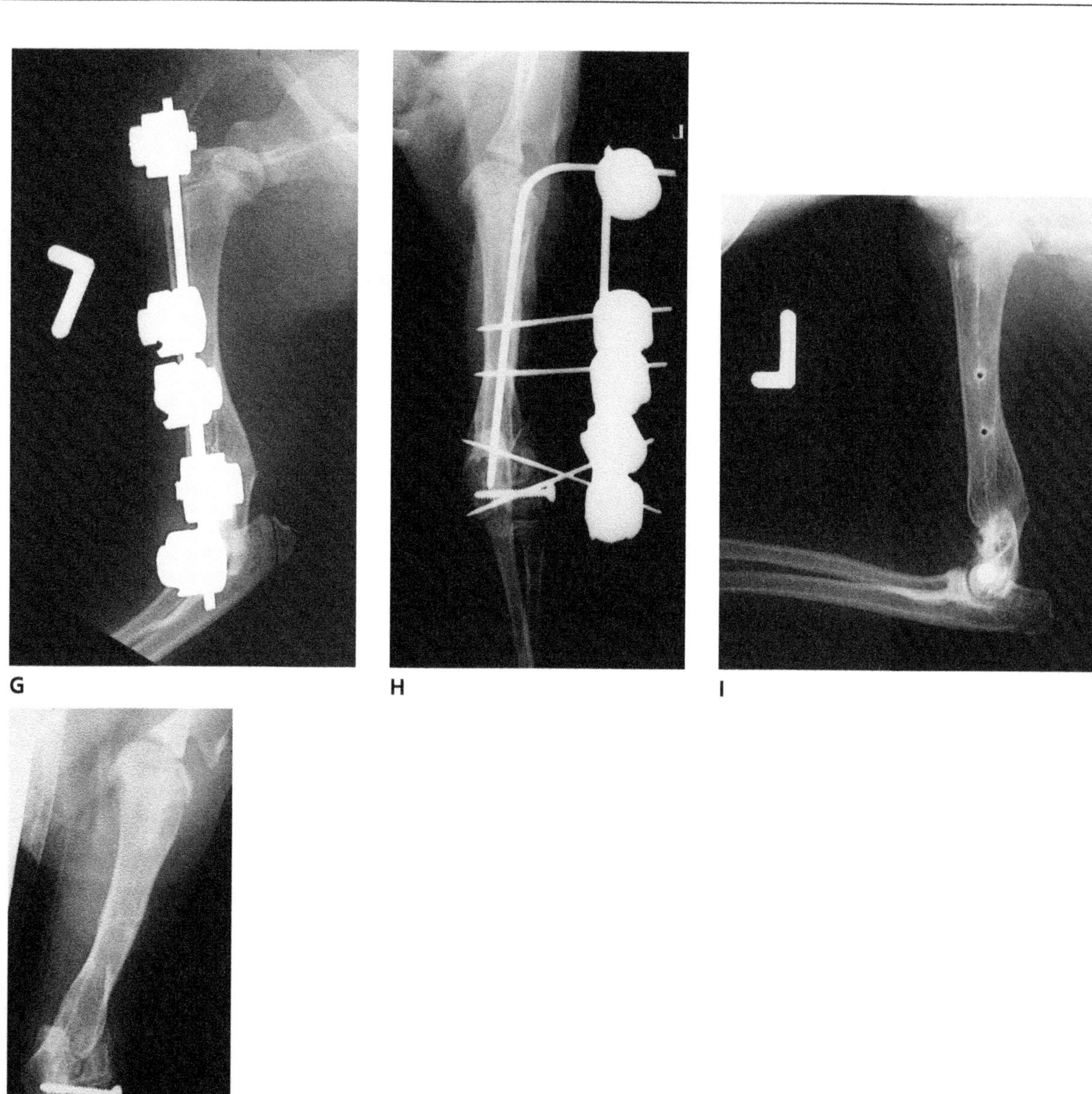

Figure 42-7 *Continued*

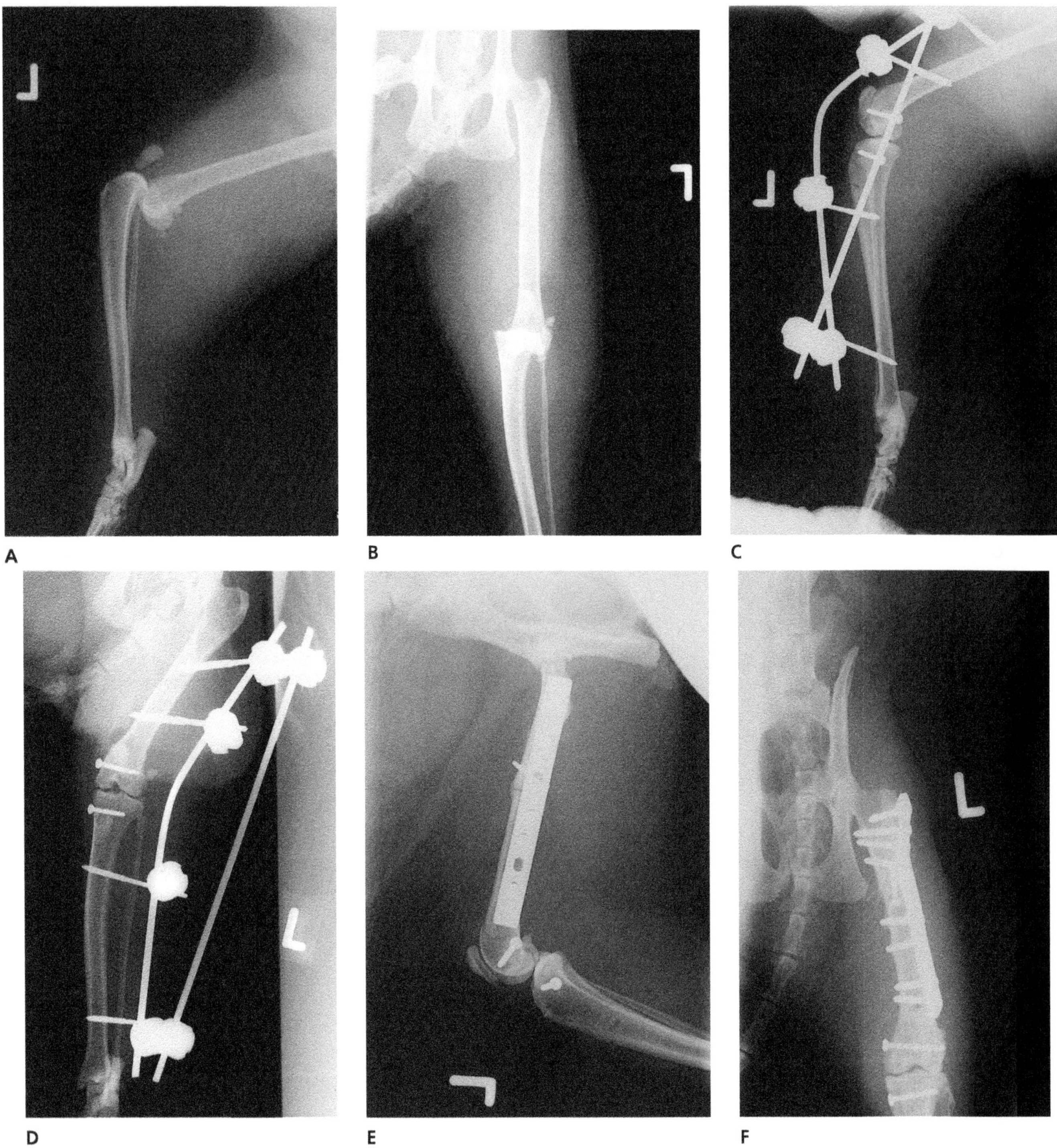

Figure 42-8 (**A**, **B**) A cat with a disrupted stifle. (**C**, **D**) The joint was explored and damaged tissue debrided, the collateral ligament rupture was repaired using two screws and a prosthetic suture and the stifle was stabilized transarticularly with pins that were too large, and a double connecting rod. After one month, a femoral fracture occurred through the most proximal pinhole. (**E**, **F**) The transarticular fixator was removed and the femur stabilized with a plate. Transarticular frames can create a long lever arm and high stresses on the thin bones of a cat.

42-8D). One month later, a fracture occurred through the most proximal pin hole in the femur. The transarticular fixator was removed at that time, and the fracture was successfully plated (Fig. 42-8E and 42-8F). It is very important to follow principles of using external skeletal fixators correctly, particularly when applying them as transarticular frames where the long lever arms create high stresses. Remember cat bones are relatively thin and transosseous pins should not be too big.

Unexpected fractures (Figure 42-9)

A 13-month-old Burmese female was presented with bilateral sacroiliac luxations that occurred spontaneously during

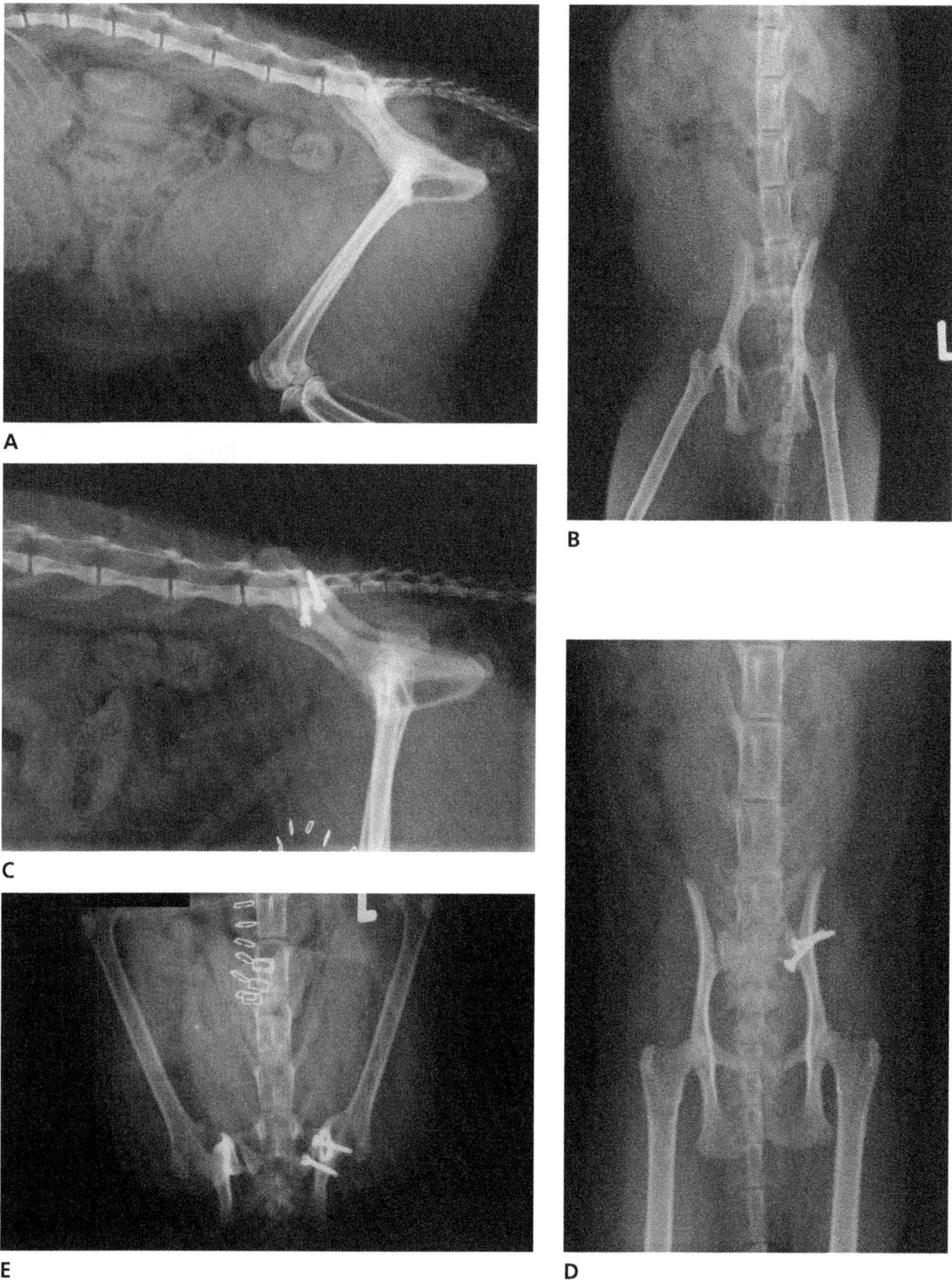

Figure 42-9 (**A**, **B**) A young Burmese cat was presented with sacroiliac luxations, which occurred during parturition. (**C**, **D**, **F**) The 2 screws do not engage into the sacral wing and the luxation is not anatomically reduced, the sacral wing remains dorsally displaced.

parturition. She presented with abnormal urine outflow control and was lame on the hindlimbs. One of the sacral wings also appeared to be luxated dorsally (Fig. 42-9A and 42-9B). A ventral approach was used to reduce and stabilize the right-sided sacroiliac luxation with 2-mm screws (Fig. 42-9C–E). The surrounding nerves (obturator and nerve roots L6 and L7) appeared contused. The reduction of the sacral wing was not anatomically reduced. Fissured or unusually displaced dorsal fragments can render the reduction difficult in such deep wounds. After surgery, the cat benefited from physiotherapy and was functioning normally 3 months postoperatively.

Conclusions

The few cases illustrated here represent daily examples of our life as small-animal veterinary surgeons. If these also happen to you during your clinical practice, please observe them carefully, learn from them, and have a permanent ambition to try to do better next time. In this way you may reach the position of a master and be the one successfully revising the errors, preventing them in future cases, and enthusing others in the art of veterinary surgery.

Index

NB: Page numbers in **bold** refer to figures and tables

A

B

C

D

E

F

G

H

I

J

K

L

M

N

O

P

Q

R

S

T

U

V

W

X

Y

Z

Printed and bound by CPI Group (UK) Ltd, Croydon, CR0 4YY

08/06/2025

01896880-0002